A Comprehensive Textbook of
OBSTETRICS AND GYNECOLOGY

A Comprehensive Textbook of
OBSTETRICS AND GYNECOLOGY

Sadhana Gupta
MBBS (Gold Medalist) MS (Gold Medalist)
FICOG FICMU FICMCH

Senior Consultant
Obstetrician and Gynecologist
Ultrasound, Infertility and In Vitro Fertilization (IVF) Specialist
Jeevan Jyoti Hospital
and
Medical Research Center
Visiting Consultant
Lalit Narayan Mishra North East Railway Hospital
Gorakhpur, Uttar Pradesh, India

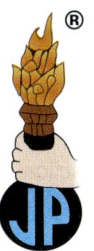

JAYPEE BROTHERS MEDICAL PUBLISHERS (P) LTD
New Delhi • St Louis • Panama City • London

Published by
Jaypee Brothers Medical Publishers (P) Ltd

Corporate Office
4838/24 Ansari Road, Daryaganj, **New Delhi** - 110002, India
Phone: +91-11-43574357, Fax: +91-11-43574314

Offices in India
- **Ahmedabad**, e-mail: ahmedabad@jaypeebrothers.com
- **Bengaluru**, e-mail: bangalore@jaypeebrothers.com
- **Chennai**, e-mail: chennai@jaypeebrothers.com
- **Delhi**, e-mail: jaypee@jaypeebrothers.com
- **Hyderabad**, e-mail: hyderabad@jaypeebrothers.com
- **Kochi**, e-mail: kochi@jaypeebrothers.com
- **Kolkata**, e-mail: kolkata@jaypeebrothers.com
- **Lucknow**, e-mail: lucknow@jaypeebrothers.com
- **Mumbai**, e-mail: mumbai@jaypeebrothers.com
- **Nagpur**, e-mail: nagpur@jaypeebrothers.com

Overseas Offices
- **North America Office, USA,** Ph: 001-636-6279734, e-mail: jaypee@jaypeebrothers.com anjulav@jaypeebrothers.com
- **Central America Office, Panama City, Panama,** Ph: 001-507-317-0160, e-mail: cservice@jphmedical.com, Website: www.jphmedical.com
- **Europe Office, UK,** Ph: +44 (0) 2031708910, e-mail: info@jpmedpub.com

A Comprehensive Textbook of Obstetrics and Gynecology

© 2011, Jaypee Brothers Medical Publishers

All rights reserved. No part of this publication should be reproduced, stored in a retrieval system, or transmitted in any form or by any means: electronic, mechanical, photocopying, recording, or otherwise, without the prior written permission of the author and the publisher.

This book has been published in good faith that the material provided by author is original. Every effort is made to ensure accuracy of material, but the publisher, printer and author will not be held responsible for any inadvertent error (s). In case of any dispute, all legal matters are to be settled under Delhi jurisdiction only.

First Edition: **2011**

ISBN 978-93-5025-112-6

Typeset at JPBMP typesetting unit

Printed at Sanat Printers, Kundli.

Dedicated to

Alma-Mater
Teachers
&
All the Teaching Moments

PREFACE

I present *A Comprehensive Textbook of Obstetrics and Gynecology* before readers with profound sense of gratitude and great satisfaction in my heart and mind.

For me, experience of writing this book emerged as communicating with all pioneers and stalwarts in the field of obstetrics and gynecology, present and past whose hard work and keen observation has contributed in progress of this subject.

This book is unique in its conception that it covers the two interrelated branches—obstetrics, i.e. science of childbirth and gynecology, i.e. science of female genital system in a single book. This will certainly help students and readers in grasping the subject as a whole. Certain topics like basic science, abortions, ectopic pregnancy, GTT, and contraception are common to both and readers will have a clear orientation by not repeating the same topic in different ways.

In section of Basic Sciences in Obstetrics and Gynecology, recent views and developments in the field with its clinical implication are included and readers will find this section challenging and interesting. The subject of General Gynecology, Obstetrics and Normal & Abnormal Labor has been explained with meticulous details as well as with simplified and rational approach.

I have tried hard to make this book comprehensive, easy to understand and give clear messages to readers in all chapters. I have carefully avoided repetition of text and tables to make subject interesting, simple and palatable for the readers and not confusing and heavy. The multiple choice questions (MCQs) have been included at the end of chapters considering the changing scenario and priorities of today's undergraduate students. In present times getting through the pre-postgraduate entrance examination is one of the prime concerns of the students. Right from the beginning while preparing for MBBS examination, if they read the subject while keeping an eye on possible MCQs, they will have definite edge in examination.

The field of obstetrics and gynecology is widening fast and there are many emerging subspecialties like endocrinology, reproductive biology, including assisted reproductive techniques, perinatal and fetal medicine, imaging and so on.

In this book all subspecialties are covered in a simple and easy-to-understand manner so that readers will have clear and updated knowledge of these subjects.

Great care has been taken in selection and quality of figures, photographs and illustrations at appropriate places which will keep the interest of readers and they will have visual memory of various clinical situations.

The language in the book has been kept simple and interesting which effectively communicates with the readers.

Almost two and a half years have been spent in writing the text of this book, editing and re-editing, selecting and preparing photographs and illustrations for this book. I acknowledge everybody who was part of this experience. It was a great learning experience and every moment was enjoyed thoroughly.

In the end I cannot resist remembering and quoting the words of my favorite writer and pioneer in obstetrics and gynecology Professor Ian Donald who asks to himself—"What motivates someone to write the textbook" and he answers "Perhaps to learn something about the subject". In these years I have understood the actual worth and meaning of his saying.

A teacher is a teacher while he/she remains a student and a doctor is said to be primarily a teacher and these things go hand-in-hand in medical profession. We hope that each one of us always remains a humble student of medicine and true teacher for our patients.

The book is being presented before readers keeping in mind that knowledge is always weightless, enjoyable, simple, and for upliftment and well being of all.

I also earnestly invite suggestions and comments from the readers about any aspect of the book to my email dr_sadhanag@yahoo.com.

I wish all readers a happy, thorough and enjoyable reading and also wish them success and achievement in their career and life.

Sadhana Gupta

ACKNOWLEDGMENTS

I present this book with great humility and first of all thank God for chosing me to write *A Comprehensive Textbook of Obstetrics and Gynecology*.

I acknowledge my teachers and seniors at my Alma-Mater institute SN Medical College, Agra from whom I learned basic skills of obstetrics and gynecology and who inculcated the habit of hard work and uncompromising approach in profession.

I acknowledge M/s Jaypee Brothers Medical Publishers (P) Ltd, New Delhi, India who not only incepted the idea of writing a combined textbook of obstetrics and gynecology but also gave me the responsibility of writing it. I also thank them for decent and esthetic formatting of the book.

It is conventional to acknowledge the family members, and I first of all acknowledge my parents who have shared my long studying hours since childhood and have been always with me in difficult times. I acknowledge my younger sister for being present in hours of needs and brother for his care and unconditional affection.

I acknowledge Shubhankur and Anindya who happen to be my sons. Interaction with Shubhankur every night about MCQs and medical education system has indirectly helped me a lot in understanding difficulty of today's medical graduates, who are supposed to answer pinpointed ways in controversies and difficult situations.

I affectionately acknowledge Anindya my younger son whose liveliness, humor and company has instilled life in time of crisis. Besides this, because of him, while writing this book I always kept in mind those students who have less time for study but their aims are high.

I acknowledge Dr PP Gupta for, perhaps, finally recognizing me as an unconventional person.

I acknowledge my hospital team especially Dr KM Singh, Chief Anesthetist for bearing with me throughout, for being always late and even then helping in taking photographs in operation theater. I lovingly acknowledge Dr Rashmi, my junior resident who has helped me a lot in hospital work and being always cheerful. I also thank Dr Achla Sinha, and Dr Pallavi, my resident doctors for their support in hospital work.

I heartily acknowledge all the patients who have patiently waited for long hours, while I spent morning hours in preparation of the book. I owe them all the skills, knowledge and every good thing in the life.

I acknowledge Mr Santosh for his dedication and hard work in preparing the illustrations for this book.

I also acknowledge my music teacher Ms Indu who has unfolded the soothing and serene world of Indian classical music to me in these two and a half years.

Lastly I acknowledge Mr Shyam who has become integral part of all my academic ventures, I thank him not only for all the dedication and concentrated work but also for being always encouraging and helping in all ways. And above all for being patient and perfectionist.

Only God destines our associations and our work. Finally, at every moment I thank and remember him for all these associations. Lastly, I pray God for his love, blessings and to make me worthy and more worthy for his work.

CONTENTS

SECTION-1
BASIC SCIENCES IN OBSTETRICS AND GYNECOLOGY

1. **Anatomy** 3
   - Anatomy of Female Genital Tract 3
   - Female Urological System 11
   - Lower Gastrointestinal Tract 13
   - Blood Vessels of Pelvis 17
   - Lymphatic Drainage of Pelvis 19
   - Pelvic Nerves 21
   - Anterior Abdominal Wall 21
   - Pelvic Skeleton 23

2. **Reproductive Physiology** 31
   - General Consideration 31
   - Basic Concept in Endocrinology 31
   - Physiology of Menstruation 35
   - Ovarian Steroidogenesis 43

3. **Conception, Fertilization and Implantation** 47

4. **Fetal Growth, Placenta and Umbilical Cord** 57
   - General Consideration 57
   - Fetal Membrane, Amniotic Fluid and Umbilical Cord 66

5. **Embryology** 71
   - General Consideration 71
   - Female Genital Tract Anomalies 75
   - Management of Specific Anomalies 76

SECTION-2
GYNECOLOGY

6. **Gynecological History and Clinical Examination** 83
   - General Consideration 83

7. **Pediatric and Adolescent Gynecology** 88
   - Puberty 89

8. **Genital Ambiguity and Intersexuality** 96
   - Intersex 96
   - Disorders of Gonadal Development 99
   - True Hermaphroditism 99

9. Amenorrhea 103
- Pathological Amenorrhea 103
- Evaluation in Case of Amenorrhea 106

10. Benign Lesions of the Vulva and Vagina 110
- General Consideration 110
- Vulvar Non-neoplastic Epithelial Disorders 113

11. Benign Disorders of the Uterine Cervix 119
General Consideration 119

12. Benign Disorders of Uterine Corpus (Fibroids, Adenomyosis and Endometrial Polyp) 123
- General Considerations 123
- Treatment 128
- Adenomyosis 131
- Endometrial Polyp 133

13. Abnormal Uterine Bleeding and Abnormalities of Menstruation 137
- Patterns of Abnormal Uterine Bleeding 137
- General Principle of Management 139
- Dysfunctional Uterine Bleeding 140
- Postmenopausal Bleeding 143
- Complications of Menstruation 144
- Dysmenorrhea 145

14. Endometriosis 148
- General Consideration 148

15. Pelvic Organ Prolapse (POP) 157

16. Urinary Incontinence 168
- Stress Urinary Incontinence 168
- Urge Incontinence 169
- Genitourinary Fistula 173
- Ureteric Injury 176
- Bladder Injury During Gynecological Surgery 176

17. Benign Adnexal Masses 178
- Ovarian Neoplasm 180
- Clinical Features of Ovarian Tumors 183
- Complications of Ovarian Tumor 185
- Management of Benign Ovarian Tumors 186

18. Gynecological Infection and STD 189
- General Consideration 189
- Vaginitis 190
- Genital Ulcer Disease 199
- Human Immunodeficiency Virus Infection 203
- Urinary Tract Infection (UTI) 208
- Acute Cystitis 208
- Acute Pyelonephritis 209

19. Pelvic Inflammatory Disease 211
- Genital Tract Tuberculosis 214
- Postoperative Infection 219

20. Infertility 222
- Guiding Principles in the Evaluation of Infertility 223
- Evaluation of Male Factors 223
- Evaluation of Female Factor 226
- Treatment Plan for Infertile Couple 230
- Female Factor Infertility 231
- Assisted Reproductive Technology 233

21. Hirsutism 236
- General Consideration 236

22. Menopause 239
- Menopause 239
- Clinical Condition Associated with Menopause 240
- Estrogen 241
- Patient Evaluation for Menopause 242
- Management of Menopause 243

23. Premalignant and Malignant Disorders of the Uterine Cervix 246
- General Consideration 246
- Epidemiological Risk Factors for CIN 247
- Clinical Findings of CIN 249
- Colposcopy 251
- Management of Histologic CIN 254
- Cancer of the Cervix 258
- Treatment 262
- Special Situation 264
- Complications of Therapy 265

24. Premalignant and Malignant Disorders of the Uterine Corpus 267
- General Consideration 267
- Endometrial Hyperplasia 268
- Endometrial Cancer 268
- Uterine Sarcoma 272

25. Premalignant and Malignant Disorders of Ovaries and Fallopian Tubes 276
- General Consideration 276
- Diagnosis of Ovarian Cancer 279
- Management of Epithelial Ovarian Cancer 282
- Malignant Neoplasm of Fallopian Tube 285

26. Premalignant and Malignant Disorders of the Vulva and Vagina 288
- General Consideration 288
- Vulvar Intraepithelial Neoplasia (VIN) 288
- Vulvar Cancer 289
- Preinvasive Disease and Cancer of the Vagina 293
- Cancer of Vagina 293

27. Gestational Trophoblastic Diseases 297
- General Consideration 297
- Persistent Gestational Trophoblastic Tumor (GTT) 300
- Metastatic Gestation Trophoblastic Tumors (Disease) 300

28. Contraception 304
- Methods of Contraception 305
- Sterilization 316

29. Breast Disease 323
- Breast Cancer 329

Section-3
Obstetrics

30. Preconceptional Counseling, Physiological Changes in Pregnancy and Antenatal Care 335
- Preconception Counseling 335
- Physiological Changes During Pregnancy: General Consideration 337
- Prenatal Care 343
- Diagnosis of Pregnancy 347
- Prenatal Diagnosis 349
- Chromosomal Abnormalities 353
- Applied Genetics 354

31. First Trimester Vaginal Bleeding 359
- Abortions 359
- Recurrent Pregnancy Loss (RPL) 363
- Septic Abortion 364
- Induced Abortion 364
- Ectopic Pregnancy 368

32. Late Pregnancy Complications 377
- Preterm Labor 377
- Preterm Premature Rupture of Membrane (PPROM) 382
- Post-term Pregnancy 385
- Intrauterine Fetal Death (IUFD) 386
- Isoimmunization and other Blood Group Incompatibility 388
- Management in Rh Negative Pregnancy 389

33. Disproportionate Fetal Growth 395
- General Consideration 395
- Intrauterine Growth Restriction 395
- Large for Gestational Age and Fetal Macrosomia 398

34. Hypertensive Disorders in Pregnancy 401
- General Consideration 401
- Management 404
- HELLP Syndrome 408
- Eclampsia 408

35. Third Trimester Bleeding 411
- General Consideration 411
- Placenta Previa 411
- Abruptio Placenta (Accidental Hemorrhage, Ablatio Placenta, Premature Separation of Placenta) 416
- Rupture of the Uterus 420

36. Multiple Pregnancy 423
- Twin 423
- Triplets and Higher Order Multiples 429

37. Disorders of Amniotic Fluid 431
- Physiology of Amniotic Fluid 431
- Polyhydramnios 432
- Oligohydramnios 433

38. Special Cases in Obstetrics 435
- Elderly Primigravida 435
- Grand Multipara 435
- Obesity 436

39. Diabetes Mellitus and Pregnancy 438
- General Considerations 438
- Pathophysiology: Glucose Metabolism in Normal and Diabetic Pregnancy 438

40. Hematological Disorders in Pregnancy 444
- Anemia 444
- Anemia in Pregnancy 445

41. Cardiac Disease in Pregnancy 453
- Specific Heart Disease During Pregnancy and Management 456
- Mechanical Heart Valves 457

42. Thyroid Dysfunction with Pregnancy 459
- General Consideration 459
- Hyperthyroidism in Pregnancy 459
- Hypothyroidism in Pregnancy 461

43. Jaundice, Hepatitis and Gastrointestinal Disorders in Pregnancy 463
- Jaundice and Hepatitis in Pregnancy 463
- Liver Problems Unique to Pregnancy 465
- HELLP Syndrome 466
- Cholelithiasis in Pregnancy 466
- Other Disorders of Gastrointestinal Tract in Pregnancy 466
- Acute Abdominal Pain Resulting from Nonobstetric Causes 466

44. Renal Disorders in Pregnancy 469
- General Consideration 469
- Urinary Tract Infections 469
- Acute Renal Failure 471
- Chronic Renal Disease 471
- Pregnancy after Renal Transplantation 472
- Adult Polycystic Kidney Disease 472

45. Nervous System Disorders in Pregnancy 473
- Epilepsy and Seizure Disorder 473
- Headache 476

46. Asthma in Pregnancy 477
- Pulmonary Disorders in Pregnancy 477
- Asthma in Pregnancy 477
- Tuberculosis 478

47. Local Abnormalities 481
- Local Gynecological Abnormalities Associated with Pregnancy 481

48. Infection During Pregnancy 488
- General Consideration 488
- TORCH infection—General Consideration 488
- Other Viral Infections in Pregnancy 490
- Human Immune Deficiency Virus 491
- Other Infections 491

49. Normal Labor 495
- General Consideration 495
- Female Pelvis 495
- Fetal Dimension and Disposition 495
- Transverse Diameter of Fetal Skull 498
- Phases of Labor (Parturition) 499
- Stages of Labor 500
- Mechanism of Labor 502
- Management of Labor 504

50. Malpresentation and Malposition 514
- Malpresentation 514
- Malposition 514
- Breech Presentation 514
- Face Presentation 522
- Brow Presentation 523
- Transverse Lie/Oblique and Shoulder Presentation 523
- Unstable Lie 524
- Compound Presentation 525
- Cord Prolapse 525
- Occipitoposterior Position 526

51. Dystocia and Cephalopelvic Disproportion 532
- Dystocia 532
- Contracted Pelvis and Cephalopelvic Disproportion 533

52. Postpartum Hemorrhage 540
- General Consideration 540
- Etiology of Postpartum Hemorrhage 541
- Management of Postpartum Hemorrhage 541
- Blood Transfusion and Fluid Replacement 545
- Secondary Postpartum Hemorrhage 546
- Retained Placenta 546

- Placenta Accreta (Adherent Placenta) 547
- Uterine Inversion 548

53. Operative Obstetrics 551
- Episiotomy 551
- Perineal Laceration 553
- Induction of Labor 553
- Operative Vaginal Delivery 555
- Forceps Operations 555
- Ventouse (Vacuum Extractor) 558
- Shoulder Dystocia 561
- Cesarean Section 563
- Vaginal Birth after Cesarean Section 567
- Dilemma of Vaginal Birth after Cesarean 568

54. Puerperium 570
- General Consideration 570
- Abnormal Puerperium 572

55. Essential of Normal Newborn Assessment and Care 576
- General Consideration 576
- Neonatal Resuscitation 579

56. Special Topics in Obstetrics 583
- Trauma in Pregnancy 587
- Assessment of Fetal Well-being 588
- Intrapartum Fetal Surveillance 592
- Obstetric Ultrasound 596

57. Critical Care Obstetric 601
- Shock in Obstetrics 601
- Septic Shock (Endotoxic Shock) 602
- Amniotic Fluid Embolism 604
- Pulmonary Thromboembolism 605

Section-4
Appendices

1. Investigations in Gynecology 609
- General Consideration 609
- Ultrasonography in Gynecology 611
- Endoscopy in Gynecology 613

2. Polycystic Ovarian Syndrome (PCOS) 618
- Introduction 618

3. Fetal Medicine 623
- General Consideration 623

4. Recurrent Pregnancy Loss and Bad Obstetrical History 625
- General Consideration 625
- Bad Obstetrical History 628

5. **Drug Use in Pregnancy** 630
6. **Psychological Aspects in Obstetrics and Gynecology** 632
   - General Consideration 632
7. **Ethicolegal Issues in Obstetrics and Gynecology** 637
   - General Consideration 637

Section-5
Annexures

1. **Medical Eligibility Criteria for Initiation and Continuation of Intrauterine Devices (IUD)** 643
2. **Medical Eligibility Criteria for Initiation and Continuation of Combined OCs/Combined Injects/Transdermal Patches and Vaginal Rings** 645
3. **Medical Eligibility Criteria for Emergency Contraceptive Pills** 646
4. **Normal Values in Pregnancy** 647
5. **Indications and Risks of Common Vaccines During Pregnancy** 649

Index *651*

Section One

Basic Sciences in Obstetrics and Gynecology

1. Anatomy

Teaching is only demonstrating that it is possible,
Learning is making it possible for yourself.

ANATOMY OF FEMALE GENITAL TRACT

An understanding of the anatomy of the female pelvis, internal and external genitalia and related structure is crucial to have clear concept of the subject of obstetrics and gynecology. It is also important to appreciate that while the basic facts of anatomy remains the same. Our understanding of specific anatomic relationship and the development of new clinical and surgical correlation continues to evolve.

Anatomy of External Genitalia

Urogenital triangle includes the external genital structure and the urethral opening. These external structures cover the superficial and deep perineal compartments and are known as vulva.

Vulva

Vulva is an ill defined area which comprises the whole of the external genitalia and conveniently includes the perineum. It is bounded anteriorly by the mons veneris (Pubis), laterally by the mons pubis and posteriorly by the perineum (Fig. 1.1).

Mons pubis: It is a traingular eminence in front of pubic bones that consist of adipose tissues covered by hair bearing skin up to its junction with the abdominal wall.

Labia majora: Labia majora is a pair of fibroadipose folds of skin that extend from mons pubis, downward and backward to meet in midline in front of the anus at the posterior fourchette. They are best developed in child-bearing period of life. In prepubertal children and in postmenopausal women the amount of subcutaneous fat in the labia majora is relatively small and the cleft between labia is prominent.

They include the terminal extension of the round ligament and occasionally a peritoneal diverticulum—the canal of Nuck. Labia majora are covered by skin with scattered hairs and are rich in sebaceous, apocrine and exocrine glands which produces a characteristic aroma and from which the rare tumor of hidreadenoma of the vulva is probably derived.

The adipose tissue is richly supported with venous plexus which may produce hematoma, if injured during childbirth. **The labia majora are homologous with the scrotum in the male.**

Labia minora: The labia minora are the folds of skin which lie on the inner aspect of the labia majora with which they merge posteriorly to form fourchette and are separated into two folds as they approach the clitoris anteriorly. The anterior folds unite to form the prepuce or hood of the clitoris and posterior fold form the frenulum of the clitoris as they attach to its inferior surface. Fourchette is a thin fold of skin, indented on separation of labia and is often torn during childbirth. Labia minora are covered by hairless skin overlying a fibroelastic stroma rich in neural and vascular elements. *The area between the posterior labia minora forms the vestibule of the vagina.*

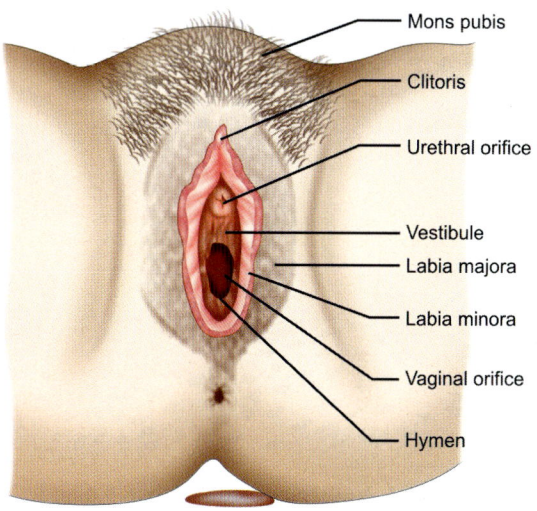

Fig. 1.1: Anatomy of external genitalia

Clitoris: It is a small cylindrical erectile organ measuring 2-3 cm in length. It consists of two crura and two corpora cavernosa and is covered by sensitive rounded tubercle (the glans). It is attached to undersurface of the symphysis pubis by the suspensory ligaments. **It is an analog to penis in the male.**

Vestibule: Vestibule is the space lying between the anterior and inner aspects of the labia minora and is bounded posteriorly by the vaginal introitus.

Vaginal orifice: Vaginal orifice is surrounded by the hymen, a variable crescentic mucous membrane that is replaced by rounded caruncle after its rupture. The opening of the duct of greater vestibular (Bartholin) gland is located on each side of the vestibule.

Urethral orifice: It is situated in the midline just in front of the vaginal orifice about 2-3 cm beneath the clitoris. The Skene (Paraurethral) gland duct presents an opening on its posterior surface.

Bartholin's gland: *Bartholin's glands are two in number and are homologous to Cowper's gland in the male.* They lie posterolaterally to the vaginal orifice embedded in the posterior part of the vestibular bulb, one on either side.

The gland measures about 10 mm in diameter and lies near the junction of the middle and posterior thirds of the labia majora. The duct of the gland is about 25 mm long and runs downwards and inwards to open at the introitus below hymen but above the attachment of the posterior end of labium minor.

It is normally impalpable when healthy but can be readily palpated between finger and thumb when enlarged by inflammation. The gland is lobulated and racemose, the acini being lined by a single layer of low columnar or cuboidal cells. The duct is lined by multilayered columnar cells but near its opening by stratified squamous epithelium (Fig. 1.2). The function of the gland is to secrete lubricating mucus during coitus. The Bartholin's gland corresponds to the bulbourethral glands of male.

Vestibular bulb: There are bilateral elongated masses of erectile tissue situated beneath the mucous membrane of the vestibule. **They are homologous to the single bulb of the penis and corpus spongiosum in male.** Each bulb lies on either side of the vaginal orifice in front of the Bartholin's gland and is incorporated with the bulbocavernosus muscle. They are likely to be injured during childbirth with brisk hemorrhage.

Vascular Connexion of Vulva

All the tissues of the vulva are highly vascular so even a minor operation in that area should not be attempted except in well-equipped settings:

i. **Arterial:** The vulva is mainly supplied by branches of *internal pudendal artery*—labial, transverse perineal artery to the vestibular bulb and deep and dorsal arteries to the clitoris. Internal pudendal artery is one of the terminal branches of the internal iliac artery. Its four parts are also served by the superficial and deep pudendal arteries which are branches of femoral artery.

ii. **Veins:** Some veins accompany corresponding arteries to the internal pudendal veins, those of the clitoris and bulb link with the vesical and vaginal plexus. The long saphenous vein also takes a share of venous return so its ligation can improve vulvar varicosities.

iii. **Lymphatics:** Lymphatic drainage is mainly to the superficial inguinal nodes and hence to the deep inguinal and external iliac nodes. Lymphatics from the deep tissues accompany the internal pudendal vessels to the internal iliac nodes.

Nerve Supply of Vulva

The skin of the mons veneris and the foreparts of the vulva are supplied by ilioinguinal nerve and the genital branch of the genitocrural nerve and the posteroinferior part by the pudendal branch from the posterior cutaneous nerve of thigh. Between these two groups the vulva is supplied by the labial and perineal branches of the pudendal nerve. The pudendal nerve supplies sensory fibers to the skin of the vulva, external urethral meatus, clitoris, perineum and lower vagina. It provides motor fibers to all the voluntary muscles including the compressor urethra, sphincter vaginae, levator ani and external anal sphincter. The skin of vulva is very sensitive and perineal injuries are especially painful. The discomfort which results from perineorrhaphy or episiotomy is mostly due to spasm in the underlying muscle.

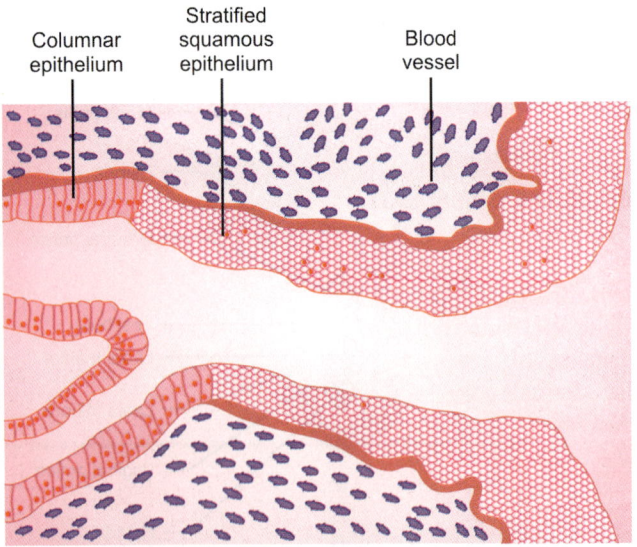

Fig. 1.2: Histology of Bartholin's gland

Internal Genital Organs

The internal genital organs in female include vagina, uterus, fallopian tubes and ovaries.

Vagina

The vagina is a hollow fibromuscular tube extending from the vulvar vestibule to the uterus. In the dorsal lithotomy position the vagina is directed posteriorly toward the sacrum but its axis is almost horizontal in the upright position. Vagina communicates interiorly with the uterine cavity and exteriorly with the vulva. It constitutes the excretory channel for the uterine secretion and menstrual blood. It is organ of copulation and for birth canal at parturition.

Vagina has anterior, posterior and two lateral walls. Vagina is attached at higher point posteriorly than anteriorly, the anterior wall measures 7 cm. The vaginal portion of the cervix projects into its upper end and forms the anterior, posterior and lateral fornices. The depth of fornices depends upon the development of the portio vaginalis of the cervix. In prepubertal girls and in elderly women where uterus is small the fornices are shallow, while in women with congenital elongation of the portio vaginalis of the cervix, the fornices are deep.

Posterior vaginal fornix is separated from the posterior cul de sac and peritoneal cavity by the vaginal wall and peritoneum. This proximity is clinically useful for diagnostic procedure of culdocentesis* and therapeutic procedure of posterior colpotomy (Fig. 1.3).**

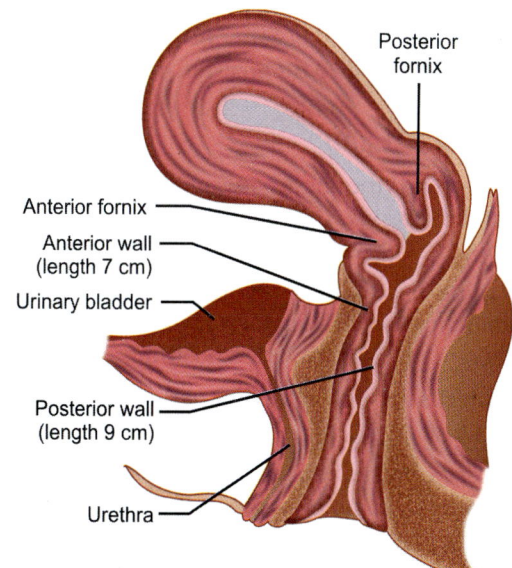

Fig. 1.3: Sagittal section of vagina

---

* Culdocentesis: A technique in which a needle is inserted posterior to the cervix through the vaginal wall into peritoneal cavity. This is used to evaluate intraperitoneal hemorrhage, pus or ascites.
** Colpotomy: It is incision into peritoneal cavity from this location (posterior to cervix, through the vaginal wall). It is done as an adjunct to laparoscopic excision of adnexal mass with removal of the mass intact through the posterior vagina.

The vagina is attached to the lateral pelvic wall with endopelvic fascial connection to the arcus tendinous (white line) which extends from the pubic bone to the ischial spine. This connection converts the vaginal lumen into the transverse slit with the anterior and posterior walls in opposition and lateral space where the two walls meet in the vaginal sulcus.

The opening of the vagina may be covered by a membrane or surrounded by a fold of connective tissue called **hymen**. This tissue is usually replaced by irregular tissue tags later in life after resumption of sexual activity and childbirth.

Vagina is not of uniform caliber. The lower vagina is a little constricted as it passes through the urogenital hiatus in the pelvic diaphragm. The upper vagina is more spacious. However, the entire vagina is characterized by its distensibility which is most evident during childbirth.

Relations of vagina: Vagina is closely applied anteriorly from below upward to—urethra, bladder neck and trigonal region. Posteriorly, the vagina is in relationship with perineal body, anal canal, lower rectum and posterior cul de sac from below upward.

Vagina is separated anteriorly from the lower urinary tract and posteriorly from gastrointestinal tract by their investing layers of fibromuscular elements known as the endopelvic fascia. Laterally, vagina is related from below upward—cavernous tissue of the vestibule, the superficial muscles of the perineum, the triangular ligament, and at about 2.5 cm from the introitus—the levator ani, lateral to which is the ischiorectal fossa. Above the levator lies the condensation of endopelvic fascia called Mackenrodt's ligament on either side. The ureter traverses this tissue in the ureteric canal and is about 12 mm anterolateral to the lateral fornix.

Superior relation: The cervix has its four fornices—anterior, posterior and two lateral. Lateral fornices are related to the uterine vessels, Mackenrodt's ligament, and the ureter. Posteriorly surrounds the pouch of Douglas where lie the uterosacral ligaments, which can be identified on vaginal examination especially if thickened by disease, as endometriosis and cancer cervix.

Histology of Vagina

1. **Mucosa:** It is nonkeratinized stratified squamous epithelium without glands, which consist of a basal layer of cuboidal cells, a middle layer of prickle cell and a superficial layer of cornified cells. Vaginal serration is derived primarily by transudation with contribution from cervical and Bartholin's gland secretions. Mucosa has a characteristic pattern of transverse ridges and furrows known as rugae. It is hormonally sensitive, responding to stimulation by estrogen with proliferation and maturation. The mucosa is colonized by mixed bacterial flora with lactobacilli predominant. Normal

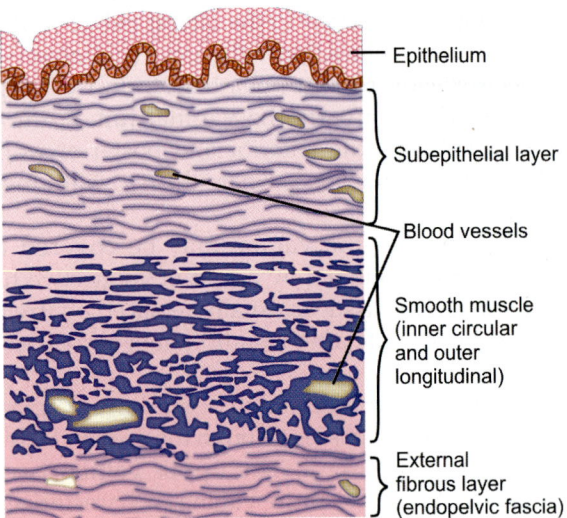

Fig. 1.4: Histology of vagina

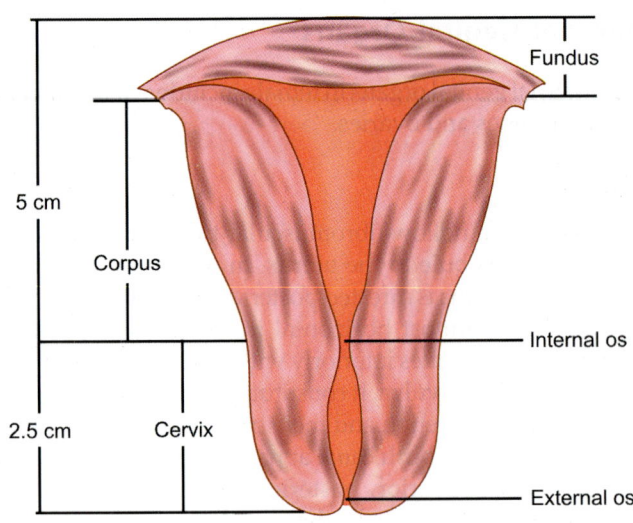

Fig. 1.5: Dimension of uterus

pH of vagina is 3.5-4.5 during reproductive life which is due to presence of lactic acid. This acidity inhibits the growth of pathogenic organism (Fig. 1.4). *Doderlein bacilli is a gram-positive, rod shaped bacilli, which grows anaerobically on acid media.* Its presence is dependent on estrogen. Its function is to convert the glycogen present in the vaginal mucosa into the lactic acid. Before puberty and after menopause due to estrogen deficiency, vaginal pH become alkaline and with deficiency of Doderlein bacilli, there is tendency for development of mixed organism infection in these age groups.

2. **Subepithelial layer** is vascular and contains much erectile tissue.
3. A **muscle layer** consist of a complex interlacing lattice of plain muscle which is external to subepithelial layer, loosely arranged in inner circular and outer longitudinal layers.
4. **Adventitia** is endopelvic fascia, adherent to the underlying muscularis.

Blood Supply

Blood supply of vagina is from the vaginal artery and branches from the uterus, middle rectal and internal pudendal arteries.

Innervation

The upper vagina is innervated from the uterovaginal plexus and distal vagina from the pudendal nerve.

Uterus

Uterus is a pear shaped fibromuscular hollow organ usually divided into a lower cervix and an upper corpus or uterine body.

Corpus (Body of Uterus)

The body of uterus varies in size and shape depending on hormonal and childbearing status. At birth the cervix and corpus are approximately equal while in adult women, the corpus is 2-3 times the size of cervix (Fig. 1.5). *Before puberty the cervix to corpus ratio is 2:1. At puberty this ratio is reversed to 1:2 and during reproductive year, cervix to corpus ratio is 1:3 or even 1:4, after menopause, the organ atrophies and portio vaginalis may eventually disappear.*

The position of the uterus in relation to other pelvic structure is variable and is generally described in terms of positioning—**Anterior, Mid position or Posterior.**

Flexion and Version

Flexion: Flexion is the angle between the long axis of uterus corpus and the cervix. It is about 120°.

Version: Version is the angle of junction of uterus with the upper vagina. It is about 90°. **Normal position is one of the anteversion and anteflexion.** In 15-20% of women uterus normally remains in retroverted position.

Body of uterus has got following parts (Fig. 1.6):

a. **Isthmus or lower uterine segment:** It is the area where endocervical canal opens into the endometrial cavity. It is annular zone, measuring 0.1-0.5 cm from top to bottom in the nonpregnant uterus. *It is limited above by the anatomical internal os and below by the histological internal os.*

The area between uterine cavity and cervical canal is anatomical internal os and the isthmus is below this. The junction between isthmus and cervical canal can only be recognized microscopically and termed as histological internal os.

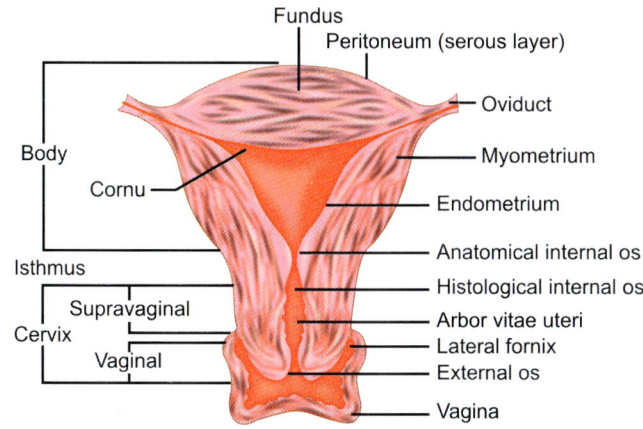

Fig. 1.6: Parts of the uterus

fibers held by connective tissues, which range in thickness from 1.5 to 2.5 cm or some other fibers of myometrium are continuous with those of fallopian tube and round ligament.

During pregnancy, three distinct layer of myometrium can be identified—outer longitudinal, middle interlacing and inner circular.

Peritoneum: It is termed serosa which covers most of corpus of uterus and the posterior cervix. The perineum is reflected onto the bladder at the level of the internal os. So the cervix of the uterus has no peritoneal covering anteriorly. Posteriorly the whole of the body of uterus and supravaginal portion of the cervix is covered by peritoneum. The peritoneum is reflected from the supravaginal portion of the cervix onto the posterior vaginal wall in the region of the posterior fornix.

Laterally, the peritoneal layer is incomplete because of the insertion of the fallopian tube, round and ovarian ligament into the uterus and below this level, the double layer of peritoneum covering the neurovascular supply to the uterus inserts into the cervix and corpus (Fig. 1.7).

b. **Uterine cornu:** On each side of the upper uterine body a funnel shaped area receives the insertion of the fallopian tube, which is called cornu.
c. **Fundus of uterus:** The part of body of uterus above the cornua is called fundus.

Endometrial cavity: Endometrial cavity is triangular in shape and represents the mucosal surface of uterine corpus. Endometrium of the body of uterus is divided into two zones:
a. Superficial epithelium which is functional layer,
b. Deeper basal layer which lies adjacent to myometrium.

The surface epithelium is a single layer of ciliated columnar epithelium and with endometrial gland, vessels and nerves forms a specialized stroma. It undergoes cyclic structural and functional changes during the reproductive years with regular shedding of the superficial endometrium and regeneration from basal layer.

Muscular layer: Muscular layer of uterus is called myometrium, which consist of interlacing smooth muscle

Cervix

Cervix is spindle shaped, measuring 2-3 cm in length bounded above by the internal os and below by the external os. The position of cervix exposed to vagina is the **Exocervix** or **Portio Vaginalis.** It has a convex round surface with a circular (in nulliparous) or slit like (in multipara) opening (the external os) into the endocervical canal. The **endocervical canal** is about 2.3 cm in length and opens proximally into the endometrial cavity at the internal os. The mucosal lining of cervix differs from that of the corpus by the absence of a submucosa. The endocervix is lined by high columnar ciliated epithelium with spindle shaped nuclei lying adjunct to the basement membrane. The glands

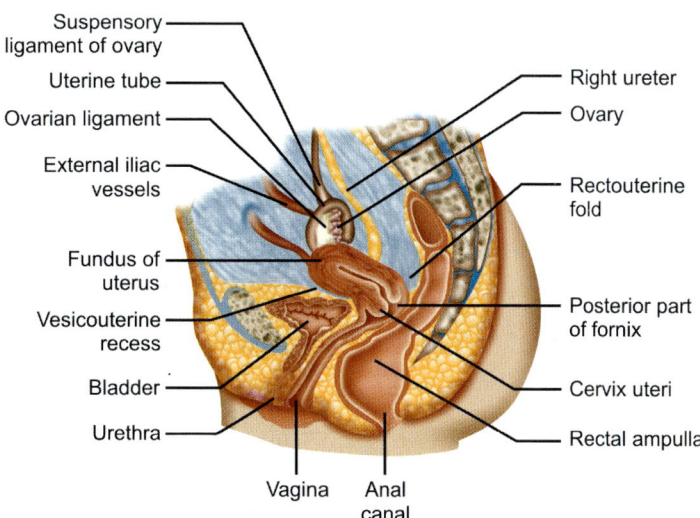

Fig.1.7: Sagittal section of human pelvis, showing relation of uterus and adnexa

are racemose in type; secrete mucus of alkaline pH with high fructose content. The direction of cilia of columnar epithelium is downwards, towards external os, so secretion collects as a plug in the cervical canal which helps against ascending infections. It is under hormonal influence. The mucous membrane lining the endocervix is thrown into folds which consist of anterior and posterior column from which radiate circumferential folds to give the appearance of true trunk and branches, so called *'arbor vitae'*.

Exocervix and portio vaginalis of cervix: It is covered by stratified squamous epithelium which extends right up to external os, where there is abrupt change to columnar type.

Transformation zone: *The intersection where the stratified squamous epithelium of exocervix and mucous secreting columnar epithelium of endocervical canal meet is called squamocolumnar junction or transformation zone.* This zone is geographically variable, dependent on hormonal stimulation as well constantly effected by infection and trauma. This dynamic interface is most vulnerable to development of squamous neoplasia. In early childhood, during pregnancy or with oral contraceptive use, columnar epithelium may extend from the endocervical canal onto the exocervix, a condition known as eversion or ectopy.

After menopause the transformation zone usually recedes entirely into the endocervical canal. Deep in the mucosa and submucosa the cervix is composed of fibrous connective tissue and a small amount of smooth muscle in circular arrangement.

Blood supply: Blood supply to the uterus is via uterine artery which anastomoses with the ovarian and vaginal arteries one on each side. Uterine artery arises directly from the anterior division of the internal iliac artery or in common with superior vesical artery.

The uterine artery cross the ureter anteriorly about 1.5 cm away at the level of internal os before it ascends up along the lateral border of the uterus in between the leaves of broad ligament (Fig. 1.8).

Nerve supply: The nerve supply to the uterus is the uterovaginal plexus:

Uterine Appendages

The uterus projects upwards from the pelvic floor into the peritoneal cavity. It carries on each side of it two folds of peritoneum which pass laterally to the pelvic wall and form the broad ligament. The fallopian tube passes outwards from the uterine cornua and lie in the upper border of the broad ligaments. The ovarian ligaments passes posteriorly and round ligament anteriorly into the uterine cornu but at a slightly lower level than fallopian tube. Round and ovarian ligament, as well the fallopian tubes are covered with peritoneum. **Fallopian tubes and ovaries collectively are referred to as the adnexa.**

Fallopian Tube

The fallopian tubes are paired hollow structure representing the proximal unfused ends of the Müllerian duct. They lie in upper margin of the broad ligament and are approximately 10 cm long (vary from 7 to 12 cm) and approximately 8 mm in diameter but the diameter diminishes near the cornu of the uterus. Each fallopian tube has got two openings—one communicates with the lateral angle of the uterine cavity called uterine opening and measure 1 mm in diameter, the other on the lateral end of the tube called pelvic opening or abdominal ostium which measures 2 mm in diameter.

The fallopian tube is divided into several portions (Fig. 1.9):
1. **Interstitial portion** (Intramural, uterine Syn): It is the narrowest portion of the tube, 1 cm in length, lies within the uterine wall and form the tubal ostia at the endometrial cavity. There are no longitudinal muscle fibers here but the circular fibers are well developed. Its internal diameter is 1 mm or less, so that only finest cannula can be passed into it during salpingostomy operation.
2. **Isthmus:** It is narrow cord tube segment closest to the uterine wall, represent 1/3rd of total length of fallopian tube, i.e. 35 mm. It is narrow but a little wider than interstitial part and its lumen has a diameter of 2 mm. It's muscle wall contain both longitudinal and circular fibers. It is covered by peritoneum except for a small inferior base area related to broad ligament.
3. **Ampulla:** It is the lateral, widest, tortuous part of tube which comprises half of length of fallopian tube (5 cm).
4. **Fimbria (Infundibulum):** It is a funnel-shaped abdominal ostia of the tube, opening into the peritoneal

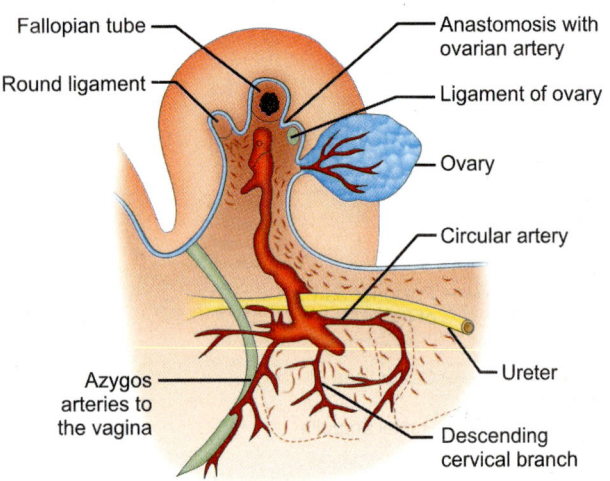

Fig. 1.8: Course of uterine artery in relation to ureter and part of uterus

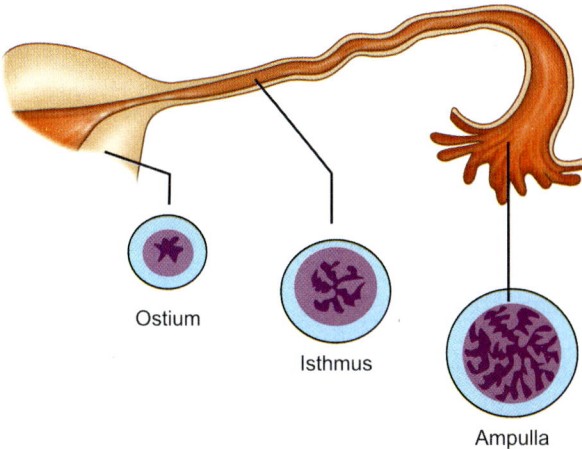

Fig. 1.9: Parts of the fallopian tube

cavity. This opening is fringed with numerous fingers like projection that provide a wide surface for ovum pickup. One fimbria is Fimbria ovarica which is larger and longer than the others and is attached to the beginning of the ovary.

Histology

It consist of three layers:
1. **Serous layer:** It consists of the mesothelium of the peritoneum which covers on all sides except all along the line of attachment of mesosalpinx. Intervening between the mesothelium and the muscle layer is a well defined subserous layer in which numerous small blood vessels and lymphatics can be demonstrated.
2. **Muscle layer:** It consists of an inner circular and outer longitudinal layer of smooth muscles. The circular fibers are best developed in isthmus. Muscular activity in the infundibulum draws the fimbria close to the ovary at the time of ovulation. The tube displays high frequency/low amplitudes and low frequency/high amplitudes contraction. The former are more characteristic of the ampulla, while the low frequency/high amplitude occur in isthmus and may propagate in either direction. Ovum transport is fast in the ampullary region but a physiological sphincter at the isthmus delays passage into the uterus for three days. Ampullary area also contains numerous (excitatory and inhibitory) adrenergic receptors.
3. **Mucosa of fallopian tube:** The fallopian tube is lined by a single layer of columnar epithelium with three types of cells: (i) Ciliated, (ii) Secretory, (iii) Resting.
   a. Function of ciliated epithelium is to propel a fluid current towards the uterus which plays some part in transport of inert ovum, which unlike sperm, has no motile power of its own. The cilia beat asynchronously at about 7 beat per second.
   b. Secretory, nonciliated cells are found throughout the tube, but are most numerous at the isthmic end. They develop microvilli and become secretory at the mid cycle.
   c. A cell intermediate in type to ciliated and secretory cells are small rod shaped **resting or peg cell**, whose purpose is not known.

Function of Fallopian Tube

Function of fallopian tube is ovum pickup, provision of physical environment for conception and transport and nourishment of fertilized ovum. Fallopian tube secretion contains pyruvate, which is an important substrate for the embryo. They contain less glucose, protein and potassium than serum.

Blood Supply

Vascular supply to the fallopian tube is the tubal branch of uterine and ovarian arteries. A anastomosing branch of uterine artery supplies the inner part and tubal branch of ovarian artery supply the main fallopian tube. Unlike the vermiform appendix, the fallopian tube does not become gangrenous when acutely inflamed, as it has two sources of blood supply, which reach it at opposite ends. Venous drainage is through the pampiniform plexus into the ovarian veins.

Innervation

The innervation to the fallopian tube is via uterovaginal plexus and ovarian plexus.

Lymphatics

The lymphatics of the fallopian tube communicate with the lymphatic of the fundus of the uterus and with those of ovary and they drain along the infundibulopelvic ligament to the aortic glands near the origin of the ovarian artery from the aorta.

Ovaries

The ovaries are paired gonadal structure that lie suspended between the pelvic walls and the uterus by the infundibulopelvic ligament laterally and uterovesical ligament medially. The ovary measures 3 cm × 1.5 cm, almond shaped, pearl grey due to a compact tunica albuginea and surface is slightly corrugated (Fig. 1.10).

The ovaries are intraperitoneal structure and not normally palpable during bimanual examination.

Relation

Ovary is attached to the posterior surface of the broad ligament by the mesovarium and occupies the ovarian fossa on the wall of the pelvis. This fossa is bounded

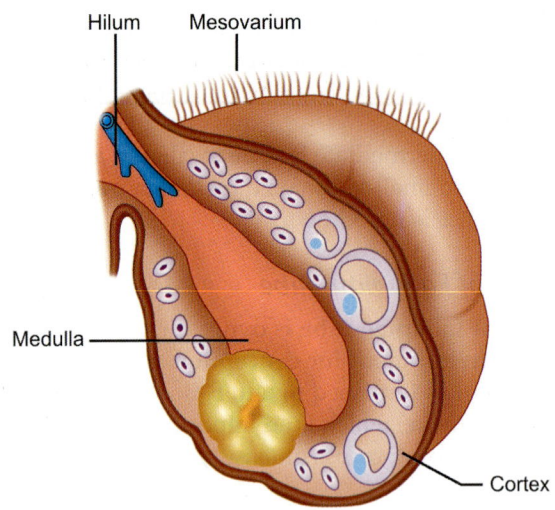

Fig. 1.10: The ovary

anteriorly by the obliterated umbilical artery and posteriorly by the ureter and the internal iliac artery and laterally to the peritoneum separating the obturator vessels and nerves.

Primary neurovascular structure reaches the ovary through the infundibulopelvic ligaments and enters through mesovarium.

Histology

The surface of the ovary is covered with a layer of cuboidal cells known as germinal epithelium which is continuous with the peritoneum at the mesovarium. Beneath this is the thin layer of condensed connective tissue, the tunica albuginea. It has a thick cortex which is composed of a specialized stroma and follicles in various stage of development or attrition (Fig. 1.11).

The medulla is highly vascular, occupies a small portion of ovary in its hilar region and is composed of fibromuscular tissue, blood vessels and nerves. There are small collections of cells called 'hilus cells' which are homologous to the interstitial cells of the testes.

Blood Supply

The blood supply to the ovary is the ovarian artery—a branch of abdominal aorta, which anastomoses with uterine artery. Venous drainage is through pampiniform plexus, which form ovarian vein which drain into inferior vena cava on the right side and left renal veins on the left side. Part of the venous blood from the placental site drains into the ovarian vein and thus may become the site of thrombophlebitis in puerperium.

Nerve Supply

The nerve supply of the ovarian plexus includes para-sympathetic, postganglionic sympathetic and autonomic afferent fibers from T_{10} segment. Ovary is sensitive to touch.

Epoophoron (Organ of Russell Miller)

It represents the cranial end of the Wolffian body. It consists of series of vertical tubules in the mesovarium and

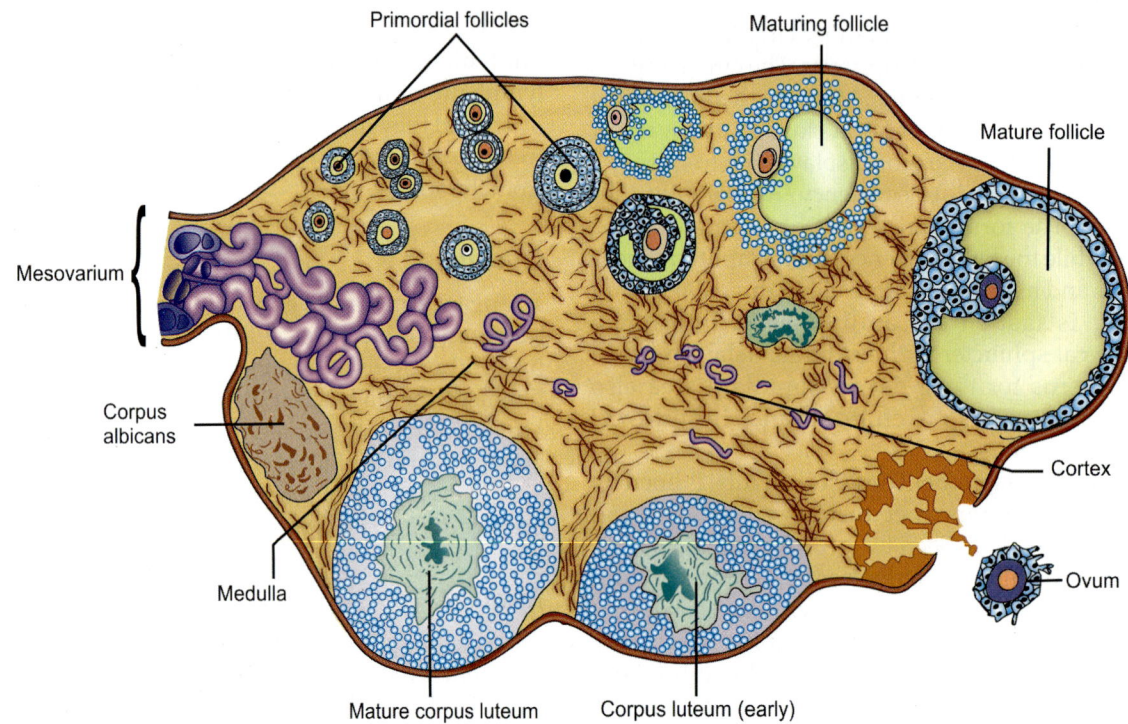

Fig. 1.11: Structure of ovary showing different stages of development of follicles

mesosalpinx between the fallopian tube above and ovary below. Each tubule is surrounded by plain muscles and is lined by cubical cells.

Paroophoron

It represents the caudal end of the Wolffian body and contains vertical tubules.

Wolffian Duct

It is an imperfect duct which runs parallel to but below the fallopian tube in the mesosalpinx, which passes downward by the side of uterus to the level of internal os, where it passes into the tissues of the cervix. From where it runs forward to reach anterior lateral aspect of the vaginal walls and may reach down up to hymen. The duct sometimes from a cyst, called *Gartner's cyst* in the broad ligament in the vagina and require surgical enucleation sometimes.

FEMALE UROLOGICAL SYSTEM

Ureter

The ureter forms as an outgrowth (metanephric diverticulum) from the lower end of the mesonephric duct. The cranial end of the diverticulum gives rise to the pelvis, calices and collecting tubules of the kidney.

The ureter is the urinary conduit, leading from the kidney to the bladder. It measures about 25 cm in length and is totally retroperitoneal in location. The abdominal part lies on the Psoas major, crosses in front of genitofemoral nerve and is crossed by the ovarian vessels. The lower half of each ureter traverses the pelvis after crossing the common iliac vessels at their bifurcation, just medial to the ovarian vessel.

The **pelvic part** follows the anterior border of the greater sciatic notch, turns medially at the ischial spine and runs above the levator ani in the base of broad ligament (Parametrium) to the base of the bladder. The ureter pierces the Mackenrodt's ligament (Parametrium) where a canal—ureteric canal is developed. It is obvious that the ureter must have a room in which its peristaltic movements can be carried out without pressure from surrounding structure and for that ureteric canal is present. In its passage through the ureteric canal, the ureter is crossed by the uterine artery and the uterine plexus of veins.

After leaving the ureteric canal, the ureter passes forwards and medially to reach the bladder, being separated from the cervix by a distance of 1-2 cm, ureter follows an oblique course through the bladder wall.

Applied Anatomy

1. The course of ureter in the pelvis is important as it is liable to get injured in gynecological surgery. The common sites of injury may be:
   a. The infundibulopelvic ligament
   b. By side of cervix
   c. Vaginal angle
   d. During pelvic peritonization
   The chances of injury are more in cases of endometriosis, pelvic inflammation or broad ligament tumors.
2. The course of ureter through the pelvis is not always constant and there is a variation also in origin of uterine artery.
3. During surgery the ureter is recognized by its pale glistening appearance and by a fine longitudinal plexus of vessels on its surface but more particularly by the peristaltic movements. It can be readily recognized by palpation between finger and thumb as a firm cord, which as it escapes gives a characteristic snap.
4. Ureter is sometimes duplicated.
5. In malignancies of the cervix with extensive involvement of the parametrium, dilatation of ureter is frequently present.

Histology

The ureter has fibrous, muscular and mucosal coats. Fibrous coat is derived from the visceral layer of the pelvic fascia. Muscularis consist of an inner longitudinal and outer circular layer of smooth muscles. The mucosa consists of the transitional epithelium.

Blood Supply

The blood supply comes from the abdominal aorta, variable with contribution from the renal, ovarian, common and internal iliac, uterine and vesical arteries.

Nerve Supply

Nerve supply is both sympathetic and parasympathetic and arises from the renal, aortic and superior and inferior hypogastric plexus (T_{10} to S_4).

Urinary Bladder

The urinary bladder is derived in part from the urogenital sinus and in part from the ends of the mesonephric ducts. It is continuous with the allantoic duct, which persist as a partly canalized fibromuscular band—the urachus, joining the apex of the bladder to the umbilicus. The bladder is a hollow organ, spherically shaped when full that stores urine.

Relations

The bladder is positioned posterior to the pubis and lower abdominal wall and anterior to the cervix, upper vagina and part of the cardinal ligament. Laterally, it is bounded by the pelvic diaphragm and obturator internus muscle.

Structure

The urinary bladder is often divided into two areas which are of physiologic significance:

The base of the bladder: Consist of urinary trigone posteriorly and a thickened area of detrusor anteriorly. The three corners of the trigone are formed by the two ureteral orifice and opening of urethra into the bladder. Base of the bladder receives alpha-adrenergic sympathetic innervation and responsible for maintaining continence.

The dome of the bladder: It is the remaining bladder area above the bladder base. It has parasympathetic innervation and is responsible for micturition.

Histology

The bladder wall has three layers: (a) Serous, (b) Muscular, (c) Mucosal. Serous layer is the peritoneal covering of the superior surface. The smooth muscle (Detrusor) has internal and external longitudinal layers and a middle circular layer. Fibers from the external layer pass with the pubovesical ligament to the pubic bones. Rather than being arranged in layers, it is composed of intermeshing muscle fibers.

The bladder mucosa is transitional cell epithelium which is loosely attached to the muscle except over the trigone where it is firmly attached.

Blood Supply

The blood supply to bladder is from the superior, middle and inferior vesical arteries and from small branches from the obturator, inferior gluteal, uterine and vaginal arteries. The veins form a plexus on inferolateral surface which drain to internal iliac veins.

Innervation

The parasympathetic nerves convey motor fibers to the detrusor (S_2-S_4 nervi erigentes). The sympathetic nerves (T_{11}, T_{12}, L_1, L_2) may have the opposite effect, but their main function is vasomotor control.

Urethra

Urethra is the vesical neck in the region of the bladder that receives and incorporates the urethral lumen. The female urethra is 4 cm long and is embedded in the anterior wall of the vagina. Its diameter is about 6 mm.

The bladder base forms an angle with the posterior wall of the urethra called *Posterior Urethrovesical (PUV) angle, which normally measures 100°*. The urethra runs downwards and forwards in close proximity of the anterior vaginal wall. About 1 cm from the lower end it pierces the triangular ligament. It ultimately opens into the vestibule about 2.5 cm below the clitoris.

Relation

The lower urinary tract and genital tracts are intimately connected anatomically and functionally. Posteriorly it is related to anterior vaginal wall to which it is loosely separated in the upper 2/3rd but firmly adherent in lower third.

Anteriorly urethra is related to posterior aspect of symphysis pubis. The upper 2/3rd is separated by loose areolar tissues, the lower 1/3rd is attached on each side of the pubic rami by fibrous tissue called pubourethral ligament.

Laterally as urethra passes through the triangular ligament, it is surrounded by compressor urethra.

Applied Anatomy

In gynecological surgery the bladder and proximal urethra can be dissected easily in midline from underlying lower uterine segment, cervix and vagina through a loose avascular plane. The distal urethra is essentially inseparable from the vagina. *Unrecognized injury to the bladder during pelvic surgery may result in the development of a vesicovaginal fistula.*

Histology

The urethral mucosa has a transitional epithelium near the bladder neck, grading to a nonkeratinized stratified squamous epithelium near the external orifice. On the posterior wall is an epithelial fold—the urethral crest.

There are numerous mucosal glands, near the lower end. The ducts of these join to form the two paraurethral (Skene's duct). **Skene's glands are homologous to prostrate in the male**, which end in an aperture lateral to the external orifice.

Chronic infection of Skene's glands, with obstruction of their ducts and cystic dilatation is believed to be an inciting factor in the development of suburethral diverticulum.

The urethra contains an inner longitudinal layer of smooth muscles and outer circularly oriented smooth muscle fibers. The smooth muscle layer is continuous with that of the bladder and there is no separate internal sphincter at the junction with the bladder. The urethra is surrounded by two layers of striated voluntary muscles. The intramural layer (external sphincter) consists of slow twitch muscle fibers which exhibit tonic activity at rest.

Blood Supply

The arterial and venous blood supply to the upper third of the urethra is associated with that of the bladder and lower two-third with that of the anterior vaginal wall and clitoris. It is from the vesical and vaginal arteries and the internal pundendal branches.

Nerve Supply

The **nerve supply** is direct from S_2-S_4. Together with the bladder neck, this layer is responsible for urethral continence at rest. The periurethral striated muscle is supplied by the perineal branch of the pudendal nerve and is responsible for augmenting urethral closure during stress events.

Physiology of Micturition and Continence

Micturition: The normal urinary bladder fills without a rise in intravesical pressure. This is the result of progressive relaxation of the detrusor smooth muscle, which occurs partly under the influence of the sympathetic nervous system. Sensation of bladder filling occur when urinary volume of 350 ml is reached with maximum capacity of 500–600 ml. Voluntary voiding is controlled by the pontine micturition center, which produces contraction of the detrusor muscle and simultaneous urethral relaxation, which continue, until the contents of the bladder have been completely expelled, leaving a negligible residual volume.

Continence

Continence of urine depends on the urethral pressure being maintained at the higher level than intravascular pressure. This is achieved by active contraction of both smooth and striated muscles of the urethral wall, with some contribution from the pelvic floor (Fig. 1.12).

When abdominal pressure rises suddenly during coughing, sneezing or straining, urethral pressure also rises to exceed abdominal pressure and prevent urine loss.

LOWER GASTROINTESTINAL TRACT

Sigmoid Colon

The sigmoid colon begins its characteristic S-shaped curve as it enters the pelvis at the left pelvic brim. The columnar mucosa and richly vascularized submucosa are surrounded by an inner circular layer of smooth muscles and their overlying longitudinal bands of muscle called tenia coli. A mesentery of varying length attach to the sigmoid to the posterior abdominal wall.

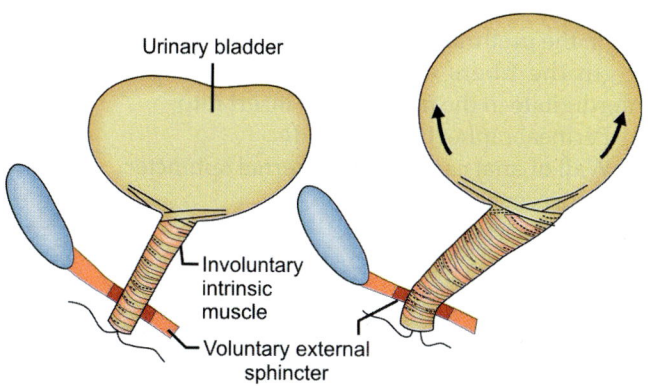

Fig. 1.12: Physiology of micturition

Blood Supply

Blood supply to sigmoid colon is from sigmoid arteries.

Innervation

The nerves to the sigmoid colon are derived from the inferior mesenteric plexus.

Rectum

The sigmoid colon loses its mesentery in the midsacral region and become the rectum about 15-20 cm above the anal opening. The rectum follows the course of the lower sacrum and coccyx and becomes entirely retroperitoneal at the level of rectouterine pouch or posterior cul-de-sac.

It continues along the pelvic curve, just posterior to the vagina until the level of anal hiatus of the pelvic diaphragm, where it takes a sharp 90° turn posteriorly and become the anal canal, separated from the vagina by the perineal body. The rectum curves twice to the left and once to the right before it passes down to continue as anal canal.

Peritoneal Covering and Relation

Rectum is covered anteriorly and laterally in its upper and one-third, only anteriorly in the middle third while whole of the posterior surface and entire lower one-third remain uncovered.

Anteriorly: From above downwards —(i) The part of rectum covered by peritoneum is related to the posterior wall of the pouch of Douglas which often contains loop of small or large bowel, (ii) The ampulla is related to posterior vaginal wall separated by rectovaginal septum, (iii) The lower part is related to perineal body.

Posteriorly: Rectum is related to the sacrum and coccyx intervened by loose areolar tissues, sacral nerve trunks and middle sacral vessels.

Laterally: From above downwards—(i) Rectum is related to uterosacral ligament, pelvic plexus of nerve and ureter, (ii) Near anorectal junction it is related to puborectalis part of levator ani, (iii) Below the muscle it is related to ischiorectal fossa.

Histology

The rectal mucosa is lined by a columnar epithelium and characterized by three transverse folds that contain mucosa, submucosa and the inner circular layer of smooth muscles.

The tenia of the sigmoid wall broadens and fuses over the rectum to form a continuous longitudinal external layer of smooth muscles to the level of the anal canal.

Anal Canal

Anal canal begins at the level of the sharp turn in the direction of the distal colon, measures 2-3 cm in length, and ends at

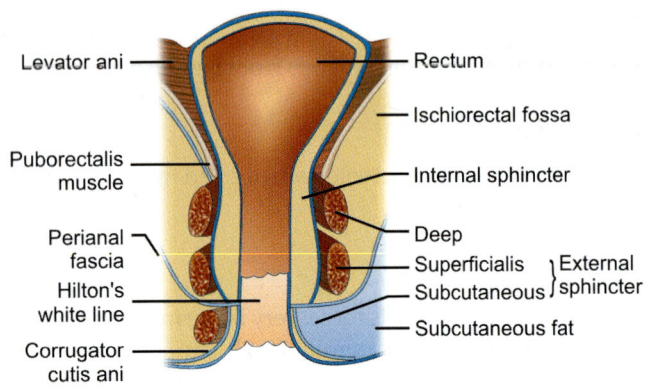

Fig. 1.13: Anatomy of rectum and anal canal with sphincters

the anal orifice. At the anorectal junction the mucosa changes to stratified squamous epithelium which is called *pectinate line* (or white line, Hilton's line synonym) which continues until the termination of the anus at the anal verge, where there is transition to perineal skin with typical skin appendages.

Relation

Anteriorly rectum is related to perineal body and posteriorly to the anococcygeal body.

Anal Sphincter

Mucosa of anal canal is surrounded by a thickened ring of circular muscle fibers that is a continuation of the circular muscles of the rectum, which is termed: (a) *Internal anal sphincter*—it is involuntary, (b) *Voluntary external anal sphincter*—it is formed by bundle of striated muscle in lower part of anal canal, it consist of three parts:
a. Subcutaneous part which is attached to skin.
b. Superficial part which starts from the perineal body and is inserted posteriorly to tip of the coccyx.
c. Deep part which is separated from the internal sphincter ani by levator ani.

Fecal continence is primarily provided by the puborectalis muscle and the internal and external anal sphincters. The puborectalis muscle surrounds the anal hiatus in the pelvic diaphragm and interdigitates posterior to the rectum to form a rectal sling. The external anal sphincter surrounds the terminal anal canal below the level of the levator ani (Fig. 1.13).

Blood Supply

The vascular supply to the rectum and anal canal is from the superior (branches of inferior mesenteric artery), middle and inferior rectal (branch of internal iliac artery). The rectum and upper one-third of anal canal has venous drainage into portal circulation via superior rectal veins. The lower one-third of the anal canal drains on both sides into inferior rectal veins.

The venous drainage is a complex submucosal plexus of vessels, that under condition of increased intra-abdominal pressure like pregnancy, ascites may dilate and become symptomatic with rectal bleeding and present as hemorrhoids.

Nerve Supply

The rectum and upper two-third of the anal canal are supplied by autonomic middle rectal plexus and inferior mesenteric plexus while the lower third of anal canal is innervated by pudendal nerve.

Applied Anatomy

Anatomic proximity of the lower gastrointestinal tract to lower genital tract makes the rectum and sphincter ani liable to injury during repair of vaginal laceration and surgery of vulva and vagina. Because of avascular nature of the rectovaginal space, it is relatively easy to dissect the rectum from the vagina in the midline.

Pelvic Floor

The pelvic floor includes all of the structure closing the pelvic outlet from the skin inferiorly to the peritoneum superiorly. It includes: (i) Pelvic peritoneum, (ii) Extraperitoneal fat and cellular tissue, (iii) Levator Ani (Pelvic diaphragm) and their fascial coats, (iv) Urogenital diaphragm (triangular coats), (v) The muscles of peritoneum and their aponeuroses, (vi) Subcutaneous fascia, (vii) Fat, (viii) Skin.

The most important of these structures are the levator ani muscles and these together with fascia which covers their upper and lower surface are collectively called the **'Pelvic Diaphragm'**. Pelvic diaphragm divides pelvic floor into a pelvic and perineal portion.

Levator Ani (Pelvic Diaphragm)

The pelvic diaphragm is spread transversely in a hammock like fashion across the true pelvis, with a central hiatus for origin the urethra, vagina and rectum. From this extensive origin the fibers sweep inferiorly and posteriorly to interdigitate in the midline and insert into:
a. Perineal raphe: Perineal body
b. Wall of anal canal: Deep external sphincter
c. Anococcygeal raphe
d. Lower part of the coccyx.

Origin

Each levator ani muscle arises from: (i) Back of the pubic rami, (ii) From the condensed fascia covering the obturator internus (white line, tendinous arch), (iii) Inner surface of ischial spine.

Each levator ani thus has two components:
1. *External component*: Which originate from the arcus tendinous, extending from the pubic bone to ischial spine. It gives rise to fibers of differing directions and includes: (a) Pubococcygeus, (b) Iliococcygeus, (c) Coccygeus
2. *Internal component*: It originates from the pubic bones above and medial to origin of the pubococcygeus and is smaller but thicker and stronger. These can be considered inner fiber of pubococcygeus. These fibers run in a sagittal direction and are divided into two portions
    i. *Pubovaginalis:* These fibers run in a perpendicular direction to the urethra, crossing the lateral vaginal wall at junction of its lower 1/3rd and upper 2/3rd to insert into the perineal body.
    ii. *Puborectalis:* Superior fibers of puborectalis sling around the rectum to the symphysis pubis, as inferior fibers insert into the lateral rectal wall between the internal and external sphincter.

Thus, these internal components of levator ani, divide the space between the two levator ani muscles into an anterior portion—the **hiatus urogenitalis** through which pass urethra and vagina and the **hiatus rectalis**, through which pass the rectum (Fig. 1.14).

The dimension of the hiatus urogenitalis depends on the two main factors: (a) Tone of levator ani muscle, (b) Existence of the decussating fibers of the puborectalis.

Fascia of Pelvic Diaphragm

The pelvic diaphragm is covered superiorly by fascia which includes a parietal and visceral component and is a continuation of the transversalis fascia. Parietal fascia has area of thickening and forms ligament, septa and gives strength and fixation for the pelvic floor (Fig. 1.15).

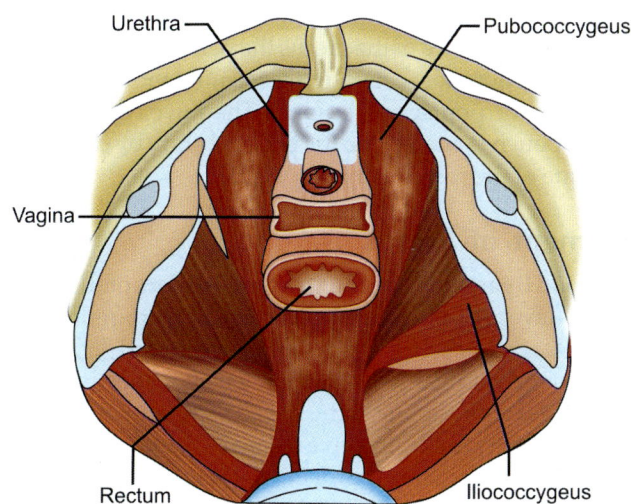

Fig. 1.14: Superior aspect of pelvic floor

The endopelvic fascia (visceral) extends medially to invest the pelvic viscera resulting in a fascial covering to the bladder, vagina, uterus and rectum. It continues laterally with the pelvic cellular tissue and neurovascular pedicles.

Nerve Supply

The muscle is supplied by 3rd and 4th sacral nerve, inferior rectal nerve and a perineal branch of pudendal nerve ($S_{2,3,4}$).

Perineal Muscles and Urogenital Diaphragm (Triangular Ligament Syn)

At a lower level in the pelvis is the urogenital diaphragm (Triangular ligament) with its two layers stretching between and attached to the inferior pubic rami. It is pierced by the dorsal vein of the clitoris which joins the retropubic urethrovesical plexus, by the urethra and the vagina. Between its fascial layers lie the: (a) Compressor urethrae, (b) The deep transverse perineal muscles, (c) Branches of internal pudendal vessel and pudendal nerve. Deep transverse perineal muscles arise from the ramus of the ischium, and are inserted partly into the sidewalls of the vagina and partly into the perineal body.

On the undersurface of the urogenital diaphragm are vestibule and Bartholin's gland and immediately superficial to these are: (a) Sphincter vaginae (bulbocavernosus), (b) Ischiocavernosus, (c) Superficial transverse perineal muscle followed by fascia and skin.

Perineal Body (Central Tendon of Perineum)

It is fibromuscular mass into which levator ani, bulbocavernosus, superficial and deep transverse perineal muscle, sphincter vaginae and external sphincter ani muscle are inserted which represent three layers of muscles of pelvic floor.

Urogenital Triangle

It contains the: (a) Termination of vagina and urethra, (b) Crura of clitoris surrounded by the ischiocavernosus muscle, (c) Bulb of the vestibule surrounded by the bulbocavernosus muscle, (d) Bartholin's gland, (e) Urogenital diaphragm, (f) Superficial and deep perineal pouches (Fig. 1.15).

Superficial perineal pouches: It is a potential space between the inferior fascia of the urogenital diaphragm and fascia of Colles. It contains the Bartholin's gland and superficial transverse perineal muscles.

Perineum

It is pyramidical in shape with its apex on a level with the junction of middle and lower third of the posterior vaginal wall.

Deep perineal pouches: It is a potential space between the two fascial layers of the urogenital diaphragm and contains

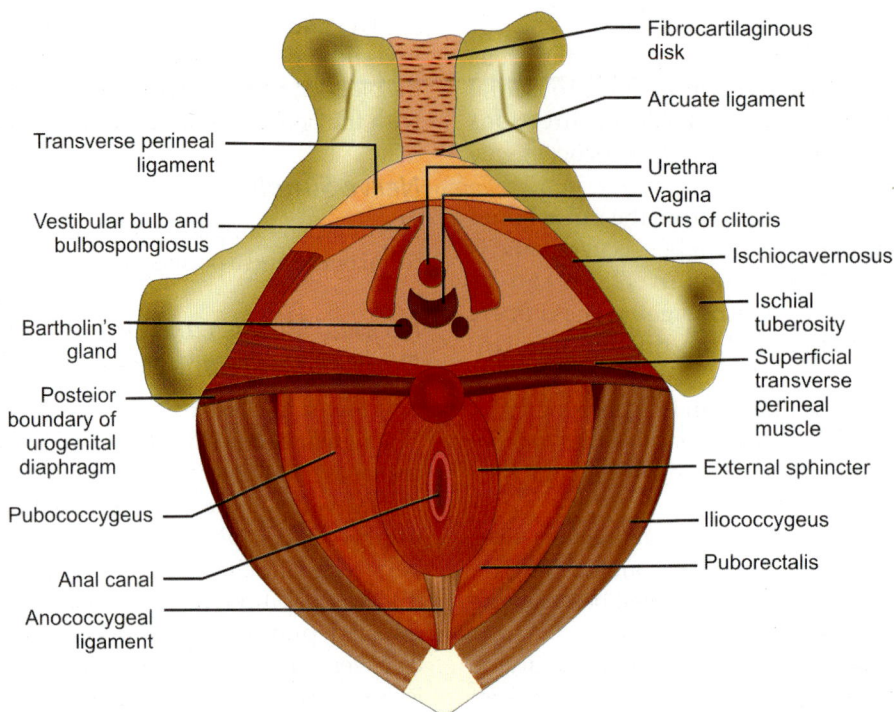

Fig. 1.15: Content of superficial perineal pouch, pelvic diaphragm, and perineal body

the membranous urethra surrounded by the external sphincter and deep transverse perineal muscles.

Perineum is situated at the lower end of trunk between the buttocks. Its bony boundaries include the lower margin of the pubic symphysis anteriorly, the tip of coccyx posteriorly and ischial tuberosity laterally. These landmarks correspond to the boundaries of the pelvic outlet. The diamond shape of the perineum is customarily divided by an imaginary line, joining the ischial tuberosities immediately in front of the anus, at the level of perineal body into an anterior urogenital and a posterior anal triangle. Perineal tear during childbirth may divide the muscles of perineal body leading to a tendency to prolapse.

The contraction of levator muscle pulls the rectum and vagina towards the symphysis pubis, the rectum is thereby kinked and closed and vaginae narrowed anteroposteriorly. The origin of levator ani is fixed from bone or white line, while insertion is movable into anococcygeal raphe and coccyx. So the contraction of the levator muscles lead to the posterior attachments being pulled towards the symphysis pubis.

During childbirth the movement of internal rotation of the presenting part is assisted by this property of the levator muscles. Uterine contraction push the presenting part down upon the levator ani (Pelvic floor) and cause the muscle to contract as a result of direct pressure of the presenting part. The lowest part of the fetus is carried forwards during the contraction of the levator muscles and because the anterior fibers of the levator ani muscles are directed inwards as well forward, the presenting part becomes rotated forwards and inwards.

Peritoneum and Ligaments of the Pelvis

1. **Peritoneal reflection (Done with anatomy of uterus):** Peritoneum covers the uterus with the exception of the anterior part of the supravaginal cervix and intravaginal cervix. From the anterior surface of the uterus the peritoneum is reflected onto the superior surface of the bladder, forming the uterovesical pouch. From the posterior surface of the uterus the peritoneum continues onto the anterior rectal surface forming the rectovaginal pouch (or pouch of Douglas). The lower extremity of this pouch is attached to the perineal body by connective tissue of the rectovaginal septum.

Ligament of Uterus

1. **Broad ligaments:** From the lateral borders of the uterus two layers of peritoneum on each side are reflected to the lateral pelvic walls forming the broad ligaments. These peritoneal folds include loose connective tissue referred to as parametrium, which merges inferiorly with extraperitoneal connective tissues.

The upper lateral border of the broad ligament forms the *infundibulopelvic fold* and contains the ovarian vessels in their course from the side wall of the pelvis. The ovary is attached to the posterior layer of the broad ligament by a short double fold of peritoneum (the mesovarium) and the portion of the broad ligaments above this is the mesosalpinx.

The top of the broad ligament envelops the fallopian tubes. Below and in front of the fallopian tube is the *round ligament* and below and behind it is the *ovarian ligament,* all enclosed in the broad ligament. Vestigial remnants of the mesonephric bodies and ducts (Wolffian duct, duct of Gartner's) are contained within the broad ligament.

Remnants of the mesonephric body lie above and lateral to the ovary (epoophoron and hydatid of Morgagni) and between the ovary and uterus (paroophoron).

The uterus is held in position by the following structures:
2. **Round ligament:** It is attached to uterine body below and in front of the fallopian tube. It is 12 cm long and passes through the broad ligament inferolaterally towards the lateral wall of the pelvis, where it crosses the psoas muscle and external iliac vessels. It hooks round the inferior epigastric arteries to the deep inguinal ring, passes through the inguinal canal and fans out into labium majus. It is composed mainly of fibrous tissues, with some smooth muscle at the uterus and some striated muscle at the labial end.
3. **Ligaments from the pelvic fascia:** The connective tissue covering the levator ani is condensed into musculofibrous bands at 3 areas (Fig. 1.16):
   a. **Transverse cervical ligament (cardinal ligament)** arising from the arcuate line on the side wall of the pelvis. It provides support to the cervix and upper vagina and contributes to the support of the bladder.
   b. **Pubocervical ligament** arising from fascia over the pubic bone and passing around the bladder neck.
   c. **Uterosacral ligament (posterior part of the cardinal ligament)** arising from the sacral promontory, providing support to the cervix and upper vagina.

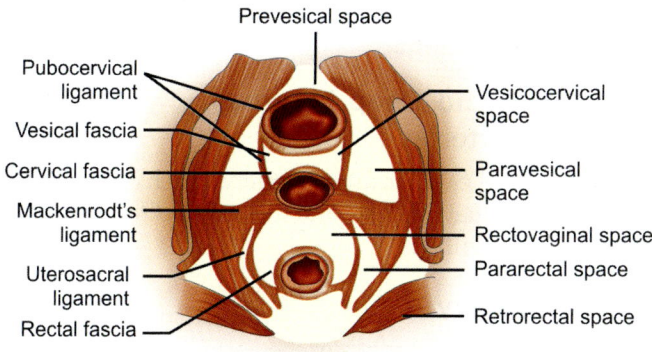

Fig. 1.16: Ligaments, fascia and spaces of uterus

BLOOD VESSELS OF PELVIS

The aorta divides at the level of fourth lumbar vertebra into two common iliac arteries and the common iliac artery divides at the level of lumbosacral intervertebral disk. Internal iliac artery arises from the bifurcation of the common iliac artery and in the fetus is the hypogastric (umbilical) artery.

From its origin the internal iliac artery descends into the pelvis as far as the greater sciatic foramen where it divides into anterior and posterior trunks. The ureter runs down its front aspect and behind it are the internal iliac veins, the lumbosacral nerve trunk and the piriformis muscle. On its outer side is the external iliac vein and lower down the obturator nerve (Fig. 1.17).

Posterior division passes through the greater sciatic foramen to supply the muscles of the buttock. While the anterior division supplies the internal pelvic organs and terminates as the internal pudendal artery. **The branches of the anterior division of the internal iliac artery are following: (i) Superior vesical, (ii) Inferior vesical, (iii) Middle hemorrhoidal (rectal), (iv) Uterine, (v) Vaginal, (vi) Obturator, (vii) Internal pudendal, (viii) Inferior gluteal (sciatic).** Last two are terminal branches.

Uterine Arteries

It arises from anterior division of internal iliac or hypogastric artery. It runs downwards and forwards along the lateral pelvic wall almost in the same direction—as ureter until it reaches the base of broad ligament.

It then turns medially and crosses the uterus anteriorly from above and at right angle to it, about 1.5-2 cm lateral to at the level of internal os. It then ascends in a tortuous course between the two layers of the broad ligament on the lateral border of the uterus giving out branches to the myometrium and anastomosing at the superior angle with the terminal portion of the ovarian artery (Fig. 1.17).

Branches to the uterus penetrate the myometrium and then turn to run parallel with the surface and divide into anterior and posterior arcuate arteries which are disposed circumferentially in the myometrium and anastomose with those from the opposite side. The uterus is therefore least vascular in the middle line which becomes the natural site for an incision.

The arcuate arteries give off the serosal branch and radial arteries which penetrate the myometrium to end as basal arteries (spiral arteries), which supply the endometrium (Fig. 1.18). Arcuate and radial arteries are coiled and the purpose of this is to reduce arterial pressure without reducing the flow, which plays important role in pregnancy.

The uterine artery also gives off branches to:
1. Ureter while crossing
2. To uterine ligaments

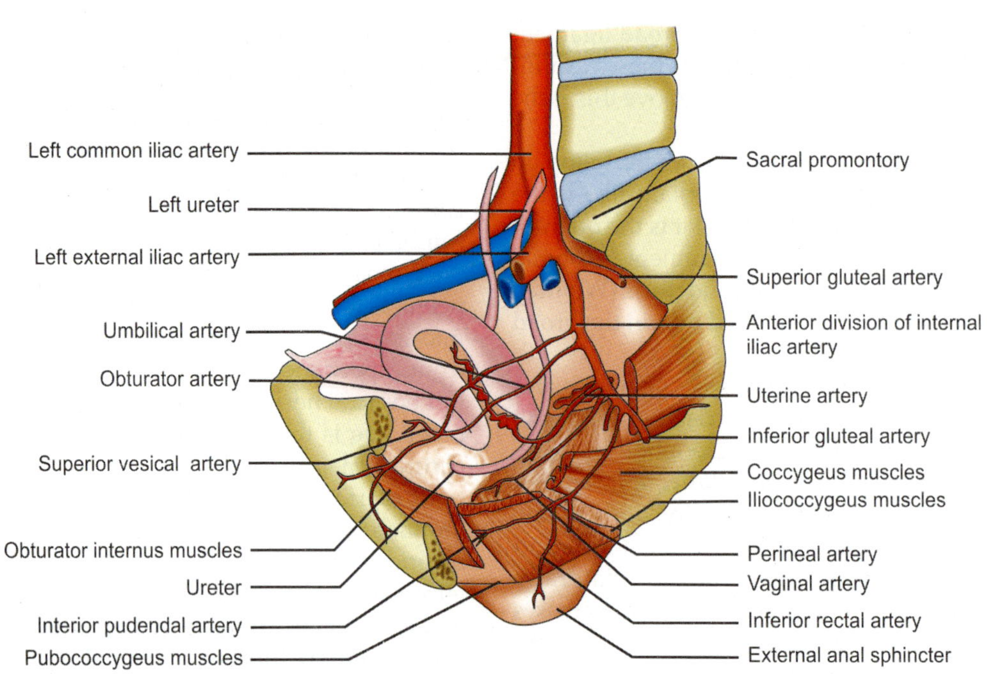

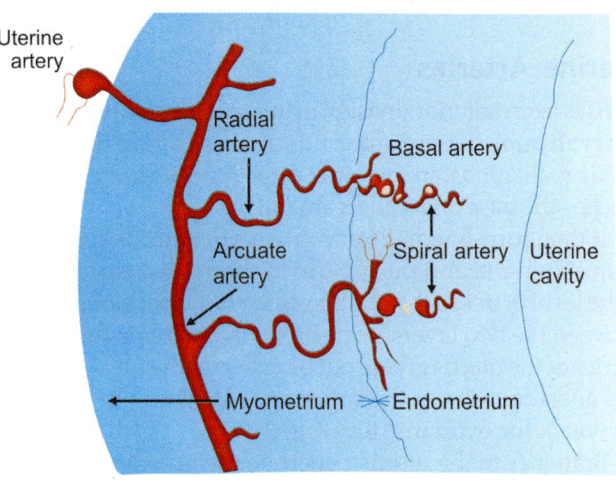

Fig. 1.17: Blood supply of the pelvis

Fig. 1.18: Course of uterine artery in myometrium

3. Circular artery to the cervix which is formed by anterior and posterior branches of the artery to the cervix on both side
4. Ovarian anastomotic branch
5. Ovarian portion of arcade gives off branches to the fallopian tube.

During pregnancy the uterine arteries hypertrophy (the luminal area increase by five times) and their course is straightened. The vaginal and ovarian arteries do not enlarge but the ovarian veins are greatly dilated.

Vaginal Arteries

The vaginal artery is usually a separate branch (or branches) of the internal iliac artery, but may come off the first part of uterine artery. It passes forwards and inwards low in the broad ligament to reach the lateral vaginal fornix. In the vaginal wall it anastomoses with the azygous branches of the circular artery to the cervix. The lower vagina is supplied from the middle and inferior rectal (hemorrhoidal) vessels and by branches from the internal pudendal artery.

Internal Pudendal Artery

Internal pudendal artery is the terminal branch of the internal iliac artery which passes out of the pelvis through the greater sciatic notch, curls round the ischial spine and returns to the lateral wall of ischial rectal fossa through the lesser sciatic notch, 4 cm above ischial tuberosity.

Together with pudendal nerve, it run forward in Alcock's canal under the lee of inferior pubic ramus and then enters between the layers of the triangular ligament to give branches to the labia, vagina, and bulb of the vestibule, perineum and various muscles. It ends as dorsal artery of the clitoris.

Superficial and Deep External Pudendal Arteries

These are branches of the femoral artery which come off just below the inguinal ligament and turn inward to supply the foreparts of the vulva.

Ovarian Artery

The ovarian artery arises from the aorta approximately at the level of renal artery. It run downwards and slightly outwards retroperitoneally and crosses the ureter to reach the brim of the pelvis where it enters the infundibulopelvic ligament.

The ovarian artery sends branches to the ovaries and to the outer part of the fallopian tube. It ends by anastomosing with the terminal part of the uterine artery after giving off a branch to cornu and the round ligament. Thus, a continuous arterial arch is formed and it is impossible to define the limits of ovarian and uterine contribution.

Pelvic Veins

The left ovarian vein ends by passing into the left renal vein. The right ovarian vein terminates into inferior vena cava. The peculiarities of the pelvic veins are that there is tendency to form plexus and plexus anastomose freely with each other and they have no valves.

In the broad ligament near the mesovarium there is a pampiniform plexus of veins which drains into the uterine and ovarian trunks. Pampiniform plexus can sometime become varicose and give rise to broad ligament varicocele.

The uterine plexus is found around the uterine artery near the uterus, the vaginal plexus around the lateral fornix of vagina, and at anorectal junction. All ultimately drain into the internal iliac veins.

The venous return from the rectum and pelvic colon enters the portal system by way of the inferior mesenteric veins. The uterine veins also communicate with the vaginal plexus and this account for low vaginal metastasis in cancer of body uterus. The vessels of bulb and clitoris link with vesical and vaginal plexus.

The pelvic plexus and veins also have communication with the presacral and lumbar channels of the vertebral plexus and thus it is possible for blood, tissue cells, emboli and organism to travel to remote parts of the body without passing through the heart and lungs. ***This explains the occurrence of metastatic growth in the spine and brain, when the primary is in the uterus***.

The collateral pathways are especially significant in late pregnancy, when the large uterus always obstructs the inferior vena cava of the woman lying on her back. It is mainly when this alternative route is inadequate and woman can have the supine hypotension syndrome.

Salient Features of Pelvic Blood Vessels

1. The pelvic vessels play an important role in pelvic support—they provide condensation of endopelvic fascia that act to reinforce the normal position of pelvic organs.
2. There is significant anatomic variation between individuals in the branching pattern of the internal iliac vessels.
3. The pelvic vasculature is a high volume, high flow system with enormous expensive capabilities throughout reproductive life.
4. The pelvic vasculature is supplied with an extensive network of collateral connection that provides a rich anastomotic communication between different major vessels system.

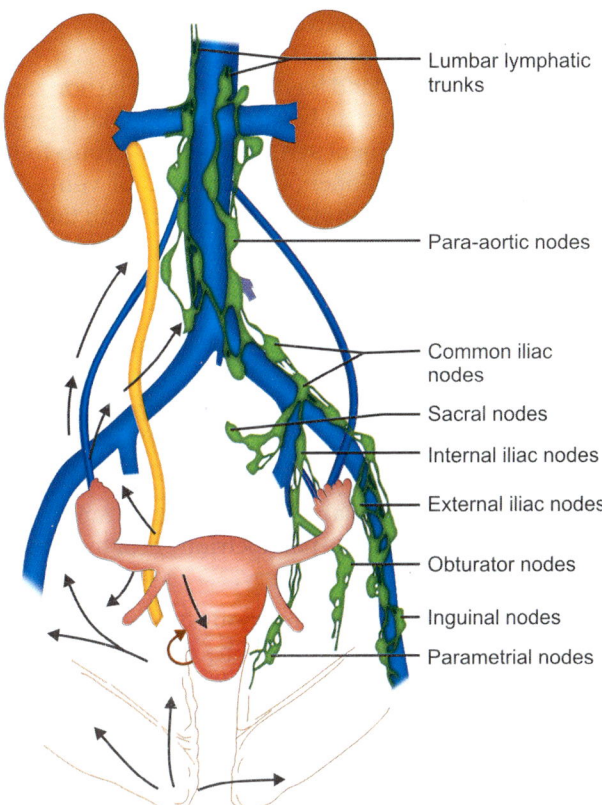

Fig. 1.19: Lymphatic drainage of pelvis

LYMPHATIC DRAINAGE OF PELVIS

The lymphatic drainage of the pelvis begins as plexus in the individual organs and generally follows the line of blood vessels. After which they are named and generally arranged in groups or chain (Fig. 1.19).

Lymph nodes in pelvis receive afferent lymphatic vessels from pelvic, peripheral, visceral and parietal structure and send efferent lymphatic to more proximal node groups.

The number of lymph nodes and their exact location though varies but major and constant group of lymph nodes are as follows:
1. Nodes at junction of internal and external iliac vein (common iliac).
2. External iliac (collecting from inguinal group of lymph nodes).
3. Internal iliac.
4. Obturator node in the obturator foramen, close to obturator vessels and nerve.
5. Ureteral node in the broad ligament near the cervix, where the uterine artery crosses over the ureter.
6. The Cloquet or Rosenmüller node—highest of deep inguinal nodes that lie within the opening of femoral canal.
7. Median and lateral sacral.

Inguinal glands: This group of glands consist of:
a. Superficial (horizontal)
b. Deep femoral gland (vertical group): The horizontal group lies superficially parallel to inguinal ligament (Poupart's ligament syn) and vertical group follow the course of saphenoid and femoral veins. The Cloquet or Rosenmüller node lies beneath the inner end of Poupart's ligament in the femoral canal between Gimbernat's ligament and the femoral vein. Inconstant deep inguinal nodes are 5 – 6 in numbers and lie on the medial side of the femoral vein, along the course of round ligament and in the tissue of mons veneris. The communication from the superficial to deep gland occurs through fossa ovalis.

The glands of the parametrium: It is of small size, inconsistently present in the parametrium, near the crossing of the ureter with the uterine artery.

Hypogastric gland (bifurcation nodes): These glands are situated below the bifurcation of the common iliac. This group contains all the regional glands for the cervix, the bladder, the upper one-third of the vagina and also for greater part of the body of the uterus. These glands may be extensively involved in carcinoma of cervix and of vagina. A further group of these glands situated in the obturator fossa often called the **obturator glands**, which is most obviously involved in carcinoma of cervix.

External iliac glands: This group of gland has three groups: (a) Lateral—lateral to external iliac artery, (b) Middle in between artery and vein, (c) Medial—medial to the vein.

These glands receive drainage from the obturator and hypogastric glands and are always involved in late cervical cancer.

Common Iliac Glands

This group is the upward continuation of the external and hypogastric group and therefore involved next after these glands.

Sacral Group

Two groups of sacral glands can be recognized—a lateral group, lying lateral to the rectum and a medial group lying in front of the promontory of the sacrum. They receive lymphatics from the cervix of the uterus and from the upper third of the vagina. The lymphatic from these glands pass directly either to inferior lumbar group or to the common iliac group.

Lumbar Group

These lymphatic glands are divided into an inferior group which lies in front of the aorta below the origin of the inferior mesenteric artery and a superior lumbar group which lies near the origin of the ovarian arteries.

The superior group of lumbar glands receive lymphatics from the ovaries and fallopian tubes as well from the inferior lumbar glands. The lymphatics from the fundus of the uterus join the ovarian lymphatics to pass to the same group.

The above group of lymphatic glands receives lymphatics 'direct' from the female generative organs and are known as the 'regional lymphatic glands' of the female genital system.

Thereafter, the lymph from the superior lumbar group of lymph nodes, passes up to cisterna chyli situated over the body of 12th thoracic vertebra. The lymph is finally carried upwards via the thoracic duct which opens into the left subclavian vein at its junction with left internal jugular vein.

Organ-wise Lymphatic Drainage of Female Reproductive System

Vulva and Perineum

The lymphatics of each side of the vulva communicate freely with each other, so for malignant disease of one labium it is proper to excise the whole vulva. Without encroaching on the inner aspect of the thigh, channels pass forward to the mons veneris and the subcutaneous tissue of the lower abdominal wall to enter the medial group of superficial inguinal nodes.

These connect with the deep inguinal (femoral) groups from which lymphatics pass to the external and ultimately to the common iliac lymph nodes.*

Vagina

The lymphatic plexus are situated in the mucosal and muscle layers. Lower vagina drains to the inguinal and femoral nodes in the same way as the vulva. The drainage of the middle and upper vagina is the same as that of cervix.

Cervix

Lymphatics from the cervix run in the broad and uterosacral ligaments and in the cellular tissue beneath these to the external and internal iliac, the obturator and sacral nodes. There is a plexus of lymphatic vessels and rarely use node in the broad ligament near the cervix.

The hypogastric and external iliac nodes communicate with those around the common iliac vessels and ultimately with the para-aortic group.

Fallopian Tube and Ovary

The intrinsic plexus of the fallopian tube are situated in the mucosal and subperitoneal layers. The fallopian tube drains in part with the fundus of uterus but mainly with the ovary. Lymphatics from the ovary accompany the ovarian vessels to reach the aortic nodes (lumbar nodes).

---

* Gland of Clocquet: It was previously thought to be the main relay gland and is said to drain the clitoris directly. Recent study shows its insignificant involvement in vulvar malignancy.

There are free anastomoses between the ovarian lymphatics of each side across the uterosacral ligament and via the subperitoneal lymphatic plexus of the fundus of uterus.

Urethra and Bladder

The external urethral meatus drains with the vulva to the inguinal nodes. The remainder of the urethra together with bladder has lymph vessels which go to external, internal and common iliac nodes.

Pelvic Colon

Lymphatic accompany the inferior mesenteric vessels to the preaortic nodes.

Anus and Rectum

The anal orifice drains to the superficial inguinal nodes and anal canal to the internal iliac group. The lymphatic drainage of lower rectum is also to the internal inguinal nodes, the lymph channels accompanying the inferior rectal and internal pudendal vessels. That of upper rectum is to the preaortic nodes, the lymph channels being associated with superior rectal vessels.

PELVIC NERVES

These are somatic and autonomic pelvic nerves.

Somatic Nerves

1. The skin of mons veneris and the foreparts of the vulva are supplied by the ilioinguinal nerve and genital branch of genitofemoral nerve both arising from L_1 and L_2 roots of the lumbar plexus.
2. The outer parts of the labia posteriorly and the perineum receive some sensory fibers from the perineal branch of posterior cutaneous nerve of the thigh.
3. The main somatic supply to the pelvic organ is pudendal nerve, which is both motor and sensory and is formed from the S_2, S_3 and S_4 roots of the sacral plexus.

Pudendal nerve leaves the pelvis through the greater sciatic notch, curls round the ischial spine and with internal pudendal vessels re-enters through lesser sciatic notch to lie on the outer wall of the ischiorectal fossa in Alcock's canal (Pudendal canal syn). Pudendal nerve supplies sensory fibers to the skin of vulva, external urethral meatus, clitoris, perineum and the lower vagina.

It provides motor fibers to all the voluntary muscles, including the compressor urethrae, sphincter vaginae, levator ani and external and sphincter.

Except in its lower part, the vagina is remarkably insensitive to ordinary stimuli. Disease such as vaginitis, ulcer with cancer and injuries including burn do not cause pain. Vaginal surgery can be carried out with minimum infiltration of local anesthetic provided the perineum and introitus are avoided, because most of the vagina is supplied by autonomic and not somatic nerves.

Autonomic Nerves

All the internal reproductive organs including the upper vagina together with urinary apparatus, rectum, and colon have only autonomic innervations. The blood vessels are controlled by their own intrinsic nerves. The autonomic nerves to these carry both sensory and motor fibers—principally adrenergic and partly cholinergic.

Sympathetic

Motor sympathetic nerves arise from D_5 and D_6 and sensory nerves arise from D_{10} to L_1 in case of sensory nerves. They pass down from the celiac plexus through intermesenteric plexus, lying retroperitoneally in front of abdominal aorta. Over the bifurcation of the aorta and promontory of the sacrum is complicated network just beneath the peritoneum, called *presacral nerve or superior hypogastric plexus*.

From superior hypogastric plexus two main chain hypogastric nerves run outwards and downwards, on each side wall of the pelvis to terminate in the inferior hypogastric plexus, which lie on either side of ampulla of rectum extending forward beneath the uterosacral and broad ligament.

It also receives fibers from the parasympathetic system, consisting of sacral fibers $S_{2,3,4}$, from here the nerve fibers pass to all the pelvic organs. The forward extension of the pelvic plexus is called the **Lee Frankenhausser plexus**. The parasympathetic fibers (nerve erigentis) are derived from the S_2, S_3 and S_4 nerves and join the hypogastric nerve of the corresponding side to form pelvic plexus. These parasympathetic fibers are mainly sensory to the cervix and lower uterus (Fig. 1.20).

From vaginal plexus the nerve fibers pass onto the uterus, upper 1/3rd of vagina, urinary bladder, ureter and rectum.

Ovarian Plexus

The fallopian tubes and ovaries are supplied by parasympathetic and sympathetic nerves which accompany the ovarian vessels and come directly from the preaortic plexus. They are both motor and sensory. The segmental supply is D_{10} and D_{11} for the ovary and D_{11} and D_{12} for the fallopian tube.

ANTERIOR ABDOMINAL WALL

It is relevant for student to know the anatomy of abdominal wall beside female reproductive system, which from the basis for different abdominal incision in obstetrical and gynecological surgery and endoscopy.

The anterior abdominal wall includes skin, superficial fascia, a muscle/aponeurosis layer, transversalis fascia and

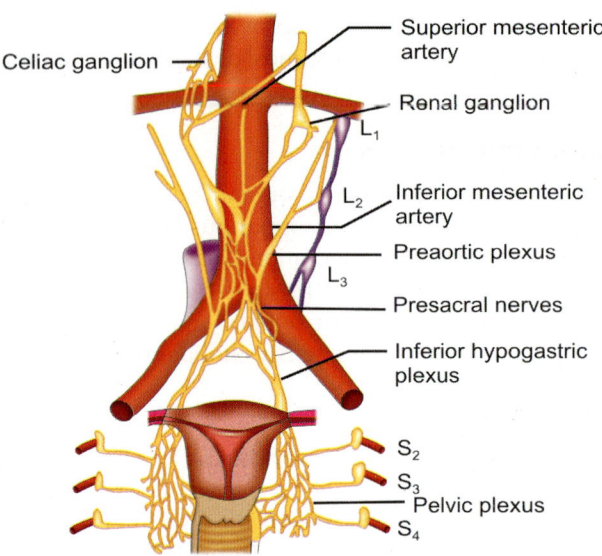

Fig. 1.20: Diagrammatic representation of pelvic innervation

peritoneum. The four main muscles are: (a) Internal oblique, (b) External oblique, (c) Transversus, (d) Rectus abdominis. All muscles are supplied by T_6 to T_{12} and L_1 (Fig. 1.21).

Muscles of Anterior Abdominal Wall

External oblique (Obliqus externus syn): It arises from the lower eight ribs. Some muscle fibers terminate on the iliac crest, the rest form an aponeurosis which ends medially in the linea alba, which is a tendinous structure extending from the xiphoid process to the pubic symphysis.

Aponeurosis ends below the pubic symphysis and pubic crest. Between the pubic tubercle and the anterior superior iliac spine the thickened margin of the aponeurosis form the **inguinal ligament**.

Inguinal Rings and Canal

Just above the pubic crest is a triangular aperture which is called superficial inguinal ring. The deep inguinal ring in the transversalis fascia lies above and lateral to superficial inguinal ring. The inguinal canal runs between these two rings and contains the round ligament (spermatic cord in the male) and the ilioinguinal nerve.

Oblique Internus Muscle

It arises from the lateral 2/3rd of the inguinal ligament, from the iliac crest, and from the thoracolumbar fascia. It inserts to the lower three to four ribs. Some fibers from the inguinal ligament arch around the round ligament of the uterus and join the aponeurosis of the transverse abdominis to form the conjoint tendon inserting into the pubic.

Transverses Abdominis

This muscle arises from the lateral third of the inguinal ligament, iliac crest, the thoracolumbar fascia and the internal aspect of the lower six cartilages. It forms an aponeurosis, the lower fibers of which contributes to the conjoint tendon, while rest of fibers blends with the linea alba in the midline.

Rectus Abdominis

Rectus abdominis arises by tendons from the pubis and is attached to the 5th to 7th costal cartilages. It has three tendinous intersections and is enclosed by the fibrous rectus sheath.

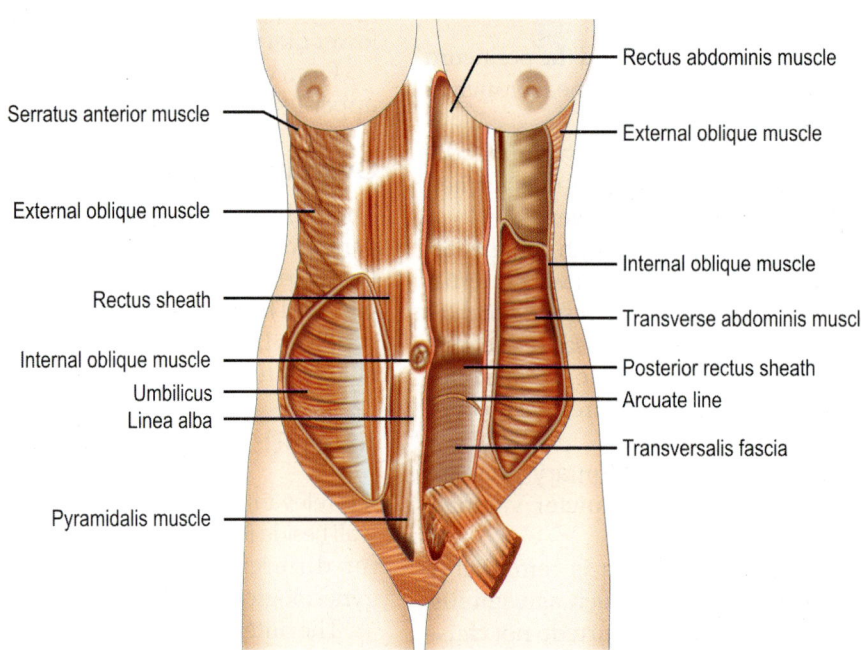

Fig. 1.21: Muscles of anterior abdominal wall

Rectus Sheath

The aponeurosis of the external and internal oblique and the transverses abdominis combines to form a sheath for the rectus abdominis and pyramidalis which fuse medially in the midline at the linea alba and laterally at the semilunar line. Above the arcuate line, the aponeurosis of the internal oblique muscle splits into anterior and posterior lamellae.

Below this line, all three layers are anterior to the body of the rectus muscle. The rectus is then curved posteriorly by the transversalis fascia, providing access to the muscles for the inferior epigastric vessels. Pyramidalis is a triangular muscle in front of the lower part of the rectus abdominis.

Nerve and Vessels

The tissues of the abdominal wall are innervated by the continuation of the inferior intercostals nerve T_4 to T_{11} and the subcostal nerve T_{12}. The inferior part of the abdominal wall is supplied by the first lumbar nerve through the iliohypogastric and ilioinguinal nerve. The primary blood supply to the anterior abdominal wall includes the following:
1. Inferior epigastric and deep circumflex iliac arteries branches of the external iliac artery.
2. The superior epigastric artery—a terminal branch of the internal thoracic artery.

The inferior epigastric artery runs superiorly in the transversalis fascia to reach the arcuate line where it enters the rectus sheath. *It is vulnerable to damage by the abdominal incision in which the rectus muscle is completely or partially transected or by excessive lateral traction on the rectus.* The superior epigastric vessels enters the rectus sheath superiorly just below the 7th costal cartilage.

Concluding Remark

Clear concepts of anatomical details lay the foundation steps of differential diagnosis, surgical approaches and techniques. Today new surgical approaches are being developed to solve old problem and new interpretation of old anatomical knowledge is being done. Surgeon has to revisit and reapply its familiar anatomy from different perspective with wide use of endoscopy or disturbed anatomic relationship in various diseases, so a clinician as well surgeons should be a perpetual students of anatomy.

PELVIC SKELETON

The skeleton of the pelvis is formed by the sacrum and coccyx, and the paired hip bones (Coxal, Innominate syn) which fuse anteriorly to form the symphysis pubis.

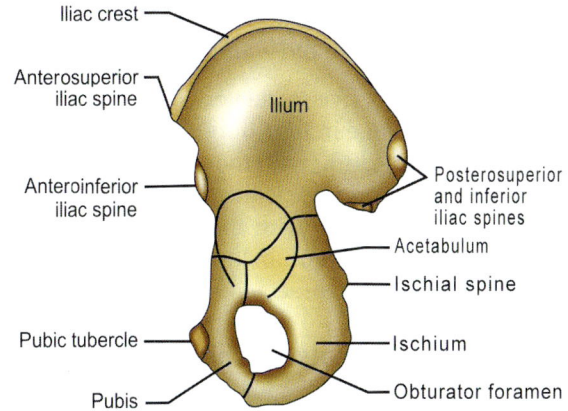

Fig. 1.22: Lateral aspect of innominate bone

The Innominate Bone

The innominate bone consists of: (a) Ilium, (b) Ischium, (c) Pubis. These components meet to form the acetabulum, a cup shaped cavity that accommodates the femoral head.

While studying for pelvic skeleton, it is mandatory that student have hip bone with them for understanding the different landmarks which are of great clinical, imaging and surgical importance (Fig. 1.22).

a. **Ilium:** Iliac crest is the most prominent feature which provides attachment to iliac fascia, abdominal muscle and fascia lata. Projections at each end of iliac crest are the anterior and posterior superior iliac spines. The medial surface presents the iliac fossa, the iliac tuberosity and auricular surface, which articulates with the sacrum.

b. **Ischium:** This consists of a body and a ramus—the body forms part of the acetabulum and the ramus fuses with the ramus of the pubis to complete the obturator foramen. Ischial spine delineates the greater and lesser sciatic notch above and below it. It has following significance:
   i. It is important clinical landmark on pervaginal examination for detection of progressive fetal descent.
   ii. It is landmark in performance of pudendal nerve block and sacrospinous ligament vaginal suspension.

Ischial tuberosity is the rounded bony prominence upon which the body rest in the sitting position.

c. **Pubis:** This consist of a body and two rami. The superior ramus joins the ilium and ischium to form the acetabulum. The inferior ramus joins the ramus of the ischium to complete the obturator foramen. The upper part of the body forms the pubic crest and pubic tubercle and the medial surface forms a cartilaginous joint with the opposite pubis (the pubic symphysis). These three parts of the innominate bones is joined by bone in the adult and cartilage in the young.

Sacrum: It consists of five sacral vertebra joined by bone in the adult and cartilage in the young. There are four sacral foramina communicating with the sacral canal. The upper border of the pelvic surface is the sacral promontory. The sacrum articulates above with the fifth lumbar vertebra, laterally with the ilium and below the coccyx, which are 3-5 fused coccygeal vertebrae.

Foramina and Canals in the Pelvis

Obturator foramina: This is bordered by ischium and pubis and is occupied by fibrous sheet—the obturator membrane. Superiorly there is a small gap (canal) which communicates between the pelvis and the thigh and carries the obturator artery, vein and nerve.

Greater sciatic foramen: This is formed by the greater sciatic notch (ilium and ischium), the sacrotuberous and sacrospinous ligaments and ischial spine. It transmits the (a) Piriformis muscles, (b) Superior and inferior gluteal nerve and vessels, (c) Internal pudendal vessels and nerve, (d) The sciatic nerve, (e) Posterior femoral cutaneous nerves, (f) Nerve to the quadratus femoris.

Lesser sciatic foramen: This is bounded by the ischium and ischial spine and by the sacrotuberous and sacrospinous ligaments. It transmits—tendon of obturator internus, internal pudendal vessel and nerve. The nerve to the obturator internus passes lateral to the internal pudendal vessels and nerve, and innervates the obturator internus on the wall of the ischiorectal fossa.

Pudendal canal: This is a sheath of fascia on the lateral wall of the ischiorectal fossa, transmitting the internal pudendal vessel and nerves.

Sacral foramina: There are four pairs of these on each of the dorsal and ventral surface of the sacrum. They communicate with the sacral canal through the intervertebral foramina and transmit the dorsal and ventral rami of the first four sacral spinal nerves.

Sacral canal: The sacral canal is formed by the vertebral foramina of the sacral vertebrae, the lower opening is the sacral hiatus. As the spinal cord ends at the first lumbar vertebrae, the sacral canal contains only nerve roots (cauda equina) and the filum terminale.

The subarachnoid space extends to the lower border of 2nd sacral vertebrae and below this the dura mater and arachnoid form a closely applied covering of the filum terminale as it descends to its attachment on the first coccygeal segment.

General Feature of the Bony Pelvis

From obstetrical point of view, it is useful to consider the bony pelvis as a whole rather than separate two bones. In both women and men the pelvis form the bony ring through which the body weight is transmitted to lower extremities but in women it has a special form that adapt the child-bearing or parturition. The sex differences in the pelvis are listed in Table 1.1.

Table 1.1: Sex difference in the pelvis	
Female	Male
Iliac blades more vertical	Iliac crest rugged
Iliac fossa shallow	
Sacrum broader and less curved	
Subpubic arch 80°-85°	50°-60°
Ischiopelvic rami marrow	Ischial spine closer
Greater sciatic notch wider	Cavity longer and more conical
Greater anteroposterior diameter especially at lower ends	

The false pelvis lies above the linea terminalis and bounded posteriorly by the lumbar vertebra and laterally by the iliac fossa. In front the boundary is formed by the lower portion of the anterior abdominal wall. The true (or lesser) pelvis consists of a cavity with upper and lower openings. The cavity of true pelvis is like obliquely truncated bent cylinder with its greatest height posteriorly. Its anterior wall at the symphysis pubis measures about 5 cm and its posterior wall about 10 cm. It is divided for systemic description into three parts: **(a) The brim, (b) The cavity, (c) The outlet** (Fig. 1.23).

The Pelvic Brim (Inlet, Upper Pelvic Strait Syn)

The pelvic brim is bounded from anteriorly to posteriorly from center of upper border of pubic symphysis, along the pubic crest, part the pubic spine to the iliopectineal eminence, thence along the iliac portion of iliopectineal line to the sacroiliac articulation, thence along the lower border of the ala of the sacrum to the center of the sacral promontory (Fig. 1.24) *(students are advised to have bony pelvis or model in hand)*. Shape of inlet of female pelvis is typically near round.

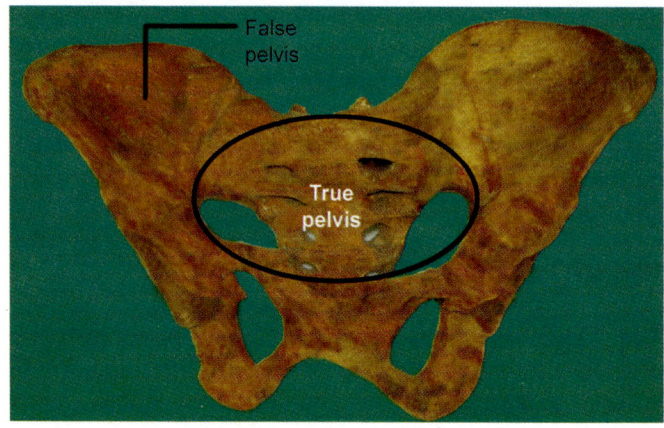

Fig. 1.23: The female pelvis

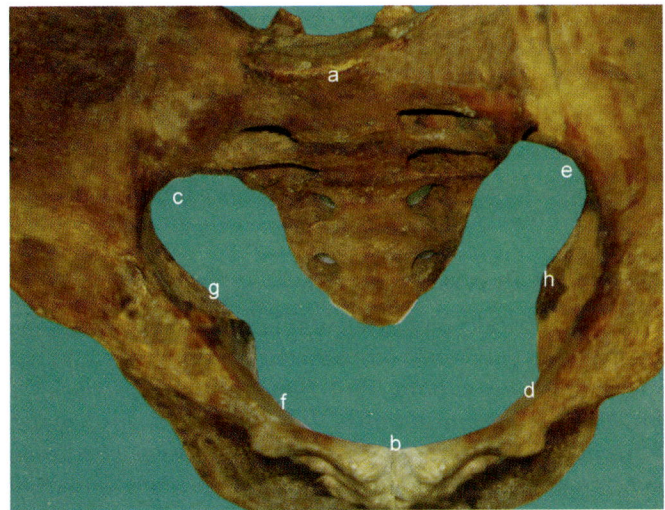

Fig. 1.24: The female pelvis—diameters of inlet (ab—Anteroposterior diameter, cd—Right oblique diameter, ef—Left oblique diameter, gh—Transverse diameter)

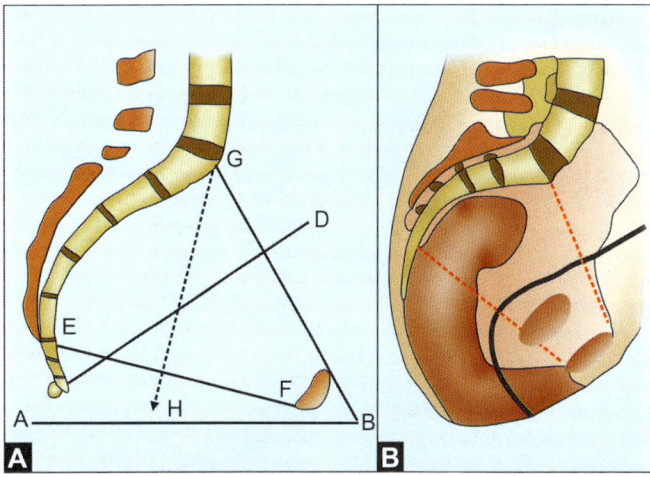

Figs 1.25A and B: The female pelvis—inclination and axis: (A) AB—Horizontal line, CD—Axis of brim, EF—Plane of obstetrical outlet, GH—Axix of obstetrical outlet; (B) Obstetrical axis

Caldwell and Moloy (1934) identified radiographically a nearly round or gynecoid pelvic inlet in approximately 50% of women).

Plane of pelvic brim is an imaginary flat surface bounded by the limits of pelvic brim. It is not strictly a mathematical plane and is therefore referred to **as superior strait**.

Inclination

Due to oblique articulation of the pelvis with the femora, the plane of pelvic brim is inclined at an acute angle of approximately 55 degrees to the horizontal surface, which is called **angle of inclination of pelvic brim (Figs 1.25A and B).**

The posterior border of the pelvic brim stands at a higher level than anterior, the sacral promontory being about 3¾ inch (9.4 cm) higher than upper border of symphysis pubis in the erect position. The fact plays an important basic for certain obstetric maneuver in breech delivery and shoulder dystocia.

When there is lumbarization of first piece of sacral vertebra there is low inclination, which has no obstetrical significance.

When there is sacralization of 5th lumbar vertebra, it is called high inclination. It has got following obstetrical significance – (a) There is delay in engagement because uterine axis fails to coincide with that of inlet, (b) It favors occipitoposterior position, (c) There is difficulty in descent of head due to long birth canal and flat sacrum which interferes in internal rotation.

Axis of Pelvic Brim

It is an imaginary straight line drawn perpendicular to the plane of the brim at its center. If it is extended upwards and downwards, this line passes through the umbilicus to coccyx. This line or axis of brim indicates the direction in which fetus passing through pelvic brim passes. It is also important that the uterine axis should coincide with the axis of the inlet so that force of uterine contraction will coincide in right direction for passage of baby through the brim (Fig. 1.25B).

Diameters of Pelvic Brim

Anteroposterior Diameter (Syn: True Conjugate, Anatomical Conjugate, Conjugate Vera):

It is the distance between the midpoint of the sacral promontory to the inner margin of upper border of symphysis pubis. *It measures 11 cm (4 ¼ inch).*

Obstetric Conjugate

It is the distance between the midpoints of the sacral promontory to prominent bony projection in the midline on the inner surface of the symphysis pubis. The point is somewhat below its upper border. It is the shortest anteroposterior diameter in the anteroposterior plane of the inlet. *It measures 10 cm (4 inch).*

Diagonal Conjugate

It is the distance between the lower border of symphysis pubis to the midpoint on the sacral promontory. *It measures 12 cm (4 ¾ inch). Diagonal conjugate is important as it can be measured clinically during per vaginal pelvic assessment in late pregnancy or labor. Obstetric conjugate is computed by subtracting 1.2 cm from the diagonal conjugate* (Fig. 1.26).

For practical purpose if the middle finger fails to reach the promontory or touches it with difficulty, it is considered that conjugate is adequate for average size fetal head to pass through.

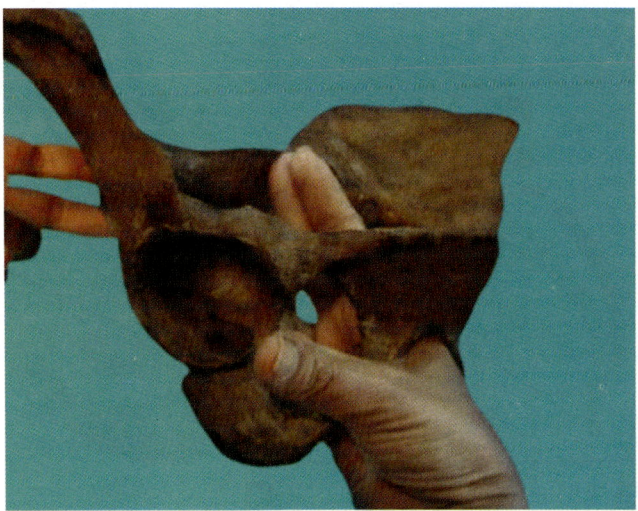

Fig. 1.26: Clinical estimation of diagonal conjugate

Transverse Diameter

It is the distance between the two farthest apart points of the pelvic brim. This line crosses the true conjugate in its middle third and divides the brim into anterior and posterior segment. Strictly speaking it is not a diameter, since it does not usually pass through center.

Oblique Diameter

There are right and left oblique diameters which are measured from the right sacroiliac articulation behind to left iliopectineal eminence on the opposite side in the front and from left sacroiliac articulation to right iliopectineal eminence irrespectively. *It measures 12 cm (4 ¾ inch).*

Mid Pelvis (Pelvic Cavity)

It is the segment of the pelvis bounded above by the inlet and below by plane of least pelvic dimension (obstetrical outlet). It forms a curved canal with a shallow anterior wall measuring 3.75 cm (1½ inch), deep posterior wall measuring 11.25 cm (4 ½ inch), and lateral walls measuring 7.5 cm (3 inch). Shape of the mid cavity is almost round in typical gynecoid pelvis.

Plane of Mid Cavity

Usually a single mid plane of cavity is described which is bounded in front by the center of the symphysis pubis and behind by the junction of 2nd and 3rd sacral vertebra. It is the plane of greatest pelvic dimensions and represents the roomiest part of the pelvic cavity.

Diameters of Mid Cavity

Anteroposterior diameter: It measures from the midpoint on the posterior surface of the symphysis pubis to the junction of 2nd and 3rd sacral vertebrae. It measures 12 cm (4 ¾ inch).

Transverse diameter: It cannot be precisely measured as the points lie over the soft tissues covering the sacrosciatic notches and obturator foramina. It measures 12 cm (4 ¾ inch).

Oblique diameter: It cannot be precisely defined. Axis of the mid plane of the cavity is represented by a line the direction of which is intermediate between those of brim and the outlet.

Outlet of Pelvis

From obstetrical point of view it is useful to consider the outlet of the pelvis as its constricted lower portion and not merely as its lower bony limit. **Bony limit or bone outlet is known as Anatomical outlet.** It is Lozenge shaped space, bounded from anterior to posterior—lower border of symphysis pubis, laterally by ischiopubic rami, the ischial tuberosities, sacrotuberous ligaments, tip of coccyx (Fig. 1.27A). These boundaries of anatomical outlet are not in a single line, they form two triangular planes, which have a common base formed by a line joining the ischial tuberosities. Apex of anterior triangle is formed by the inferior border of the pubic arch and that of posterior triangle by the tip of coccyx.

Obstetrical Outlet

It forms a shallow bony segment which is bounded above at the level of ischial spine, which is known as narrow pelvic plane and below by the anatomical outlet (Fig. 1.27B).

Diameter of Anatomical Outlet

a. *Anteroposterior:* It extends from the lower border of the pubic symphysis to tip of coccyx. *It measures 11.5 cm when coccyx is in normal position and 13 cm (5 ¼ inch) when coccyx is pushed back by the head in second stage of labor.*
b. *Transverse (Intertuberous diameter syn):* It measures between inner border of two ischial tuberosity measuring 11 cm (4 ¼ inch). Oblique diameter cannot be defined as between ischial tuberosity and the coccygeal border the pelvic outlet is filled in with the soft structure only and these diameters are skeletal.
c. *Posterior sagittal diameter:* It is the anteroposterior distance between the sacrococcygeal joint and midpoint of transverse diameter of anatomical outlet. It measures 8.5 cm (3 ½ inch). *It is clinically measured by the distance between sacrococcygeal joint and anterior margin of anus.*

So the obstetrical outlet must be clearly distinguished from anatomical outlet. Its anterior wall is defective at pubic arch, its lateral walls are formed by ischial bones and the posterior wall is made up of whole of coccyx.

Narrow Pelvic Plane (Plane of Least Pelvic Dimension Syn)

It is an imaginary flat surface bounded in front by the lower border of the symphysis pubis, laterally by the tips of ischial

Chapter - 1 ♦ Anatomy

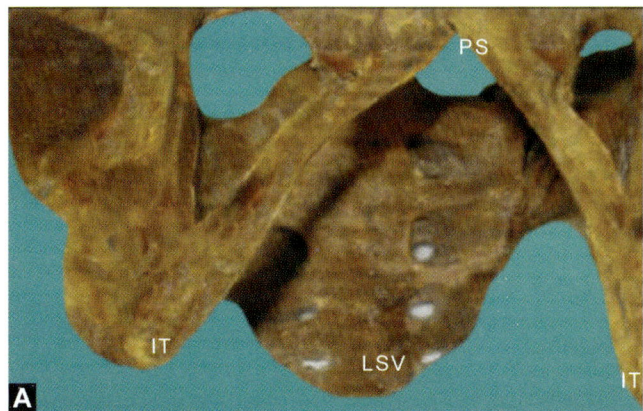

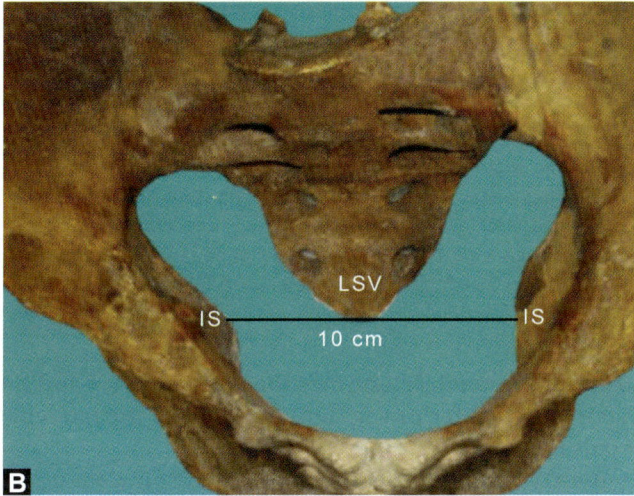

Figs 1.27A and B: The female pelvis—anatomical and obstetrical outlet (PS—Pubic symphysis, IT—Ischial tuberosity, LSV—Last sacral vertebra, IS—Ischial spine)

spines and posteriorly by the lower border of the last sacral vertebra. Its shape is anteroposteriorly oval and measures 10.7 cm (4.3 inch).

It is general agreement to refer it as plane of outlet. **Axis of narrow pelvic plane** is represented by a line joining the center of its plane with the sacral promontory, the direction of which is nearly vertical than the axis of brim.

Diameter of Narrow Pelvic Plane

Anteroposterior diameter: It extends from the inferior border of pubic symphysis to the tip of sacrum, *measuring 11 cm (4 ¼ inch).*

Transverse diameter (bispinous): It is the distance between two ischial spines *measuring 10.5 cm (4 1/5 inch).*

Posterior sagittal: It is the distance between the tip of sacrum and the midpoint of bispinous diameter, *measure 5 cm (2 inch).*

Obstetrical Significance of Narrow Pelvic Plane

Narrow pelvic plane is the useful landmark for following reasons:
a. It corresponds to the site of origin of levator ani muscles (Pelvic diaphragm).
b. It marks the beginning of forward curve of pelvic axis.
c. Ischial spines are easily felt on pervaginal examination. So it is an important landmark for clinical documentation of descent of presenting part in assessment of progress of labor. For example, if head has reached up to ischial spine, it is certain that head is engaged in the pelvic brim.
d. At this level completion of internal rotation of head takes place.
e. It is a landmark used for pudendal nerve block.

Other Obstetrical Significant Landmarks

a. *Subpubic angle:* It is formed by the approximation of the two descending pubic rami. In gynecoid pelvis, it measures approximately 85°.
b. *Pubic arch:* It is formed by descending rami of both the sides. At the level of 2 cm below the apex of subpubic arch it measures 6 cm. Clinically, it is assessed by placing the finger of hand side by side.

Waste Space of Morris

In gynecoid pelvis the subpubic arch is rounded and fetal head is well placed under the pubic arch. But in narrow pubic arch as found in android pelvis, the fetal head is displaced backwards and there is less room available for head. This distance between the lower border of symphysis pubis and the circumferences of the head is termed—**waste space of Morris, which should not exceed 1 cm in proportionate pelvis**.

When waste space of Morris is more than 1 cm, the anterior point of the anteroposterior diameter of the outlet extends below the symphysis pubis on the pubic rami for distance equivalent to the waste space of Morris. The distance between above point and the sacrum is called **available anteroposterior diameter of the outlet.** Through this available anteroposterior diameter the fetal head escapes out of the bony outlet (Figs 1.28A to C).

Axis of Pelvis

By uniting the axis of the three planes of pelvic brim, mid cavity and the outlet, a line is formed which traverse the center of the canal of the bony pelvis. It is uniformly curved, with anterior concavity. It is directed at first downwards and backwards (corresponding to axis of brim) than gradually more and more forwards (corresponding to axis

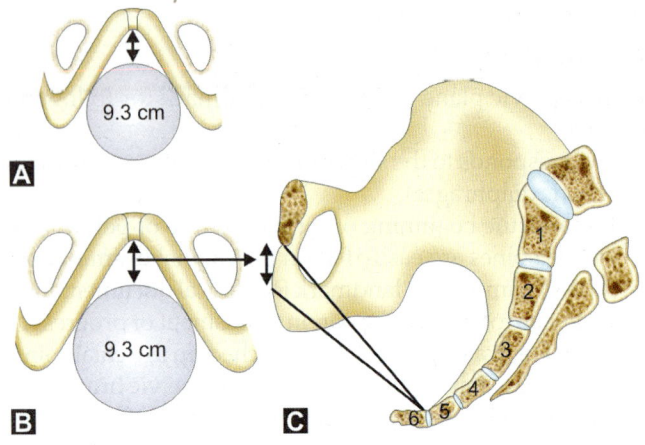

Figs 1.28A to C: Diagrammatic representation of: (A) Normal pubic arch; (B) Waste space of Morris; (C) Available anteroposterior diameter of the outlet

	Table 1.2: Diameter of bony pelvis		
	Anteroposterior	Transverse	Oblique
Inlet (Pelvic brim)	11 cm ± 0.5 cm Anterior sagittal 7 cm Posterior sagittal 4 cm	12.8 cm ± 0.5 cm	11.8 cm ± 0.3 cm
A. Outlet (Obstetrical)	11.0 cm ± 0.5 cm	Interspinous 10.7 cm ± .3 cm	
B. Anatomical Outlet	13 cm	Interspinous 10.7 cm ± 0.3 cm Intertuberous 12.5 ± 0.5 cm	

- Subpubic angle = 80° ± 5°
- These diameters are reduced by soft structure lining the pelvic walls and viscera. For example, iliopsoas and obturator internus muscles reducing the transverse and oblique diameter of brim, pelvic colon in left oblique diameter of brim and cavity, urethra diminish anteroposterior diameter of outlet.

of cavity and then outlet) until it reaches the axis of the outlet, where it has anterior concavity. This line is known as **anatomical axis of the pelvis or curve of Carus** (Figs 1.25A and B).

Obstetrical Axis

Fetus passing through the pelvis does not follow the anatomical axis because pelvic cavity is almost cylindrical in its upper three fourth parts, so head descends in axis of pelvic inlet till level of ischial spines and than curves forward near the narrow pelvic plane.

This line represents obstetrical pelvic axis, which represent the real path of head through the pelvis. This line is straight in upper part and curved only in its lower portion.

Summarization of diameter of bone pelvis is in Table 1.2.*

Pelvic Shapes

Coldwell and Molloy (1933, 34) used special methods of stereoradiography which enabled them to study the architecture of pelvic in life size accurately. Coldwell and Molloy classification is still considered the gold standard for obstetrics and anticipating various difficulties and complications in different types of pelvis.

This classification is based on measurement of the greatest transverse diameter of the inlet and its division into anterior and posterior segment. **The character of posterior segment determines the type of pelvis and the characters of anterior segment determines the tendency of pelvis.**

Both type as well tendency are not pure but determined because many pelvis are not pure but mixed type.

However, the four parent types of pelvis are:
a. Gynecoid
b. Anthropoid
c. Android
d. Platypelloid

Gynecoid pelvis is found in approximately 50% of women and intuitively suited for delivery of most fetuses. In contrast in android pelvis the posterior sagittal diameter at the inlet is much shorter than the anterior sagittal diameter, which limits the use of the posterior space by the fetal head. Beside, the anterior portion is narrow and triangular. **So the extreme android pelvic passage has a poor prognosis for vaginal delivery.**

In the **anthropoid** pelvis the anteroposterior diameter of the inlet is greater than transverse, which results in a narrow and somewhat pointed anterior segment. Anthropoid pelvis and its variant are found in approximately one third of the women.

The **platypelloid** pelvis has a flattened gynecoid shape with short anteroposterior and wide transverse diameter.

Table 1.3 summarizes the different characteristics of four types of pelvis.

---

* The pelvic measurements given are average when measured radiologically and vary within a limited degree. The conversion of centimeters into inches is approximate.

CHAPTER - 1 ♦ Anatomy

Table 1.3: Feature of various types of pelvis (Coldwell and Molloy—1933)

	Gynecoid	Android	Anthropoid	Platypelloid
Shape of brim	Well rounded	Triangle with base towards sacrum	Oval	Flat
Relation of hind pelvis and fore pelvis	Area of hind pelvis is only somewhat less than that of fore pelvis limiting use of posterior space by fetal head	Postsagittal segment or hind pelvis is shorter	Hind pelvis and fore pelvis are almost equal	Short anteroposterior and transverse diameter
Sidewall	No convergence or parallel	Convergent downwards		Divergent downwards
Ischial spines	Not prominent	Often prominent	No distinguished feature	Not prominent
Subpubic angle	Not ≥ 85°	Narrow		> than 90°
Subpubic arch	Normal	Narrow		Wide
Sacral angle	Exceeds 90°	more than 90°		> than 90°
Labor complication	Normal	• Persistent occipito-posteior position of head • Less tendency to injury to bladder neck	• Direct occipito-posterior or anterior • Face to pubes delivery	• At brim difficulty in engagement • Outlet dystocia • Asynclitism is usually present sometimes resulting in secondary face presentation • Tendency to bladder neck injury
Approximate incidence	50%	19%	27%	4%
Body build	Feminine	Thick and heavy built somewhat masculine	Tall, long headed, wide shouldered	Average height

- Intermediate form are more common that pure parent type
- Slight degree of contraction in any of non-gynecoid group have more difficulty in labor than in more perfectly adapted female type.

MULTIPLE CHOICE QUESTIONS

1. Lymphatics from clitoris drain into
   a. Superficial inguinal lymph node
   b. Deep inguinal lymph node
   c. Lymph node of cloquet
   d. Obturator lymph node
   Ans. a, b, c.

2. All of the following pelvic structure support the vagina *except*:
   a. Perineal body
   b. Pelvic diaphragm
   c. Levator ani
   d. Infundibulopelvic
   Ans. d

3. All of the following are classified as primary supports of uterus *except*:
   a. Transcervical ligament
   b. Pubocervical ligament
   c. Uterosacral ligament
   d. Broad ligament
   Ans. d

4. Peg cells are seen in:
   a. Vagina
   b. Fallopian tube
   c. Vulva
   d. Uterus
   Ans. b

5. Epithelial lining of Bartholin's duct is:
   a. Columnar
   b. Transitional
   c. Cuboidal
   d. Squamous
   Ans. a

6. The mucosal lining of vagina is composed of:
   a. Ciliated columnar
   b. Pseudostratified columnar
   c. Stratified squamous keratinized
   d. Transitional
   Ans. c

7. Bartholin's duct opens into:
   a. Labia majora
   b. Labia minora
   c. Lower vagina
   d. Groove between labia minora and hymen
   Ans. d

8. Corpus cervix ratio up to 10 years of age:
   a. 3:2
   b. 2:1
   c. 3:1
   d. 1:2
   Ans. d

9. The length of fallopian tube is:
   a. 8-10 cm
   b. 10-12 cm
   c. 15 cm
   d. None
   Ans. b

2. Reproductive Physiology

The way you decide to think has a dramatic effect on your chemistry & physiology.

GENERAL CONSIDERATION

The reproductive process in women is a complex and highly evolved interaction of many components. The carefully orchestrated series of events that contributes to a normal ovulatory menstrual cycle requires precise timing and regulation of hormonal input from the central nervous system, the pituitary gland and the ovary. Disruption of this balance can result in various type of menstrual disorders, infertility, pregnancy loss, which are major gynecological problems faced by gynecologist. To effectively diagnose and manage these conditions, it is critical that gynecologist understand the normal physiology of menstrual cycle.

BASIC CONCEPT IN ENDOCRINOLOGY

Neuroendocrinology: Neuroendocrinology represents facts of fields of medicine **endocrinology**—which is study of hormones and **neurosciences**—which is study of action of neurons. The discovery of neurons that transmit impulses and secrete their products into the vascular system to function as hormones themselves, a process known as neurosecretion demonstrates that the two systems are intimately linked.

Hypothalamus—Functional Anatomy

Hypothalamus is small neural structure situated at the base of the brain above the optic chiasma and below the third ventricle. It is connected directly to the pituitary gland and is the part of the brain that is the source of many pituitary secretions. Anatomically, hypothalamus has three zones:

i. Paraventricular (Adjacent to third ventricle)
ii. Medial (Primarily cell bodies)
iii. Lateral (Primarily axonal)

Each zone is further subdivided into structure known as **nuclei** which represents location of concentration of similar types of neuronal cell bodies. T**he paraventricular** and **supraoptic** centers synthesize the posterior pituitary hormones. Ventromedial nuclei control satiety (Fig. 2.1). Median eminence contains terminals of many peptide secreting neurons whose cell bodies are situated in the hypothalamic centers. These nerves terminals are closely applied to the looped capillaries in this region and contain the pituitary releasing and inhibiting hormones.

The activity of the central nervous system is converted into chemical signals and the hypothalamus with adrenal medulla and pineal gland is referred to as a

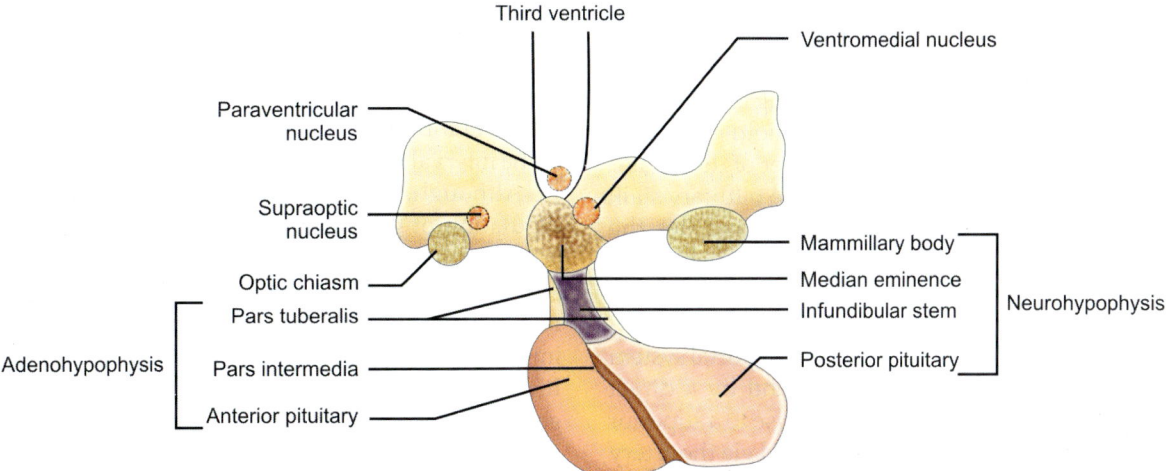

Fig. 2.1: Functional anatomy of the hypothalamus and pituitary

neuroendocrine transducer. In addition, the portal vessels in the median eminence are connected to the fluid of third ventricle by specialized ciliated ependymal cells called **tanycytes**. Hypothalamus can be influenced by higher cortical centers especially the temporal lobe. Emotional upsets are known to stimulate or depress HP axis. Thus, hypothalamus is not an isolated structure within the CNS, but it has multiple interconnections with other region in the brain.

Beside this several level of feed back to the hypothalamus exist and are known as long, short and ultrashort feedback loop. The long feedback loop is composed of endocrine input from circulating hormones, e.g. feedback of androgen and estrogen onto steroid receptor is present in the hypothalamus. Similarly, pituitary hormones may feedback to the hypothalamus and serve important regulatory function in **short** loop feedback. Finally, hypothalamic secretion may directly feedback to the hypothalamus itself in an **ultrashort** feedback loop (Figs 2.2A to C).

The major hypothalamic hormones and factors effecting anterior pituitary cells are summarized in Table 2.1.

Table 2.1: Hypothalamic hormones and its effects on anterior pituitary

Hypothalamic hormone	Effect on anterior pituitary
1. Gonadotropic releasing hormonal (GnRH) decapeptide	Release of LH and FSH
2. Thyrotropin releasing hormone (Tripeptide)	Release of TSH and prolactin
3. Somatostatin (Growth hormone inhibiting hormones) 14 amino acid	Inhibition of growth hormone
4. Corticotropin releasing hormone (CRH)—42 amino acid	Release of ACTH
5. Growth hormone releasing hormone (40 amino acid)	Release of growth hormone
6. Prolactin inhibiting factor (dopamine)	Inhibition of prolactin and growth hormone

Pituitary—Anatomy and Embryology

The anterior pituitary forms from Rathe's pouch, an upward evagination of the ectoderm of the pharyngeal roof. The pituitary lies in a depression in the sphenoid—the sella turcica. The sella turcica is covered by a layer of duramater (the diaphragmatic sella) through which the pituitary stalk passes. Immediately above the pituitary gland lies the hypothalamus and in front of this is the optic chiasma. Cavernosus sinus and ocular motor nerves are above and lateral.

The pituitary is supplied with blood by the portal system originating in the hypothalamus (80%) and by a direct arterial supply. The internal carotid gives rise to a superior pituitary artery (which supplies the stalk and via the artery of the tubercula—the posterior pituitary) and an inferior pituitary artery. The pituitary increases in weight by 30-50% during pregnancy due to an increase in prolactin secreting cells. The pituitary is divided into three region or lobes—**Anterior, Intermediate, and Posterior.**

Anterior pituitary—(Adenohypophysis syn) is quite different structurally from the **posterior neural pituitary (neurohypophysis syn)** which is direct physical extension of the hypothalamus.

Adenohypophysis is not composed of neural tissue, as is the posterior pituitary and does not have direct neural connection to the hypothalamus. Instead a unique anatomic relationship exists that combines elements of neural production and endocrine secretion. Adenohypophysis itself has no direct arterial blood supply. Its major source of blood flow are portal vessels which is also its source of hypothalamic input. *Blood flow in these portal vessels is primarily from the hypothalamus to the pituitary. Blood flow to posterior pituitary is via superior, middle and inferior hypophyseal arteries.*

Reproductive Hormones

Gonadotropic Releasing Hormones

Luteinizing hormone releasing hormone (LHRH) GnRH are Syn: It is the controlling factor for gonadotropic secretion. It is a decapeptide produced by neurons with cell bodies primarily in the arcuate nuclei of the hypothalamus.

Pulsatile Secretion

GnRH is unique among releasing hormone in that it simultaneously regulates the secretion of two hormones – FSH and LH. It is also unique among the body hormones because it must be secreted in a pulsatile fashion to be effective and the pulsatile release of GnRH influences the release of the two gonadotropins. *GnRH has an extremely short half-life of only 2-4 minutes as a result of rapid proteolytic cleavage.* The pulsatile secretion of GnRH varies in both frequency and amplitude throughout the menstrual cycle and is tightly regulated. The follicular phase is characterized by frequent small amplitude pulse of GnRH secretion. In the late follicular phase, there is increase in LH frequency and amplitude of pulses. During luteal phase there is a progressive lengthening of the interval between pulses.

Although, GnRH is primarily involved in endocrine regulation of gonadotropin secretion from the pituitary, it is now apparent that this molecule has autocrine and paracrine function throughout the body. Beside GnRH is involved not only in release of stored LH and FSH but it is of importance in maintaining the synthesis of gonadotropins. It has been demonstrated that repeated exposure of the gonadotropins to GnRH seems essential for the adequate pituitary stores. This response has been termed **self-priming**.

Chapter −2 ♦ Reproductive Physiology

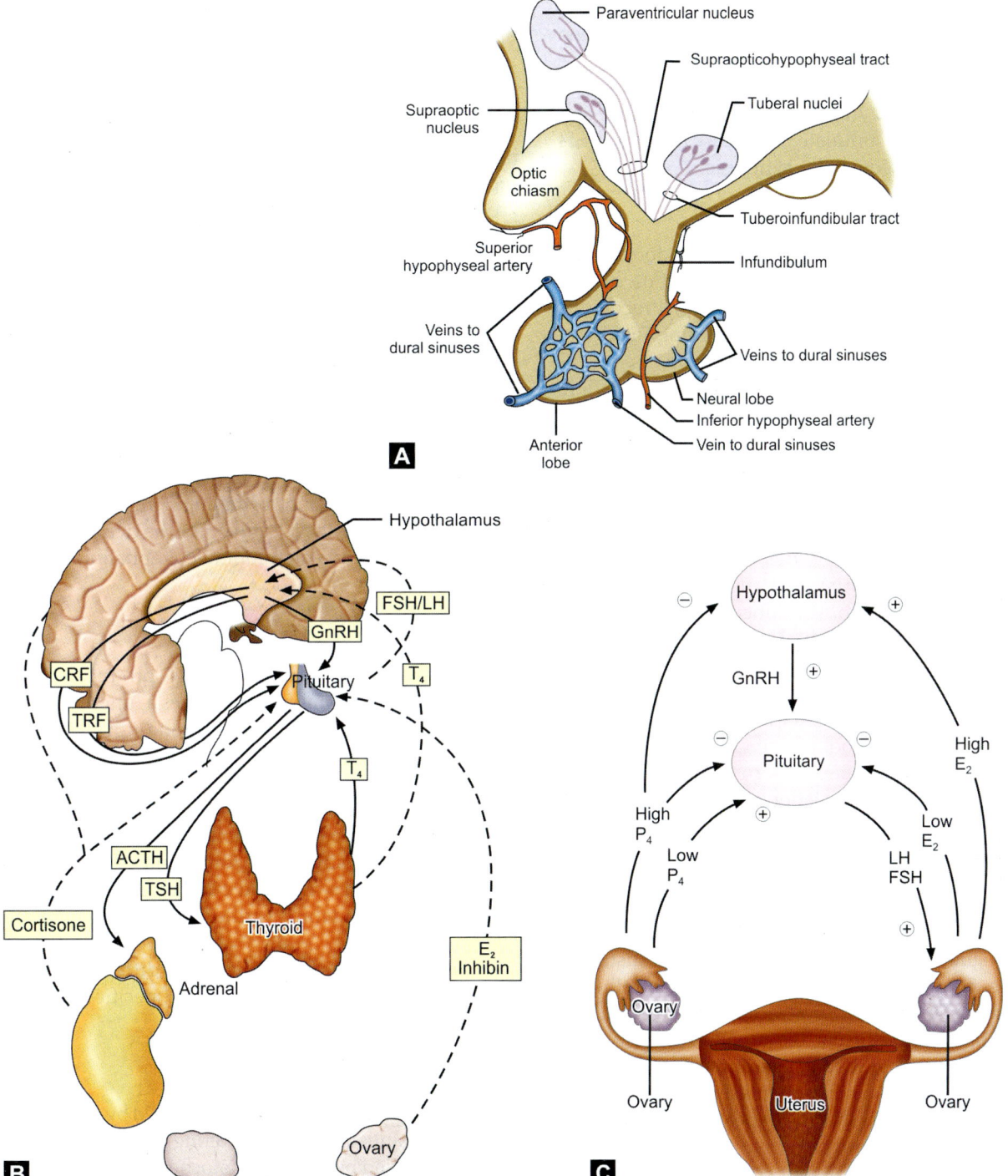

Figs 2.2A to C: (A) Hypothalamus and its neurological connections; (B) Hypothalamus and its connections with pituitary, thyroid, adrenal and ovary; (C) Hypothalamopituitary ovarian axis showing positive and negative feedback of hormones

GnRH—Agonist and Antagonist (Structure and Function)

The short half-life of GnRH is due to rapid cleavage of the bonds between amino acids 5-6, 6-7 and 9-10. By altering amino acids at these positions, analog of GnRH can be synthesized with different properties. Substitution of amino acids at the six positions or replacement of the C-terminal glycine amide (inhibiting degradation) produces agonist.

Function—Mechanism of Action of GnRH on Pituitary Cells

GnRH binds to the specific receptors on the cell membrane of the gonadotropins. Within a second there is activation of the enzyme, adenylcyclase which catalyzes the conversions of ATP to cyclic AMP. CAMP receptor-protein complex then activate protein kinase C. Intracellular free Ca^{++} concentrates increases. Protein kinase C causes phosphorylation and activation of specific enzymes. Ca^{++}, protein kinase C and CAMP then interact to stimulate the release of stored FSH and LH and their subsequent biosynthesis.

Clinical Application

This suppression of pituitary secretion of gonadotropin by a GnRH agonist can be used for treatment of: (1) Endometriosis, (2) Uterine leiomyoma, (3) Precocious puberty, (4) Prevention of menstrual bleeding in special clinical situations, e.g. thrombocytopenic patients, down-regulation *in vitro* fertilization, prior to follicle stimulation, (5) Various tumors contain receptors for GnRH, as breast, pancreas, prostrates ovary, so they may be a potential treatment, (6) Shrinkage of endometrium prior to endometrial ablation.

Administration of GnRH Analog

GnRH agonist is administered in following ways: (a) Intramuscular injection, (b) Subcutaneous injection, (c) Intranasal absorption. An initial agonist action (so called Flare effect) is associated with an increase in the circulatory level of FSH and LH. This response is greatest in the early follicular phase when GnRH and estradiol have combined to create a large reserve pool of gonadotropins. After 1-3 weeks in continuous release, there is suppression of gonadotropins and downregulation of the pituitary, which produce a hypogonadotropic hypogonadic state. **On continuous infusion of GnRH the gonadotropin secretion is inhibited, because the receptors are saturated and are unable to stimulate the release of second messenger. This is known as desensitization or downregulation.** The initial response is due to desensitization whereas the sustained response is due to loss of receptors and uncoupling of effector system. Furthermore, postreceptor mechanism lead to secretion of biologically inactive gonadotropin.

GnRH analog is degraded in gastrointestinal tract so it is given—intravenously, intramuscularly, intranasaly and subcutaneously. Due to its short life repeated administration at short interval is mandatory.

- Drugs available are as follows:
  - Nafarelin 400 μg, intranasaly daily for 6 months
  - Buserelin 300 μg, tds daily, subcutaneously for 5 days
  - Depot injection of Goserelin, intramuscularly or implant 3.6 mg monthly
  - Leupride depot 3.75 mg, I/m monthly for 5 months.

Side Effects of GnRH

(a) Insomnia, (b) Nausea, (c) Osteoporosis caused by estrogen deficiency, (d) Decrease breast size, (e) Myalgia/edema, (f) Decreased libido, (g) Decreased in high density lipoprotein (HDL and increase in cholesterol by 10% each).

Endogenous Opioids and Effects on GnRH

The endogenous opioids are three related families of naturally occurring substances produced in the CNS that represent the natural ligands for the opioid receptors. There are three major classes of endogenous opioids.

Endorphins

They are named endorphin because of their endogenous morphin like activity. These substances are produced in the hypothalamus from the precursor POMC (pro-opiomelanocortin) and have diverse activities including regulation of temperature, appetite, mood and behavior.

Enkephalin

They function in regulation of the autonomic nervous system. Proenkephalin A is the precursor for the two enkephalin of primary importance-methionine-enkephalin and lucine-enkephalin.

Dynorphin

Dynorphin are endogenous opioids, produced from the precursor proenkaphalin B that serves a function similar to that of endorphin, producing behavioral effect and exhibiting a high analgesic potency. The endogenous opioid plays a significant role in the regulation of hypothalamic pituitary junction.

Endorphins appear to inhibit GnRH release within the hypothalamus resulting in inhibition of gonadotropin secretion. Ovarian sex steroid can increase the secretion of central endorphin which further depresses gonadotropin level.

Variation of endorphin level in different phases of menstrual cycle, contribute to cycle specific symptom of ovulatory women.

Pituitary Hormone Secretion

The anterior pituitary cells are surrounded by a rich network of capillary sinusoids. Cells secreting individual hormones can be identified by immunohistochemistry. Identification by classic staining reaction (acidophil) is inaccurate and now not considered.

The **anterior pituitary** is responsible for the secretion of the following hormone releasing factors:
(1) FSH, (2) LH, (3) TSH, (4) ACTH, (5) GH, (6) Prolactin.

Posterior Pituitary Gland (Neurohypophysis)

The posterior pituitary (Neurohypophysis) is a neuro-secretory gland. The cell bodies lie in hypothalamus and axon terminal make up the stalk and gland itself.

The axon terminals are closely associated with capillaries as a neurohemal organ.

Oxytocin: Postpituitary secretes nanopeptide hormone (containing nine amino acids)—oxytocin and vasopressin. Both are secreted by the supraoptic and periventricular nuclei of the hypothalamus. The hormones are transported as granules up to nerve axons and stored in the axon terminals prior to release. The granules contain the active hormone and carrier protein—neurophysin, both of which arise from same large precursor molecule. Oxytocin has two main actions:
a. Stimulation of the uterus in labor and controlling bleeding in third stage of labor.
b. Stimulation of the myoepithelial cells of the breast to cause milk ejection.

Arginine vasopressin: It is also a nanopeptide with two amino acid composition different from that of oxytocin. It is mainly produced by supraoptic nuclei. The main physiological action of arginine vasopressin (Antidiuretic hormone) is to increase the permeability of renal collecting system to water. Its secretion is controlled by the osmotic pressure of extracellular fluid via osmoreceptors in the hypothalamus. It is stimulated by nicotine and inhibited by alcohol. The pressor effect of vasopressin is of no significance under normal circumstances, but substantial elevation may be seen in acute events as hemorrhage and anoxia.

Gonadotropin

The gonadotropin FSH and LH are produced by anterior pituitary gonadotropin cells and are responsible for ovarian follicle stimulation. Both are glycoprotein that share identical alpha subunit and differ only in structure of their α subunit, which confer receptor specificity.

Thyroid stimulating hormone and placental human chorionic gonadotropin (hCG) also share identical subunit with gonadotropin. So, the synthesis of the α subunit is the rate regulating step in gonadotropin biosynthesis.

The gonadotropins have molecular weight of around 28,000. They are metabolized in the liver and kidney and a significant fraction is excreted in urine. *LH has a half-life of around 20 minutes and FSH about twice this.* FSH controls the (a) ripening of primordial follicles, (b) in conjunction with luteinizing hormones, activates the secretion of estrogen.

LH in conjunction with FSH (a) activates the secretion of estrogen, (b) it brings about the maturation of the ovum and causes ovulation, (c) LH stimulate the completion of the reduction division of the oocyte, (d) following ovulation it produces luteinization of the granulosa and theca cells and initiates progesterone secretion.

Pattern of gonadotropin secretion in the menstrual cycle: In most of the menstrual cycle, gonadotropins are controlled by a negative feedback of estrogen (and to a lesser extent of progesterone). **So LH and FSH are at their lowest level during luteal phase of cycle when steroid levels are highest and their level tend to rise during menstruation as steroid level fall (Fig. 2.2C).**

During the follicular phase, FSH level are suppressed but LH level remain steady. Shortly before ovulation, there is a surge of LH with a simultaneous smaller FSH rise. This is due to positive feedback from the relatively high estrogen level in the late follicular phase.

PHYSIOLOGY OF MENSTRUATION

Menstruation is the periodic and cyclical discharge of blood, mucus and cellular debris from the uterine mucosa, which occurs due to progesterone withdrawal after ovulation in nonfertile cycles. It occurs in response to changes in the hormonal production by the ovaries, which themselves are governed by the pituitary and hypothalamus.

Menstruation takes place at approximately 21-35 days interval between menarche (onset of menstruation) and menopause (cessation of menstruation), with 2-6 days of flow and an **average blood loss of 20-60 ml**. The extremes of reproductive life (after menarche and perimenopause) are characterized by a higher percentage of anovulatory or irregularly timed cycle.

Normal Menstrual Cycle

The normal human menstrual cycle can be divided into two segments:
a. Ovarian cycle
b. Uterine cycle

Ovarian cycle is further subdivided into *follicular and luteal phase.*

Uterine cycle is divided into corresponding *proliferative and secretory phase.*

Follicular Phase

Hormonal feedback promotes the orderly development of a single dominant follicle, which should be mature at midcycle and prepared for ovulation. The average length of the human follicular phase ranges from 10 to 14 days and variability in the length causes most variation in total cycle length of menstrual cycle.

Luteal Phase

It is the phase from ovulation to onset of menstruation and has an average length of 14 days.

Ovarian Follicular Development

The ovary has two functional roles—first gametogenesis and second hormonogenesis. In **fetal life** gonads contain 6-7 million oogonia at 16-20 weeks of gestation. Only 1-2 million survive to reach neonatal life.

At puberty: only 300,000 of the original 6-7 million oocytes are available for ovulation. Of **these only 400-500 will be ultimately released during ovulation.**

By the time of **menopause**, the ovary will be composed primarily by dense stromal tissue with only rare interspersed oocyte remaining.*

Meiotic Arrest of Oocyte and Resumption

Meiosis is the reduction division of germ cells. It has four phases—**Prophase, Metaphase, Anaphase and Telophase.**

The prophase of meiosis is divided into five stages: **(i) Leptotene, (ii) Zygotene, (iii) Pachytene, (iv) Diplotene, (v) Diakinesis.**

When developing oogonia begins to enter meiotic prophase first, they are known as primary oocytes, which starts at around 8 weeks of gestation. Oogonia that enter meiosis will survive the atresia which occurs during fetal life.

The oocytes arrested in late diplotene stage will remain till time of ovulation. The mechanism for this mitotic stasis is probably caused by oocyte maturation inhibitor (OMI) produced by granulosa cells, which enters oocyte via gap junction connecting the oocyte and its surrounding cummulus.

When ovulation occurs with midcycle LH surge, the gap junctions are disrupted, granulosa cell lose connection with oocyte and meiosis I is allowed to resume (Fig. 2.3).

Follicular Development

It is a dynamic process that continues from menarche until menopause. The process is designed to allow the monthly

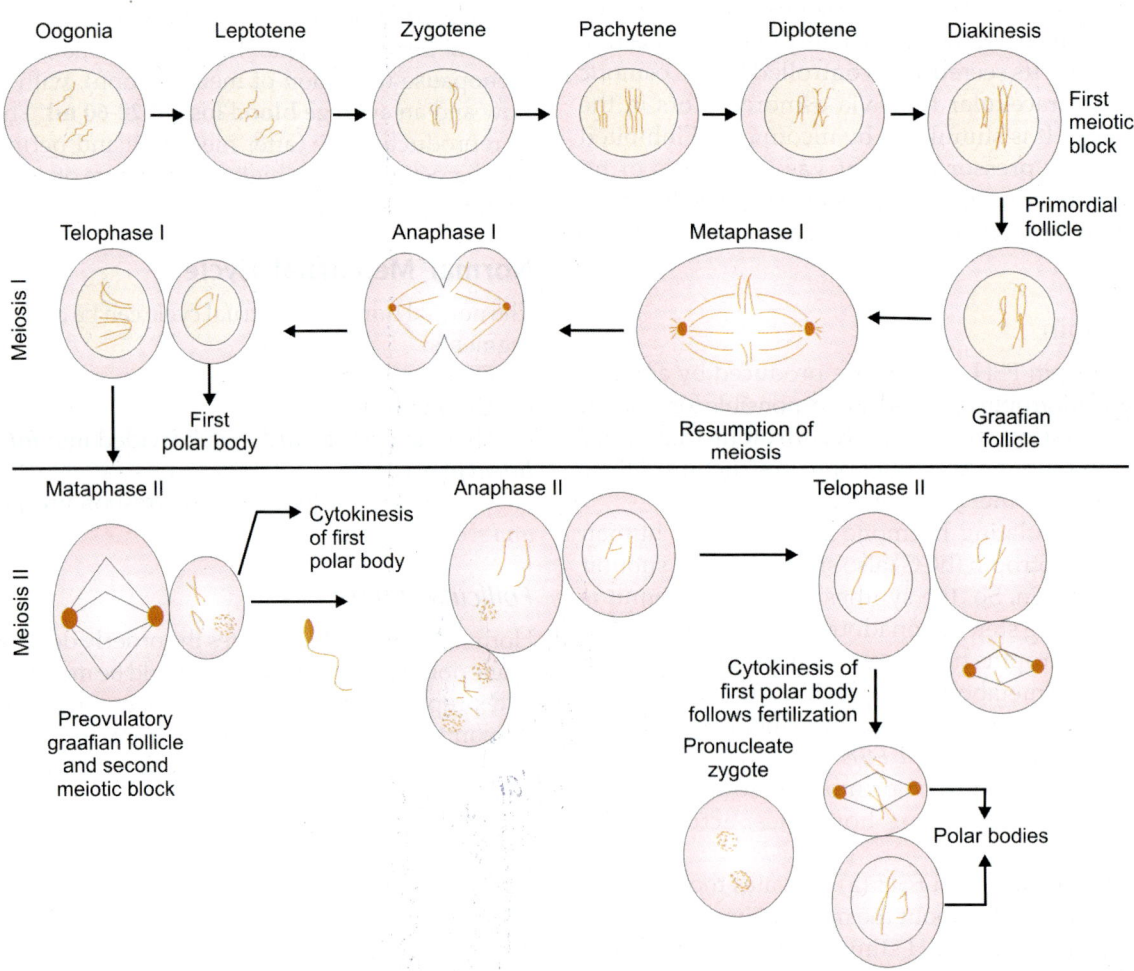

Fig. 2.3: Oocyte maturation development and gamete interaction during human fertilization

---

* A central dogma of reproductive biology is that in mammalian fetus there is no capacity for oocyte production.

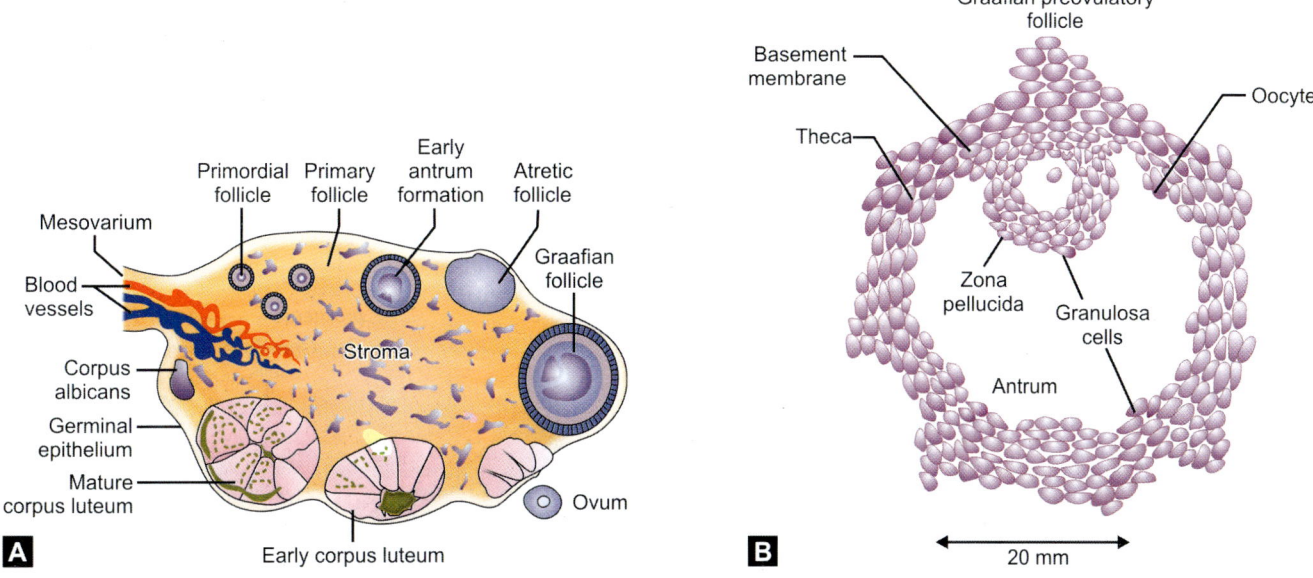

Figs 2.4A and B: (A) Sequencial stages of follicular development and corpus luteum in ovary; (B) Graafian follicle

recruitment of a cohort of follicles and ultimately to release a single mature dominant follicle during ovulation each month.*

Stages of follicular development are as follows: (a) Primordial follicle, (b) Preantral follicle, (c) Preovulatory follicle, (d) Ovulation, (e) Luteal phase (Figs 2.4A and B).

Approximately 85 days are required for primordial follicle to grow and become a preantral stage. From preantral to preovulatory stage it takes 14 days, which occurs during follicular phase of ovarian cycle. The initial stage of follicular development is independent of hormonal stimulation. Development beyond preantral stage is stimulated by pituitary gonadotropins (FSH and LH) which orchestrate the whole events of ovarian and menstrual cycle. If there is no correct and coordinated hormonal mileu, the follicles undergo atresia. Even though anatomically there are two ovaries, it functions as a single unit.

Primordial follicle: The initial recruitment and growth of primordial follicle is gonadotropin independent and affects a cohort over several months. Some 3 months before ovulation, about 300 follicles are recruited for development. Only 30 of these become gonadotropin dependent and will commence rapid growth at the beginning of menstrual cycle.

Shortly after initial recruitment FSH assumes control of follicular differentiation and growth and allows a cohort of follicles to continue differentiation. The decline in luteal phase estrogen, progesterone and inhibin A production by the new fading corpus luteum from the previous cycle allows the increase in FSH that stimulates this follicular growth.

This is the point where there is shift from gonadotropin independent to gonadotropin dependent growth. Under which influence there is growth of oocyte and expansion of the single layer of follicular granulosa cells into a multilayer of cuboidal cells.

Preantral follicle: During the several days following the breakdown of the corpus luteum, growth of the cohort of follicles continues by the stimulus of FSH. There is predominant change in the oocyte, which is enlarged out of proportion to the size of follicle. This enlarging oocyte secretes a glycoprotein rich substance—zona pellucida, which separates oocyte from the granulosa cells except at gap junction.

The flattened outer single layer pregranulosa cells become cuboidal and multilayered which is called granulosa cells. Simultaneously there is noticeable beginning of differentiation of the theca interna layer of ovarian stroma surrounding the follicle.

Both cell types theca interna and granulosa cells function synergistically to produce estrogens that are secreted into systemic circulation. The hormonogenesis is functionally compartmentalized, within the follicle as 'Two

---

* Postnatally because oocyte enters diplotene resting stage of meiosis in the fetus, and persist in this stage until ovulation. So, DNA, RNA, and protein necessary for development of preimplantation embryo will have been synthesized by this stage.

At the diplotene stage, a single layer of 8-10 granulosa cells surround the oogonia to form the primordial follicle. The oogonia that fail to become properly surrounded by granulosa cell undergo atresia. The rest proceed with follicular development. So, most oocytes are lost during fetal development and remaining follicles are used up steadily throughout the intervening years until menopause.

With research in stem cell, there has been challenge to this theory. The survivor of germline stem cells responsible for this oocyte development appears to reside in the bone marrow.

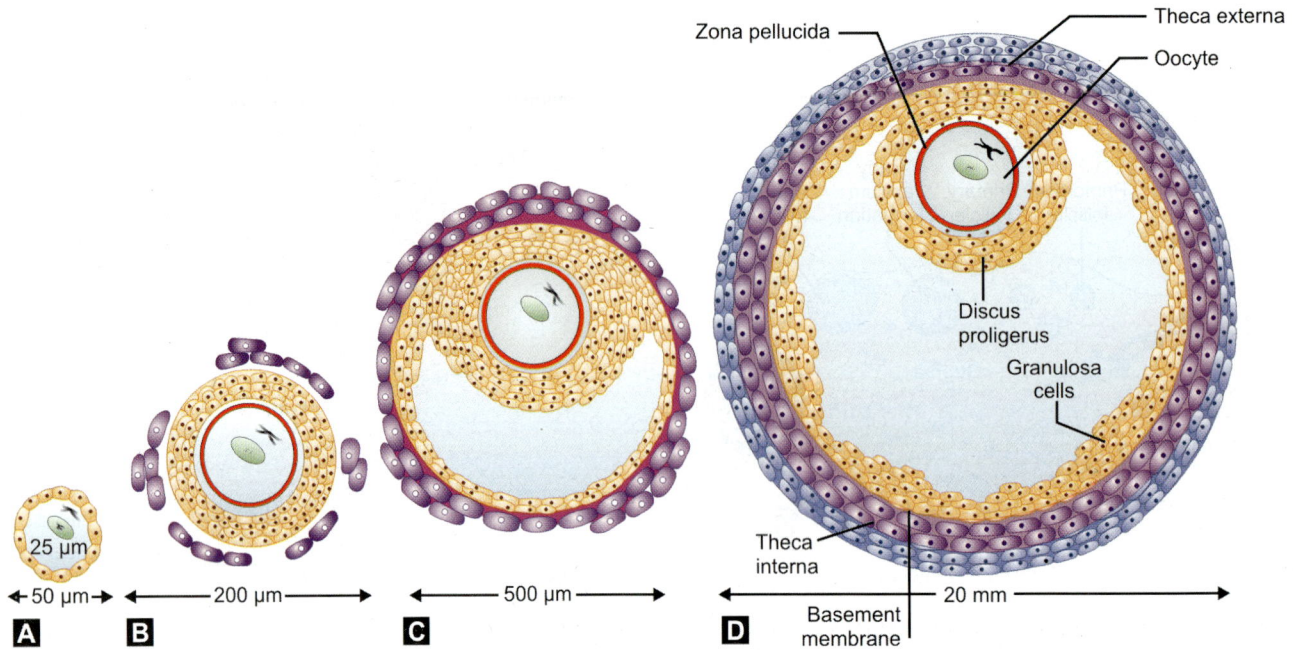

Figs 2.5A to D: Different stages of follicular development: (A) Primordial follicle; (B) Preantral follicle; (C) Antral follicle; (D) Preovulatory follicle

cell Two Gonadotropin Systems". *In preantral and central follicles, LH receptors are present only on the theca cells and FSH receptors only on granulosa cells.*

In response to LH, the theca cells are stimulated to produce androgens. The FSH induces aromatization in the granulosa cells, which converts the thecally derived androgens into estrogen.

Androgen production within the follicle may also regulate the development of the preantral follicles. Low level of androgen enhances aromatization and increases estrogen production. In contrast high androgen production inhibits aromatization and produces follicular atresia.

Meanwhile, as the peripheral estrogen level rises, it negatively feeds back on the pituitary and hypothalamus to decrease circulating FSH levels. Increased ovarian production of inhibin B further decreases FSH production.

The falling FSH level that occurs with the progression of the follicular phase represents a threat to continued follicular growth. The resulting adverse environment can be withstood only by follicles with a selective advantage for binding the diminishing FSH molecules that is those with the greatest number of FSH receptors.

So, the dominant follicle can be perceived as the one with a richly estrogenic microenvironment and the most FSH receptors. As follicle grows and develops, the follicle continues to produce estrogen, resulting in further lowering of circulating FSH and creating a more adverse environment for competing follicles.

The process continues until all members of the initial cohort, with the exception of the single dominant follicle, have suffered atresia. The stage is then set for ovulation.

Preovulatory follicle: Preovulatory follicles are characterized by a fluid filled antrum that is composed of plasma with granulosa cell secretions. This is called **graafian follicle,** which is named after the Dutch physician and anatomist **Reynair de graaf** (1641-1673).

There is accelerated growth of all the components of follicles of the preantral phase. The granulosa cell grows faster than the theca cells. There is production of follicular fluid which is primarily an ultrafiltrate of blood from the vessels within theca interna. The fluid filled space is formed amidst the granulosa cells. The space coalesces to form an antrum (Figs 2.5A to D).

One follicle with highest antral concentration of estrogen and lowest androgen (estrogen ratio) and whose granulosa cells contain maximum receptor for FSH, becomes the dominant follicle. The dominant follicle controls the endocrine mileu, as it prepares itself, the reproductive tract and hypothalamic pituitary axis for ovulation.

In dominant follicle there is marked enlargement of the granulosa cells with lipid inclusion. The granulosa cells surround the ovum to form cumulus oophorous or discus proligerous which in fact anchors the ovum to the wall of the follicle. The cells adjacent to the ovum are arranged radially and is called corona radiata.

Rising estrogen levels have a negative feedback effect on FSH secretion. Conversely LH undergoes biphasic regulation by circulating estrogen. At lower concentrations estrogen inhibit LH secretion. At higher level, however estrogen enhances LH release.

This stimulation requires a sustained high level of estrogen (200 pg/ml) for more than 48 hours. Once the rising

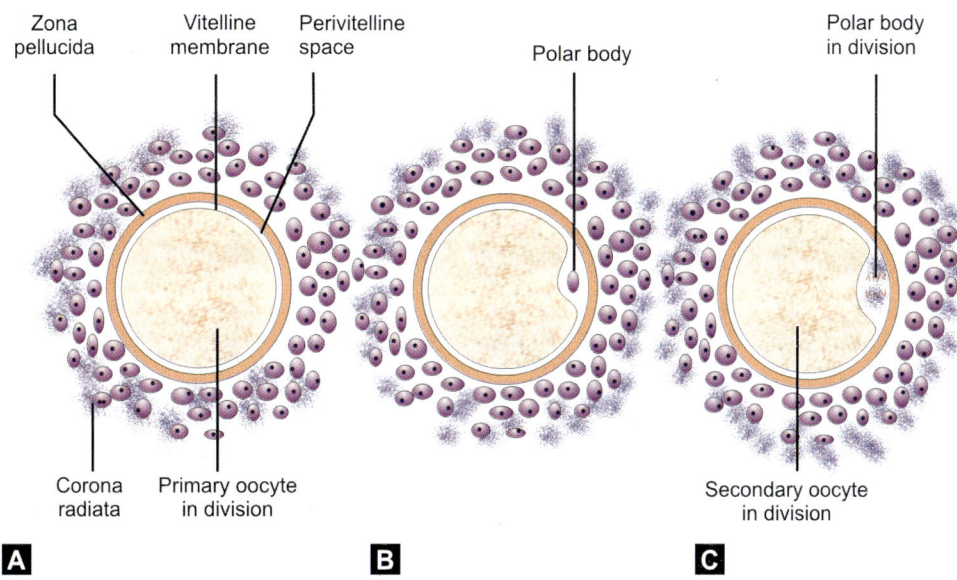

Figs 2.6A to C: Resumption of meiosis in primary and secondary oocyte

estrogen level produces positive feedback, a substantial surge in LH secretion occurs. Concomitant to these events, the local estrogen—FSH interaction in the dominant follicle induce LH receptors on the granulosa cells.

Thus, exposure to high level of LH results in specific three major events:
1. Resumption of meiosis (Figs 2.6A to C).
2. Luteinization of the granulosa and theca cells walls with increased production of progesterone.
3. Extrusion of the mature oocyte about 36 hours after the beginning of the LH surge.

In general, ovulation will occur in the single mature or graafian follicle 10-12 hours after the LH peak or 34-36 hours after the initial rise in midcycle. It is significant that today it is understood that sex steroids are not the only gonadotropin regulation of follicular development. Two related granulosa cell derived peptides—**inhibin A and inhibin B play opposing roles in pituitary feedback.** Inhibin B is secreted primarily in the follicular phase and is stimulated by FSH, whereas inhibin A is mainly active in the luteal phase. Both form of inhibin act to inhibit FSH synthesis and release.

The second peptide activin stimulates FSH release from the pituitary gland and potentiates its action in the ovary.*

Ovulation

The dominant follicle shortly before ovulation, reaches the surface of the ovary. The cummulus becomes detached from the wall so that the ovum with the surrounding cells (corona radiata) floats freely in the liquor follicles. The oocyte completes the first meiotic division with extrusion of the first polar body which is pushed to the perivitelline space. Midcycle LH surge causes a dramatic increase in local concentration of prostaglandin and proteolytic enzymes in the follicular wall. These substances progressively weaken the follicular wall and ultimately allow a perforation to form. Ovulation most likely represents a slow extrusion of the oocyte through this opening in the follicle rather than a rupture of the follicular structure. The stigma is soon closed by a plug of plasma. Unless fertilized the ovum survives only 12-24 hours and then disintegrates in the tube without leaving any trace (Figs 2.7A to C).

Menstruation is unrelated to ovulation and anovular menstruation is quite common during adolescence, following childbirth and in women approaching menopause.

Luteal Phase

The corpus luteum is formed immediately after ovulation as a result of the following changes:
1. The follicle collapse after extrusion of the ovum and fluid and the central cavity fills with blood and fibrin.
2. The basement membrane separating the granulosa from the theca disappears and thecal capillaries enter the granulosa in response to secretion of angiogenic factors such as vascular endothelial growth factor.
3. The cytoplasm of the granulosa and theca cell hypertrophies, with accumulation of lipid droplet and characteristic yellow lutein pigment for which the structure is named. Proliferation of the smooth endoplasmic reticulum and mitochondria of granulosa lutein and theca luteum cells occurs.

---

* It is likely that there are numerous other intraovarian regulators similar to inhibin and activin, each of which may play a key role in promoting normal ovulatory process. Some of these are follistatin, insulin like growth factor (ICFI), Epidermal growth factor (EGF), Interleukin I, OMI, renin angiotensin.

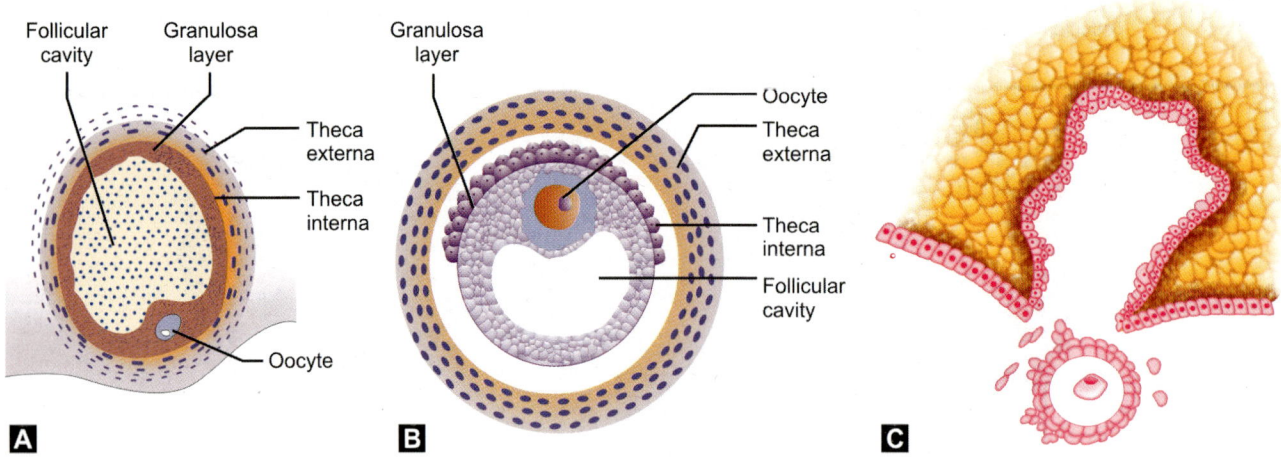

Figs 2.7A to C: (A) Mature graafian follicle; (B and C) Ovulation

4. Degeneration (apoptosis and formation of a corpus albicans begins after 10 days unless a pregnancy occurs.
Luteinization of human follicles may sometimes occur without extrusion of ovum.

Hormonal Function and Regulation

The hormonal changes of the luteal phase are characterized by series of negative feedback interaction designed to lead to regression of the corpus luteum if pregnancy does not occur. Progesterone production increases rapidly after extraction of the ovum, although it begins to rise shortly before ovulation. Estrogen production, which declines about 20 hours before ovulation recovers within a day. Both hormones peak after 6-8 days (Figs 2.8A and B).

Corpus luteal function depends both qualitatively and quantitatively on normal development of the granulosa and theca cells during the preceding follicular phase and require gonadotropin support, notably from LH and to a much lesser extent from FSH. The number of LH receptors reaches a maximum during the mid luteal phase. The corpus luteum can be sustained artificially by injection of hCG for at least 21 days beyond the expected time of the period.

In nonconceptual cycle, luteolysis is probably programmed to occur at the cellular level and is initiated automatically at the time of ovulation. Luteolysis begins with shunting of blood away from the corpus luteum, following which lysosome initiates a process of lipolysis.

Corpus Luteum

After ovulation ruptured graafian follicle develop into corpus luteum. It undergoes following stage:
a. Stage of proliferation.
b. Stage of vascularization.
c. Stage of maturation.
d. Stage of regression.

Corpus Luteum of Pregnancy

There is a surge of hyperplasia of all the layers between 23rd to 28th day due to chronic gonadotropin hCG. hCG like LH will stimulate the corpus luteum to secrete progesterone. The corpus luteum grows to 2-3 cm at about 8th week of pregnancy and looks bright orange and later yellow.

Menopausal Ovary

Apart from certain stains of rodents, the menopause is confined to the human species and does not occur in other primates. Follicle numbers decline at a steady rate up to age of approximately 37-40 years, after which there is accelerated loss until the menopause.

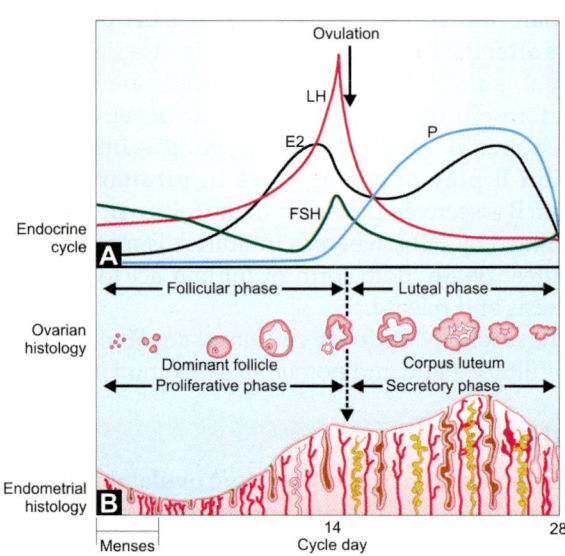

Figs 2.8A and B: Physiology of menstrual cycle: (A) Cyclic change of FSH, LH estradiol and progesterone; (B) Correlation between ovarian and endometrial cycle

Several hundred primordial follicles remain in the ovary, but these are insensitive to the action of gonadotropins and subsequent development is arrested at early age. Estradiol production is low after the menopause. However, the ovarian stroma continues to secrete androstenedione and circulating estrone levels are maintained by peripheral conversion of androstenedione.

Follicular Atresia

Follicular atresia is continued process starting at 20 weeks of intrauterine life and ends around menopause. The probable and various causes of follicular atresia can be summarized as follows:
  i. Oogonia which fails to develop granulosa cell layer envelope.
  ii. Follicles which do not enter the germ cell meiotic division.
  iii. Follicle either not rescued by FSH or not having estrogen induced FSH receptors.
  iv. Follicles losing FSH receptors either due to negative feedback effect of estrogen secreted by dominant follicle or due to high androgen estrogen ratio.
  v. Genetic as in chromosomal aberration.
  vi. Apoptosis programmed cell death.

Cyclic Changes of the Endometrium in Menstrual Cycle

The endometrium is the special epithelial lining of that part of the cavity of the uterus which lies above the level of internal os. In 1907, variation in the histological structure of the endometrium during the menstrual cycle was studied by Hitschmann and Adler, further work was done by Noyes, Hertig and Rock in 1950. Endometrium has two principle components: (a) Glandular epithelium, (b) Supporting stromal cells.

Cyclic histological changes in endometrium proceed in an orderly fashion in response to cyclic hormonal production by the ovaries.

During menstrual cycle, the endometrial epithelium differentiates to form following functional zones:
1. Stratum (Decidua) basalis
2. Decidua functionalis which is composed of:
   a. Stratum spongiosum: It is a deeply situated intermediate zone.
   b. Stratum compactum: Superficial compact zone

Decidua basalis is deepest region of the endometrium. It does not undergo significant change in menstrual cycle but is a source of endometrial regeneration after each menstrual bleeding. The endometrial events can be divided into three phase:
a. Proliferative phase
b. Secretory phase
c. Menstrual phase

Proliferative Phase

By convention, the first day of vaginal bleeding is called day 1 of the menstrual cycle. The phase of the menstrual cycle which starts when regeneration of menstruating endometrium is complete and last for 10-14 days of 28 days cycle is referred to as the proliferative or estrogenic phase. The ovarian follicular phase corresponds to menstrual proliferative phase of endometrial cycle.

At the start of proliferative phase, the endometrium is relatively thin (1-2 mm). Under influence of rising plasma estrogen level there is reconstruction and growth of both glandular and stromal component of endometrium, which peaks at 8 – 10 days of cycle, corresponding to peak estrogen level. During proliferative phase, endometrium grows from approximately 0.5 to 3-5 mm in height. Histologically these proliferating glands have multiple mitotic cells and their organization changes from a low columnar epithelium in early proliferative phase to pseudostratified pattern before ovulation. In this phase, the stroma is a dense compact layer and vascular structure is infrequently seen (Fig. 2.9).

Secretory Phase

In an average 28 days cycle, ovulation occurs on cycle day 14 within 48–70 hours after ovulation. The onset of progesterone secretion from corpus luteum acts upon the estrogen primed endometrium to convert it to actively secreting tissue. So, in contrast to the proliferative phase, the secretory phase of the menstrual cycle is characterized by the cellular effects of progesterone in addition to estrogen.

In general progesterone effect antagonizes to those of estrogen and there is a progressive decrease in the endometrial cells estrogen receptor concentration. So during

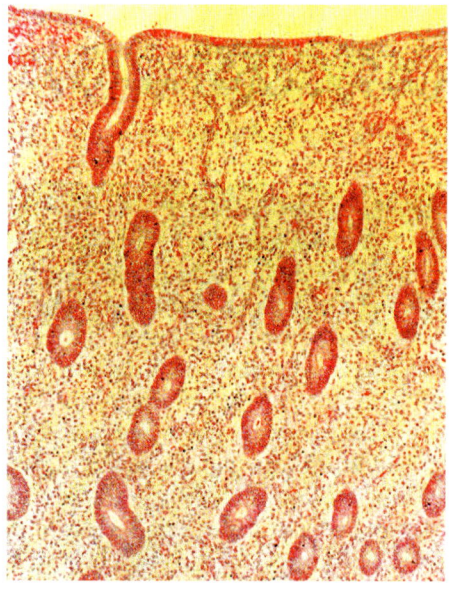

Fig. 2.9: Histological picture of proliferative endometrium

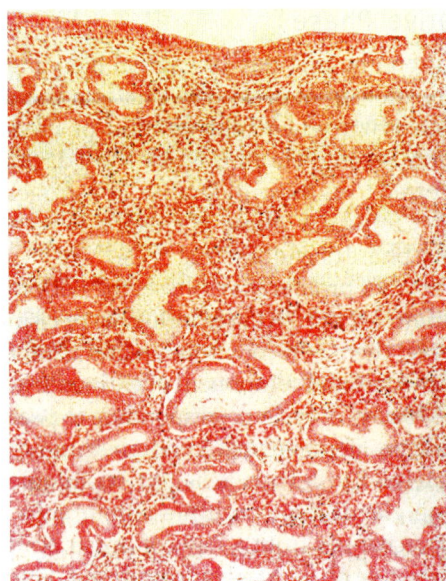

Fig. 2.10: Histological picture of secretory endometrium

this phase, estrogen induced DNA synthesis and cellular mitosis is antagonized.

The most characteristic sign of this phase is found in the glands. Glandular epithelium develops. Spherical translucent area appears between the nuclei and the basement membrane which contains the precursor of glandular secretion. This characteristic appearance is called subnuclear vacuolation. This is presumptive evidence of ovulation and progesterone activity and persists until about the 21st day of the cycle. The fluid in subnuclear vacuoles consists of mucus and glycogen, whose function is presumably to provide nutrition to the fertilized ovum. This phase of subnuclear vacuolation is followed by an increase in intracellular secretion which pushes the nucleus to the basement membrane and fills the cell. So, subnuclear vacuolation migrates past the nucleus to the surface of the cell. In later part of secretory phase the inner border of the epithelium cells become irregular through the discharge of the secretion into the lumina of the glands. So, just before menstruation glands are full of coagulated secretion which stains deeply with eosin (Fig. 2.10). The secretory phase is also characterized by change in shape of glands. The glands become crenated and assume a characteristic corkscrew shaped form and finally saw toothed form. The stroma of the secretory phase remains unchanged histologically until about 17th postovulatory day. After that there is a progressive increase in stromal edema and vascularity with maximal stromal edema in the late secretory phase. The spiral arteries become clearly visible, and then they progressively lengthen and coil during rest of the secretory phase. These changes give the stroma a reticular appearance. By around day 24, an eosinophilic staining pattern is visible in the perivascular stroma, known as "**cuffing**". Eosinophilic staining then progresses to form islands in the stroma followed by areas of confluence. This staining pattern of the edematous stroma is termed '**pseudodecidual**' because of its similarity to the pattern found in pregnancy.

About 2 days before menstrual bleed there is a dramatic increase in the number of polymorphonuclear lymphocytes that migrate from the vascular system. So, the leukocytic infiltration heralds the collapse of the endometrial stroma and onset of the menstrual flow.

At the end of secretory phase, the endometrium measures 8 to 10 mm in thickness. Endometrial thickness can be measured ultrasonically which is useful for patient on infertility treatment.*

Menstrual Phase

If there is no implantation of embryo, glandular secretion ceases and irregular breakdown of the decidua functionalis occurs. The resultant shedding of this layer of the endometrium is called menstrual bleeding. The presumed cause of shedding of decidua functionalis is degeneration of corpus luteum and resultant stopping of estrogen and progesterone hormone. With withdrawal of estrogen and progesterone, there is profound spiral artery vascular spasm that leads to endometrial ischemia. At the same time there is a breakdown of lysosome and release of proteolytic enzyme, which further promote local tissue destruction.

Prostaglandin ($PGF_{2\alpha}$) is a potent vasoconstrictor, causing further arteriolar vasospasm and endometrial ischemia. $PGF_{2\alpha}$ also encourage myometrial contraction that decrease local uterine wall blood flow and keep in physically expelling sloughing endometrial tissue from the uterus. The decidua functionalis of endometrium is shed, during menstrual bleeding, leaving the decidua basalis as the source of subsequent endometrial growth.

Active degeneration of decidua functionalis layer of endometrium seems to be restricted to the first-two days of menstruation. The subsequent bleeding is the result of oozing from the capillaries of the denuded stroma.

---

* Dating of endometrium: The secretory change of endometrium have long been thought to allow assessment of the normalcy of endometrial development. Traditional thinking held that any discrepancy of more than 2 days between chronologic and histological date indicated a pathological condition termed "Luteal Phase Defect", which has been correlated with infertility as well early pregnancy loss.

But recent randomized observational study of fertile women and large prospective multicentric trials showed that histological dating of the endometrium does not discriminate between fertile and infertile women and today the consensus is that endometrial biopsy has no role in uterine evaluation of infertility and early pregnancy loss.

Regeneration

Regeneration of the denuded epithelium starts before the stoppage of menstrual bleeding and is completed 48 hours after the end of menstruation. Repair is brought about by the glandular epithelium growing over the base stroma.

Hormone Variation and Correlation of Endometrial and Ovarian Cycle

> At the start of menstrual cycle level of gonadal steroids are low and have been decreasing since, the end of the luteal phase of the pervious cycle.
> ↓
> With degeneration of corpus luteum, FSH level begin to rise and cohort of growing follicle is recruited.
> ↓
> Follicles secrete increasing level of estrogen which provides negative feedback on pituitary FSH secretion. FSH secretion begins to wane by the midpoint of follicular phase, also added by inhibin B produced by growing follicle.
> ↓
> At the end of follicular phase FSH induced LH receptors are present on granulosa cells and with LH stimulation, modulate secretion of progesterone.
> ↓
> After sufficient degree of estrogen stimulation, the pituitary LH surge is triggered, which is the proximate cause of ovulation that occurs after 24-36 hours.
> ↓
> The estrogen level decrease through early luteal phase from just before ovulation to mid luteal phase, when it begins to rise again as a result of corpus luteum secretion.
> ↓
> Progesterone level rise precipitously after ovulation and is a presumptive evidence of ovulation. It produces secretory changes in the uterine endometrium.
> ↓
> Progesterone, estrogen and inhibin A acts centrally to suppress gonadotropin secretion and new follicular growth.
> ↓
> With degeneration of corpus luteum, estrogen and progesterone level wane, there is degeneration of decidua functionalis of endometrium in form of menstrual bleeding and setting the stage for the next cycle.

OVARIAN STEROIDOGENESIS

The functions of the ovary are ovulation and production of hormones that is steroidogenesis. The principal hormones secreted from the ovary are:
a. Estrogen.
b. Progesterone.
c. Androgens.
d. Inhibin.

The basis of hormonal activity in preantral to preovulatory follicle is described as the *"Two cell two gonadotropin"* hypothesis. This theory establishes that two cells, theca cells and granulosa cells produce different hormones under the influence of two gonadotropins that is LH and FSH. Within the theca Cells, LH stimulates the production of androgen from cholesterol. Within the granulosa cells, FSH stimulates the conversion of thecally derived androgen to estrogen by process of aromatization (Fig. 2.11).

In addition to its effect on aromatization, FSH is also responsible for the proliferation of granulosa cells. Androgen production within the follicle may also regulate the development of preantral follicle. Low levels of androgens enhance aromatization and therefore increase estrogen production. In contrast high androgen levels inhibit aromatization and produce follicular atresia.

Estrogen

Natural estrogen are C-18 steroid. The **main sources of estrogen** are granulosa cells of the follicle and a relatively small quantity from the theca cells and ovarian stroma. Secondary sources of estrogen are adrenal gland and peripheral tissue particularly skin and fat by conversion of androstenedione. This is an important source of estrogen in the male (50%) and on postmenopausal female.

Metabolism of Estrogen

Estrogen is secreted as estradiol. **Estradiol** is the most potent and binds more avidly to the receptor than weaker estrogen as estriol. Estradiol binds to albumin (19%) and in addition there are specific binding proteins in plasma. Estradiol (E2) and testosterone bind to the same binding protein called sex hormone binding globulin (SHBG). This is a high affinity low capacity β glycoprotein synthesized by the liver. SHBG binds approximately 70-80% of E2 in blood and only 1% is free and biologically active. **Estriol** (E3) is not bound to SHBG, 30% is bound to albumin. Metabolism of estrogen takes places principally in the liver. The steroid molecules are conjugated with glucuronide to form water soluble products which are excreted in urine or bile. A small proportion of E2 is converted to E3 prior to conjugation. Deconjugation by intestinal bacteria leads to reabsorption (enterohepatic circulation). The half life of circulating estrogen is 5-25 minutes. Total daily production of estradiol is approximately 50 µg during early follicular phase, reaching 150-300 µg at time of ovulation. After ovulation there is sharp fall, and rises again to about 150-200 µg/ml in luteal phase.

Action of Estrogen

a. **Secondary sexual character:** The hormone is responsive for feminine body configuration, skin and hair texture, etc.
b. **Specific action on genital tract:**
   i. Growth of vulva.
   ii. Breast development.

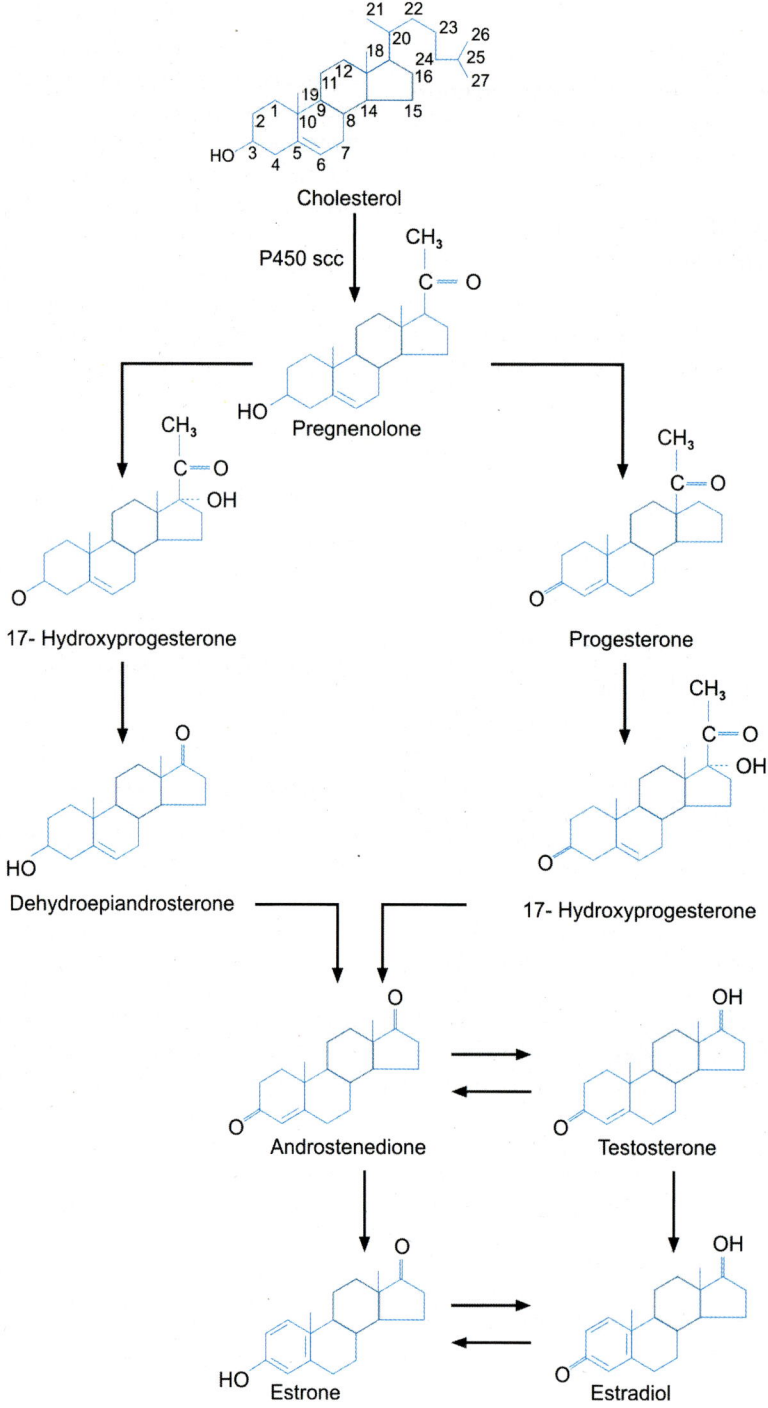

Fig. 2.11: Ovarian steroidogenesis

    iii. Growth of body of uterus.
    iv. Hypertrophy of vaginal wall, increased glycogen content and resulting decrease in pH.
c. **Bones:** It induces fusion of epiphysis and change in shape of bony pelvis.
d. **Menstrual function:** It causes negative and positive feedback on pituitary and hypothalamus. Estrogen induces proliferative phase of endometrium and together with progesterone promote secretory changes.
e. **Maturation of oocyte:** It is dependent on high blood concentration of estrogen.
f. **Physiological and anatomical changes in pregnancy:** Estrogen causes breast development and hypertrophy and hyperplasia of the myometrium.

g. **Metabolic effects:**
   i. Calcification of bone.
   ii. Possible increase in renin and angiotensin.
   iii. Diminished peripheral glucose uptake.
   iv. Increased thyroxine, cortisol and SHBG.
   v. Increase in cholesterol and triglycerides.
   vi. Decrease in high density lipoprotein.
   vii. Increase in factors VII, VIII, IX and X.
   viii. Decrease in fibrinolysis.
   ix. Inhibition of conversion of tryptophan to serotonin.

Tissues that react to estrogen have a specific intranuclear receptor protein. Estrogen bind to this protein, the complex binds and activates DNA. Among protein produced in this way is the progesterone receptor. Thus, the effect of progesterone is dependent on estrogen priming. Strong estrogen as estradiol binds more avidly to the receptor than weaker estrogen as estriol. Antiestrogen agent as progestogen and clomiphene citrate depletes the estrogen receptor.

Progesterone

The progesterone is secreted from the luteinized theca granulosa cells of the corpus luteum. A trace amount is secreted from the theca granulosa cell of the follicle and the ovarian stroma.

Metabolism

Daily production of progesterone is *2-3 mg in follicular phase and 20-30 mg in luteal phase*. 70% of circulating progesterone is bound to cortisol binding globulin. Progesterone is metabolized to variety of products including pregnanediol. These metabolites are converted by the liver to water soluble glucuronide or sulfate. About 20% of progesterone is excreted as pregnanediol glucuronide.

Action

The intracellular progesterone receptor which is induced by the action of estrogen acts similarly to the estrogen receptor. Progesterone depends on the presence of estrogen in order to exert its biological effects. These are:
a. **Vagina:** Large superficial cells with small pyknotic nuclei are replaced by small cells and large nuclei.
b. **Cervical mucus:** Becomes thicker, opaque and less abundant.
c. **Endometrium:** In endometrium induces secretory changes.
d. **Uterus:** Progesterone produces myohyperplasia and causes low frequency high amplitude contraction. The threshold for uterus excitation is increased.
e. **Other smooth muscles:** General relaxant effect.
f. **Breast:** Along with estrogen promote glandular development.
g. **Metabolic effect:** Progesterone is thermogenic, opposes the sodium retaining effect of aldosterone, increases the respiratory minute volume and thus reduces alveolar and blood pCO_2. It has catabolic effect resulting in increased urinary nitrogen excretion.

Testosterone (Androgen)

The androgens are produced in the ovary by all three types of cells—stroma, theca and granulosa cells but mainly by the theca interna of the follicle. The production of androgen is primarily under control of LH. The main androgens secreted are: ***Dehydroepiandrosterone, androstenedione and testosterone.***

Metabolism

Plasma level of androstenedione is 1.3-1.5 ng/ml, testosterone is 0.3-0.6 ng/ml and of SHBG 38-103 nmol/l. 80-85% androgen are bound to SHBG, 10-15% to albumin and only 1% of testosterone is free. In male 2% of testosterone is free.

The principal site of metabolism is liver. Androgens are partially metabolized to androsterone and etiocholanolone prior to excretion in urine as water soluble sulfate or glucuronide.

Action

Androgens exert their effect by binding to an intracellular receptor. In most tissues testosterone binds very weakly to the receptor and must first be converted to dihydrotestosterone (DHT) by enzyme 5 α reductase. **DHT is 100 time more potent than the parent compound.** In normal female its role is less clear but together with androstenedione, it is responsible for development of pubic hair and axillary hair. In male testosterone is responsible for secondary sexual development and development of male psychology.

Peptide—Inhibin and Activin

Although folliculogenesis and ovulation can be explained in terms of interaction between pituitary gonadotropins and sex steroids, it is becoming clear that other autocrine or paracrine mediator also play a role. One of the most important of these is inhibin.

Inhibin

It is produced by granulosa cells within the ovary. It attenuates FSH production by pituitary by a negative feedback and within the ovary it enhances LH induced androgen synthesis. The production of inhibin is one of the mechanism by which FSH levels are reduced below a threshold at which only the dominant follicle can respond ensuring atresia of the remaining follicle.

Activin

It is a peptide that is structurally related to inhibin. It is produced by granulosa cells of antral follicle and by the pituitary gland. The action of activin is almost opposite to that of inhibin in that it augments pituitary FSH secretion and increases FSH binding to granulosa cells.

Relaxin

It is secreted from the preovulatory follicle and corpus luteum. It probably facilitates follicular rupture during ovulation.

Insulin Like Growth Factor

IgF-I and IgF-II act as peracrine regulator. Circulating levels do not change during the menstrual cycle but follicular fluid levels increase toward ovulation, with the highest level found in dominant follicle. IgF- I is produced by theca cells under the action of LH. Within the theca, IgF-I augments the stimulatory effects of FSH on mitosis, aromatase activity and inhibin production. In the preovulatory follicle IgF-I enhances LH induced progesterone production from granulosa cells. Following ovulation, IgF-II is produced from luteinized granulosa cells and acts in an autocrine manner to augment LH induced proliferators of granulosa cells.

MULTIPLE CHOICE QUESTIONS

1. The ovarian cycle is initiated by:
   a. FSH
   b. Estrogen
   c. LH
   d. Progesterone
   Ans. a

2. The corpus luteum secretes:
   a. Estrogen
   b. Progesterone
   c. Both
   d. None
   Ans. c

3. The probable source of relaxin is:
   a. Ovary
   b. Adrenal cortex
   c. Bartholin gland
   d. Anterior pituitary
   Ans. a

4. All are features of inhibin, *except*:
   a. Nonsteroidal water soluble protein
   b. Secreted by graafian follicle
   c. Stimulate FSH secretion
   d. Increased secretion occurs in PCOD
   Ans. c

5. Ovulation in a female with a 38 days cycle occurs:
   a. 14th day
   b. 8th day
   c. 24th day
   d. 30th day
   Ans. c

6. Ovulation occurs due to:
   a. Midcycle FSH surge
   b. High prolactin level
   c. Decreased T_3 and T_4 level
   d. Midcycle LH surge
   Ans. a, d

7. Ferning of cervical mucus depends on:
   a. Estrogen
   b. Progesterone
   c. LH
   d. FSH
   Ans. a

8. Corkscrew shaped endometrial gland is seen in:
   a. Early proliferative phase
   b. Late proliferative phase
   c. Early secretory phase
   d. Late secretory phase
   Ans. d

9. Which of the following is the earliest change in the endometrium after ovulation:
   a. Secretion in the lumina of the endometrial glands
   b. Subnuclear vacuolation
   c. Corkscrew shaped glands
   d. Stromal cell become edematous, enlarged and polyhedral
   Ans. b

10. In the absence of fertilization and implantation, the corpus luteum persist for:
    a. 2-3 days
    b. 6-8 days
    c. 12-14 days
    d. 28-30 days
    Ans. c

3 Conception, Fertilization and Implantation

A baby is God's opinion that the world should go on.

INTRODUCTION

Life begins when an oocyte is fertilized by sperm. The union of egg and sperm at fertilization is one of the most important process in biology.

Gametogenesis is the process involved in the maturation of two highly specialized cells (spermatozoon in male and ovum in the female) before they unite to form zygote.

Oogenesis

The process involved in development of mature ovum is called **oogenesis**. The primitive germ cells take their origin from the yolk sac at about the end of 3rd week of intrauterine life and their migration to the developing gonadal ridge is completed round about the end of 4th week. In female gonads the germ cells undergo a number of rapid mitotic divisions and differentiate into **Oogonia**. The numbers of oogonia are maximum at 20th week, which number about 7 million. While the majority of oogonia continue to divide, some enter into the prophase of first meiotic division and are called **primary oocytes**. Primary oocyte is surrounded by flat cells and is called **primordial follicle** which are present in the cortex of the ovary. After birth there is no more mitotic division and all oogonia are replaced by the primary oocytes which have finished the prophase of the first meiotic division and remain in the resting phase (**dictyotene stage**) between prophase and metaphase. **Total number of primary oocyte at birth is approximately 2 million.**

Maturation of oocyte is reduction of the number of chromosomes to half. Before the onset of first meiotic division, the primary oocyte doubles its DNA by replication, so they have double amount of normal protein content. There are 22 pairs of autosomes which determine the body characteristics and one pair of sex chromosomes named XX. The first stage of maturation occurs with full maturation of the ovarian follicle just prior to ovulation. **Final maturation occurs only after fertilization.**

The primary oocyte undergoes **first meiotic division** giving rise to secondary oocyte and one polar body. The **secondary oocyte** contains haploid number of chromosomes (23X) and nearly all the cytoplasm. Small **polar body** contains half of chromosomes (23X) but only scanty cytoplasm. *Ovulation occurs just after the formation of secondary oocytes* (Fig. 3.1B).

The secondary oocyte completes the second meiotic division only after fertilization by the sperm in the fallopian tube. It results again in formation of 2 daughter cells. Larger one is called **mature ovum** containing (23X) and smaller one is called **second polar body** containing same number of chromosomes. The first polar body may also undergo the second meiotic division. In the absence of fertilization, the secondary oocyte does not complete the second meiotic division and degenerates as such.

Structure of Mature Ovum

A fully mature ovum is the largest cell in the body measuring 130 µm in diameter. It consists of cytoplasm and a nucleus with eccentric nucleolus and contains 23X chromosomes. During fertilization, the nucleus is converted into a female pronucleus. The ovum is surrounded by a cell membrane called *vitelline membrane*. There is an outer transparent mucoprotein envelope called Zona pellucida. In between vitelline membrane and Zona pellucida there is a narrow space called, **perivitelline space** which accommodates the polar bodies. After escape from primordial follicle, oocyte retains a covering of granulosa cells known as *corona radiata*, which is derived from *cumulus oophorous* (refer Figs 2.4A and B).

Spermatogenesis

Spermatogenesis is the production of mature sperm. It occurs in the seminiferous tubules of the testis. The primordial germ cells divide to produce spermatogonia, the precursor of mature sperm. At onset of puberty the spermatogonia located at the basal lamina of the

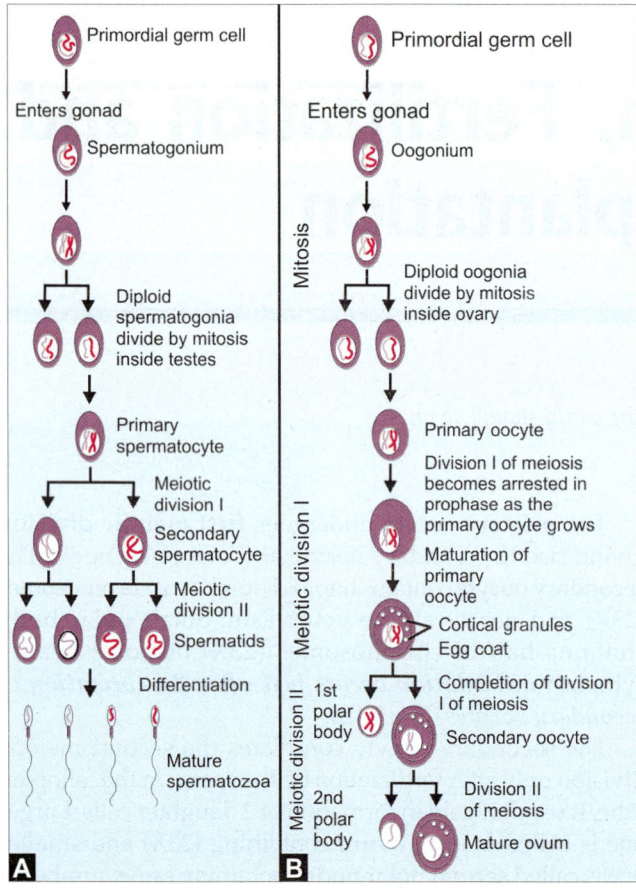

Figs 3.1A and B: (A) Various stages of spermatogenesis; (B) Oogenesis

This compact structure of the sperm is important for its motility.

The production of spermatozoa in the testis requires the presence of germ cells and their transformation and maturation is under the control of hypothalamic and pituitary hormones and testicular androgens.

The Mature Sperm

Spermatozoa are produced at the onset of puberty in boys. Thereafter, the seminiferous tubules of the testis will go on producing sperms daily until 60 years of age and beyond. Following spermatogenesis, the spermatozoa pass through seminiferous tubule to rete testis, on to the vasa differentia, the head of the epididymis and hence, 12 days later to the tail of epididymis. The transport of mature sperm is facilitated via muscular activity within the epididymis and vas. The seminal fluid is made up from secretion of bulbourethral gland, seminal vesicle, the prostrate and epidymal fluid. During this time the sperm acquire motility and undergo the final biochemical changes that give them ability to fertilize the ovum.

The sperm has complex structure. It contains haploid number of chromosomes (22 + X or Y). It is few microns long. It has **head** which consist principally of the condensed nucleus and acrosomal cap. Acrosome is rich in enzyme. **Tail** gives the motility and propulsion while the mid piece acts as energy source. At the time of intercourse, million of sperms are deposited in vagina (Fig. 3.2). Seminal fluid containing sperm coagulates immediately following ejaculation. Under normal circumstances it liquefies within 20 minutes. The basic pH of the seminal fluid protects the spermatozoa from acidity of vagina. They travel in all

seminiferous tubercle begin to divide mitotically to produce primary spermatocytes.

Primary spermatocytes remain in *stage of prophase of the first meiotic division* for long time (16 days). Each spermatocytes contains 22 pair of autosomes and one pair of sex chromosomes named XY. With completion of first meiotic division, two secondary spermatocytes are formed having equal share of cytoplasm and haploid number of chromosomes either 23X or 23Y. Immediately after there is second meiotic division with formation of 4 spermatids, each containing haploid numbers of chromosomes, two with 23X and two with 23Y (Fig. 3.1A). **Spermiogenesis** is the differentiation of round spermatids to motile spermatozoa. In this process a series of morphological changes occur which produce motile sperms and takes about 61 days. The most visible change is the reduction in size and formation of tail, which allows the sperm cell to swim. The chromosomes in the sperm cells are almost crystallized by a special set of sperm specific proteins called protamines. In fact this protamine induced condensation of the sperm chromosome is so extensive that the size of sperm nucleus is about one thirtieth of the size of the mature human egg.

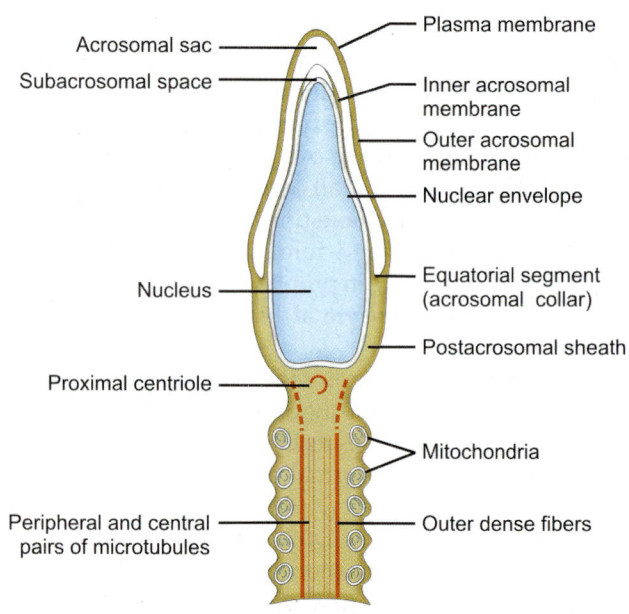

Fig. 3.2: Outline of mature spermatozoa

directions, some through the cervix, where in midcycle the molecules of cervical mucus untangle their barbed fence like morphology to assume straight lines.

Fertilization

At time of ovulation, the secondary oocyte with adhering cells of the cumulus oophorous is freed from ovary. This oocyte is then released in peritoneal cavity. The fimbriated end of the fallopian tube, possibly excited by chemotaxis, closes to embrace the ovary like a hand holding a rugby football. So, virtually the egg has no transperitoneal passage.

The oocyte is transported through fallopian tube to the uterus by tubal peristalsis as well directional movement of cilia. Ciliary action is more important in ampulla. **Fertilization usually occurs at the ampullary end of the fallopian tube, within 12-24 hours of the oocyte production.** So, spermatozoa must be present in the fallopian tube at the time of oocyte arrival.

A few sperm reach each fallopian tube where they swim counter current, the first arriving near the oocyte within 30 minutes of intercourse. Two changes occur before spermatozoa are able to fertilize the ovum—first the **capacitation,** which occurs in fallopian tube, taking time of 5-6 hours. In this there are no obvious morphological changes, but there is an increase in motility. The life span of spermatozoa is greatly reduced to 18 hours. The cell membrane overlying the acrosome is depolarized and calcium enters the cell. Substances in the lower genital tract of both male and female inhibit capacitation.

Second is **Acrosome Reaction:** This begins with a swelling of acrosome after that multiple area of fusion appears between the plasma and outer acrosomal membranes. Gaps develop where the membranes have fused and finally membrane disappears altogether. During acrosome reaction Hyaluronidase and proteinase enzyme are released, which enable the sperm to penetrate the corona radiata of the oocyte. The sperm attaches to receptors on the zona pellucida. A trypsin like acrosomal enzyme called acrosin is then activated and enables spermatozoa to penetrate the zone pellucida to reach the perivitelline space (Fig. 3.3).

After a brief interval, one sperm attaches to receptors on the cell membrane (vitelline membrane) of the secondary oocyte, causing depolarization of the membrane. *Oscillogen*— A sperm protein induces oscillation of calcium ions into and out of the cell. Cortical granules move closer to the cell surface and discharge a substance which changes the density of the zona pellucida and mask the surface receptor, which finally block polyspermy.

As soon as the sperm has entered the ooplasm, meiosis is resumed in the oocyte. This results in extrusion of the second polar body which unlike the first contains no granules. The remaining chromosomes are surrounded by a nuclear membrane to form the **female pronucleus.** Head and neck of the spermatozoa become male pronucleus containing haploid number of chromosomes (23X) or 23Y. The sperm nuclear envelope breaks down. The chromatin decondenses and swells to form the male pronucleus. This contains very prominent nucleoli.

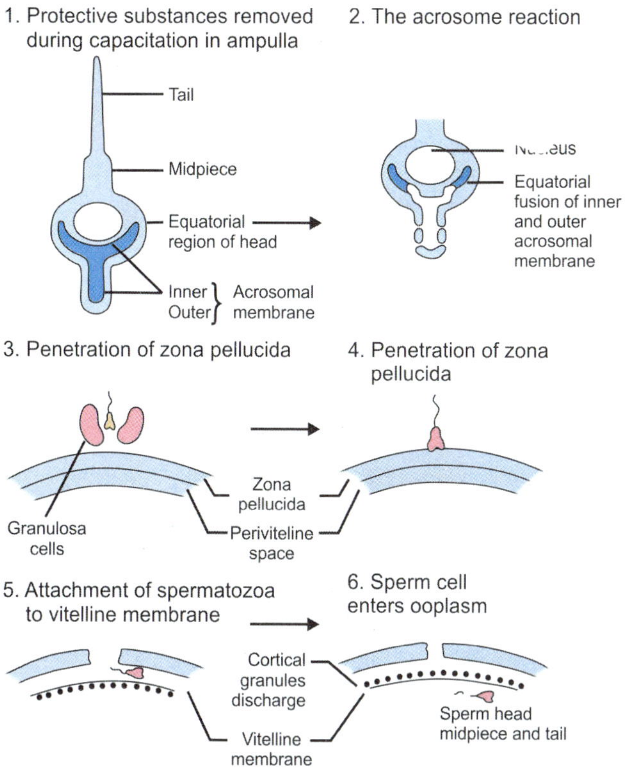

Fig. 3.3: Stages of sperm maturation in the female reproductive tract leading to fertilization

The two pronucleus approach each other—**karyogamy.** The nuclear membranes break down and the two gamete fuse with pairing of homologous chromosome—**syngamy.** The first mitotic division begins. Initial development of the embryo is directed from the cytoplasm. Replacement of the pronuclei by an adult nucleus does not preclude embryonic development.

The zygote thus formed, contains both the paternal and maternal genetic material. Sex of the child is determined by the pattern of the sex chromosome supplied by the spermatozoon. If the spermatozoon contains 'X' chromosome, a female embryo 46XX is formed. If it contains 'Y' chromosome, a male embryo 46XY is formed.

Cleavage of Embryo—The Morula and Blastocyst

The first cleavage of zygote takes place in the ampulla of fallopian tube within 30 hours of fertilization. The second division occurs at right angle to the first. Division occurs every 12 hours and is synchronous i.e division occurs simultaneously in all cells until the 16 cells stage (Fig. 3.4).

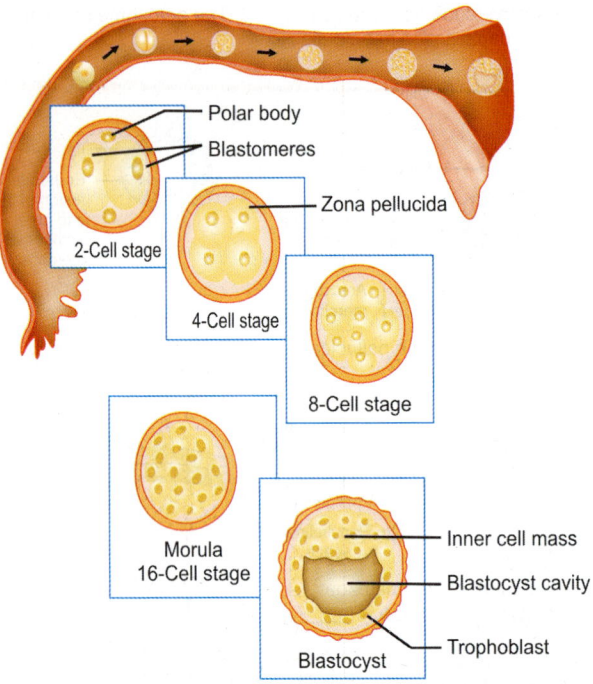

Fig. 3.4: Zygote cleavage and formation of blastocyst

Daughter cells formed by the cleaving embryo are called **blastomere.** These blastomeres are **totipotent** (i.e. can develop in any direction) until the eight cell stage. Until the end of first cleaving, development is directed by RNA transcribed from DNA of the oocyte. After eight cell stage, the surface of the cells has microvilli and cellular organelles are found at the apex of the cells. This subcellular distribution of organelles precedes differentiation in the embryo as a whole. As the blastomeres continue to divide a solid mulberry like ball of cells, referred to as **morula** is produced. The morula enters the uterine cavity about 3 days after fertilization at 8 cell stage and further division results in 16 and then a 32 cell morula. The outer cells of the morula become tightly adherent to each other with the formation of desmosomes and gap junction—(**compaction**). Fluid collect between this layer and the deeper blastomeres, thus **blastocyst is** formed. **Blastocyst cons**ists of—(A) An outer layer which will form the trophoblast, (B) Blastocoelic fluid, (C) Inner cell mass (Fig. 3.4).

The total size of the blastocyst is the same as that of the secondary oocyte (about 100 μm in diameter). It remains encased within the zona pellucida until shortly before implantation. The trophoblast is divided into mural and polar area. Polar trophoblast is in contact with the inner cell mass. New trophoblast cells are generated from this area. **In contrast to the post implantation embryo, the preimplantation morula and blastocyst are very resistant to teratogenic agents such as radiation and chemicals which either have no effect or are immediately lethal.**

As the embryo enlarges from the 2-cells stage, the mitochondria enlarge and develop more internal folds. Numerous microvilli appear on the surface but the endoplasmic reticulum does not become prominent until the 16-cell stage when protein synthesis increases.

Till 8-cell stage oxygen consumption is low, after which metabolic rate increases rapidly. Pyruvate is principal energy substrate instead of glucose. The sex chromosome of female fetus (XX) remains active until the blastocyst stage. One of them then becomes inactive in a highly condensed form so called—**Barr body**.

Implantations of the Blastocyst and Early Development of the Placenta and Embryo

Implantation of the embryo into the wall of the uterus is a common feature of all mammalians. In human implantation occur 6 or 7 days after fertilization. Successful implantation requires a receptive endometrium that has been appropriately primed with estrogen and progesterone.

Receptivity of uterus towards blastocyst is limited to 20-24 days of the ovarian endometrial cycle. The ability of blastocyst to adhere to the epithelium is mediated by cell surface receptors at the implantation site which interact with receptors on the blastocyst. This receptive epithelium results from the postovulatory production of estrogen and progesterone by the corpus luteum. If blastocyst approaches the endometrium after cycle day 24, the potential for adhesion is less because of synthesis of anti adhesive glycoprotein which prevents receptive interaction. After 2-3 days in the uterine lumen implantation begins. Implantation has following stages:

1. **Apposition:** The polar trophoblast comes into contact with the endometrium. Under the influence of a trypsin like enzyme from the blastocyst, the endometrium increases mitosis and produces **pinopods,** i.e. protrusions from the endometrial surface. Pinopods withdraw fluid from the lumen by **pinocytosis**. When apposition is completed the microvilli of both trophoblast and endometrial surface interdigitate and the pinopods are withdrawn.
2. **Adhesion:** The microvilli disappear and production of sticky glycoprotein leads to contact over a large surface area.
3. **Penetration:** Contraction of microfilaments in the trophoblast permits the blastocyst to migrate between endometrial cells. Simultaneously syncytiotrophoblast forms and synthesis of trophoblast specific protein like SPI and HCG begins. Decidual cells form in the endometrial stroma which are large cells rich in glycogen and lipid.

Biology of Trophoblast

The formation of the human placenta begins with the **trophectoderm,** which is the first tissue to differentiate at the morula stage of development, giving rise to a layer of trophoblast cells encircling the blastocyst. From the early blastocyst to term placenta, the trophoblast plays critical and most valuable role at the fetal maternal surface. It is **invasive**, thus causes attachment of the blastocyst to deciduas. It provides **nutrition** to the conceptus and it functions as an endocrine organ in pregnancy which is essential to maternal physiological adaptation and maintenance of pregnancy.

Differentiation of Trophoblast

By 8th day postfertilization, after initial implantation of the blastocyst, the trophoblast has differentiation into: (A) Inner layer of primitive mononuclear cytotrophoblast or **Langhan's layer**. (B) Outer primitive layer of multinucleated synctium called **syncytiotrophoblast**.

The cytotrophoblast are germinal cells for the synctium. The synctium acts as the primary secretory component within the placenta. The cytotrophoblast has ability to undergo DNA synthesis and mitosis, a well demarcated cell border and single nucleus. The syncytiotrophoblast lack these characteristics.

The synctium has no individual cells, only a continuous synctial lining in which cytoplasm is amorphous without cell borders and nuclei are multiple and diverse in size and shape. Because of absence of cell border, transport across the syncytiotrophoblast is facilitated as transport is not dependent on the participation of individual cells. When implantation is complete, the cytotrophoblast further differentiates along the main pathways giving rise to villous and extravillous cytotrophoblast (Figs 3.5 and 3.6).

Villous cytotrophoblast line the villous stem and primarily function in the transport of oxygen and nutrient between the fetus and mother. The extravillous trophoblast migrates into the decidua and myometrium and also penetrate maternal vasculature. It comes in contact with various types of maternal cells.

Interstitial extravillous trophoblast invades the maternal decidua eventually penetrating the myometrium to form placental bed giant cells and surrounds the maternal spiral arteries. The **endovascular** extravillous trophoblast penetrates the lumen of the spiral arteries.

The Decidua of the Endometrium

The decidua is a specialized highly modified endometrium of pregnancy and is a function of hemochorial placentation. William Hunter the 18th century British Gynecologist provided the first scientific description of the membrane decidua. *Membrane denoted its gross anatomical appearance, word deciduas was added with analogy to deciduous leaves to indicate an ephemeral nature and the fact that it is shed from the rest of uterus after child birth.* Decidualization is the

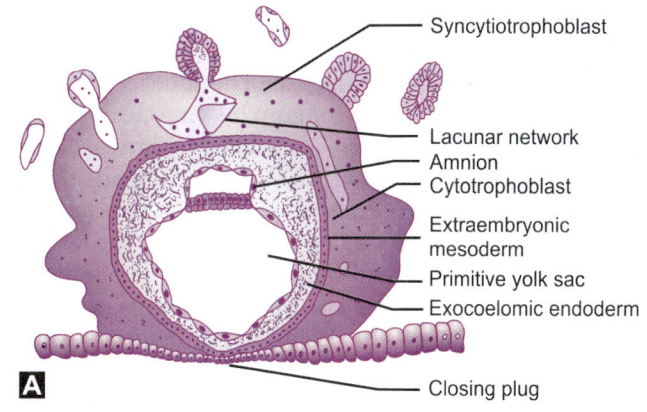

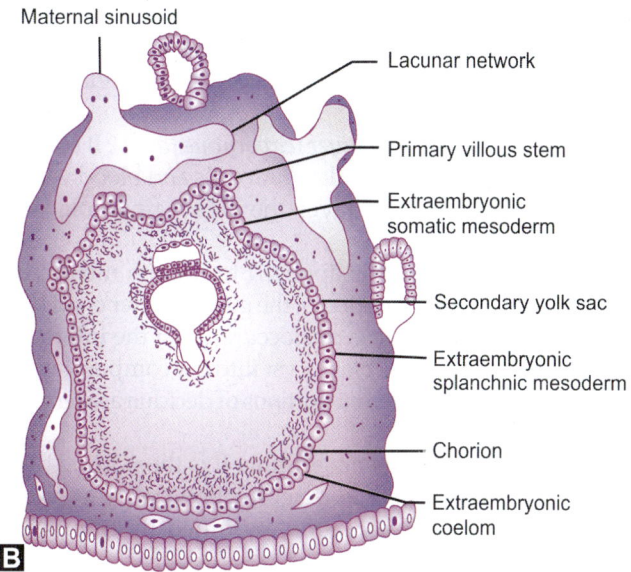

Figs 3.6A and B: (A) At 10 days formation of lacunae communicating with maternal blood vessels and start of formation of extra-amniotic mesoderm; (B) Extraembryonic coelom formation, secondary yolk sac forming from primary yolk sac, the trophoblast and mesoderm together form chorion

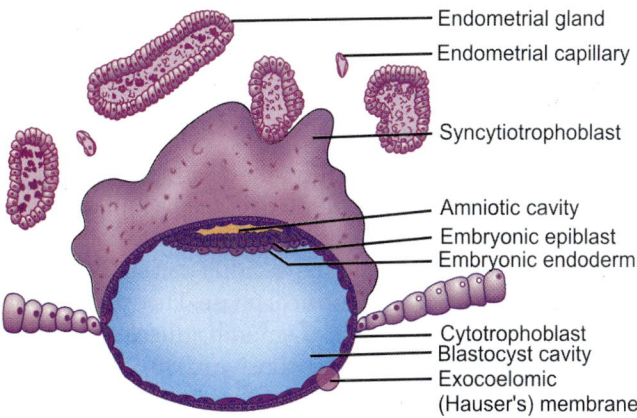

Fig. 3.5: Implanting embryo at 8 days

transformation of secretory endometrium to decidua. It is dependent on the action of estrogen and progesterone and factors secreted by the implanting blastocyst during trophoblast invasion.

The success of the unique semiallograft is of great scientific interest as this process harbor insight leading to more successful transplantation surgery and even immunological treatment of neoplasia.

Decidual Reaction

The increased structural and secretory activity of the endometrium that is brought about in response to progesterone following implantation is known as decidual reaction. **Predecidual** changes start during mid luteal phase in endometrial stromal cell close to spiral arteries and arterioles, from where spread in waves throughout the mucosa of the uterus and after that from the site of implantation.

The endometrial stromal cells enlarge to form polygonal or round decidual cells. The nucleus of decidual cell becomes round and vesicular. The cytoplasm become clear, slightly basophilic and surrounded by a translucent membrane. Each mature decidual cell is surrounded by a pericellular membrane. Thus the human decidual cells clearly build walls around themselves and possibly around the fetus.

The pericellular membrane matrix: (a) Provides for attachment of cytotrophoblast through cellular adhesion molecules, (b) Protects the decidual cells against selected enzymes of the cytotrophoblast.

Decidual Structure

The well developed decidua differentiate into three layers –
a. *Superficial compact layer (stratum compactum):* It consists of compact mass of decidual cells, gland duct and duct capillaries.
b. *Intermediate spongy layer (cavernous layer):* It contains dilated uterine glands, decidual cells and blood vessels. Through cavernous layer the cleavage of placental separation occurs.
c. *Thin basal layer:* It is apposed to uterine muscle and contains the basal portion of the glands. After child birth, regeneration of mucus coat occurs. After the **interstitial implantation** of the blastocyst into the compact layer of the decidua the different portions of decidua are renamed (Fig. 3.7)
   i. **Decidua basalis or serotina:** It is the portion of the decidua which is directly beneath the site of blastocyst implantation, modified by trophoblast invasion.
   ii. **Decidua capsularis (reflexa):** The portion of decidua which overlies the enlarging blastocyst and initially separating it from the rest of the uterine cavity is called decidua capsularis. It is most prominent during the second month of pregnancy and consists of decidua cells covered by a single layer of flattened epithelial cells without traces of glands. Internally decidua capsularis contacts the avascular extraembryonic fetal membrane —**the chorion laeve.**
   iii. **Decidua parietalis or vera:** The rest of the decidua lining the uterine cavity outside the site of implantation is decidua vera.

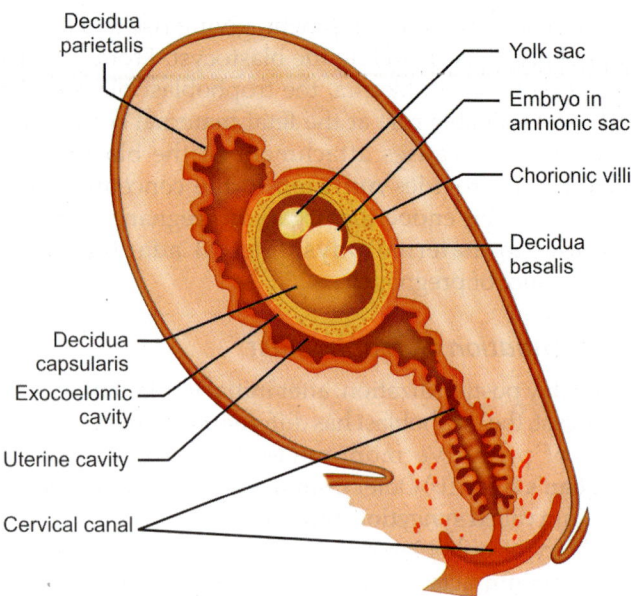

Fig. 3.7: Three portion of decidua (basalis, capsularis, parietalis) decidualized endometrium covering the early embryo

During the early weeks of pregnancy the gestational sac does not fill the entire uterine cavity so there is a space between the decidua capsularis and deciduas parietalis. By 14-16 weeks, the gestational sac expands enough to fill the uterine cavity with fusion of the deciduas capsularis and parietalis.The uterine cavity is functionally obliterated. In early pregnancy the decidua begins to thicken, eventually attaining a depth of 5-10 mm. Later in pregnancy, as the fetus grows and amniotic fluid expands, the thickness of the deciduas decreases probably because of the pressure exerted by the expanding uterine contents. Decidua basalis retains the characteristic appearance till term and becomes the maternal position of the placenta.

Decidual Blood Supply

As a consequence of implantation, the decidual blood supply is changed. The blood supply to decidua capsularis is lost as the embryo fetus grows and expands into the uterine cavity. The blood supply to the decidua parietalis through the spiral arteries persist like luteal phase. The spiral arteries of decidua parietalis retain a smooth muscles wall and endothelium so they remain responsive to vasoactive agents acting on the smooth muscles or the endothelial cells of these vessels.

The spiral arteriole and arteries of decidua basalis are invaded by the cytotrophoblast and during this process the walls of the vessels in the decidua basalis are destroyed. So these vascular conduits of maternal blood, which become the uteroplacental vessels, are not responsive to vasoactive agents. In contrast fetal chorionic vessels, which transport blood between the placenta and the fetus, contain smooth muscles and respond to vasoactive agents.

Early Trophoblast Invasion

With the process of opposition, adhesion and penetration, the invading trophoblast burrow deeper into the endometrium. By 10th day post fertilization, the blastocyst becomes totally encased within the endometrium. This active mechanism of erosion and invasion into the endometrium by trophoblast cells simulates characteristics of metastasizing malignant cells (Fig. 3.5).

At 9 days of development, the wall of the blastocyst facing towards the uterine lumen is a single layer of flattened cells. The opposite, thicker wall comprises two zones—the **trophoblast** and the embryo forming **inner cell mass**. The inner cell mass is called **embryonic disc**. It is differentiated into a thick plate of primitive **ectoderm** and an underlying layer of **endoderm**. The endoderm gives rise to cells that migrate onto the inner layer of the mural trophoblast. The two layers from **Hauser's membranes** (Fig. 3.5).

The amniotic cavity forms between cytotrophoblast and the epithelial layer of the embryonic disc. The embryonic mesenchyme first appears as isolated cells within the cavity of the blastocyst. When the cavity is completely lined with mesoderm, the blastocoelic cavity is now called the **primary yolk sac**. The **secondary yolk sac** forms by collapse of the endodermal lining of the primary yolk sac. The **extraembryonic coelom** forms in the site of the primary yolk sac and surrounds the yolk sac, embryonic disc and amnion (Figs 3.6A and B).

A layer of mesoderm separates the endoderm of the extraembryonic coelom from the underlying structure. The mesoderm between the amnion and trophoblast is called **the embryonic stalk**, which serve to join the embryo to the nutrient **chorion** and later develops into **the umbilical cord**.

At the time of the first missed period the embryonic disc is still bilaminar, but a node of epithelial cells, the primitive streak is forming at the caudal end. It is only 0.55 mm in size but by this stage the placenta and membranes have undergone extensive development. The spatial identity of cells during embryogenesis appears to be directed by a group of homeiotic genes, which have in common a sequence of DNA referred to as **the homeobox**.

Lacunae formation within the syncytiotrophoblast: About 12 days after conception, the Syncytiotrophoblast of the trophoblast shell is permeated by a system of inter communicating channels of trophoblastic lacunae or small cavities. As embryo enlarges, more decidua basalis is invaded by the basal syncytiotrophoblast, which also includes the wall of superficial decidual capillaries, so these lacunae develop a brush border and fuse with maternal capillaries, yielding blood filled space, which will become the **intervillous space** (Fig. 3.8).*

Organization of Placenta

The placenta is formed from (a) Chorion, (b) Decidua basalis covered by amnion. Placenta is hemochorial or hemochorioendothelial. Hemo refers to maternal blood which directly bathes the syncytiotrophoblast; chorion is for chorion placenta which is separated from fetal blood by endothelial wall of fetal capillaries, which trasverse the villous core.

Development of Villous System

At 12th day, primary villous stem are formed with a lining of syncytiotrophoblast and a core of cytotrophoblast and mesoderm. The cytotrophoblast grows as 'column' through the syncytiotrophoblast to make contact with maternal decidua and then forms a shell enclosing the lacunae and syncytiotrophoblast (Fig. 3.8).

---

* When there is failure of angiogenesis in villi, the villi become distended with fluid and form vesicles.

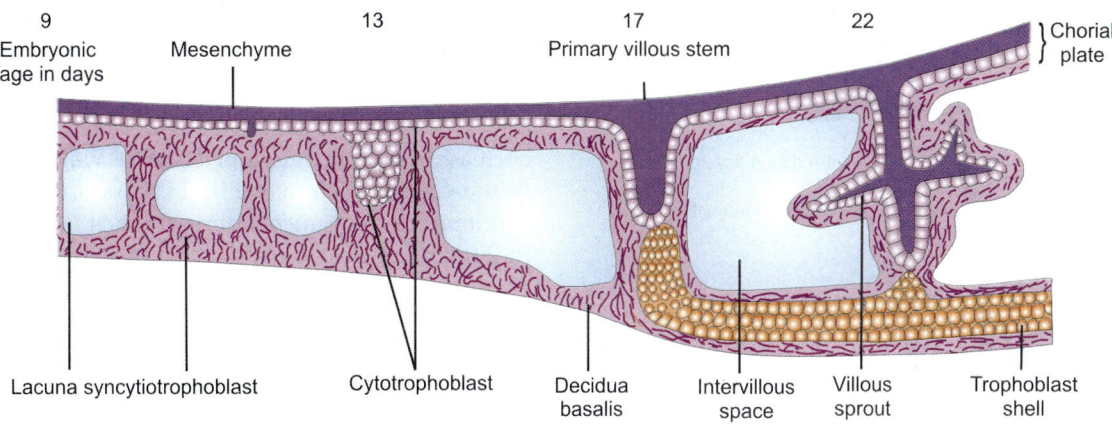

Fig. 3.8: Formation of stem villi and primary placental villi

Primary stem villi are formed with a lining of syncytiotrophoblast and a cord of cytotrophoblast surrounded by lacunar spaces which later form intervillous space. **Mesenchymal cord**, derived from extraembryonic mesoderm, invade the solid trophoblast columns forming **the secondary villi.**

After angiogenesis occurs from the mesenchymal core, the resulting villi are termed **tertiary**. Maternal venous sinuses are trapped early in the process of implantation, but it is only 14th or 15th day after fertilization, that maternal arterial blood enters the intervillous space (Fig. 3.9).

By about 17th day, fetal blood vessels are functional and a placental circulation is established. The fetal placental circulation is completed when the blood vessels of the embryo are connected with the chorionic blood vessels.

After day 21, the villi adjacent to the uterine cavity degenerate to form **the chorion laeve. T**his process is complete by 8-10 weeks. The villi on the decidual side are called **chorion frondosum,** which proliferate to form the placenta. Growth occurs by fresh villous formation from the villous stems and progressive arborisation of previously formed villi. The villous stem themselves undergo further division. The primary stems break up into a number of secondary stem villi just below the chorial plate. After a short lateral course these give rise to tertiary stems which sweep down through the intervillous space and turn back on themselves near the maternal surface. From these tertiary stems placental villi arise.

Further demands of fetal metabolism require swifter exchange at the placenta. These demands are met by:

(a) Longer and larger villi, (b) Branching of villi, (c) Absorption of Langhan's layer so that syncytiotrophoblast is in direct contact with blood capillary, (d) Syncytiotrophoblast thinned and nuclei migrate from areas over capillaries where exchange actually occurs, (e) Localized dome like swelling occurs on the villi protruding into the intervillous space. These areas are especially thin walled and are probably the site of much of the gas exchange.

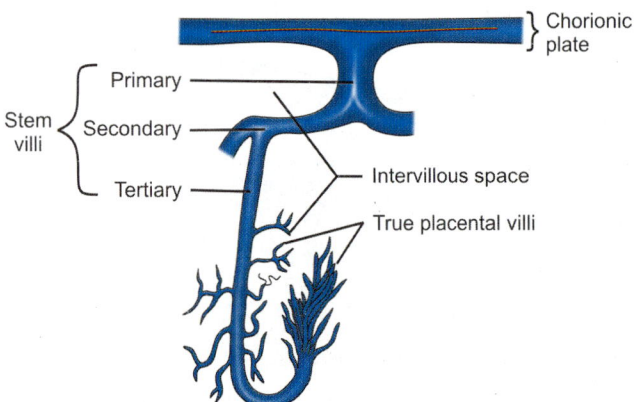

Fig. 3.9: Formation of tertiary stem villi

Villi are like fronds of seaweed under water as the maternal blood circulates around them. The number of stem villi does not increase after the 12th week; hence the number of lobule of placenta is now fixed.

By 12 weeks the placenta achieves its definitive form and thickness because subsequent growth is circumferential. In the beginning the placental growth is more rapid than that of the fetus, by 17th week they have equal weight. **By term the placenta is one-sixth of the fetal weight.**

Fetal and Maternal Blood Circulation in the Mature Placenta

Placental circulation consist of following two independent system: **(a) Uteroplacental** circulation, **(b) Fetoplacental** circulation.

Fetal Circulation

Deoxygenated or venous like fetal blood flows to the placenta through the two umbilical arteries. Umbilical arteries enter the chorionic plate underneath the amnion, each supply one half of the placenta. At site of the umbilical cord joining the placenta, the umbilical vessels branch repeatedly beneath the amnion and again within the dividing, primary, secondary and tertiary villi, finally forms capillary network in the terminal divisions.

The blood flows into the corresponding venous channels either through the terminal capillary network or through the shunts. Blood with significantly higher oxygen concentration returns from the placenta to the fetus through a single umbilical vein. The branch of umbilical vessels that traverses along the fetal surface of the placenta in the chorionic plate are termed—*chorionic vessels.* **Chorionic vessels are responsive to vasoactive substances but in all ways—anatomically, morphologically, histologically and functionally, they are unique chorionic arteries always cross over chorionic vein**.

In 65% of placenta, the chorion arteries have a pattern of disperse type branching while in remaining 35% arteries radiate to the edge of the placenta without narrowing. In both type these are end arteries, which supply one cotyledon, as each branch turn downwards to pierces the chorionic plate.

The perforating branches of surface arteries, which pass through chorionic plate, are calle**d truncal** arteries. Truncal artery penetrate through the chorionic plate, there is a decrease in smooth muscle of the vessel wall and an increase in the caliber of the vessel. This loss of smooth muscle continues as the truncal arteries branch into the rami and the smooth muscle loss also occur in vein.*

---

* Before 10 weeks there is no end diastolic flow within the umbilical artery at the end of fetal cardiac cycle. At 10 weeks, end diastolic flow appears and is maintained throughout normal pregnancies. Clinically this finding is recorded with Doppler ultrasonography as an assessment of fetal well being.

Maternal Circulation

Fetal homeostasis is dependent on an efficient maternal placental circulation. Studies done by Ramsey and Harris (1966), explained the physiological basis of placental circulation which is as follows:

Maternal blood enters through the basal plate and is driven high up towards the chorionic plate by maternal arterial pressure before lateral dispersion occurs. After bathing the external microvillous surface of the chorionic villi, the maternal blood drains back through venous surface in the basal plate and enters the uterine veins. Thus maternal blood traverses the placenta randomly without preformed channels with force of maternal arterial pressure. At term about 120 spiral arteries enter into intervillous space. The process of trophoblastic invasion of the spiral arteries convert spiral arteries into low resistance, large bore uteroplacental vessels which can accommodate the massive increase in uterine perfusion in pregnancy.

Generally the spiral arteries are perpendicular to uterine wall, while the veins are parallel. Due to this the veins are occluded during uterine contraction. This prevents squeezing of essential maternal blood from the intervillous space. So during contraction, somewhat larger volume of blood is available for exchange even though the rate of flow is decreased. By Doppler velocimetry, it is shown that diastolic flow velocity in spiral artery is decreased during the uterine contraction. So, principal factors regulating blood flow in the intervillous space are:
a. Maternal arterial blood pressure.
b. Intrauterine pressure.
c. The pattern of uterine contraction.
d. Factor that act specifically on the arterial wall.

The blood in the intervillous space is prevented from clotting by fibrinolytic enzyme of the trophoblast.

Microchimerism

A variety of fetal cell type may persist in mother's body for years to decade after a pregnancy. It is called **microchimerism**. It shows that placenta does not maintain absolute integrity of the fetal and maternal circulation. It is exemplified clinically by some situations:
a. Erythrocyte D–antigen isoimmunization and occurrence of erythroblastosis fetalis (will be discussed in chapter of Rh negative pregnancy.
b. Clinical consequence of fetal cells in mother may cause maternal autoimmune disease as scleroderma, thyroiditis and thyroid failure, maternal cutaneus eruptions.

Immunological Aspect of the Fetomaternal Surface

Since 50 years, many hypothesis have been proposed to explain the survival of the semiallogenic fetal graft. Some are as follows:

a. Antigenic immaturity of embryo fetus but transplantation (HLA) antigen is demonstrated very early in embryonic life.
b. Decreased immunological responsiveness of the pregnant woman but no evidence has proved it.
c. The uterus (decidua) is an immunological privileged tissue site.

But this would preclude well documented advanced ectopic pregnancy. So the acceptance and survival of the conception in the maternal uterus should be attributed to the immunological peculiarity of the trophoblast, not the decidua.

The HLA genes (Human Leukocyte Antigens) are the human analogue of major histocompatibility complex. The HLA genes are the product of multiple genetic loci of MHC located within the short arm of choromosomes. There are 17 HLA class 1 genes including three classical genes HLA-A, B and C that encode the major class I transplantation antigens. Three other class 1 genes designated HLA-E, F and G encode class Ib H_2A antigens.

Normal implantation is dependent on controlled trophoblastic invasion of maternal endometrium—deciduas and the spiral arteries. Trophoblast invasion should proceed far enough to provide for normal fetal growth and development and at the same time there should be some mechanism to regulate this depth of trophoblast invasion. **Uterine Large Granular Lymphocytes (LGLC) and the unique expression of 3 specific HLA class I genes in extravillous cytotrophoblast act to allow and finally to limit the process of trophoblastic invasion.**

Uterine Large Granular Lymphocytes (LGLC) are believed to originate in the bone marrow and belong to natural killer cell lineage. They are the predominant leucocytes present in midluteal phase of endometrium at the time of implantation. Their infiltration is increased by progesterone as well stromal cell production of IL-15 and prolactin. If there is no conception, nuclei of uterine LGL begin to disintegrate. If there is blastocyst implantation, LGL cells persist in large numbers in the decidua during early weeks of pregnancy. In first trimester many LGL are close to extravillous macrophage colony-stimulating factor (GM-CSR) which may function to forestall trophoblastic apoptosis. So LGL can bear the primary responsibility for immunosurveillance in deciduas.

MULTIPLE CHOICE QUESTIONS

1. Implantation occurs on the:
   a. 4th day
   b. 6th day
   c. 3rd day
   d. 8th day
   Ans. d

SECTION -1 ♦ Basic Sciences in Obstetrics and Gynecology

2. At birth, oocytes are in which stage of development?
   a. Prophase of 1st meiotic diversion
   b. Oogonia
   c. Telophase of 2nd meiotic division
   d. Resting phase between prophase and metaphase of 1st meiotic division

   Ans. d

3. Common site of fertilization is:
   a. Isthmic
   b. Ampulla
   c. Infundibulum
   d. Interstitial

   Ans. b

4. By which day after fertilization is placental circulation established?
   a. 11th day
   b. 13th day
   c. 15th day
   d. 21st day

   Ans. d

4. Fetal Growth, Placenta and Umbilical Cord

Follow faithfully, inward leads you on.

GENERAL CONSIDERATION

In contemporary obstetrical practice, the status of the fetus is that of second patient, who should be given the same meticulous care that obstetrician provides for the pregnant women. Virtually conception—embryo and fetus is a dynamic force in pregnancy unit. The conceptus plays an active and vast role in process of implantation, maternal recognition of pregnancy, immunological acceptance, endocrine function, nutrition and parturition.

Prenatal development of the fetus can be distinguished in following periods:

a. **Ovular period or germinal period:** It last for first two weeks following ovulation.
b. **Embryonic period**: The embryonic period commences at the beginning of the 3rd week after ovulation and fertilization, which coincides in time with the expected date of next menstrual cycle. End of embryonic period is arbitrarily designated by most embryologists at eight weeks after fertilization. At this time embryo fetus is nearly 4 cm **long** (Figs 4.1A and B).
c. **Further development of embryo:** At this time embryonic disk is well defined. A longitudinal thickening of posterior part of the embryonic disk develops as the **primitive streak**. Cells spread out laterally from this to form layer of mesoderm separating the endoderm and ectoderm (Figs 4.2A and B). These three germ cell layers then give rise to the various organs and tissues. The **ectoderm** develops into the entire nervous system, epidermis and lens of the eye. The **endoderm** develops into the lining of the intestinal and respiratory tract and associated organ (Liver, thyroid, pancreas and lungs). The **mesoderm** gives origin to the dermis, skeleton, connective tissues, muscles, vascular, and urogenital systems. The cavity that later divides the somatic and visceral sheets of intraembryonic mesoderm is the **coelom**. The primitive streak becomes prominent during the third week postconceptional (5th week gestational age). This is an important event during which a number of developmental landmarks are generated. For example, *the primitive streak determines symmetry and defines the cephalic and caudal poles of the embryo.* Definition

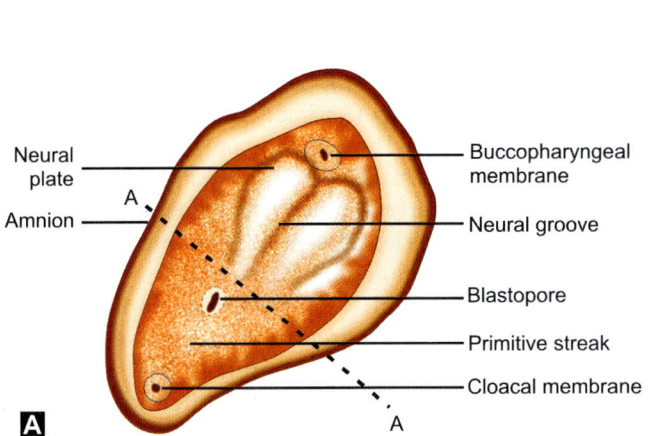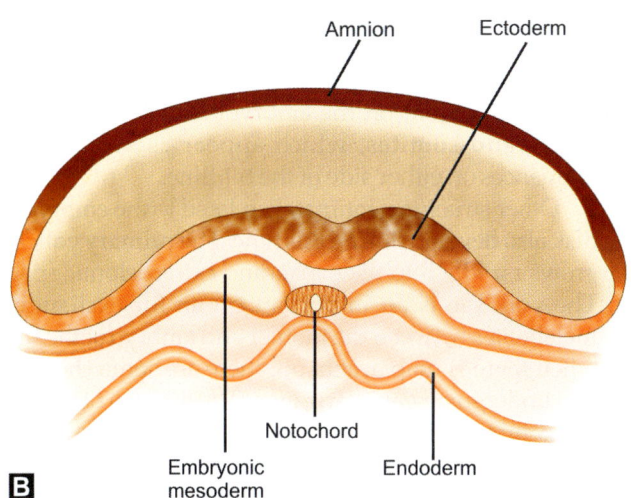

Figs 4.1A and B: (A) Dorsal aspect of 18 days presomite embryo; (B) Section of the presomite embryo at 18 days at A-A level

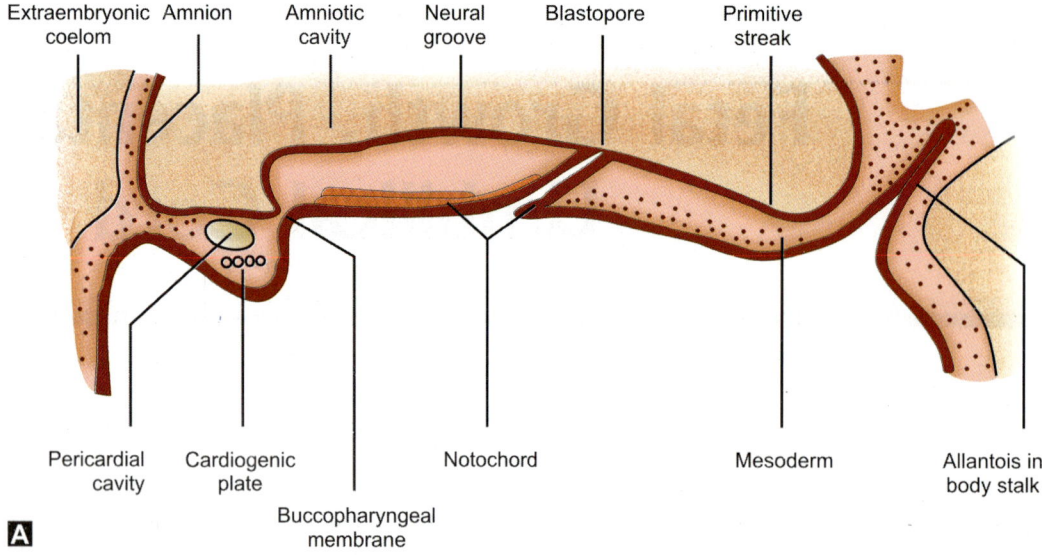

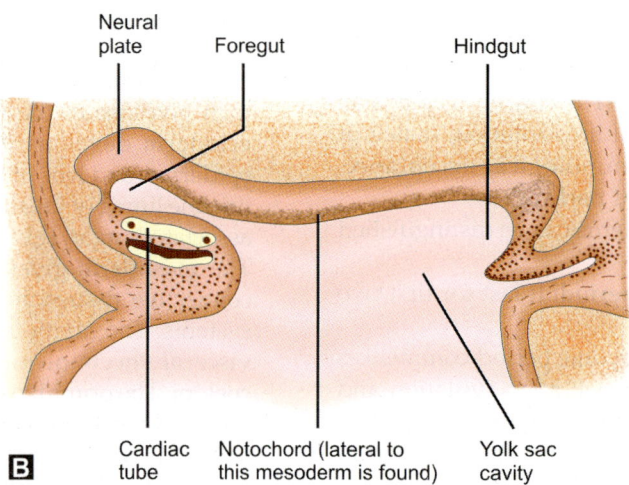

Figs 4.2A and B: (A) Longitudinal section of presomite embryo; (B) Longitudinal section of 7 somite embryo (24 days embryo)

of symmetry, polarity and laterality at outset of organogenesis is fundamental for appropriate organ system topology and number of genes participates in this initial step. During third week two other structures become apparent on the embryonic disk—the **neural plates and somites**, which appear as symmetrical eminences on either side of the midline.

Other structures intimately related to the embryonic disk also develop during this time. The **primary yolk sac** grows rapidly into the expanding extracoelomic space. The yolk sac is an important organ for exchanging metabolites between the mother and embryo at the time when there is no placenta but there are some chorionic villi undergoing vascularization. The lifespan of the yolk sac is limited. It is fully developed by 32 days and its complex wall starts degenerating by end of 6 week. The **amniotic membrane** is another extraembryonic element which by day 17 is closely opposed to the embryonic disk.

During 4th week the embryonic disk folds into an embryonic cylindric. Within which is a craniocaudal, blind ending tube which has three parts—**the foregut, midgut opened to the developing yolk sac, and the hindgut. This stage marks the start of organogenesis**. The first organ to become apparent is the heart in shape of forward buckling loop. Cardiac activity is evident by **day 22** after fertilization. The development of nervous system takes place at this stage of development. By end of 4th week the central nervous system has defined segments, the primary brain vesicles prosencephalon, mesencephalon and rhombencephalon (Figs 4.2A and B).

Towards end of 4th week, the foregut septates along the midline into the respiratory and digestive primitive elements. The ventral pancreatic bud migrates posteriorly to fuse with dorsal pancreatic bud. The lower respiratory system appears as septation of the foregut occurs. Two lung buds are evident at end of 4th week.

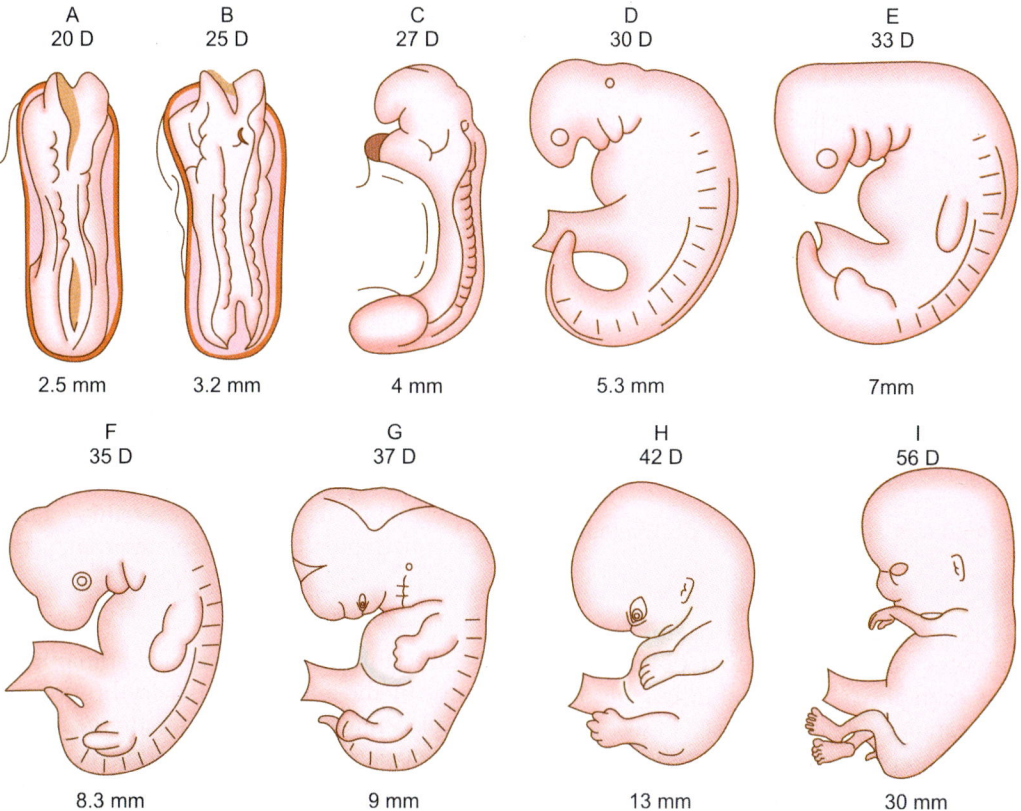

Fig. 4.3: Sequential changes during the development of external form in a normal human embryo from day 20 to day 56

By days 26 the mesonephric duct and mesonephros differentiate. At 28 days, ureteric buds and the metanephric blastema are defined structure. So it can be said that by the end of the 4th week, almost all organ systems though immature can be defined (Fig. 4.3).

d. **Fetus:** Fetal period begins after eight weeks following conception and ends in delivery. Development during the fetal period of gestation consists of growth and maturation of structure that were formed during the embryonic period. Normal fetal growth is characterized by cellular hyperplasia followed by hyperplasia and hypertrophy and lastly by hypertrophy alone. **The fetal growth is controlled by genetic factor in the first half and by environment factors in the second half of pregnancy. Fetal growth is predominantly controlled by IGF-1, insulin and other growth factors.**

Fetal Physiology and Organ System

Nutrition

Following fertilization, in early post fertilization period, the nutrition is stored in the deutoplasm within the cytoplasm and a very small part is derived from the tubal and uterine secretion. Following implantation and before the establishment of uteroplacental circulation, the nutrition is derived from the eroded decidua by diffusion and later from stagnant blood in the trophoblastic lacunae. From third week onwards, fetal circulation is established and nutrition is obtained by active and passive transfer.

Fetal Blood

Fetal Hemopoiesis

In the early embryo hemopoiesis is seen in yolk sac. By 10th week of gestation the liver becomes the major site of erythropoiesis. The great enlargement of the early fetal liver is due to erythropoietic function. Gradually the red cell production is mainly in spleen and bone marrow and near term the bone marrow is the major site of red cell production. In early fetal period the erythropoiesis is megaloblastic but near term it becomes normoblastic (Fig. 4.4).

Fetal Hemoglobin

Most hemoglobin in the fetus is HbF, which has two γ chains ($\alpha 2, \gamma 2$) in place of adult hemoglobin (HbF) ($\alpha 2, \beta 2$) and Hb A2 ($\alpha 2, \delta 2$). γ chains are made by two genes which make two slightly different forms of γ chain. While β chains are identical and come from a single gene.

90% of fetal hemoglobin is HbF between 10 and 28 weeks of gestation. From 28 to 34 weeks a change from

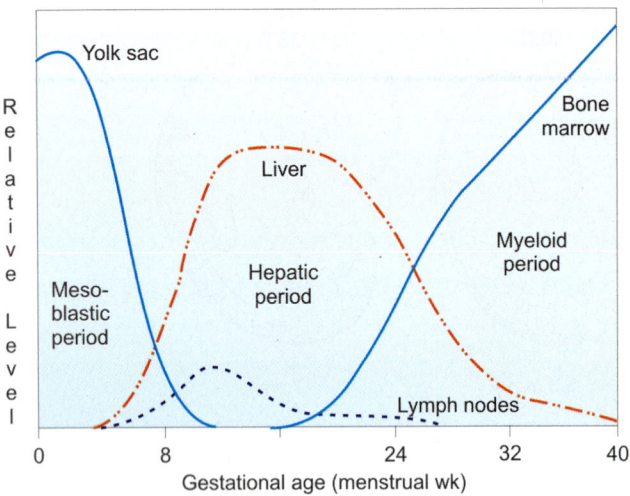

Fig. 4.4: Fetal hemopoiesis at various stages of development

($\alpha2, \gamma2$) to ($\alpha2, \beta2$) begins. By term the ratio of HbF to HbA is 80:20 and by 6 months only 1% of hemoglobin is HbF. In normal adult less than 1% of hemoglobin is HbF. Fetal hemoglobin is a tetramer protein, composed of two copies each of two different peptide chains. The types of chain determine the type of hemoglobin produced. α and β chain make up normal adult hemoglobin A.

During embryonic and fetal life, a variety of α and β chain precursor are produced which results in the serial production of several different embryonic hemoglobin. The genes that direct production of the various embryonic versions of these chains are arranged in the order in which they are temporarily activated on chromosomes 11 (β type chains) and 16 (α type chain).

Each of three genes is turned on and then off during fetal life, until the α and β genes, which direct the production of hemoglobin A, are permanently activated. In yolk sac hemoglobin Gower1, Gower2, and Portland are made. In liver hemoglobin F is produced and in bone marrow normal hemoglobin A appears in fetal red blood cells and is present in progressively greater amounts as the fetus matures. At term about 75–80% of the total hemoglobin is of fetal type – HbF. Between 6 and 12 months after birth, the fetal hemoglobin is completely replaced by adult hemoglobin. Glucocorticosteroids mediate the switch from fetal to adult hemoglobin and effect is irreversible.

The fetal hemoglobin has got a greater affinity to oxygen due to lower binding of 2-3 diphosphoglycerate as compared to adult hemoglobin. Fetal hemoglobin is resistant to alkali in the formation of alkaline hematin.

Fetal Blood Volume

Total fetoplacental blood volume is 125 ml/kg body weight of the fetus. The red cells of fetus develop their group antigen quite early and the presence of Rh factor has been demonstrated in the fetal blood at approximately 38 days after conception. The lifespan of fetal RBC is about 2/3rd of the adult RBC, i.e. about 80 days.

Fetal Coagulation Factor

The fetus starts producing normal adult type procoagulant, fibrinolytic and anticoagulant proteins by about 12 weeks, at quite reduced level. So the concentrations of several coagulation factors at birth are markedly below the levels that develop within a few weeks of life. So factors II, VII, IX, X, Xi, XII, XII and fibrinogen are markedly low in cord blood. Without prophylactic treatment, the vitamin K dependent coagulation factors usually decrease even further during the first few days after birth, which may lead sometimes to hemorrhage in newborn.

Cord blood levels of iron, ferritin, vitamin B_{12}, folic acid are consistently higher than maternal blood.

Fetal Erythropoiesis

Fetal erythropoiesis is controlled primarily by erythropoietin made by the fetus. Maternal erythropoietin does not cross the placenta. Fetal erythropoietin production is influenced by testosterone, estrogen, prostaglandin, thyroid hormone and lipoprotein. Fetal liver is an important site of erythropoietin production, till renal production starts.

Leukocyte

Leukocytes appear after 2 months of gestational age. The lymphocytes are divided into two distinct populations:
a. Thymus derived (T lymphocytes)
b. Bone marrow derived (B lymphocytes)

In each group there are long and short lived lymphocytes. The T cells account for 60-80% of lymphocyte present in the thoracic duct, lymph nodes and blood. The long lived T cells are present in blood stream, while the short lived T cells are located mainly in the thymus, bone marrow and spleen.

B lymphocytes are found in perilymphoid organs, lymph nodes, thymus independent areas around germinal centers and in small amount in peripheral blood. The fetus however rarely forms antibody because of relatively sterile environment. Maternal immunoglobulin (IgG) crosses the placenta from the 12th week onwards to give the fetus a passive immunity, which increases with increase in gestation period. At term fetal IgG level is 10% higher than the mother.

In contrast IgM response to antigenic stimulant is dominant in the fetus and remains so for weeks to month in the newborn. Very little IgM is produced by normal healthy fetus and that produced may include antibody to maternal lymphocytes.

Increased levels of IgM are found in newborn with congenital infections such as rubella, cytomegalovirus or toxoplasmosis. Serum IgM level in umbilical cord blood and identification of specific antibodies may be useful in diagnosis of intrauterine infection. Adult levels of IgM are normally attained by 9 months of age.

Fetal Blood Cells

Fetal blood cells are larger than maternal cells and possess the i antigen, which is replaced by the I antigen after birth. They are more resistant than adult cells to osmotic alkali and acid lysis, have a shorter lifespan and have lower levels of 2–3 diphosphoglyceric acid and carbonic anhydrase. Fetal cells have no surface ABO antigen until after birth.

Fetal Pulmonary System

Fetal lung is an outgrowth of the primitive foregut. Like the branching of tree, lung development proceed along an established timetable that apparently can not be expedited or influenced by antenatal or neonatal therapy. So limits of viability appear to be determined by the usual process of pulmonary growth.

There are three essential stage of lung development:

Pseudoglandular stage: It entails the growth of intrasegmental bronchial tree between the 5th and 17th week.

Canalicular stage: It entails from 16th to 25th week, in which the bronchial cartilage plate extend peripherally. Each terminal bronchiole gives rise to several respiratory bronchioles and each of these in turn divides into multiple saccular ducts.

Terminal sac stage: In which the alveoli gives rise to primitive pulmonary alveoli called the terminal sacs. At birth only 15% of the adult numbers of alveoli are present and thus lung continues to grow, adding more alveoli, from *late fetal life up to about 8 years.**

Fetal Respiration

Respiratory muscles develop early and movements of the fetal chest wall have been detected by ultrasound as early as 11 weeks. Fetal breathing occurs for 15% of the observation time in the second trimester rising to 30% in the third trimester. Time spent in breathing increases after meals and decrease after alcohol ingestion and during labor.

---

* Various insults can upset this process and timing of the insult determines the outcome. For example, if there is renal agenesis, there is no amniotic fluid from the beginning of lung growth, and major defect occur in all the three stages. If there is premature rupture of membrane before 20 weeks, there is usually normal bronchial branching and cartilage development but has immature alveoli. Membrane rupture occurring after 24 weeks may have little long-term effect on pulmonary structure.

Surfactant

Lung alveoli are lined by a group of phospholipids known collectively as surfactant. Surfactant prevents collapse of small alveoli during expiration by lowering surface tension or by acting at an internal molecular splint.

The surfactant is continuously replaced by synthesis from type II alveolar cells, which make up 10% of the lung parenchyma. Surfactant is produced on microsomes and stored in 1.5 µg osmiophilic lamellar bodies.

The 80% of total phospholipids is dipalmitoyl-phosphatidylcholine (DPPC, Lecithin). **There is a surge of lecithin production at 35-36 weeks of fetal life. This surge can be promoted by steroids, growth retardation, and prolonged rupture of membrane. It is delayed in diabetes.**

Before activation of this pathway fetal lung is functionally immature and premature delivery is associated with respiratory distress syndrome. Other phospholipids which are included in surfactant are—sphingomyelin, phosphatidylglycerol and phosphatidyl inositol. Sphingomyelin production reaches a peak at about 32 weeks and diminishes after 35 weeks. As some lung fluid is excreted into amniotic fluid, **so lecithin/ sphingomyelin ratio provides a measure of lung maturity.** The action of lecithin is dependent on phosphatidylinositol (secreted early in the second trimester) and phosphatidylglycerol (secreted mainly in last 5 weeks of pregnancy). The relative deficiency of phosphatidylglycerol in diabetic pregnancy may lead to development of RDS despites a "mature" lecithin/sphingomyelin ratio (more than 2).

During late fetal life, the alveoli are characterized by water to tissue interface. The intact lamellar bodies are secreted from the lung and swept into the amniotic fluid during fetal breathing movement. At birth with the first breath, air to tissue interface is produced in the lung alveoli. *Surfactant uncoils from the lamellar bodies and it then spreads to line the alveoli to prevent alveolar collapse during expiration.* So it is the capacity for fetal lung to produce surfactant and not the actual laying down of this material in the lung *in utero* that establishes fetal lung maturity.

Fetal Urinary System

Two primitive urinary systems: Pronephros and **Mesonephros** precede the development of metanephros. The pronephros involutes by two weeks; mesonephros produces urine at fifth weeks and degenerates by 11-12 weeks. Failure of these two structures either to form or to regress may result in anamolous development of the definitive urinary system. Between 9 and 12 weeks, the ureteric bud and nephrogenic blastema interact to produce the metanephros. The kidney and ureter develop from intermediate mesoderm. The bladder and urethra develop from urogenital sinus. The bladder also develops partly from allantois. By 14 weeks, loop of Henle is functional and resorption occurs. New nephrons continue to be formed until 36 weeks. In preterm infants nephrons continue to be formed after birth.

The fetal kidney starts producing **urine at 12 weeks**. By 18 weeks they are producing 7–14 ml/day and at term this increase to 27 ml/hr or 650 ml/day. Maternally administered furosemide increase fetal urine formation and uteroplacental insufficiency decrease it. Kidneys are not essential for survival *in utero*, but are important in the control of composition and volume of amniotic fluid. So the abnormalities that cause chronic anuria are usually associated with oligohydramnios and pulmonary hypoplasia.

Fetal Gastrointestinal Tract

Fetal gut differentiates from endoderm by 6 weeks after conception. Swallowing movements are present by 14 weeks and full suckling reflex by 28 weeks. Secretion of bile and digestive enzyme begins at 12 weeks. Meconium is present by 16 weeks and consists of desquamated intestinal cells, lanugo, scalp, hairs, and vernix. The dark green black appearance is caused by pigments especially biliverdin.

Meconium passage can result from normal bowel peristalsis in the mature fetus or from vagal stimulation. It can also occur when hypoxia stimulates arginin vasopressin release from the fetal pituitary gland.

Fetal Skin

At 16th week, lanugo which is soft colorless hairs appears but near term almost completely disappears. Sebaceous glands appear at 20th week and sweat glands somewhat later. Vernix caseosa is found by secretion of the sebaceous glands mixed with the exfoliated epidermal cells which abundantly present on fetal skin at time of birth. The horny layer of the epidermis is absent before 20th week, which favors transudation from fetal capillaries into the liquor amni.

Endocrine System

The fetal endocrine system is functional for sometime before the central nervous system reaches a state of maturity competent to perform many functions associated with homeostasis. The fetal endocrine system does not necessarily mimic that of the adult but nonetheless may be one of the first homeostatic systems to develop.

Fetal Pituitary

It develops from two different sources – (**anterior pituitary**) **adenohypophysis** develops from the **oral ectoderm**. Rathke's pouch and **neurohypophysis (Posterior Pituitary)** develops from the **neuroectoderm**.

Thyroid Physiology in Fetus and Neonate

The human fetal thyroid gland develops the capacity to concentrate iodine and synthesize hormone between 8 and 10 weeks of gestation. At the same time the pituitary begins to synthesize TSH. By 12–14 week, the development of pituitary thyroid system is complete. Level of TSH and T4 are low until an abrupt rise occur at 20 weeks which correlates with maturation of the hypothalamus and development of the pituitary portal vascular system, which make releasing hormones available to the pituitary gland.

T4 rises rapidly and exceeds maternal values at term. However, total T3 and free T3 level are low throughout gestation and level of RT3 are elevated. Paralleling the rise in T4 like T3, this compound is derived predominantly from conversion of T4 in peripheral tissues. *The increased production of T4 in fetal life is compensated by rapid conversion to inactive RT3, allowing the fetus to conserve its full resources. The fetal pattern of low T3 and high RT3 is similar to that seen with calorie malnutrition.*

After delivery TSH peaks at 30 minutes of age followed by a T3 peak at 24 hours and a T4 peak at 24–48 hours. The T3 increase is independent of the TSH surge and related to cord cutting and sudden exposure of fetus to cold world. High RT3 level present for 3–5 days after delivery, then reach normal values by 2 weeks.

Fetal Adrenal Gland

The fetal adrenal cortex is differentiated by 8–9 weeks gestational age into a thick inner fetal zone and a thin outer definitive zone, which is source of cortisol and forerunner of the adult cortex. Early in pregnancy, adrenal growth and development are remarkable and the gland achieves a size equal to or larger than that of kidney by the end of first trimester.

After 20–24 weeks, the adrenal gland slowly decrease in size until a second spurt in growth begins at about 34–35 weeks. The gland remains proportionately larger than the adult adrenal glands. After delivery the fetal zone (about 80% of the bulk of gland) rapidly involutes to be replaced by simultaneous expansion of the adrenal cortex composed of the zona glomerulosa, the zone fasciculata and zone reticularis, which expands again during adrenarche at puberty. Thus, the specific steroidogenic characteristics of the fetus are associated with a specific adrenal morphology that is dependent on specific factors present during intrauterine life.

Fetal Circulation

The major variants in the fetal cardiovascular system are explained by the presence of umbilical placental circulation and the absence of significant pulmonary circulation. In addition the fetal heart chambers work in parallel, not in series, which effectively supplies the brain and heart with more highly oxygenated blood than the rest of the body.

Oxygen and nutrient material required for fetal growth and maturation are delivered to the fetus from the placenta by the single umbilical vein. The vein then divides into the ductus venosus and portal sinus. The ductus venosus is the major branch of the umbilical vein and traverses the liver to enter the inferior vena cava directly. Ductus venosus does not supply oxygen to the intervening tissues. It carries well oxygenated blood directly to the heart. While the portal sinuses carries blood to the hepatic veins primarily on the left side of the liver, where oxygen is extracted. The relatively deoxygenated blood from the liver then flows back into the inferior vena cava, which also receives less oxygenated blood returning from the lower body. So the oxygen content of blood delivered to the heart from the inferior vena cava is thus lower than that leaving the placenta.

In contrast to postnatal life, the ventricles of the fetal heart work in parallel not in series. Well oxygenated blood enters the left ventricle which supplies the heart and brain. Less oxygenated blood enters the right ventricle, which supplies the rest of the body. The two separate circulations are maintained by the structure of the right atrium, which effectively directs entering blood to either left atrium or the right ventricle, depending on its oxygen content via foramen ovale. This separation of blood according to its oxygen content is facilitated by the pattern of blood flow in the inferior vena cava. The well oxygenated blood tend to course along the medial aspect of the inferior vena cava and less oxygenated blood stays along the vessels walls, facilitating their shunting into opposite sides of the heart. Once this blood enters the atrium, the configuration of the upper interatrial septum called the crista dividens is such that it preferentially shunts the well oxygenated blood from the medial side of inferior vena cava and the ductus venous through the foramen ovale into the left heart and then the heart and brain. After these tissues have extracted needed oxygen, the resulting less oxygenated blood returns to the right heart through the superior vena cava.

The less oxygenated blood coursing along the lateral wall of the inferior vena cava enters the right atrium and is deflected through the tricuspid valve to the right ventricle. The superior vena cava courses inferiorly and anteriorly as it enters the right atrium, ensuring that less well oxygenated blood returning from the brain and upper body also will be shunted directly to the right ventricle. The ostium of the coronary sinus lies just superior to the tricuspid valve so that less oxygenated blood from the heart also return to the right ventricle. Because of this blood flow pattern, blood in right ventricle is 15–20% less saturated than blood in the left ventricle.

Almost 90% of blood of right ventricle is then shunted through the ductus arteriosus to the descending aorta. The high pulmonary vascular resistance and the comparatively lower resistance in the ductus arteriosus and the umbilical placental vasculature ensure that about 15% of the right ventricle output and 8% the combined ventricular output goes to the lungs. Thus, 1/3rd of the blood passing through the ductus arteriosus is delivered to the body. The remaining right ventricular output returns to the placenta through the two hypogastric arteries which distally becomes the umbilical arteries. In the placenta, this blood picks up oxygen and other nutrients and is then recirculated back through the umbilical veins (Fig. 4.5).

At Birth

The cessation of umbilical blood flow causes a fall in pressure in the right atrium and closure of foramen ovale. Ventilation of the lung opens the pulmonary circulation and the ductus arteriosus closes as a direct effect of increasing PO_2. Prior to birth the ductus arteriosus remains patent due to production of PGE2 and prostacyclin which act as local vasodilator. With functional closure of the ductus arteriosus and the expansion of the lungs, blood leaving the right ventricle preferentially enters the pulmonary vasculature to become oxygenated before it returns to the left heart, virtually instantaneously at the time of birth. The ventricles which had worked in parallel in fetal life, now effectively works in series.

The more distal portion of the hypogastric arteries courses from the level of the bladder along the abdominal

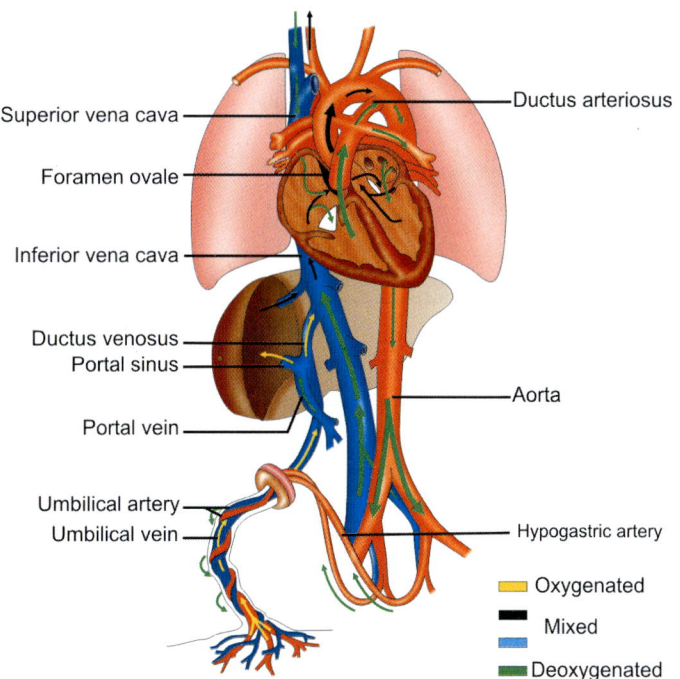

Fig. 4.5: Fetal circulation: There is presence of three main vascular shunts: Ductus venosus, foramen ovale, ductus arteriosus. Oxygenation is provided by placenta in intrauterine life

wall to the umbilical ring and into the cord as the umbilical arteries undergo atrophy and obliteration within 3–4 days after birth. This becomes the **umbilical ligament**, while the intra-abdominal remnants of the umbilical vein form the **ligamentum teres**. The ductus venosus constricts by 10–96 hours after birth and is anatomically closed by 2–3 weeks, which results in the formation of the **ligamentum venosum**. The pathway of fetal blood is summarized in Table 4.1 and Figure 4.5.

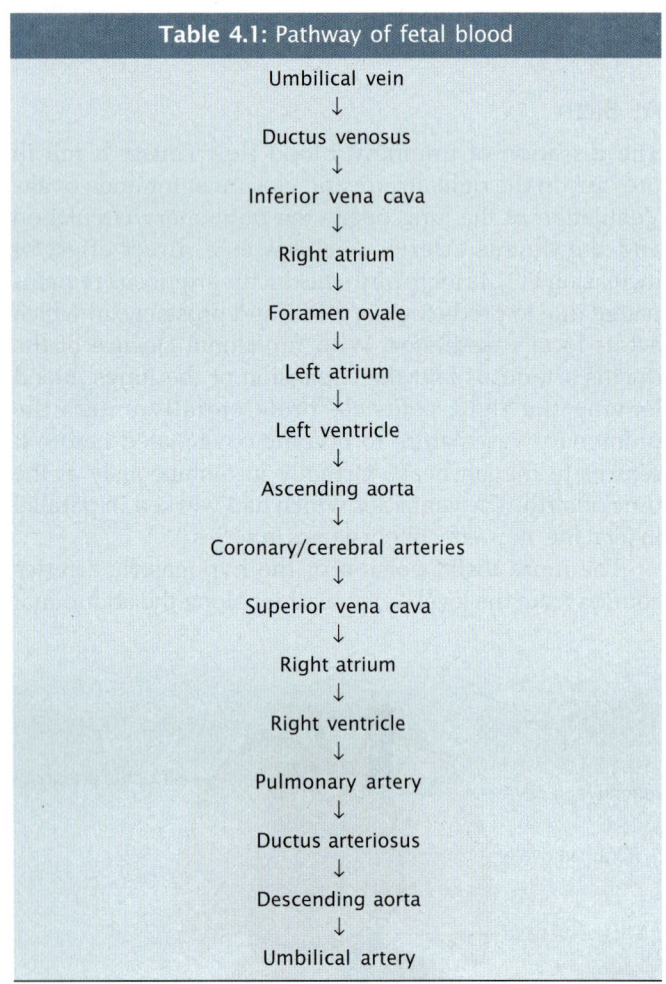

Table 4.1: Pathway of fetal blood

Umbilical vein ↓ Ductus venosus ↓ Inferior vena cava ↓ Right atrium ↓ Foramen ovale ↓ Left atrium ↓ Left ventricle ↓ Ascending aorta ↓ Coronary/cerebral arteries ↓ Superior vena cava ↓ Right atrium ↓ Right ventricle ↓ Pulmonary artery ↓ Ductus arteriosus ↓ Descending aorta ↓ Umbilical artery

Fetal Nervous System

The spinal cord extends along the entire length of the vertebral column in the embryo. After that spinal cord grows more slowly. By 24 weeks the spinal cord extends to S1, at birth to L3 and in the adult to L1. Myelination of the spinal cord begins in the middle of gestation and continues through the first year of life.

Synaptic function is developed by 8 weeks. At 10 weeks, local stimuli may evolve squinting, opening of mouth, incomplete finger closure, and flexion of the toe. **Swallowing is evident at 14-16 weeks.** Rudimentary taste buds are present at 7 weeks and mature receptors are present by 12 weeks. During 3rd trimester, integration of nervous and muscular function proceeds rapidly. The internal, middle and external component of the ear are well developed by mid pregnancy. The fetus apparently hears some sounds *in utero* as early as 24–26 weeks. By 28 weeks, the eye is sensitive to light, but perception of form and color is not complete to until long after birth.

Functions of Placenta

a. Transfer of nutrients and waste products between the mother and fetus by following:
   i. Nutritive
   ii. Excretory
   iii. Respiratory function
b. Placenta as a barrier
c. Placenta as a endocrine organ
d. Immunological

The main functions of placenta are:

1. **Nutritive:** The fetus usually receives its nutrient from maternal blood and only in cases of inadequate nutrition of mother, depletion of maternal tissue storages occurs. The main nutrients are:
   a. **Glucose:** It is the principal source of energy which is transferred to the fetus by facilitated diffusion. Usually fetal glucose level is lower than that of mother which indicates rapid rate of glucose utilization by the fetus.
   b. **Lipids:** In early pregnancy triglycerides and fatty acids are directly transported from the mother to fetus and probably synthesized by fetus in late pregnancy. Essential fatty acids are transferred more than the nonessential fatty acids. Cholesterol is directly transferred. So fetal fat has a dual origin.
   c. **Amino acids:** Amino acids are transferred to fetus by active transport through ATPase enzyme mechanism. Some protein like IgG crosses the placenta by endocytosis. Amino acid concentration is higher in fetal blood than that of maternal blood. Fetal protein are synthesized from the transferred amino acid and level is lower than in mother.
   d. **Water and electrolytes:** Electrolyte like sodium, K^+, chloride cross through the fetal membrane by simple diffusion, while calcium, phosphorus and iron cross by active transport against concentration gradient as their levels are higher in fetal than in maternal blood. Water soluble vitamins are transferred by active transport slowly so fat soluble vitamins are at low concentration in fetal blood.
   e. **Hormones:** Thyroid, placental lactogen, insulin, steroid from the adrenal cross the placenta at a very slow rate, so that their concentration in fetal plasma are quiet lower than in maternal plasma. *Paratharmone as well calcium does not cross the placenta*

2. **Excretory:** Waste products from the fetus like urea, uric acid are excreted into maternal blood by simple diffusion.

3. **Respiratory function:** Although the fetal respiratory movements are observed as early as 11 weeks there is no gaseous exchange. Intake of oxygen and output of carbon dioxide take place by simple diffusion across the fetal membrane. Partial pressure gradient is the driving force for exchange between maternal and fetal circulation. The oxygen supply to the fetus is at the rate of 8 ml/kg/min, which is achieved with cord blood flow of 165-330 ml/minute.
4. **Placenta as a barrier:** In general substance of high molecular weight more than 500 Daltons are not transferred from maternal to fetal blood through placental barrier but there are exceptions and layer molecules can be transferred through placenta by pinocytosis. Antibody and antigen in immunological quantities can traverse across the fetal membrane in both the direction. Maternal infection by virus, bacteria, or protozoa as well almost any drug used in pregnancy can cross the placenta barrier and may effect the fetus.
5. **Placenta as endocrine organ:** The placenta has a function of endocrine organ making various hormones that regulates the following:
   a. *Rate of growth of fetus:* First directly and later indirectly through control of placental blood supply.
   b. *Suppress activity of uterus to prevent premature delivery* and at correct time encourages labor contraction.
   c. *Activity of other organs* like breast, pelvic ligaments in pregnancy.

It is to be emphasized that the production of steroid and protein hormones by human trophoblast is greater in amount and diversity than that of any other single endocrine tissue in mammalian physiology. **Syncytiotrophoblast are the principal site of protein and steroid hormones in pregnancy.**

These products are considered to play an important part in adjusting maternal metabolism during pregnancy. So it is understandable that another remarkable feature of human pregnancy is the success of physiological adaptation of pregnant women to the unique endocrine mileu.

The main factors controlling the secretion of placental products (and hence maternal levels) are the functional mass of the trophoblast and uteroplacental blood flow. So maternal level of placental products usually correlates with the weight of the placenta and fetus. Table 4.2 summarizes products of placenta.

Table 4.2: Product of placenta

1. Steroid	Progesterone, estrogens (estrone, estradiol, estriol)
2. Protein hormones	Placental lactogen, chorionic gonadotropin (hCG) ACTH Hypothalamic like—releasing hormones, e.g. CRH, GnRH, TRH, GHRH
3. Enzymes	Heat stable Alkaline phosphatase (HASP), Oxytocinase (Cystine amino peptidase), Histaminase Other nonspecific enzymes
4. Proteins	Pregnancy specific β, glycoprotein, Pregnancy associated plasma protein (PAPPA) Placental protein 5 (PP5) Other protein identified immunologically but with no clearly defined biological function

Function of Steroid Hormone (Estrogen and Progesterone)

It is actually difficult to separate their function from one another:
1. Both play critical role in maintenance of pregnancy. Estrogen causes hypertrophy and hyperplasia of the uterine myometrium. Progesterone along with estrogen stimulates growth of uterus, causes decidual changes of the endometrium required for implantation and inhibits myometrial contraction.
2. Estrogen and progesterone both are required for the adaptation of the maternal organ to the constantly increasing demands of the growing fetus.
3. Hypertrophy and proliferation of ducts of breast are due to estrogen, while those of a lobuloalveolar systems are due to combined action of estrogen and progesterone.
4. Estrogen sensitizes the myometrium to oxytocin and prostaglandins and ripens the cervix, while progesterone maintains uterine quiescence by stabilizing lysosomal membrane and inhibiting prostaglandin synthesis.
5. Estrogen with progesterone combined cause inhibition of cyclic fluctuating activity of gonadotropin—gonadal axis thereby preserving gonadal function.
6. Progesterone with hCG and decimal cortical inhibits. T-lymphocyte mediated tissue rejection and protects the conceptus.

Human Placental Lactogen (HPL)

Placental lactogen (mol weight 2,16,000, half-life 15 min), has a single chain of 191 amino acids, two disulphide bonds and no carbohydrate residue. HPL is chemically and functionally similar to pituitary growth hormones and prolactin, but has less biological activity.

The level of HPL in maternal blood show a progressive rise with a plateau after 35 weeks, and only small amounts are excreted in urine.

Function of HPL: HPL has probable action in a number of metabolic processes. These include:
1. **Maternal lipolysis:** It increases in the level of circulating free fatty acids, thus providing a source of energy for maternal metabolism and fetal nutrition.

2. **An anti-insulin or diabetogenic:** Leading to an increase in maternal level of insulin, which favors protein synthesis and provides a readily available source of amino acids for transport to the fetus.
3. **A potent angiogenic hormone:** It also may play an important role in the formation of fetal vasculature.

Human Chorionic Gonadotropin (hCG)

The hCG—so called pregnancy hormone is a glycoprotein, which has biological activity very similar to luteinizing hormone (LH). LH and hCG both act via the plasma membrane LH—hCG receptor.

Chemical characteristic of hCG: It is glycoprotein, has molecular weight of 38,400, half-life 5 hours (fast component) and slow component has half of 24 hours. It consist of two chains of amino acids (α and β) which are linked by non-covalent bonds. α subunit is the common subunit of all the glycoprotein hormones (LH, FSH, TSH, hCG), whereas the β subunit is similar to that of LH, but with an additional 30 amino acids at the carboxy terminus. *So the immune assay directed to the β subunits is specific for hCG.*

The major excretory product in urine is a fragment of β subunit, known as β core. This product is measured by many pregnancy tests.

Biological function of hCG:
1. The best known biological function of hCG is maintenance of corpus luteum. hCG may be the luteotropic signal from the early embryo that prevents the normal degeneration of corpus luteum.
2. hCG has weak thyrotrophic activity.
3. hCG has immunosuppressive activity, which may inhibit the maternal process of immunorejection of the fetus as a homograft.
4. It stimulates adrenal and placental steroid synthesis.
5. hCG stimulates Leydig cells of the male fetus to produce testosterone in conjunction with fetal pituitary gonadotropins. Thus, it is indirectly involved in the development of male external genitals.

Concentration of hCG in serum and urine: The intact hCG molecule is detectable in plasma of pregnant women about 7–9 days after the midcycle surge of LH that precedes ovulation. Thus, probably hCG enters maternal blood at the time of blastocyst implantation. Blood level of hCG increases rapidly, doubles every 2 days, with max level is attained at 8–10 weeks gestation. After that maternal plasma level of hCG begins to decline and a nadir is reached by about 20 weeks. Plasma levels of hCG are maintained at this level for rest of gestation. hCG disappears from the circulation within 15 days following delivery.

Maternal urine hCG also can be monitored, and is composed of a variety of degradation products. The primary form of hCG in urine is the terminal degradation product of hCG, the β core fragment. Its concentration has the same pattern as that in maternal plasma. But the so called β subunit antibody used in most pregnancy tests reacts with both intact hCG, the major form in the plasma and with fragments of hCG, major form formed in urine.

Pregnancy Associated Plasma Protein (PAPP)

PAPP is secreted by syncytiotrophoblast. It acts as a immunosuppressant in pregnancy.

Early Pregnancy Factor (EPF)

It is a protein, which is produced by the activated platelets and other maternal tissues. It is detectable in maternal circulation 6–24 hours after conception. EPF is immunosuppressant and prevents rejection of the conceptus.

Pregnancy Specific β-1 Glycoprotein (PS β-1G)

It is produced by the trophoblast cells. It is detectable in maternal serum 18–20 days after ovulation. PS β-1G is a potent immunosuppressant of lymphocyte proliferation and prevents rejection of conceptus.

Other placental protein hormones:
1. Chorionic adrenocorticotropin.
2. Relaxin.
3. Parathyroid hormone related protein (PTH – rp).
4. Growth hormone variant (GHV).

Hypothalamic Like Releasing Hormones

For each of the known hypothalamic releasing or inhibiting hormones described GnRH, TRH, CRH, GHRH and Somatostatin—there is an analogous hormone produced in human placenta. Many investigators have proposed that these substances in placental tissues are indicative of a hierarchy of control in the synthesis of chorionic trophic agents. Following hypothalamic like releasing hormones secreted by placenta has been identified:
 i. Gonadotropin releasing hormones (GnRH).
 ii. Corticotrophic releasing hormone (CRH).
 iii. Growth hormone-releasing hormone (GHRH).

Other placental peptide hormones:
 i. Leptin.
 ii. Neuropeptide.
 iii. Inhibin and activin.

FETAL MEMBRANE, AMNIOTIC FLUID AND UMBILICAL CORD

Fetal membrane consist of two layers: (a) Outer chorion, (b) Inner amnion.

Chorion

The main layer of chorion is the trophoblast, which arises as a single layer of cells surrounding the blastocyst. The chorion has four layers:

a. Cellular layer (fibroblast).
b. Reticular layer.
c. Basement membrane.
d. Trophoblast.

The trophoblast is a two to ten cell thick layer, lying immediately adjacent to the decidua which is in continuation with the placental trophoblast. No synctium is apparent, although obliterated chorionic villi may be recognizable. In nonplacental areas, at the term pregnancy, chorion contains no vessels or nerves.

Amnion

The amnion at term is a tough and tenacious nonpliable membrane. It is the innermost fetal membrane and is contiguous with amniotic fluid. Amnion provides almost all of the tensile strength of the fetal membranes so the development of the components of the amnion that protects against its rupture or tearing is vitally important to successful pregnancy outcome.

Development of Amnion

Early in the process of implantation a space develops between the embryonic cell mass and adjacent trophoblast. Small cells that line this inner surface of trophoblast have been called angiogenic cells, which is the precursor of amniotic epithelium. Thus, human amnion is first identifiable at 7–8 days of embryo development.

Initially it is a minute vesicle, after that the amnion develops into a small sac, which covers the dorsal surface of the embryo. As gradually the amnion enlarges and engulfs the growing embryo which prolapses into its cavity.

Gradual distention of the amniotic sac finally brings the sac into contact with the interior surface of the chorion leavae. Apposition of the nearest of chorion laevae and amnion near the end of the first trimester then causes an obliteration of the extraembryonic coelom.

The amnion and chorion leavae, though are a little adherent, but they are never intimately connected and usually can be separated easily even at term gestational age.

Structure of Amnion

Amnion has five layers:
a. Cuboidal epithelium with a microvillous surface and prominent intracellular canal and numerous vacuoles.
b. Basement membrane.
c. Compact layer.
d. Fibroblast layer.
e. Spongy layer.

There are no blood vessels, lymphatics or nerves.

Amniotic Fluid

In early pregnancy, the amniotic fluid is a transudate of fetal serum via fetal skin and umbilical cord. From second trimester onwards there are contribution from fetal urine, fetal swallowing (500 ml/day) and excretion of lung fluids. Throughout pregnancy there is a fairly free exchange of fluid with the mother via the membranes.

Origin and Circulation of Amniotic Fluid

In early first trimester the amniotic fluid is produced by the **amniotic membrane** by a process of active transportation of electrolytes with passive osmotic diffusion of water.

In late first trimester and early second trimester other pathways develop for amniotic fluid production and absorption. This includes movement of fluid across the chorion frondosum and across the fetal skin. The exchange across the **fetal skin** continues up to 24 weeks until keratinization is complete. Around the same time, fetal **swallowing and urination** begin and progressively become major routes of amniotic fluid consumption and production respectively. At 25 weeks the **fetal urine** production is 100 ml/day, which increases to 600 ml/day at term. The fetus swallows 200–500 ml/day at term.

The **fetal respiratory tract** provides another route of production and consumption of amniotic fluid. There is a net flow of fluid from the respiratory epithelium into the amniotic cavity. With increasing contribution from fetal urine output the amniotic fluid become hypotonic with increasing concentration of urea and creatinine.

Volume

Amniotic fluid increases slowly from about 50 ml at 12 weeks, 250 ml at 16 weeks to 800 ml at 28 weeks and 1000 ml at 34 weeks. It therefore decreases to 800 ml at 40 weeks.

The amniotic fluid volume correlates with maternal plasma volume. Maternal dehydration is associated with oligohydramnios which returns to normal with hydration of the mother.

In post-term pregnancy, there is further reduction of amniotic fluid volume to extent of about 200 ml at 43 weeks.

Physical Feature

The amniotic fluid is faintly alkaline with low specific gravity of 1010. It becomes highly hypotonic to maternal serum at term pregnancy. In early pregnancy, amniotic fluid is color less. Near term, it becomes pale straw colored due to the presence of exfoliated lanugo and epidermal cells from the fetal skins or may be turbid due to presence of vernix caseosa.

Composition of Amniotic Fluid

In the first half of pregnancy, the composition of the fluid is almost identical to transudate of plasma. But in late pregnancy, the composition is altered mainly due to contamination of fetal urinary metabolite.

Composition of amniotic fluid is summarized in Table 4.3.

Table 4.3: Feature of composition of amniotic fluid	
Salts	Sodium and osmolality full progressively urea and creatinine increase
Protein	Total rise to 26 weeks Levels around 1/10 of fetal serum. No fibrinogen α Fetoprotein peak at 10-12 weeks
Lipids	Half the lipids are fatty acids towards term include lecithesis (Long surfactant)
Hormones	Similar to found in maternal Blood but in lower concentration Renin level are 20 times higher than maternal level Insulin level increase throughout pregnancy and are many times higher in the presence of maternal diabetes
Bilirubin	Decrease progressively in 3rd trimester
Water	Transfer (exchange) of 250 ml/hr with mother and 150 ml/hr with fetus
Cells	Cells are more abundant with female fetus- Epithelial like (E cells) Amniotic fluid cells (AF cells) F cells (Fibroblast cells) Glial cells
Antibacterial cells	Zinc associated, B lysine, lysozynes, peroxidase and α Interferon α

Function of Amniotic Fluid

Amniotic fluid has manifold function:

During Pregnancy

1. It surrounds the fetus and cushions it against the wall of the gravid uterus protecting it from external trauma.
2. It plays a crucial role in the development and maturation of fetal lung.
3. It provides space and enables the fetus to move it, facilitates joint development and prevents contractures.
4. It helps in maintaining fetal body temperature and plays a part in homeostasis of fluid electrolytes.

During Labor

1. During uterine contraction, amniotic fluid prevents excessive interference with placental circulation if the membranes are intact.
2. The amniotic fluid forms the hydrostatic wedge with amnion and chorion which facilitates dilatation of cervix.
3. It flushes the birth canal at the end of first stage of labor and by its bacterial action protects the fetus as well prevents ascending infection to uterine cavity.

The Umbilical Cord

The umbilical cord forms the connecting link between the fetus and the placenta through which the fetal blood flows to and from the placenta.

Development of Cord

The yolk sac and the umbilical vesicle into which it develops are quite prominent early in pregnancy. At first the embryo is a flattened disk interposed between amnion and yolk sac. Because the dorsal surface grows faster than the ventral surface in association with the elongation of the neural tube, the embryo bulges into the amniotic sac and the dorsal part of the yolk sac is incorporated into the body of the embryo to form the gut.

The allantoic diverticulum projects into the base of the body stalk from the caudal wall of the yolk sac and later from the anterior wall of the hindgut. With advancement of gestation the yolk sac becomes gradually small and its pedicle becomes relatively longer. By middle of third month the expanding amnion obliterates the exocoelom; it fuses with the chorion laeve and covers the bulging placental disk and the lateral surface of the body stalk. This body stalk is now called umbilical cord or fines.

Remnants of the exocoelom in the anterior portion of the cord may contain loops of intestine which continue to develop outside the embryo. Although loops are later on withdrawn into the peritoneal cavity, the apex of the midgut loop retains its connection with the attenuated villous duct.

Cord Structure

Umbilical cord extends from the fetal umbilicus to the fetal surface of the placenta or chorionic plate anatomically; the umbilical cord can be regarded as component of fetal membranes.

Its exterior is dull white, moist, covered with amnion, through which three umbilical vessels are seen. Its average length is 55 cm (range of 30–100 cm) and its diameter is 0.8 to 2.0 cm cord. Length less than 30 cm is considered abnormally short.

The cord has initially four vessels, two arteries and two veins. The arteries are derived from the internal iliac arteries of the fetus and carry the venous blood from the fetus to the placenta. Out of two umbilical veins, the right umbilical vein disappears by the 4th month, leaving one vein which carries oxygenated blood from the placenta to the fetus. The two arteries are smaller in diameter than two veins.

The vessels contained in the cord are characterized by spiraling or twisting. The spiraling may occur in a clockwise (dextra) or anticlockwise (senistral) direction. The anticlockwise pattern is present in 50–90% of cases. Spiraling may serve to prevent clamping. Folding and tortuousity of the vessels, which are longer than the length of cord, create nodulations on the surface which are called false knots. So these false knots essentially varies.

The umbilical arteries do not possess internal elastic laminas but have developed muscular coat which help in effective closure of the arteries due to reflex spasm after birth of the baby. Both the arteries and vein do not possess vasovasorum.

Blood Flow

Blood flows from the umbilical vein by two routes: (a) The ductus venosus, which empties directly into the inferior vena cava, (b) Numerous smaller opening into fetal hepatic circulation, and then into inferior vena cava by the hepatic veins. The blood takes the path of least resistance through these alternate routes.

Fetal Attachment of Umbilical Cord

In the early period, the cord is attached to the ventral surface of the embryo close to the caudal extremity, but as the coelom closes and the yolk sac is atrophied, the cord attachment is moved permanently to the center of the abdomen at 4th month.

Placental Attachment of Umbilical Cord

It is inconsistent and may be:
a. Central.
b. Eccentric—between center and edge of the placenta.
c. Marginal.
d. Velematous—on chorion laeve, at a varying distance away from the margin of the placenta.

Term Placenta

In the first trimester growth of placenta is more rapid than that of fetus but by approximately 17 weeks postconception, placental and fetal weights are equal. At term the placental weight is roughly one sixth of fetal weight.

Gross Anatomy of Term Placenta

The average placenta at term is 185 mm in diameter, 25 mm in thickness and have a weight of 500 gm. Viewed from maternal surface the placenta is rough and spongy. Maternal blood gives a dull red color. There are 15-20 slightly elevated convex areas which are termed **lobes or cotyledons**, which are limited by fissures. Each fissure is occupied by decidual septum. The total number of lobes remains the same throughout gestation and individual lobe continues to grow. The growth is less in final weeks of gestation. Numerous small gestation spots are visible which are due to calcium deposition in degenerated areas. Fetal surface is covered by smooth and glistening amnion with the umbilical cord attached to its center (Figs 4.6A and B). Branches of the umbilical vessels beneath the amnion are seen as they radiate from the insertion of umbilical cord. The amnion can be peeled off from underlying chorion except at insertion of cord. **At term about 4/5 of the placenta is of fetal origin.**

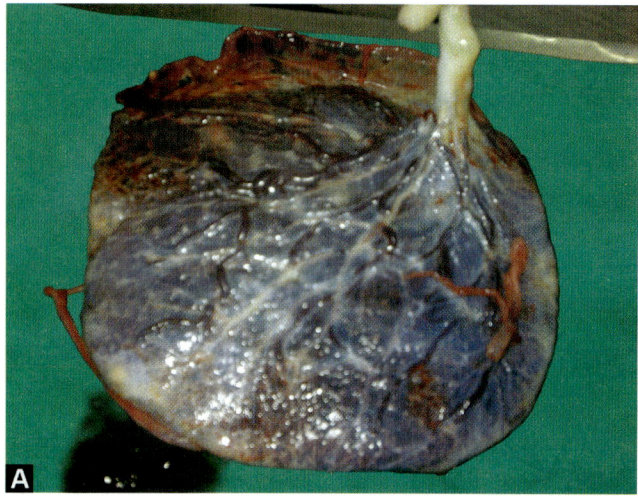
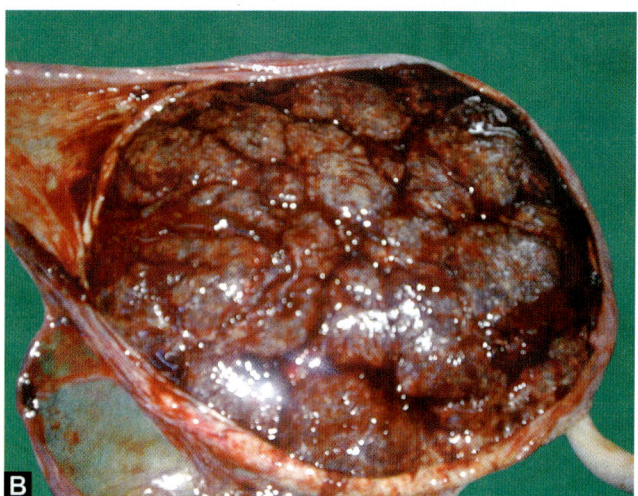

Figs 4.6A and B: (A) Term placenta fetal surface; (B) Maternal surface

Margin of term placenta: Peripheral margin of placenta is limited by the fused basal and chorionic plates and is continuous with the chorion laevae and amnion. **Thus, the chorion and placenta are one structure but the placenta is specialized part of chorion.**

Attachment of Placenta

The placenta is usually attached to the upper part of the body of the uterus encroaching to the fundus adjacent to the anterior and posterior wall with equal frequency. If the placenta is attached to lower uterine segment it is called **placenta praevia** and can cause second or third trimester vaginal bleeding.

Separation of Placenta

Placenta separates after birth of the baby through layer of decidua spongiosum.

Placental Ageing

Placenta has a limited lifespan, so it undergoes degenerative changes as a mark of senescence. This ageing process involves both the fetal and maternal components. These changes are as follows:

Villi Changes

a. *Appearance of syncytial knots*: These are seen due to decreased thickness of syncytium and aggregation of syncytium in small areas on the sides of villi.
b. Partial disappearance of Langerhans cell
c. Decrease in the stromal cell including Hofbaur's cell.
d. Obliteration of some vessels and dilatation of capillaries.
e. Thickening of basement layer of fetal endothelium and cytotrophoblast.
f. Deposition of fibrin on surface of villi.

Decidual Changes

There is area of fibrinoid degeneration where trophoblast cell meet the decidua. This zone is called *Nitabuch layers*. This layer limits further invasion of the decidua by trophoblast and absent in cases of adherent placenta (Placenta accreta).

Intervillous Space

The syncytium covering the villi and extending into the decidua or intravillous space undergoes fibrinoid degeneration and form a mass entangling variable number of villi. These are called **white infarct**, which vary in size from few mm to a cm or more. Calcification or cyst formation may occur which is usually found near the placental margin. There may be inconsistent deposition of fibrin called Rohr's striae at the bottom of intervillous space.

MULTIPLE CHOICE QUESTIONS

1. The zone of fibrinoid degeneration where the trophoblast and decidua meet is:
    a. Fold of Hoboken
    b. Nitabuch's layer
    c. Parietal deciduas
    d. Chorion
    Ans. b
2. Ligamentum teres is formed after:
    a. Obliteration of umbilical vein
    b. Obliteration of ductus venosus
    c. Obliteration of ductus arteriosus
    d. Obliteration of hypogastric artery
    Ans. a
3. hCG is secreted by:
    a. Trophoblast cells
    b. Amniotic membranes
    c. Fetal yolk sac
    d. Hypothalamus
    Ans. a
4. Weight of the placenta at term is …% of fetus:
    a. 10
    b. 20
    c. 30
    d. 45
    Ans. b
5. Urine formation in intrauterine life starts at:
    a. 3 months
    b. 4 months
    c. 5 months
    d. 6 months
    Ans. a
6. Oxygenated blood from placenta to heart *in utero* is by:
    a. Umbilical vein
    b. IVC
    c. Ductus arteriosus
    d. None of the above
    Ans. a

5

Embryology

Always be—Work in Progress.

GENERAL CONSIDERATION

The reproductive organs in the female (as also in the male) consist of gonads, external genitalia and internal duct system between gonads and external genitalia. There is close relationship between the genital glands, the urinary organs and the uterus and its appendages during early intrauterine life.

Female urinary and genital tract are closely related anatomically as well embryologically. Both are derived largely from primitive mesoderm and endoderm and there is evidence that the embryologic urinary system has an important induction influence on the developing genital system. About 10% of infants are born with some abnormality of genitourinary system and anomalies of one system are often mirrored by anomalies in another system.

Besides this, developmental defect may play a significant role in differential diagnosis of certain clinical signs and symptoms and have special implication in pelvic surgery. Thus, it is important for gynecologist to have a basic understanding of embryology of genitourinary system.

Urinary System

The kidney, renal collecting system and ureter derive from the longitudinal mass of mesoderm (known as **nephrogenic cord**) found on each side of the primitive aorta. The pronephros or first kidney is rudimentary and non-functional, which is succeeded by middle kidney or mesonephros which probably function for a short-time before regressing, but mesonephric or Wolffian duct is important because:

a. It grows caudally in the developing embryo to open for the first time an excretory channel into the primitive cloacae and the outside world.
b. It serves as the starting point for development of the metanephros which becomes the definitive kidney.
c. It ultimately differentiates into the sexual duct system in the male.
d. Although regressing in female fetus, mesonephric duct may have direct role in development of paramesonephric duct or Müllerian duct.

Development of the "**Metanephros**" is initiated by the ureteric buds, which sprout from the distal mesonephric duct. These buds extend upwards and penetrate the position of the nephrogenic cord known as "**Metanephric Blastema**". The ureteric bud begins to branch sequentially with each growing tip covered by metanephric blastema.

The metanephric blastema ultimately forms the renal function unit (Nephron) and the ureteric buds become the collecting duct system of kidney which is collecting tubules, minor and major calyces, renal pelvis and ureters. It is important that these primitive tubules are interdependent on induction influences from each other.

The kidney initially lies in the pelvis but subsequently ascends to their permanent location, rotates almost 90° in the process as the more caudal part of the embryo in effect grows away from them. Blood supply of kidney which first arises as branch of the middle sacral and common iliac arteries, comes from progressively higher branches of the aorta until the definitive renal arteries form and then previous vessel regress.

Bladder and Urethra

The cloaca forms as the result of dilatation of the opening to the fetal exterior. The cloaca is partitioned by the mesenchymal urorectal septum into an anterior urogenital sinus and a posterior rectum.

The bladder and urethra form the most superior portion of the urogenital sinus with surrounding mesenchyme contributing to their muscular and serosal layers. The remaining inferior urogenital sinus is known as "**Phallic or Definitive Urogenital Sinus**".

At the same time (simultaneously) the distal mesonephric ducts and attached ureteric buds are incorporated into the posterior bladder wall in the area that will become the bladder trigone.

As a result of the absorption process, the mesonephric duct ultimately opens independently into the urogenital sinus below the bladder neck. The allantois is vestigial diverticulum of the hindgut that extends into the umbilicus and is continuous with bladder. It becomes a fibrous band known as **"Urachus or Median Umbilical Ligament"** (Fig. 5.1).

Genital System

Genetic sex is determined at fertilization. The early genital system is indistinguishable between the two sexes in embryonic stage so termed **indifferent** stage. Clinically sex is not apparent, until about 12th week of embryonic life.

Sex differentiation depends on the elaboration of *testis determining factor* and subsequently *androgen* by the male gonad. Female development has been called the basic developmental path of the human embryo requiring not estrogen but the absence of testosterone.

The hindgut appears about the 20th postovulatory day. The intermediate mesoderm develops adjacent to the midline dorsal mesentery of the gut, extending through the length of body cavity, i.e. coelom. *A part of this intermediate cell mass medial to the mesonephros (Primitive Kidney) proliferates to form the gonadal ridges* (Fig. 5.1).

Primordial germ cells that are subsequently capable of meiosis, separate out from the pool of the somatic cells that are capable only of mitosis.

These germ cells are present in the allantoic diverticulum and the adjacent parts of the yolk sac in 17–20 days embryo. From here they migrate through the dorsal mesentery of the hindgut, reaching the gonadal ridge in the human embryo at 35 days. The cause of this migration of the germ cell is yet unknown.

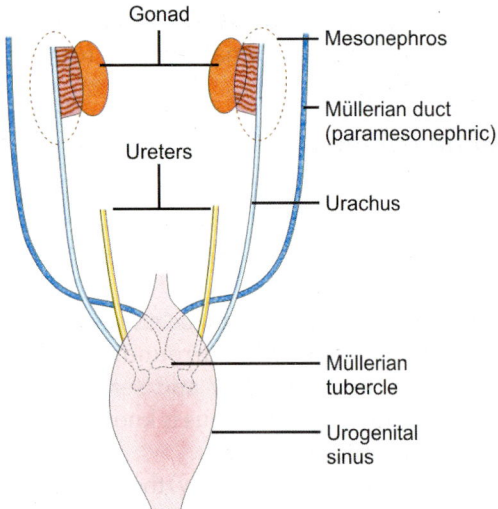

Fig. 5.1: Formation of Müllerian and Wolffian duct system and their entrance into the urogenital sinus

The area to which the germ cells migrate is referred to as the **indifferent gonad,** until gonadal sex is established. At 35 days the indifferent gonad is formed by the primordial germ cell, cells from the overlying coelomic epithelium and the cells of adjacent mesonephros. The germ cells now undergo rapid mitotic proliferation and are enclosed by extensions of the coelomic epithelium (sex cords) and the mesonephric ducts.

Müllerian Duct (Paramesonephric Duct)

In 1830, Johannes Muller described a cord on the outer aspect of the Wolffian body; named Müllerian cord, now referred as **paramesonephric duct**. It appears at about 40 days. Each paramesonephric duct begins as a thickening and an invagination of the coelomic epithelium on the lateral aspect of the intermediate mesoderm. It extends caudally as a solid rod of cells and is associated with and initially lateral to the mesonephric duct. The ducts are interdependent. *The paramesonephric duct will not develop if the mesonephric duct is absent.*

As the paramesonephric cord of cell continues its descent, a lumen appears in its cranial position in continuity with intraembryonic body cavity. The lumen extends caudally, as the duct passes ventral to the mesonephric duct, comes in close association with each other and reaches the posterior aspect of the urogenital sinus. The two sides of Müllerian duct grow caudally and then medially to fuse in the midline. They contact the urogenital sinus in the region of posterior urethra at a slight thickening known as **sinusal tubercle (Figs 5.2A and B)**.

Gonadal Differentiation

Male and female embryos are morphologically indistinguishable till 42 days. Subsequent sexual development is controlled by the presence or absence of testis determining factors, encoded on the Y chromosome and elaborated by the somatic sex cord cells. *Testis determining factor causes the degeneration of the gonadal cortex and differentiation of the medullary region of the gonad into Sertoli cells.*

The Sertoli cells secrete a glycoprotein known as "Anti-Müllerian Hormone (AMH)" which causes regression of the paramesonephric duct systems in the male embryo and is the likely signal for differentiation of Leydig cells from the surrounding mesenchyme.

The Leydig cells produce testosterone and with the converting enzyme 5 alpha reductase-dihydrotestosterone. Testosterone is responsible for evolution of the mesonephric (Wolffian) duct system into the vas deferens, epididymis, ejaculatory duct, and seminal vesicle.

At puberty, testosterone leads to spermatogenesis and changes in primary and secondary sex characteristics.

Dihydrotestosterone triggers the development of the male external genitalia, the prostrate and bulbourethral glands. *In absence of testis determining factors, the medulla regresses and the cortical sex cord breaks up into isolated cell clusters (The primordial follicle).*

Development of Ovary

The transformation of the indifferent gonad into an embryonic ovary occurs gradually before 45 and 55 days. A gonad with the germ cells in meiosis is always an ovary since meiotic division does not occur in the testis until puberty.

The germ cells differentiate into oogonia and enter the first meiotic division as *primary oocyte* at which point development is arrested until puberty. Meiosis II occurs at fertilization. During early fetal stage, the ovaries contain 5 million germ cells which along with sex cords from the coelomic epithelium remain in the superficial part of the ovary, the future cortex. The cord loses contact with the surface forming small groups of cells each with a germ cell– **a primitive follicle (Fig. 5.2C)**.

Descent of Ovary into the Pelvis

Meanwhile the ovary descends extraperitoneally, its descent controlled by the suspensory ligament that connects it to its site of origin on the genital ridge—**The gubernaculums** (Figs 5.2A to C). The gubernaculum is the inferior continuation of the genital mesentery that becomes attached to the uterine cornu forming the proximal ovarian ligament and continues as the distal round ligament passing through the original canal and ending in the labium majus. *The total number of germ cells in the ovary decline to about two million at birth and only 4, 00,000 oocytes remain at the onset of puberty. Of these 400 will be ovulated during reproductive life, the remaining 99.9% undergoing atresia.*

Female Genital Tract Differentiation

At the end of the embryonic period the fetus has gonads, recognizable as either testes or ovaries, but possess both the mesonephric duct and the paramesonephric ducts. The subsequent differentiation of the duct is governed by fetal testicular hormones. In male fetus Müllerian duct regression begins under the influence of the "Anti-Müllerian Hormone" at 50–60 days while the mesonephric ducts are stabilized under the influence of testosterone between 56 and 70 days.

In contrast, the absence of testicular hormone in the female fetus allows the stabilization of Müllerian duct and regression of the mesonephric ducts to take place. In at least 1/4th of adult women *remnant of mesonephric duct may be found in mesovarium as epoophoron, paraphoron or along the lateral wall of the uterus or vagina as gartner duct cyst.* The first and second portion of Müllerian ducts eventually form the fimbria and the fallopian tube while the distal segments form the uterus and upper vagina. It is the growth

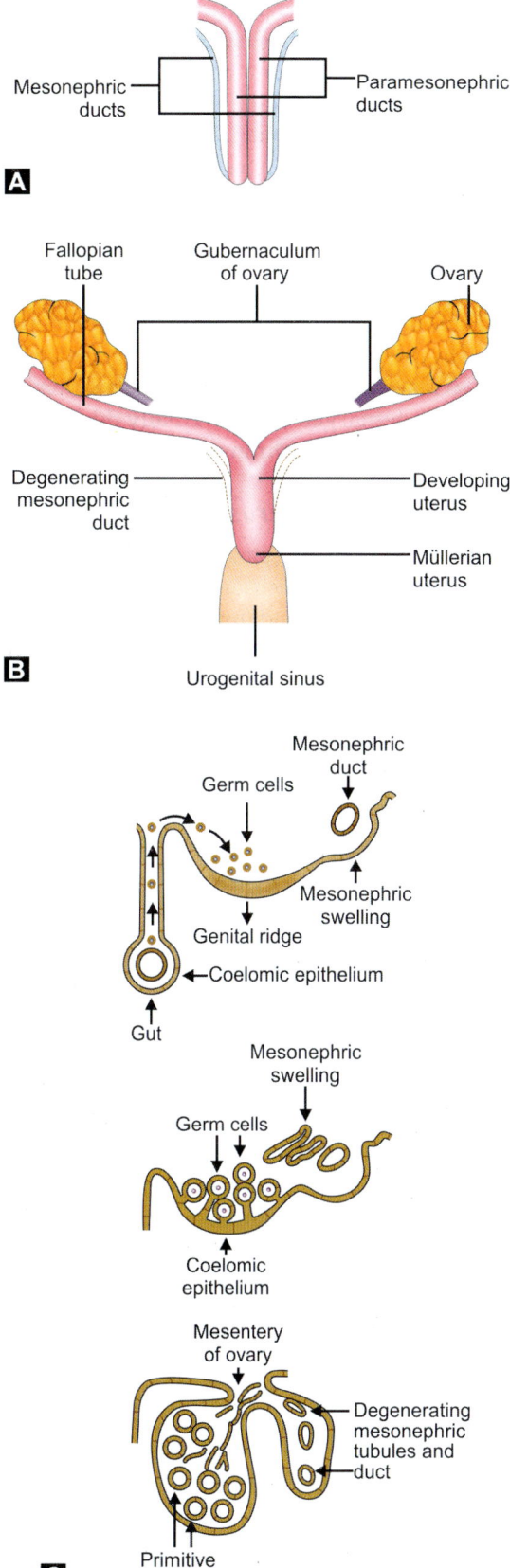

Figs 5.2A to C: (A) Caudal growth of paramesonephric duct; (B) Fusion to form uterus and fallopian tube; (C) Development of ovary

of the vaginal plate in conjunction with the sinovaginal bulb that results in the restructuring of the urogenital sinus from a long narrow tube to a broad flat vestibule. These changes result in the positioning of the female urethra down to the future perineum. Canalization of the vaginal plate begins caudally and continues in a cephalad direction, creating the lower vagina. Canalization is complete by the fifth month of gestation. The distal most portion of the sinovaginal bulb proliferates to form the hymenal tissue. The hymen becomes perforated before birth.

The basic sequence of change from the bipotential state is directed by chromosomal sex determined gonad formation, which then favors the development of male or female duct systems and external genitalia. **So finally this depends on endocrine effect and not chromosomal sex.**

Development of the Uterus

The inferior fused portion of paramesonephric duct becomes the uterovaginal canal, which later becomes the epithelium and glands of the uterus and upper vagina. The Müllerian duct fuse, forming the uterus around 63 days, the median septum being completely reabsorbed by 80 days, forming a single uterovaginal canal.

While the complete failure of fusion between the ducts results in a **diadelphic uterus**, a partial failure results in an **arcuate or bicornuate uterus**, and a failure of septal resorption results in variants ranging from a **subseptate to septate uterus**.

The uterus at birth and during childhood is devoid of flexion and version, these characteristic developing at puberty. The cranial unfused part of the paramesonephric ducts open into the coelomic (future peritoneal cavity) and becomes the fallopian tube.

The fusion of paramesonephric ducts bring together two folds of peritoneum, which become the broad ligament and divide the pelvic cavity into a posterior rectouterine and anterior vesicouterine punch or cul-de-sac. Between the leaves of broad ligament, mesenchyme proliferates and differentiates into loose areolar tissues and smooth muscles.

Development of the Vagina

The vagina forms in the third month of embryonic life. There is general agreement that the vagina originates as a composite formed partly from the Müllerian ducts and partly from urogenital sinus. The Müllerian tubercle is the point of contact between the Müllerian ducts and the urogenital sinus. While the uterovaginal canal is forming, the endodermal tissue of the sinusal tubercle begins to proliferate, forming a pair of "**Sinovaginal bulb**, which becomes the inferior 20% of the vagina".

The most inferior portion of the uterovaginal canal becomes occluded by a solid core of tissue called **vaginal plate**, the origin of which is unclear. Over the subsequent two months, this tissue elongation and canalization by process of central desquamation and the peripherals cells become the vaginal epithelium. **The fibromuscular wall of the vagina originates from the mesoderm of the uterovaginal canal.**

Accessory Genital Glands

The female accessory genital glands develop as outgrowth from the urethra (Paraurethral or Skene's) and the definite urogenital sinus (greater vestibular or Bartholin).

Development of the External Genitalia

The external genitalia develops in the area bound by the body stalk above and the tail below, the sex of the external genitalia being unrecognizable till the 12th week. Early in fifth week of embryonic life, folds of tissue form on each side of the cloacae and meet anteriorly in the midline to form the genital tubercle (Fig. 5.3).

With the division of the cloaca by the urorectal septum and consequent formation of the perineum, these cloacal folds are known anteriorly as **urogenital folds** and posteriorly as the **anal folds**. The genital tubercle begins to enlarge in the female embryo, the growth gradually slows to become clitoris and the urogenital fold forms the labia minora. In male embryo the genital tubercle continues to grow to form the penis and the urogenital fold are fused to enclose the penile urethra.

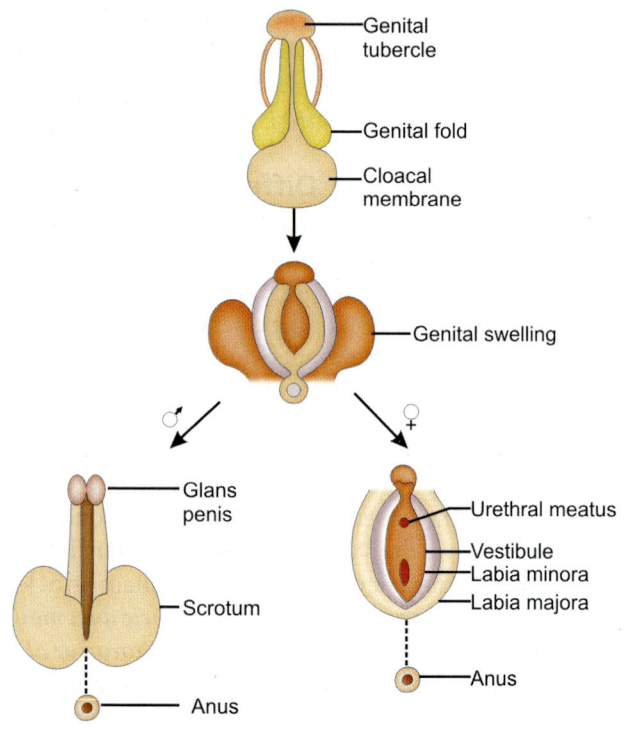

Fig. 5.3: Development of external genitalia

Lateral to urogenital folds, another pair of swelling develops known in the indifferent stage as *labioscrotal swelling*. In the absence of androgens, they remain largely unfused to become the labia majora and genital fold develop into labia minora. The definitive urogenital sinus gives rise to the vaginal vestibule, into which urethra, vagina and greater vestibular glands opens.

Malformation and Maldevelopment of Genital Tract

Developmental abnormalities of the urinary and genital systems can be explained and understood by a consideration of female and male embryologic development. Following main principle govern the practical approach to malformation of genital tract:

i. The Müllerian and Wolffian ducts are so closely linked embryologically that gross malformation of the uterus and vagina are commonly associated with congenital anomalies of the kidney and ureter.
ii. The development of the gonad is separate from that of the ducts. Normal and functional ovaries are therefore usually present when the vagina, uterus and fallopian tube are absent or malformed.
iii. Gross malformation such as absence of the uterus and vagina may be associated with anomalies in the sex chromosome make up of the individual. There is also some evidence that less severe malformation such as bicornuate uterus can be genetically determined, the trait being passed from mother to daughter.
iv. Because of the intertwined development of these two systems, urinary anomalies can be associated with genital tract anomalies.

Urinary Tract Anomalies

Urinary tract anomalies arise from defect in the ureteric buds. The **metanephric blastema,** and their **inductive interaction with each other**.

Renal Agenesis

It occurs when one or both ureteric bud fail to form or degenerate and the metanephric blastema is therefore not induced to differentiate into nephrons. Bilateral renal agenesis is incompatible with postnatal survivors, but infant with one budding usually survives with compensatory hypertrophy of single kidney.

Unilateral renal agenesis is often associated with absence or abnormality of fallopian tube, ureter or vagina – the paramesonephric duct derivative.

Abnormalities of Renal Position

Abnormality of renal position results from disturbance in the normal ascent of kidney. A malrotated pelvic kidney is the most common. A horse shoe shaped kidney is found when the kidneys are fused across the midline. It occurs one in 600 individuals. Horseshoe kidney is lower than usual because its normal ascent is prevented by the root of inferior mesenteric artery.

Duplication of Upper Ureter and Renal Pelvis

It results from primitive bifurcation of the ureteric bud.

FEMALE GENITAL TRACT ANOMALIES

There can be several anomalies—Jone's classification is listed below:

1. As early development of the genital system is similar in both sexes, congenital defect in sexual developments tend to present clinically as ambiguous external genitalia, the condition known as **Intersex or Hermaphroditism.** It may be true hermaphroditism where individuals have both ovaries and testicular tissues commonly as composite ovotestes, and occasionally with an ovary on one side and a testis on the other or Pseudohermaphroditism when the genetic sex indicates one sex, whereas the external genitalia has characteristics of the other sex.
2. **Aplasia:** Failure of organ to develop.
3. **Hypoplasia:** Organs are rudimentary.
4. **Afusia:** Partial or complete failure of canalization of these ducts leading to varying degrees of gynatresia.
5. Müllerian duct anomalies.
6. **Developmental defect of urogenital sinus:** Manifest in the form of defective development of the urinary bladder, hymen and the perineum.

Disorders of Development of Müllerian System

Incidence of Müllerian tract anomalies are 0.16%. These are believed to result because of :

a. Improper fusion of the paramesonephric duct.
b. Incomplete development of one paramesonephric duct.
c. Failure of part of the paramesonephric duct on one or both sides to develop.
d. Absent or incomplete canalization of vaginal plate.

Those girls, who have mature secondary sex characteristics and any of a number of disorders of the outflow tract and uterus, often termed **Müllerian Agenesis and Dysgensis**. The basic classification of Müllerian tract include:

a. Agenesis/hypoplasia
b. Vertical fusion (canalization) defect
c. Lateral fusion (duplication) defect.

The American Society of Reproduction Medicine (ASRM) formerly American Fertility Society has adopted a classification system of Müllerian anomalies.

The ASRM classification does not include vaginal anomalies but allows for the inclusion of a description of associated vaginal, tubal or urinary anomalies (Box 5.1). Others have suggested classification system for vaginal anomalies (Box 5.2):

> **Box 5.1:** Classification of Müllerian anomalies according to ASRM classification system
>
> **Type I—Müllerian Agenesis or Hypoplasia**
> a. Vaginal
> b. Cervical
> c. Fundal
> d. Tubal
> e. Combined
>
> **Type II—Unicornuate Uterus**
> a. Communicating (endometrial cavity present)
> b. Noncommunicating/endometrial cavity present
> c. Horn without endometrial cavity
> d. No rudimentary horn
>
> **Type III—Uterus Didelphys**
>
> **Type IV—Uterus Bicornuate**
> a. Complete (division down to internal os)
> b. Partial
>
> **Type V—Septate Uterus**
> a. Complete (Septum to internal os)
> b. Partial
>
> **Type VI—Arcuate**
>
> **Type VII—DES Related Anomalies**
> a. T shaped uterus
> b. T shaped with dilated horns
> c. T shaped
>
> Disorder of the outflow tract and uterus often occurs as a part of syndrome of malformation that includes abnormalities of the skeletal and renal system (Rokitansky-Kuster-Hauser syndrome). Familial aggregate of the most common disorders of Müllerian differentiation in girls are Müllerian aplasia and incomplete Müllerian Fusion which are best explained on the basis of polygenic and multifactorial inheritance.

> **Box 5.2:** Classification for vaginal anomalies
>
> | Classification | Feature |
> |---|---|
> | Class I | Transverse |
> | | a. Obstructing |
> | | b. Nonobstructing |
> | Class II | Longitudinal |
> | | a. Obstructing |
> | | b. Nonobstructing |
> | Class III | Stenosis |
> | | Iatrogenic |

Clinical Presentation

a. **Ovarian agenesis/dysgenesis:** It leads to Turner's syndrome (Chromosome 45X0) and this will present as primary amenorrhea, and has special characteristic like short stature web neck.

b. **Uterus:** Uterus anomalies like Didelphys, bicornuate, arcuate, septate, subseptate uterus, do not cause any problem. However, in childbearing age, it may cause increased incidence of abortion, preterm labor, malpresentation. Coexisting vaginal septum can cause dyspareunia. PAP smears must be taken separately from each cervix during course of gynecological examination and if women opt for use of IUD for contraception, a separate IUD will have to be inserted in each of the horn. Partial fusion resulting in bicornuate uterus and septate uterus cause the following obstetrical and gynecological problems:
  i. Habitual abortion
  ii. Preterm labor
  iii. Persistent and recurrent malpresentation.

c. **Vagina:** Noncanalization of vagina leads to cryptomenorrhea and may present as primary amenorrhea during adolescent age. There will be cyclical pain because of menses which is colleted above the noncanalized vagina. If there is only imperforate hymen then the bulge is exterior. At this stage there can be retention of urine also along with primary amenorrhea.

Investigation

The diagnostic methods of determining the exact nature of the anomalies have now progressed much beyond the clinical examination, bimanual palpation, D & C and hysterosalpingography. Now diagnostic hysteroscopy and laparoscopy, abdominal and vaginal sonography and MRI imaging of the pelvic organs are used as diagnostic modality to enhance the clinician capability to pick up many more minor anomalies, hitherto missed.

It is now agreed that MRI and endovaginal sonography (sometimes with sonohysterography) are as accurate as invasive technique like HSCo, laparoscopy and hysteroscopy.*

MANAGEMENT OF SPECIFIC ANOMALIES

Imperforate Hymen

It is the most common obstetric anomaly of female reproductive tract. The diagnosis of imperforate hymen should be made at birth. At birth a bulge from the mucocolpos may be evident as there is an increase in vaginal secretion during the newborn period because of maternal estradiol stimulation. If the imperforate hymen is not diagnosed, the mucus will more likely to resorb and the bulge will no longer be present. The thin membrane of the imperforate hymen can be visualized within the hymenal ring.

---

* MRI can be helpful in determining the anatomy in case of complicated obstetrical anomalies, and many consider it the 'Gold Standard' for imaging of anomalies of reproductive tract. But it is to be kept in mind that even with MRI, an unestrogenized normally small prepubertal uterus may be difficult to image. MRI is especially useful in determining the presence or absence of the cervix in complex anomalies or the presence of functioning endometrium in cases of a noncommunicating, obstructed rudimentary uterine horn.

But usually the girls present at puberty with complaint of primary amenorrhea, and cyclic colicky abdominal pain. A bluish bulging hymen and a vagina distended with blood may be found on general inspection and rectoabdominal palpation.

As the vagina gets progressively and increasingly distended with the menstrual blood, pressure symptoms follow. Difficulty during micturition finally ends up with urinary retention. If the condition is neglected, the increasing vaginal distention progresses beyond the hematocolpos to hematosalpinx and hematometra with irreparable damage to the genital structure and development of endometriosis (Fig. 5.4).

Diagnosis

Physical examination: A bluish bulging hymen and vagina distended with blood may be found on general inspection and rectoabdominal palpation. A hypogastric or suprapubic bulge is often obvious.

D/D is full bladder, ovarian cyst, appendicular mass, matted loops of bowel and omentum encysted ascites due to tuberculosis. A pelvic ultrasound scan helps to establish diagnosis. USG scan of upper abdomen will reveal any associated renal anomalies.

Pelvic and abdominal MRI is done only if the diagnosis of imperforate hymen is not absolutely certain based on physical examination or pelvic USG finding.

Treatment

A. A cruciate incision along the diagonal diameter of the hymen rather than anterior or posterior, avoiding injury to the urethra is given. It is enlarged and an excess hymenal tissue is removed and blood is evacuated.
B. The vaginal epithelium then is sutured to the hymenal ring using interrupted stitches with fine absorbable suture (4-0 polyglycolic acid) to prevent recurrence.
C. Lidocaine 2% jelly can be applied to suture line. *Aspiration or puncture of mucocolpos or hematocolpos without definitive enlargement of the vaginal orifice should be avoided because a pyocolpos or ascending infection may develop. Pelvic examination should not be done since it will cause ascending infection.*

Vaginal Aplasia (Agenesis of Lower Vagina/ Segmental Vaginal Agenesis)

Congenital aplasia of the vagina is rare. Incidence is 1:4000–15000 women. Failure of the vagina to canalize may be partial or complete. Generally the uterus accompanying this anomaly is rudimentary and nonfunctional. In 7-8% of cases a functioning uterus may be present when vaginal aplasia is associated with hematometra.

Vaginal aplasia with absence of uterus is encountered in testicular feminizing syndrome and the **Rokitansky-Kuster-Hauser syndrome**, which may be associated in 20-30% of cases with rib and skeletal abnormalities in addition to urinary and genital abnormalities (Fig. 5.5).

Ovaries function normally, the development of secondary sex character is normal but sexual intercourse is not possible.

Treatment

Surgery is the most effective method of treatment for vaginal agenesis. Choosing the proper time to perform a vaginoplasty is of paramount importance. Surgical treatment should be considered only when the patient wishes to become sexually active and is highly motivated to use a vaginal prosthesis for several months postoperatively.

Preoperative Evaluation

Routine preoperative evaluation should include Intravenous pyelography and renal ultrasound to exclude

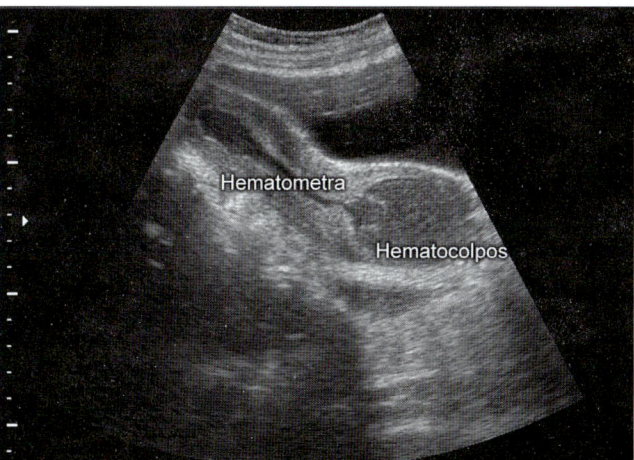

Fig. 5.4: Ultrasound image showing imperforate hymen with hematocolpos and hematometra

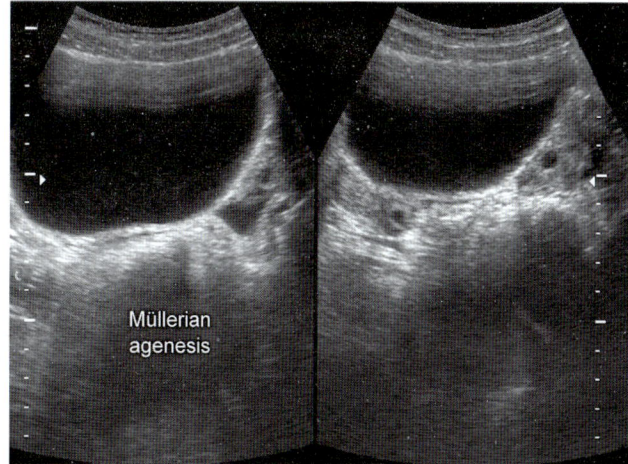

Fig. 5.5: Ultrasound image showing absent uterus with ovary present in Müllerian agenesis

urinary tract anomalies. Presence of pelvic kidney is important in planning conservative surgery since its presence may limit the amount of potential space. These patients are selected for construction of artificial vaginal either by McIndoe's operation or the more simple William vaginoplasty. The vagina thus provided is generally both psychologically and functionally satisfactory.

Disorder of Uterus

Uterus didelphys: When the two Müllerian ducts fail to fuse along the whole of their length and they develop normally and remain separate, uterus didelphys result. In this the two vagina open at the vulva where a vaginal septum can be seen. A cervix lies at the top of each vagina and two parts of the uterus above the level of cervixes are completely separate since there is no fusion at any point between one two halves of uterus body (Fig. 5.6A). There can be single vagina with double uterus if there is partial fusion from müllerian duct (Fig. 5.6B).

Treatment

Women with nonobstructive didelphys uterus usually are not candidates for surgical unification. Strassman procedure of metroplasty is not done in modern gynecology. Since, unification was causing higher incidence of rupture of uterus during subsequent pregnancy.

Bicornuate uterus: The uterine fundus is deeply indented. The level of indentation can be complete, partial or arcuate. The vagina is usually normal (Figs 5.6C and D).
Unicornuate uterus: A unicornuate uterus is a single horned uterus that has a single round ligament and fallopian tube. The other hemiuterus, round ligaments and fallopian tube are usually absent. Variation of hemiuterus can occur with existence of noncommunicating uterus horns with or without active endometrium. Single asymmetric uterus communicates with a single cervix and a normal vagina. Associated renal anomalies are common. *Patient with a unicornuate uterus are at increased risk of infertility, endometriosis, premature labor, and breech presentation* (Fig. 5.6F).
Septate uterus: In case of uterine septum, the external surface of the uterus appears to have a normal configuration, but there are two endometrial cavities. Septum is considered *complete* if it extends to the internal os, thus dividing the endometrial cavity and termed *partial* if it does not or *segmented* which results in partial communication between the endometrial cavities. As fertility does not appear to be significantly compromised its presence alone is not an indication for surgery (Fig. 5.6E).

Transvaginal ultrasound is a useful aid for diagnosing septate uterus with sensitivity of 100% and specificity of 80%.

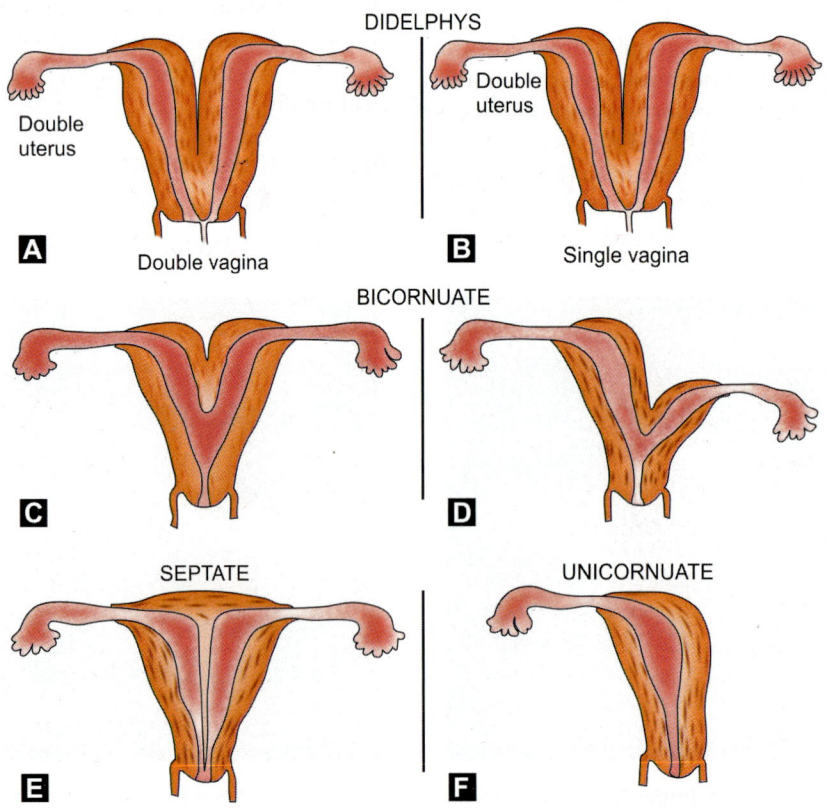

Figs 5.6A to F: Different types of Müllerian anomalies

Surgical Management of Septate Uterus

Traditional transabdominal Tompkins metroplasty has been replaced by operative hysteroscopy. **The surgical approach utilizes concurrent laparoscopy and hysteroscopy.** Laparoscopy is essential to the success of the surgery. It helps in confirming the diagnosis of septate uterus and reducing the risk of uterine perforation during septal incision.

Postoperative Management

Postoperative placement of IUCD for a month is controversial. Conjugated estrogen (1.25 mg/d for 25 d) and progesterone (10 mg/d, 21-25 d) are frequently prescribed postoperatively to promote epithelialization. At one month postoperative follow-up examination is recommended. Either hysteroscopy or hysterosalpingography can be performed to assess the uterine cavity. Ultrasound can also be performed. The risk of pelvic adhesion is limited and recovery is rapid with no prolonged postoperative delay in conception.

Hysteroscopic metroplasty allows vaginal delivery, obviating the need for subsequent cesarean section, as was recommended using the transabdominal approach.

Conclusion

Müllerian duct anomalies are a morphological diverse group of congenital disorder involving the female reproductive tract. Establishing an accurate diagnosis is essential for patient management and planning treatment strategies. Usually uterus septa or anomalies do not require active measure of surgery. Vaginal reconstruction operations have a place if vagina is absent.

MULTIPLE CHOICE QUESTIONS

1. Ovary develops from:
    a. Müllerian duct
    b. Genital ridge
    c. Genital tubercle
    d. Mesonephric duct
    Ans. b
2. What is epoophoron:
    a. Vestigial structure of urogenital sinus
    b. Remnants of Wolffian duct
    c. Un-fused portion of Müllerian duct
    d. Urogenital sinus
    Ans. b
3. Clitoris develops from:
    a. Urogenital sinus
    b. Labioscrotal swelling
    c. Genital folds
    d. Genital tubercle
    Ans. d
4. Scrotum is analogous to:
    a. Labia minora
    b. Labia majora
    c. Uterus
    d. Vagina
    Ans. b
5. Primary oocytes:
    a. Is formed after single meiotic division
    b. Maximum in number in 5 months fetus
    c. Is in prophase arrest
    d. Also called as blastocyst
    Ans. b, c
6. Cervix develops from:
    a. Wolffian duct
    b. Müllerian duct
    c. Mesonephros
    d. Metanephros
    Ans. b
7. Paraovarian cyst develops from:
    a. Wolffian duct
    b. Müllerian duct
    c. Gartner's duct
    d. Pronephros
    Ans. a
8. Complete failure of Müllerian duct fusion will result is:
    a. Uterine didelphys
    b. Arcuate uterus
    c. Subseptate uterus
    d. Unicornuate uterus
    Ans. a
9. Vaginal atresia is associated with:
    a. Uterine atresia
    b. Exostrophy of bladder
    c. Imperforate hymen
    d. Ovarian atrophy
    Ans. a
10. In complete Müllerian duct aplasia all of the following are likely to be absent, *except*:
    a. Ovaries
    b. Fallopian tubes
    c. Uterus
    d. Vagina
    Ans. a

Section Two

Gynecology

6. Gynecological History and Clinical Examination

To listen is to hear with one's heart.

GENERAL CONSIDERATION

The Gynecology (from the Greek word, Gynaec meaning women and Logos, means discourse) pertains to disease of women and is generally used for disease related to female genital organs. For majority of women, gynecologist often is both specialist and primary care provider and as such has the responsibility to prevent and treat a wide variety of diseases. The initial approach to the gynecologic patient and the general diagnostic procedure available for the examination of gynecologic complaints are presented here.

History Taking

The onus of eliciting a good, relevant and informative history lies on the clinician. To adequately evaluate the gynecologic patient, it is important to establish a rapport during history taking. The following outline varies from the routine medical history because in evaluating the gynecologic patient, the problem often can be classified, if the history is obtained in the following order:

Age: Knowledge of the patient age sets the tone for the complaint and approach to the patient. The problem and approach to them vary at different stages in a woman's life (pubescence, adolescence, childbearing years, premenopausal and postmenopausal years). Name, place of residence help us to know the patient's background and to identify some of risk factors.

Presenting symptom: This may help us to understand the underlying problem and to organize one's thoughts to probe further. One should always keep in mind that all patients do not have classical clinical presentation and more than one pathology or disorder may be present in the same patient. Chief complaint usually is best elicited by asking what kind of problem you are having. The patient should be interrupted only to clarify certain points that may be unclear.

Present illness: Each of the problem patient describes must be obtained in detail by questioning regarding what exactly the problem is, where exactly the problem is occurring, the date and time of onset, whether the symptoms are abating or getting worse, the duration of symptoms, when they do occur, and how these symptoms are related to or influence other events in her life.

It is important to maintain eye contact with the patient. The doctor should judiciously adjust the level of terminology according to the patient's knowledge and vocabulary. Communicating with the patient in this manner may help the physician obtain an accurate history and establish rapport. In addition to physiologic events and life cycle, symptoms described could be related to starting a new job, the beginning of a new relationship, new medication and any emotional change in the patient life.

Past history: After elaborating the history of chief complaint, the following history should be elicited specifically in a gynecologic patient:
a. Contraceptive use
b. Medication and habit
c. Other medical and psychiatric illness
d. History of surgical operation if any
e. Allergy to drug or specific food
f. Bleeding and thrombotic diathesis.

Obstetrical history: The obstetrical history includes each of the patient's pregnancies listed in chronologic order. The date of birth, sex and weight of the offspring, duration of pregnancy, length of labor, type of delivery, type of anesthetic and any complication should be included in history.

Gynecological history: The first item in gynecological past history is the **menstrual history**—age at menarche, interval between periods, duration of flow, amount and character of flow, degree of discomfort and age at menopause. The menstrual history often gives the clue to diagnosis. A prior history of reproductive tract infection needs to be detailed. Any treatment or admission to the hospital for treatment of salpingitis, endometriosis or tubo-ovarian abscess must be carefully documented. A gynecologist should elicit the impact of these processes in relation to ectopic pregnancy, infertility and type of contraception. It is also important to document exposure to

Human Immunodeficiency Virus (HIV), Hepatitis, Herpes virus, Chlamydia and Papilloma virus.

Sexual history: The sexual history should be an integral part of any general gynecologic history. In taking a sexual history, the physician must be nonjudgmental and not embarrassed or critical.

Social history: Knowledge of the type of work the patient does, the educational background, and her community activities may assist in ascertaining the patient's relationship to her environment. The patient's involvement with her own health care should be carefully elicited including her attention and knowledge concerning diet, health screening examination, recreation, and degree of regular physical exercise.

Family history: The patient's family history should include the state of health of immediate relatives—parents, siblings, grandparents and offspring. The incidence of familial heart disease, hypertension, renal or vascular disease, diabetes mellitus (insulin dependent or non-insulin dependent), vascular accident, and hematology abnormalities should be ascertained. Family history of breast, ovarian and colon cancer is important to elicit. It is important to relate the time of menopause in the mother or grandmother and to ascertain a history of osteoporosis.

Physical Examination

The physical examination is most useful if it is conducted in an environment that is esthetically pleasing to the patient. Adequate gowning and draping assist in preventing embarrassment. It is highly recommended that physician explains the steps and acts that will be taken, especially during the pelvic examination, when the patient might not like a direct eye contact with the physician.

General Examination

If the gynecologist is the primary care physician for the patient, a general physical examination should be performed. A complete examination provides the work information, demonstrates the physician thoroughness and establishes rapport with the patient.

General Evaluation

a. **Vital signs:** Patient's height, weight and blood pressure examination should be part of every gynecological check-up. Looking for color, edema, examination of chest and auscultation of lung and heart are important to exclude any cardiac or pulmonary problem.
b. **Abdominal examination:** The patient should be lying completely supine, and relaxed, the knees may be slightly flexed and supported as an aid to relaxation of the abdominal muscles.
   Inspection: There may be an obvious distension or mass. The presence of surgical scars, dilated veins or striae gravidarum should be noted. It is important specifically to examine the umbilicus for laparoscopy scars and just above symphysis pubis for Pfannensteil scar (incision used for cesarean section, hysterectomy, etc.), which can be missed. The patient should be asked to raise her head or cough and any hernia or divaricating of the rectus muscle will be evident (Fig. 6.1).

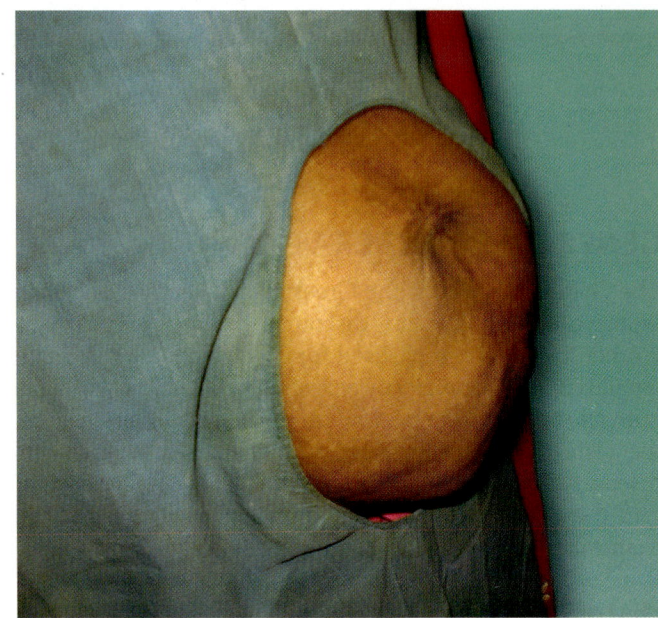

Fig. 6.1: Incisional hernia—Note the bulge of abdominal wall which becomes more prominent on coughing

Palpation of the entire abdomen gently at first, then more firmly as indicated, should detect rigidity, voluntary guarding, masses and tenderness. If the patient complains of abdominal pain or if unexpected tenderness is elicited, the examiner should ask her to indicate the point of maximal pain or tenderness with one finger. Suprapubic palpation is designed to detect uterus, ovarian or urinary bladder enlargement.

A painful area should be left until last for deep palpation, otherwise the entire abdomen can be guarded voluntarily. As a final part of the abdominal examination the physician should carefully check for abnormality of the abdominal organs – liver, gallbladder, spleen, kidney and intestines. If a mass is present but it is possible to palpate below it, it is more likely to be an abdominal mass rather than a pelvic mass. It is important to remember that one of the **characteristics of a pelvic mass is that one cannot palpate below it.** Finally the patient should be examined for inguinal hernia and lymph nodes.

Percussion of the abdomen should be performed to identify organ enlargement, tumor or ascites. In the

7
Pediatric and Adolescent Gynecology

Don't be afraid of going slowly, Be afraid of standing still.

INTRODUCTION

Pediatric gynecology is a unique subspecialty. Gynecologic disorders in children can differ greatly from those encountered in the adult female.

Common Problems in Pediatric Gynecology

Labial Adhesion

Labial adhesion develops in 1-5% of prepubertal girls and in approximately 10% of female infants within the first year of life. Adhesion between labia minora begins as a small posterior midline fusion which may remain asymptomatic and minor isolated finding, or may progress towards the clitoris to completely close the vaginal orifice (Figs 7.1A and B).

The cause of labial adhesion is unknown but probably relates to low estrogen level. It is important to differentiate labial fusion from congenital absence of the vagina. Asymptomatic minimal to moderate labial fusion do not require treatment. Symptomatic fusion may be treated with short course of estrogen cream, applied twice daily for 7-10 days.

If medical treatment fails or if severe urinary symptoms exist, surgical separation of labia is indicated. It can be done as an office procedure using 1-2% topical lidocaine gel. Recurrence of labial adhesion is common until puberty because of low estrogen level. Following puberty, the condition resolves spontaneously. Improved perineal hygiene and removal of vulvar irritation may help prevent recurrences.

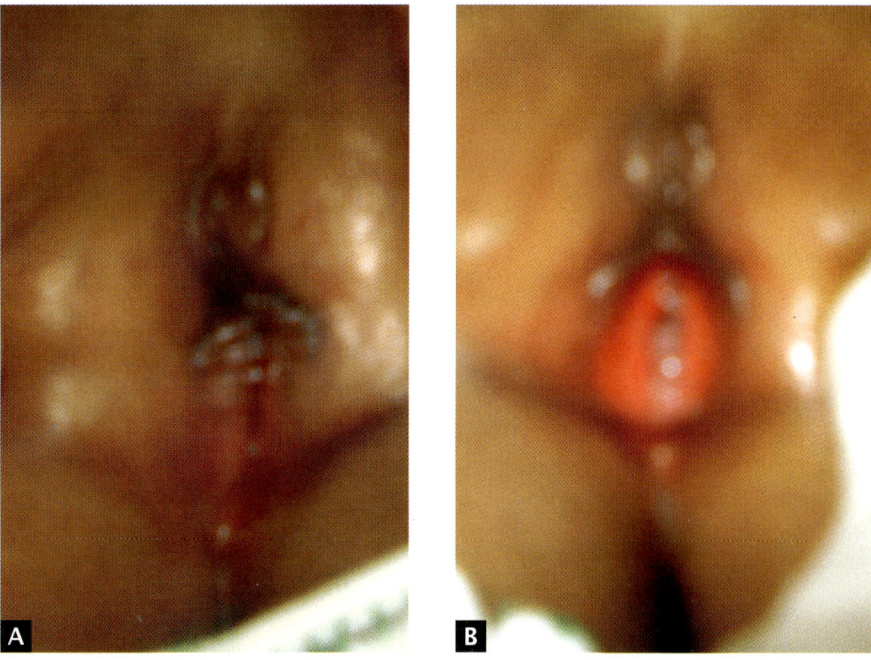

Figs 7.1A and B: (A) Labial adhesion in a one year old child; (B) Corrected labial adhesion

Chapter -6 ♦ Gynecological History and Clinical Examination

Rectal Examination

Lower genital tract is anatomically and embryologically closely related to the rectum and anal canal. Hence per rectal examination forms an important ancillary examination for a gynecologist.

In virgins, as vaginal examination is avoided, a per-rectal examination with well-lubricated anesthetic gel can be used for a bimanual assessment of the pelvic structure. A rectal examination is very useful adjunct examination when there is any palpable pathology in the pouch of Douglas. It often allows the ovaries to be more easily identified.

In parametritis and endometriosis, the uterosacral ligaments are often thickened, nodular and tender. This examination is often performed by gynecologist and is very useful in assessing pathologies in the rectovaginal septum and the parametrium.

Combined rectovaginal examination is done in which the middle finger of the right hand is inserted into the rectum whereas the index finger of the same hand is inserted into the vagina. **In cancer cervix, rectovaginal examination will help us in the clinical staging of the disease**. If the two fingers can not be approximated together it may indicate that tumor may have spread to uterosacral and cardinal ligaments.

In ovarian malignancy, rectovaginal examination may give us a clue about the fixity of the tumor and possible tumor deposits in the pouch of Douglas.

Breast Examination

While examining the heart and lungs the breast can be inspected for development of secondary sexual characters, any abnormality or disparity, development, presence of nipple abnormalities like retracted nipple or any signs of infection. In all women of age 30 or more, breast should be palpated as a routine to exclude any tumor formation. If there is specific complaint of pain or lump, examination should be thorough to exclude any lump, fibroadenoma, or fibroadenosis. Axillary lymph glands should be palpated as a routine. Galactorrhea should be looked for in women who are infertile and have complaint of oligomenorrhea.

Conclusion

Good history and thorough examination should be considered as the pillars of good clinical practice. They form very important piece of the clinical jigsaw puzzle. Hence, it is important to make every effort to identify useful piece of information from both history and examination as to enable us to get an idea about broader picture. This helps the clinician to choose the right and appropriate investigation for the patients and make an optimum management plan.

available—Cusco's and Sim's (Figs 6.2A and B), which are routinely used in clinical practice. In these various sizes are available to accommodate vaginal length and laxity. Prior to insertion the labia minora are gently separated and the urethra is identified. Because of urethral sensitivity the speculum is inserted below the meatus.

Alternatively, prior to speculum placements, the index finger may be placed in the vagina and pressure placed against the bulbocavernosus muscles. Woman is encouraged to relax her posterior wall muscles, to improve comfort with speculum insertion. It is helpful for women undergoing their first examination or those with heightened anxiety. With speculum insertion the vagina commonly is contracted and women may note pressure or discomfort. A pause at this point typically is followed by vaginal muscle relaxation. As the speculum blade is completely inserted, it is angled 30° downwards to reach the cervix. Commonly the uterus lies in an anteverted position and the face of cervix lies against the posterior vaginal wall. As the speculum is opened, the ectocervix is identified. Vaginal wall and cervix are inspected for masses, ulceration or unhealthy discharge.

At the same time a Pap smear is obtained and additional swab for culture or microscopic evaluation may also be collected.

The Sim's vaginal speculum with anterior vaginal wall retractor can be used for pelvic examination. Asking the patient to elevate leg close to the abdomen increases the ease of speculum examination for the patient as well clinician in dorsal position.

Bimanual Examination of the Uterus and the Adnexa

Patient should preferably have an empty bladder prior to procedure. After separating the labia with the thumb and index finger of the left hand, two fingers of the right hand are introduced into the vagina with palmer surface facing up. Throughout the whole examination, the clinician should observe the patient's face to notice any sign of pain or discomfort. The position and consistency of cervix is felt. The left hand is placed on the abdomen and the bimanual examination is commenced and pelvic organs are examined between the abdominal and vaginal fingers. The vaginal hand is often termed *"Passive"* and the abdominal hand *"Active"* because vaginal fingers should be kept stationary. The pelvic organs are *"pushed" w*ith the abdominal hand towards the vaginal hand, so that they could be felt. At times, when faced with an obese patient the cervix and uterus may have to be "pushed' up by the fingers in the vagina to help palpate them (Fig. 6.4A).

Once uterus is felt and its size, shape, mobility is confirmed, the vaginal fingers are moved to the right fornix of the vagina and abdominal hand is moved to the right iliac fossa to feel the right adnexa. The same procedure is repeated on the left side (Fig. 6.4B). The contents of the pouch of Douglas are examined by sweeping the vaginal fingers across the posterior fornix and lifting any contents to be palpated by the hand on the abdomen. If the uterus is not felt it may be retroverted. So it is important to carry out the bimanual examination with the vaginal fingers in the posterior fornix. **During examination of posterior fornix if the nodules can be felt in pouch of Douglas, they may be indicative of endometriosis or ovarian malignancy. Usually uterine masses move with the cervix and pushing the mass upward will make the cervix move upwards from the vaginal fingers. A pedunculated fibroid may be an exception to this rule. Likewise ovarian masses will be felt to move separately.** If there are adhesion between the ovarian mass and the uterus, it may move enmasse. This is specially seen with endometrioma or inflammatory tubo adnexal mass.

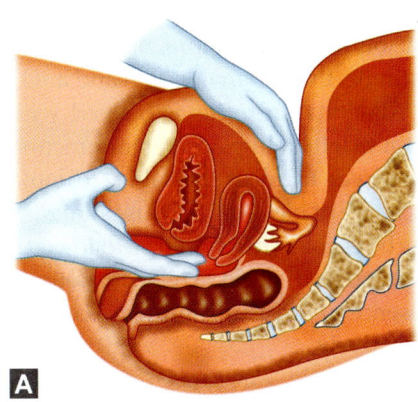 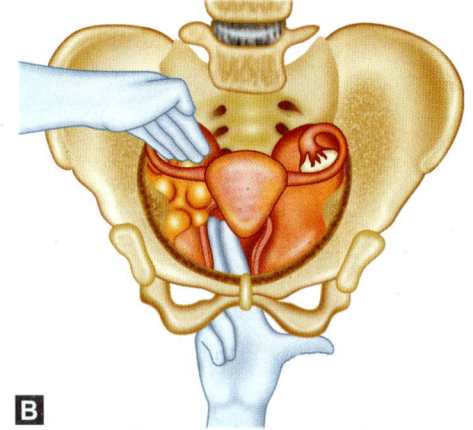

Figs 6.4A and B: Bimanual pelvic examination to palpate pelvic organs between both hands: (A) Bimanual pelvic examination, assessing uterine size; (B) Examination of lateral fornix

recumbent position ascites fluid will settle down into a horseshoe shape and dullness in the flanks can be demonstrated. As the patient moves over to her side, the dullness will move to her lowermost side, this is known as *shifting dullness*. *A fluid thrill* can also be elicited. *Auscultation* Usually auscultation is not required for the gynecological examination. But if a patient presents with acute abdomen with bowel obstruction or postoperative patient with illness, bowel sound auscultation is important. If patient is suspected to have pregnancy, auscultation of fetal heart sound is important finding.

c. **Pelvic examination:** The pelvic examination is the most crucial and challenging part of gynecological examination, though it may be omitted in virgins and adolescent. The pelvic examination is feared by many women, so it must be conducted in such a way as to allay her anxieties. The empathic physician usually finds that patient is relaxed by the time the history has been obtained and a painless and non-embarrassing general examination performed. Relaxing surroundings, a nurse or attendant chaperone if indicated, warm instruments, gentle unhurried manner with continued explanation and reassurance are helpful in securing patient relaxation and cooperation. Occasionally an ultrasound examination may be helpful in ascertaining whether the pelvic organs are normal in size and configuration in patients who cannot adequately relax the abdominal muscles. If a more definitive pelvic examination is essential, it can be performed with the patient anesthetized.

d. **Position:** Most commonly in the clinical setting patients are examined in the **dorsal** position, in which they lie on their back with the legs flexed at the knee joint. This gives a good exposure of the perineum and the introitus and facilitates use of Cusco's or Sim's speculum (Figs 6.2A and B). An alternative is the **lateral** position, which may

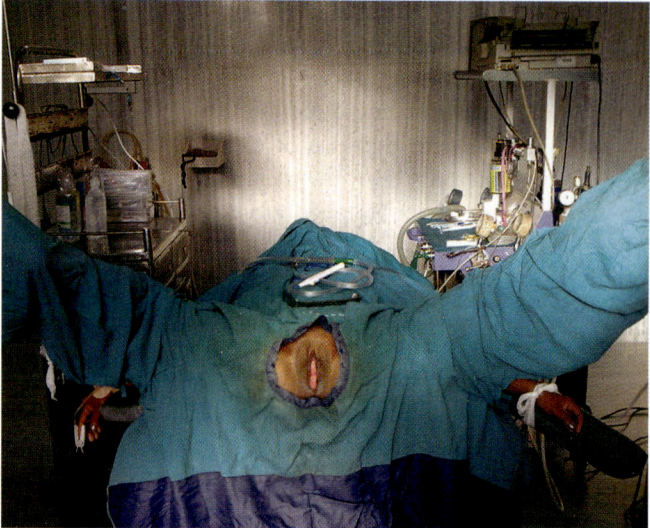

Fig. 6.3: Lithotomy position

be acceptable to some women, especially teenagers. Sim's position is variant of lateral position, in which the inner (left) leg is kept extended whereas the outer (right) leg is flexed. **Lithotomy** position with its various modifications is used especially when various procedures are carried out – this is a modified dorsal position, in which legs are held in stirrups with the thighs abducted and flexed to increase space and exposure (Fig. 6.3).

e. **Technique:** Pelvic examination is essentially composed of three steps:
   a. Inspection of the external genitalia
   b. Visualization of the vagina and cervix with speculum
   c. Bimanual examination of the uterus and the adnexa

Inspection of External Genitalia

It is prudent to be systematic in describing the external genitalia. One can start with labia majora and move inwards commenting on the appearance of each structure. One should note and document appearance of pubic hair distribution, labia majora, minora, clitoris, urethral orifice, vestibule, the perianal region and anal verge.

After that introitus is opened with thumb and index finger of left hand placed at the junction of upper two third and lower third of the labia, to look for any abnormal discharge or bleeding. At this point rectocele or urethrocele may be visible. This should be followed by asking the patient to cough and strain. These maneuvers may unmask the presence of stress incontinence or utero vaginal prolapse respectively.

Speculum Examination

Speculum examination should ideally precede bimanual vaginal examination. The common types of specula are

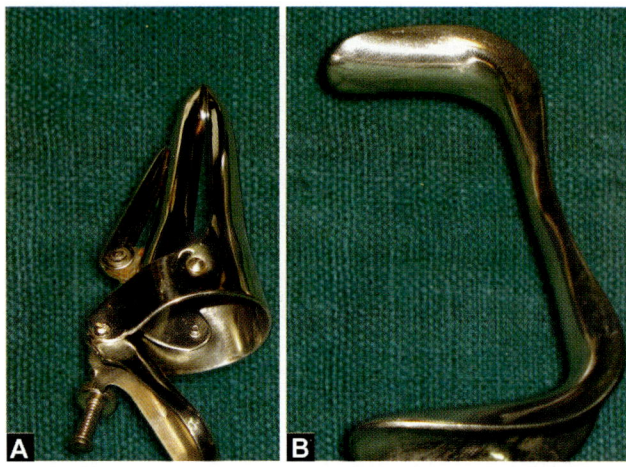

Figs 6.2A and B: (A) Cusco's self-retaining speculum; (B) Sim's posterior vaginal wall speculum

Vulvo Vaginitis

Pruritis vulva and vulvovaginitis are common gynecologic disorders in children. 75% of vulvovaginitis in this age group is nonspecific. The reasons of susceptibility of child to vulvovaginitis are — the prepubertal vulva is thin without labial fat pad and pubic hair. Unestrogenized vagina has high pH range which favors bacterial growth. Close proximity to anus predisposes to contamination and often suboptimal perineal hygiene.

Diagnosis

Diagnosis is suspected by the typical appearance of inflamed tissue. A wet mount preparation reveals numerous leukocytes. Culture of vaginal secretions sometimes identifies the offending organism.

Treatment

Most cases of nonspecific vulvovaginitis resolves with improvement in hygiene and avoidance of irritation including soap. **Amoxicillin** (20-40 mg/kg in three divided doses) is effective against a variety of potentially pathogenic organism in nonspecific vulvovaginitis. *If infection is severe, a short course of topical estrogen cream* is given to promote healing of vulvar and vaginal tissues.

In recurrent infections refractory to treatment or associated with fowl smelling bloody discharge, vaginoscopy is necessary to exclude a foreign body or tumor.

Genital Trauma

The children have increased risk of trauma due to lack of labial fat and increased physical activities. Usually most injuries to vulva are blunt, minor and accidental. Sharp object penetration may cause sometimes serious injury to vulvovaginal area. In many cases of genital trauma sexual or physical abuse should also be considered.

Ovarian Tumors

Ovarian tumors are the most common neoplasm found in childhood. They may be found incidentally during abdominal examination or during sonographic examination for some other indications. Enlarging cyst may cause increased abdominal girth or chronic pain. Hormone secreting cyst may lead to isosexual or heterosexual precocious puberty. Sometimes rupture, hemorrhage, or torsion may precipitate acute abdominal pain, similar to that seen in adults. Most of the tumors are benign but approximately 1% of all malignant tumors in this age group are of ovarian origin.

Management

Small simple ovarian cyst without septation or internal echoes may be monitored with serial sonographic examination. Most cysts less than 5 cm in size resolve within 1–4 months. **Persistent or enlarging cyst warrant surgical intervention and laparoscopy is the preferred method.** Optimal management includes fertility sparing ovarian cystectomy with preservation of any normal ovarian tissue.

Vaginal Bleeding

Neonates may present with vaginal bleeding during the first week of life due to withdrawal of maternal estrogen at birth. Bleeding typically resolves after a few days. However pubertal bleeding in a child often warrants careful evaluation. In children causes of vaginal bleeding are: (a) Foreign body, (b) Genital tumors, (c) Urethral prolapse, (d) Lichen scleroses, (e) Vulvovaginitis, (f) Condyloma acuminata, (g) Trauma, (h) Precocious puberty, (i) Exogenous hormone use.

Premature Thelarche

Thelarche may begin before the age of 8 years in some girls and is most commonly seen in girls aged less than 2 years. This early breast maturation is termed premature thelarche. It is to be differentiated from precocious puberty in that it is benign, self-limited and develop in isolation without other signs of pubertal development.

Management

Usually monitoring body growth and breast changes alone may suffice, but in those with increased height, weight, or with other pubertal changes, additional testing for precocious puberty is warranted.

PUBERTY

Puberty is the period during which secondary sexual characteristics develop and the capability of sexual reproduction is attained. **It is characterized by marked neuroendocrine and physiologic changes in the reproductive systems, culminating in mature secondary sexual characteristic and in girls ability to ovulate and menstruate.** Significant increase in somatic growth as well dramatic psychosocial changes also characterize puberty. It is important to note that changes in growth and psychosocial development do not always parallel the reproductive changes and this can lead to misunderstanding regarding an individual's maturity.

Timing of Puberty

The major determinant of timing of the onset of puberty is genetic. There is concordance of the age of menarche in mother daughter pair and between sisters and in one ethnic population. Other factors influencing the onset of puberty are:
a. General health and nutrition
b. Geographic location

Section -2 ♦ Gynecology

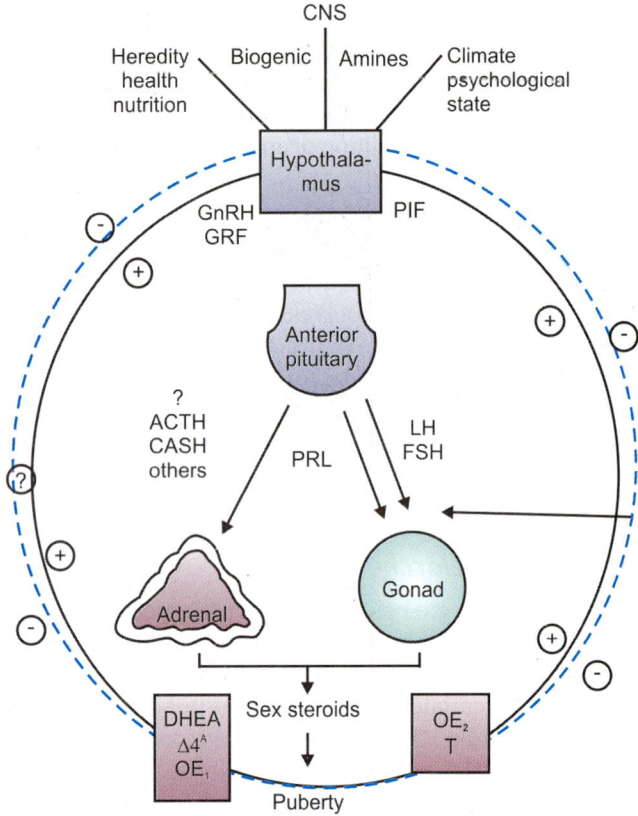

Fig. 7.2: Neuroendocrinological control of puberty

c. Exposure to light
d. Psychologic factors.

Children close to equator, at lower altitude, in urban areas and mildly obese children start menstruation earlier than those in northern latitude, urban areas and non-obese children.

Adolescence

Adolescence is the span of human growth extending from immaturity of childhood to the physical and psychological maturity of adulthood. This period extends from 10 to 20 years of age. Puberty marks the beginning of adolescence.

Prepubertal Period

As puberty approaches, three critical changes in the low endocrine homeostatic function of childhood emerge:
a. **Adrenarche:** Causing growth of pubic and axillary hairs due to increased production of adrenal androgen.
b. **Decreasing repression of the gonadostat:** Puberty does not represent simply final complete development of hypothalamic pituitary gonadal axis (HPG). HPG axis is intact as early as 20 weeks of life. LH and FSH level peak at 20 week of gestation and then are suppressed by maternal estrogen. Immediate postpartum, LH and FSH level flare for 1-2 years and then are suppressed until puberty either by exquisite sensitivity to very low level of estrogen or by a central inhibiting factor. **In late prepubertal period, there is derepression of the central nervous system**—Pituitary gonadostat and progressive responsiveness of the anterior pituitary to exogenous GnRH and follicle reactivity to FSH and LH.
c. Alteration and amplification of GnRH gonadotropins and gonadotropins ovarian steroid interaction (Fig. 7.2).

Puberty Period

Maturation of the hypothalamic pituitary axis initiates puberty. The hypothalamus begins to secrete Gonadotropin releasing hormone (GnRH) in pulses during sleep and eventually followed by similar pulses of less amplitude occurring throughout the 24 hours a day. GnRH pulses stimulate the pituitary gland to secrete pulses of gonadotropins of which there is Luteinizing hormone (LH) predominance. In response to increased secretion of gonadotropins there is increased secretion of gonadal hormones that lead to the progressive development of secondary sexual characteristic and gametogenesis.

When episodic peak of estradiol occurs—there is menarche. By mid to late puberty, maturation of the positive feedback relationship between estradiol and LH is established, leading to ovulatory cycles. It is postulated that a critical body weight (≥ 45 kg) must be reached by a girl to achieve menarche. The shift in body composition to a greater percent of fat (from 16% to 23.5%) can be possibly more important, causing earlier menarche in moderately obese girls. The **identification of Leptin** has also revitalized the importance of a relationship between body fat and reproductive function. Leptin is a peptide secreted in adipose tissue that circulates in the blood bound to a family of proteins. It acts on the central nervous system which regulates eating behavior and energy balance. Leptin level increases during childhood until the onset of puberty, suggesting that a threshold level of leptin and critical amount of adipose tissue (source of leptin) is necessary for puberty to begin. After puberty leptin level in boys return to prepubertal range. In girl leptin levels are higher than boys and decrease with increasing tanner stages of puberty.

Stages of Pubertal Development in Girls

The changes associated with puberty occur in an orderly sequence over a definitive time frame. Any deviation from this sequence or time frame should be regarded as abnormal. The first sign of puberty is often said to be breast budding—called *thelarche around age of 10*. There is increase in linear growth velocity, 1-2 years prior to thelarche. Thelarche is followed by *pubic hair development— adrenarche at age of 11, attainment of peak growth velocity (9 cm/year) at age 12, and menstruation (menarche) at age 13*.

Tanner Staging

Dr JM Tanner proposed a 5-stage system to grade breast and pubic hair development in girls and genital and pubic hair development in boys (Tables 7.1 and 7.2).

Age Limit for Pubertal Changes

The onset of puberty is said to be normal if it occurs within 2.5 standard deviations from the mean. The generally accepted range is in between 8-14 years. **Girls with no secondary sexual characteristic by age 14 years should have a work up as should girls with normal secondary sexual characteristics but no menstrual period by age of 16 years.** Isolated breast or pubic hair development without other signs of puberty may occur and does not require extensive evaluation but does warrant observation to exclude the possibility of precocious puberty. Premature thelarche usually occurs in the first several years of life. **Premature adrenarche has been considered a possible early sign of polycystic ovary syndrome later in life.**

Aberrations of Pubertal Development

It can be classified in four broad categories:
1. Delayed or interrupted puberty
2. Asynchronous pubertal development
3. Precocious puberty
4. Heterosexual puberty.

Delayed or Interrupted Puberty Workup

The history and physical examination with particular attention to growth are most important in the evaluation of individuals with delayed puberty. Pubertal delay is much more common in boys than in girls. It is also to be remembered that puberty may be delayed in any child suffering from any severe chronic disease like malnutrition, tuberculosis, cardiac disease, cystic fibrosis, so chronic illness should be excluded during the history and physical examination.

In brief, patients with delayed puberty are classified by: (a) Presence or absence of breast development which is sign of estrogen production, and (b) By the presence or absence of uterus (absent when anti-müllerian hormone from testicular tissue is produced).

If breast development is absent, an FSH level is done to diagnose ovarian failure, (high FSH level, or hypergonadotropic ovarian failure). If uterine development is absent, a testosterone level and karyotype will distinguish uterovaginal agenesis from androgen insensitivity syndrome. In presence of both breast and uterine development workup is identical to secondary amenorrhea.

Causes of Delayed Puberty

The most common cause of primary amenorrhea and delayed puberty is gonadal dysgenesis (usually Turner syndrome), followed by uterovaginal agenesis and androgen

Table 7.1: Tanner stages of pubertal development in girls

Stage	Breast development	Pubic hair development
Stage 1 (Prepubertal)	Elevation of papilla only	No pubic hair
Stage 2	Breast budding	Scattered labial hair
Stage 3	Enlargement of breast without areola separation	Hair spreading to mons pubis
Stage 4	Secondary mould formed by areola	Slight lateral spread. Thick adult type hair
Stage 5	Mature breast with adult contour of breast and areola	Hairs on medial thighs, adult in type and distributed in classic inverse triangle

Table 7.2: Tanner stages of pubertal development in boys

Stage	Genital development	Pubic hair development
Stage 1	Prepubertal testicular length < 2.5 cm	Prepubertal no pubic hair
Stage 2	Testes >2.5 cm in longest diameter scrotum thinning and reddening	Sparse growth of slightly curly pubic hair
Stage 3	Growth of penis in width and length and further growth of testes	Thicker, curlier hair spread to mons pubis
Stage 4	Penis further enlarged, testes larger with darker scrotal colors	Adult type hair do not spread medial thighs
Stage 5	Genitalia adult in size and shape	Adult type hairs spread on medial thighs

In all cases Tanner Stage I is prepubertal and Tanner Stage V is complete maturation.

Table 7.3: Cause of delayed pubertal abnormalities

Hypergonadotropic hypogonadism
    Ovarian failure: Abnormal karyotype
    Ovarian failure: Normal karyotype
        46 xx
        46 xy
Hypogonadotropic hypogonadism
    Reversible
        Physiologic delay
        Weight loss/anorexia
        Primary hypothyroidism
        Congenital adrenal hyperplasia
        Cushing syndrome
        Prolactinoma
    Irreversible
        GnRH deficiency
        Hypopituitarism
        Congenital CNS defects
        Other pituitary adenomas
        Craniopharyngioma
        Malignant pituitary tumor
Eugonadism
    Mullerian agenesis
    Vaginal septum
    Imperforate hymen
    Androgen insensitivity syndrome
    Inappropriate positive feedback

insensitivity syndrome. Hypothyroidism, anorexia nervosa, extreme exercise, chronic illnesses are also common cause of delayed puberty. The causes of delayed pubertal development are summarized in Table 7.3.

Management of Delayed Puberty

The first priority in therapy is removal or correction of primary etiology when possible. *Thyroid therapy for hypothyroidism, growth hormone for isolated growth hormone deficiency and treatment of ileitis are examples of specific therapy.* In XY individuals properly timed gonadectomy followed by sex hormone treatment is required.

Treatment in Hypogonadism

Hormone therapy initiates and sustains maturation and function of secondary sexual character. It promotes achieving full height potential. In adolescent increase in bone density is very important and so hormone treatment is recommended which should confirm to physiology of early stages of puberty. The recommended dosages are as follows:
- Start with 0.3 mg conjugated estrogen or 0.5 mg estradiol daily.
- After 6 months to 1 year with 0.625 mg conjugated estrogen or 1.0 mg estradiol daily and 5 mg medroxyprogesterone acetate or equivalent progestin for the last 14 days of each month.

Patient with Physiologic Delay

Reassurance that anticipated development will occur is the only management especially if there is family history of delayed puberty. However, early hormone treatment is sometimes needed to minimize psychological stress. Usually, patients with only physiologic delay of puberty continue development on their own when bone age has advanced to 13 years. If one is sexually active, it is wise to use oral contraception for hormone therapy. Treatment with pulsatile GnRH is both a logical and effective means of inducing a physiologic puberty but it is expensive, technically difficult and cumbersome.

Precocious Puberty

If one accepts the mean ± 2.5 standard deviation as encompassing the normal range, then pubertal changes before the age of 8 and menarche before age of 10 are regarded as precocious. Certainly thelarche and adrenarche before age of 6 warrant evaluation. *Isosexual* precocious puberty is premature pubertal development compatible with the individual's genetic sex. *Heterosexual Precocious puberty* refers to pubertal changes occurring opposite to the patient genetic sex and in girls denotes excessive androgen production from adrenal gland or ovaries. Isosexual problems are far more common than heterosexual one. *Traditionally* Precocious puberty is divided into two classifications:

1. ***GnRH-dependent precocious puberty (Complete, isosexual, central or true):*** These all terms refer to early activation of hypothalamopituitary gonadal axis.
2. ***GnRH independent precocious puberty (Incomplete, isosexual, or heterosexual, peripheral, or precocious pseudopuberty):*** Sexual maturation in these cases is due to extrapituitary secretion of Human Chorionic Gonadotropins (hCG) or sex steroid secretion so this mechanism is GnRH-independent.

In clinical practice, these classifications are of little practical value, because they are finally diagnosed only after a comprehensive evaluation. Precocity is five times more common in girls than boys. In almost 75% of girls precocity is idiopathic as opposed to 40% for boys. Nevertheless in face of any precocious development, the clinician is obliged to rule out a serious disease process in central or peripheral sites.

Box 7.1 summarizes the classification and relative occurrence of precocious puberty. *Idiopathic GnRH dependent precocity* is idiopathic and treated with GnRH agonist. *Tumors of CNS* are the most common cause of GnRH dependent precocious puberty. Hemartomas are most common CNS tumors which are treated by surgery, radiation and GnRh agonist. The most common cause of GnRH independent precocious puberty is *functional ovarian* cyst like granulosa

Box 7.1: Causes of precocious puberty

GnRH-Dependent (True Precocity)
  Idiopathic
  CNS problem
GnRH-Independent (Precocious Pseudopuberty)
  Ovarian (cyst or tumor)
  McCune-Albright syndrome
  Adrenal feminizing
  Adrenal masculinizing
  Ectopic gonadotropin production

cell tumors, which should be removed surgically. *Primary hypothyroidism is the only form of precocious puberty, in which bone age is delayed instead of advanced.*

McCune Albright Syndrome or (Polyostotic fibrous dysplasia) is characterized by multiple cystic bone lesions, café-au-lait spots and precocious puberty. Autonomous estrogen production from the ovary due to a genetic mutation in the gonadotropins receptor that renders it constitutionaly activated, results in precocious puberty. This syndrome is treated with testolactone (an aromatase inhibitor).

Workup of Patients with Precocious Puberty

History and Physical Examination

The patient and her parents should be asked about growth and pubertal milestone, family history of reproductive abnormalities, the possibility of exogenous hormonal drug ingestion, symptoms of thyroid disease, neurological symptoms or a history of CNS insults. On *physical examination*, height, weight, and the percentile for age should be assessed. Tanner staging, a neurologic and thyroid examination, a skin examination, looking for café-au-lait spots, and an abdominal examination and pelvic/ rectal examination looking for any pelvic masses should be the integral part of clinical examination.

Laboratory and Radiological Investigation

1. Bone age should always be assessed in evaluation; most important radiographic test is a *left wrist bone X-ray*.
2. Basal FSH, LH, TSH and hCG assays: In true precocity FSH and LH levels are in pubertal range (>7.5 IU/lit. and >15 IU/lit) respectively. Low or pubertal level of gonadotropins indicates the need to determine circulatory estradiol concentration in isosexual precocity. Increased estradiol level suggests estrogen secreting neoplasm. If estradiol level is compatible with degree of pubertal development, evaluation of CNS by MRI or CT scanning is warranted. Primary hypothyroidism has to be ruled out as the cause of precocious puberty. In heterosexual cases DHEAS, 17 hydroxyprogesterone and testosterone is measured to rule out adrenal or ovarian tumors or congenital adrenal hyperplasia.
3. Pelvic ultrasound or CT for ovarian or adrenal mass.
4. MRI of CNS looking for CNS tumors.
5. A skull radiograph can detect multiple cystic lesions which is a characteristic of McCune Albright syndrome. Clinically the nature of precocity also detects certain diagnostic priorities:
1. First is to rule out life-threatening disease like neoplasm of CNS, ovary and adrenal.
2. Define the velocity of process.
3. Isolated nonendocrine cause of vaginal bleeding like trauma, foreign body, vaginitis or genital neoplasm must be excluded.

Management of Precocious Development

The objective of management and treatment of precocious puberty are:
1. Diagnosis and treatment of intracranial disease
2. Arrest maturation until normal pubertal age
3. Attenuation and diminishing of established precocious characteristics
4. Maximize eventual adult height
5. Facilitate the avoidance of abuse and reduction of emotional problem and provide contraception if necessary.

GnRH Agonist

GnRh agonist treatment produces an initial short term 'flare' stimulation of gonadotropins release followed by desensitization and down regulation, causing a profound reduction in gonadotropin steroid production and biologic effects.

There is substantial regression of pubertal changes causing amenorrhea. Final bone height is increased. Maximal achievement of height requires early onset of treatment and long duration of treatment. The decision to treat with GnRH agonist is based primarily on the predicted adult height and progression of pubertal development. *Dosage of GnRH agonist treatment is monitored by measuring estradiol level, which should be maintained less than 10 pg/ml – a prepubertal range.* Treatment is maintained until the epiphysis is fused or until appropriate pubertal and chronologic ages are matched.

For GnRH dependent true isosexual puberty— *cyproterone acetate, medroxyprogesterone acetate injection as well as tablet, and danazol* has been tried, but they have undesirable side effects and bone maturation and growth was not sufficiently controlled.

GnRH Independent Precocious Puberty

In these cases primary treatment is directed towards suppression of gonadal steroidogenesis. Medroxy progesterone acetate in depot form or aromatase inhibitor can be administered for precocious pubertal changes.

But in these cases treatment is aimed at curing the underlying disorders. Neurological excision of hypothalamic, pituitary, cerebral, or pineal tumor must be individualized in each patient. If an ovarian or adrenal tumor is identified, surgical excision is the treatment of choice. With primary hypothyroidism, thyroid replacement prevents further progression of sexual precocity. If adrenal hyperplasia is identified, treatment with glucocorticoids and/or mineralocorticoid prevents further progression of pubertal development.

Psychosocial Problem

Careful consideration must be given to management of psychosocial problem in all children with precocious puberty as these children are behaviorally, intellectually and psychologically of their chronological age. Patient and teacher should be counseled and especial care in studies and home will help a lot in supporting them. Possibility of sexual abuse should be explained to guardians as well children with steps for prevention.

Prognosis

Prognosis depends on the underlying cause. With primary hypothyroidism the prognosis is excellent. Patient with benign ovarian and adnexal tumor after removal has good prognosis, while malignant carcinoma has poor prognosis. In the same way among CNS causes, prognosis depends on nature and location of tumor. However, with exception of short stature, as an adult, the prognosis for idiopathic sexual precocity remains good, if the children enter adult life without psychosexual scars.

Growth Problem in Normal Adolescents

Adolescents are very sensitive about excessive or insufficient growth. So their concern should not be dismissed lightly and psychological support and reassurance are key factors in the management of such problems. A willingness to listen to problem, together with adult to adult attitude, will place the adolescent clinician relationship at the proper level of mutual respect.

Investigation

The basic and essential laboratory procedure is a **left hand X-ray for bone age**. The Bayley Pinneau table predicts future adult height, utilizing bone age and present height.

Short Stature Management

Thorough medical history and physical examination is done to rule out the usual disorders with short stature like *malnutrition, chronic urinary tract disease, chronic infection, hypothyroidism, mental illness, panhypopituitarism, and gonadal dysgenesis*. In history height and weight of parents, siblings and relatives should be obtained along with dietary history, daily activities and sleep habits.

Normal history and examination in an individual with a bone age only 1 year behind the chronological age suggest a constitutional pattern that does not require treatment. It is helpful to point out that X-ray indicates that individual has 1 year or more of unused potential in which to catch up with her friends.

Hormone Therapy

Hormone treatment can be considered when there is continued failure of growth in the absence of disease. With recombinant growth hormone, there can be average gain of about 5–6 cm with 2 years of therapy, but response is inconsistent. GnRH agonist or aromatase inhibitor can be added with growth hormone. It has to be kept in mind that treatment is every expensive.

In female adolescent with gonadal failure, estrogen can be used to stimulate epiphyseal growth, bringing the bone age to match the chronological age. Conjugated estrogen (0.3 mg) or estradiol (0.5 mg) administered daily are effective in hypogonadal individual. Hormone treatment can be discontinued when the bone age matches the chronological age.

Anabolic androgenic steroid are illegally utilized by both adolescent male and female to increase athletic performance and even to look better. Response to these steroid ranges from increased libido, virilization and menstrual dysfunction in women to liver disease, impotence, and oligospermia with risk of psychological dependence in male.

Tall Stature

This is rarely problems in boys. Sports and some jobs provide a ready outlet. But girls who are the daughter of very tall parents may come for help. A hand wrist X-ray for bone age is necessary. The degree of development of secondary sexual character is important, because the more mature a girl is, less effective treatment is in influencing her eventual height.

Treatment

High doses of estrogen have been used effectively to increase the rate of bone maturation and shorten the ultimate height in appropriately selected girls. Treatment should begin as early as 8 or 9 years, certainly before the age of 12. Parental participation in decision is essential and they must be informed of possible problem of menorrhagia, breast symptom and water retention.

MULTIPLE CHOICE QUESTIONS

1. The sequence of development of puberty in girls:
    a. Thelarche, Pubarche, Menarche
    b. Pubarche, Thelarche, Menarche

Chapter -7 ♦ Pediatric and Adolescent Gynecology

    c. Pubarche, Menarche, Thelarche
    d. Menarche, Thelarche, Pubarche
  Ans. a
2. The first sign of puberty in girls is:
    a. Breast budding
    b. Growth spirit (peak height velocity)
    c. Menarche
    d. Pubic and axillary hair growth
  Ans. a
3. Gynecomastia is seen in:
    a. Secondary syphilis
    b. Lepromatous leprosy
    c. HIV
    d. Klinefelter's syndrome
  Ans. b, d
4. Sexual infantilism is associated with:
    a. Pituitary tumor
    b. Gonadal aplasia
    c. Dwarfism
    d. All
  Ans. d
5. Gonadal sex of the fetus is determined by:
    a. Secretion of testosterone
    b. Secretion of anti-Müllerian hormone
    c. Sex determining region on the Y chromosome
    d. Secretion of estrogen
  Ans. b
6. In polycystic ovarian disease all of the following are seen, *except*:
    a. Endometrial carcinoma
    b. Increased FSH
    c. Streak ovaries
    d. Insulin resistance
  Ans. b, c
7. Increased LH:FSH ratio is found in:
    a. Premature menopause
    b. Sheehan's syndrome
    c. Polycystic ovary syndrome
    d. Turner's syndrome
  Ans. c
8. A 15-year-old young girl present in emergency with acute pain in lower abdomen. She has not attained menarche history of cyclic pain for the last 6 months and she has not attained her menarche yet. On local examination a tense bulge in the region of hymen is seen. The most probable diagnosis is:
    a. Rokitansky–Busterk-Hauser syndrome
    b. Testicular feminization
    c. Imperforate hymen
    d. Asherman's syndrome
  Ans. c
9. DES causes the following defects, *except*:
    a. Renal anamolies
    b. Perifimbrial cyst
    c. T-shaped uterus
    d. Vaginal adenosis
  Ans. a
10. Ideal age for repair of vaginal agenesis:
    a. 6 months
    b. 3 years
    c. At puberty
    d. Before marriage
  Ans. d
11. Commonest cause of primary amenorrhea is:
    a. Genital tuberculosis
    b. Ovarian dysgenesis
    c. Mullerian duct anomalies
    d. Hypothyroidism
  Ans. b

8 Genital Ambiguity and Intersexuality

*Life is for one generation, Good name is for ever. Medicine includes real experiments
which are spontaneous, and not included by physicians.*

Genital Ambiguity at Birth

Because of concern of parents and the need to prevent life-threatening complications, prompt and proper evaluation of infant is warranted, if infant has ambiguous genitalia. The initial evaluation is as follows:
1. Cytogenic and endocrine studies: Karyotyping is must. Nowadays probe for many specific inherited disorders are available.
2. Exclude congenital adrenal hyperplasia: By serum level of sodium, potassium, and 17α hydroxyprogesterone and urinary excretion of 17 ketosteroid, pregnanetriol and tetrahydrodeoxycortisol. It is most common cause of genital ambiguity and infant should be monitored closely to prevent development of dehydration, hyponatremia and hyperkalemia.
3. Anti-Müllerian hormone: It can be measured as it is elevated in boys and undetectable in girls for first sexual year.

Physical Signs

In normal boys there is only a single midline frenulum on the ventral side of the phallus. In normal girls there are two frenula lateral to midline. A girl with clitoral enlargement still has two frenula and a boy with hypospadias has a single midline frenulum or several irregular fibrous bands.

The location or consistency of the gonads may be helpful. A gonad located in labial or inguinal regions almost always contains testicular tissue. A testis is generally softer than an ovary or a streak gonad.

Diagnosis and Management

In a newborn, who presents a problem of correct sex assignment, it is better to delay than to reverse the sex assignment at a later date. It is important to be supportive of these parents. Physician should emphasize that child should undergo normal psychosexual development regardless of the sex of rearing selected. Genital ambiguity is usually identified at birth, though it may not be recognized for several years. Questions about changing the sex of rearing may arise, which may be done before 2 years of age without psychologically damaging the child. Though surgery is warranted, but has not always been successful.

Teratogens

Maternal ingestion of synthetic steroid and danazol can cause the ambiguous genitalia.

INTERSEX

Intersexuality may be defined as the presence of both male and female external and or internal genital organs in the same individual causing confusion in the diagnosis of true sex. The incidence is about 2 in 1000. Embryologic development of gonad has already been described in chapter of basic sciences. In determination of sex, following factors are to be considered:
 i. Genetic sex
 ii. Chromosomal sex
 iii. External and internal anatomic sex
 iv. Gonadal sex,
 v. Hormonal sex
 vi. Psychologic sex
 vii. Sex of rearing

In newborn, as just described, the diagnosis of apparent sex is determined by the appearance of the external genital organs. In adolescence beside appearance of external genitalia secondary sexual character, psychogenic sex and sex of rearing have to be taken in account.

The schematic representation of development of gonad is summarized in Box 8.1.

Box 8.1: Representation of development of gonad

1. The SRY gene directs the gonad to become a testes
2. The absence of SRY genes allows the gonad to become an ovary
3. The presence or absence of androgen determines external genital development
4. The presence of gonadal testosterone production leads to Wolffian duct differentiation into vas deferens, epididymis and seminal vesicle
5. The presence of gonadal AMH production leads to Mullerian duct regression

Classification and Nomenclature of Abnormal Sexual Differentiation

The standard classification of individual with intersexuality or hermaphroditism proceeds according to gonadal morphology.

I. True hermaphrodite - Possess both ovarian and testicular tissue
II. Male pseudohermaphrodite - Has testis but external and sometimes internal genitalia on female phenotypic aspect
III. Female pseudohermaphrodite - Has ovaries, but genital development displays masculine characteristics

Disorders of fetal endocrinology are summarized in Table 8.1.

Table 8.1: Disorders of fetal endocrinology

1. Masculinized females (Female pseudohermaphroditism)
   a. Congenital adrenal hyperplasia
      i. 21 hydroxylase deficiency
      ii. 11 α hydroxylase deficiency
      iii. 3 α hydroxysteroid dehydrogenase deficiency
   b. Elevated androgen in maternal circulation
      i. Drug intake
      ii. Maternal disease
      iii. Aromatase (P 450 arom) deficiency
2. Incompletely masculinized males (Male pseudohermaphroditism)
   a. Androgen insensitivity syndrome
   b. 5 α reductase deficiency
   c. Testosterone biosynthesis defects
   d. Gonadotropin resistant testes
   e. Anti-Müllerian hormone deficiency
3. Disorders of gonadal development
   a. Male pseudohermaphroditism
      i. Primary gonadal defect—Swyer's syndrome
      ii. Anorchia
   b. True hermaphroditism
   c. Gonadal dysgenesis
      i. Turner's syndrome
      ii. Mosaicism
      iii. Normal karyotype—Noman syndrome

Masculinized Female

Masculinized females possess ovaries and are female by genetic sex (XX) but external genitalia are not those of a normal female. Of all infants with ambiguous genitalia, 40-45% have adrenal hyperplasia.

Congenital Adrenal Hyperplasia (Adrenogenital Syndrome)

This is an autosomal recessive disorder, which is result of a deficiency in one of the multiple enzymes required for adrenal synthesis of cortisol like 21 hydroxylase deficiency (95%), 11 hydroxylase or 3α hydroxysteroid dehydrogenase. Due to various enzyme deficiencies, there is lack of cortisol production resulting in excess of ACTH production from the pituitary. ACTH, in turn, stimulates the adrenal to produce excess androgens with virilization of female offspring. An associated aldosterone deficiency may lead to excess salt depletion. The girls are potentially fertile.

Diagnosis

At birth the infants have ambiguous genitalia. There can be enlarged clitoris, presence of penile urethra, fused labia minora. During infancy, if there is no serious electrolyte disturbance, children grow more rapidly than other. But epiphysial closure occurs by age 10 and these people are much shorter than normal as adult. Process of virilization occurs at early age. Acne may develop early. Puberty never occurs with absence of thelarche and menarche.

Investigation

a. Sonography: Uterus, fallopian tubes and ovaries are present.
b. Sex chromatin: Shows female karyotyping 46 xx and positive Barr body.
c. Serum estimation: 17 hydroxyprogesterone is elevated beyond 800 ng/ml. There can be low sodium and chloride and raised potassium.
d. Urinary excretion: Urinary excretion of pregnanetriol and 17 ketosteroid are markedly elevated.

Treatment

Treatment of adrenal hyperplasia is to supply the deficient hormone that is cortisol. This decreases ACTH secretion and lowers production of androgenic precursors. The addition of salt retaining hormone to glucocorticoid therapy has improved the control of the disease. The drug of choice is hydrocortisone 10 mg per day and 9 fluorohydrocortisone 100 µg/day. Optimal regulation of ACTH secretion requires administration of hydrocortisone in 3 divided doses and Prednisolone twice a day. 17 OHP level should be maintained in range of 100-1000 ng/day, so avoiding both under and over treatment.

Normal reproduction is possible with replacement therapy of cortisol deficiency. Fertility is only slightly reduced, and maintenance steroid dose usually does not need to be changed during pregnancy. During labor additional parenteral steroid is needed. Aside from liability associated with genetic transmission of this syndrome, the children born to patients with adrenal hyperplasia have been normal. The newborn should be closely observed for adrenal insufficiency due to steroid crossover.

Treatment Problem

Over treatment causes Cushing's syndrome, osteopenia and poor growth. Under treatment is associated with short stature.

Masculinization due to Elevated Androgen in Maternal Circulation

Masculinization of female fetus can be sometimes produced by exogenous intake of androgenic substance as progestin and danazol. The majority of these cases result from antenatal maternal treatment of threatened or recurrent miscarriage with various progestin compounds. There is no evidence of therapeutic benefit of progestin other than progesterone or 17α hydroxyprogesterone acetate and should not be administered to pregnant women. This iatrogenic virilization is not progressive, blood steroid are not elevated and no hormonal therapy is needed. Subsequent development will be normal. Therefore, surgical correction of abnormalities in the external genitalia is the only indicated treatment.

Incompletely masculinized males: Incompletely masculinized males are male by genetic sex (XY) and possess testicles, but the external genitalia are not normally male; so called male pseudohermaphrodite. It occurs in following ways:
a. Defective response in androgen dependent tissues: Androgen insensitivity syndrome—complete and incomplete
b. 5 α reductase deficiency
c. Aromatase (P450 arm) deficiency abnormal androgen synthesis.

Androgen Insensitivity Syndrome

It accounts for about 10% of all cases of primary amenorrhea, the third most common cause after gonadal dysgenesis and congenital absence of vagina. It is inherited as an X-linked recessive gene. In this end organ does not respond to androgens, because of either lack of androgen cytosol receptor or defective/mutated receptors so androgen induction of Wolffian duct development does not occur.

Salient feature of complete androgen insensitivity syndrome: Clinical features:
a. They are phenotypically and psychologically female.
b. Diagnosis is likely when an individual presents with primary amenorrhea, absent pubic and axillary hairs, short vagina and absent cervix and uterus, but breast development occurs because of total absence of androgen influence.
c. Gonads which are testis are either placed in the labia or inguinal canal or intra-abdominal so children with inguinal hernia or inguinal mass should be suspected of androgen insensitivity.

Investigation

a. Sex chromatin negative, and karyotype is 46-'XY'.
b. High LH, normal to elevated FSH, normal to slightly elevated male testosterone levels and high estradiol for men.

Management

As there is no androgen response, these infants should be reared as females. Gonadectomy should be performed at the age of 16 - 18 years to allow endogenous hormonal changes and smooth transition through puberty. Postoperative hormone therapy can be a simple daily 0.625 mg conjugated estrogen or 1.0 mg estradiol administration. Dose can be adjusted, if vaginal lubrication and an acidic pH is not maintained or if loss of bone density is documented. It is advocated that truthful education of syndrome with appropriate psychological counseling of patients and parents should be done. Detection of this syndrome demands careful investigation for other affected family members.

Incomplete Androgen Insensitivity

It is X-linked recessive trait and encompasses a spectrum of disorder. Reifenstein syndrome is now applied to all the intermediate forms. The clinical presentation ranges from complete failure of virilization to essential complete phenotypic masculinization.

Clinical Presentation

1. Sex assignment at birth can be a problem, because of ambiguous genitalia, like mild cliteromegaly and slight labial fusion.
2. Karyotype is male X-Y, distinguishing it from other feminizing syndrome.
3. Presentation can be undervirilized subfertile male having azoospermia or severe oligospermia.
4. Hormonal levels are like complete androgen insensitivity.

Reductase Deficiency

It is familial incomplete male (46 XY) autosomal recessive trait of male pseudohermaphroditism. It is characterized by severe perineal hypospadias and underdevelopment of vagina.

Diagnosis

1. Karyotype X-Y
2. Elevated testosterone/dihydrotestosterone ratio.

Management

Sex assignment is usually female. Gonadectomy is necessary to avoid neoplasia as well virilization at puberty. But on the other hand early correction of cryptorchidism and hypospadias can preserve fertility and allow a male life.

Abnormal Androgen Synthesis

Defective male development can stem from a secretory failure of testis during the critical period of sex differentiation. It accounts for 4% of male pseudohermaphroditism and can occur because of one of following:
a. Defects in testicular steroidogenesis.
b. Gonadotropins resistant testis.
c. Congenital lipoid adrenal hyperplasia.
d. Defective synthesis, secretion or response to anti-Müllerian hormone.

DISORDERS OF GONADAL DEVELOPMENT

The proper development and eventual function of the gonad depends on presence of germ cells, the appropriate sex chromosome contribution and appropriate gonadal ridge somatic cells. Abnormalities in this can cause following disorders.
a. **Bilateral dysgenesis of the testis (Swyer syndrome):** Affected individual has an 'XY' karyotype, but normal infantile female external and internal genitalia (Fig. 8.1). There are fibrous bands in place of gonads causing primary amenorrhea and lack of secondary sexual development at puberty.
   Fibrous bands should be removed as soon as the diagnosis is made. Estrogen and progestin sequential therapy supports female secondary sex development.
b. **Anorchia:** Disappearing testis syndrome: In this early testis function occurs but not sustained in sufficient amount or duration to develop a normal size phallus. Affected 'XY' individual has infantile unambiguous male external genitalia and male Wolffian duct and back Mullerian duct. Sex assignment depends on extent of external genitalia development.

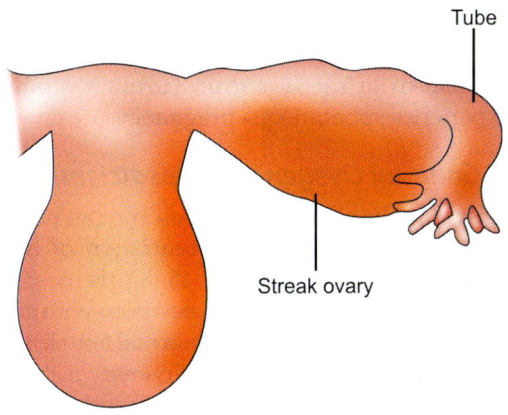

Fig. 8.1: Fibrous band in place of ovary

TRUE HERMAPHRODITISM

Hermaphrodite - (the Greek god with bisexual attitude) - was the son/daughter of Hermes the God of athletics, secrets and occult Philosophy and Aphrodite the goddess of love. Pliny (23-79 AD) was the first to apply the true hermaphrodite term to humans, in his massive work—Historia Naturalis. Abnormal sexual differentiation can occur as a result of:
a. Mixture of gonadal sex (true hermaphroditism)
b. Completely uncertainty of gonadal sex (gonadal sex with some virilization). A true hermaphrodite possesses both ovarian and testicular tissue either in one gonad (ovotestis) or side by side. Gonadal malignancies have been reported in 5% of true hermaphroditism. 70% are genetic female ('XX'), few are 'XY' and rest are mosaics.

In the majority, external genitalia are ambiguous, with sufficient male character to allow male sex assignment. But 3/4th develops gynecomastia and 50% menstruate after puberty.

Gonadal Dysgenesis

The term gonadal dysgenesis is frequently used to describe all subject with female genitalia, normal mullerian structure and streak gonads with either 46 XX or 46 'XY' karyotype.

Turner's Syndrome

Streak gonads due to an abnormality in or absence of one of the X chromosomes in all cell lines is called Turner's syndrome. It was first described by HH Turner in 1938 in annual meeting of the association for the Study of Internal Secretion.

Causes

The most common cause is nondisjunction during meiosis. Approximately, 60% of Turner patient has total loss of one X-chromosome; the remainders have structural abnormality or mosaicism of one of X-chromosome. Maternal X is retained in nearly 70% and paternal X in the rest.

Salient features of Turner's syndrome (Fig. 8.2):
1. Female gender identification is unambiguous
2. Spontaneous puberty is reported in 10-20% and spontaneous menarche in 2-5% of girls with Turner's syndrome.
3. Phenotypically female with:
   a. Short stature, sexual infantilism, streak gonads.
   b. Webbed neck, high arched palate, cubitus vulgus, broad shield like chest, with widely spaced nipples, a low hairline on neck, short 4th metacarpal bone, short legs, and renal abnormalities.
   c. Autoimmune disorders are common as Hashimoto's thyroiditis, Addison's disease, alopecia and vitiligo.

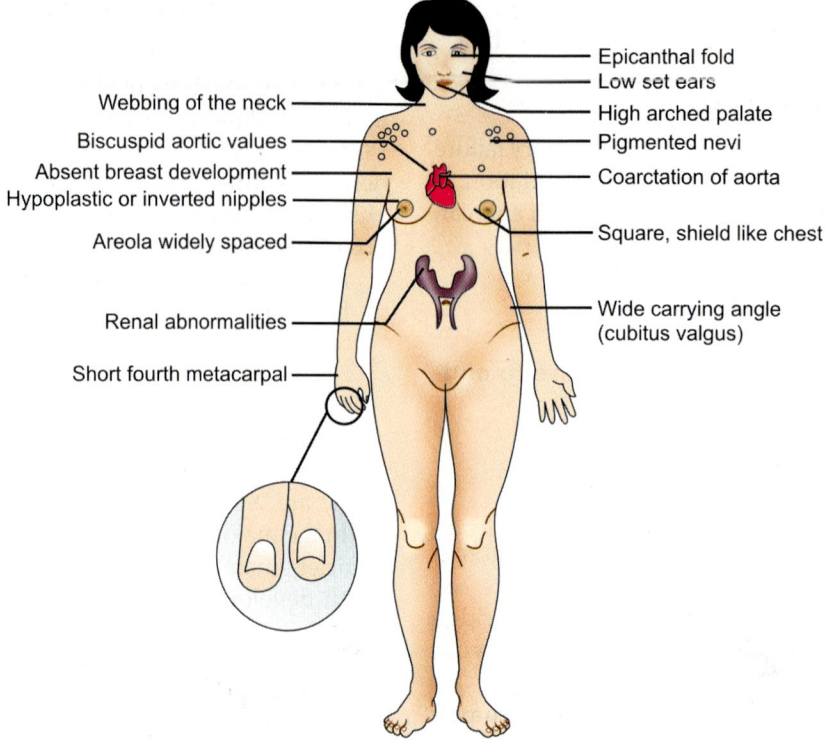

Fig. 8.2: Features of Turner's syndrome

   d. They can have mild insulin resistance, and prone to Keloid formation.
   e. 20% patients have cardiovascular abnormalities like coarctation of aorta, bicuspid aortic valvular, mitral valve prolapse and aortic aneurysm. Rupture of dissection of the aorta in pregnancy achieved with oocyte donation is a complication associated with a mortality rate of about 2%. Women with Turner's syndrome should be screened with echocardiography before planning pregnancy.
   f. They have normal intelligence but can have characteristic cognitive profile like difficulty in mathematical problems, visual motor coordination.

Treatment of Turner's Syndrome

   i. To increase final adult height, use of exogenous recombinant GH can be used and 4-16 cm gain of height can be achieved, especially if early started at 2 - 8 years of age. Weekly doses of GH of 0.375 mg/kg dd in 7 daily doses are typical.
   ii. To promote sexual maturation, therapy with exogenous estrogen should be initiated, when patient is psychologically ready at about 12-13 years of age. Low dose estrogen can be introduced at this time without compromising final adult height.
   iii. Progestin (5-10 mg medroxyprogesterone acetate or 200 mg micronized progesterone) can be added for 12-14 days every 1-2 months to prevent endometrial hyperplasia after patient first experience vaginal bleeding or after 6 months of unopposed estrogen.
   iv. The dose of estrogen is increased slowly over 1-2 years.
   v. They should be carefully monitored for hypertension.
   vi. The patient and their parents should be adequately counseled.
   vii. Calcium and vitamin supplementation is strongly recommended.
   viii. Contraception advice must be given if pregnancy is risk. A low dose oral contraceptive is a good choice for hormonal support and contraception.
   ix. Usually women require oocyte donation, but in mosaicism or rarely classic Turner's syndrome can experience spontaneous pregnancy.

Mixed Gonadal Dysgenesis (Mosaicism)

Mosaicism involving the Y-chromosome can be associated with abnormalities of sex differentiation of the variety of karyotypes possible—45 'X' / 46 'XY' is most common. Clinical presentations range from newborn with ambiguous genitalia to normal fertile male or normal female phenotype with bilateral streak gonads. The diversity is presumed to reflect the relative proportion of 45 'X' and 46 'XY' cells in the gonadal ridge.

Table 8.2: Key points of intersex condition feature

Intersex condition	Karyotype	External genitalia	Internal genitalia	Special features
Congenital adrenal hyperplasia (CAH)	XX	Masculinized	Uterus and ovaries	**Coexisting** glucocorticoid deficiency requiring steroid replacement
Complete androgen insensitivity syndrome (CAIS)	XY	Female	Testes	Absent pubic and axillary hair, at risk of osteoporosis, gonadal malignancy risk until after 50 years of age
Swyer's syndrome	XY	Female	Streak gonads and uterus	High risk of gonadal malignancy, poor breast development, normal axillary and pubic hair
5α reductase deficiency	XY	Female or Ambiguous at birth, Masculinizing at puberty	Testes	If testes in site 60-80% undergo change of gender from female to male in puberty
17α hydroxysteroid dehydrogenase type 3 deficiency	XY	Variable	Testes	As above
True hermaphroditism	71% XX 20% XX/XY 7% XY 2% other	Often ambiguous	Mix of ovary and or testes/ovotestes uterus or male duct	Fertility is sometimes reported

In typical mixed gonadal dysgenesis, usually there is a streak gonad on one side and dysgenetic or normal appearing testis on the other side of abdomen.

Management

The decision to initiate therapy in patient with gonadal dysgenesis should be based on circulating FSH level. Levels in the normal range for patient's age imply the presence of functional gonad.

Gonadal tissue having Y-chromosome component in phenotypic female require removal as soon as the diagnosis is made to avoid the risk of malignant gonadal tumors. It can be accomplished by experienced laparoscopist, with option of laparotomy if gonads prove to be inaccessible. Uterus and fallopian tubes should be preserved for the possibility of pregnancy with donor oocytes.

The key points of all the intersex conditions are summarize in Table 8.2.

MULTIPLE CHOICE QUESTIONS

1. The most common cause of female pseudohermaphroditism:
   a. Virilizing ovarian tumor
   b. Ovarian dysgenesis
   c. Exogenous androgen
   d. Congenital adrenal hyperplasia

   Ans. d

2. What is the appropriate advice for a mother with previous history of delivering a child with congenital adrenal hyperplasia?
   a. To start prednisolone after chorion villous sampling
   b. To start steroid before conception
   c. To start steroid as soon as pregnancy is confirmed
   d. To start after USG examination

   Ans. c

3. A patient of 47 XXY karyotype presents with feature of hypogonadism likely diagnosis is:
   a. Turner's syndrome
   b. Klinefelter's syndrome

c. Edward's syndrome
d. Down syndrome
Ans. b

4. All are seen in testicular feminization syndrome, *except*:
   a. 46 XY
   b. Primary amenorrhea
   c. Short stature
   d. Vagina may be present
   Ans. c

5. The chromosomal component in person with Klinefelter's syndrome is:
   a. 45 XX
   b. 45 XXY
   c. 46 XY
   d. 47 XXY
   Ans. d

6. Gonadal sex in fetus is determined by:
   a. Secretion of testosterone
   b. Secretion of anti-Müllerian hormone
   c. Sex determining region on Y-chromosome
   d. Secretion of estrogen
   Ans. c

7. Sexual infantilism is associated with:
   a. Pituitary tumor
   b. Gonadal aplexia
   c. Dwarfism
   d. All
   Ans. d

8. Barr body is seen in:
   a. Turner's syndrome
   b. Klinefelter's syndrome
   c. Testicular feminization
   d. 46 XY
   Ans. b

9. Characteristic of XO chromosome defect is:
   a. Short stature
   b. Infertility
   c. Widely spaced nipple
   d. All
   Ans. d

10. 16-year-old female presents with primary amenorrhea with bilateral inguinal hernia. She has normal sexual development with no pubic hair. USG shows no uterus and ovarian and a blind vagina. Diagnosis is:
    a. Turner's syndrome
    b. Müllerian agenesis
    c. STAR syndrome
    d. Androgen insensitivity
    Ans. d

11. Androgens insensitivity syndrome. True is:
    a. Phenotypically may be complete female
    b. Predominantly ovarian component in gonads
    c. Always in female
    d. Testis formed abnormally and receptors are normal
    Ans. a

12. A 16-year-old female presents with primary amenorrhea. Examination shows a short blind vagina with absent uterus. The next investigation of choice is:
    a. IVP
    b. Gonadotropin level
    c. Serum prolactin
    d. Karyotype
    Ans. d

9 Amenorrhea

Once a problem is solved,
Its simplicity is amazing.

INTRODUCTION

Evaluation and management of a patient with amenorrhea is a common practice in gynecology and prevalence of pathologic amenorrhea ranges from 3-4% in reproductive aged population.

Definition

Any patient fulfilling the following criteria should be evaluated as having the clinical problem of amenorrhea:
1. No menstrual period by age of 14 in the absence of growth or development of secondary sexual character.
2. No menstrual period by age 16, regardless of the presence of normal growth and development with secondary sex character.
3. In a women who has been menstruating, the absence of period for a length of time equivalent to a total of at least 3 of the previous cyclic interval or 6 months of amenorrhea.

Traditionally amenorrhea has classically been defined as primary (No prior menstruation) or secondary (cessation of menstruation) but this distinction may lead to diagnostic error and should be avoided. There are following basic factors involved in the onset and continuation of normal menstruation:
1. Normal female chromosomal pattern (46 'XX').
2. Coordinated hypothalamic pituitary ovarian axis.
3. Anatomical presence and patency of the outflow tract.
4. Responsive endometrium.
5. Active support of thyroid and adrenal gland.

Physiologic

Amenorrhea occurs in women's life before puberty, during pregnancy and lactation and following menopause. Pregnancy is the most common cause of amenorrhea and must be considered in every patient presenting the evaluation of amenorrhea.

PATHOLOGICAL AMENORRHEA

Numerous classifications have been developed with their strength and weakness. A useful classification in outlined in Table 9.1.

Table 9.1: Classification of cause of amenorrhea

1. Hormonal
   A. Hypergonadotropic hypogonadism
      i. Premature ovarian failure
      ii. Inherited
         a. Chromosomal (gonadal dysgenesis)
         b. Single gene disorder
      iii. Acquired
         a. Infectious
         b. Autoimmune
         c. Iatrogenic
         d. Environmental
         e. Idiopathic
   B. Hypogonadotropic hypogonadism
      i. Hypothalamic disorder
         a. Inherited
            - Idiopathic hypogonadotropic hypogonadism (IHH)
            - Kallman's syndrome
         b. Acquired
            - Functional
            - Eating disorders
            - Excessive exercise
            - Stress
         c. Destructive process
            - Tumor
            - Radiation
            - Infection
            - Infiltrative disease
2. Disorder of anterior pituitary
   A. Inherited
      i. Pituitary hypoplasia
   B. Acquired
      i. Adenoma
      ii. Prolactinoma
   C. Destructive
      i. Radiation
      ii. Trauma

Contd.

Contd.
        iii. Sheehan's syndrome
        iv. Infiltrative disease
  3. Chronic disease
     A. End stage kidney disease
     B. Liver disease
     C. Malignancy
     D. Acquired immunodeficiency syndrome
     E. Malabsorption syndrome
  4. Eugonadotropic amenorrhea
     A. Inherited
        i. Polycystic ovarian syndrome
        ii. Late onset congenital adrenal hyperplasia
        iii. Ovarian tumor (steroid producing)
     B. Acquired
        i. Hyperprolactinemia
        ii. Thyroid disease
        iii. Cushing syndrome
        iv. Acromegaly
  5. Anatomic
     A. Inherited
        i. Müllerian agenesis
        ii. Vaginal septum
        iii. Cervical atresia
        iv. Imperforate hymen
        v. Labial fusion
     B. Acquired
        i. Intrauterine synechia (Asherman syndrome)
        ii. Dilatation and curettage
        iii. Infection—tuberculosis
        iv. Cervical stenosis

Anatomic Disorders

Anatomic abnormality that may present as amenorrhea can broadly be viewed as:
a. Inherited
b. Acquired disorder of the outflow tract.

a. **Inherited:** These are frequent causes of amenorrhea in adolescent and pelvic anatomy is abnormal in approximately 15% women with primary amenorrhea.

Figure 9.1 depicts the range of anatomic defects that may present with amenorrhea. Any transverse blockage of the müllerian system will cause amenorrhea. Causes of out flow obstruction are: (1) Imperforate hymen, (2) Transverse vaginal septum.

Patients with these anomalies have a 46 'XX' Karyotype, female secondary sexual characteristic and normal ovarian function. So amount of uterine bleeding is normal, but typical path for outflow is obstructed or absent.

Accumulation of menstrual blood behind an obstruction frequently results in cyclic abdominal pain or palpable abdominal mass. There is risk of development of endometriosis with complication of chronic pain and infertility.

In complete **müllerian agenesis** often called Mayer Rokitansky Kuster: Hauser syndrome, patients fail to develop any müllerian structure and on examination are found to have only a vaginal dimple. Incidence is

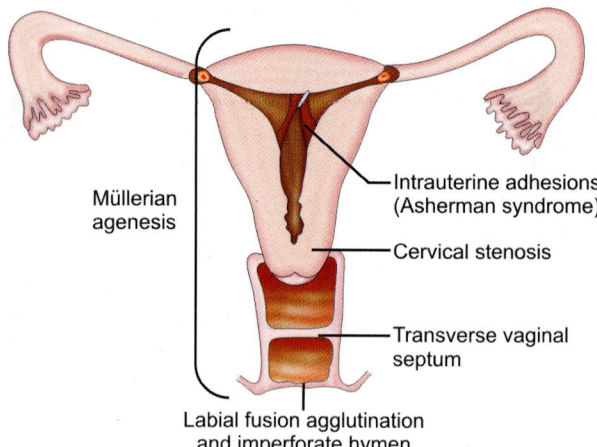

Fig. 9.1: Sites of defects in vagina and uterus causing amenorrhea

1 in 5000, 2nd only to gonadal dysgenesis as a cause of primary amenorrhea.

b. **Acquired:**
   a. Obstruction due to stenosis of cervix after conization, electrosurgery or cryosurgery
   b. *Asherman syndrome*: It is caused by intrauterine synechiae. It may present as amenorrhea, hypomenorrhea or recurrent pregnancy loss.

Etiopathogenesis of Acquired Disorder of Outflow Tract

The endometrium is divided into a functional layer, which lines the endometrial cavity and a basal layer which regenerates the functional layer with each menstrual cycle. Destruction of basal endometrium prevents endometrial thickening in response to ovarian steroid. So, no tissue is produced and shedded, when steroid hormone level fall at the end of luteal phase.

This may follow vigorous curettage after postpartum hemorrhage, miscarriage, or therapeutic abortion complicated with infection. Syndrome can also occur after myomectomy, cesarean section, IUD related infection, or metroplasty. **In developing countries tubercular endometritis is relatively common cause of amenorrhea and infertility**. If these patients are surgically treated and achieve pregnancy, there is increased risk of uterine rupture or placenta accreta.

Endocrine Disorders

Hypergonadotropic Hypogonadism (Premature Ovarian Failure)

This term refer when ovarian function is decreased or absent (Hypogonadism) due to lack of negative feedback, the gonadotropins LH and FSH have increased levels (Hypergonadotropic). So this category implies primary dysfunction at the level of the ovary, not centrally at hypothalamus pituitary level.

Clinical Presentation

In a woman before 40 years there are symptoms of hypoestrogenism and increased FSH level grater than 40 m IU/ml obtained at least 1 month apart. There is generalized sclerosis of ovary or only primordial follicles with the progression.

Causes of premature ovarian failure:

1. *Heritable disorders:*
   a. *Chromosomal defects*: Gonadal dysgenesis is most frequent cause of premature ovarian failure. In this disorder a normal complement of germ cells is present in early fetal ovary, oocytes undergo atresia and the ovary is replaced by fibrous streak. They can have normal or abnormal karyotype. Abnormal karyotype with Turner syndrome can present as primary amenorrhea and infertility. They contribute 2/3rd of gonadal dysgenesis.
   b. *Normal karyotype*: In remaining 1/3rd of patients with gonadal dysgenesis will have a normal karyotype (46 'XX' or 46 'XY') and are said to have pure gonadal dysgenesis. It is poorly understood but is likely due to single gene defect or destruction of gonadal tissue in uterus, perhaps by infection or toxin.
2. *Specific gene defect:*
   a. Mutation in single gene like CYPI7 results in decreased 17α hydroxylase and 17,20 lyase activity, thereby preventing the production of cortisol, androgens and estrogens. These patients have sexual infantilism (lack of breast and hairs development and small uterus) and primary amenorrhea due to lack of estrogen.
   b. Mutation in LH and FSH receptors can cause premature ovarian failure. These mutations prevent normal response to circulating gonadotropins so called resistant ovary syndrome.
   c. Galactosemia inherited as autosomal recessive trait is rare cause of POF.
3. *Acquired:* Hypergonadotropic hypogonadism can be acquired by following:
   a. Autoimmune disease: Auto immune disorder are estimated to account for 40% of POF cases. **It may be one component of polyglandular failure together with hypothyroidism, adrenal insufficiency or other auto immune disorders such as systemic lupus erythematosus.** In addition POF has been associated with myasthenia gravis, idiopathic thrombocytopenic perpura, rheumatoid arthritis, vitiligo, and autoimmune haemolytic anemia.
   b. *Iatrogenic:* Iatrogenic ovarian failure is a relatively common presentation—like surgical excision of significant portion of ovaries following pelvic radiation, or chemotherapy, for treatment of malignancies. A wide variety of environmental toxins like cigarette smoking, heavy metals, solvents, pesticide and industrial chemicals have a clear detrimental effect on follicular health.

Hypogonadotropic Hypogonadism

It implies that primary abnormality is in the hypothalamic pituitary axis. A decrease in gonadotropic stimulation of the ovaries leads to loss of ovarian hormone production. Generally in these patients LH and FSH level are low, but usually in detectable range (< 5 m IU/ml), but may be absent as occurs in Kallmann's syndrome.

Disorders of the Hypothalamus

A. Inherited anomalies
  a. *Kallmann's syndrome:* It is X linked autosomal dominant or autosomal recessive disorder. It is due to mutation in the gene which encodes fibroblastic growth factor receptor 1. Kallmann's syndrome is associated with defect in the ability to smell (*Hyposmia or anosmia*). Kallmann patient have normal complement of GnRH neurons but these neurons fails to migrate and remain in nasal epithelium. So local secreted GnRH fails to stimulate gonadotropins secretion by the anterior pituitary gland. Marked decrease in estrogen cause lack of breast development and menstrual cycle.
  b. Other idiopathic hypogonadotropic hypogonadism (IHH).

B. Acquired hypothalamic dysfunction: Functional disorders of hypothalamic amenorrhea are more common. This diagnosis encompasses three main categories

a. *Eating disorder:* Anorexia nervosa and Bulimia both can result in amenorrhea. Anorexia nervosa is associated with severe caloric restriction, weight loss, self-induced vomiting, excessive use of laxative and compulsive exercise. Weight loss is generally less severe in bulimic women, who eat in binges, and than purge to maintain weight.
b. *Exercise induced amenorrhea:* This is most commonly seen in women whose exercise regimen is associated with significant loss of fat as ballet, gymnastics.
c. *Stress induced amenorrhea:* This may be associated with clearly traumatic life events as death of family member or divorce.
d. *Pseudocyesis:* It is Rare. This diagnosis should be considered in women presenting with amenorrhea and pregnancy symptoms. *Pseudocyesis exemplifies the ability of the mind to control physiologic process.* A common link in these patients is a history of severe grief. Psychiatric treatment is generally required to treat the associated depression.

C. Anatomic destruction: Any process that destroys the hypothalamus can impair GnRH secretion and lead to the development of hypogonadotropic hypogonadism and amenorrhea, e.g. CNS tumor associated with amenorrhea include craniopharyngioma, germinomas, endodermal sinus tumor and glioma as well metastatic lesion. Craniopharyngioma are most common and located in suprasellar region and patient frequently present with headache and visual changes.

Disorders of Anterior Pituitary Gland

A. Inherited abnormalities of pituitary gland: Inherited disorders are uncommon and involve mutation in genes that encode the LH or FSH subunit or the GnRH receptors.

B. Acquired pituitary dysfunction: Most pituitary dysfunction is acquired after menarche and therefore women present with normal pubertal development followed by secondary amenorrhea.

Pituitary tumors: Pituitary adenomas are most common cause of acquired pituitary dysfunction. The most common adenoma secrete prolactin, however, altered secretion of any pituitary derived hormone can result in amenorrhea. The women can present with only hyperprolactinemia or associated with galactorrhea. Pituitary tumors also may indirectly alter gonadotropic function via pressure effect. The tumor mass may compress neighboring gonadotropes or may damage the pituitary stalk, disrupting dopamine inhibition of prolactin secretion.

Alteration in function of pituitary gland: Pituitary function can be disrupted by inflammation, infiltrative disease or metastatic lesion. In addition there can be loss of pituitary function following surgical or radiation treatment of pituitary adenoma.

Sheehan's syndrome: It refers to panhypopituitarism that develops after massive postpartum hemorrhage complicated by hypotension. In most severe form, patient develops shock and pituitary apoplexy. Loss of gonadotropic activity results in anovulation and subsequent amenorrhea. Damage to other pituitary cells may present as failure to lactate, loss of sexual and axillary hair, hypothyroidism and adrenal insufficiency. The pituitary cell types are differentially sensitive to damage. Prolactin secretion deficiency is the most common followed by loss of gonadotropins and growth hormone release, loss of ACTH and least commonly by decrease in thyroid stimulating hormone.

Other causes of hypogonadotropic hypogonadism: It is observed in wide variety of chronic disease including end stage kidney disease, liver disease, malignancies, acquired immunodeficiency syndrome and malabsorption syndrome.

C. Eugonadotropic amenorrhea: There are number of diseases that produce amenorrhea which are not associated with significantly abnormal gonadotropin levels. In these patients chronic steroid secretion interferes with the normal feedback between the ovary and hypothalamic pituitary axis. The lack of cyclicity interferes with normal oocyte maturation, and menstruation failure occurs. . **This is in contrast to the patient with ovarian failure or hypothalamic pituitary failure in which estrogen is low**. This distinction is useful in evaluation and treatment. There can be following presentations:

a. *Polycystic ovary syndrome:* It is by far the commonest cause of chronic anovulation with estrogen present. Presentation can be varied ranging from occasional ovulatory cycles to menometrorrhagia secondary to unopposed estrogen stimulation of the endometrium to complete amenorrhea. Amenorrhea in PCOS is attributed to atrophic effects of androgen on endometrial proliferation. An elevated ratio of LH: FSH level (> 2-fold) is noted in most patients.

b. *Adult onset congenital adrenal hyperplasia:* It is due to mutation in CYP21 gene, which encodes the 21 hydroxylase enzyme. These patients are unable to convert an adequate percentage of progesterone to cortisol and aldosterone, thus increasing the production of androgens. Likes PCOS, elevated androgens level blunt oocyte maturation and thereby result in anovulation and amenorrhea.

c. *Ovarian tumors:* It is uncommon. Sex steroid stromal tumors with production of either estrogen or androgen can cause chronic anovulation.

d. *Hyperprolactinemia and hypothyroidism:* Thyroid disease is relatively common cause of oligomenorrhea associated with normal gonadotropins. Classically hypothyroidism is stated to cause amenorrhea while hyperthyroidism is implicated in menorrhagia. Hyperprolactinemia can be primary, like in prolactin secreting tumors, or may be secondary due to an elevation in TRH. In secondary hyperprolactinemia, prolactin levels are generally relatively less than 100 ng/ml (generally level are relatively low than primary hyperprolactinemia). Increase in circulating prolactin results in compensatory increase in central dopamine, which alters GnRH secretion and prevents ovulation. Drugs that stimulate hyperprolactinemia are antipsychotic as haloperidol, tricyclic antidepressant, antihypertensive, antianxiety drugs, etc.

EVALUATION IN CASE OF AMENORRHEA

History-Taking

The evaluation of menstrual abnormalities should start with questions regarding pubertal development, any regular menstrual cyclicity and its pattern, and whether development of amenorrhea is correlated with pelvic infection, surgery, radiation, chemotherapy or other illness,

In addition a thorough medical history and any surgery especially prior pelvic surgery should be obtained.

A focused review of symptom is helpful. New onset headache or visual change may suggest a tumor of central nervous system. *Spontaneous bilateral discharge from breast is consistent with diagnosis of hyperprolactinemia.* Thyroid disease may be associated with heat or cold intolerance or weight changes. Hot flushes and vaginal dryness suggest hypergonadotropic hypogonadism or POF. Hirsutism and acne are seen with PCOS and late onset CAH. *Cyclic pelvic pain would suggest a reproductive tract outlet obstruction.* Family history of POF, autoimmune disease would suggest an increased risk for POF. Social history should investigate exposure to environmental toxins like cigarettes and any antipsychotic drugs.

Physical Examination

A thorough physical examination will frequently provide a diagnosis. *General appearance* is helpful. In eating disorders there is low body mass index with loss of teeth enamel due to recurrent vomiting. Phenotype of Turner syndrome should be evaluated. Midline facial defect as cleft palate are consistent with a developmental defect of the anterior pituitary gland.

Visual field changes and other visual defect may be indication of a tumor in the pituitary gland or central nervous system. Skin should be inspected for acanthosis nigricans, hirsutism or acne which may indicate PCOS or other causes of hyperandrogenism. Hypothyroidism may present as enlarged thyroid gland, delayed reflex and bradycardia. *Bilateral galactorrhea* implies the hyperprolactinemia.

Genitalia examination should start with noting hair pattern. Sparse or absent female pubic hair may be lack of adrenarche or androgen insensitivity syndrome. While elevated androgen level will result in a male pattern of genital hair growth. Evidence of estrogen production includes a pink moist vagina and cervical mucus. Müllerian anomalies can be examined by rectal examination. Hematocolpos suggest normal ovarian and endometrial function.

Laboratory Testing

1. *Exclude pregnancy:* By urinary or serum β-hCG level.
2. *Progesterone withdrawal:* Classically patients are given exogenous progesterone like 10 mg oral medrox progesterone for 5 days and monitored for progesterone withdrawal bleed. **A positive test** is any bleeding within 2-10 days of the test. In positive test a woman is assumed to produce estrogen and to have an intact endometrium and patent outflow tract. If bleeding does not follow **(Negative test)**, a patient is given estrogen followed by progesterone treatment. If a woman again fails to bleed, then an anatomic abnormality is diagnosed.
3. *Serum hormone level:* It is more reasonable to begin with hormonal evaluation in any women found to have a normal pelvic examination.
4. *Follicle stimulating hormone (FSH):* FSH level differentiates hypergonadotropic and hypogonadotropic form of hypogonadism. **An elevated FSH level strongly suggests premature ovarian failure.** Two FSH level > 40 mIU/mL obtained at interval of one month is diagnostic. Estriol level at the same time can be measured, which are low. If FSH level is low, then estimation should be repeated with additional LH level to confirm hypogonadotropic hypogonadism. In these cases GnRH stimulation test can be done.
5. *Prolactin and thyroid stimulating hormone:* Both hormone should be measured simultaneously because of close relationship between thyroid disease and prolactin level.
6. *Testosterone:* It is measured in any women with suspected PCOS or signs of clinical excess of androgen. Mild increase is coexistent with PCOS, but value > 200 ng/dl is consistent with presence of an ovarian tumors and added sonography is needed.
7. *Dehydroepiandrosterone sulfate:* High normal or mild increased level are associated with PCOS, while adrenal adenoma may produce circulating DHEAS level above 700 μg/dl, and MRI and CT of adrenal is warranted.
8. *Other serum testing:* If there is suggestion of eating disorder, serum electrolyte should be immediately preformed as electrolyte imbalance is life threatening. An ECG should also be added. Women with PCOS should be screened for insulin resistance and lipid abnormalities and repeated every few years.
9. *Radiological evaluation:* Any patients with hypogonadotropic hypogonadism should be assumed to have an anatomic abnormality unless proven otherwise by imaging of the brain and pituitary gland with MRI or a CT scan. **So functional hypothalamic amenorrhea due to stress, exercise or eating disorder is a diagnosis of exclusion.** USG is indicated in all cases to exclude pregnancy, presence or absence of uterus, ovaries, and blood collection in müllerian system, PCOS and any ovarian tumor and to know associated renal tract abnormality.
10. *Chromosomal analysis:* Patients with gonadal dysgenesis as Turner syndrome should be considered for karyotype testing. Though classic teaching suggest that this test is unnecessary after age of 30. A 'Y' cell line requires bilateral oophorectomy because of increased risk for malignancy. Many specialist advice karyotyping for all women with POF, who are shorter than 60 inches or and with family history of POF.

Investigation for Specific Disorders

a. *Premature ovarian failure:* For etiology testing for autoimmune disease can be done.
b. *Anatomic disorders:* To be confirmed with hysterosalpingography and USG. Saline infusion

sonography is excellent for detection of intrauterine synechiae or developmental anomalies.

Malformation of other organ system should be searched in patient with müllerian agenesis like urinary tract, spine.

Treatment

The treatment of amenorrhea depends on the etiology as well as the aim of the patient such as desire to treat hirsutism or to become pregnant. Anatomical abnormalities like imperforate hymen, vaginal septum require surgical correction. CNS tumor may require surgical resection after careful evaluation.

Hypothyroidism should be treated with thyroid replacement and Hyperprolactinemia with dopamine agonist like bromocriptine or cabergoline. Macroadenoma may require surgery.

Estrogen Replacement

Individuals with amenorrhea associated with all forms of gonadal failure (Hypo as Hypergonadotropic) need cyclic estrogen and progestin therapy to initiate mature and maintain secondary sexual characteristic. *Prevention of osteoporosis is an additional benefit of estrogen therapy.* Therapy is usually started with 0.625 mg/day conjugated estrogen or 1 mg/day of estradiol. If patient is short in stature, higher dose should not be used in an attempt to prevent premature closure of the epiphysis. Estrogen can be given daily in combination with progestin or progesterone to prevent unopposed estrogen stimulation of the endometrium in patients with a uterus. Younger women may be given combined oral contraceptive pills. For most patients therapy is continued until normal age of menopause, which is 45-48 years.

If 17α hydroxylase deficiency is confirmed treatment is instituted with corticosteroid replacement as well as estrogens.

Specific therapies are directed towards eating disorder, stress and exercise amenorrhea, malnutrition and chronic disease. In patient with eating disorders, psychiatric intervention is imperative due to significant morbidity and mortality with this diagnosis. Elite athlete may choose not to alter their exercise regimen and well therefore require estrogen treatment. If the patient has physiological delay of puberty, the only management is reassurance.

Polycystic Ovaries

Treatment of PCO may include cyclic progesterone or oral contraceptives or other forms of estrogen progesterone treatment. Patient with insulin resistance can be given insulin sensitizing agents as metformin. Hyperandrogenism due to PCOS may be treated with oral contraceptive and or spiranolactone.

Option for infertility treatment in cases of amenorrhea: If woman desire conception, treatment may require modification.

a. Adequate treatment of hyperprolactinemia and thyroid-disease results in ovulation and normal fertility.
b. Surgical correction of anatomic abnormality. But if correction is not possible, surrogacy can be considered.
c. POF patient require IVF with donor oocytes.
d. Hypogonadotropic hypogonadism typically require GnRH or gonadotropins from an infertility specialist. It is to be emphasized that there is risk of death in pregnant patients with Turner syndrome resulting from dissection of coarctation of aorta and rupture. *So before treatment option of donor oocyte, careful counseling and investigation should be undertaken.*
e. PCOS patient frequently ovulate with clomiphene citrate or aromatase inhibitor.

Patient Education

In amenorrhea the patient should be adequately counseled about their diagnosis, the long-term implication of the diagnosis and the treatment. The potential for child-bearing should also be discussed. The benefits of therapy, its limitation and side effects should be explained to these women.

MULTIPLE CHOICE QUESTIONS

1. Commonest cause of female pseudohermaphroditism:
   a. Virilizing ovarian tumor
   b. Ovarian dysgenesis
   c. Exogenous androgen
   d. Congenital adrenal hyperplasia
   Ans. d
2. What is the appropriate advice for a mother with previous history of delivering a child with congenital adrenal hyperplasia.
   a. To start prednisolone after chorion villous sampling
   b. To start steroid before conception
   c. To start steroid as soon as pregnancy is confirmed
   d. To start after USG examination
   Ans. c
3. A patient of 47 XX Y karyotype presents with feature of hypogonadism likely diagnosis is:
   a. Turner syndrome
   b. Klinefelter's syndrome
   c. Edward's syndrome
   d. Down's syndrome
   Ans. b
4. All are seen in testicular feminization syndrome, *except*:
   a. 46 XY
   b. Primary amenorrhea
   c. Short stature
   d. Vagina may be present
   Ans. c
5. The chromosomal component in person with Klinefelter syndrome is:
   a. 45 XX.
   b. 45 XXY.

Chapter -9 ♦ Amenorrhea

   c. 46 XY.
   d. 47 XXY.
   Ans. d.
6. Gonadal sex in fetus is determined by:
   a. Secretion of testosterone
   b. Secretion of anti-müllerian hormone
   c. Sex determining region on Y chromosome
   d. Secretion of estrogen
   Ans. c
7. Sexual infantilism is associated with:
   a. Pitutary tumor
   b. Gonadal aplexia
   c. Dwarfism
   d. All
   Ans. d
8. Barr body is seen in:
   a. Turner syndrome
   b. Kleinfelter syndrome
   c. Testicular feminization
   d. 46 XY
   Ans. b
9. Characteristic of XO chromosome defect is:
   a. Short stature
   b. Infertility
   c. Widely spaced nipple
   d. All
   Ans. d
10. 16 year ole female presents with primary amenorrhea with bilateral inguinal hernia. She has normal sexual development with no pubic hair. USG shows no uterus and ovarian and a blind vagina. Diagnosis is:
    a. Turner's syndrome
    b. Müllerian agenesis
    c. STAR syndrome
    d. Androgen insensitivity
    Ans. d
11. Androgens insensitivity syndrome. True is:
    a. Phenotypically may be complete female
    b. Predominantly ovarian component in gonads
    c. Always in female
    d. Testis formed abnormally and receptors are normal
    Ans. a
12. A 16 years old female presents with primary amenorrhea. Examination shows a short blind vagina with absent uterus. The next investigation of choice is:
    a. IVF
    b. Gonadotropin level
    c. Serum prolactin
    d. Karyotype
    Ans. d

10. Benign Lesions of the Vulva and Vagina

Our mind is a jungle,
Proper education converts it in a garden.

GENERAL CONSIDERATION

Benign vulvar and vaginal disorder are common gynecological conditions. These disorders may present with significant clinical symptoms or may be asymptomatic and noted only during routine examination.

This chapter reviews the predisposing factors that contribute to the development of these disorders as well as evaluation, diagnosis and treatment of the different benign vulvovaginal disorders.

Anatomy and Physiology

Anatomy is described in the earlier chapters. The development of vulvar and vaginal disorder is influenced in part by presence or absence of endogenous and exogenous estrogen. Estrogen thickens the vaginal epithelium and results in presence of large quantities of glycogen in epithelial cells which results in production of lactic acid. The acid environment (pH 3.5–4.0) promotes the growth of normal vaginal flora, chiefly lactobacilli and acidogenic *corynebacteria*.

The absence of endogenous estrogen in prepubertal girls results in a thin vaginal epithelium, which predisposes this age group most commonly to bacterial infections. In postmenopausal women endogenous estrogen production declines, the cells of the vaginal epithelium and vulvar skin lose glycogen and vaginal acidity declines. The resulting atrophic vaginal and vulvar tissue is prone to trauma and infections and the lactobacilli are replaced by a mixed flora consisting chiefly of pathogenic cocci.

Vulvar irritation also occurs with urinary and fecal soiling, which can be an underlying factor in this age group.

Vulvar Disorders

They are classified in Table 10.1

Table 10.1: Benign lesions of vulva

I. Vascular and lymphatic disease
   - Varicosity
   - Hematoma
   - Hemangioma
   - Edema
   - Granulosa pyogenicum
   - Lymphangioma

II. Vulvar manifestation of systemic disease
   - Leukemia
   - Dermatological disorders, e.g.
     - disseminated lupus erythematosus
     - pemphigus vulgaris
     - contact dermatitis, psoriasis
   - Obesity
   - Diabetes mellitus
   - Bechet's syndrome

III. Viral infection
   - Herpes genitalis
   - Herpes zoster
   - Molluscum contagiosum
   - Condyloma acuminatum

IV. Infestation of the vulva
   - Pediculosis pubis
   - Scabies, Enterobiasis

V. Fungal infection of vulva
   - Candidiasis, fungal dermatitis

VI. Vulvar non-neoplastic epithelial disorders
   - Lichen sclerosis, squamous cell hyperplasia
   - Other dermatosis, lichen planus, lichen simplex

VII. Benign cystic tumors
   - Epidermal cyst
   - Sebaceous cyst
   - Apocrine sweat gland cyst
   - Skene duct cyst
   - Urethral diverticulum, inguinal hernia
   - Gartner's duct cyst, Bartholian duct cyst and abscess

VIII. Benign solid tumor
   - Acrochordon
   - Pigmented nevi
   - Leiomyoma, Fibroma, Lipoma
   - Neurofibroma
   - Granular cell myoblastoma

Vulvar Varicosity

Vulvar varicosity may involve one or more vein which may be aggravated during pregnancy. Symptomatic vulvar varices in patients who are not pregnant are uncommon and may signify an underlying vascular disease in the pelvis either primary or secondary to tumors in the pelvis. Whatever is the cause, varicosity can cause considerable discomfort consisting of pain, pruritis and sense of heaviness.

On examination, one can see dilated plexus of veins, which is best seen in standing position. Sometimes rupture of a vulvar varicosity during pregnancy may cause profuse hemorrhage. There may be pain and tenderness if there is acute phlebitis or thrombosis.

Treatment

Treatment is seldom necessary although symptoms might be quite severe during pregnancy. Supporting clothing give adequate relief, pregnancy management is guided by standard obstetric care. Persistent postpartum cases can be treated with injection of a sclerosing agent.

Hematoma

The vulva has rich blood supply predominantly from the pudendal vessels. If vessel is improvised spontaneously or by trauma, during delivery or by blunt object like bicycle stand, horn of animal, significant bleeding and hematoma formation can occur because of the distensible nature of the vulvar tissue (Figs 10.1A and B). Following trauma, an icepack should be applied. If hematoma continues to expand than the hematoma should be incised, clots are evacuated and any bleeders should be ligated. The wound is packed and left open or closed with a drain in place, if required. Pack is removed after 24–48 hours. Antibiotics are administered depending on the initiating event and contamination in the area.

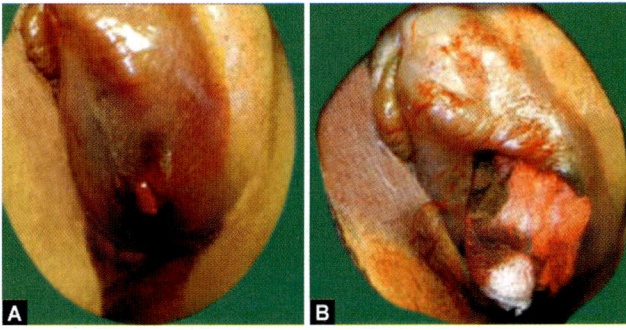

Figs 10.1A and B: (A) Vulvar hematoma; (B) Hematoma drained and packed

Edema

The loose integument of the vulva predisposes to the development of edema. Severe generalized vulvar edema may represent an underlying illness such as pre-eclampsia or eclampsia, severe anemia, congestive heart failure, nephrotic syndrome. Acute edema may sometimes develop from a systemic or local allergic reaction.

Vascular or lymphatic obstruction may be caused by underlying neoplasm or infection as Lymphogranuloma venerum which can cause extensive lymphatic obstruction and gross deformity of vulvar tissues.

Accidental trauma from a bicycle accident (saddle injury) or kick to pudendum may cause painful swelling. After acute trauma ice packs should be applied immediately to reduce development of significant edema. Warm packs or warm sitz bath may then be applied after 1–2 days to help resolve associated inflammation or hematoma.

Granuloma Pyogenicum

Pyogenic granuloma is considered to be a variant of a capillary hemangioma. It is usually single, raised and dull red. If size is less than 3 cm. it tends to bleed easily if traumatized. Wide excisional biopsy is indicated to alleviate symptoms and to rule out malignant melanoma.

Hemangioma

a. **Senile:** Senile (cherry) hemangioma usually are multiple, small, dark, blue, asymptomatic papules discovered incidentally during examination of the older patients. Excision biopsy is needed only if the hemangioma bleeds repeatedly. A cryosurgical probe or carbon dioxide laser can also be used.
b. **Childhood:** Childhood hemangiomas usually are diagnosed in the first few months of life. They may vary in size from small strawberry hemangioma to large cavernous one. Usually they become static or regress without therapy after approximately age of 18 months. Most of these hemangiomas can be observed without therapy, larger ones may require treatment with cryosurgery, argon laser therapy.
c. **Lymphangioma:** Lymphangioma are tumors of the lymphatic vessels. Lymphangioma cavernosum may cause a diffuse enlargement of one side of the vulva and perineum. A tumor which is sufficiently enlarged should be surgically excised. Lymphangioma simplex tumors (circumscription tumors) usually are small, soft, white, or purple nodules or small wart like lesion most commonly seen on labia majora. They are usually asymptomatic and do not require excision, unless intense pruritis and excoriation are present. And are not alleviated with topical measure.

Vulvar Manifestation of Systemic Disease

1. *Dermatological disorders:* Recurrent ulceration of the mucous membranes of the mouth and vagina may be a manifestation of *disseminated lupus erythematosus*. Bulbous eruption of apparently normal skin and mucus membrane surface of vulva may be one of the first signs of pemphigus vulgaris. *Contact dermatitis* is an inflammatory response of the vulvar tissue to agents that may either be locally irritating or induce sensitivity on contact. The local reaction to a systemically administered drug is called *dermatitis medicamentosa*. *Psoriasis* is a chronic relapsing dermatosis that may also affect the scalp, extensor surface of the extremities, the trunk and vulva. The vulvar skin may be the only body surface affected. Primary lesion of psoriasis is typically erythematous, sharply demarcated lesion, resembling Candidial infection. **Treatment** is *topical corticosteroids*.
2. *Obesity:* Acanthosis nigricans is a benign hyper-pigmented lesion characterized by papillomatous hypertrophy. It may be associated with an underlying adenocarcinoma. Pseudoacanthosis nigricans is a benign process that may appear on the skin of the vulva and inner thigh in obese and darkly pigmented women. In these women glucose intolerance, insulin resistance, chronic anovulation, and androgen disorders may be associated. *Intertrigo* is an inflammatory reaction involving the genitocrural folds or the skin under the abdominal panniculus. It is common in obese patients caused by persistent moistness of the skin surface. There may be superimposed superficial fungal or bacterial infection. **Treatment** measures are to promote dryness as wearing absorbent cotton undergarments and dusting with corn starch powder.
3. *Diabetes mellitus:* Diabetes mellitus is the systemic disease most commonly associated with chronic pruritus vulva. Diabetes vulvitis is caused by a chronic vulvovaginal candidiasis. A diagnosis of diabetes should be confirmed or excluded with glucose tolerance test in any patient who responds poorly to antifungal treatment or who has recurrent fungal infections. In uncontrolled diabetes, the vulvar epithelium often undergoes lichenification and secondary bacterial infection. Treatment is controlling the diabetes and specific therapy for the bacterial or fungal infection. Suppressive antifungal therapy using Fluconazole should be initiated in diabetic patients with recurrent vulvovaginal candidiasis.
4. *Bechet's syndrome:* It is a rare inflammatory disorder of unknown cause characterized by recurrent oral and genital ulceration and uveitis. Treatment is only palliative care. Topical and systemic corticosteroids provide the most consistent relief. Patient may require long term management by a dermatologist.
5. *Lukemia:* Rarely nodular inflammation and ulceration of vulva and rectovaginal septum occur with acute leukemia.

Viral Infection

Genital herpes virus: It is sexually transmitted infection with incubation period of first attack in usually 2–10 days. Lesions are initially vesicular but rupture to form single, multiple or grouped shallow, tender ulcers, 1-2 mm in diameter. Lesions are most common on the labia majora and minora, clitoris, perineum and perianal areas.

Treatment

Acyclovir is the drug of choice for treatment of outbreaks. However it does not influence rate of recurrence.

Human papilloma virus: It is sexually transmitted with incubation period ranging from 3 weeks to 8 months. HPV virus manifests on the vulva as genital warts. Commonly warts are papular, appearing as small raised, rounded lesion, usually multiple. Sometimes present as 'Condylomata acuminata', which are irregular fleshy vascular tumors affecting any part of the vulva. Treatment is **repeat application of Trichloroacetic acid, Podophyllin, topical Imiquinod (Aldara), Cryotherapy or laser therapy.**

Infestation of Vulva

Pediculosis Pubis

The crab louse (Phthirus pubis) is transmitted through sexual contact or from shared infected bedding or clothing. Treatment consists of **Permethrin 1% cream, Lindane 1% shampoo or Pyrethrin with Piperonyl Butoxide.** Lindane is not recommended for pregnant or lactating women or for children younger than two years. All contacts should be treated and contact clothing should be sterilized.

Scabies

Sarcoptes scabiei causes intractable itching and excoriation of the skin surface in the vicinity of minute skin burrows, where parasites have deposited ova. The itch mite is transmitted often directly from infected persons. The patient should take a hot soapy bath, scrubbing the burrowes and encrusted areas thoroughly.

Treatment consists of Permethrin cream (5%) which should be applied to the entire body from the neck down, with particular attention to the hands, wrist, axilla, breast and anogenital regions. It should be washed off after 8–14 hours. Alternatively Lindane 1% in lotion or cream form can be applied in a thin layer on all areas of the body and washed off after 8 hours. All contacts or persons in the family must be treated in the same way to prevent reinfection. All potentially infected clothing or bedding should be washed or dry cleaned. Therapy should be repeated in 10–14 days if new lesion develops.

Enterobiasis (Pinworm, Seatworm)

Enterobiasis vermicularis infection is common in children. Nocturnal perineal itching is described by patient and perianal excoriation may be observed. Diagnosis can be confirmed by microscopic examination for ova and adhesive tape sticked to lesions which are examined under microscope for ova.

For prevention, patient should wash their hands and scrub their nails following each defecation. Underclothes must be boiled. Ammoniated mercury ointment to the perianal regions relieves itching. Pinworm is treated with systemic treatment with **Pyrantel pamoate, Mebendazole, or Pyrvinium pamoate.**

Other Infections of the Vulva

Tuberculosis (Vulvovaginal lupus vulgaris): Pudendal tuberculosis is manifested by chronic, normally painful, exudative 'sores' that are tender, reddish, moderately raised firm and nodules with central apple jelly like contents. There can be induration and sinus formation. Systemic antituberculous therapy should be given with local Burrow's solution (aluminum acetate solution).

Furunculosis: Vulvar folliculitis is caused by a staphylococcal infection of hair follicles. Furunculosis occurs if the infection spreads into perifollicular tissues producing localized cellulitis.

A furuncle begins as a hard, tender, and subcutaneous nodule that rupture through the skin, discharging blood and purulent maternal. After that lesion heal. Minor infections can be treated by application of topical antibiotic lesion. Deeper infection can be brought to a head with hot soaps after which the pustules should be incised and drained. If there is extensive Furunculosis systemic antibiotic are warranted.

Hydradenitis

Hydradenitis suppurativa is a refractory process of the apocrine sweat glands usually associated with staphylococci or streptococcal infection. The apocrine sweat glands of the vulva become active following puberty. Inspissation of secretory material and secondary infection may be related to occlusion of the ducts. Initially, multiple pruritic subcutaneous nodules appear that eventually develop into abscesses and rupture.

Treatment early in the disease consist of drainage and administration of antibiotic according to organism culture and sensitivity. Long term therapy with isoretinon may be considered. Antiandrogenic therapy with cyproterone acetate or ethinyl estradiol may be an alternative but highly effective treatment.

Erysipelas

Erysipelas is a rapidly spreading erythematous lesion of the skin, which is caused by invasion of superficial lymphatics by β-hemolytic streptococcus. Though erysipelas of vulva is very rare and is commonly seen after trauma to the vulva or a surgical procedure.

Systemic symptoms are chills, fever, and malaise associated with an erythematous vulvitis. **Treatment** is systemic penicillin or tetracycline in large dosages.

VULVAR NON-NEOPLASTIC EPITHELIAL DISORDERS

Vulvar dystrophies represent a spectrum of atrophic and hypertrophic lesions caused by a variety of stimuli resulting in circumscribed or diffuse white lesions. These lesions present classically with intense pruritis with or without pain and vulvar epithelial changes. Differentiating in between these disorders and ruling out an underlying malignant process require histopathological diagnosis. The risk of underlying malignancy is less than 5%. The patients must be examined periodically and multiple biopsies may be needed. Toludine blue test helps in identifying areas of maximum epithelial hyperactivity for taking site selected biopsy.

International Society for the Study of Vulvovaginal Disease (ISSVD), characterized following lesions:
1. Lichen sclerosis
2. Squamous cell hyperplasia
3. Other dermatosis.

Lichen Sclerosis

Lichen sclerosis is a benign, chronic inflammatory process and the most common vulvar dermatologic disorder. Its **etiology** is not known. Multifactorial process is most likely involved in its development. Estrogen deficiency, autoimmunity, genetic and familial tendency has been implicated in its etiopathogenesis. **Clinical feature** during **acute phase**—the lesion may appear red or purple and classically involves the non hair bearing areas of the vulva, perineum and perianal area in an hourglass pattern. The patient experiences intense pruritis leading to scratch cycle, ulceration and ultimately scar formation. Pruritis is thought to result from inflammation of local terminal nerve fibers.

With **chronic disease**, the skin is thin, wrinkled and white and has a *cigarette paper appearance*. The vulvar structure contracts with agglutination of the labia minora and prepuce and introital stenosis (Figs 10.2A and B). Symptoms of pain including dyspareunia occur mostly from decreased skin elasticity with loss of elastin from the upper dermis.

Thus, although skin atrophy may ultimately develop, the underlying disease is inflammatory in nature. Consequently areas of dysplasia may develop so suspicious

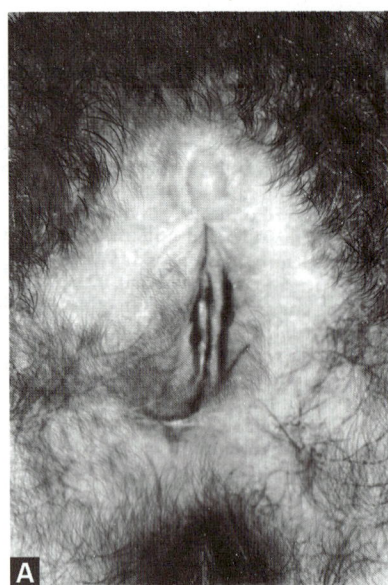

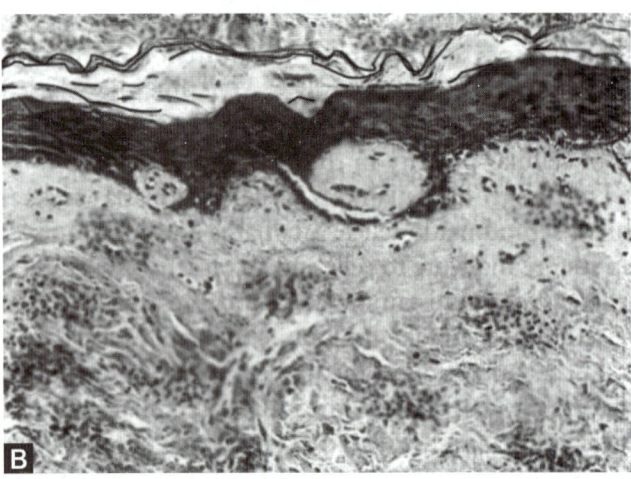

Figs 10.2A and B: (A) Advance lesion of lichen sclerosis; (B) Microscopic appearance of lichen sclerosis

area must be biopsied. Repeat biopsy should be taken as indicated because of possible 4-6% risk of developing squamous cell carcinoma.

Differential Diagnosis

a. *Vitiligo:* Produces a depigmented pattern like lichen sclerosis but vulvar architecture is normal with vitiligo.
b. *Estrogen deficient atrophy:* It leads to thinning of epidermis with labial adhesion and dyspareunia. If local therapy with estrogen does not show improvement a vulvar biopsy should be done.

Treatment

Treatment involves initially stopping the itching scratch cycle, and minimizing dermal inflammation. Ultrapotent steroid cream or ointment are most effective. **Clobetasol propionate** 0.05% twice daily for one month and then daily for 3 months, has 75% success rate. An oral antihistamine agent can be added at bed time. 2% testosterone and progesterone cream has been used but they are minimally effective and should not be used as a first line therapy. In addition, patient should be told to avoid tight undergarments, daily cleaning with mild soap and use of hair dryer to keep the vulvar skin dry.

Squamous Cell Hyperplasia

It is also known as hyperplastic dystrophy, atopic dermatitis, atopic eczema, and neurodermatitis.

Etiopathogenesis

Chronic trauma secondary to rubbing, scratching or vulvo vaginal infection elicits lichenification, a protective response of the involved skin which causes epithelial thickening and hyperkeratosis.

Clinical Feature

During active phase, the lesions may be red and moist and demonstrate evidence of secondary infection. This is exacerbated by the accompanying pruritis which lead to rubbing and scratching, at times may be involuntary.

As epithelial thickening develops, the environment of the vulva causes maceration and a raised while lesion may be circumscribed or diffuse and may involve any portion of the vulva, adjacent thighs, perineum or perianal skin.

Vulvar Biopsy

Thickened white plaques on the vulva should typically prompt vulvar biopsy to exclude pre invasive or invasive lesions. Biopsy is performed with Keye's punch biopsy instruments. This tool has an open, circular sharp edged tip that is designed to remove a vertical core of tissue when pressed against the skin. Once the dermis has been cut, fine dissecting scissors are used to undermine the circular biopsy and free it.

Keye's punches are available in a variety of diameter ranging from 2 mm to 6 mm. Following excision, bleeding may be controlled with direct pressure, silver nitrate stick or Monsel's solution (Fig. 10.3).

Management

Biopsy must be performed to eliminate intraepithelial neoplasm or invasive tumors. In squamous cell hyperplasia, histology demonstrates hyperkeratosis and acanthosis producing epithelial thickening and elongated rete pegs, while atypical hyperplasia or cancer is characterized by nuclear pleomorphesim and loss of cellular polarity in the epithelium.

Treatment is symptomatic. Sitz bath and lubricant help to restore moisture of cells and reconstruct the epithelial barrier. **Oral antihistaminics or antidepressant (selective**

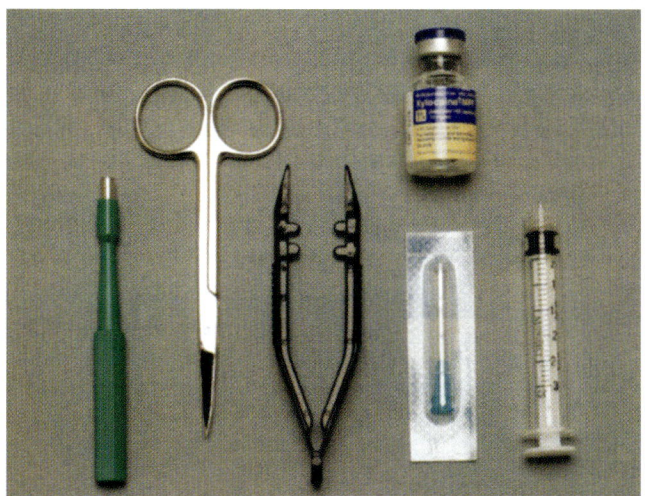

Fig. 10.3: Equipment of vulvar biopsy

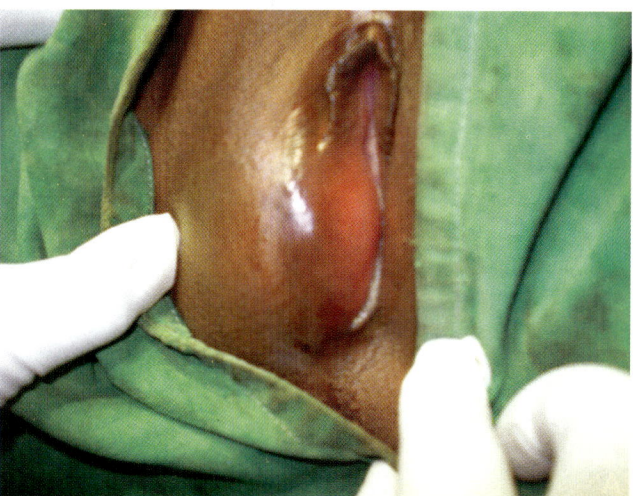

Fig. 10.4: Bartholin's abscess

serotonin reuptake inhibitors) may help relieve pruritis. Local application of medium potency topical steroid twice per day can decrease inflammation and pruritis. Vulvar epithelium takes at least 6 weeks to heal. In intractable lesion, subcutaneous intralesional injection of steroid can be considered.

Lichen Planus

Incidence and Etiopathogenesis

Lichen planus is an uncommon disease that involves both cutaneous and mucosal surface. It equally affects men and women between ages of 30–60 years. Etiology is unknown. It is believed to be related to cell related auto immunity to basal keratinocytes.

Clinical Features

Women complain of chronic vaginal discharge with intense pruritis, dyspareunia and postcoital bleeding. On examination there can be one of the following variants:
  i. Erosive lichen planus
 ii. Papulosquamous lichen planus
iii. Hypertrophic lichen planus.

Additionally classical picture with lichen planus is violaceous, flat topped papules on the skin most commonly present on flexor surface of extremities, trunk or buccal mucosa. Women with a genital lesion suspicious for lichen planus require a thorough dermatologic survey to seek extragenital lesion and vice versa. Nearly one fourth of women with oral lesion will have vulvovaginal involvement.

Treatment

Out of three variant, erosive lichen planus is the most difficult to treat, as course of unusual erosive lichen planus is one of exacerbations with slow healing. Treatment is mainly topical using fluorinated corticosteroids or ultrapotent corticosteroids for the vulva and hydrocortisone foam for the vagina (colofoam).

In case of severe pruritis and intensive mucocutaneous involvement, systemic steroids should be used. Recently topical treatment with tacrolimus 0.1% has been tried with success.

Lichen Simplex Chronicus

It is another chronic inflammatory process of the vulva that presents as white lesion associated with vulvar itching. Biopsy is generally necessary for the diagnosis. Histologically the features are similar to these of squamous cell hyperplasia. Treatment is medium strength topical corticosteroid cream.

Cystic Vulvar Tumors

Bartholin's gland duct cyst and abscess: Bartholin's gland and duct are located deep in the posterior third of each labium majors. They produce mucus to moisten vulva and vagina. Obstruction of this gland's duct can lead to cystic enlargement. This accounts for nearly 2% of all new gynecological admission. Cyst if secondarily infected can result in abscess formation (Fig. 10.4).

Symptoms: Most Bartholin's gland cyst are small and asymptomatic except for minor discomfort. Acute symptoms ordinarily results from infection which leads to pain, tenderness and dyspareunia. The surrounding tissues become edematous and inflamed. A mass is usually palpable which is tender and fluctuant and warrant prompt treatment.

Treatment

The treatment is excision of Bartholin's gland or marsupialization. In marsupialization, an incision is made over cyst and epithelial lining is sutured to the skin. The opened end eventually shrinks (Figs 10.5A and B).

Others

Others infrequently found cystic vulvar tumors should be considered in differential diagnosis:
　i. Skene's duct cyst or urethral diverticulum
　ii. Inguinal hernia
　iii. Gartner's duct cyst

Benign Solid Tumors of Vulva

A benign solid tumor may be an incidental finding or it may cause symptom of irritation or bleeding. The diagnosis should be established by excision or biopsy to rule out an underlying malignancy.

Acrochordon

Commonly known as a skin tag, acrochordons are benign polypoid fibroepithelial lesions. Acrochordons are soft, devoid of hair, sessile or pedunculated tumor of the vulvar skin. The tumor does not become malignant (Fig. 10.6).

Treatment

Surgical excisional biopsy in the office setting is ordinarily adequate therapy.

Pigmented Nevus

Pigmented nevus on the vulvar skin may be flat, slightly elevated, papillomatous, dome shaped or pedunculated.

Treatment

Treatment is primarily conservative with close observation in asymptomatic individuals. If lesions become palpable with subsequent irritation and bleeding, surgical excision is diagnostic as well therapeutic.

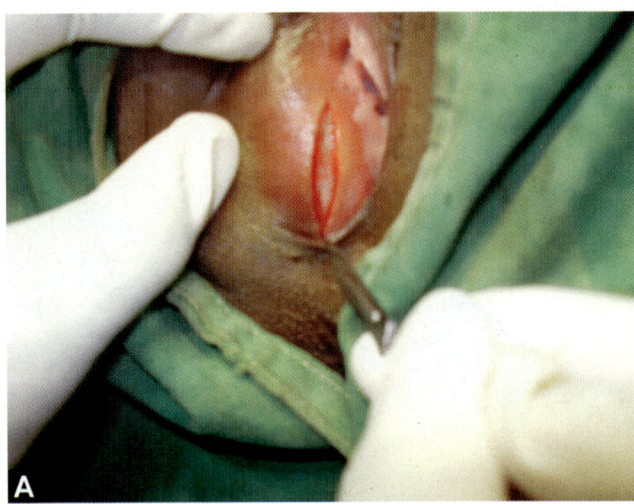
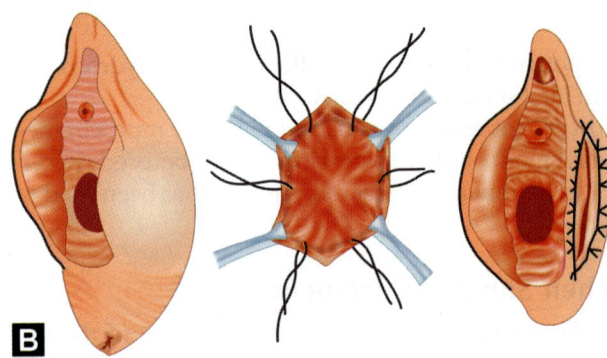

Figs 10.5A and B: (A) Incision given on Bartholin's abscess; (B) Diagrammatic representation of Marsupialization of Bartholin cyst

Epidermal inclusion cyst: Cyst of epidermal origin are lined with squamous epithelium and filled with oily material and desquamated epithelial cells. Epidermal inclusion cyst arise usually from occlusion of pilosebaceous ducts and some times may result from traumatic suturing of skin fragments during closure of the vulvar mucosa and skin after trauma or episiotomy. Usually these cyst are small, solitary and asymptomatic.

Apocrine Sweat Gland Cyst

Apocrine sweat glands are numerous in the skin on the labia majora and of mons pubis. They become functional after puberty. Occlusion of the duct with keratin results in extremely pruritic, microcystic disease called Fox Fordyce disease.

　Chronic infection in the apocrine glands, usually with staphylococci or streptococcus results in multiple painful subcutaneous abscess and draining sinuses. This condition is called 'Hydradenitis Suppurativa, which is generally treated with a broad spectrum antibiotic.

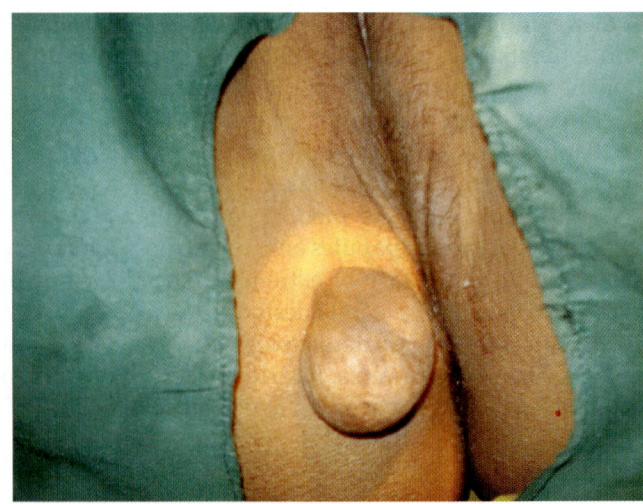

Fig. 10.6: Acrochordon vulva

Leiomyoma, Fibroma and Lipoma

They are tumors of mesodermal origins. Vulvar leiomyoma are extremely rare tumors. They arise either from smooth muscle within the vulvar erectile tissue or transmigration through round ligament. Surgical excision to exclude leiomyosarcoma is warranted.

Fibroma

Fibroma is rare benign tumor (0.03%). Fibroma arises from deep connective tissues by proliferation of fibroblasts. Lesion varies in size from 0.6 to 8 cm, primarily found on labium majora. Surgical excision is the primary treatment for symptomatic lesion.

Lipoma

A large, soft sessile or pedunculated mass composed of mature adipose cells is termed lipoma. Like fibroma, lipoma is kept under observation. If symptomatic, prompt surgical excision is needed. Lipoma lacks a fibrous connective tissue capsule and complete dissection may be complicated by bleeding requiring larger incision.

Granular Cell Myoblastoma (Schwannoma)

Granular cell myoblastoma is usually a solitary, painless, slow growing, infiltrating but benign tumor of neural sheath origin. It is most commonly found in the tongue or integument, although approximately 7% involve the vulva.

They present as small subcutaneous nodules varying from 1-4 cm in size. With increasing size they erode through the surface and result in ulceration which can be confused with cancer.

Treatment

Wide local excision is necessary. The area of resection must be periodically examined and secondary excision performed promptly if recurrence is suspected.

Vulvar Pain Syndrome (Vulvodynia)

Vulvodynia is defined by ISSVD as vulvar discomfort, most often described as burning pain, occurring in the absence of relevant visible finding or a specific clinically identifiable neurologic disorder. The pain of vulvodynia is described:
a. Spontaneous (unprovoked).
b. Provoked as finger tip pressure, tampon, and sexual intercourse.

Incidence

Incidence is not known, which is explained on the fact that there is an average delay of 4 years in reaching the appropriate diagnosis and by under-reporting of patients.

Etiology

The precise etiology is unknown. Although, many factors have been investigated, the process is multifactorial and requires an interdisciplinary approach to treatment.

Diagnosis

Vulvodynia refers to vulvar discomfort of at lest 3 – 6 months duration without an identifiable cause. Many women with localized vulvodynia complain of burning, itching, or cutting pain, which may follow a touch stimulus (called Allodynia) as wearing tight clothing or after pelvic examination. Sensations are intermittent and even episodic with premenstrual exacerbation.

History taking should be elaborate to identify frequently associated condition or risk factors as irritable bowel syndrome, interstitial cystitis, psychological disorders, relationship discord and prior infection as herpes simplex or zoster. Past surgical procedures are noted as they may cause injury to pudendal nerve. Additionally clinician should inquire about recurrent candidiasis, prior genital trauma including child birth injury, current hygienic practices, cosmetic use and sexual history. Importantly prior therapies should be documented to avoid unnecessary treatment repetition.

Physical Examination

By definition, vulvodynia lacks identifying physical markers. So, a thorough examination is first required to exclude other possible pathologies. Inspection of external vulva is followed by examination of the vestibule to search for foci of erythema. Colposcopic investigation of vulva and directed biopsy will exclude other pathology.

Systemic pain mapping of the vestibule, perineum and inner thigh is completed and serves as a reference to assess treatment success. A cotton swab is used to check allodynia and hyperesthesia subsequently. The wooden stick is broken to form a sharp point to retest the same areas. The severity of pain on a 5 or 10 point scale should be recorded and followed over time.

Management of Vulvodynia

Although numerous medical options are available for treatment, the success of many of these modalities is not substantiated by properly conducted study. In general a combination of multiple medical forms of therapy may be required to stabilize and improve patient symptoms. In the absence of improvement with medical treatment, surgical excision is option.

Medical Therapy

Vulvar care: Gentle vulvar care is first step. Use of cotton undergarments, avoidance of vulvar irritants, restoration of the barrier function and appropriate lubrication during intercourse are the mainstays of vulvar care.

Biofeedback and physician therapy: If components of back pain, muscle spasm or vaginismus are present, trained vulvar physical therapies can improve symptoms.

Topical medication: Generous amount of 5% Lidocaine ointment applied to the vestibule has been shown to significantly decrease dyspareunia. Long term use may lead to healing by minimizing feed back pain amplification. Topical estradiol application has yielded mixed results.

Oral medication: The two major classes of oral medication formed to help in treatment of vulvodynia are:
a. Antidepressant
b. Anticonvulsant

Tricyclic antidepressants have become first line agent in treatment of vulvodynia. Amitriptyline started between 5–25 mg orally and increased as needed by 10–25 mg weekly give the best results.

Max dosage should be 150–200 mg. It is important that women should continue to take drugs as there is nearly 4 week lag required to achieve significant pain relief. Cases resistant to Tricyclic antidepressant may be treated with the anticonvulsant—*Gabapentin* or *Carbamazepine*. Gabapentin is started in a dose of 100 mg orally three times a day and gradually increased in 6 – 8 weeks to a max dose of 3600 mg. After reaching this dose pain is reassessed after 1–2 weeks.

Intralesional Injection

In case of localized vulvodynia, trigger point injection using a combination of steroids and anesthetic can be injected directly into the lesion.

Surgical Therapy

The women who fail to improve despite aggressive therapy are candidates for surgical intervention. The options are:

a. Vestibulectomy with vaginal advancement (70% success).
b. Perineoplasty: It is extensive and only considered if significant perineal scarring is suspected to contribute to dyspareunia.

MULTIPLE CHOICE QUESTIONS

1. Mycotic vulvovaginitis is due to:
   a. Candida.
   b. Aspergillus.
   c. Cryptococcus.
   d. Pseudomonas.

   Ans. a

2. Fungal vulvitis is associated with:
   a. Tuberculosis.
   b. Lymphoma.
   c. Diabetes.
   d. Sulfonamides.

   Ans. c

3. Which of the following about lymphatics of vulva is true:
   a. Do not cross the labiocrural fold.
   b. Traverse labia from medial to lateral.
   c. Drain directly into deep femoral glands.
   d. Do not freely communicate with each other.

   Ans. b

4. Middle aged women with recurrent pain and swelling in the vulva:
   a. Hydradenitis.
   b. Bartholin's cyst.
   c. Hematoma.
   d. Sebaceous cyst.

   Ans. b

5. Women presents with fluctuant swelling on the introitus. The best treatment is:
   a. Marsupialization.
   b. Incision and drainage.
   c. Surgical resection.
   d. Aspiration.

   Ans. a

11. Benign Disorders of the Uterine Cervix

There are in fact two things—Science and opinion,
The former begets knowledge,
The later ignorance.

GENERAL CONSIDERATION

Benign disorders of uterine cervix are of the common presenting problems in gynecology OPD. Proper knowledge of these disorders is essential for evaluation and management with particular emphasis to differentiate it from dysplastic and neoplastic condition.

Eversion (Ectropion)

The squamocolumnar junction (SCJ) is the border between the columnar epithelium of the endocervix and the squamous epithelium of the ectocervix. Endocervical tissue in some women may move out from the endocervical canal in a process termed as **Eversion or ectropion** (Fig. 11.1). It is caused by laceration due to childbirth injury, and superimposed chronic cervicitis.

Ectropion can be detected by digital and per speculum examination, as the external os is patulous and lower part of cervical canal can be felt and seen. In these cases, to perform an adequate Pap smear, the clinician must identify the circumferential path of squamocolumnar junction (SCJ) prior to sampling. Trachelorrhaphy can be done in selected cases.

Nebothian Cyst

Mucus secreting columnar cell line the endocervical canal. During squamous metaplasia, squamous epithelium may cover part of glandular cells, predisposing them to accumulation of secretion. With this benign process smooth, clear or yellow glandular elevations are visible during routine per speculum examination. Nebothian cyst requires no further therapy.

Cervical Tears

Cervical tears most frequently occur after vaginal delivery but can also occur after dilatation and curettage and use of resectoscope in hysteroscopy surgery. With delivery the most common tears occur at 3 and 6'o clock positions or it may be irregular stellate type. Most lacerations can be easily repaired with suture technique. Often tear is asymptomatic and does not require repair.

Benign Neoplasm of the Cervix

Microglandular Hyperplasia of the Endocervical Mucosa

Microglandular hyperplasia (MGH) usually occurs in women of reproductive age, but 6% of known cases are detected in postmenopausal women.

Etiopathogenesis

MGH has been associated with hormonal stimulus of oral contraceptive use, pregnancy and inflammation.

Clinical Picture

It appears as exuberant granular tissue within the cervical canal, often extruding beyond the cervical os.

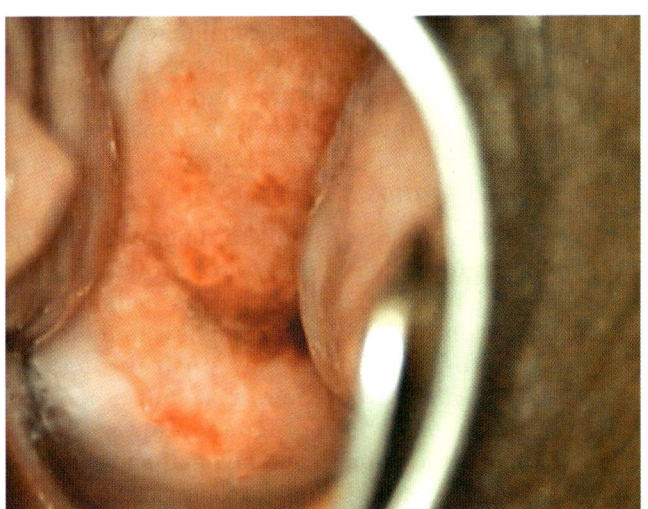

Fig. 11.1: Colposcopic view of ectropion

Histology

It present as a collection of closely packed cystic spaces lined by non-neoplastic columnar epithelium and filled with mucus.

Treatment

Excisional biopsy should always be performed to differentiate it from cancer.

Cervical Polyp

Cervical polyps are small, pedunculated as well sessile neoplasm of the cervix. Most originate from endocervix; a few arise from the portio vaginalis (Fig. 11.2).

Etiopathogenesis

Polyp arises as a result of focal hyperplasia of the endocervix in response to chronic inflammation or hormonal stimulation or local vascular congestion of cervical blood vessels. Polyps are often found in association with endometrial hyperplasia, suggesting role of hyperestrogenism in its etiology.

Pathology

Endocervical polyp usually are red, flame shaped, fragile growth varying in size from few mm to 2–3 cm. These polyps usually are attached to the endocervical mucosa near the external os by a narrow pedicle but occasionally the base is broad.

On the microscopic examination, the stroma of a polyp is composed of fibrous connective tissue containing numerous small vessels in the center. There is often extravasation of blood and marked infiltration by leukocytes. The surface epithelium resembles that of the endocervix varying from typical picket fence columnar cell to areas that show squamous metaplasia and mature stratified squamous epithelium.

Ectocervical polyps are pale, fish colored smooth and rounded or elongated, often pedunculated. They arise from the portio and are less likely to bleed than endocervical polyp. They are covered by stratified squamous epithelium.

Clinical Findings

Symptoms

Intermenstrual bleeding, postcoital bleeding and postmenstrual bleeding are the most common symptoms of cervical polyp. There may be leukorrhea and hypermenorrhea. Infertility may be traceable to cervical polyp and cervicitis.

Signs

Per speculum examination shows a smooth, red, finger-like projection from the cervical canal. Generally, they are too soft to be felt on pervaginal examination.

Imaging

Polyps high in endocervical canal may be demonstrated by hysterosalpingogram or saline infusion sonohysterography. They often are significant findings in otherwise idiopathic infertility.

Lab Finding

Vaginal cytology will reveal sign of infection and often mildly atypical cells. Blood and urine study are not helpful.

Special Examination

A polyp high in the endocervical canal may be seen with the aid of special endocervical speculum or by hysteroscopy. Some polyps are found at the time of diagnostic D & C in investigation of abnormal bleeding.

Differential Diagnosis

Typical polyps are not difficult to diagnose by gross inspection but ulcerated and atypical growth must be distinguished from *small submucous pedunculated myomas* or *endometrial polyps* arising low in the uterus. *The products of conception* may push through the cervix and resemble a polypoid mass but other signs and symptoms of recent pregnancy are generally absent. **Condyloma, submucous myoma, and polypoid carcinoma** are diagnosed by microscopic examination.

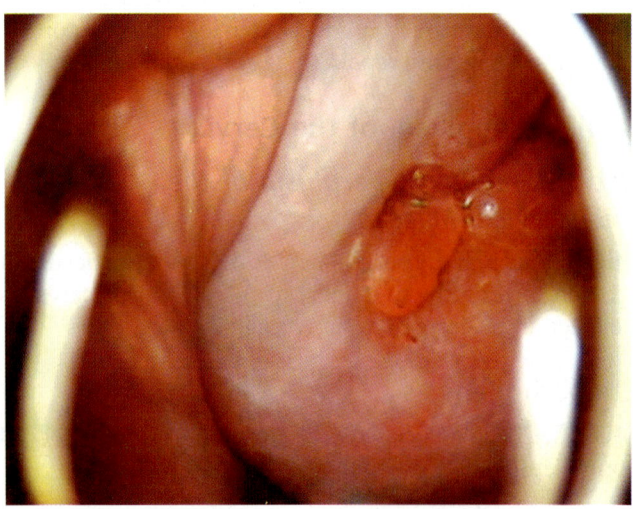

Fig. 11.2: Cervical polyp

Complication

Infection

Cervical polyp may be infected by *Staphylococcus, Streptococcus* or other pathogens, following instrumentation. Broad spectrum antibiotic should be administered. It is also unwise to remove a large polyp and then perform a hysterectomy, after few days because there is chance of pelvic peritonitis after hysterectomy. A delay of several weeks or 1 month between polypectomy and hysterectomy is recommended.

Malignant Change

Incidence of malignant change in a cervical polyp is **less than 1%**. Squamous cell carcinoma is the most common. Endometrial cancer may involve the polyp secondarily.

Treatment

Medical measures: Appropriate testing for cervical discharge should be performed as indicated and treatment of infection should be given.

Surgical measures: In the presence of slender stalk, polyp removal can be done in office setting by a continuous twisting of the lesion with ring forceps. Twisting leads to occlusion of supporting vessels and avulsion of the mass. A thick pedicled polyp is best treated by surgical excision. Excised cervical polyp must be sent for histopathologic evaluation to exclude malignancy.

Cervical Ectopy (Erosion)

Cervical erosion or ectopy is the condition in which the squamous covering of the vaginal portion of the cervix is replaced by columnar epithelium, which is continuous with that lining the endocervix. It is not an ulcer (Fig. 11.3).

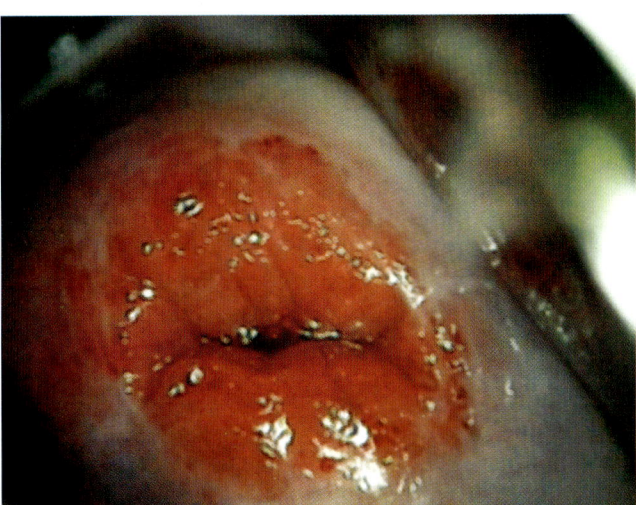

Fig. 11.3: Cervical erosion

Etiology

Congenital

Towards the ends of intrauterine life columnar epithelium grows down from the cervical canal and in one-third of all newborn female children extends to some degree over vaginal portion of the cervix. This condition persists for only a few days, until the level of estrogen derived from the mother falls and the congenital erosion heals spontaneously.

Acquired

Hormonal dependent: The squamocolumnar junction is not static and it moves outwards with high estrogen level like in pill users and pregnancy. SCJ returns back to normal position after 3 months following delivery and earlier after stopping pill usage.

Infection: Infection is not the primary cause, but chronic cervicitis may be associated or infection may superimpose on ectopy because of delicate columnar epithelium, which is more vulnerable to trauma and infection.

Pathogenesis

In the active phase of ectopy the SCJ moves out from the os. The columnar epithelium of the endocervix is continued while covering the ectocervix replacing the squamous epithelium. This replaced epithelium can be arranged in following pattern:

a. Flat type: Columnar epithelium arranged in a single layer.
b. Follicular ectopy: May be so hyperplastic as to fold inwards.
c. Papillary ectopy: Columnar epithelium heaped up to fold inward and outwards.

Underneath the epithelium, there are evidence of round cell infiltration and glandular proliferation. When ectopy heals, the SCJ gradually moves towards the external os. The squamous epithelium goes beneath the columnar epithelium until it reaches at or near to its original position at the external os. The columnar epithelium gradually disintegrates. Alternatively, the replacement occurs by squamous metaplasia of the columnar cells. Ectopy is not to be considered as precancerous but the squamous columnar junction is vulnerable to malignant changes.

Clinical Features

Symptoms: Lesion may be asymptomatic. Vaginal discharge, contact bleeding especially among pill users and in pregnancy can be presenting symptoms. Associated cervicitis may cause backache, pelvic pain and at times infertility.

Signs: On per speculum examination, there is bright red area surrounding and extending beyond the external os in the ectocervix. The lesion may be smooth or having small capillary folds. On rubbing with gauze piece, there may be multiple oozing spots. On touch, erosion is soft and granular, giving rise to grating sensation.

Differential Diagnosis

Ectropion, tubercular vulva, primary sore and early carcinoma has to be differentiated by clinical examination and confirmed by histopathological examination.

Management of Erosion

In all cases cytological examination must be done from cervical smear to exclude dysplasia or malignancy. In doubtful cases colposcopy and cervical biopsy should be done. In asymptomatic cases, no treatment is needed.

In symptomatic cases with persistent vaginal discharge- **cryosurgery, thermal cautery or laser vaporization ca**n be done. These methods are based on the principle of destruction of the columnar epithelium to be followed by its healing by the squamous epithelium. During pregnancy and early puerperium, the treatment should be withheld for at least 12 weeks postpartum. In pills users, the 'pill' should be stopped.

Cervical Stenosis

Cervical stenosis can be congenital, inflammatory, neoplastic or surgical. It may be partial or totally occlusive.

Etiology

a. In majority of cases cervical stenosis is caused by extensive surgical manipulation of the cervix – Electrocoagulation, cryotherapy, laser vaporization, conization or cervical amputation, or radiation therapy.
b. In postmenopausal women, it may be caused by estrogen deficiency.

Symptoms

Cervical stenosis can cause marked to complete obstruction of menstrual blood resulting in development of hematometra. There is amenorrhea, with abdominal discomfort felt at time of menstruation. On **examination** one can feel soft, slightly tender mid pelvic mass. In postmenopausal women there may be pyometra and should always raise the suspicion of associated endometrial carcinoma.

Diagnosis

Hematometra and pyometra can be readily confirmed by pelvic ultrasonography.

Treatment

Cautious dilatation of the cervix is recommended, with drainage of entrapped fluid. Culture and sensitivity test should be performed and treated with appropriate antibiotic coverage. Cervical or endometrial tissue or both should be obtained for histopathology to rule out cancer.

Removal of cicatrix by laser vaporization and loop excision has been effective in case of postconization stenosis.

12. Benign Disorders of Uterine Corpus (Fibroids, Adenomyosis and Endometrial Polyp)

Only a man who is familiar with the art and science of the past,
Is competent to aid in the progress of future.

GENERAL CONSIDERATIONS

Leiomyoma of uterus also called as myoma, or fibroids are the most common benign tumors of the female reproductive tract. The most frequently quoted prevalence is that they affect between 20% and 25% of women above the age of 30 years. Most leiomyomas are diagnosed in women in their 40's. Usually most myomas tend to regress following menopause. Incidence of symptomatic fibroid in hospital outpatient is about 3%. In black women incidence is very high (10%) and is more common in nulliparous.

Uterine leiomyomas are benign monoclonal neoplasm arising from smooth muscle cells in the uterine wall. They contain an increased amount of extracellular collagen and elastin. A thin pseudocapsule composed of areolar tissue and compressed muscle fibers surrounds the tumor.

Although usually myomas are asymptomatic, they can produce a wide variety of problems like menorrhagia and metrorrhagia, dysmenorrhea, pelvic pain and infertility. Menorrhagia due to fibroid is one of the most common indications for hysterectomy.

Pathogenesis

The cause of uterine enlargement is not known. Studies suggest that each individual leiomyoma is unicellular in origin (Monoclonal). Although there is no evidence that estrogen causes leiomyoma, estrogens are certainly implicated in growth of myoma. Leiomyomata contain estrogen receptors in higher concentration than the surrounding myometrium but in lower concentration than the endometrium. Progesterone increases the mitotic activity of myoma in young women and it may allow tumor enlargement by increasing the production of extracellular matrix. So leiomyoma may increase in size with estrogen therapy and during pregnancy, but not always. There is speculation that leiomyoma growth in pregnancy is related to synergistic activity of estradiol and human placental lactogen.

Myomas usually decrease in size after menopause. Beside this multiple chromosomal abnormalities are detected in approximately 50% of leiomyoma by cytogenic analysis, particularly chromosome 6 or 7. It is suggested that abnormal cellular proliferation may be due to this genetic potential. A positive family history is often present. Polypeptide growth factors can stimulate the growth of leiomyoma either directly or via estrogen.

Classification and Pathophysiology

Leiomyomata are usually multiple, discrete and either spherical or irregularly lobulated. Their pseudocapsule usually clearly demarcates them from the surrounding myometrium. On *gross examination* in transverse section, myomas are buff colored, rounded, smooth and usually firm and lighter in color than the myometrium. On *microscopy* nonstriated muscle fibers are arranged in interlacing bundles of varying size running in different directions (whorled appearance). Individual cells are spindle shaped, have elongated nuclei and uniform in size. Varying amount of connective tissues is intermixed with the smooth muscles bundles (Fig. 12.1).

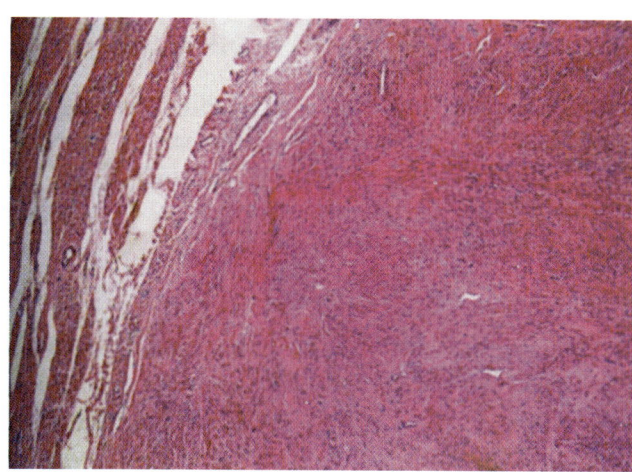

Fig. 12.1: The microscopic appearance of fibroid

Leiomyomata are sharply demarcated from surrounding normal musculature by a pseudocapsule of areolar tissue and compressed myometrium. The arterial density of a leiomyoma is less than that of the surrounding myometrium; small arteries that supply the tumors are less tortuous than are adjacent radial arteries. The arteries penetrate the myoma randomly on its surface and are oriented in the direction of the muscle bundles. One or two major vessels may be found in the base of pedicle.

Classification

Uterus leiomyomata originates in the myometrium and are classified by anatomic location (Fig. 12.2).

Interstitial or Intramural (75%)

Intramural or interstitial myoma lie within the uterine wall, giving it a variable consistency. They may be pushed outwards or inwards, but in about 70% leiomyoma persist in that position.

Subserous or Subperitoneal (15%)

These myomas may lie just at the serosal surface of the uterus or may bulge outwards from the myometrium. The subserous myoma may become pedunculated. If such a tumor acquires an extrauterine blood supply from the omental vessels, its pedicle may atrophy and resort. The tumor is then named as *parasitic*.

Subserous tumors arising laterally between the two peritoneal layers of the broad ligament and called *broad ligament myoma*, which may lead to compression of the ureter and or pelvic blood supply.

Submucous Leiomyoma (5%)

Submucous leiomyoma lie just beneath the endometrium and tend to compress it as they grow towards the uterine lumen. Their impact on the endometrium and its blood supply most often leads to irregular uterine bleeding. These leiomyoma may develop pedicles and protrude fully into the uterus cavity. Occasionally, they pass through the cervical canal, while still attached within the corpus by a long stalk. When this happens, there can be torsion or infection, which must be taken into consideration before treatment.

Secondary Changes

There may be areas of hyalinization, cystic changes, calcification, hemorrhage, fat or inflammation with leiomyomata. These secondary alterations are histologically and radiologically interesting but usually have little clinical significance.

Benign Degeneration

It consists of following:

Atrophic: Sign and symptoms regress or disappear as tumor size decreases at menopause or after pregnancy.

Hyaline: Mature or old leiomyoma are white but contain yellow, soft and often gelatinous areas of hyaline change. It is usually asymptomatic.

Cystic: Liquefaction follows extreme hyalinization and physical stress may cause sudden evacuation of fluid content into uterus, peritoneal cavity or the retroperitoneal space.

Fatty degeneration: It is usually found at or after menopause. Fat globules are deposited mainly in the muscle cell. This is asymptomatic and follows hyaline and cystic degeneration.

Calcific (calcareous) degeneration (10%): Subserous leiomyomata are most commonly affected by circulatory deprivation which causes precipitation of calcium carbonate and phosphate with the tumors.

Septic: Circulatory inadequacy may cause necrosis of the central portion of tumors followed by infection or following delivery or abortion. Acute pain, tenderness and fever result.

Carneus or red degeneration: It occurs in a large fibroid mainly during second half of pregnancy and puerperium. Venous thrombosis and congestion with interstitial hemorrhage are responsible for the color of a leiomyomata undergoing red degeneration.

During pregnancy, edema and hypertrophy of the myometrium occurs. The physiological changes in the leiomyoma are not the same as in the myometrium.

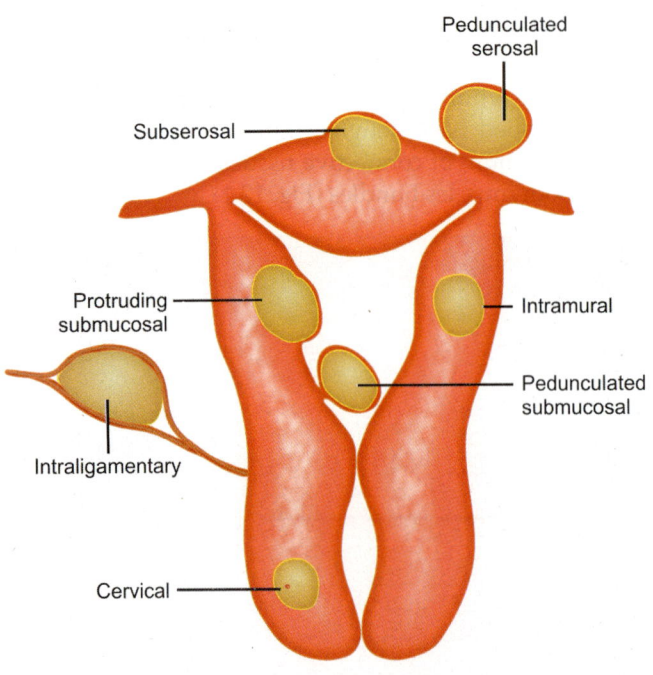

Fig. 12.2: Various locations of fibromyoma

Resultant anatomic discrepancy impedes the blood supply resulting in aseptic degeneration and infarction. This process is usually accompanied by pain, but is self-limited. Potential complication of degeneration in pregnancy is preterm labor and rarely initiation of disseminated intravascular coagulation.

Metastasizing leiomyomata: Rarely myomas spread beyond the uterus to distant location such as peritoneum, distant vasculature, and lung. Histologically these leiomyoma appear benign and have a low mitotic rate, often they are asymptomatic. Most women with these tumors give history of prior dilation and curettage (D & C) myomectomy or hysterectomy, suggesting the possibility of surgically induced vascular spread of leiomyoma cell.

Another theory suggests a multifocal origin from smooth muscle in blood vessels anywhere in the body.

Vascular changes: Dilatation of the vessels (telangiectasis) or dilatation of the lymphatic channels (lymphangiectasis) inside the myoma may occur. The cause is not known.

Sarcomatous changes: Sarcomatous change may occur in less than 0.1% cases. The usual type is leiomyosarcoma. If there is sudden rapid enlargement of fibroid or fibroid with menopausal bleeding or recurrences of fibroid polyp, one should have clinical suspicion for sarcomatous change. To the naked eye a sarcomatous myoma is yellowish gray in color and hemorrhagic. The consistency is soft and friable and not firm like a smooth myoma. Another important sign is the non-encapsulation of the tumor. Sarcoma is highly malignant and spread via the blood stream.

Secondary changes in pelvic organs: The presence of myoma causes hyperplasia of the myometrial wall. The cavity of the uterus is often distorted and enlarged. The endometrium tends to be thicker due to endometrial hyperplasia. The ovaries may be enlarged, cystic and hyperemic with evidence of salpingo-oophoritis in about 15% of cases.

Clinical Features

There are a variety of clinical manifestations of leiomyomas of the uterus ranging from asymptomatic pelvic masses to symptomatic tumor characterized by abnormal uterine bleeding, pain and pressure. In addition, secondary features such as spontaneous abortion, obstetric problem and infertility may be the presenting feature.

Most Women (75%) with Fibroid Remain Asymptomatic

The symptoms are related to anatomic type and size of tumor. The site is more important than the size. A small submucous fibroid may produce more symptom than a big subserous fibroid.

Abnormal Uterine Bleeding

Abnormal uterine bleeding is the most common and most important clinical manifestation of leiomyoma being present in up to 30% of patients. This can produce iron deficiency anemia which may not be improved even with iron therapy, if bleeding is heavy and protracted.

Most common type of abnormal uterine bleeding is prolonged heavy menses (**menorrhagia**), premenstrual spotting, or prolonged light staining following menses. However, any type of abnormal bleeding is possible.

The pathophysiology underlying this bleeding may relate to dilatation of venules. Downregulation of local vasoactive growth factors are also thought to promote vasodilatation. When engorged venules are disrupted at time of menstrual sloughing, bleeding from markedly dilated venules overwhelms usual hemostatic mechanism.

Increased uterine surface, associated endometrial hyperplasia, pelvic congestion and *interference with normal uterine contractility* are other proposed mechanism for menorrhagia.

Bleeding from a submucous leiomyoma may occur from interruption of the blood supply to the endometrium, distortion and congestion of the surrounding vessels, particularly the veins or ulceration of the overlying endometrium. Thus **metrorrhagia** (intermenstrual bleeding) may be associated with presence of submucous myoma, torn vessels from sloughing base of a polyp and also if there is associated endometrial carcinoma. Any intermenstrual or irregular bleeding should be comprehensively investigated despite presence of leiomyoma.

Pain

There can be **congestive dysmenorrhea** due to associated pelvic congestion or endometriosis and **spasmodic dysmenorrhea,** if uterus tries to expel in cases of pedunculated fibroid or polyp.

Leiomyomata may cause pain when vascular compromise occurs. Thus pain may result from degeneration associated with vascular occlusion, infection, torsion of a pedunculated tumors or myometrial contraction to expel a submucous myoma from the uterine cavity. The pain associated with infection from torsion or red degeneration can be excruciating and produced a clinical picture consistent with acute abdomen.

Large tumor may produce a sensation of heaviness or fullness in the pelvic area, feeling of mass in the pelvic or feeling of mass palpable through the abdominal wall. Myomas that become impacted within the bony pelvis may press on nerves and create pain radiating to back or lower extremities. Dyspareunia may result depending on the position of tumors and the pressure they exert on the vaginal walls.

Pressure Effect

Pressure effects are uncommon and difficult to directly relate to leiomyomata, unless the tumors are very large. Intramural or intraligamentous leiomyomata may distort or obstruct other organs. Parasitic tumors may cause intestinal obstruction if they are large or involve omentum or bowel.

Cervical tumor may cause serosanguinous vaginal discharge, vaginal bleeding, dyspareunia and infertility. Large tumors may fill the true pelvis and displace or compress the ureters, bladder or rectum.

Compression of surrounding structure may result in urinary symptom or hydroureter. Large tumors may cause pelvic congestion and lower extremity edema or constipation.

Infertility

The relationship between fibroid and infertility remains uncertain. Between 27% and 40% of women with multiple leiomyomas are reported to be infertile but other causes of infertility are present in the majority of cases. When fibroids are entirely or mostly endocavitary, there is strong reason to support the use of surgery to improve fertility.

It is estimated that 2–3% of infertility cases are due to solely to their leiomyomas. Presumed causes are occlusion of tubal ostia and disruption of the normal uterine contraction which propel sperm or ova. Distortion of the endometrial cavity may diminish implantation and sperm transport.

Spontaneous Abortion

The incidence of spontaneous abortion secondary to leiomyoma is unknown, but the incidence is two times than in normal pregnant women.

Diagnosis

Clinical Signs

General examination may reveal varying degree of anemia depending upon the magnitude and duration of menstrual blood loss. Most myomas are detected by routine *bimanual examination* of the uterus, which reveals an enlarged uterus, regular or bossy depending upon the number and size of the tumors. The cervix moves with the swelling which is not separate from the uterus, unless it is pedunculated. Uterine retroflexion and retroversion may obscure the physical examination diagnosis of even medium size leiomyomata. If cervix is pulled up behind the symphysis, large fibroids are usually implicated.

In *cervical fibroid*, the normal uterus is perched on top of the tumor. The broad ligament fibroid displaces the uterus to the opposite side. In *myomatous polyp* the cervical os is open and its lower pole felt. Submucous myoma may produce symmetrical enlargement of the uterus and at times it is difficult to diagnose accurately.

Investigation

Laboratory finding: Anemia is a common consequence of leiomyoma due to excessive uterine bleeding and depletion of iron reserve. Leukocytosis, fever and an elevated ESR may be present with acute degeneration or infection.

Imaging: Pelvic ultrasound examinations are useful in confirming the diagnosis of leiomyoma. Although ultrasound examination should never be a substitute for a thorough pelvic examination, it can be extremely helpful in identifying leiomyomata, detailing the cause of other pelvic masses and identifying pregnancy. Moreover, ultrasonography can be particularly useful in obese individuals. On USG myoma shows specific feature of a well-defined rounded tumor, hypoechoic with cystic spaces if degeneration has occurred (Figs 12.3A to C).

Preoperative ultrasound checks the number, location and size of fibroids, which is important for myomectomy operation. USG is also useful in the follow-up of fibroid after menopause and following GnRH therapy. Saline sonohysterography can identify submucosal myoma that may be missed on ultrasound.

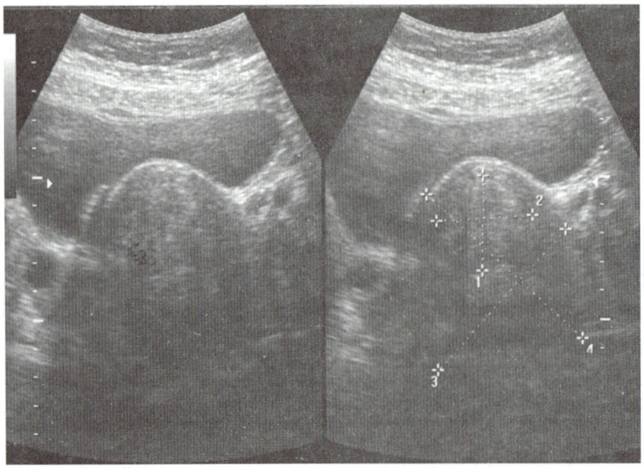

Fig. 12.3A: Ultrasound image of interstitial myoma

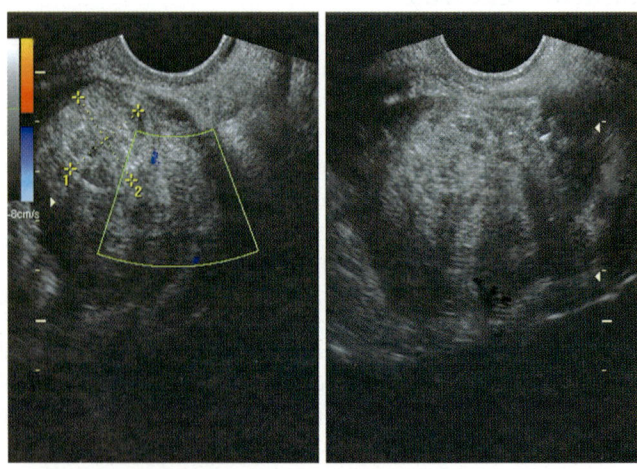

Fig. 12.3B: Ultrasound image of submucous myoma

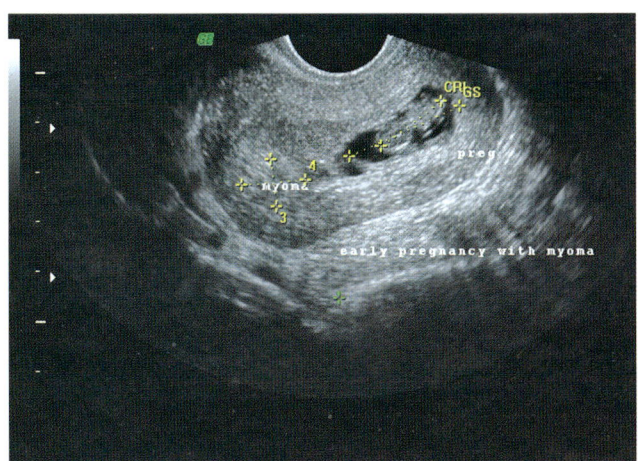

Fig. 12.3C: Early pregnancy with myoma

Hydroureter and hydronephrotic changes can be diagnosed with USG. Leiomyomas have characteristic vascular pattern which can be identified by color flow Doppler. A peripheral rim of vascularity from which a few vessels arise to penetrate into the center of tumor is traditionally seen.

Hysterosalpingography may be useful in detecting an intrauterine leiomyoma in infertile patient besides evaluating fallopian tube anatomy and function. **CT scan** is not very useful but **MRI** is accurate in identifying adenomyosis and sarcoma. **Intravenous pyelography** is required in *broad ligament fibroid* to check the anatomy and pathology of ureter and to identify a pelvic kidney.

Special examination: **Hysteroscopy** may assist in identifying and may also be used for removal of submucous leiomyoma. **Laparoscopy** is often definitive in establishing the precise origin of leiomyoma and is increasing being used for myomectomy.

Differential Diagnosis

The diagnosis of uterine myoma with clinical examination and ultrasound is usually not difficult, although any pelvic mass, including pregnancy can be mistaken for leiomyoma. So in differential diagnosis the other causes of uterine enlargement and abnormal uterine bleeding should be considered and evaluated.

Pelvic Mass

The following should be kept in mind:

Benign ovarian tumor: A subserous or pedunculated fibroid may resemble ovarian tumor as abnormal uterine bleeding may not be present in all cases of fibroid. Though ultrasound will help in diagnosing but at times the true nature of the tumor is revealed only at laparotomy.

Malignant ovarian tumor: One of the grave errors is to mistake a malignant ovarian tumor for the uterine fibroid and in case of doubt laparotomy should be performed.

Chronic ectopic pregnancy and chronic PID: Adnexa, omentum or bowel adherent to the uterus may be erroneously diagnosed as leiomyomata. Careful history taking is important. Because a fetus *in utero* or outside utero may exist within an obviously myomatous uterus, a pregnancy test should be obtained in all women of child bearing age with a suspected pelvic mass. In chronic PID, inflammatory masses are slightly tender and the uterus is normal size and fixed.

Endometriosis/chocolate cyst: Careful history taking, presence of normal size uterus adherent to pelvic mass in endometriosis differentiate from fibroid. However, laparoscopy is gold standard for diagnosis of endometriosis.

Adenomyosis: Adenomyosis shares the clinical feature of uterine fibroma. Adenomyomatous uterus is often tender. Ultrasound confirms the diagnosis.

Hematometra, congenital anomalies, myometrial hypertrophy can be differentiated by ultrasound.

Pelvic kidney: History is different in pelvic kidney. The tumor is fixed, behind the normal sized uterus. Ultrasound will reveal absence of the abdominal kidney and IVP will locate the pelvic kidney.

Abnormal Uterine Bleeding

The definitive diagnosis in cases of uterine bleeding usually can be established by endometrial biopsy or fractional D & C. Some form of endometrial evaluation should be considered essential in the workup of any patient with abnormal bleeding or a pelvic mass particularly those over age 35 years in whom endometrial cancer may be serious concern. It is important to remember that even in the presence of uterine leiomyoma other conditions can coexist and must be ruled out before definitive therapy is undertaken.

Chronic Inversion of Uterus

It is often associated with fibroid polyp. The sounding of uterine cavity and laparoscopy are mandatory prior to surgical excision to avoid uterine perforation.

Complications
Myoma and Pregnancy

Leiomyoma can cause infertility because it interferes with implantation of the fertilized ovum, it hinders the ascent of spermatozoa by distorting the uterus and fallopian tube and there may be associated disturbance of ovulation.

However, leiomyomata have been reported as a sole cause in less than 3% of cases of infertility and approximately two-third of women with uterine leiomyoma and otherwise unexplained infertility conceive after myomectomy and approximately half of those women go to deliver term infant.

During **2nd and 3rd trimester** of pregnancy, myoma may increase in size and undergo vascular deprivation and subsequent degenerative changes. This may cause acute abdomen due to red degeneration and as well can initiate preterm labor.

During **labor,** leiomyoma may cause uterine inertia, fetal malpresentation or obstruction of the birth canal. In general, leiomyomas tend to rise out of the pelvis, as the pregnancy progresses and vaginal delivery may be accomplished. Nevertheless, a large cervical or isthmic myoma may be immobile and may necessitate cesarean delivery. Leiomyoma may interfere with effective uterine contraction immediately after delivery and can cause postpartum hemorrhage.

Complications in Nonpregnant Women

Heavy bleeding with anemia is the most common complication of myomas. **Urinary or bowel obstruction** from large or parasitic myoma is much less common. **Malignant transformation** is rare. Ureteral injury or ligation is a well-recognized complication of surgery for leiomyoma particularly cervical.

TREATMENT

Choice of treatment in leiomyomata depends on the patient's symptoms, age, parity, pregnancy status, reproductive plans and general health as well as the size and location of leiomyomas. Before resorting to any treatment other causes of pelvic masses must be ruled out.

Asymptomatic Fibroid

Small and asymptomatic uterine fibroids do not require removal. Regardless of the size, asymptomatic leiomyomata usually can be managed expectantly by annual pelvic examination (ACOG, 2001). If assessment of the Adnexa is hindered by the uterine size or contour, annual sonographic surveillance can be recommended.
It is justifiable to operate on symptomless tumors if:
a. It is larger than 12–14 weeks of pregnancy.
b. It is growing rapidly.
c. It is subserous and pedunculated and prone to torsion of its pedicle.
d. It is likely to complicate future pregnancy.
e. There is doubt about its nature.
f. In case of infertility, single or multiple tiny subserous leiomyomata are best left undisturbed but intramural or submucous tumors, even of moderate size, deserve removal if no other cause is found.
g. An asymptomatic fibroid causing pressure on the ureter. in broad ligament fibroid and pressure on bladder.

Emergency Measures

In certain situations, emergency and vigorous measures are required. Blood transfusion may be needed to correct severe anemia, and usually in these cases surgery is indicated when patient becomes hemodynamically stable.

Emergency surgery is indicated for infected leiomyoma, acute torsion or intestinal obstruction caused by a pedunculated parasitic myoma.

Specific Measures

Medical therapy: Medical therapy is preferred in certain situation. In addition because leiomyoma typically regress postmenopausally, some women choose medical treatment to relieve symptoms in anticipation of menopause. The situation where medical treatment is required to relieve/reduce symptoms or as a preoperative preparation are:
a. To improve menorrhagia and to correct anemia before surgery.
b. To minimize the size and vascularity of tumor in order to facilitate surgery.
c. As an alternative to surgery in premenopausal women or women with high risk factor for surgery.
d. Where postponement of surgery is planned temporarily.

Choice of medical treatment depends on the aim of treatment, cost of drug and therapeutic effectiveness of drug.

Following drugs can be used for symptomatic fibroid:

Nonsteroidal Anti-inflammatory Drugs (NSAIDs)

Role of NSAIDs for leiomyomata related uterine bleeding is less clear and their use as sole agent for leiomyomata related menorrhagia is not supported.

Hormonal Therapy

RU486 (Mifepristone): 10–25 mg daily for 3 months, causes amenorrhea and shrinkage of tumors by 50% but long-term therapy should be avoided, as it causes endometrial hyperplasia.

Danazol: 400-800 mg daily for 3 to 6 months reduces the size of tumor. It minimizes blood loss or even produces amenorrhea by its antigonadotropin and androgen agonist action. But development of androgenic side effect like hair growth, voice change as well cost of treatment precludes its routine use.

GnRH analogs: GnRH agonist induces hypogonadism through pituitary desensitization, downregulation of receptors and inhibition of gonadotropins. GnRH treatment of uterine fibroids for 3 months usually will achieve maximal shrinkage of the myomatous uterus to approximately 38–60% of its volume and amenorrhea with resulting improvement in hematological parameters.

But GnRH treatment is costly, there are hypoestrogenic side effects and bone loss especially with treatment for more than 6 months and there is rapid resumption of uterine volume and menses upon discontinuation of therapy. So its use is only limited to following situations:
a. Control acute bleeding from leiomyoma.
b. Improving preoperative hematocrit level.
c. As a temporary preoperative measure till surgery schedule or menopause.
d. Shrinkage of myoma sufficiently to allow vaginal hysterectomy or laparoscopic myomectomy or hysterectomy. Drug commonly used are **goserelin, luprolin, buserelin or nafarelin.**

GnRH antagonist: They also cause immediate suppression of pituitary and ovaries. But experience of these drugs is limited. These profound hypoestrogenic effects are similar to those of GnRH agonist. But they avoid the initial gonadotropins flare and have a more rapid action.

Oral contraceptive pills: Oral contraceptive pills are commonly used to control abnormal uterine bleeding but they do not appear to be effective in treatment of fibroids. But they are therapeutically effective in treating coexisting condition such as pelvic pain, or anovulatory bleeding which may otherwise be contributed to leiomyoma.

Levonorgesterol releasing intrauterine system: Small observational studies have shown good results with use of levonorgesterol releasing intrauterine device for treatment of menorrhagia related to multiple smaller leiomyomatas.

Surgical Measures

Surgery is the mainstay of treatment of leiomyomas. Imaging most often must be accompanied by endometrial evaluation to rule out other pelvic neoplastic process. Before surgery all patients should undergo cervical Papanicolaou's smear test and evaluation of the endometrium if bleeding is irregular. Before definitive surgery, necessary blood volume should be replenished. Mechanical and antibiotic bowel preparation can be used when difficult pelvic surgery is anticipated. The techniques used are – conventional myomectomy and hysterectomy.

Myomectomy

Myomectomy is an option for symptomatic women who wish to preserve fertility or conserve the uterus. It is also considered for improving reproductive outcome in infertility and recurrent pregnancy loss in selected cases. There is a risk of recurrence of development of future leiomyomas. Five years postmyomectomy 50–60% of patients will have new myomas on ultrasound and 25% will require a second major surgery.

Couple should undergo a thorough infertility evaluation before the women undergoes myomectomy to improve fertility. Myomectomy can be performed by following routes:
(a) Abdominal (Laparotomy), (b) Vaginal myomectomy, (c) Endoscopy – Laparoscopy, Hysteroscopy.

Preoperative Requisite
a. Hemoglobin should be restored as myomectomy causes much more blood loss during surgery as compared to hysterectomy.
b. In infertility, other causes of infertility including male partner should be excluded.
c. Written consent for possibility of hysterectomy should be taken in difficult unforeseen circumstances. Preferred time is preovulatory period to reduce blood loss during surgery.

Technique

Abdominal myomectomy: An incision preferably over the anterior wall of the uterus is given, and as many fibroids as possible are removed through minimal tunneling incisions. Preoperative hemorrhage is minimized with myomectomy clamp over uterine vessels or diluted 20 units of vasopressin injection in myoma. Myoma bed is thoroughly obliterated with several catgut sutures to avoid reactionary hemorrhage (Figs 12.4A to D).

Vaginal myomectomy: A pedunculated submucous myoma protruding into the vagina can sometimes be removed vaginally. A moderate size fibroid can be removed with sponge forceps and twisting. This is useful if other tumors do not obviously require removal. If the pedunculated myoma cannot be removed vaginally, carefully biopsy should be performed to rule out leiomyosarcoma or a mixed mesodermal sarcoma; both of these tumors are known to protrude through the cervix in older women and may be clinically indistinguishable from an infarcted prolapsed myoma.

Hysteroscopic myomectomy: Hysteroscopic myomectomy has become possible in submucous fibroids not removable by the simple vaginal route. The fibroid is excised either by cautery, laser, or by resectoscope. It is best done under laparoscopic guidance to avoid uterine perforation.

Laparoscopic myomectomy: Laparoscopic myomectomy is being performed by experts in cases of a pedunculated fibroid and submucous fibroid not exceeding 10 cm in size. Unipolar, bipolar cautery and laser have been employed to remove fibroma and obtain hemostasis. The fibroma is then retrieved through posterior colpotomy, minilaparotomy or by morcellation.

Though these minimal invasive procedures are liberalizing the surgical indications for myomectomy, the strength of uterine scar is controversial and scar rupture has been reported even at 33 weeks gestation. Patients desiring fertility should be counseled carefully regarding these risks. Beside laparoscopic myomectomy can cause more bleeding.

SECTION -2 ♦ Gynecology

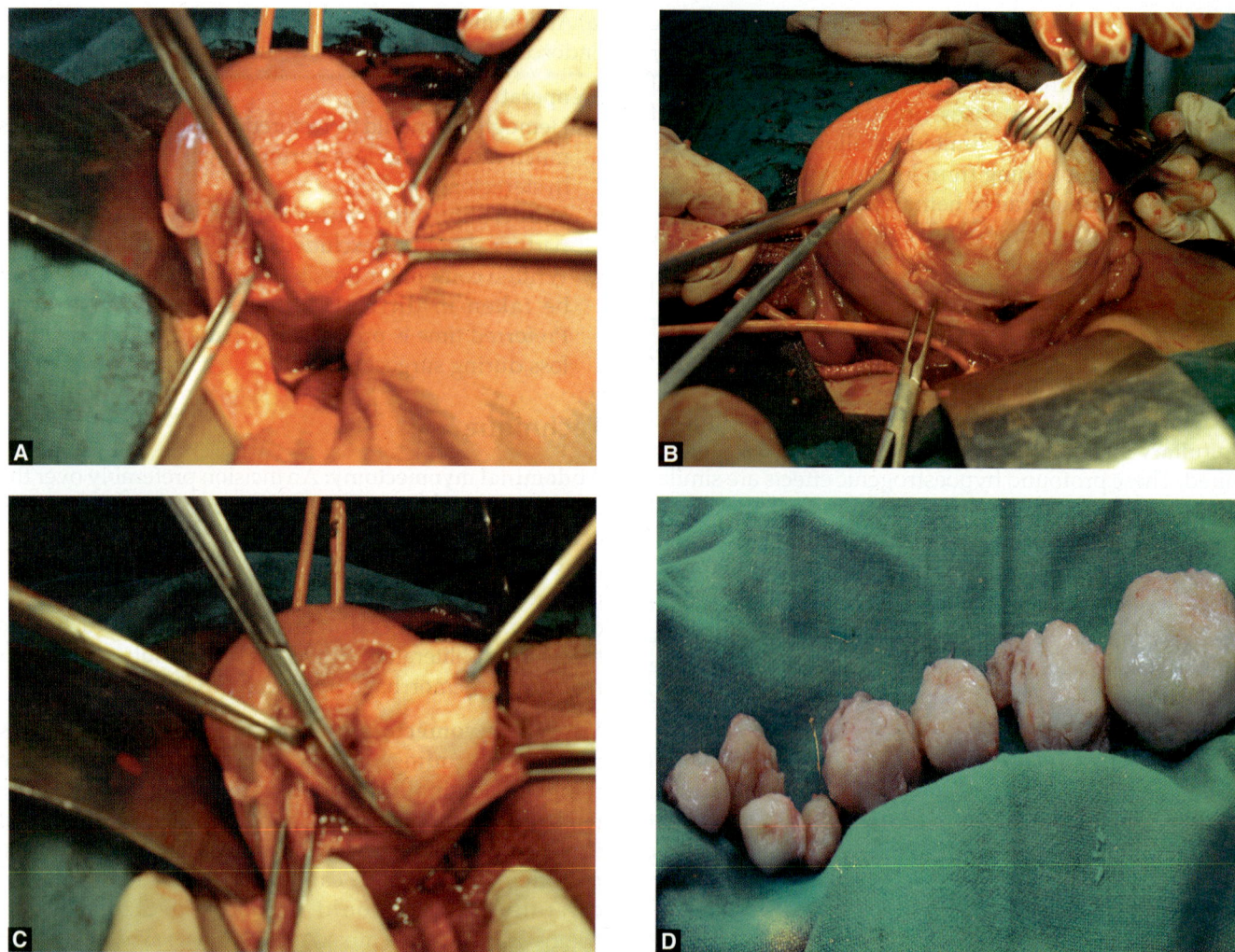

Figs 12.4A to D: (A) Incision into capsule of myoma; (B) Dissection of myoma bed; (C) Enucleation of myoma; (D) Multiple myoma removed

Myomectomy during pregnancy: Surgical intervention for properly diagnosed uterine fibroids should normally be avoided in pregnancy. The only indication for myomectomy in pregnancy is torsion of a pedunculated fibroid in which transaction and hemostasis of the stalk can be achieved with relative safety. Similarly myomectomy has traditionally been discouraged during cesarean section, except perhaps to facilitate access to the lower uterine segment.

Hysterectomy

Leiomyomas are the most common indication for hysterectomy with a cumulative risk of 7% for all women between 25- and 45-year-old. Hysterectomy eliminates the symptoms and recurrence. Uterus with small myomas may be removed by total vaginal hysterectomy especially if vaginal relaxation is present, where pelvic floor repair can be done simultaneously. In case of bigger fibroids, preoperative treatment with GnRH analog may facilitate vaginal hysterectomy.

When there are multiple tumors, intraligamentary myomas, total abdominal hysterectomy is indicated. Ovaries are generally preserved in premenopausal women. There is no consensus about the virtue of conserving or removing ovaries in postmenopausal women. In certain clinical situations like severe pelvic inflammatory disease, endometriosis or in any technical problem, subtotal hysterectomy can be performed. Steps of abdominal hysterectomy are illustrated in Figures 12.6A to H.

Uterine Fibroid Embolization

Embolic occlusion of the uterine arteries is an alternative to major surgery in premenopausal women not desiring fertility but who wish to retain their uterus. In this procedure an arteriogram is performed to identify the blood supply to the fibroid. A catheter is then advanced into the

Endometrial Ablation

For women not desiring fertility, ablation of the endometrium may control symptoms of bleeding. The procedure is more effective when combined with myolysis.

Myolysis

This is the technique of laparoscopic thermal coagulation of leiomyoma. It does not require suturing and is easy to perform. But localized tissue destruction may contribute to increase postoperative adhesion or chances of rupture during pregnancy.

Magnetic Resonance Guided Focused Ultrasound Surgery

This method was approved by FDA in 2004 for treatment of leiomyoma, in premenopausal women who have completed childbearing. This is an outpatient procedure, in which MRI is used for real time thermal monitoring of the thermoablative technique. In this technique multiple waves of ultrasound energy destroy a small volume of tissue. Experience of this method is very limited.

ADENOMYOSIS

Adenomyosis is defined by the presence of endometrial glands and stroma within the myometrium of the uterus, i.e. beneath the basement membrane. It may exist as either diffuse disease detected at hysterectomy only by microscopy or as distinct nodules, known as **adenomyoma**.

Adenomyosis is generally thought to affect 20% of women although meticulous sectioning of hysterectomy specimens has range of 20–60% incidence of adenomyosis.

Pathogenesis

The pathogenesis of adenomyosis is unknown. The most widely held theory regarding adenomyosis development describes the **downward invagination of the endometrial basalis layer** deeply into the myometrium. The endometrial myometrial interface is unique from most mucosal muscular interfaces is that it lacks an intervening submucosa. Mechanisms which initiate deep myometrial invasion are not known but it is thought that postpartum endometritis or vigorous curettage might cause the initial break in the normal boundary allowing endomyometrial invasion of the endometrium.

Another theory of **metaplastic origin** speculates an arrest of pluripotent Müllerian cells in the myometrium and later *de novo* development of endometrial glands in this site. This theory provides explanation for endometrial rest that has been identified in the rectovaginal septum far from the uterine endometrium and myometrium. **Estrogen and progesterone** likely play a role in its development and maintenance as adenomyosis develops during reproductive years and regresses after menopause.

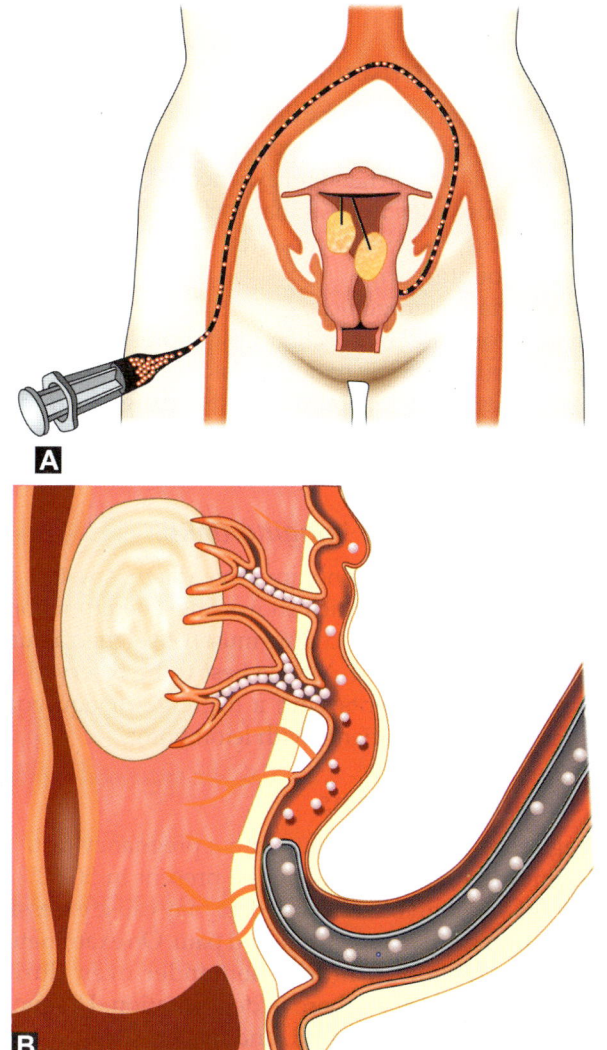

Figs 12.5A and B: Diagram showing uterine artery embolization

distal uterine artery under fluoroscopic guidance, usually through the right femoral artery. The artery is infused with an embolizing agent (Polyvenyl alcohol particles or tris acryl gelatin microspheres) until flow ceases. Usually procedure lasts for one hour (Figs 12.5A and B). As a result of leiomyoma necrosis, there can be significant postmenopausal symptoms, which are termed post-embolization syndrome. This lasts for 2-7 days and is classically marked by pelvic pain and cramping, nausea and vomiting, low grade fever and malaise of varying intensity. Management strategies include oral, intravenous, epidural or patient controlled analgesia regimen. Sufficient collateral circulation is present from the ovarian arteries to sustain normal uterine metabolic requirements.

Observational studies suggest that treatment is as effective as hysterectomy or myomectomy with more frequent minor complication, fewer major complications and shorter hospital stays. Leiomyoma recurrence rate with embolization is 10–15% as compared to 20–50% after myomectomy.

Pathology

On gross inspection, the uterus is uniformly enlarged and boggy but it rarely exceeds that of 12 weeks pregnancy. The surface contour is smooth and regular, uterine texture is softened and reddish myometrial discoloration is common. The cut uterine surface appears spongy with focal areas of hemorrhage.

Microscopic pattern is one of endometrial islands scattered throughout the myometrium at a distance of least 1 low power field from the basement membrane of the endometrium. Myometrial hypertrophy and hyperplasia are almost invariably apparent around the endometrial islets. The ectopic endometrium usually has an immature proliferative pattern. If the degree of involvement is marked, the embedded endometrium may show cyclic changes identical to those of normal endometrium. Although both adenomyosis and endometriosis are disorders of ectopic endometrium, the two diseases are unrelated though both frequently coexist.

Clinical Features

Symptoms and Signs

One-third of patients with adenomyosis are asymptomatic. The classic patient with adenomyosis is a parous middle aged woman with menorrhagia and dysmenorrhea who has a symmetrically enlarged uterus.

Menorrhagia

In 70% of women there is complaint of menorrhagia. The increased surface area of the endometrium, associated endometrial hyperplasia and inadequate uterine contraction contribute to menorrhagia. There is direct correlation between the degree of involvement of adenomyosis as opposed to depth of penetration, vascularity of the uterus and occurrence of menorrhagia.

Dysmenorrhea

Dysmenorrhea is present in 30% of women. Dysmenorrhea is directly related to the depth of penetration and degree of involvement. It probably results from myometrial contraction invoked by premenstrual swelling and menstrual bleeding in endometrial islands.

Sign

Abdominal examination may reveal a hypogastric mass arising out of the pelvis and occupying the midline. Uterine size usually does not exceed 12-14 weeks pregnant uterus. Pelvic examination reveal uniformly enlarged, slightly softened uterus, which may be tender premenstrually – **Halban's sign.**

Imaging

Transvaginal Ultrasound (TVUS)

As transabdominal sonography does not consistently identify the often subtle myometrial changes of adenomyosis. Imaging with TVS is preferred. In hands of experienced sonographers, finding of diffuse adenomyosis may include:

a. Anterior or posterior myometrial wall appear thicker than its counterpart.
b. Myometrial heterogenicity.
c. Small myometrial hypoechoic cyst, representing cystic glands within ectopic endometrial foci.
d. Linear striated projection extending from the endometrium into the myometrium.

Magnetic Resonance Imaging (MRI)

MRI is the most accurate noninvasive diagnostic test for detecting adenomyosis which shows thickened functional zone. But the cost of the procedure must be weighed against the information gathered. MRI is best to be reserved for the symptomatic patients with a negative or equivocal sonogram or for the patients with leiomyoma.

Differential Diagnosis

a. **Pregnancy** can be ruled out with a pregnancy test.
b. **Submucous leiomyoma** may be present in 50-60% of cases of adenomyosis. Leiomyoma may cause excessive and progressive menorrhagia and pain. On examination uterus is usually firm and nontender even during menstruation, unless there is degeneration. Diagnosis is confirmed by ultrasound, and hysteroscopy.
c. **Endometrial cancer** is diagnosed by endometrial biopsy or curettage.
d. **Pelvic congestion syndrome (Taylor's syndrome):** It is characterized by chronic complaints of continuous pelvic pain and menometrorrhagia. In some cases the uterus is enlarged, symptomatic and minimally softened. Cervix may be cyanotic and patulous. At operation the pelvic vessels may appear enlarged and tortuous.
e. **Pelvic endometriosis** is marked by premenstrual and intermenstrual dysmenorrhea, adherent adnexal masses and shotty cul-de-sac or uterosacral ligament nodulation. It can be often associated with adenomyosis.

Prevention

Adenomyosis cannot be prevented.

Complications

a. Chronic severe anemia may result from persistent menorrhagia.

b. When the stromal component of endometrium without glands invades the myometrium, the resulting tumor is referred to as endolymphatic stromal myosis, or stromatosis. This entity is not dependent on ovarian hormonal production and therefore is not truly comparable to adenomyosis.
c. Primary adenocarcinoma has rarely been observed in islands of aberrant endometrium within myometrium.

Treatment

Hysterectomy

Hysterectomy is the only definitive treatment of adenomyosis and it is also the only method for establishing the diagnosis with certainty (Figs 12.6A to H). Decision of conservation of ovary depends on patient's age. If there are obvious ovarian lesions or generalized pelvic endometriosis ovaries should be removed.

Uterine artery embolization has also been used to reduce symptoms for some women and success rate varies widely and ranges from 25 to 90%.

Medical Treatment

a. NSAID can be given for menorrhagia.
b. Oral contraceptives are usually not effective.
c. GnRH agonist can provide temporarily relief of symptoms if the focus of adenomyosis is estrogen and progesterone receptor positive.
d. Progesterone releasing intrauterine contraceptive device has been found useful in reducing symptoms of adenomyosis in some studies.

Prognosis

Hysterectomy is curative.
Ovaries should be removed.

ENDOMETRIAL POLYP

'Polyp' is a general descriptive term for any mass of tissue that projects outwards or away from the surface of surrounding tissue. An endometrial polyp is a hyperplastic overgrowth of endometrial glands visible as a spheroidal or cylindric structures that may be either pedunculated (attached by a slender stalk) or sessile (relatively broad based).

Incidence

Benign endometrial polyps are rare among women younger than 20 years. Their incidence increases directly with age, peaks in the fifth decade and slowly decreases after menopause. Risk factors are hypertension and obesity. Higher incidence of endometrial polyp is noted in patients undergoing Tamoxifen therapy.

Pathology

Grossly: An endometrial polyp is a smooth, red or brown ovoid body with a velvety texture, ranging from a few millimeters to many centimeters in widest diameter.

Microscopy: The endometrial polyp consists of: (a) Generally dense fibrous tissues – the stroma, (b) Impressively large and thick walled vascular channels, (c) Gland like spaces of variable sizes and shapes lined with endometrial epithelium.

The relative amount of these three components varies considerably. The surface of an intact polyp in a functioning uterus usually is covered by a layer of endometrium resembling that of the remainder of the endometrial surface but beneath this exterior are glandular components that are seemingly much older but apparently do not participate in menstrual shedding.

Secondary Changes in Polyp

a. There can be squamous metaplasia of surface epithelium.

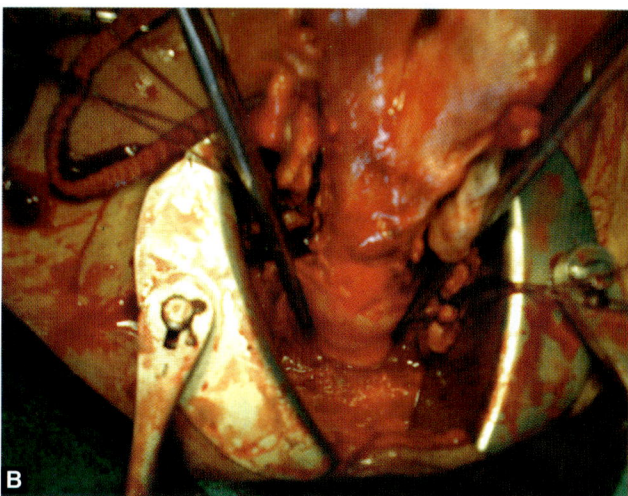

Figs 12.6 A and B

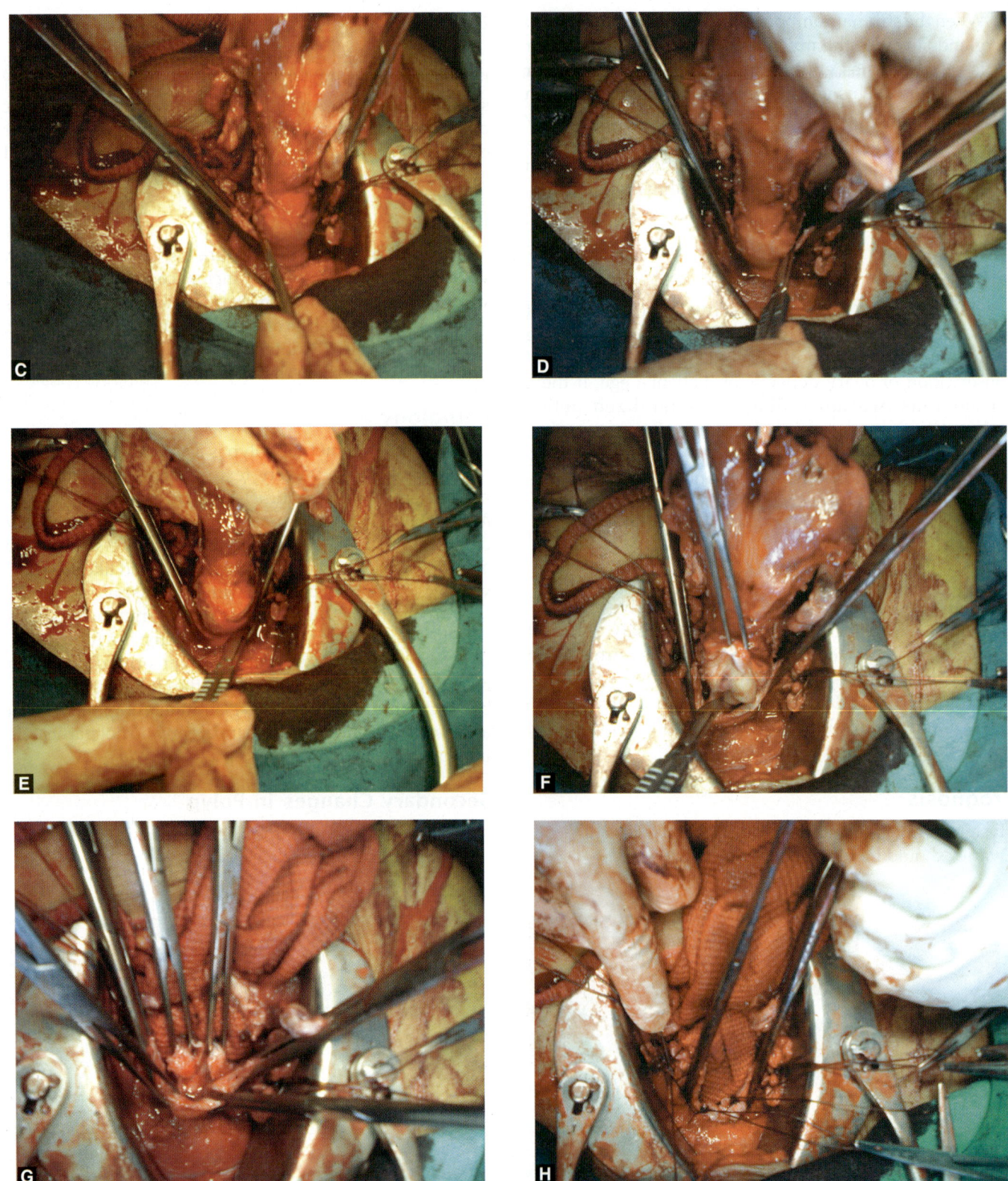

Figs 12.6C and H

Figs 12.6A to H: Steps of abdominal hysterectomy: (A) Clamping of fundal structure (Fallopian tube, round ligament and ovarian ligament; (B)—Clamping and ligation of uterine artery; (C) Clamping of paracervical ligament; (D) Ligation of paracervical ligament; (E and F) Incision on vault of vagina and delivery of cervix; (G) Suturing of vaginal vault; (H) All ligated pedicles are seen and tied with ligature of vaginal vault to reduce the chances of vault prolapse

b. Adenocarcinoma may develop within an otherwise benign polyp usually at some distance from its base or pedicle. At the same time a benign polyp may exist in an area of endometrial carcinoma. So *recovery of a harmless appearing polyp from the bleeding uterus in postmenopausal women does not assure that a more serious lesion does not exist elsewhere in the cavity.*
c. Pedunculated adenomyomas: Polyp that contains interlacing bands of smooth muscle are called pedunculated adenomyomas.
d. Multiple polyposis: In case of hyperplasia of the endometrium, the abundant overgrowth of tissue may produce a gross pattern called multiple polyposis. Curettage of such lesion may suggest the presence of adenocarcinoma because of unexpectedly large volume of tissue.

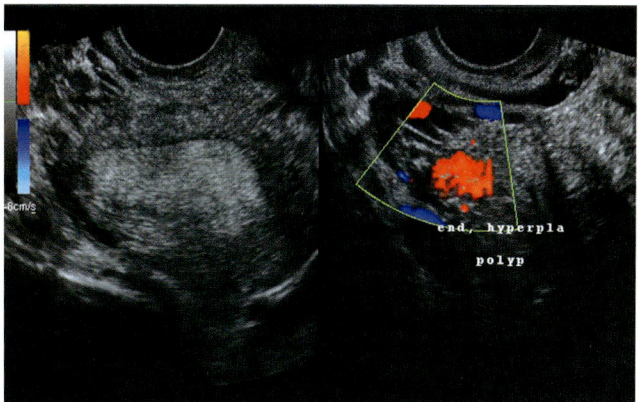

Fig. 12.7: Ultrasound image of endometrial polyp

Clinical Findings

Metrorrhagia, i.e. irregular bleeding is the most common presentation of symptomatic polyp occurring in half of patients. Menorrhagia, postmenopausal bleeding or prolapsed mass may also be presenting complaint. Polyp may be the source of minor premenstrual or postmenstrual bleeding, allegedly because the dependent top of the polyp is the first endometrial area to degenerate and last to obtain a new epithelial covering and cease bleeding after menstrual slough.

In the postmenopausal women bleeding from polyp is usually light and is often described as staining or spotting. A polyp should be suspected when bleeding continues following a D & C that has produced only benign normal tissue.

Imaging

Sonohysterography (transvaginal ultrasound added with saline infusion in endometrial cavity by pediatric Foley's catheter) is the most useful imaging modality for diagnosing polyps. Polyp appears as a homogeneous hyperechoic intracavitary mass on both transvaginal ultrasound and sonohysterogram (Fig. 12.7).

Polyp may be evident on hysterosalpingogram as irregularities in the outline of uterine cavity or as filling defect. However, hysterosalpingography has largely been replaced by office hysteroscopy and saline hysterography. No imaging modality can reliably distinguish between benign and malignant polyp.

Treatment

Surgical Excision

Hysteroscopic resection of polyp followed by curettage is the gold standard for diagnosis and treatment of symptomatic polyp as small polyps can be missed on blind curettage. Direct visualization of polyp by hysteroscopy has greatly aided in their identification and removal. Direct visualization of the endometrium and selected biopsies can rule out endometrial atypia or dysplasia.

If hysteroscopy is not available and a blind curettage is planned, the endometrial cavity must be explored separately using a grasping forceps preferably at the beginning of curettage procedure. Despite this precaution polyps are frequently missed and remain in the uterus after curettage and discovered later when menorrhagia persists and hysterectomy is performed. Sometimes only a portion of polyp is removed by curettage, and brisk bleeding continues postoperatively from the residual portion of the lesion. **In all cases a fractional curettage should follow any non-visualizing attempt at polyp removal to rule out endometrial carcinoma (Fig. 12.8).**

A polyp should be labeled as such, preserved separately in fixative solutions and sent to pathology laboratory as a separate specimen, because it may be the most significant portion of the tissue sample. If it is mixed with other part of curettage material; it is not assured that polyp specimen will be part of material chosen for histologic screening. Hysteroscopic resection of polyp

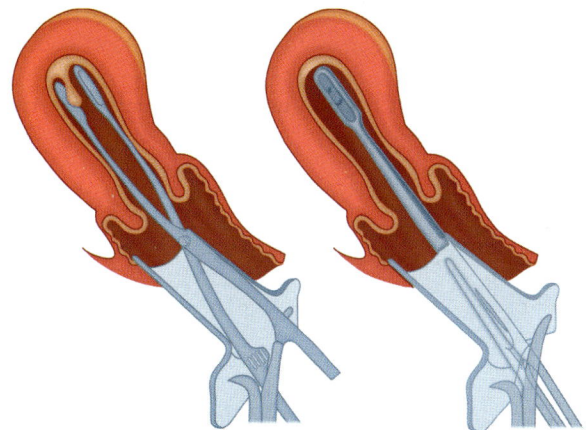

Fig. 12.8: Removal of endometrial polyp by use of polyp forceps

prior to intrauterine insemination, in infertility patients has been associated with a significantly higher pregnancy rate (63% vs 28% in control) even when the polyp is asymptomatic. So infertility patient should be offered excision of polyp before initiating assisted reproductive technologies.

Medical Therapy

GnRH agonist may be useful for short-term treatment of polyps but symptoms tend to recur after cessation of treatment. Progestin therapy may also cause some regression. Prospective studies have also shown that some polyp less than 1 cm regress spontaneously.

Hysterectomy

Usually simple excision is adequate for a benign polyp but if area of carcinoma or sarcoma is discovered hysterectomy should be performed. Besides, in a premenopausal patient persistence of abnormal uterine bleeding after removal of an apparently benign polyp may require further diagnostic step and more invasive treatment.

Prognosis

Removal of polyp is curative treatment, but recurrence is frequent. Hysterectomy is of course definitive treatment but usually unnecessary, if cancer has been ruled out.

MULTIPLE CHOICE QUESTIONS

1. Fibroids cause all, *except*:
   a. Menstrual irregularities
   b. Infertility
   c. Abdominal mass
   d. Amenorrhea
   Ans. d
2. To start with, all fibroids are:
   a. Interstitial
   b. Submucous
   c. Ovarian
   d. Subserous
   Ans. a
3. The percentage of myoma undergoing malignant transformation:
   a. 10%
   b. 5%
   c. 1%
   d. 0.5%
   Ans. d
4. Red degeneration of fibroid is due to:
   a. Thrombosis of veins
   b. Infection
   c. Gangrene
   d. Rupture of capsule
   Ans. a
5. Which statement is not true about red degeneration of myoma?
   a. It occurs commonly during pregnancy
   b. Immediate surgical intervention is needed
   c. Due to interference with blood supply
   d. Treated with analgesics
   Ans. b
6. Uterine fibroid is associated with:
   a. PID
   b. Ovarian cancer
   c. Amenorrhea
   d. Endometriosis
   Ans. d
7. Fundal myoma commonly presents as:
   a. Inversion of uterus
   b. Menorrhagia
   c. Urinary retention
   d. Dysmenorrhea
   Ans. b
8. All drugs can reduce the size of fibroids, *except*:
   a. Danazol
   b. GnRH
   c. RU-486
   d. Estrogen
   Ans. d
9. Treatment of choice in a 45 years old, multipara with a single fibroid in uterus of 12 weeks size and asymptomatic:
   a. Hysterectomy
   b. Myomectomy
   c. Hysteroscopic removal
   d. No treatment indicated
   Ans. a
10. Treatment of choice in a perimenopausal women with bleeding P/V due to multiple fibroids is:
    a. TAH with BSA
    b. TAH
    c. Vaginal hysterectomy
    d. Enucleation of fibroids
    Ans. b
11. Which one of the following is the definitive treatment of adenomyosis?
    a. LNG – Intrauterine device
    b. GnRH analog
    c. Danazol
    d. Hysterectomy
    Ans. d

13
Abnormal Uterine Bleeding and Abnormalities of Menstruation

The great end of life is not knowledge but action.

General Consideration

Regular cyclic menstruation results from the choreographed relationship between the endometrium and its regulating factors. (See Basic Sciences) Change in either of these frequently results in abnormal bleeding. Cause of this bleeding may be abnormal menstrual bleeding and bleeding due to other causes such as pregnancy, systemic disease or cancer. So abnormal uterine bleeding is a common gynecologic complaint that may affect female of all ages.

PATTERNS OF ABNORMAL UTERINE BLEEDING

The standard classification for patterns of abnormal bleeding recognizes following patterns:

Menorrhagia (Hypermenorrhea): It is excessive or prolonged bleeding at regular intervals. The presence of clot may not be abnormal, but may signify excessive bleeding. Gushing or open faucet bleeding is always abnormal. In objective term it is a blood loss greater than 80 ml per cycle.

Hypomenorrhea (Cryptomenorrhea): It is unusually light menstrual flow, sometimes only spotting.

Metrorrhagia (Intermenstrual bleeding): It is bleeding that occurs at any time between menstrual period.

Polymenorrhea: It is frequent regular bleeding that occurs at interval of less than 21 days.

Oligomenorrhea: It describes menstrual period that occurs more than 35 days apart. **Amenorrhea** is diagnosed if no menstrual period occurs for more than 6 months.

Menometrorrhagia: It is bleeding that occurs at irregular intervals. Any condition that causes intermenstrual bleeding can eventually lead to menometrorrhagia.

Postmenopausal bleeding: Bleeding that occurs more than 1 year after menopause, or at irregular intervals while on hormone replacement therapy.

Incidence

Abnormal uterine bleeding affects 10–30% of reproductive aged women and up to 50% of perimenopausal women. Factors that affect this incidence most are age and reproductive status. Uterine bleeding is uncommon in prepubertal girls and postmenopausal women whereas incidence of abnormal uterine bleeding increases significantly in adolescent, perimenopausal and reproductive age group. Recognition and awareness of most common etiologies of bleeding within these groups helps in diagnosis and treatment.

Causes of Abnormal Uterine Bleeding

Causes of abnormal bleeding can be listed in Box 13.1:

Box 13.1: Causes of abnormal uterine bleeding

(i) **Pregnancy related**
  a. Miscarriage
  b. Ectopic pregnancy
  c. Gestational trophoblastic disease
(ii) **Infection**
  a. Cervicitis
  b. Endometritis
(iii) **Neoplasm**
  a. Cervical dysplasia/carcinoma
  b. Endometrial hyperplasia/polyp, carcinoma
  c. Submucous leiomyoma
  d. Estrogen producing ovarian tumor
(iv) **Systemic disease**
  a. Thyroid disease
  b. Liver disease
  c. Coagulation disorder
  d. Sepsis
(v) **Iatrogenic**
  a. Oral contraceptive
  b. Progestin only contraceptives
  c. Intrauterine device
  d. Hormone replacement therapy
  e. Steroids

Evaluation of Abnormal Uterine Bleeding

Detailed history, physical examination, cytologic examination, pelvic ultrasound and blood test are the first steps in the evaluation of abnormal uterine bleeding.

History

A careful menstrual history is the single most useful tool in differentiating anovulatory bleeding from other causes. Detailed information regarding **intermenstrual interval**, volume (heavy, light, variable), **duration** (normal or prolonged, consistent or variable), **onset** of abnormal menses (perimenarcheal, sudden, gradual), **temporal associations** (postcoital, postpartum, postpill, weight gain or loss), **associated symptoms** (premenstrual monilinia, dysmenorrhea, dyspareunia, galactorrhea, hirsutism), underlying **systemic illness** (renal, hepatic, hematopoietic, thyroid) and **medications** (hormonal, anticoagulant) can provide important clues and help to quickly determine whether additional evaluation is needed before treatment begins.

Physical Examination

Physical examination should exclude visible **vaginal or cervical lesion** and define **uterine size** (normal or enlarged), **contours** (smooth and symmetrical or irregular), **consistency** (firm or soft) and **tenderness.** Figure 13.1 summarizes the main causes of abnormal uterine bleeding.

Laboratory Test

They are helpful but are not always necessary. A sensitive **urine pregnancy test** can quickly exclude any realistic possibility that the bleeding is related to an accident or complication of pregnancy. A **complete blood count** to exclude anemia and thrombocytopenia should be done in women with history of prolonged or extensively heavy bleeding.

A well-timed **serum progesterone** determination during the luteal phase of the cycle can help to document ovulation or anovulation. When doubt exists, any value greater than 3 ng/ml provides reliable evidence of ovulation. However, in poorly documented or too frequent bleeding episode, proper timing for progesterone measurement can be difficult to determine.

In anovulatory women a **serum thyroid stimulating hormone** (TSH) level can quickly exclude any associated thyroid disorder. In adolescent, those with a suspicious personal or family history and with unexplained menorrhagia, suspicion of bleeding disorder is sufficient indication for screening **coagulation studies. Liver or renal function tests** are indicated only for those with known or strongly suspected disease.

Cytologic Examination

Both cervical and endometrial cancers can cause abnormal bleeding and evidence for these tumors can often be found with Pap smear screening. The most frequent abnormal cytologic result gives indication of squamous cell pathology and may reflect cervicitis, intraepithelial neoplasia or cancer.

Less commonly atypical glandular or endometrial cells may be found. Any of these may suggest the cause of bleeding and depending on the cytologic result, colposcopy or endometrial biopsy or both may be indicated.

Pelvic Ultrasound Scan

Pelvic ultrasound examination has become an integral part of the gynecologic pelvic examination. This scan can be performed either transvaginally or transabdominally. The transvaginal examination is performed with an empty bladder and enables a closer look with greater details at the pelvic organs. Transabdominal examination is performed with full bladder and enables a wider but less discriminative examination of the pelvis. The ultrasound scan can add many details to the physical evaluation, as description of uterine lining, its width and regularity and presence of intramuscular or submucous fibroids, intrauterine polyp, and adnexal mass.

Persistent thick and irregular endometrium is one of the preoperative predictors of endometrial pathology and warrants further evaluation and tissue biopsy.

Sonohysterography is a modified pelvic scan in which saline is injected by a thin catheter into the uterus. It increases significantly the sensitivity of transvaginal ultrasonography and has been used to evaluate the endometrial cavity for polyp, fibroid and other abnormalities.

Endometrial Biopsy

TVS, cytology and history of duration of exposure to unopposed estrogen stimulation directs the necessity of endometrial biopsy. Endometrial biopsy is unnecessary when the endometrial thickness is less than 5 mm. Biopsy

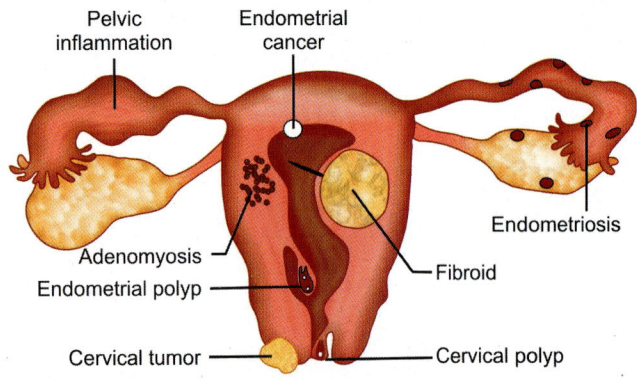

Fig. 13.1: Diagram explaining various causes of abnormal uterine bleeding

is indicated when the clinical history suggests long-term unopposed estrogen exposure even when endometrial thickness is normal (5-12 mm) and biopsy should be performed when endometrial thickness is greater than 12 mm even when clinical suspicion of disease is low. Instrument for endometrial biopsy includes use of Novak suction curette, Duncan curette, the Kevorkian curette or pipette.

Hysteroscopy

It is done with an instrument which uses an endoscopic camera in the telescope. Hysteroscope is passed through the cervix into endometrial cavity. It allows direct visualization of the cavity. Because of its higher diagnostic accuracy and suitability for outpatient investigation, hysteroscopy is increasingly being used replacing dilatation and curettage for evaluation of AUB (Fig. 13.2).

Hysteroscopy is currently regarded as the gold standard for evaluation of pathology in uterine cavity. Resection attachments allow immediate capabilities to remove or biopsy lesions. But it is an invasive procedure, has greater cost and there are potential anesthetic and surgical risk, which preclude its routine use.

Use of 3.5 mm mini-hysteroscope instead of conventional 5 mm endoscope significantly decrease patient discomfort and can be performed in office settings. But still major intrauterine pathologies generally require more traditional operative hysteroscopy using instruments having a larger caliber and greater capabilities.

Dilatation and Curettage

For many years D & C has been regarded as the gold standard for diagnosis of AUB. It can be performed with patient under local anesthetic, almost always in an

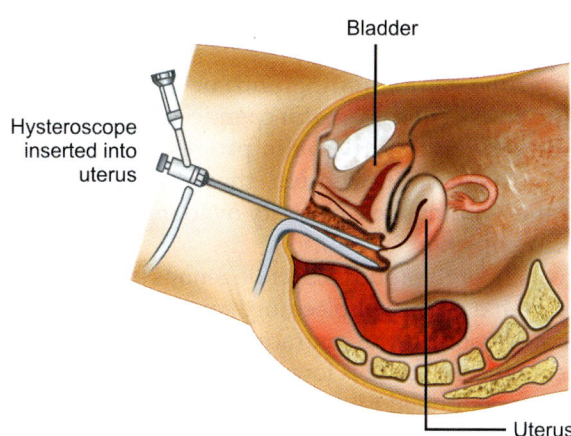

Fig. 13.2: Hysteroscopic evaluation in abnormal uterine bleeding

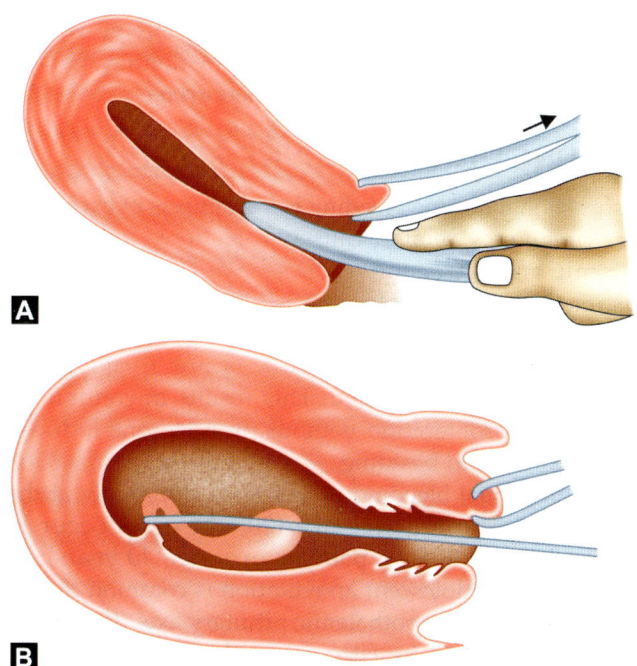

Figs 13.3A and B: (A) Dilatation and curettage for AUB; (B) Removal of polyp in AUB

outpatient setting (Figs 13.3A and B). General anesthetic allows more thorough pelvic examination, more precise evaluation of pelvic masses and more complete curettage. Nonetheless D & C is a blind procedure, and its accuracy particularly when the cause of AUB is a focal lesion, such as polyp, is debatable.

GENERAL PRINCIPLE OF MANAGEMENT

In making the diagnosis, it is important not to assume the obvious. A careful history, physical evaluation and appropriately directed investigation are essential for a definitive diagnosis. Improved diagnostic technique and treatment have resulted in markedly decreased use of hysterectomy to treat abnormal uterine bleeding pattern.

If pathologic cause can be excluded, there is no significant risk for cancer development and if there is no accurate life-threatening hemorrhage, most patients can be treated with hormone preparation. **Myomectomy in selected** case can be offered. For menorrhagia, *many drugs* are available (described in dysfunctional uterine bleeding).

Abnormal Bleeding Due to Nongynecological Cause

Nongynecological cause must be ruled out. Besides, gynecologic and nongynecologic causes of bleeding may coexist. Systemic disease should be diagnosed and treated, e.g. Myxedema usually causes amenorrhea but less severe hypothyroidism is associated with increased uterine bleeding. Blood dyscrasias and coagulation abnormalities can also produce gynecologic bleeding. Extreme weight loss due to eating disorder, exercise or dieting may be associated with anovulation and amenorrhea.

DYSFUNCTIONAL UTERINE BLEEDING

Dysfunctional uterine bleeding is a diagnosis of exclusion after pregnancy related causes, infections, neoplastic, systemic and iatrogenic causes have been ruled out. Dysfunctional uterine bleeding is bleeding as a result of anovulation or oligoanovulation. The ovary produces estrogens but a corpus luteum is not formed and progesterone is not secreted. This results in continuous endometrial proliferation without progesterone induced desquamation and bleeding.

Dysfunctional bleeding occurs most commonly at the extremes of reproductive age (20% of cases occur in adolescents and 40% in patients over age 40 years). In perimenarchal adolescent anovulation is common due to immaturity of the hypothalamic pituitary axis. The axis is unable to respond to estrogen with an LH surge. In perimenopausal women it is related to declining ovarian function.

Diagnosis of dysfunctional uterine bleeding is made by history, absence of ovulatory temperature changes, low serum progesterone, and results of endometrial sampling in the older women. Structural abnormality like fibroid, polyp should be ruled out by ultrasonography.

Major Causes of Anovulation

a. **Physiologic**
   a. Adolescence
   b. Perimenopause
   c. Lactation
   d. Pregnancy
b. **Pathologic**
   a. Hyperandrogenic states
   b. Hyperprolactinemia
   c. Hypothyroidism
   d. Premature ovarian failure.

Ovulatory Dysfunctional Uterine Bleeding

Ovulatory dysfunctional uterine bleeding is caused by predominantly from vascular dilatation alone. In women with ovulatory DUB, it is thought that vessels supplying the endometrium have decreased vascular tone and therefore increased rates of blood loss resulting from vasodilatation. Prostaglandins are strongly suggested for provoking this change in vascular tone.

Treatment

Anovulatory Bleeding

The immediate objective of medical therapy for anovulatory bleeding is to restore or induce the natural control mechanism that are not operating in orderly synchronous growth development and shedding of a structurally stable endometrium. Just as progesterone is the dominant and controlling influence in normal menstrual cycle, **progestins are the mainstay of treatment for anovulatory bleeding.**

Progestin Therapy

Anovulatory bleeding is which as stated above is more common in adolescent and perimenopausal years, but may occur at any time. The usual clinical presentation is oligomenorrhea with episodes of heavy or prolonged bleeding. In most of these situations progesterone therapy will control anovulatory bleeding, once uterine pathology has been excluded. Cyclic progestin therapy restores the normal sequence of endometrial steroid hormone stimulation – *estrogen, followed by estrogen plus progesterone, followed by withdrawal bleeding.*

Mode of Action of Progestins

Progestins are powerful antiestrogen. Progesterone stimulates 17α hydroxysteroid dehydrogenase and sulfotransferase activity, which work in concert to convert estradiol to estrone sulfate which is rapidly cleared from the body. Progestin further antagonizes estrogen action by inhibiting estrogen induction of its own receptors. There is antimitotic, growth limiting effect of progesterone and progestin on the endometrium.

Dosage schedule: In treatment of oligomenorrhea in anovulatory women with episodic abnormal bleeding orderly predictable progesterone withdrawal bleeding can be induced by cyclic treatment with an orally active progestin like *medroxyprogesterone acetate 5–10 mg daily for 2 weeks every month,* starting from 15–16 days after onset of last menstrual cycle. If menses do not follow progestin withdrawal, the possibility of more profound ovulatory dysfunction associated with grossly low estrogen levels must be considered, and additional evaluation is indicated.

Estrogen Progestin Contraceptive

In women who are ovulating and/or want to avoid pregnancy, an estrogen progestin contraceptive is a better choice. Because standard cyclic progestin treatment regimens are not contraceptive, they do not reliably suppress the hypothalamic pituitary ovarian axis and will not prevent ovulation.

Oral contraceptives suppress endogenous function and give predictable pattern of bleeding. Any of the low dose monophasic combined oral contraceptive may be used (one pill twice daily). The dose is lowered after a few days and lower dose is continued for next few cycles. When readily available a transvaginal ultrasound examination before start of treatment can help to confirm the diagnostic impression (as finding of uniformly increased endometrial thickness) and minimize the risk of unsuccessful treatment with continued heavy bleeding.

With either OC's or pure progestin treatment, further diagnostic evaluation is indicated when treatment is unsuccessful.

Maintenance Therapy

a. After the menstruation that follows estrogen progestin withdrawal, maintenance therapy with a standard cyclic low dose combination estrogen progestin contraceptive can begin. A gradual but steady decline in volume and duration of flow and associated dysmenorrhea with each successive cycle can be expected and is reassuring. In women with normal uterus, oral contraceptive reduces menstrual flow by 60% from that in natural cycle.

b. **Depot medroxyprogesterone acetate (Depot provera DMPA)** in the dose used for contraceptive, 150 mg intramuscular every 3 months can be a useful option for maintenance therapy in women, who have difficulty with or cannot take estrogen progestin contraceptive due to medical or other reasons. But it is to be noted that it has no place in the acute management of abnormal bleeding. Once given, it cannot be withdrawn. And if unsuccessful, its effect can be difficult to overcome.

c. **Estrogen therapy:** Intermittent vaginal spotting frequently is associated with marginal or quiet low levels of estrogen stimulation, so it is termed as estrogen breakthrough bleeding. Under such circumstances, the endometrium is extremely thin and beneficial effect of progestin treatment cannot be achieved because estrogen levels are insufficient to stimulate the growth that serves as the foundation for the action of progestins.

Again transvaginal ultrasound can helps to guide the choice of treatment by defining the endometrial thickness and revealing any other cause of bleeding. When endometrium is attenuated or grossly denuded and bleeding is acute and heavy, high dose estrogen therapy should be administered. In those patients when bleeding demands hospitalization and careful observation, intravenous estrogen therapy (25 mg conjugated equine estrogen every 4 hours until bleeding subsides or for 24 hours) can be very effective. The mechanism of action responsible for the efficacy of intravenous estrogen is unclear but has been attributed to stimulation of clotting at the capillary level.

When bleeding is less profuse and emergent but still quite heavy, high dose oral estrogen treatment – 1.25 mg conjugated estrogen, or 2.0 mg micronized estradiol (Progynova) every 4-6 hours for 24 hours is generally effective, tapering to once daily dose for another 7-10 days after bleeding is controlled. Less acute or lighter intermittent nuisance bleeding generally responds well to the single daily dose (1.25 mg conjugated estrogen or 2.0 mg micronized estradiol for 7-10 days).

For best results, all such initial estrogen therapy should be followed by treatment with progestin or estrogen progestin contraceptive to stabilize the estrogen stimulated endometrial growth. Estrogen therapy is also the logical and best choice for management of episodic progesterone breakthrough bleeding as commonly observed in women receiving low dose estrogen progestin contraceptive or depot form of progestin therapy (Injectable or implants). In these cases, a short interval of added estrogen (conjugated estrogen 1.25 mg or micronized estradiol 2.0 mg daily for 7-10 days) is generally highly effective.

Estrogen Therapy and Risk of Thromboembolism

High doses of estrogen are associated with an increased risk for thromboembolism. *More than one oral contraceptive pill per day or several doses of oral or intravenous estrogen within a single 24 hours interval must be considered as high doses.*

It is important to emphasize that while in young women and adolescent above hormonal treatment is quite effective, in premenopausal women more care must be given to excluding pathologic causes because of the possibility of endometrial cancer. The initial evaluation should be complemented by hysteroscopy and endometrial biopsy and should clearly establish anovulatory or asynchronous cycle before start of hormonal therapy. **Again recurrence of abnormal bleeding demands further evaluation.**

Nonspecific Treatment for Abnormal Menstrual Bleeding

A specific cause for heavy or prolonged menstrual bleeding in ovulatory women cannot always be identified. Local defects in endometrial hemostasis are presumed responsible. Under such circumstances the problem of DUB can still be effectively managed using variety of nonspecific medical and surgical therapies.

Nonsteroidal Anti-inflammatory Drugs

Prostaglandins have important action on the endometrial vasculature and in endometrial hemostasis. The concentration of PGE_2 and $PGE_2\alpha$ increase progressively in human endometrium during the menstrual cycle and are found in high concentration in menstrual endometrium. Nonsteroidal anti-inflammatory drugs (NSAIDs) inhibit PG synthesis and decrease menstrual blood loss. NSAID may alter the balance between thromboxane A2 (A vasoconstrictor and promoter of platelet aggregation) and prostacyclin (PGF_2) a vasodilator and inhibitor of platelet aggregation.

Though the exact mechanism is unclear, NSAIDs reduce blood loss by approximately 20–40% and to a greater extent in those with excessive bleeding. Naproxen, Mefenamic acid have been most extensively used.

Treatment with NSAIDs might be considered the first line therapy for ovulatory women with heavy menstrual bleeding and no demonstrable pathology: NSAIDs are started with onset of bleeding and continued for 3-5 days as necessary. They also provide relief from dysmenorrhea.

Oral Contraceptives

Oral contraceptive can be used to reduce menstrual blood loss in ovulatory women with heavy menstrual bleeding, regardless of whether their menorrhagia is associated with pathology (myoma, adenomyosis) or unexplained. In women with unexplained menorrhagia oral contraceptive can be expected to reduce bleeding by approximately 40%. *Seasonale* is combined oral contraceptive taken for 84 days with gap of 6 days. It acts as contraception as well reduced frequency of menstrual bleeding.

Levonorgesterel IUD

The levonorgesterel releasing intrauterine device has a reservoir containing 52 mg LNG mixed with polydimethylsiloxane that controls the rate of hormone release. For contraceptive purpose the device can remain in place for 10 years. By LNG-IUD, menstrual blood loss in women with heavy menstrual bleeding can be reduced by 75-95% due to progestin induced decidualization of the endometrium. The LNG-IUD is an attractive and alternative option for ovulatory women with heavy menstrual bleeding and women with intractable bleeding associated with chronic illness like renal function. Higher cost of the device is limiting factor for its common use.

Gonadotropins Releasing Hormone Agonist

Treatment with gonadotropins releasing hormone agonist (GnRH) can achieve short-term relief from abnormal uterine bleeding and can be used effectively as a preoperative adjunct in women awaiting conservative (myomectomy, endometrial ablation) or definitive surgery (hysterectomy) for abnormal bleeding. GnRH analog treatment is also useful in the management of abnormal menstrual bleeding that may follow organ transplantation, where the toxicity of immunosuppressive drugs makes use of sex steroids less desirable. As stated in previous chapter, the expense and side effects resulting from estrogen deficiency (hot flushes, bone mineral depletion) make GnRH a an unattractive long-term strategy for treatment of abnormal bleeding.

Other Medical Treatment Strategies:
a. Tranexamic acid is an antifibrinolytic agent used for treatment of menorrhagia. It is more effective than NSAID therapy but rather large dose (2-6 gm daily) is required. Incidences of gastrointestinal side effects and intermenstrual bleeding are relatively high.
b. Danazol (200 mg daily) is more effective than NSAID, progestin and oral contraceptive for treatment of heavy menstrual bleeding. But the long-term treatment is required, cost is high, and there are associated androgenic side effects. All factors make it unacceptable to most women.
c. Ormeloxifene: Selective estrogen receptor modulator. This is antiestrogenic drug, agonist to bone and cardiovascular system. It has been tried in DUB with success rate of 50%.

Surgical Measures in Dysfunctional Uterine Bleeding

a. *Dilatation and curettage:* In hemodynamically unstable women, fluid resuscitation and operative dilatation and curettage is the most effective way to stop uncontrollable uterine bleeding in the absence of any apparent organic pathology. The mechanism of the effect of curettage is not entirely clear but surgical denudation of the basal layer of the endometrium is presumed to actively stimulate all of the normal processes involved in cessation of normal menstrual bleeding – local clotting mechanism, vasoconstriction of basal arterioles and rapid re-epithelialization.

b. *Endometrial ablation:* Persistent bleeding despite treatment is both frustrating and concerning. In patients who want to avoid surgery or poor candidate for major surgery, endometrial ablation is another choice for management of unexplained menorrhagia. When medical treatments are rejected, unsuccessful or poorly tolerated endometrial ablation can be performed to selectively destroy the basalis layer of the endometrium. The following methods of endometrial ablation are in use:

   (i) **Hysteroscopically** directed thermal ablation using a roller ball or resectoscope (Figs 13.4A and B).
   (ii) **Hysteroscopic** Na:YAG (Neodymium, yttrium aluminum garnet) laser photovaporization.
   (iii) **Thermal balloon ablation:** A latex balloon is inserted into the uterus and filled with 5% dextrose which is then heated to 87°C and circulated for 8 minutes.
   (iv) **Hydrothermal ablation:** Normal saline that has been superheated to 80-90°C flows into the uterus through an insulated sheath under direct hysteroscopic visualization. Intrauterine pressure never exceeds 55 mm Hg – well below the 70-75 mm Hg (opening pressure of the fallopian tube), to ensure that fluid does not pass into the peritoneal cavity.
   (v) **Microwave endometrial ablation:** Microwave energy is delivered through an 8 mm intrauterine applicator. Once the tip is activated, a temperature of 95°C is achieved and the temperature display is

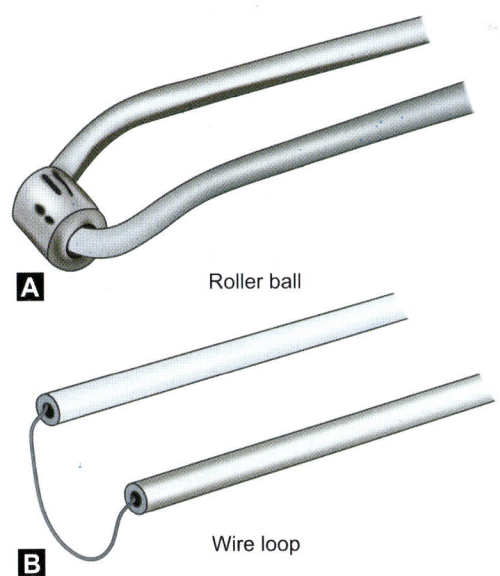

Figs 13.4A and B: (A) Roller ball; (B) Wire. Used for hysteroscopic endometrial ablation

used to monitor the ablation process as the surgeon moves the probe laterally from one cornua to another and then to the midline. The average treatment time is 1-4 minutes and is determined by the size of the uterus and the thickness of the endometrium. Studies have shown a success rate of 70-90%. There are legitimate concerns that endometrial carcinoma might be inadvertently treated by endometrial ablation or procedure might obliterate portion where uterine cavity leave isolated, residual islands of endometrium in which adenocarcinoma could develop and go unrecognized in the absence of bleeding. These observations emphasize the importance of thorough preoperative evaluation to include endometrial biopsy and proper patient selection for ablation procedure. **Endometrial ablation is not recommended for women at high risk for endometrial cancer.**

(vi) **Hysterectomy:** Hysterectomy continues to be the definitive therapy for patients who are not assisted by other methods.

POSTMENOPAUSAL BLEEDING

Postmenopausal bleeding may be defined as bleeding that occurs after 12 months of amenorrhea or at irregular intervals while on hormone replacement therapy. If amenorrhea occurs in younger person with diagnosis of premature ovarian failure or menopause, episodes of bleeding can be classified as postmenopausal. In this situation follicle stimulating hormone (FSH) levels are particularly helpful in the differential diagnosis of menopausal versus hypothalamic amenorrhea. An FSH level greater than 30 mIU/ml is highly suggestive of menopause.

Incidence

The incidence of postmenopausal bleeding in the age group of 50–55 years is reported to be 1.3% and at 70–75 years nearly 0.2%.

Approach to Diagnosis

Postmenopausal bleeding is more likely to be caused by pathologic disease than is bleeding in younger women and must always be investigated. Nongynecological causes must be excluded as patient may be unable to determine the site of bleeding by proper evaluation. Neither functional nor *dysfunctional bleeding* should occur after menopause. Although pathologic disorders are more likely, other causes may occur. These may be as follows:

1. **Benign condition:**
   a. Senile endometritis
   b. Atrophic endometrium
   c. Vulvar dystrophies
   d. Endometrial polyps
   e. Cervical polyps, cervical erosion
   f. Hormone replacement therapy
   g. Trauma
   h. Retained foreign body as pessary or IUCD
   i. Decubitus ulcer
2. **Malignant conditions:**
   a. Endometrial carcinoma
   b. Carcinoma cervix
   c. Carcinoma vagina, vulva
   d. Carcinoma fallopian tube
   e. Secondary tumors

Exogenous Hormone Replacement Therapy

The increasing use of hormone replacement therapy in postmenopausal women, to improve quality of life makes its special mention necessary. Regular menstrual bleeding may resume if they take HRT agents cyclically. Not uncommonly these patients present with vaginal bleeding as many as 6–12 months after initiation of hormone replacement therapy. If bleeding is still occurring by that time further investigation is warranted to determine its etiology. If endometrium hyperplasia is found on TVS endometrial biopsy must be taken to see presence of atypia and treatment should be started by increasing the progesterone component or by hysterectomy.

Vaginal Atrophy and Vaginal and Vulvar Lesions

Bleeding from the lower reproductive tract almost always is related to vaginal atrophy with or without trauma. Examination reveals thin tissue with ecchymosis. With vulvar dystrophies a white area and cracking of the skin of vulva may be present. Cytologic study from cervix and vagina reveals immature epithelial cell with or without inflammation. Vulvar lesion requires further diagnostic evaluation (Details in Chapter 10).

Benign and Malignant Tumors of the Reproductive Tract

Exclusion of benign and malignant tumor of reproductive tract requires a detailed history, thorough clinical examination that includes local, per speculum examination, bimanual pelvic examination and per rectal examination in selected case. Pelvic ultrasonography is extremely useful in **evaluation of thickness of endometrium and diagnosis of ovarian tumors and in differentiation between uterine myoma and adnexal tumors.**

Fractional curettage under anesthetic was the standard method of assessing postmenopausal bleeding. For this PAP smear, endocervical curettage with endometrial sampling and if needed endometrial curettage is performed. **Hysteroscopy** performed in office setting or operating room may prove helpful in locating endometrial polyp or fluid that could be missed by fractional curettage.

Treatment

Treatment of postmenopausal bleeding is directed towards the organic condition detected. If no cause is detected and there is minimal bleeding, careful observation is mandatory. In case of recurrent episodes of postmenopausal bleeding, it is better to perform hysterectomy with bilateral salpingo-oophorectomy, even when diagnosis cannot be established by endometrial sampling.

COMPLICATIONS OF MENSTRUATION

Premenstrual Syndrome

The first published description of premenstrual syndrome was in 1931 and syndrome was given the name PMS by Dalton in 1953. Speroff defines it as a *"Constellation of symptoms that occurs in cyclic pattern, always in the same phase of the menstrual cycle, interfering with work or lifestyle and followed by a period entirely free of symptoms"*. When these symptoms disrupt daily functioning, they are clustered under the name *Premenstrual Dysphoric Disorder* (PMDD).

Pathogenesis

The etiology of symptom complex of PMS is not known, although several theories have been proposed. The proposed theories are **estrogen progesterone imbalance, excess aldosterone, hypoglycemia, hyperprolactinemia and psychogenic factors**. A **hormonal imbalance previously** was thought to be related to clinical manifestation of PMS/PMDD, but in most recent consensus, **physiologic ovarian function** is believed to be the trigger. The thought is supported by the efficacy of ovarian cyclicity suppression either medically or surgically in eliminating premenstrual complaint. Sex steroid also interacts with the renin angiotensin aldosterone system (RAAS) to alter electrolyte and fluid balance. The antimineralocorticoid properties of progesterone and possible estrogen activation of the RAAS system may explain PMS symptoms of bloating and weight gain. Recent experience with selective serotonin receptor inhibitors (SSRIs) suggest that **serotonin may play a significant role** in the disease either as a primary cause or as secondary effect. Many of the symptoms of other mood disorders resembling the feature of PMS/PMDD have been associated with seratonergic dysfunction.

Diagnosis

No objective screening and diagnostic test for PMS and PMDD are available, thus special attention must be paid to the patient's medical history. Thyroid disease, anemia, underlying psychiatric conditions can mimic PMS/PMDD and must be ruled out. The patient is instructed to chart her symptoms for at least two symptomatic cycles. The classic criteria for PMS require that the patients have symptoms in the luteal phase and symptoms free period of at least seven days in the first half of the cycle, for a minimum of two consecutive symptomatic cycles.

For criteria of PMDD, women must have a chief complaint of at least one of the following – **Irritability, Tension, Dysphasia, or Mood liability**, and **five of eleven of the following – Depressed mood, Anxiety, Affected liability, Irritability, Decreased interest in daily activities, concentration difficulties, lack of energy, change in appetite or food cravings, sleep disturbance, or physical symptoms, e.g. breast tenderness, bloating.**

Treatment

Lifestyle Modification

Treatment of PMS/PMDD depends on the severity of the symptoms. For some women, *change in eating habits* – limiting caffeine, alcohol, tobacco and chocolate intake and eating small frequent meals high in complex carbohydrates may be sufficient. Decreasing sodium intake reduces edema. Stress management, cognitive behavioral therapy and aerobic exercise have all been shown to improve symptoms. Low risk symptomatic pharmacologic treatment:
a. Calcium carbonate (1000 – 1200 mg/day) for bloating, food craving and pain.
b. Magnesium (200 – 360 mg/day) for water retention.

c. Vitamin B$_6$ and vitamin E.
d. Nonsteroidal anti-inflammatory drugs (NSAIDs).
e. Spironolactone for cyclic edema.
f. Bromocriptine for mastalgia.

For symptoms of severe PMS and PMDD, further pharmacologic intervention may be necessary.

Pharmacological Treatment

a. Low risk symptomatic treatment as mentioned above
b. Psychotropic medication are effective are – (a) SSRI, (b) Despiramine, (c) L-tryptophan.

Selective serotonin receptor inhibitor (SSRI) have minimal side effects and provide symptomatic improvement in more than 60% of patient. Treatment should be given 14 days prior to the onset of menstruation and continued through the end of the cycle. Fluoxetine 20 mg daily is usually adequate in most of women. Anxiolytics as alprazolam and buspirone also have been shown to be effective but their side effects and potential for dependence must be seriously considered.

Other Treatment Option

Use of oral **contraceptive** has been suggested because they suppress ovulation, but they have not been found to be effective. **GnRH** agonist leads to temporarily medical menopause but their limitations lie in high cost, hypoestrogenic state and risk for osteoporosis. Add back therapy with estrogen and progesterone may obviate these problems. **Bromocriptine** 5 mg/day during luteal phase and **Danazol** may improve mastalgia.

Surgical Treatment

Finally bilateral oophorectomy is a definitive surgical treatment option. But it is too invasive therapy. If it is considered estrogen replacement would be recommended.

Besides, there is important role of clinician patient relationship and interaction in management of premenstrual syndrome.

DYSMENORRHEA

Dysmenorrhea is pelvic pain associated with menstrual periods, described usually as cramping in nature. Dysmenorrhea can also be accompanied by many other systemic symptoms including light headedness, insomnia, and gastrointestinal symptoms such as nausea, vomiting and diarrhea.

Types of Dysmenorrhea

There are following types:
a. Primary (No organic cause)
b. Secondary (Pathologic causes)
c. Membranous

Primary dysmenorrhea is not associated with identifiable pathology. This chapter will focus mainly on primary dysmenorrhea.

Secondary dysmenorrhea can be caused by a number of gynecologic conditions. The common conditions associated with secondary dysmenorrhea are uterine myoma, adenomyosis, endometriosis and pelvic infection.

Membranous dysmenorrhea is rare. It causes intense cramping pain due to passage of cast of endometrium through an undilated cervix.

Another cause of dysmenorrhea that should be considered is cramping due to presence of an intrauterine contraceptive device.

Pathogenesis

Dysmenorrhea has long been known to be associated with ovulatory cycles. The principal cause seems to be increased production of prostaglandin F$_2\alpha$. PGF$_2\alpha$ causes uterine cramping and is the mechanism for the systemic symptoms (i.e. nausea, diarrhea, and headache) associated with dysmenorrhea.

Increased leukotriene level is proved to be a contributing factor. **Vasopressin** was thought to be an aggravating agent. **Atosiban** – a vasopressin antagonist has found to be of no effect on menstrual pain. **Psychological factors** are important, including attitudes passed from mother to daughter. Girls should receive accurate information about menstruation before menarche, provided by parents, teachers, physicians or counselor. **Emotional anxiety** due to academic or social demands may be a cofactor.

Management of Dysmenorrhea

Evaluation

Symptoms and Signs

The history and physical examination are the major tools in the evaluation of dysmenorrhea. History is essential to define type of dysmenorrhea – primary or secondary and gynecological or nongynecological causes of dysmenorrhea. History taking should include – timing of pain, other symptoms associated with pain, relieving and aggravating factors. Pelvic examination is needed if symptoms persist despite imperial treatment.

Investigation

1. In women with risk for PID cultures for *Chlamydia trachomatais* and *N. gonorrhoeae* are indicated and high vaginal swab for other pathogens should be taken.
2. If pelvic examination is abnormal and an organic cause is likely, pelvic ultrasound should be performed.
3. Endoscopy: If necessary in the some cases, if there is possibility of Asherman's syndrome or cervical stenosis,

hysteroscopy can be used to investigate. Likewise in suspected cases of endometriosis and in patients unresponsive to imperical therapy laparoscopy can be considered. But these are infrequent conditions and usually not needed routinely.

Treatment

Both primary and secondary dysmenorrhea can be managed medically at least initially. The mainstay of treatment are NSAIDs and oral contraceptives.

1. **NSAIDs:** These drugs decrease prostaglandin production which help in improving symptoms. Naproxen, Ibuprofen, Mefenamic acid are reasonably effective. Cyclooxygenase (COX-2) inhibitor such as Valedecoxib 20-40 mg/day is equally effective, has fewer gastrointestinal effects but more costly. The drugs must be used at the earliest onset of symptoms, usually at the onset and sometimes 1-2 days prior to bleeding or cramping. Because once the pain has been established, antiprostaglandins are not nearly as effective as with early use.
2. **Oral contraceptives:** Cyclic administration of oral contraceptive usually in the lowest doses prevents pain in most of the patients who are not responsive with antiprostaglandin or cannot tolerate them. The mechanism of pain relief may be related to anovulation or altered endometrium resulting in decreased prostaglandin production. In women not requiring contraception, oral contraceptives are given for 6-12 months. Many women continue to be free of pain even after discontinuation of treatment. NSAIDs act synergistically with OC pills to improve dysmenorrhea.
3. **Gonadotropin releasing hormone agonist and androgens:** The estrogen releasing effect of these agents lead to endometrial atrophy and decreased prostaglandin production. But their use is associated with substantial side effects and treatment is much costly.
4. **Non-medical and adjuvant treatment:** Diet change, massage, exercise, direct application of heating pad to lower abdomen may help some patient. Alternative medical therapy such as acupuncture and hypnosis have also been tried. Diets low in fat and meat products have been shown to decrease serum sex binding globulin and decrease the duration and intensity of dysmenorrhea.

Surgical treatment: Cases of dysmenorrhea refractory to conservative treatment are unusual. They should have proper work up and should be offered treatment of underlying pathology. Laparoscopic uterosacral ligament division and presacral neurectomy are infrequently done and have limited evidence for benefit.

MULTIPLE CHOICE QUESTIONS

1. Postmenopausal bleeding is associated with all *except*:
    a. Cancer cervix
    b. CIN
    c. Cancer ovary
    d. Endometrial cancer
    Ans. b
2. A 45-year-old woman presents with history of polymenorrhea for last six months. The first line of management is:
    a. Hysterectomy
    b. Progesterone for 3 cycles
    c. Diagnostic curettage
    d. Oral contraceptive for 3 cycles
    Ans. c
3. Which of the following is not indicated in menorrhagia is:
    a. NSAIDs
    b. Clomiphene
    c. Norethisterone
    d. Tranexamic acid
    Ans. b
4. Treatment for 32 years old multipara with dysfunctional uterine bleeding is:
    a. Progesterone
    b. Danazol
    c. Prostaglandins
    d. Endometrial ablation
    Ans. a
5. A 45-year-old female presenting with dysmenorrhea and menorrhagia most probably has:
    a. DUB
    b. Endometriosis
    c. Fibroid
    d. Endometrial cancer
    Ans. b,c
6. The most common histological findings of endometrium in DUB is:
    a. Hypertrophic
    b. Hyperplastic
    c. Cystic glandular hyperplasia
    d. Dysplastic
    Ans. b
7. Most common cause of puberty menorrhagia is:
    a. Anovulation
    b. Malignancy
    c. Endometriosis
    d. Bleeding disorder
    Ans. a
8. Average blood loss in normal menstruation is:
    a. 50 ml
    b. 80 ml

Chapter – 13 ♦ Abnormal Uterine Bleeding and Abnormalities of Menstruation

    c. 100 ml
    d. 120 ml
Ans. a

9. Menorrhagia is defined as blood loss per vaginum more than:
    a. 80 ml
    b. 110 ml
    c. 150 ml
    d. 50 ml
Ans. a

10. Initial evaluation in adolescent with abnormal uterine bleeding:
    a. Hemogram
    b. Platelet count
    c. USG
    d. D & C
Ans. a,b,c

11. The treatment of DUB in young women is:
    a. Hormones
    b. Radiotherapy
    c. D & C
    d. Hysterectomy
Ans. a

12. Most common cause of postmenopausal bleeding in India is:
    a. Cancer endometrium
    b. Cancer cervix
    c. Cancer vulva
    d. Ovarian tumor
Ans. b

13. Evaluation of a patient with postmenopausal bleeding is done by:
    a. PAP smear
    b. USG
    c. Endometrial biopsy
    d. Dilatation and curettage
Ans. c

14 Endometriosis

One who combines the knowledge of physiology and surgery, in addition to the artistic side of subject, reaches the highest ideal in medicine.

GENERAL CONSIDERATION

Endometriosis is a disorder in which hormonally responsive endometrial tissue is found outside the uterus. In adenomyosis, endometrial tissue is found within the uterine myometrium. The high prevalence of endometriosis, its progressive nature, its impact on quality life as it relates to both pelvic pain and infertility and difficulty in controlling the symptoms and course of disease makes this a frustrating disease entity. The disease owns a unique pathology of a benign proliferative growth yet having the propensity to invade the normal surrounding tissues.

Incidence

Incidence of endometriosis is difficult to quantify as surgery is required for its diagnosis. It is estimated to be present in 3-10% of women in the reproductive age group and 25-35% of infertile women. It is seen in 1-2% of women undergoing sterilization or sterilization reversal, in 10% of hysterectomy surgeries, in 16-31% of laparoscopies and in 53% of adolescents with pelvic pain severe enough to warrant surgical evaluation. It has been suggested that frequency of this disease has increased in recent years and factors as environmental pollution has been implicated. Besides this greater use of diagnostic laparoscopy may be the reason for apparent increase in incidence of endometriosis.

Pathogenesis

The cause of endometriosis is unknown. Theories for histogenesis are as follows:

a. *Metastatic theory:* This theory ascribes endometriosis to implantation following retrograde menstruation into the peritoneal cavity, lymphatic dissemination or hematogenous spread of endometrial tissue or iatrogenic dissemination due to some operative procedure. Location of endometriosis in dependent portion of body, the ability of endometrial cells to implant, an increased incidence of endometriosis in patients with uterine or vaginal outlet obstruction, and identification of endometriosis at distant sites outside the abdominal cavity support this theory.

b. *Embryonic cell rest and coelomic metaplasia theory:* According to this theory, there is *de novo* development of endometrial tissue outside the uterus. There is common origin of embryonic tissue for ovarian germinal epithelium, Müllerian epithelium, and peritoneal mesothelium. It is proposed that these cells undergo de differentiation back to their primitive origin and then transform into endometrial cells.

c. *Induction theory:* The induction theory proposes that some hormonal or biologic factors may induce the differentiation of undifferentiated cells into the endometrial tissue.

d. *Role of immune system:* Evidence indicates that altered humoral and cell mediated immunity plays a role in pathogenesis of endometriosis. The activity of natural killer cells may be reduced and deficient cellular immunity may cause an inability to recognize endometrial tissue in abnormal locations. Endometriosis may occur when the deficiency in cellular immunity allows menstrual tissue to implant and grow on the peritoneum. Altered macrophage capacity to induce cytolysis of ectopic endometrial cells along with increased ability of this tissue to survive, proliferate, invade, and induce angiogenesis along with impaired cell apoptosis may be the etiology of endometriosis. Evidence indicates increased concentration of leukocytes and macrophage in the ectopic endometrium and the peritoneal cavity, which secrete growth factors and cytokines into the peritoneal fluid. These cytokines and growth factors are postulated to lead to proliferation of the endometriotic implants and inflammatory reaction. Patients with endometriosis have been shown to have a higher rate of autoimmune inflammatory disorders compared to general population.

e. *Genetic influence:* Studies have found 7–9% incidence of endometriosis in first degree female relatives as compared to 1–2% control population. Possible role of

HLA B7 allele has been revealed which inhibits cytotoxic activity of natural killer like T lymphocytes, suggesting that growth of ectopic endometrial cells might be under genetic control.

f. *Hormonal dependence:* Estrogen hormone can have a causative role in endometriosis. Endometriosis implants have been shown to express aromatase and 17α hydroxysteroid dehydrogenase type 1, which converts androstenedione to estrone and of estrone to estradiol respectively. At the same time implants are deficient in 17α hydroxysteroid dehydrogenase type 2 which inactivates estrogen. So the endometriotic implants are exposed to estrogenic environment. Furthermore, the locally produced estrogens within endometriotic lesion may exert their biologic effect within the same tissue or cell in which they are produced, a process which is termed as **intracrinology**.

In contrast normal endometrium does not express aromatase and has elevated level of 17α hydroxysteroid dehydrogenase type 2 in response to progesterone, which ensures that estrogenic effects are attenuated in response to progesterone. As a result progesterone antagonizes the estrogen effects in normal endometrium during the luteal phase of the menstrual cycle. Endometriosis, however manifest a relative progesterone resistant state which prevents attenuation of estrogen stimulation in this tissue. Estradiol produced in response to increased aromatase activity subsequently augments PGE_2 production by stimulating cyclooxygenase type 2 (COX-2) enzymes in uterine endothelial cells. This creates a positive feedback loop and potentiates estrogenic effect on proliferation of endometriosis. This concept is basis for pharmacologic inhibition of aromatase activity in cases of endometriosis that are refractory to standard therapy.

Pathology

The gross appearance of endometriosis at laparotomy or laparoscopy is usually quite characteristic and to an experienced surgeon is sufficient for diagnosis. There are following stages and type of appearance:
a. The smallest and earliest implants are red, petechial lesion on the peritoneal surface
b. With further growth menstrual like detritus accumulate within the lesion, giving it a cystic, dark brown, dark blue or black appearance. The surrounding peritoneal surface becomes thickened and scarred giving *powder burn* appearance of 5–10 mm.
c. With progression of disease number and size of lesion increase, there can be extensive adhesions.
d. In ovary, there can be chocolate cyst or endometrioma of several centimeters.
e. Nonclassical appearance can be clear vesicles, white or yellow spots or nodules, circular folds of peritoneum (Pockets), even visually normal peritoneum.

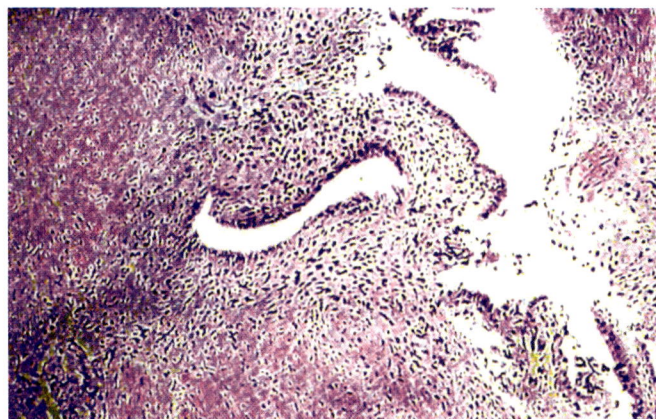

Fig. 14.1: Histology of endometriotic nodule showing fibrous tissue and endometriotic gland

Distribution of Lesion

Distribution of endometriotic lesions exhibits a characteristic pattern. Solitary lesions are possible, but multiple implantations are the rule. The most common site of disease is **ovary (50%) followed by uterine cul de sac, uterosacral ligaments, uterus, fallopian tubes, sigmoid colon, and appendix and round ligaments** respectively (Figs 14.2A and B). In order of frequency implants may occur over the bowel, bladder and uterus. Rarely they erode into underlying tissue and cause blood in the stool or urine or their associated adhesions result in strictures and obstruction of these organs.

Endometriosis is seen in the umbilicus following operation, in the laparotomy scars, in the tubal stumps following sterilization operation, in the amputated stump of cervix and in the scars of vulva and perineum. Very rarely endometriosis is found distant from the pelvis as lung, brain and kidney. Pleural implantations are associated with recurrent right pneumothorax at the time of menstruation, termed **catamednial pneumothorax**. Lesions in the central nervous system can cause **catamenial seizure**.

Microscopic Appearance

The microscopic finding shows tissues histologically resembling endometrial gland and stroma. The normal endometrial appearance is seen in early lesion. With advanced disease cyst formation and fibrosis is seen. The wall of the implant is lined by monolayer of cells. Blood is present inside the cyst, and hemosiderin laden macrophages are found in the cyst wall (Fig. 14.1).

Diagnosis

Clinical Presentation

The symptoms vary according to sites and do not correlate well with the extent of the disease. The classic symptoms complex includes **pelvic pain, dyspareunia, menorrhagia and infertility**. About 30% of patients are asymptomatic.

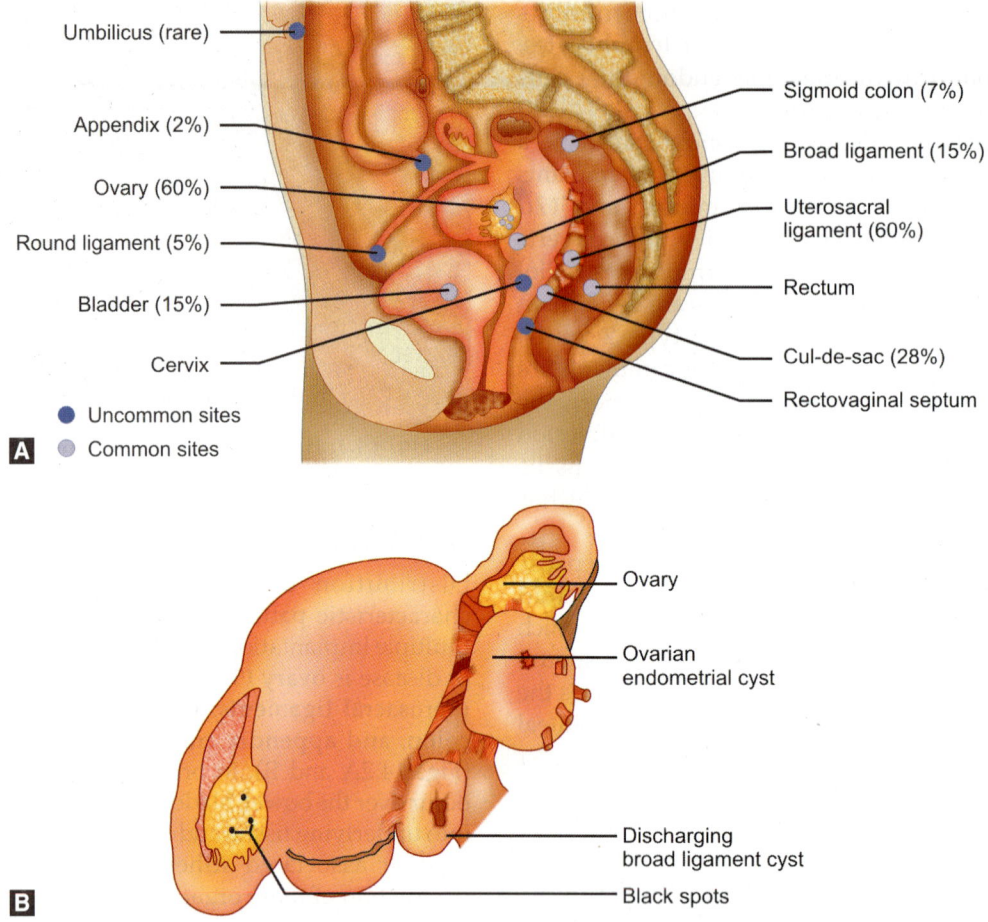

Figs 14.2A and B: Usual distribution of endometriotic lesion

Pelvic pain: Pelvic pain usually occurs cyclically just prior to or with menses and located unilaterally or bilaterally in the lower quadrants. With progression of disease, there is increased pain specifically in the week before menses. With severe disease, pain is present throughout the month. The pain is produced by pressure and inflammation within and around the lesion, by traction on adhesion associated with lesion, by number of implants and their proximity to nerves and other sensitive structures and by the mass effect of large lesions.

Infertility: The effect of scarring and adhesion disturbs the pelvic architecture and affects oocyte transport from the ovary to the tube. The peritoneal environment affects the oocyte and sperm. In presence of endometriosis, peritoneal fluid inhibits sperm function. Deep dyspareunia can be indirect cause of subfertility resulting in reduced coital frequency. Sperm inactivation occurs due to antibodies and phagocytosis. Besides this there can be early pregnancy failure due to luteal phase deficiency and prostaglandin induced immune reactions. This affects 30-40% of women with endometriosis.

Dyspareunia: It is noted with an immobile fixed uterus. This is usually present with severe disease.

Rectal discomfort at tenesmus: It is related to posterior cul de sac scarring and immobility.

Abnormal uterine bleeding: Premenstrual spotting may occur. Menorrhagia is common with adenomyosis and irregular bleeding may occur with cervical or vaginal lesions. Polymenorrhea is noted with ovarian involvement (10–30%).

Other symptoms: Urological symptoms like frequency and dysuria and rarely hematuria during menstruation may result from bladder or urethral involvement. Scar endometriosis can cause cyclical pain and enlargement of scar site and pulmonary lesion cause cyclical hemoptysis.

Physical Findings

Classically pelvic examination reveals tender nodules in the posterior vaginal fornix and pain upon uterine motion. The uterus may be fixed and retroverted due to cul-de-sac adhesion and tender adnexal mass may be felt because of the presence of endometriomas. Careful inspection may reveal implants in healed wounds, especially episiotomy and cesarean section incision, in the vaginal fornix and cervix. Biopsy may be required to prove that the lesions are due to endometriosis.

Investigation

a. *Imaging:* Ultrasonography is not much helpful in diagnosis. TVS can detect ovarian endometriomas (Fig. 14.3). TVS and endorectal ultrasound are found better for rectosigmoid endometriosis.
b. *CT and MRI:* These are expensive and usually of not much help in diagnosis. MRI can be advantageous as compared to ultrasound only when there are ovarian cysts or invasion of surrounding organs such as the bowel, bladder or rectovaginal septum.
c. *Serum marker CA-125:* Cancer antigen 125 is often elevated in women with endometriosis. But this is elevated in other pelvic disease also so has little specificity in diagnosis. However, it is helpful to assess the therapeutic response and follow-up of cases in evaluation for recurrences.
d. *Laparoscopy:* **Double puncture laparoscopy is gold standard diagnosis** of endometriosis. The wide spectrum of the disease has to be appreciated. The macroscopic black and blue black lesion are characteristics but the red, red pink, yellow brown, white and clear vesicular lesion along with peritoneal defects, fibrosis and scaring should be observed and documented (Fig. 14.4). There can also be microscopic implants, which can only be appreciated after histological diagnosis of biopsies of normal appearing surface peritoneum (Figs 14.2A and B).

Differential Diagnosis

The varied presentation of endometriosis mandate that it should be considered in differential diagnosis of virtually all pelvic disease. In particular, the pain, infertility and adhesion found in endometriosis must be distinguished from similar symptoms accompanying **pelvic inflammatory disease and pelvic tumors**. Usually the clear diagnosis requires operative evaluation. Table 14.1 summarizes the conditions which should be considered prior to surgical exploration.

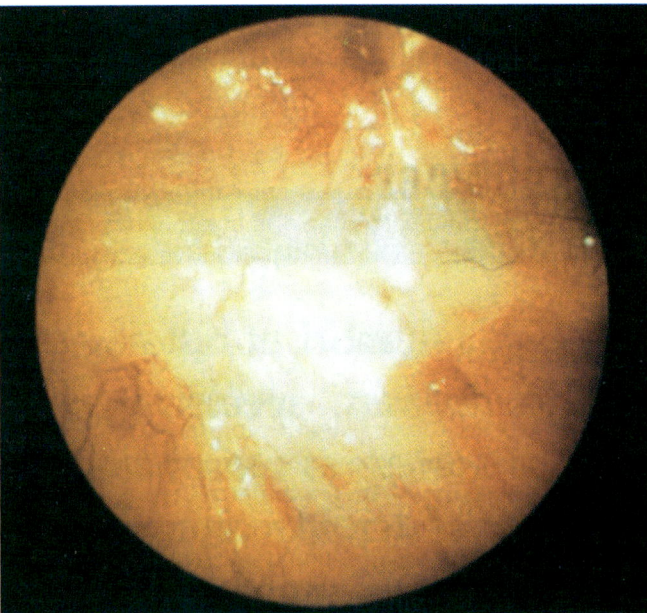

Fig. 14.4: Laparoscopic appearance of endometriosis— Red lesion

Table 14.1: Differential diagnosis of endometriosis	
Gynecological	Pelvic inflammatory disease
	Tubo-ovarian abscess
	Salpingitis and endometritis
	Hemorrhagic ovarian cyst
	Ovarian torsion
	Degenerating leiomyoma
Non-gynecological	Cystic and chronic urinary tract infection
	Renal calculi
	Inflammatory bowel disease
	Irritable bowel syndrome
	Diverticulitis musculoskeletal disorder
	Mesenteric lymphadenitis

A patient with a persistent adnexal mass larger than 5 cm should never be presumed to have an endometrioma even if endometriosis has been diagnosed previously. Such mass requires surgical diagnosis.

Complications

True complications of endometriosis are few. Implants over the bowel or ureter may cause obstruction and silent impairment of renal function. Endometrioma can cause ovarian torsion or they can rupture and spill their irritating contents into the peritoneal cavity resulting in

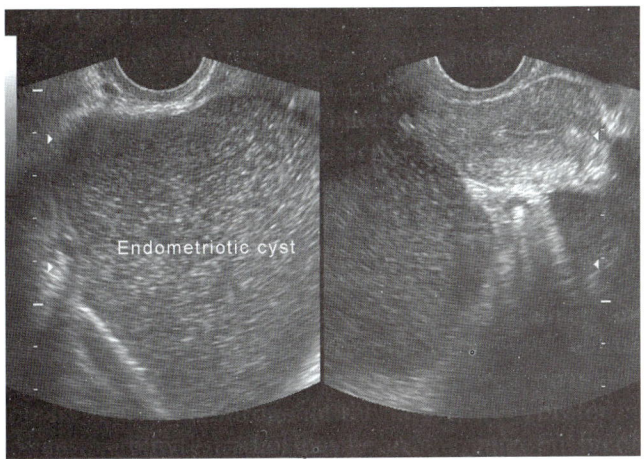

Fig. 14.3: Ultrasound image showing endometriotic cyst

chemical peritonitis and acute abdomen. Excision of endometriosis causing catamenial seizures or pneumothorax may be necessary.

Prevention

Prevention of endometriosis is not currently possible. A more thorough understanding of the pathophysiology of endometriosis is required before preventive strategies can be devised.

Classification

The staging system is the revised American Society for Reproductive Medicine classification of endometriosis. The staging is done postoperatively, documenting the extent and location of the endometriotic implants and adhesions. This is to be noted that this system does not correlate with severity of pain but is mainly designed to predict the chance of pregnancy. Staging is summarized in Table 14.2.

Treatment

Treatment options are decided by the patient's desire for future fertility, her symptoms, stage of her disease and to some extent her age. It must be emphasized again that therapy for endometriosis requires operative inspection of the lesions for correct diagnosis and staging, and to ensure that the patient's symptoms are attributable to endometriosis only.

Expectant Management

In asymptomatic patient, those with mild discomfort, or infertile women with minimal or mild endometriosis, expectant management may be appropriate. Though endometriosis is believed to be a progressive disease, no evidence shows that treating an asymptomatic patient will prevent or ameliorate the onset of symptoms later. There are many reports who found that expectant management of infertile women with minimal or mild endometriosis is as successful as medical or surgical therapies (Table 14.3).

Table 14.2: Staging of endometriosis (Revised American Society for Reproductive Medicine)

		<1cm	1-3cm	>3cm
Peritoneum	ENDOMETRIOSIS			
	Superficial	1	2	4
	Deep	2	4	6
Ovary	Superficial	1	2	4
	Deep	4	16	20
	L Superficial	1	2	4
	Deep	4	16	20
	Posterior cul-de-sac obliteration	Partial	Complete	
		4	40	

		<1/3 Enclosure	1/3-2/3 Enclosure	>2/3 Enclosure
Ovary	ADHESIONS			
	R Filmy	1	2	4
	Dense	4	8	16
	L Filmy	1	2	4
	Dense	4	8	16
Tube	R Filmy	1	2	4
	Dense	4*	8*	16
	L Filmy	1	2	4
	Dense	4*	8*	16

* If the fimbriated end of the fallopian tube is completely enclosed, change the point assignment to 16.

Additional Endometriosis
_____
_____

Associated Pathology
_____
_____

L — To be used with normal tubes and ovaries — R

L — To be used with abnormal tubes and ovaries — R

Table 14.3: The management of endometriosis			
Stage	Characteristics	Diagnosis	Treatment
I,II	**Minimal, Mild** Small surface nodules with no scaring or peritubal adhesions	Only by laparoscopy in investigation of infertility	At most, electrocautery or CO_2 laser to lesions Do not give hormones
III	**Moderate** Small scattered surface lesions with scarring; ovarian endometriomata, <2.5 cm, few periovarian or peritubal adhesions; in the cul-de-sac or uterosacral ligaments	Often symptoms but confirmation by laparoscopy needed	Electrocautery or CO_2 laser to lesions Hormones Conservative surgery if hormones fail to relieve symptoms
IV	**Severe** Ovarian endometriomata >2.5 cm marked adhesions of ovary or tubes, cul-de-sac obliteration	Symptoms and signs Laparotomy confirms	Conservative surgery Hormones Hysterectomy and salpingo-ophorectomy
V	**Very Severe** Stage III plus involvement of bowel, bladder, ureter, etc.	Laparotomy Barium enema IVP	Surgery Hormones, if surgery incomplete

Analgesic Anti-inflammatory

NSAIDs are appropriate sole therapy for the patients who have mild premenstrual pain from minimal endometriosis, no abnormalities on pelvic examination and no desire to conceive in near future.

Hormonal Therapy

Hormonal therapy involves suppression of ovarian estradiol production, decreasing the stimulus for endometriosis growth and proliferation. Ectopic endometrial tissue growth is retarded and with decreased hormonal activity, atrophy and or decidualization occur.

Combined oral contraceptive pills: Oral contraceptive pills containing estrogen and progesterone are a good choice for patients with minimal or mild symptoms. Oral contraceptive pills are prescribed either cyclically or continuously for 6–12 months. It has shown to be effective in decreasing dysmenorrhoea and may retard progression of endometriosis. Low dose COCS (containing 20 µg ethinyl estradiol) have not found superior to conventional dose COCS for treatment of endometriosis and may lead to higher rates of abnormal bleeding.

Progestins: They also cause decidualization in the endometriotic tissue. Oral medroxyprogesterone can be prescribed as 10–30 mg daily dose. An alternative regiment is Norethindrone acetate 5 mg daily or megestrol acetate prescribed as 40 mg daily dose. Depot medroxyprogesterone acetate 150 mg I/M can also be given as a single injection every 3 months. In a few small studies Levonogesterel releasing intrauterine device has been shown to relieve pelvic pain and dysmenorrhea. 80% of women treated with progestin have partial or complete relief of pain.

Danazol: It is a synthetic derivative of *17 alpha ethinyl testosterone*, inhibits multiple enzymes in steroidogenesis, as well as cytosolic hormone receptors. This leads to high androgen, low estrogen environment that reduces activity of all endometrial tissue and endometriosis. The dosage of Danazol is 400–800 mg/day in divided doses for 6 months. Side effects are androgenic like acne, oily skin, deepening voice, weight gain, edema and adverse plasma lipoprotein change. Pain relief is achieved in up to 90% of patient taking Danazol. Its use is precluded due to its high cost, androgenic side effects, adverse effect on fertility and high recurrence rate (up to 40%).

Gestrinone: It is 19 nortestosterone derivative and has progestogenic and antiprogestogenic activity. It predominantly induces a progesterone withdrawal effect and decreases the numbers of estrogen and progesterone receptors. Gestrinone equals the effectiveness of Danazol and GnRh agonist for endometriosis related pain relief but has fewer androgenic and hypoestrogenic side effects. Dose of Gestrinone is 2.5–10 mg weekly, given daily or 3 times weekly.

GnRH agonist: Gonadotropins releasing hormones agonist are analo of 10 amino acid peptides hormone GnRH. With continuous administration of GnRH analo suppression of gonadotropins secretion occurs, resulting in elimination of ovarian steroidogenesis and suppression of endometrial implants. The goal is to maintain reduced level of serum oestrogen (30–40 pg/ml) so that growth of endometriosis is suppressed.

Dosage of GnRH agonist: I/M as Leuprolide acetate depot 3.75 mg once per month. Intranasally as Nafarelin 400-800 mg daily, or Goserelin 3.6 mg once per month. Endometriosis related pain is relieved in most cases by 2nd or 3rd month of therapy (Table 14.4).

Table 14.4: Gonadotropin releasing hormone agonist for treatment of endometriosis	
Depot Preparation	Intranasal Preparation
Goserelin 3.6 mg S/C	Nafarelin 200 mg BD
Leuprorelin 3.75 mg I/m or S/C	Buserelin 200 mg TDS
Triptorelin 3.75 mg I/m	

Adverse effect of GnRH agonist: GnRH agonist induced hypoestrogenic state causes hot flushes, insomnia, reduced libido, vaginal dryness, and headache. Particular concerning adverse effect is loss of bone mineral density. Because of increased risk of osteoporosis, GnRH analog therapy is limited to maximum period of six months. Additionally, estrogen in the form of combined oral contraceptive (COC) or 0.625 mg conjugated estrogen (premarin) with 5 mg of norethindrone acetate may be added to GnRH agonist therapy to counteract the bone loss and is termed add back therapy.

Aromatase inhibitors: As described in theories of endometriosis endometrial tissue locally produces aromatase, the enzyme responsible for estrogen synthesis. In endometriotic tissue estrogen may be produced locally through aromatization of circulating androgens, which explains the postmenopausal endometriosis. Aromatase inhibitors have not been studied extensively in endometriosis. Phase II trial of drug Anastrozole 1 mg daily, Letrozol 2.5 mg has revealed significant pain reduction. These drugs also have hypoestrogenic side effects as GnRH agonist but hold promise in severe refractory cases of endometriosis.

None of the drug treatments described will prevent recurrence of endometriosis once therapy has been stopped, though there may be a period of some months between stopping treatment and re-emergence of symptoms. No medical treatment has been shown to improve subsequent fertility. Beside this, it is important to consider that except combined oral contraceptive pills, no drug is proper contraceptive agent and patient should be advised to use barrier contraception to avoid the potential teratogenic effect of drugs such as danazol if they are at risk of becoming pregnant.

Surgical Treatment Options

The objective of surgical treatment of endometriosis is to restore normal anatomic relationship, to excise or destroy all visible disease to the maximum extent, to prevent or delay recurrence of disease. **For women who hope to restore or preserve fertility having moderate or severe endometriosis that distorts the reproductive anatomy, surgery is the treatment of choice, because medical treatment cannot achieve these goals.** When disease is less severe, medical treatment can effectively control pain in majority of cases, but has no effect on fertility. *Surgery is at least as effective as medical treatment for relieving pain and can also improve fertility.*

Laparotomy vs Laparoscopy

Although surgery for the treatment of endometriosis can be performed via laparotomy or laparoscopy, technical developments in instrumentation and technique generally allow the endoscopic approach in all, excepting those who require extensive adhesiolysis or bowel resection. Highly skilled surgeons can accomplish even these objectives. **Laparoscopy offers the advantage of better visualization, less tissue trauma and desiccation, smaller incision and speedier postoperatively recovery.** Postoperative adhesion and complications are also less as compared to laparotomy.

Types of Surgery

The conservative surgery in endometriosis is intended for:
a. To ablate as many endometrial deposits as possible.
b. To restructure pelvic anatomy by adhesiolysis.
c. To destroy endometrial deposits in the ovary.
d. To deal with sensory nerve pathways.

Conservative surgery: Peritoneal implants of endometriosis can be ablated with unipolar or bipolar electrosurgical instruments or laser or excised by sharp dissection. Opinion regarding superiority of one method over another are strongly held but not substantiated by the result of any direct comparisons. Those favoring excision over ablation emphasize that because the depth of disease in ablation cannot be determined, the risk that treatment may be inadequate is greater when disease is ablated rather than excised. **Excision is preferable to simple lysis because adhesion will frequently contain the disease.** Strict adherence to microsurgical principles that is use of magnification, minimum tissue trauma, and exposure and meticulous hemostasis is must.

a. *Ovarian endometriosis:* Superficial ovarian lesion can be vaporized. Small ovarian endometrioma (< 3 cm in diameters) can be aspirated and irrigated. Large (> 3 cm in diameter) ovarian endometrioma should be aspirated, followed by incision and removal of cyst wall from the ovarian cortex. *To prevent recurrence, the cyst wall of endometrioma must be removed, and normal ovarian tissue must be preserved.* Based on current evidence ovarian cystectomy appears to be the method of choice.

b. *Adhesiolysis:* The removal of endometriotic related adhesion (adhesiolysis) should be performed carefully. Though there is tendency to adhesion reformation.

c. *Pre-and posthormonal treatment:* In patients with severe endometriosis it has been recommended that surgical treatment should be preceded by a three-months course of medical treatment to reduce vascularization and nodular size. Though RCT have failed to show a significant difference in ease of surgery after preoperative hormonal treatment. The idea of postoperative hormonal therapy is to destroy the lesion left behind after surgery and to control the pain. But it does not improve fertility and best avoided.

d. *Deep rectovaginal and rectosigmoid endometriosis:* The surgical excision of endometriosis at these sites is difficult and can be associated with major complication. Postoperative bowel perforation with peritonitis has been reported in 2–3% of cases.

e. *Presacral neurectomy:* Transaction of presacral nerve within the interiliac triangle has been tried to relieve chronic pelvic pain in recurrent endometriosis. But it should only be tried in selected cases, as efficacy of this treatment is not established.

f. *Definitive surgery:* If the women do not desire future child bearing and have severe disease or symptoms, definitive surgery is appropriate and often curative. This entails total abdominal hysterectomy, bilateral salpingo-ophorectomy and excision of removing adhesion or implants. If endometriosis remains after excision, postoperative medical therapy may be indicated. After this or complete excision, hormone replacement therapy is indicated. Estrogen progestin therapy can be used without reactivating the endometriosis, but individualization of therapy is required.

The management protocol of endometriosis has been summarized in Flow chart 14.1 and Table 14.3.

Assisted Reproductive Techniques

Infertile women with endometriosis, who are older, or who have not responded to other therapies for infertility, can undergo assisted reproduction, such as ovulation induction with intrauterine insemination or *in vitro* fertilization (IVF). However, women with endometriosis undergoing IVF were found to have significantly lower pregnancy rates, fertilization rates, implantation rates, mean number of oocytes retrieved, as compared to women with tubal factor infertility. The need to treat women surgically or medically prior to starting an IVF cycle remains unclear.

Prognosis

Proper counseling of patients with endometriosis requires attention to several aspects of the disorder. Primary importance is the initial operative staging of the disease to obtain adequate information on which future decision about therapies is based. Besides this, the patient's symptom and desire for child bearing dictate appropriate therapy. Most patients can be reassured to obtain significant pain relief. Long-term concerns are more guarded, because all current therapies offer relief but not cure. After conservative surgery reported recurrence rate vary greatly but usually 10% in 3 years and 35% in 5 years. Pregnancy delays but does not preclude recurrence. Recurrence rates after medical treatment vary and are similar to or higher than those reported following surgical treatment.

Conservative surgery prevents the necessity of hysterectomy in majority of cases. But the cause of endometriosis in any individual cannot be predicted at present, and future treatment options should greatly improve upon what is offered now.

MULTIPLE CHOICE QUESTIONS

1. Endometriosis is explained by:
    a. Sampson's implantation of theory
    b. Metaplastic epithelium
    c. Histogenesis by induction
    d. Coelomic metaplasia theory
   Ans. a, c, d
2. The best method for diagnosis of endometriosis is:
    a. Laparoscopy
    b. Ultrasound
    c. MRI
    d. Serum CA-125
   Ans. a
3. Endometriosis is commonly associated with:
    a. Bilateral chocolate cyst of ovary
    b. Adenomyosis
    c. Fibroid uterus
    d. Luteal cyst
   Ans. a
4. Ovarian reserve tests are:
    a. LH
    b. FSH
    c. Plasma progesterone
    d. Endometrial biopsy
   Ans. b
5. Which of the following is the drug of choice to treat endometriosis?
    a. Testosterone propionate
    b. Norethisterone
    c. Medroxyprogesterone
    d. Danazol
   Ans. d
6. Treatment of adenomyosis:
    a. Estrogen
    b. Estrogen and progesterone
    c. Total hysterectomy
    d. Laser
   Ans. c
7. Commonest manifestation of endometriosis is:
    a. Infertility
    b. Pain
    c. Bleeding
    d. Leukorrhea
   Ans. b

Flow chart 14.1: Management protocol for endometriosis

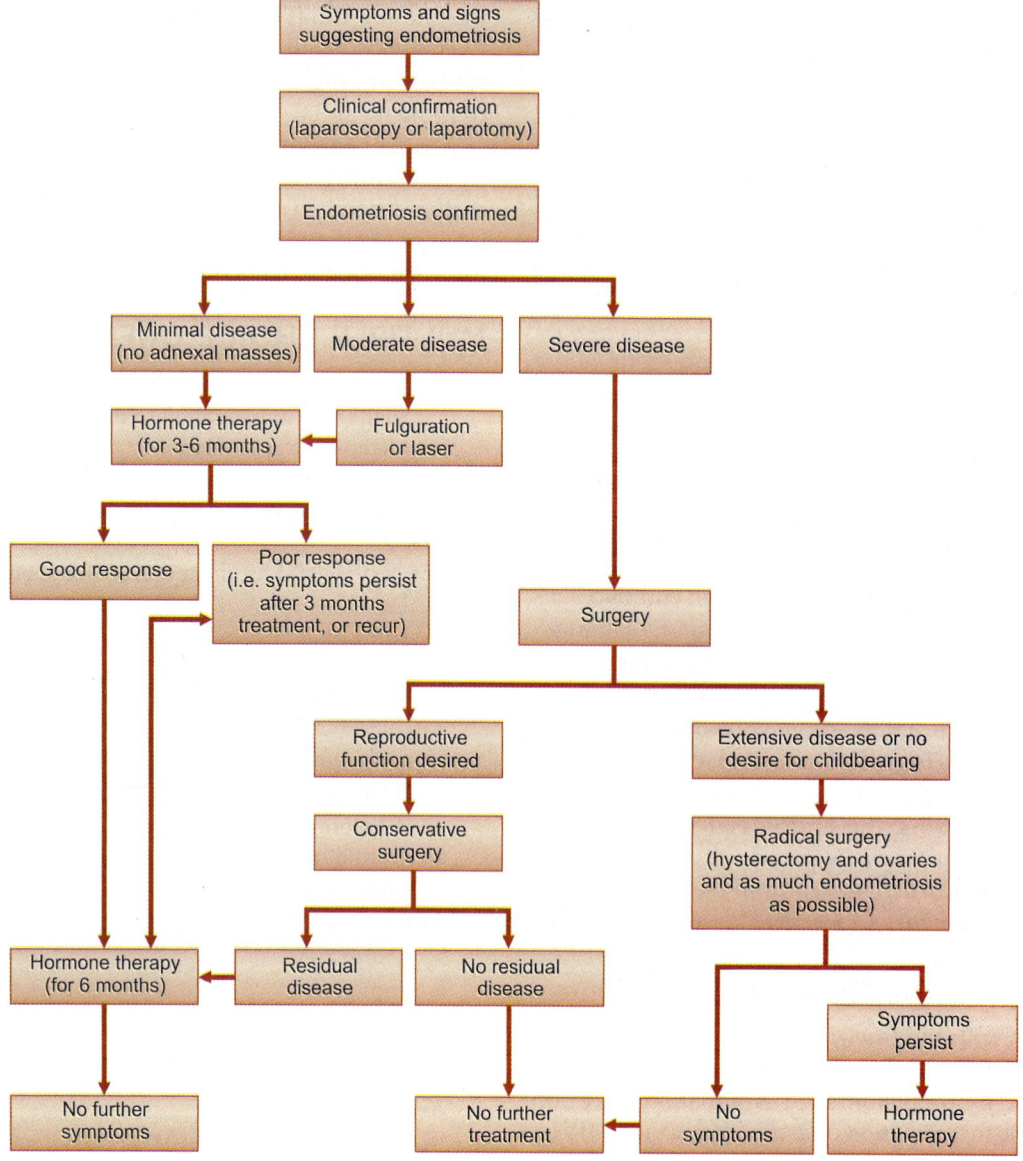

8. Treatment of a case of endometriosis at a younger age group:
   a. Progestin
   b. Danazol
   c. GnRH analog
   d. Hysterectomy with oophorectomy
   Ans. c

9. Which is not used in treatment of endometriosis?
   a. Danazol
   b. Tamoxifen
   c. Medroxyprogesterone
   d. GnRH analog
   Ans. b

10. A 40-year-old primiparous woman suspected to be suffering from endometriosis is subjected to diagnostic laparoscopy, which shows normal uterus, bilateral chocolate cyst of ovary, endometrial deposit in round ligament, both fallopian tubes with dense adhesion on pouch of Douglas. Treatment of choice is:
    a. Danazol therapy
    b. Progesterone therapy
    c. Fulguration of endometrial deposit
    d. Total hysterectomy with bilateral salpingo-oophorectomy
    Ans. d

15 Pelvic Organ Prolapse (POP)

A physician should never appear to be in hurry, and never absent minded.

INTRODUCTION

A prolapse is a downward or forward displacement of one of the pelvic organs from its location. Conventionally, the prolapse is referred to displacement of bladder, the uterus or rectum.

Incidence

Pelvic organ prolapse is very common but accurate prevalence rates are unknown. It has been estimated that up to 50% of all parous women lose some pelvic support and 10-20% of them seek advice for care of prolapse. Prolapse is one of the most common indications for gynecologic surgery. Women have an approximately 11% risk of undergoing surgery to repair pelvic organ prolapse or urinary incontinence in their lifetime. Anterior pelvic organ prolapse is 34.3%, posterior wall prolapse is 18.6% and uterine prolapse is 14.3%.

Classification

The genital prolapse is broadly grouped into: (a) Vaginal prolapse, (b) Uterine prolapse. While vaginal prolapse can occur independently without uterine descent, the uterine prolapse is usually associated with variable degree of vaginal descent. Pelvic support defects can be classified by their anatomic location (Figs 15.1A to E).

Anterior Vaginal Wall Defect

a. *Anterior vaginal prolapse:* It describes a defect of upper two-third of the anterior vaginal wall where urinary bladder is associated with prolapse. It is also known as cystocoel.
b. *Urethrocele:* It is distal or lower third of anterior vaginal wall defect where urethra is associated with prolapse. It may be independent or usually along with cystocele so called cystourethrocele.
c. *Paravaginal/midline/transverse prolapse:* It indicates the location of anterior vaginal wall defect.

Apical Prolapse

a. Uterine prolapse
b. Vaginal vault prolapse (Posthysterectomy or secondary vault prolapse)
c. *Enterocele:* It describes an apical vaginal wall defect in which bowel or omentum or both are contained within the prolapsed segment. Traction enterocele is secondary to uterovaginal prolapse. Pulsion enterocele is secondary to chronically raised intra-abdominal pressure.

Posterior Vaginal Wall

a. *Relaxed perineum:* Torn perineal body produces gaping introitus with bulge of the lower part of the posterior vaginal wall.
b. *Rectocele:* There is laxity of the middle 1/3rd of the posterior vaginal wall.

Description and Staging of Pelvic Organ Prolapse

Two general classifications are used to describe and document the severity of pelvic organ prolapse.

Baden Walker Halfway System

Descent of anterior vaginal wall, posterior vaginal wall or apical prolapse can be graded with this system. It takes hymen as reference point and as follows:

Grade 0 - Normal position for each respective site
Grade 1 - Descent halfway to hymen
Grade 2 - Descent to the hymen
Grade 3 - Descent halfway past the hymen (Fig. 15.2A)
Grade 4 - Maximum possible descent for each site (Fig. 15.2B).

Although it is not as accurate or informative as current POP-Q system, it is adequate for clinical use if each compartment (anterior, apical or posterior) is evaluated.

SECTION -2 ◆ Gynecology

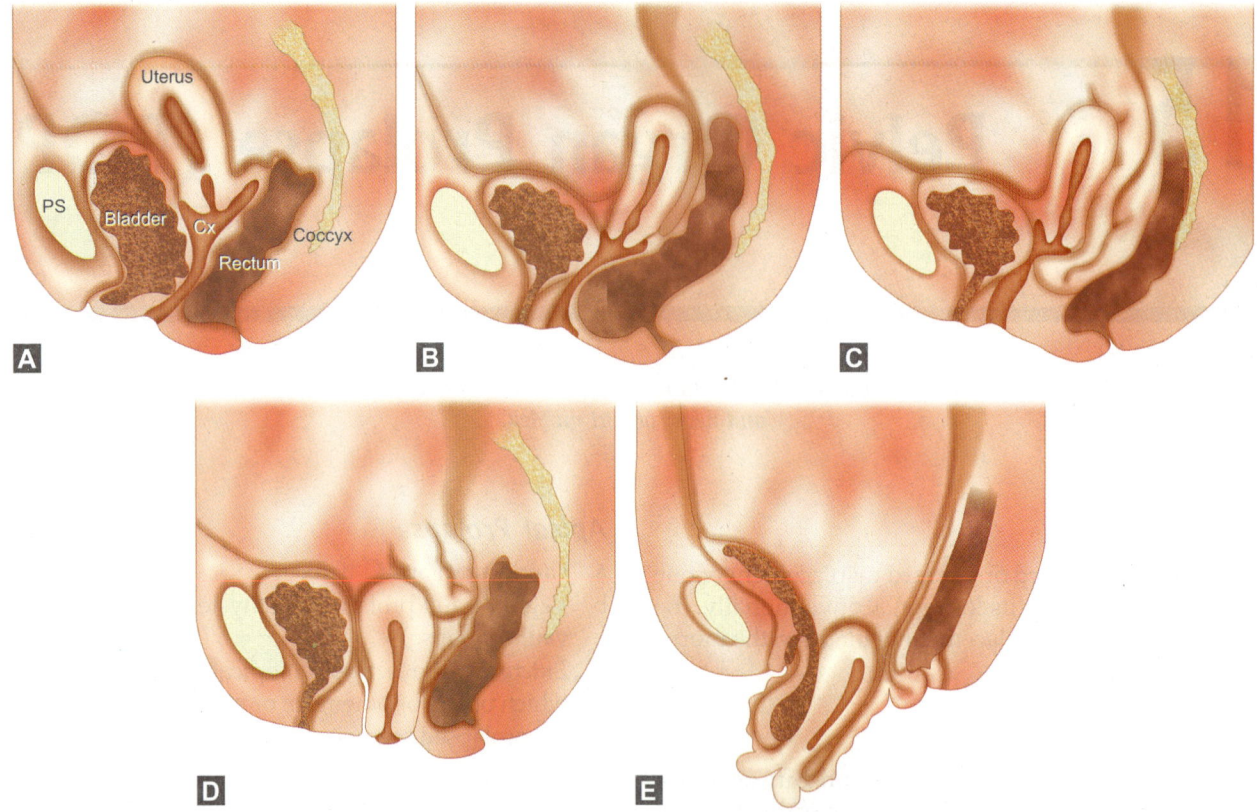

Figs 15.1A to E: Types of prolapse: (A) Cystrourethrocele; (B) Rectocele; (C) Enterocele; (D) Uterine prolapse; (E) Procidentia

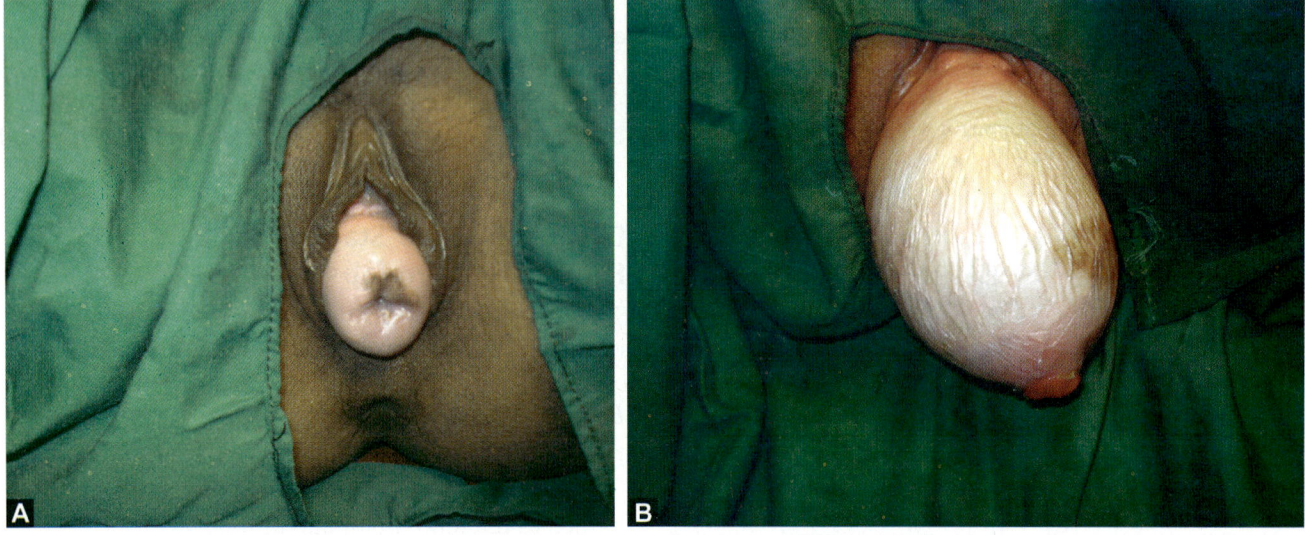

Figs 15.2A and B: (A) Grade III prolapse showing keratinizing change; (B) Grade IV prolapse showing decubitus ulcer

Pelvic Organ Prolapse-Quantification (POP-Q)

In 1996, International Continence Society defined a system of pelvic organ prolapse (POP-Q). This standardized quantification system facilitates communication between physician in practice and research and enables progression of these conditions to be followed accurately. In this system, anatomic description of specific sites in the vagina is used in place of traditional terms. The system identifies nine locations in the vagina and vulva in centimeters relative to the hymen, which are used to assign stage 0-4 of prolapse at its most advanced site.

The following six points are located. All POP-Q points except total vaginal length (TVL), are measured during patient vasalva maneuvers and should reflect maximum protrusion.

Chapter - 15 ♦ Pelvic Organ Prolapse (POP)

Box 15.1: Six points of POP-Q system

Vaginal wall points	Description	Range
Anterior vaginal points		
Aa	Midline of anterior vaginal wall, 3 cm proximal to external urethral meatus correspond to proximal location of urethrovesical crease	− 3 to + 3 cm
Ba	Most dependent portion of rest of anterior wall	− 3 cm in absence of prolapse to + TVL
Apical vaginal points		
Point C	Most distal edge of cervix or the leading cervix or the leading edge of vaginal cuff after hysterectomy	± TVL
Point D	Location of posterior fornix in a women having cervix. Omitted if cervix is absent. Represent level of uterosacral ligament attachment to proximal posterior cervix	± TVL or Omitted
Posterior vaginal wall point		
Point Ap	Point in the midline of the posterior vaginal wall that lies 3 cm proximal to the hymen	− 3 to + 3 cm
Point Bp	Most dependent portion of rest of posterior wall	
Other		
Genital hiatus (gh)	Measured from the middle of external urethral meatus to midline of posterior hymenal ring	
Perineal body	Measured from the posterior margin of genital hiatus to mid anal opening	

Box 15.1 defines six points of POP-Q system representing anatomic landmarks of evaluation of POP.

Documentation of POP-Q

With the hymenal plane defined as zero, the anatomic position of these points from the hymen is measured in centimeters. Points above or proximal to the hymen are described in negative number (Fig. 15.3). The point measurement can be organized using 3 by 3 grid. Depending on measurement of points, following stages of POP-Q is defined:

Stage 0 - No prolapse is demonstrated
Aa, Ap, Ba, Bp are all - 3 cm
Point C is between TVL and TVL − 2 cm

Stage 1 - The most distal portion of prolapse is > 1 cm above the level of hymen (Quantitation value is < − 1 cm)

Stage 2 - The most distal portion of prolapse is < 1 cm proximal or distal to the plane of hymen (Quantitation value is ≥ − 1 cm but ≤ +1cm)

Stage 3 - The distal portion of prolapse is > 1 cm below plane of hymen, but protrudes no further than 2 cm less than the total vaginal length in cm (Quantitation value is > + 1 cm but < + (TVL − 2) cm

Stage 4 - Complete to nearly complete eversion of vagina. The most distal portion of prolapse protrudes to at least > + TVL − 2 cm

Its quantitation value is ≥ + (TVL − 2) cm. In most instances the leading edge of stage IV prolapse will be the cervix or vaginal cuff scar.

Old system of degree of uterus prolapse: It is shown in Box 15.2.

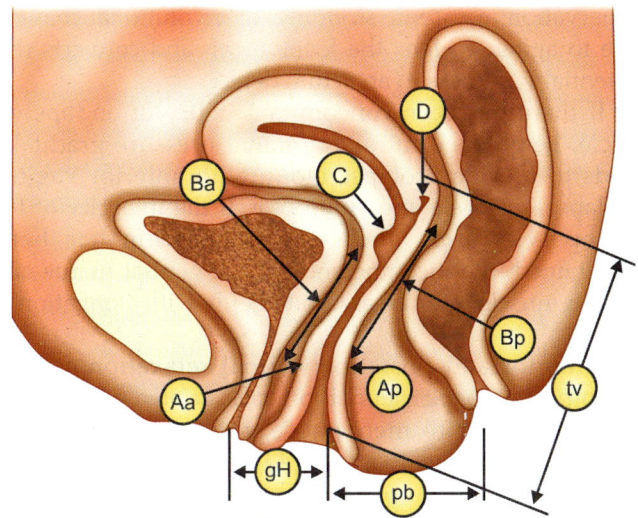

Fig. 15.3: Anatomical landmarks used during pelvic organ prolapse quantification

Box 15.2: Uterine descent

Degree	Description
1°	Cervix below ischial spine
2°	Cervix up to the introitus
3°	Cervix outside introitus
4° (Procidentia)	All of uterus outside introitus

Etiology and Risk Factors

The etiology of pelvic floor disorders is more likely to be multifactorial. Box 15.3 summarizes risk factor for pelvic organ prolapse (POP).

Box 15.3: Risk factors associated with POP

```
Pregnancy
Vaginal delivery
Menopause — (a) Aging, (b) Hypoestrogenic
Chronic raised intra-abdominal pressure
Pelvic floor trauma
Genetic factor
Hysterectomy
Spina bifida
```

Multiparity: Vaginal child birth is most frequently cited risk factor (Swift, 2005). Moreover the risk of POP is increased 1.2 times with each vaginal delivery.

Other Obstetrical Related Risk

Although vaginal delivery is implicated in women's lifetime risk for POP, specific obstetric risk factor remains controversial. These include macrosomia, prolonged 2nd stage of labor, episiotomy, forceps delivery, and sphincter laceration, etc. Each is a proposed risk factor, although not definitely proven.

According to current recommendation, elective forceps delivery and episiotomy to shorten second stage labor is not advocated because of lack of evidence of benefit and their potential for maternal and fetal harm. Likewise elective cesarean delivery is not advised to reduce incidence of POP in community.

Age

Advancing age is also implicated in the development of POP. In women aged 20-59 years, the incidence of POP roughly doubles with each decade. The increased incidence may result from degenerative process, as well hypoestrogenism.

Race

Black and Asian women have lower risk as compared to Hispanic women.

Increased Abdominal Pressure

Chronically increased intra-abdominal pressure caused by any factor like obesity, chronic constipation, chronic coughing, and repeated weight lifting can increase the risk of developing POP.

Risk Factors for Nulliparous Prolapse

Prolapse seen in unmarried or nulliparous women is attributed to spina bifida occulta or split pelvis which results in inherent weakness of the pelvic floor support. Women with connective tissue disorders like Marfan's syndrome, Ehlers-Danlos syndrome are more likely to develop POP.

Pathophysiology

Pelvic organ support is maintained by complex interaction between levator ani muscle, vagina and pelvic floor connective tissue. It closes the pelvic outlet and surrounds the external vaginal opening, the urethra and anal canal. Levator ani (include puborectalis, pubococcygeus, iliococcygeus muscles) and coccygeus muscle form pelvic floor. These muscles create a hammock like sling between the pubes and coccyx and are attached laterally along the pelvic side walls. The levator ani muscle is tonically contracted providing a firm shelf posteriorly to support the pelvic contents and aiding with urinary and fecal continence.

Endopelvic fascia is a loose network of connective tissue containing small vessels, lymphatics and nerves which surround the pelvic organ and the vagina. Thicker areas of endopelvic fascia in the pelvis are described as ligaments, called cardinal and uterosacral ligament (details chapter basic sciences), which help to support the uterus and cervix. The supported endopelvic fascia that separates the vagina from the bladder and from the rectum is called pubovesical and rectovaginal fascia respectively.

The urogenital hiatus (anterior levator muscle gap) which permits the urethra, vagina and anus to emerge from the pelvis is a site of potential weakness. Attenuation of the pubococcygeal and puborectal portion of levator muscles, both as a result of direct injury into 2nd stage of labor, or newer injury due to stretching in labor or denervation in chronic straining, or involutional changes due to aging, widens the levator gap and converts this potential weakness to an actual defect.

If there has been concomitant injury of endopelvic fascia, heightened intra-abdominal pressure gradually leads to uterine prolapse along with anterior vaginal prolapse, rectocele and enterocele. If the integrity of the endopelvic fascia and its condensation has been maintained, the incompetency of the genital hiatus and levator muscles may be associated only with elongation of cervix.

Anterior and posterior vaginal relaxation as well incompetence of perineum is often associated with uterine prolapse. Prior to menopause, the prolapsed uterus hypertrophies and is engorged and flaccid. After the menopause, the uterus atrophies. In procidentia, the vaginal mucosa thickens and cornifies, resembling skin. Recently it is suggested that primary problem in genitourinary prolapse is increased collagen degradation causing a decrease in the mechanical strength of supporting fascia.

Secondary Change in POP

Vagina

a. Vaginal mucosa becomes stretched and if exposed to air, becomes thickened and dry with surface keratinization (see Fig. 15.2A). Pigmentation can also be present.
b. **Decubitus ulcer** (see Fig. 15.2B) is a trophic ulcer, always found at the dependent part of prolapsed mass. It is due to decreased circulation due to narrowing of uterine vessels by stretching effect with additional keratinization, cracks. Superimposed friction and infection cause finally sloughing and ulceration. The reduction of prolapse into vagina and daily packing heals the ulcer in 1-2 weeks. Decubitus ulcer needs to be differentiated from cancer cervix by cytology and biopsy.

Cervix

a. **Portio vaginalis:** In vaginal part of the cervix there is chronic congestion, which may lead to hyperplasia and hypertrophy of the fibromuscular glandular components. So vaginal part of cervix becomes hypertrophied and congested. If there is added infection there is purulent or blood stained discharge.
b. **Supravaginal part:** If the supravaginal part of cervix is well-supported by Mackenrodt's ligament, but the vaginal portion of the cervix prolapse with vagina; the supravaginal portion gets stretched and elongated. It is usually in 2nd and 3rd degree prolapse of uterus. In procidentia, the entire uterus slides with vagina, and hence cervix retains its normal length.

Urinary System

In a big cystocele there is hypertrophy of the bladder wall and trabeculation due to sharp angulation of the urethra. Incomplete evacuation of urine may cause recurrent cystitis. In procidentia there can be kinking of distal ureter and cause hydroureter and hydronephrosis if prolapse is not surgically corrected.

Incarceration of Prolapse

It is uncommonly encountered when due to edema, and congestion there is irreducible prolapse. Head low posture, ice packing or packing with magnesium sulphate reduces the edema, enabling the prolapse to be reduced.

Diagnosis

Symptoms

The symptoms of POP are in general not unique to any particular vaginal defect. Usually the symptoms are reflection of only the most prominent point of prolapse. Most women complain only when the prolapse reaches near the vaginal opening. A critical concept is that the functional complaints may not always relate to anatomical findings.

Mild forms of prolapse are usually asymptomatic and identified only on physical examination. The most common symptom of prolapse is a bulge of tissue protruding from the vaginal opening. It may interfere with sitting or walking. Some women with POP report pelvic pressure, especially after prolonged standing.

Prolapse may interfere with coitus. Long standing prolapse that protrudes beyond the introitus may result in ulceration and bleeding from the prolapsed vaginal skin. Advanced forms of prolapse may also cause difficulty with urination or defecation and urinary or fecal incontinence are often associated with the disorder.

Clinical Findings

Physical Examination

Physical examination begins with full body system evaluation to identify pathology outside the pelvis. Systemic condition like cardiovascular, respiratory may affect approach to treatment. Examination for POP should begin in dorsal lithotomy position and vulva and perineum are examined for sign of vulvar or vaginal atrophy, lesion or other abnormalities.

As prolapse is a dynamic condition which changes with gravity and intra-abdominal pressure, patient can be encouraged to perform Valsalva's maneuver, so the full extent of the prolapse can be ascertained. If findings are inconsistent even with Valsalva's maneuver, it may be helpful to perform a standing, squatting, straining examination with the empty bladder. In evaluating patient it is useful to divide the pelvis into specific compartments.

POP-Q Examination

a. The genital hiatus (gh) and perineal body (pb) are measured during Valsalva's maneuver.
b. Total vaginal length (TVL) is then measured by placing the marked ring forceps at the vaginal apex and noting the distance to hymen.
c. A bivalve speculum is inserted at the vaginal apex and points C and B are measured.
d. A split speculum then used to displace the posterior vaginal wall and allows for visualization of anterior wall and measurement of points Aa and Ba.
e. The split speculum is then rotated to 180° to displace the anterior wall and postwall is examined and points Ap and Bp are measured. If posterior wall descends, attempts are made to differentiate in rectocele and enterocele. Enterocele can only be definitively be diagnosed by observing small bowel peristalsis behind the vaginal wall. Standing rectovaginal examination may be needed to confirm the diagnosis.

f. Evaluation of urinary function is also important with POP especially with anterior compartment prolapse. With prolapse of the anterior vagina, the urethra may kink and can cause incomplete emptying of urine. Post-void residual volume over 100 ml is considered elevated and may indicate more sophisticated testing. Urethral kinking can mask underlying stress urinary incontinence. Reduction of prolapse during examination and asking patient to strain may confirm or exclude stress urinary incontinence. This is referred as potential stress incontinence and should be offered with an anti-incontinence procedure at the same time if surgery is being done for POP.

Investigation

The laboratory investigation includes: (a) Blood hemoglobin, (b) Urine routine and culture examination, (c) Renal function test, (d) Blood sugar, (e) X-ray chest, (f) ECG.

Diagnostic imaging of pelvis in women with POP is not routinely performed. If clinically indicated following tests may be performed by urogynecologist: (a) Fluoroscopic video cystourethrography (VCUG), (b) Ultrasound of pelvis, (c) Defecography if suspected intussusception or rectal mucosa prolapse. MRI is only for research purpose for knowledge and understanding of functional pelvic support.

Differential Diagnosis

Prolapse of vagina is generally a straight forward diagnosis. However, less common disease entities may present as bulge in the vagina:

a. Tumors of urethra and bladder are much more indurated and fixed then anterior vaginal prolapse.
b. Urethral diverticulum is usually more focal and painful. Compression may express some purulent material from the urethral meatus. Urethroscopy helps in diagnosis.
c. Anterolateral defect can represent embryologic remnants as Gartner's duct cyst.
d. Skene's and Bartholin gland can enlarge to form cyst or abscess.
e. Congenital elongation of cervix is differentiated from the POP as vaginal portion of the cervix is elongated and there is no accompanying vaginal prolapse. The fornices are deep, not shallow.
f. Cervical fibroid polyp can be identified as cervix is high up in its normal anatomical position.
g. *Chronic inversion:* It is recognized as cervix is further up, uterus cannot be defined. Uterine sound will confirm the diagnosis. On laparoscopy, there will be fundal depression and absence of uterine fundus in the pelvis.

Prevention of POP

Prevention of genital prolapse is the focus of much debate. Avoiding multiparty, spacing between child births, proper supervision of second stage of labor, adequate puerperal care, prevention of obesity as well malnutrition are general measures to be adopted by society and health systems.

Antepartum, intrapartum and postpartum exercise especially designed to strengthen levator and perineal muscle group often helps to improve or maintain pelvic support. Hormone replacement therapy following menopause may help to maintain the tone and vitality of pelvic musculofascial tissues and can prevent or postpone POP.

Treatment

POP, except in certain situations is a condition that impacts only the quality of life. So the extent and type of treatment should reflect and be commensurate the degree of negative impact on the quality of life patient experiences. Patient perception is also a critical component. Common reasons to provide treatment are when women's daily function is impaired because of the prolapse.

Conservative Measures

Primary Treatment

Pessary are supportive vaginal devices, usually made from inert material such as silicone. They are designed to be placed into the vagina, to retain and hold pelvic structure in their normal positions. Pessaries are used when surgery is not elected or contraindicated. They can also be used as temporary treatment in a patient awaiting a surgical procedure. Pessaries are effective in relieving symptoms of POP. A wide variety of pessaries shape and size are available. Commonly used are ring, doughnut and Gellhorn pessaries (Figs 15.4A and B).

Precaution with Pessary

a. A careful fitting by an experienced health care provider is important to avoid complication related to poor sizing, urethral obstruction or vaginal erosion.
b. The pessary must be removed and cleaned regularly either by patient or her health care provider at period of 2-3 months.

Side effects of pessary are urinary tract and vaginal infection, vaginal odor, discharge and bleeding. Some women with severe laxity of the pelvic floor may not be able to retain a pessary successfully.

Surgical Measures

The type of surgery offered to the patient with prolapse depends on the age of patient, her reproductive desires, her general condition and degree of POP. Procedures for prolapse can be broadly categorized into three groups.

a. **Restorative:** Which use the patient's endogenous support structure.
b. **Compensatory:** Which attempt to replace deficient support with permanent graft material.

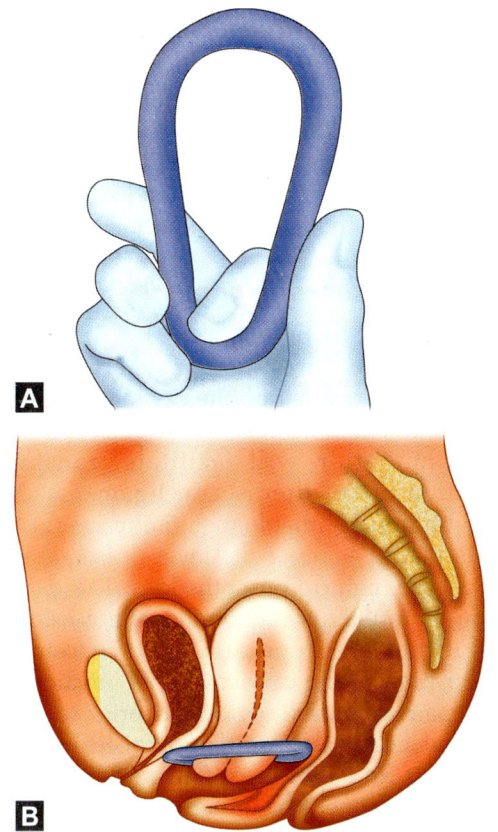

Figs 15.4A and B: (A) Ring pessary; (B) Inserted ring pessary

Table 15.1: Common surgical procedure for treatment of pelvic organ prolapse		
Defect location	Clinical condition	Procedure
Anterior	Cystocele	Anterior colporrhaphy Paravaginal repair
Superior (Apical)	Uterine prolapse	Hysterectomy (Fig. 15.5C) Colpocleisis
	Enterocele	Vaginal enterocele repair Mccall culdoplasty Abdominal enterocele repair

c. **Obliterative:** Which close or partially close the vagina.

Most procedures are performed via vaginal approach, although they may also be performed through an abdominal incision or laparoscopically. Typically several procedures are combined, since prolapse tends to occur at more than one site in most patients. Table 15.1 summarizes various surgical methods according to type of prolapse.

Though these groupings are somewhat arbitrary and not entirely exclusive. The commonly performed operations are as follows:

Anterior vaginal colporrhaphy: It is one of the most common surgical treatments for anterior vaginal prolapse. It is a vaginal approach that involves dissecting the vaginal epithelium from the underlying fibromuscular connective tissue and bladder (Figs 15.5A and B), then plicating the vaginal musculature across the midline. Excess vaginal epithelium is excised and wound closed. Recurrence up to 52% has been reported. Modifications involving permanent suture material and most recently graft material have been introduced for better results.

Paravaginal Repair

Paravaginal repair is performed for anterior vaginal prolapse that is confirmed to be a result of detachment of the pubocervical fascia from its lateral attachment at the white line (arcus tendineus fascia pelvis) either at one or both sides. It is confirmed preoperatively by noting loss of the lateral sulci and lack of rugation over the epithelium along the base of the bladder and elongation of the anterior vaginal wall.

Clinically vaginal examination using a speculum reveals a preponderance of the prolapse lateralized to one side as speculum is withdrawn. Besides this, a ring forceps can be used by gently exerting anterior traction along the vaginal sulci. If the defect is reduced then the defect is peravaginal and can be approached with a paravaginal repair technique.

In these cases repair should be done by fixing the endopelvic fascia to the arcus tendineus fascia (white line) of the pelvis. This may be done retropubically through the space of Retzius or vaginally.

Posterior Vaginal Prolapse

There are two main surgical methods of posterior vaginal defect.

Traditional Repair

Posterior midline incision is given in vagina often high to level of posterior fornix. The vaginal epithelium is separated off the underlying fibromuscular layer and endopelvic fascia. Plication of levator ani muscle and bulk lateral plication of tissues oversewing the rectovaginal fascia is done. There is no attempt at identifying specific fascial defect. In **alternative method of rectocele** repair, discrete defect in rectovaginal fascia are identified and repaired. After separating the vaginal epithelium off the underlying rectovaginal fascia as in traditional method, the surgeon inserts a finger of nondominant hand into the rectum to inspect the rectovaginal fascia for defect. These defects are then repaired with interrupted suture to plicate over the rectal wall. In this levator ani is not plicated as this may result in bandlike stricture over the posterior wall, causing dyspareunia.*

Perineorrhaphy is generally combined with posterior vaginal repair. This procedure restores the perineal body and reduces the vaginal outlet to more normal caliber. Re-approximation of the superficial transverse perineal muscle and bulbocavernosus muscle rebuilds the perineum and lengthens the distance between vaginal opening and anal verge.

Apical Vaginal Repair

Prolapse of the vaginal apex includes: (a) Uterine prolapse, (b) Post-hysterectomy vaginal cuff prolapse, (c) Enterocele. There is a growing appreciation that supports of the vaginal apex provides the cornerstone for a successful prolapse repair. The vaginal apex can be re-suspended with a number of procedures:
a. Sacrospinous ligament fixation
b. Uterosacral ligament vaginal vault suspension
c. Abdominal sacropexy

Sacrospinous Ligament Fixation

Technique

The vaginal apex is suspended to the sacrospinous ligament unilaterally or bilaterally using a vaginal extraperitoneal approach. In this technique vaginal mucosa is separated from the rectovaginal tissues and the associated enterocele is identified and repaired. Perforation through right or left rectal pillar is accomplished by directing blunt dissection towards the ischial spine through the loose areolar tissue. Sacrospinous ligament is identified 2-3 cm medial to ischial spine and 2 or more unabsorbable or delayed absorbable ligature is passed through the ligaments to the submucosal apex of the vagina. Tying the suture brings the vaginal apex to sacrospinous ligament and posterior colporrhaphy is then performed.

Complication

Bilateral vaginal connection to both sacrospinous ligaments may result in excessive lateral stretching of the vaginal apex or posterior impingements on the distal sigmoid colon. Gluteal and posterior leg pain is a potential complication of this procedure, it requires a skilled surgeon.

---

* It is difficult to achieve optimal results when the paravaginal repair is used in combination with traditional central repair because of creation of tension on opposing suture lines. When large central defects coexist with lateral defects one option is an extensive central repair accompanied by a good apical support procedure.

Iliococcygeal Vaginal Suspension

Iliococcygeal vaginal suspension involves the attachment, usually bilaterally, of the vaginal apex to the iliococcygeus muscle and fascia. In this extraperitoneal access is achieved via the posterior vagina. It is generally a safe procedure, requiring a posterior vaginal incision in the midline with wide dissection of the overlying epithelium.

Bilateral Uterosacral Ligament Suspension

This technique can be done at the time of vaginal hysterectomy or to correct post-hysterectomy apical cuff prolapse. After entrance into the peritoneum is complete, traction on the ipsilateral posterior vaginal wall with rectal digital examination will facilitate transperitoneal identification of the uterosacral ligaments. Now two sutures with nonabsorbable material in lateral to medial fashion is placed—one at the level of ischial spine and another a little high up on both sides. These sutures are then brought to the ipsilateral vaginal apices. Fixation of the cuff at this level reproduces cuff placement to the normal position of the cervicovaginal junction. Anterior vaginal repair should be performed prior to tying down the vaginal cuff. Risk of this procedure is medial displacement and kinking of ureter (up to 11%), so cystoscopic assessment of ureteral function without and with tension on the fixation sutures, prior to tying down the vaginal apices should be done. If there is compromised ureteral flow, removal of suture on the affected side should be done.

Abdominal Sacrocolpopexy

Vaginal vault suspension can also be performed abdominally by laparotomy or by laparoscopy by attaching vaginal cuff to the sacral promontory. It is an excellent primary procedure for apical vaginal prolapse and enterocele. **It is the procedure of choice for those who are already having an abdominal approach for hysterectomy or for other indication.**

In this procedure, by laparotomy or by laparoscope cul de sac and peritoneum overlying the sacrum is visualized. A window in the peritoneum over sacral promontory is created and permanent sutures are placed through the anterior longitudinal ligament, approximately at level of S1. The vaginal cuff is then exposed by dissecting off the overlying peritoneum. Fixation of Y shaped graft over anterior and posterior vagina is done. This Y shaped graft is then brought posteriorly along the hollow of sacrum and affixed to the anterior longitudinal ligament suture, overriding the sacral promontory.

Many different graft types have been described. Synthetic grafts have higher erosion complication rates than biologic graft. But biologic grafts have high failure rate when placed at apex. As graft technologies evolve, identification of the optimal graft material that maximizes durability and compatibility may materialize. Besides graft complications, operative hemorrhage is significant risk. Specifically during placement of sacral suture laceration of sacral vein may be problematic.

Obliterating Vaginal Operation (Colpocleisis and Le Fort Operation)

These procedures involve removing excessive vaginal epithelium, suturing anterior and posterior wall together, obliterating the vaginal vault and effectively closing the vagina. These operations are technically easier, require less operative time, and offer superior success rate. They are appropriate for elderly or medically compromised patient, who have no future desire for coital activity.

Fothergill's Manchester operation and vaginal hysterectomy are few operations which have been traditionally performed since years for POP. In recent years role of these operations in treatment of POP is critically reviewed.

Fothergill's Repair (Manchester Operation)

In this anterior and posterior colpoperineorrhaphy is combined with amputation of cervix, suturing of cut end of Mackenrodt's ligament in front of the cervix and covering raw area of amputated cervix with vaginal mucosa (Strumdorf's suture) (Figs 15.5A to F). This operation is suitable for women in reproductive age group. However, fertility is somewhat reduced and there can be incompetent cervical os and resultant risk of abortion and preterm delivery.

Vaginal Hysterectomy

Vaginal hysterectomy with anterior and posterior colpoperineorrhaphy is recommended in clinical practice over age of 40 years, who are not keen on retaining their child bearing and menstrual function. If there is associated abnormal uterine bleeding, fibroid, adenomyosis this age can be relaxed up to 35 years (Figs 15.6A to E). However, in European countries, hysterectomy is rarely performed

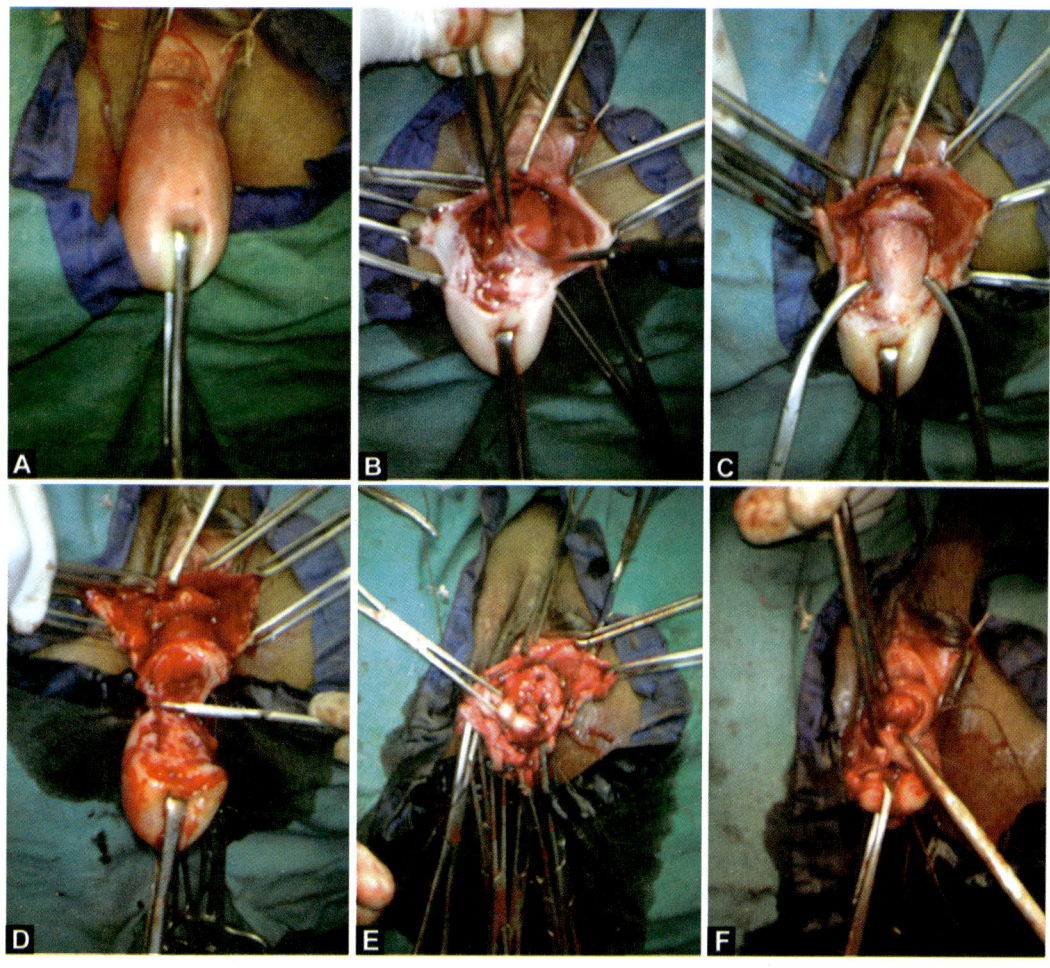

Figs 15.5A to F: Steps of Fothergill's operation: (A) Holding of cervix; (B) Dissection of vaginal fascia from vesical fascia; (C) Clamping and suturing of Mackenrodt's ligament; (D) Amputation of cervix; (E and F) Application of posterior and anterior Strumdorf's suture

Section -2 ♦ Gynecology

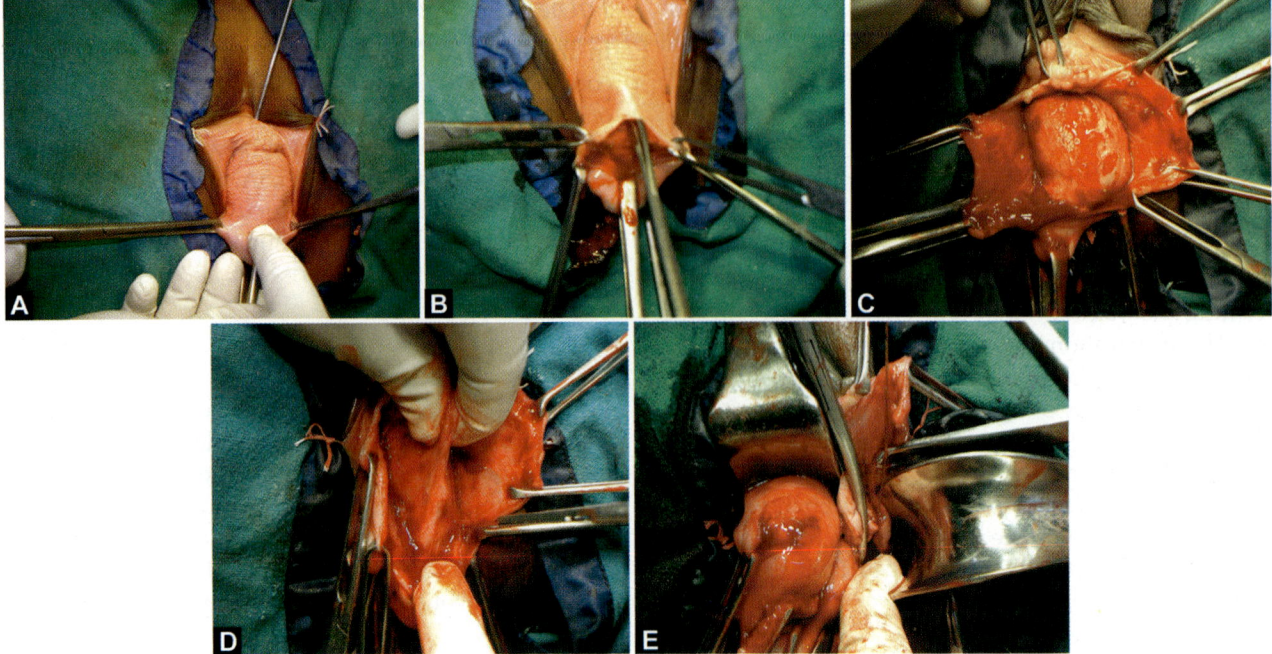

Figs 15.6A to E: (A) Demarcation of various landmark—vaginal edge, bladder sulcus, urethral sulcus; (B and C) Dissection of vaginal fascia from vesical fascia; (D) Identification of vesicouterine ligament; (E) Vaginal hysterectomy being performed for POP

during pelvic floor reconstruction while in United States and India hysterectomy is often performed concurrently with prolapse surgery.

If apical or uterine prolapse is present, hysterectomy will more readily allow the vaginal apex to be suspended with the above described apical suspension procedures. Alternatively if apical or cervical prolapse is not present, hysterectomy need not to be incorporated into prolapse repair.

Procedure of Vaginal Hysterectomy

A cervical incision is performed and the utero vesical fold and pouch of Douglas opened. The uterosacral and cardinal ligament are divided and ligated first, followed by uterine pedicles and finally the tuboovarian and round ligament (Figs 15.6A to E). The sequence can be reversed also, according to ease of surgeon. In case of procidentia care should be taken to avoid kinking of ureters which are often dragged into lower positions than normal. After closure of the pelvic peritoneum, the upper pedicles are tied in the midline to give support for the vaginal vault. In the same way uterosacral ligaments are tied posteriorly to obliterate potential enterocele space. The vaginal epithelium is then closed with interrupted sutures.

MULTIPLE CHOICE QUESTIONS

1. Most common genital prolapse is:
    a. Cystocele
    b. Procidentia
    c. Rectocele
    d. Enterocele
    Ans. a
2. Presence of decubitus ulcer in prolapse indicates:
    a. Infection
    b. Circulatory disturbance
    c. Malignancy
    d. Mechanical trauma
    Ans. b
3. Urinary incontinence in uterovaginal prolapse is mostly due to:
    a. Detrusor instability
    b. Stress incontinence
    c. Urge incontinence
    d. True incontinence
    Ans. B
4. Cystocele is formed by which part of urinary bladder:
    a. Superior surface
    b. Base
    c. Trigone
    d. Posterior
    Ans. b
5. A 25-year-old nulliparous women with 3rd degree uterine descent but no cystocele or rectocele or enterocele is best treated by:
    a. Fothergill operation
    b. Abdominal sling operation
    c. Amputation of cervix and pelvic reconstruction
    d. Le Fort's colpocleisis
    Ans. b

Chapter – 15 ♦ Pelvic Organ Prolapse (POP)

6. A 28-year-old woman, with para 3, with 2nd degree prolapse, the treatment of choice is:
   a. Fothergill's operation
   b. Wertheim's operation
   c. Pelvic floor exercise
   d. Vaginal hysterectomy with pelvic repair
   Ans. a

7. The treatment of choice for decubitus ulcer is:
   a. Bed rest
   b. Reduction with tampoon
   c. Antiseptic dressing
   d. Antibiotic
   Ans. b

8. In Fothergill's operation the following are undertaken, *except*:
   a. Amputation of cervix
   b. Anterior colporrhaphy
   c. Colpoperineorrhaphy
   d. Plication of round ligament
   Ans. d

16. Urinary Incontinence

The art of winning a patient's confidence lies in the art of listening.
A patient is always more anxious to talk than to listen.

General Consideration

Urinary incontinence is defined as involuntary urine loss that is a social or hygienic problem. Urinary incontinence is 2-3 times more common in women than in men and prevalence increases with age. Its presence has a significant effect on the quality of life of women.

Physiology of Micturition

Continence

The urinary bladder is a storage organ of urine with the capacity to accommodate large increase in urine volume with minimal or no increase in intravesical pressure. The ability to maintain urine storage with convenient and socially acceptable voluntary emptying is continence. Continence requires the complex coordination of multiple components. Simplistically during filling urethral contraction is coordinated with bladder relaxation and urine is stored. While during voiding the urethra relaxes and bladder contracts. An alteration of this mechanism can cause incontinence. The urinary bladder displays the phenomena of adaptation to increased urinary volume. Intravesical pressure remains below 10 cm H_2O until over 500 ml of urine is contained. Urethral pressure is maintained by internal sphincter made up of longitudinal and circular plain muscles and elastic tissues. External sphincter is made up of striated muscles. Usually urethral pressure is much greater than intravesical pressure so it ensures continence (Figs 16.1A and B). Beside this, sympathetic and parasympathetic innervations plays important role. The parasympathetic nerve fibers from S2–S4 stimulates detrusor contraction and the sympathetic fibers T1–L2 stimulate contraction of bladder neck and urethra. Voluntary control of micturition is controlled by the central nervous system. Cortical control of detrusor muscles rests in the supramedial portion of the frontal lobes and in the genu of the corpus collosum.

Epidemiology

Most epidemiologic studies indicate prevalence of 25-55%. But data are limited by the fact that most women do not seek medical attention for this condition. The most common condition is stress incontinence which represents 29-75% of cases. Detrusor over activity accounts for up to 33% of incontinence cases, whereas the remainder is attributable to mixed forms.

STRESS URINARY INCONTINENCE

Stress urinary incontinence occurs during period of increased intra-abdominal pressure like straining coughing or exercise, when the intra vesical pressure rises higher

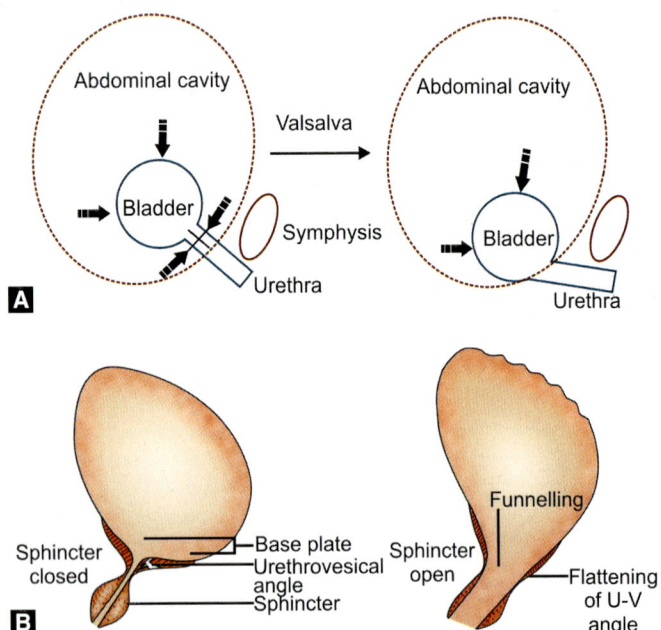

Figs 16.1A and B: On left in normal support, increased intra-abdominal pressure is equally distributed to contralateral sides of bladder and urethra. On right in poor urethral support, there is alteration of urethrovesical angle with resulting incontinence

than the pressure that urethral closure mechanism can withstand.

Pathogenesis

Stress urinary incontinence can result in two ways:
a. **Urethral hypermobility:** Urethral hypermobility following child birth is the most common cause of genuine stress incontinence. Normally the vagina is attached bilaterally to the pelvic diaphragm providing a stable base on which the bladder neck and urethra rest. This positioning allows increase in intra-abdominal pressure to be transmitted equally to the bladder and urethra which maintain urethral closure and continence. *When there is urethral hypermobility, there is descent of the proximal urethra and bladder neck in a way that these structures are no longer compressed against the vagina during increased intra-abdominal pressure and leakage of urine occurs.*
b. **Weakness of internal urethral sphincter:** In certain group of patients there is weakness of internal urethral sphincter which results in intrinsic sphincter deficiency. In these women SUI occurs with minimal exertion or even at rest. This is found in women with advanced age, prior bladder neck surgery and radiation treatment.

URGE INCONTINENCE

Urge urinary incontinence is the involuntarily leakage of urine accompanied by or immediately preceded by urgency. This is a symptom based diagnosis and may or may not be caused by detrusor overactivity, which is a urodynamic observation characterized by involuntary detrusor contractions during the filling phase. Detrusor overactivity is quantified by cause and can be:
a. *Neurogenic detrusor overactivity—Detrusor hyperreflexia:* When a neurological condition is found like cardiovascular disease, multiple sclerosis or spinal cord injury.
b. *Idiopathic detrusor overactivity—Detrusor instability:* When there is no definite cause. The term overactive bladder syndrome also includes women with symptoms of urgency, frequency and urge incontinence. It is referred to *OAB – dry*, when women with these symptoms do not leak urine and *OAB wet* when it is accompanied by incontinence.
c. *Mixed incontinence:* Women with mixed incontinence have symptoms of both stress and urge urinary incontinence. Younger women are more likely to have stress incontinence alone whereas in older women mixed and urge incontinence predominate.
d. *Continuous incontinence:* This is continuous leakage of urine such as that caused by genitourinary fistula. These fistulas may be congenital or may follow difficult delivery, pelvic surgery or radiation.

Diagnosis or Evaluation

The initial evaluation of patients with incontinence requires a systemic approach to consider possible cause.

History

A thorough medical history should be obtained. History may reveal systemic illness as diabetes mellitus (producing osmotic diuresis) vascular insufficiency (leading to incontinence at night), chronic pulmonary disease or a wide variety of neurologic conditions.

Quality of Life Measures

Physician should ask carefully that how the incontinence specifically affects their lives and to what degree the incontinence disturb their day to day activities.

Physical Examination

a. **General examination:** For neurological and systemic disorders.
b. **Pelvic examination:** In patients with SI, there is typically pelvic relaxation. A pelvic mass also may contribute to GSI. In coughing with full bladder, it is frequently possible to demonstrate GSI. Vaginal atrophy in postmenopausal women can be detected.

Simple Test

Voiding Diary

A woman should complete a urinary diary for a thorough record of voiding habits. Patients are instructed to record for three days the volume of each oral fluid intake, volume of urine with each void, episode of urinary leakage and provokers of urinary incontinence, episodes and time of sleep and awakening. This historical information gained is a valuable diagnostic tool and also can be used later on to provide an assessment of treatment efficacy.

Urine Analysis

Examination of urine by dipstick testing sugar, protein and microscopy is done to exclude infection and hematuria. If urinary tract infection is documented by microscopy or culture it is to see whether urinary tract symptoms improved with eradication of bacteriuria. If hematuria as well bacteriuria is found, the urine is rechecked after treatment of urinary tract infection. If there is hematuria in the absence of bacteriuria, it may need further evaluation to rule out kidney or bladder tumors.

Post Void Residual Volume

Measurement of post void residual urine is an easy initial test to begin after the patient void. *In general there should be less than 50 ml of urine in the bladder.* Post void residual urine is measured by ultrasound or catheterizing the patient in the office after patient is asked to void the urine. A patient with an elevated post void residual urine > than 100–200 ml may have an underlying neurologic disorder. The presence of an elevated post void residual urine is a relative contraindication to surgical treatment of GSI and to anticholinergic medication for detrusor instability.

Cough Stress Test

Patient is examined with full bladder and involuntary egress of urine is checked at the time of cough. Stress incontinence should be documented in supine as well standing position. However, the physical findings must be considered in context of patient's clinical history.

Urodynamics

Urodynamic study is any test that provides objective evidence about lower urinary tract infection. So post void urine is also urodynamic study. Further urodynamic study is recommended:
a. If diagnosis is uncertain.
b. Surgery is being considered.
c. Patient has hematuria in absence of infection.
d. Increased PVR.
e. Any neurologic condition.
f. Prior failed surgical attempts at correction.

Following test can be performed:
1. *Cystometrogram:* It involves filling the bladder to measure volume pressure relationships. As the bladder is filled to its normal capacity of 300-500 ml, the pressure inside the bladder should remain low. The patient usually experiences the first urge to void at 150-200 ml. **Patients with detrusor instability have reduced bladder capacity (< 300 ml)** and demonstrate urinary incontinence that is associated with involuntary bladder contraction (Pressure increase above baseline). In patients with GSI, **incontinence is demonstrated on coughing or Valsalva maneuver.** Leak point pressure that is the intravesical pressure at which leakage is noted, is generally less than 60 cm of water pressure if intrinsic sphincter deficiency is present.
2. *Uroflowmetry:* In this the women is asked to empty their bladder into a pan connected to a flowmeter. It can be performed to measure detrusor pressure and flow rate to evaluate for voiding dysfunction.
3. *Multichannel urodynamics:* These urologic tests can simultaneously record urethral, vesical and intra-abdominal pressure as well as electromyographic activity of the pelvic musculature. It should be done in patients with SI prior to surgical correction and in patients with urge incontinence not responsive to medical therapy (Fig. 16.2).

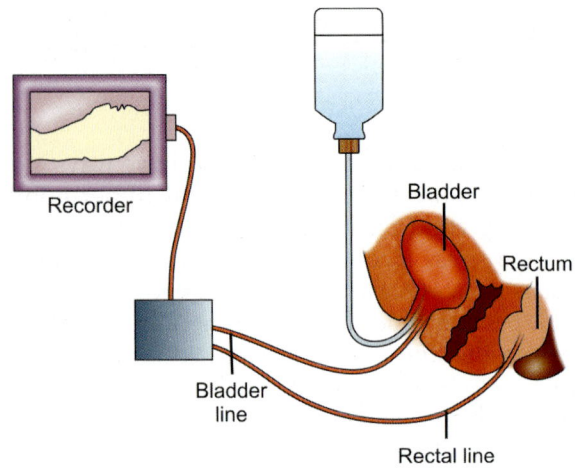

Fig. 16.2: Multichannel urodynamics

4. *Q test and Marshall test:* Q test and Marshall test are less helpful in differentiating between GSI and DI and has high false positive or negative rate. In Q test, a sterile Q tip swab is placed in the urethra to a depth of 3 cm to evaluate the angle between the urethra and bladder. **In positive test the angle of the Q tip changes by > 35° on Valsalva maneuver.** It is considered to be evidence of poor bladder neck support. In *Marshall test* **pelvic support is assessed.** The tips of a Kelly clamp are placed on each side of the urethra to restore the urethra to its normal anatomic positions. If incontinence is corrected the test is believed to be positive for GSI and patient is judged a good candidate for surgical correction. However, current studies show that the Marshall test causes obstruction of the urethra and is not helpful in differentiating between GSI and DI.
5. *Bonney's test:* In Bonney's test two fingers are placed in the vagina at the urethrovesical junction on either side of urethra and the bladder neck region is elevated. On straining or coughing absence of leakage of urine shows, that bladder neck elevation surgery will prove beneficial to the patient.
6. *Cystourethroscopy:* Endoscopic evaluation is an invaluable adjunct for the diagnosis and management of the urogynecologic patient.

Treatment

The treatment of urinary incontinence can be either non surgical or surgical. The approach to treatment is based on the clinical findings and the degree of discomfort experienced by the patient, who should be fully informed of the risk and expected outcome.

Lifestyle Changes

Lifestyle intervention can decrease stress urinary incontinence in many women. Weight loss in obese women decreases leakage. Postural changes such as crossing the legs during period of increased intra-abdominal pressure often prevent stress urinary incontinence. Avoidance of smoking and caffeine can be considered but has no proven value in control of symptoms.

Physical Therapy

The Cochrane incontinence group concluded that pelvic floor muscle training is consistently better than no treatment or placebo treatment for stress incontinence and should be offered as first line conservative management for women. The pelvic floor muscle exercise (Kegel exercise) should be supervised and done regularly for adequate duration 3-4 times per week. Electrical stimulator via probe placement in vagina and rectum has given mixed result but may be more helpful in women with overactive bladder.

Behavioral Therapy and Bladder Training

Bladder training focuses on modifying bladder function by changing voiding habits. Behavioral therapy focuses on improving voluntary control rather than bladder function. Behavioral modification includes fluid intake regulation, improving accessibility to toilet for patients with limited mobility and change of medication as diuretic. Patients with neurogenic detrusor overactivity do not respond to behavioral therapy because the problem is in neural pathways.

Pessary and Urethral Inserts

Incontinence pessaries are designed to reduce downward excursion or funneling of the urethrovesical junction. This provides bladder neck support and help to reduce incontinence. As an alternative to pessary urethral insert may also be considered for GSI. The *Fem soft* insert is currently commercially available. They are placed into urethra by the patient and removed before a void after which a new sterile one is reinserted. However, not all women are appropriate candidate for pessaries nor will all desire long-term management of incontinence or prolapse with these devices.

Medical Treatment

Stress Incontinence

The tone of the urethra and bladder neck is maintained in large part by α adrenergic activity from the sympathetic nervous system. So drug tried are—Imipramine—which has a concomitant relaxing effect on the detrusor. Ephedrine, Pseudoephedrine, Phenylpropalamine and Norepinephrine has been tried.

Use of HRT

Conjugated estrogen with or without progestin can be prescribed for prevention or relief of urinary incontinence as per current recommendation.

Recently **Duloxetine** selective serotonin and norepinephrine receptor inhibitor has been evaluated for treatment of SUI. It promotes urine storage by relaxing the bladder and increasing outlet resistance. In initial trials drugs has been found to improve symptoms. Previously Phenylpropalamine (PPA) was used to treat SUI but now FDA has reclassified PPA in category II and considered it as generally not safe or effective.

Urge Incontinence and Overactive Bladder

Anticholinergic Medication

These drugs exert their effect on the bladder by blocking the activity of acetylcholine at muscarinic receptor sites. But muscarinic receptors are not limited to the bladder. So side effects with these drugs may be significant. Of these, dry mouth, constipation and blurry vision are the most common. So drug selection should be tailored and efficacy is balanced against tolerability. Drugs include *Tolterodine, Oxybutynin and Imipramine*. Oxybutynin should be started with a lower dose and increased as needed to a higher and more frequent dose according to patient symptoms and needs. A two weeks trial is sufficient to determine effectiveness.

Most side effects of Oxybutynin result from its secondary metabolite that follows its liver metabolism, so transdermal patch has been designed which is applied twice weekly to the abdomen, hip or buttock. *Imipramine* is less effective than Tolerodine and Oxybutynin, but displays α adrenergic as well as anticholinergic characteristic so it is occasionally prescribed for those with mixed urinary incontinence. Importantly, doses of Imipramine used to treat incontinence are significantly lower than those used to treat depressive or chronic pain. It has good effect in nocturia and nocturnal enuresis. The starting dose is 25 mg at bed time, which may be increased to 75 mg. In the elderly Imipramine should be used cautiously because it increases the risk of hip fracture presumably related to the potential side effects of orthostatic hypertension.

Surgical Treatment

Surgical treatment should be offered for moderate to severe incontinence. SI is not a life threatening condition but related to quality of life concerns and the decision to operate must be based on the patient's symptoms and the impact on daily life. **Medical management and behavioral therapy should be first line management.** Surgery should be reserved for only those women when above measures fail to improve incontinence above tolerable threshold.

Surgical treatment of GSI can be divided into two groups:
a. Procedure that restore the anatomic support of the proximal urethra and the urethrovesical junction in women with hypermobility and normal intrinsic urethral sphincter.

b. Procedure designed to compensate for a poorly functioning urethral sphincter (intrinsic sphincter deficiency).

Surgical Treatment of Intrinsic Sphincter Deficiency

Periurethral bulking agent: For this a sling is placed under the urethra to support it. Periurethral collagen injection under local anesthesia is used to treat intrinsic sphincter deficiency.

Surgical Treatment of Anatomic Stress Incontinence

a. *Anterior repair:* Anterior colporrhaphy with Kelly plication is one of the oldest methods of surgical correction used for cystocoel. The technique involves vaginal dissection of the epithelium below the bladder and bladder neck, identifying the perivesical fascia and pubocervical fascia and plicating each side over the mid line. The Kelly plication involves specific support at bladder. It is not considered as an effective cure for stress incontinence.

b. *Needle urethropexy:* It was introduced by Armand Pereyra. Many authors have published alteration of this technique. In this vagina is incised, dissected, periurethral tissue is mobilized, space of Retzius entered (Retropubic space) and a needle ligature carrier is padded from a small abdominal incision into the vaginal incision. The periurethral tissue and fascia is identified, secured through delayed absorbable suture (Vicryl, Dexon), and brought through retropubically and secured above the abdominal rectus fascia. In this manner the bladder neck is elevated and continence is restored.

c. *Abdominal retropubic urethropexy (Colposuspension):* Marshall Marchette–Krantz (MMK) and Burch Colposuspension are the two classic retropubic surgeries for incontinence. Many modifications have been also described. All operation share the following characteristics:
  i. Operation is performed through an open low abdominal incision or with laparoscopically assisted exposure of the space of Retzius.
  ii. Attachment of the periurethral or perivesical endopelvic fascia to some other supporting structure in the anterior pelvis. In MMK operation the periurethral fascia is attached to back of the pubic symphysis. In BURCH Colposuspension bladder neck fascia is attached to ileopectineal ligament (Cooper's ligament) (Fig. 16.3).

d. *Pubovaginal sling:* In this surgery, a strip of either rectus fascia or fascia lata is placed under the bladder neck through the retropubic space. The ends are secured at the level of rectus abdominis muscle. This surgery is a standard procedure for SUI (Fig. 16.4).

e. *Midurethral sling:* In this procedure, synthetic minimally invasive mesh is placed at midurethral level. They are classified based on route of placement:
  i. Tension free vaginal tape (TVT): Retropubic method.
  ii. Transobturator tape (TOT)—Transobturator method: They are considered effective and recovery is rapid. Short term cure rate is claimed to be 90% but long term data are still not available. Surgeon should be aware that most new devices for urinary

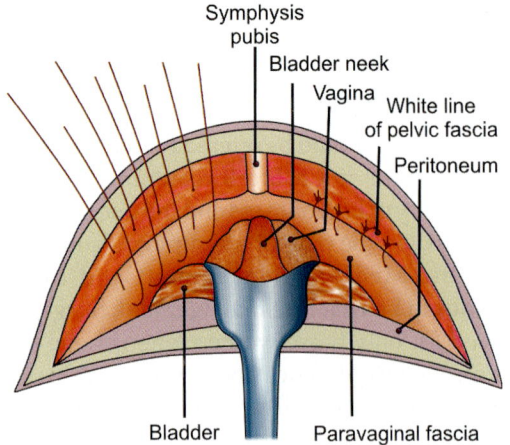

Fig. 16.3: Illustration showing BURCH colposuspension operation; bladder neck fascia is attached to ileopectineal ligament

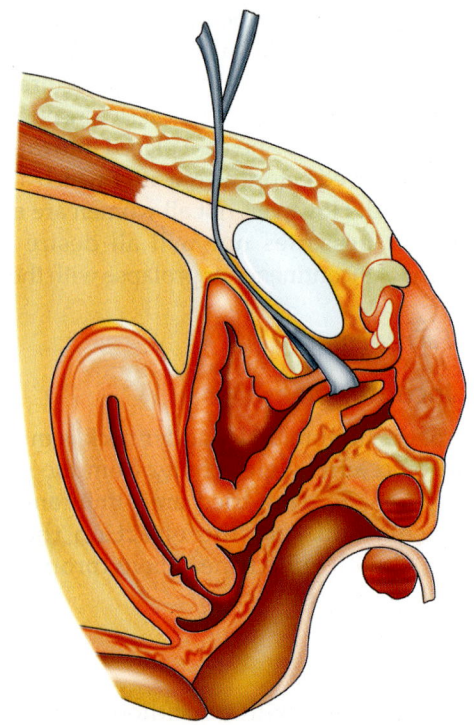

Fig. 16.4: Suburethral sling—Fascia located at bladder neck with the ends of the sling tied to rectus fascia

incontinence are not tested in clinical trials before they are marketed.

f. In modification of TVT procedure a 3-4 inch strip of polypropylene synthetic mesh is placed directly below the mid urethra through a small vaginal incision.

General Risk of Incontinence Surgery

In choosing surgical management surgeon must weigh the chance of cure against the chance of severe complications. The complication can be:
a. Bladder injury.
b. Urinary retention.
c. Vascular injury.
d. Hematoma formation.
e. Graft erosion is unique to graft surgery and rate depends largely on the type of graft used.
f. Urinary tract infection.
g. De novo voiding dysfunction as urgency when new onset detrusor overactivity occurs after surgery for incontinence. Cystoscopy should be considered to rule out a foreign body in the bladder in this situation.

Surgical Treatment of Detrusor Overactivity

Even with development of newer anticholinergic medication with fewer side effects, there is still a select group of patients with overactive bladder who remain refractory to standard medical and behavioral treatment. Following surgical treatment can be considered in carefully selected cases and refractory cases.

Sacral Neuromodulation

The outpatient surgically implanted device contains a pulse generator and electrical leads that are placed into the sacral foramina to modulate innervations to the bladder and pelvic floor. In this treatment in the first phase a percutaneous nerve evaluation test is performed to determine the response. These who respond are then implanted with permanent electrode lead adjacent to the third sacral nerve root connected to a pulse generator. Success rate is nearly 80%. It is minimally invasive and typically completed in a day surgery settings. Still 30% of patients require further surgical revision because of pain or other complication at the generator or implant site.

Botox Injection

In this via cystoscopy at 15-30 different detrusor muscles sites, Botulinum toxin is injected under direct visualization, sparing the bladder trigone and urethral orifice. This toxin acts on peripheral cholinergic nerve endings to inhibit calcium mediated release of acetylcholine.

GENITOURINARY FISTULA

A genitourinary fistula is defined as an abnormal communication between the urinary (ureter, bladder and urethra) and the genital (uterus, cervix and vagina) systems. The incidence is 0.5-3% amongst gynecological admissions in referral hospitals. However, incidence is much less in developed countries.

Etiology

1. *Congenital:* Genitourinary fistula—rare
2. *Acquired:* Most vesicovaginal fistula follow either obstetric trauma or pelvic surgery:
   a. **Obstetrical:** In poor and developing countries the most common cause is obstetrical, constituting 80-90% of cases. The fistula may be ischemic or following trauma.
      i. Ischemic vesicovaginal fistula results from prolonged compression effect on the bladder base between the head and symphysis pubis in obstructed labor. It results in ischemic necrosis with superimposed infection and sloughing. Ischemic fistula takes few days (3-7) following delivery to produce such type of fistula.
      ii. Traumatic fistula may be caused by injudicious use of instruments like forceps.
      iii. Abdominal surgery: In repeat cesarean section or hysterectomy, the injury may be direct or ischemic following a part of bladder well being caught in the suture.
   b. **Pelvic surgery:** In developed countries, iatrogenic injury during pelvic surgery is responsible for 90% of vesicovaginal fistula. Accepted incidence of fistula formation after pelvic surgery is 0.1-2%. 80-90% of genitourinary fistulas are related to surgery by obstetrician, gynecologist, and rest result from procedures performed by urologist and general surgeons. Because most genitourinary fistulas have an operative etiology, prevention and intraoperative recognition of lower urinary tract injury is important. Imperative use of intraoperative cystoscopy in suspected lower urinary tract injury improves the detection rate of lower urinary tact injuries.
   c. **Other causes:** Although, surgical and obstetric causes account for most urinary fistula, other uncommon causes are as follows:
      i. **Radiation:** Radiation therapy induces an endarteritis, which leads to tissue necrosis and subsequent potential fistula formation.
      ii. **Malignancy:** Advanced carcinoma of the cervix, vagina or bladder may produce fistula by direct spread.

iii. **Trauma and foreign body:** Trauma sustained during coital injury or assault can result in fistula. Foreign bodies like neglected pessary, vesical calculi are also documented cause. During sling surgeries for incontinence, placement of the synthetic mesh under excess tension may contribute to increased tissue stress and necrosis and eventually may lead to fistula formation.

iv. **Miscellaneous:** Other rare cause of fistula formation include infection as Lymphogranuloma venereum, urinary tuberculosis, pelvic inflammation, and syphilis, inflammatory bowel disease and autoimmune disease.

Clinical Presentation—Symptoms

Vesicovaginal fistula classically presents with complaint of continuous urinary leakage 7-10 days after difficult delivery or 1-3 weeks after recent operation commonly hysterectomy. Other less specific symptoms of genitourinary fistula include fever, pain, illness and bladder irritability.

History

A thorough history regarding obstetric deliveries, prior surgeries, previous management of fistula and pelvic surgery or radiation therapy should be documented.

Physical Examination

1. *Direct visualization:* It identifies the defect. A meticulous assessment for other fistulous tract should be performed and their location and size is noted. It is mandatory to differentiate from stress urinary incontinence or vaginal discharge.

2. *Dye instillation:* In some instances, physical examination is unrevealing in presence of incontinence. In these cases *three swab test* should be done. In the test gauge is packed sequentially into vaginal canal. A diluted solution of methylene blue or indigocarmine is instilled into urinary bladder in a retrograde fashion using a catheter. After 15-30 minutes the gauge is removed serially and inspected for the presence of dye. **If inner most gauge is colored—it indicates proximal or high location, if outermost dye is colored—it shows distal fistula.** If distally placed gauge is stained with dye, it should be confirmed that it is not contaminated by stress incontinence (Fig. 16.5).

3. *Cystourethroscopy:* It is a valuable adjunct for diagnostic evaluation. It allows localization of the fistula, determination of its proximity to the urethral orifice and assessment of surrounding bladder mucosa viability.

4. *Urethral involvement:* Concomitant urethral involvement is estimated to complicate 10-15% of vesicovaginal fistula and should be excluded in diagnostic evaluation.
    a. *Intravenous urography:* Can be done to assess integrity of the upper collecting system and urethral involvement in the fistula.
    b. *Phenazopyridine hydrocholoride (Pyridium):* It can be used with three swab test to determine urethral involvement. Pyridium 200 mg orally is taken a few hours before the test and gauge is packed serially high, middle and lower part of vagina. If the most proximal sponge is colored with orange dye (as drug stains the urine orange), ureteral involvement us suspected. If both orange and blue dye is seen then both the bladder and ureter are typically involved.
    c. *Voiding cystourethrography:* This radiologic study can demonstrate leakage into the vagina and help to confirm the presence, location and number of fistula tract.

Treatment

Conservative

Occasionally genitourinary fistula may spontaneously close during continuous bladder drainage using an indwelling urinary catheter. An attempt at conservative treatment should be usually done. However, most urinary fistulas ultimately require surgical intervention.

Surgical Treatment

General principles of fistula repair are fundamentally as follows:
a. Timely repair.
b. Adequate mobilization of layers.

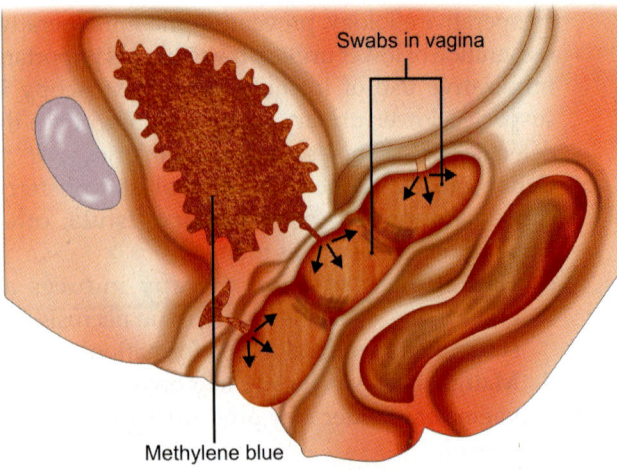

Fig. 16.5: Three swab test

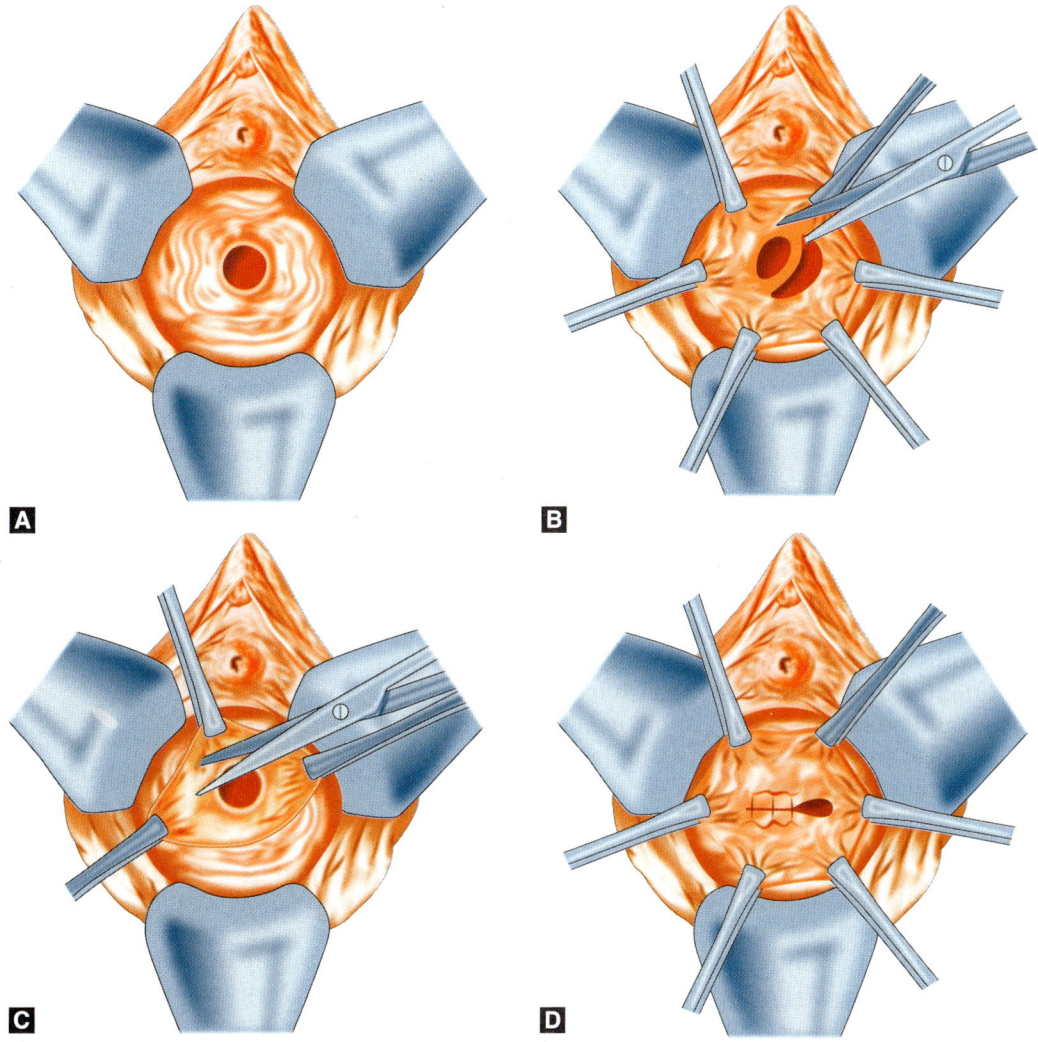

Figs 16.6A to D: Classical method of repair of vesicovaginal fistula: (A) Exposure of fistula; (B) Dissection of vaginal epithelium from the fistula to mobilize the tissue; (C) Excision of fistula tract; (D) Interrupted absorbable suture is placed in extramucosal situation

  c. Tension free closure.
  d. Assessment of adequate surrounding tissue viability.
  e. Postoperative bladder drainage.

Timing of repair: Traditional teaching recommends delayed repair of fistula at 3-6 months after injury. But now it is recommended that unless there is severe infection or acute signs of inflammation, waiting is not necessary. Fistula identified within first 24-48 hours of surgery can be safely repaired immediately with success rate of 90-100%.

Route of surgical repair:
1. *Vaginal:* The transvaginal approach is associated with shorter operative time, decreased blood loss, less morbidity and shorter hospital stay. There are following techniques:
   a. *Classical technique:* In this fistula, tract is excised. After excision of fistula, the vaginal epithelium is undermined and mobilized widely. The bladder mucosa is closed followed by two layers of fibromuscular tissues of bladder. A watertight repair is confirmed and vaginal epithelium is reapproximated (Figs 16.6A to D).
   b. *Latzko technique:* It is like a partial colpocleisis. Surgically most proximal portion of the anterior and posterior vaginal wall is approached and thus upper most vagina is partially obliterated.
2. *Abdominal approach:* This approach is used in following situations:
   a. The fistula is located proximally in a narrow vagina.
   b. It is in close proximity to the ureteral orifice.
   c. A concomitant ureteric fistula is present.
   d. Previous failed attempts.
   e. Vaginal walls are rigid with little mobility.
   f. The fistula is large or complex in configuration.
   g. There is a need for abdominal interposition graft.

In this approach fistula is reached through surgically cystotomy (opening of urinary bladder). Bladder mucosa is dissected off the vaginal mucosa, and mobilized for approximately 1.5 cm in all directions. After adequate mobilization, the fistula site is closed in layers.

3. *Interpositional flaps:* In some cases when intervening tissue for fistula closure are weak and poorly vascularized, various tissue flaps may be placed vaginally or abdominally between the bladder and vagina to lend support and blood supply.

Special Postoperative Care

Bladder is drained through indwelling catheter for 10-14 days. The patient is advised to pass urine frequently after removal of catheter. Coitus is deferred for at least three months and pregnancy is deferred for at least one year. Delivery in next pregnancy should be by elective cesarean section.

Failed repair: If VVF repair fails, repair should again be tried after three months. The fistula may become smaller and the second attempt may be successful. Advice of urologic surgeon should be sought. As last resort, urinary diversion has to be opted in which ureters are implanted into the pelvic colon or ileal bladder.

Urethrovaginal Fistula

Causes of urethrovaginal fistula are same as that of vesicovaginal fistula. Small isolated urethrovaginal fistula may be caused by operative injury during anterior colporrhaphy, urethroplasty, and sling operation.

Diagnosis

The patient has got urge to pass urine but the urine dribbles out into the vagina during the act of micturition. Three swab test can be done to confirm the diagnosis.

Treatment

Surgical repair is done in two layers like VVF repair. In cases of complete destruction of the urethra, reconstruction of urethra is to be performed.

URETERIC INJURY

The incidence of ureteric injury in hysterectomy is 0.03-6.0%. Risk factors are altered pelvic anatomy from malignancy, prior surgery and enlarged uterus or adhesions from endometriosis or prior pelvic inflammatory disease.

Site and Causes

Common Site of Ureteric Injury

a. Clamping the uterine artery at level of internal cervical os, 1.5 cm lateral to cervix where uterine artery cross the ureter from above.
b. Suturing the vaginal cuff.
c. Ligating the infundibulopelvic ligament during adnexa removal.
d. Suturing the uterosacral ligament during culdoplasty.
e. Placing suspensory sutures during colposuspension.
f. Any congenital malformation (duplex ureter) makes it more vulnerable to injury at any of these sites.

Identification

Ideally injuries should be recognized intraoperatively because those repaired at time of initial surgery are associated with improved repair and low patient morbidity. Injury can be apparently visible and may be identified with cystoscopy. Intravenous administration of 5 ml ampoule of indigocarmine dye aids in detection of ureter injury. Cystoscopy can detect 90% of unsuspected ureteral injury and 85% of unsuspected bladder injuries. Alternatively, intraoperative ureteral catheterization or intravenous pyelography may be used to isolate lesions. Injuries however may be unsuspected and diagnosed following surgery. *Women have complaints of flank pain, fever and costovertebral angle tenderness.* Ureterovaginal fistula, ileus, urine peritonitis and pyelonephritis may be noted. **To increase early detection liberal use of intraoperative cystoscopy has been advocated.**

BLADDER INJURY DURING GYNECOLOGICAL SURGERY

Bladder injury is more frequent than ureteric injury during gynecological surgery and includes perforation by sutures or laceration. *Incidence is 1-2% of hysterectomy* and is associated more commonly with vaginal approach.

Risk Factors

a. Prior cesarean delivery with scarring between the bladder and anterior uterus.
b. Prior pelvic reconstruction surgery.

Sites of Injury

a. Initial abdominal entry when incising the anterior parietal peritoneum.
b. Dissection within the space of Retzius.
c. Dissection of vaginal epithelium when performing anterior colporrhaphy.
d. Hysterectomy when dissecting the vesicouterine fold.
e. When entering or suturing vagina during hysterectomy.

Diagnosis

It is identified at time of surgery when a gush of clear fluid into the operative fluid is seen. Laceration is confirmed with seeing the bulb of Foley's catheter or installation of sterile dye through a Foley's catheter into the bladder. Cystoscopy can be done to define bladder injury and exclude concurrent ureteral injury or identify the sutures placed through the bladder mucosa.

The administration of indigocarmine dye several minutes before cystoscopy aids in diagnosis.

Management

Repair at the time of primary surgery is performed. It lowers the risk of postoperative vesicovaginal fistula formation. Ureteral patency is confirmed. The bladder is closed with 2 or 3 layer running suture using a 3-0 absorbable or delayed absorbable suture. The first layer inverts the mucosa into the bladder and subsequent layer reapproximate muscularis of bladder. Postoperatively indwelling catheterization is done for 7-10 days.

MULTIPLE CHOICE QUESTIONS

1. Most common cause of vesicovaginal fistula in India is:
   a. Gynecological surgery
   b. Irradiation
   c. Obstructed labor
   d. Trauma
   Ans. c

2. Which surgical procedure has the highest incidence of ureter injury?
   a. Vaginal hysterectomy
   b. Abdominal hysterectomy
   c. Wertheim's hysterectomy
   d. Anterior colporrhaphy
   Ans. c

3. A female on 7th day of hysterectomy develops fever, burning micturition and continuous urinary dribbling. She can also pass urine voluntarily. The diagnosis is:
   a. Vesicovaginal fistula
   b. Urge incontinence
   c. Stress incontinence
   d. Ureteric vaginal fistula
   Ans. d

4. A 55-years-old woman has recurrent urinary retention after a hysterectomy done for a huge fibroid. The most likely cause is:
   a. Atrophic and stenotic urethra
   b. Lumbar disc prolapse
   c. Injury to bladder neck
   d. Injury to hypogastric plexus
   Ans. d

5. The cause of retention of urine in obstetric and gynecology is/are:
   a. Impacted ovarian tumor
   b. Retroversion
   c. Hematocolpos
   d. All
   Ans. d

6. Bonney's test is used to demonstrate:
   a. Stress incontinence
   b. Urge incontinence
   c. Fibroid
   d. True incontinence
   Ans. a

7. Ureterovaginal fistula formation is common at:
   a. Infundibulopelvic ligament
   b. Vaginal vault
   c. Distal to uterine artery near vaginal vault
   d. Distal to uterine artery in cardinal ligament
   Ans. a

8. Marshal-Marchetti Kront surgery is done for:
   a. Stress incontinence
   b. Urge incontinence
   c. VVF
   d. Bladder obstruction
   Ans. a

9. Important postoperative management in case of VVF are:
   a. Continuous bladder drainage
   b. Antibiotic
   c. Complete bed rest
   d. Early ambulation
   Ans. a

17 Benign Adnexal Masses

The wise man is always anxious to learn,
But never anxious to teach.

General Consideration

Benign adnexal masses are common in women in the reproductive age group and are caused by physiologic cyst or benign neoplasm. The management of these benign masses is dictated by their presentation. Operative intervention is indicated when a patient is symptomatic because of hemorrhage of a ruptured cyst or torsion.

Most adnexal mass are however discovered incidentally and risk of malignancy must always be assessed and excluded with relevant investigation like ultrasound, Doppler flow studies, laparoscopic directed biopsies. When malignancy is not suspected, expectant management is indicated as many of these cyst are physiologic in nature and are expected to regress overtime. Patients should be re-evaluated 6 weeks after initial presentation preferably postmenstrually. Persistent masses should be considered potentially benign or malignant neoplasm that warrants operative evaluation.

About two-third of ovarian tumors are encountered during the reproductive years. Most ovarian tumors (80-85%) are benign and two-third of these occur in women between 20 and 40 years of age.

Physiologic Enlargement

Functional Cyst

Follicular cyst: Follicular cyst is the most common functional cyst and varies in diameter from 3 to 8 cm. Follicular cyst results from failure in ovulation, usually secondary to disturbances in the release of pituitary gonadotropins. The fluid of the incompletely developed follicle is not reabsorbed producing an enlarged follicular cyst.

Histology

Follicular cysts are lined by an inner layer of granulosa cells and an outer layer of theca interna cells that may or may not be luteinized.

Symptoms

Typically they are asymptomatic. Large cysts may cause pelvic pain, dyspareunia and occasional abnormal uterine bleeding.

Treatment

Most follicular cyst disappears spontaneously by 60 days without treatment. Use of oral contraceptive pills have often been recommended to help establish a normal rhythm. But recent data show that this practice may not produce more rapid resolution than expectant management.

Corpus Luteum (Granulosa Lutein) Cyst

These are thin walled unilocular cyst ranging from 3-11 cm in size. Following normal ovulation the granulosa cells lining the follicle become luteinized. In the stage of vascularization blood accumulates in the central cavity producing the corpus hemorrhagicum. Resorption of the blood then results in a corpus luteum, which is defined as a cyst when it grows larger than 3 cm (Fig. 17.1).

Symptoms

A persistent corpus luteal cyst may cause local pain and tenderness. It can also be associated with either amenorrhea or delayed menstruation thus can simulate the clinical picture of an ectopic pregnancy.

A corpus luteal cyst may rupture leading to a hemoperitoneum and require surgical management. Patient taking anticoagulant therapy are at particular risk for rupture. Most rupture occurs on cycle day 20-26.

Treatment

Unless acute complications develop, symptomatic therapy is indicated. Like follicular cyst, corpus luteal cysts usually regress after 1-2 months in menstruating patients. Oral contraceptive pills have been recommended but may be of questionable benefit.

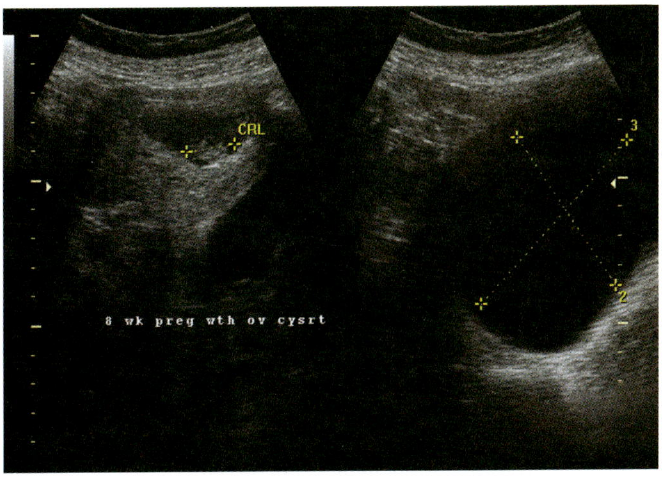

Fig. 17.1: Ultrasound showing 8 weeks pregnancy with cystic ovary

Theca Lutein Cyst

Elevated level of chorionic gonadotropins can produce theca lutein cyst and thus are seen in patients with hydatdiform mole or choriocarcinoma and in patient undergoing chorionic gonadotropins or clomiphene therapy. Rarely they are seen in normal pregnancy.

Pathology

The cysts are lined by theca cells that may or may not be luteinized and they may or may not have granulosa cells. They are filled with clear straw colored fluid.

Symptoms

Abdominal symptoms are minimum although a sense of pelvic heaviness or aching may be described. Rupture of cyst may result in intraperitoneal bleeding. There are associated continued signs and symptoms of pregnancy especially hyperemesis.

Treatment

The cyst disappears spontaneously following termination of molar pregnancy, treatment of the choriocarcinoma or discontinuation of fertility therapy. Such resolution may take months to occur. Surgery is undertaken only in event of complication like torsion and hemorrhage.

Endometrioma

In women with endometriosis ovarian endometriotic cyst can develop and grow up to 6-8 cm. These endometriomas are also referred to as chocolate cyst because they contain thick, brown, blood debris inside.

Hyperthecosis

Hyperthecosis or thecomatosis commonly produces no gross enlargement of the ovary. Thus, the lesions are demonstrable only by histologic examination of the excised gonad. In the premenopausal women hyperthecosis is associated with virilization and clinical findings similar to those seen in polycystic ovarian disease. These alterations may also be associated with postmenopausal bleeding and endometrial hyperplasia.

Polycystic Ovarian Syndrome (Stein-Leventhal Syndrome)

Polycystic ovarian syndrome (PCOS) is a multisystem endocrinopathy with ovarian expression of metabolic disturbances and a wide spectrum of clinical feature as hyperandrogenism and obesity along with metabolic disorders, secondary amenorrhea or oligomenorrhea and infertility.

It has a prevalence of 5-10%. 50% of patients are hirsute and 30-75% are obese. A presumptive diagnosis of PCOS can often be made based on the history and initial examination. The syndrome can be diagnosed if at least two of the following conditions are present:
a. Oligomenorrhea or amenorrhea.
b. Hyperandrogenism.
c. Polycystic ovaries on ultrasound.
d. Raised LH and low FSH/LH ratio.

The disease has genetic and familial tendency and may be autosomal dominant inherited.

Pathogenesis

PCOS is presumably related to hypothalamic pituitary dysfunction and insulin resistance. A primary contribution to the problem has not been clearly defined.

Pathology

Microscopically, the ovaries are often enlarged with a thick capsule. The surface may be lobulated but the peritoneal surface is free of adhesions.

Investigations

Ultrasound

Ultrasound shows multiple cyst (more than 10 in numbers), 0.5 - 1 mm, and rarely up to 20 mm in size are located along the surface of the ovary giving a 'Necklace' appearance on ultrasound. These are atretic follicle. The ovarian volume is enlarged to more than 8 CC or 9 CC due to stromal hyperplasia (Fig. 17.2).

Low FSH/LH ratio and raised testosterone, androstenedione and dehydroepiandrosterone will be observed. Fasting insulin level is more than 10 m IU/ml in insulin resistant case.

Laparoscopy can be diagnostic as well sometimes can play a therapeutic role if cysts are cauterized.

Treatment

Recognition of immediate and long-term sequelae of PCOS needs early and adequate treatment of this disease.

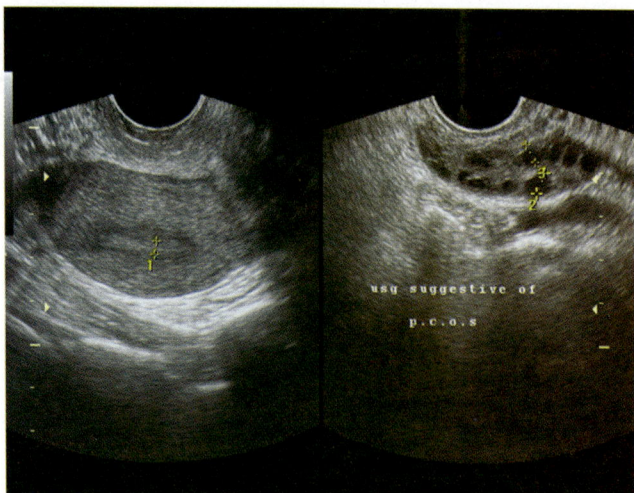

Fig. 17.2: Ultrasound image showing polycystic ovaries

Long-term sequelae are diabetes, hypertension, hyperlipidemia and endometrial cancer.

Following modalities or combination of treatment can be applied according to patient age, reproductive desires, concern for cosmetic appearance, and associated metabolic disorder:

Weight Loss

Even a small reduction in body weight as little as 2-7% is associated with improved ovulatory function and restoring hormonal mileu.

Hirsutism

Hirsutism can be treated with any agent that lowers androgen level. Oral contraceptive pills particularly with cyproterone acetate are typically the first choice in patients not desiring pregnancy.

Infertility

In infertile women, PCOS respond often to clomiphene citrate. In clomiphene failure or resistant cases experienced clinician can add human gonadotropins to produce the desired ovulation.

Metformin

Metformin is lately extensively used as insulin sensitizers. It reduces insulin level, delay glucose absorption and liver production of glucose (Liver neoglucolysis). By reducing the level of insulin Metformin reduces the level of testosterone and increases sex hormone binding globulins. It also improves ovulation rate.

Contraindications to use of Metformin are—hepatic disease, renal disease and cardiorespiratory dysfunction. Dosage is started from 500 mg OD to TDS. Long acting 1 gm is also available, to be taken on bed time.

Progestational Agents

As patients with PCOS are chronically anovulatory, the endometrium is stimulated by estrogen alone. Thus endometrial hyperplasia, both typical and atypical and endometrial carcinoma are more frequent in patient with PCOS associated with long-term anovulation. Many of these markedly atypical endometrial features can be reversed by large doses of progestational agent such as megesterol acetate 40-60 mg/day for 3-4 months. Follow-up endometrial biopsy is mandatory to determine endometrial response and subsequent recurrence. Details of PCOS are mentioned in Appendix 2.

Luteoma of Pregnancy

Tumor like nodules of lutein cells may form in the ovaries during pregnancy and are often both multifocal and bilateral.
Clinically: They appear ominous to the obstetrician who become aware of them only when abdomen is opened at time of cesarean delivery.
Microscopy: The lutein is formed of sheets of large luteinized cells with abundant cytoplasm and relatively uniform nuclei with occasional mitosis.
Treatment: A confirmatory biopsy can be done and follow-up will reveal total regression within few months.

OVARIAN NEOPLASM

Ovarian tumor is not a single entity but a complex wide spectrum of neoplasm involving a variety of histological tissues ranging from epithelial tissues, connective tissue, specialized hormone secreting to germinal and embryonic cells. Incidence of ovarian tumor amongst gynecologic admission varies from 1 to 3%. About 75-80% of these are benign.
Classification: In an attempt to standardize the nomenclature used in describing the diverse varieties of tumors, the World Health Organization (WHO) devised a classification listing nine major groups for benign and malignant tumors (Table 17.1).

Epithelial Tumors

Epithelial tumors constitute approximately 60-80% of all true ovarian neoplasm. They include: (a) Serous, (b) Mucinous, (c) Endometrioid, (d) Clear cell, (e) Transitional cell (Brenner) tumor, (f) Stromal tumor with an epithelial element, (g) Undifferentiated and unclassified.

The epithelium of these tumors arise from a common anlage—(That is the first accumulation of cells in an embryo; the beginning of an organized tissue, organ, or part) the mesothelium lining the coelomic cavity and ovarian surface.

Table 17:1: International histological classification of epithelial ovarian tumor	
Histological type	Cellular type
Serous	
a. Benign	Endosalpingeal
b. Borderline	
c. Malignant	
Mucinous	
a. Benign	Endocervical
b. Borderline	
c. Malignant	
Endometrioid	
a. Benign	Endometrial
b. Borderline	
c. Malignant	
Clear Cell Mesonepheroid	
a. Benign	Mullerian
b. Borderline	
c. Malignant	
Brenner	
a. Benign	Transitional
b. Borderline	
c. Malignant	
Mixed Epithelial	
a. Benign	Mixed
b. Borderline	
c. Malignant	
Undifferentiated	Anaplastic
Unclassified	Mesothelium

This basic thesis explains the similarity of the epithelia of upper genital tract - endocervix, endometrium, and endosalpinx to those found in the ovarian tumors.

Most tumors presumably arise from invaginated surface epithelium and proliferation or malignant degeneration in the epithelial lining of the resulting surface inclusion cyst. The epithelial tumors are classified as the basis of their histologic appearance.

Serous Tumors

Serous tumors occur in all age group and accounts for approximately 30% of all epithelial ovarian neoplasm. Of these 70% are benign, 15% borderline and 20-25% are malignant. Low grade neoplasms generally are found in patients in their 20s and 30s, whereas their anaplastic counterparts occur more commonly in perimenopausal and postmenopausal women.

Pathology

Naked eye appearance: Serous cystadenoma are benign lesions, commonly unilocular, with a smooth surface and containing thin clear yellow fluid.

Microscopic examination: The cells lining the cyst are a mixed population of ciliated and secretory cells similar to those

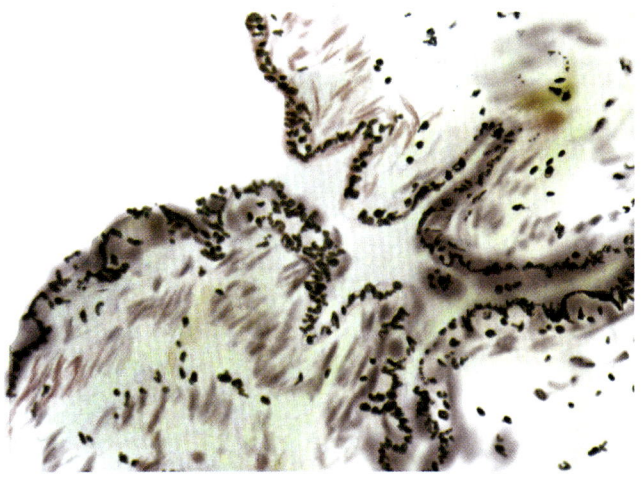

Fig 17.3: Histology of serous cystadenoma

of endosalpinx. Focal proliferation of the underlying stroma may produce firm papillary projections into the cyst, forming a cystadenofibroma. It is important to study histopathologically these papillary projections to rule out malignant foci (Fig. 17.3).

Symptoms: Serous tumors may grow large enough to fill the abdominal cavity but usually they are smaller than their mucinous counterpart.

Mucinous Tumor

Mucinous tumors account for approximately 10-20% of all epithelial ovarian neoplasm of which approximately 75-85% are benign.

Pathology

They are usually smooth walled. Tumors are generally multilocular and mucinous containing locules which appear blue through the tense capsule. The internal surface is lined by tall columnar cells with dark basally situated nuclei and mucinous cytoplasm. The epithelium of mucinous cyst resembles that of the endocervix in approximately 50% of cases. In the other 50% mucin containing goblet cells resembling intestinal epithelial cells are present (Figs 17.4A to C).

It is important that histologic appearance may vary greatly from area-to-area, some area appear benign, other of low malignant potential or frankly malignant. Hence, sampling must be more extensive than in typically serous tumors. Beside this metastases from primary tumors may simulate that of mucinous cystadenoma.

Clinical Feature

They are the largest tumors found in the human body. They are generally asymptomatic and patient present as abdominal mass or nonspecific abdominal discomfort. In postmenopausal women luteinization of the stroma rarely

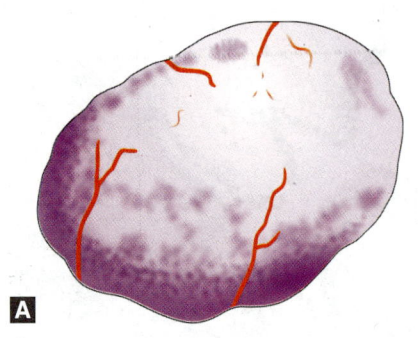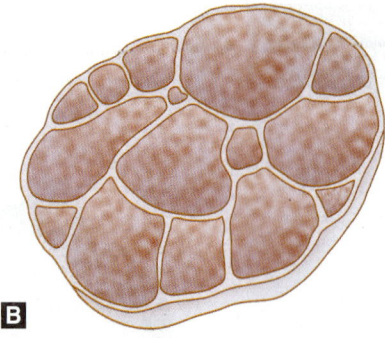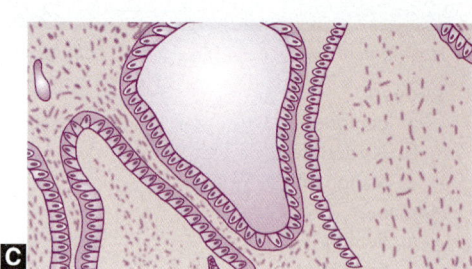

Figs 17.4A to C: (A) Gross picture of mucinous cystadenoma; (B) Cut surface of mucinous cystadenoma; (C) Histological picture of cystadenoma

may result in hormone production usually estrogen, leading to associated endometrial hyperplasia with vaginal bleeding.

Endometrioid Lesions

Endometrioid tumors are characterized by proliferation of benign nonspecific stroma in which bland endometrial type gland may be found. The only clearly recognizable benign endometrioid tumors are the uncommon benign endometrioid adenofibroma and proliferative endometrioid adenofibroma. If the epithelial growth is exuberant but cytology is benign, it is termed a proliferation rather than a low malignant potential. Prognosis is good. Endometriosis of ovary is a benign tumor like condition not a true neoplasm.

Transitional Cell (Brenner) Tumor

Transitional cell tumors are adenofibroma in which the proliferating epithelial element has a transitional cell appearance which represents metaplasia. Brenner tumors account for 1-2% of primary ovarian tumor, 98% are benign, and 95% are unilateral.

Pathology

Usually small but may reach up to 5-8 cm in diameter and present as adnexal mass. *On cut section* - they are firm and pale yellow or white. *On microscopy* - the epithelium composed of nests of cells with ovoid nuclei with a prominent longitudinal groove (called Coffee bean nucleus) (Fig. 17.5).

Sex Cord Stromal Tumor (Mesenchymoma)

Sex cord stromal tumor originate either from the sex cord of the embryonic gonad or from stroma of the ovary.

Thecoma

This type of tumor can occur at any age although they are most commonly found in postmenopausal women. Size range from nonpalpable to more than 20 cm in size and constitute 2% of all ovarian tumor.

Histology

The mass is filled with lipid containing cells similar to theca cells. Tumor can produce estrogen and cause dysfunctional uterine bleeding or postmenopausal bleeding. Occasionally they present as adenocarcinoma of the endometrium due to unopposed estrogen production by the tumor. They are rarely bilateral and rarely malignant.

Fibroma

Fibroma produces no hormone. They can occur at any age but usually in perimenopausal age group. Size ranges from nonpalpable to greater than 20 cm.

Pathology

On gross appearance they appear multinodular and whorled. *On microscopy* - they are formed from bundles of collagen producing spindle cells. Fibroma can be a part of Meigs'

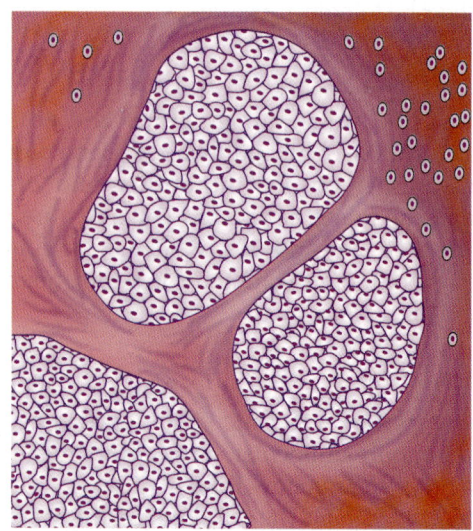

Fig. 17.5: Histological feature of Brenner tumor

syndrome in which patient has fibroma in concert with ascites and hydrothorax.

Hilus Cell Tumor

Hilus cell tumors are a subset of Leydig cell tumors which originate from the ovarian hilum or less frequently from the ovarian stroma. They secrete male hormone so can present as hirsutism, virilization and menstrual irregularities.

Pathology

They rarely attain a palpable size. On histology, group of Sertoli cells containing eosinophilic cytoplasm and lipochrome pigments are found. *For the tumor to be defined as Leydig cell neoplasm elongated eosinophilic crystalloid of Reinke must be found.*

Germ Cell Tumor

Mature Teratoma (Dermoid Cyst)

Mature cystic teratoma or dermoid cyst arises from the germ cells arrested after the first meiotic division. They may contain any of the three germ layers - ectoderm, mesoderm or endoderm. These layers typically form tissues that are foreign to the ovary and that have a disorganized structure and haphazard collection of tissues such as hair, fat, bone and teeth. **Term dermoid was given because of the prevalence of dermal elements in these cysts.**

Incidence

Dermoid cyst constitutes 40-50% of all benign ovarian neoplasm and 97% of teratoma.

Symptoms

They are usually asymptomatic unless complications such as torsion occur which is common complication in 15 - 20% and rupture which is uncommon complication (1%).

Diagnosis

Transvaginal ultrasound is quite accurate as hair and sebum create highly reflective irregular solid components within fluid containing masses.

Pathology

On gross examination dermoid cyst is of moderate size and capsule is tense and smooth. on cut section- the content is predominantly sebaceous material with hair.

On microscopic examination: Endodermal or mesodermal derivative may be found but ectodermal elements usually predominate. The cyst is typically lined with keratinized squamous epithelium and contains abundant sebaceous and sweat glands. Hair and fatty secretion are commonly found within. The Rokitansky protuberance is usually where the most varied tissue types are found and is alone a common site of malignant transformation. Malignant transformation develops only in 1-3% of cases.

Struma Ovary

Though most mature teratoma contain cells from all germ cell layers, a subset of monodermal teratoma exist. Those tumors composed mostly or entirely of thyroid tissue. These are called Struma ovarii. Struma ovarii account for only 3% of all teratoma and only 5% of these will produce symptom of thyrotoxicosis.

CLINICAL FEATURES OF OVARIAN TUMORS

Symptoms

Presentation of benign tumors can be one or more of the following:
a. Asymptomatic.
b. Pain.
c. Abdominal swelling.
d. Pressure effects.
e. Menstrual disturbance.
f. Hormonal effect.

Usually the tumor causes no symptoms and is found *incidentally.* In a benign ovarian tumor the patient's attention is first directed to the abdominal swelling.

Acute *abdominal pain* can develop if ovarian tumors undergo torsion, rupture, hemorrhage or infection with torsion. The woman develops sudden acute pain in abdomen with vomiting, low grade fever and may have sign of shock. *On examination* the cyst is tense and tender. Immediate laparotomy is required to remove the tumor. Pressure from the tumor can produce bowel or bladder symptoms. In extreme cases it can produce edema of legs, varicose veins and hemorrhoids. Menstrual disturbance is associated with hormone secreting tumors.

Physical Sign

Usually the general condition is unaffected. In huge mucinous cystadenoma the patient can have cachectic look due to protein loss.

On inspection: The abdominal wall can be seen to move over the swelling, visibly noted on deep inspiration. The tumors are symmetrically situated in abdomen.

On palpation: The upper and lateral limit of tumor are well defined but lower pole is difficult to reach, which suggest pelvic origin of tumors. Surface is smooth, and usually cystic. Solid tumors like fibroma, thecoma, Brenner tumors are common. The tumor is freely mobile from side to side but has restricted mobility from above down unless the pedicle is too long. Surface can be smooth or lobulated, depending upon the length of tumor.

On percussion: Percussion note is dull in center and resonant in the flanks (in ascites it is reversed). A fluid thrill may be elicited when the walls are thin and content is watery. Coexisting ascites is present in ovarian fibroma.

Bimanual Pelvic Examination

Uterus can be felt separately from the tumor and tumor does not move with movement of cervix. The lower pole of the cyst can be felt through the fornix. It is difficult to identify a huge cyst by bimanual examination as the findings are obscured.

Investigation

The following investigation may be employed to confirm the diagnosis.

Ultrasound

Transabdominal scan first should always be performed to have a panoramic view of pelvic organ and to look for ascites or free fluid in abdominal cavity, liver, stomach, lymph nodes to look for any abnormality. In small cyst transvaginal sonography gives more detailed feature of tumor. **A benign cyst characteristically is unilateral, unilocular or multilocular with a thin wall and thin septa of less than 5 mm in a multilocular cyst.**

Color flow Doppler imaging further helps to distinguish between benign and malignant tumor. Neovascularization and low pulsatile index suggest increased blood flow in suspected malignant tumor. Ultrasound score for malignancy is calculated by giving one point for each of the following findings:
a. Multilocular cyst.
b. Solid areas.
c. Bilateral lesions.
d. Metastasis.
e. Ascites.

Pelvic X-ray Abdomen

Radiograph of abdomen/pelvis may demonstrate a soft tissue shadow or teeth in a dermoid.

CT and MRI

CT and MRI are useful in differentiating between dermoid cyst, hemorrhagic cyst, fibroma, endometriosis and hydrosalpinx. In suspected malignancy CT, MRI identifies the spread of tumor and enlargement of pelvic and para-aortic lymph nodes more than 1 cm. This helps in planning surgery and postoperative radiotherapy or chemotherapy.

Tumor Markers

CA-125 and NB/70k are tumor markers which are useful in follow-up of certain ovarian tumors. CA-125 antigen is expressed by epithelial ovarian tumors and therefore its levels are markedly elevated in women with epithelial ovarian malignancies. CA-125 more than 35 U/ml should raise the suspicion of malignancy in menopausal women. It is important to remember that CA-125 determinants is also expressed by various other pathologic and normal tissues of mullerian origin, as endometriosis, uterus leiomyomas, pregnancy, pelvic infection like tuberculosis and menstruation. As all these condition are more likely to occur in menstruating women, CA-125 levels are less specific to ovarian cancer in the premenopausal age group. Some studies have defined alogrithm for risk of malignancy index (RMI). **RMI is the product of serum CA-125 level (in unit/ml), the ultrasound score (0,1,3) and menopausal status (1- premenopausal, 3 - postmenopausal). The RMI provides a means of triaging women for referral to a gynecological oncologist.**

βhCG

βhCG can be performed to rule out cysts associated with pregnancy or ectopic pregnancy. If levels of βhCG are unusually elevated there is an increased suspicion for molar pregnancy or choriocarcinoma.

α fetoprotein is elevated in germ cell tumor.

Lactate dehydrogenase is elevated with dysgerminoma.

Laparoscopy

Laparoscopy can be sometimes helpful in differentiating painful cystic mass with disturbed ectopic pregnancy.

Laparotomy

If the clinical and ancillary aid fails to diagnose the mass sometimes laparotomy is justified to arrive at a diagnosis.

Cytology

When the patient presents with ascites or pleural effusion cytological examination of the aspirated fluid is done for malignant cells.

Differential Diagnosis

Differential diagnosis of benign ovarian tumor is summarized in a Table 17.2. The common clinical situation can be differentiated from benign ovarian tumor as follows:

Hormonal

Causes of menstrual irregularities, precocious puberty and postmenopausal bleeding.

Full Bladder

To exclude full bladder one should always examine the patient with empty bladder or if necessary even catheterization should be done.

CHAPTER - 17 ♦ Benign Adnexal Masses

Table 17.2: Differential diagnosis of benign ovarian tumors	
Clinical feature	Differential diagnosis
Pain	a. Ectopic pregnancy
	b. Spontaneous abortion
	c. Pelvic inflammatory disease
	d. Nongynecological cause like appendicitis, Meckel's diverticulum Diverticulitis
Abdominal swelling	a. Pregnancy
	b. Fibroid uterus
	c. Full bladder
	d. Distended bowel
	e. Ovarian cancer
	f. Colorectal cancer

Pregnancy

Pregnancy should be excluded by relevant clinical findings like presence of fetal body part and fetal heart and should be confirmed with ultrasound.

Fibroid

Pedunculated subserous myoma or degenerated myoma can be mistaken for ovarian cyst. Ultrasound helps in diagnosis. In either condition laparotomy is indicated.

Ectopic Gestation

Chronic ectopic gestation can be confused with ovarian mass. Ultrasound, βhCG level and sometimes laparoscopy help in diagnosis.

Encysted Peritonitis

Encysted mass is usually irregular not movable with ill defined margins and usually situated high up. It can be confirmed with clinical signs of tuberculosis. Ultrasonography and diagnostic curettage can confirm the diagnosis.

Ascites

In ascites there is fullness in flanks on percussion; flanks are dull with resonance in the center. There may be presence of fluid thrill and positive shifting dullness. While in ovarian cyst the percussion note over the tumors is dull whereas both flanks are resonant.

Pelvic Inflammatory Disease

It can be differentiated by symptoms and sign of pelvic inflammatory disease. Ultrasound and hematological investigation can confirm the diagnosis.

COMPLICATIONS OF OVARIAN TUMOR

Axial Rotation (Ovarian Torsion)

Ovarian torsion is the most common complication having incidence of 12%. It is common in dermoid cyst, cyst having long pedicle or free mobility like pseudomucinous cystadenoma or paraovarian cyst. The etiology of torsion is obscure. It is suggested that, some vigorous or violent movement initiates the twist which cause venous occlusion and partial arterial compression. It initiates intermittent forcible arterial pulsation which further aggravates the axial rotation until it become complete. The rotation occurs towards midline. It can lead to ischemia and interstitial hemorrhage. The cyst can become tense and may rupture or bowel may adhere to twisted cyst.

Symptoms and Signs

Severe acute abdominal pain is usually the presenting symptoms. On examination patient is in agony and there will be tender, tense cystic lump with restricted mobility in lower abdomen arising from the pelvis. On pelvic examination the true cystic mass will be felt separate from the uterus.

Treatment

Ovarian torsion is a gynecologic emergency and requires prompt surgical management. To suppress pain analgesic is given. Most cases can be managed laparoscopically in young women. For whom fertility and preservation of ovarian function is desired, conservative treatment with untwisting of adnexa and ovarian cystectomy is performed. However, this mode of surgical management requires prompt diagnosis and investigation to avoid strangulation and necrosis of torsed tissues.

If strangulation and necrosis do occur, salpingo-oophorectomy should be done either via laparotomy or laparoscopically according to facility and expertise.

Rupture

Rupture of ovarian cyst may be result of direct trauma or spontaneous. Traumatic rupture results from direct blow on abdomen due to accident, violence or during labor, when a cyst is impacted in pouch of douglas in advance of the presenting part. Spontaneous rupture occur in rapidly growing mucinous cystadenomas because epithelial element of the tumor grow so rapidly that the connective tissue of the capsule are unable to keep with them and there is spontaneous rupture. It also occurs following intracystic hemorrhage or in papillary variety or in malignancy.

Infection

It is infrequent. Infection of cyst can occur in following situations:
a. After acute salpingitis.
b. Cyst is infected during puerperium, as part of an ascending genital tract infection.
c. Following axial rotation.

Infected ovarian tumors are always adherent to adjacent viscera.

Ovarian Tumor and Pregnancy

One pregnancy in 1500 is complicated by clinically detectable ovarian tumor measuring more than 15 mm in diameter. The size of tumor may not change during the pregnancy but the growing uterus may displace it so it becomes more obvious. Rarely torsion and rupture may occur. Beside this ovarian tumor may become incarcerated in the cul-de-sac and obstruct the birth canal (Fig. 17.6).

Pseudomyxoma Peritonei

Pseudomyxoma peritonei usually occurs with mucinous cystadenoma of the ovary but also has been reported with a mucocele of gallbladder, appendix and intestinal malignancy. In this peritoneal mesothelium is converted into high columnar epithelium, which secretes mucinous material into the peritoneal cavity.

The prognosis of pseudomyxoma peritonei is bad even after salpingo-oophorectomy as the peritoneal mesothelium cells continue to secrete mucin.

MANAGEMENT OF BENIGN OVARIAN TUMORS

Expectant Management

Functional ovarian cysts are usually functional and most regress spontaneously, within six months of identification. For postmenopausal women with a simple ovarian cyst expectant management can be done only if following criteria are met:
a. Sonographic evidence of a thin walled unilocular cyst.
b. Cyst diameter less than 5 cm.
c. No cyst enlargement during follow-up.
d. Normal serum CA 125 level.

Surgical Excision

Any patient with an adnexal mass more than 10 cm in size require surgical exploration because functional cyst rarely exceed 7-8 cm. Preferred treatment is surgical excision with careful exploration of the abdominal contents.

Cystectomy vs Oophorectomy

The decision for one surgical technique depends upon lesion size, age and intraoperative findings, for, e.g. in

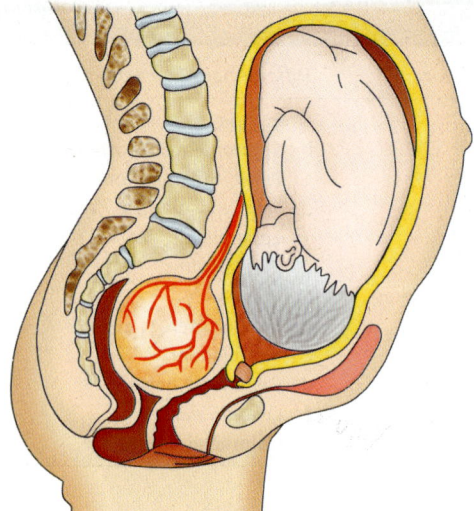

Fig. 17.6: Ovarian cyst obstructing the birth canal

premenopausal women smaller lesions generally require only cystectomy with preservation of reproductive function. Larger lesion may necessitate oophorectomy because of difficulty with cyst enucleation without rupture and greater risk of malignancy in larger cyst (Figs 17.7A and B).

In postmenopausal women oophorectomy is performed because the risk of cancer is high and benefits to ovarian salvage is limited. Clinical, ultrasonological finding and laparotomy findings suggestive of malignancy will dictate further actions. Multiple small lesions studding the peritoneal surface, ascites and exophytic growth extending from the ovarian capsule should prompt appropriate clinical staging and treatment of ovarian cancer.

Laparotomy vs Minilaparotomy vs Laparoscopy

Laparoscopy

The surgical approach for cyst excision is also guided by clinical feature. Laparoscopy has many advantages but it generally has been underused for management of ovarian cyst. Concern of increased rate of cyst rupture with the risk for tumor spill has restricted the surgeon to use this modality. But nowadays in very low risk malignant neoplasm laparoscopy is being increasingly preferred.

Minilaparotomy

For small or moderate size cyst laparotomy incision can be minimized. Although minilaparotomy typically offers shorter operative time, lower rates of cyst rupture and cost saving as compared with laparoscopy or laparotomy, this

Chapter – 17 ♦ Benign Adnexal Masses

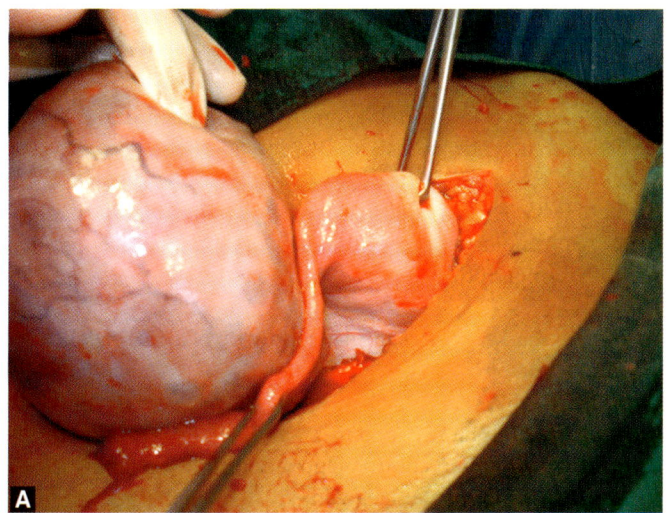 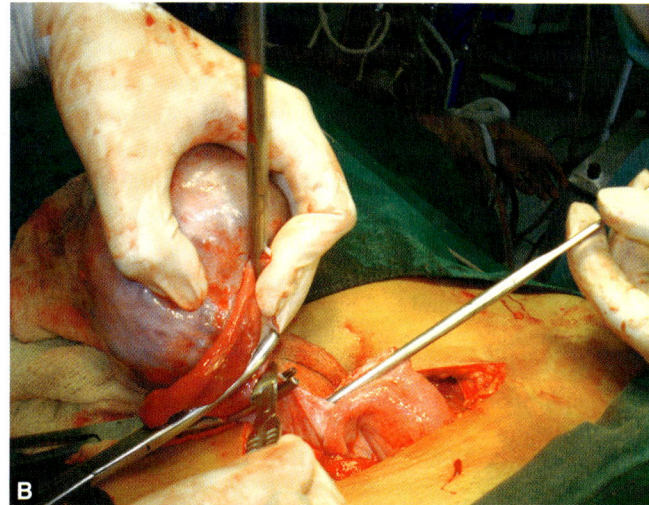

Figs 17.7A and B: Operation of oophorectomy: (A) Solid ovarian cyst; (B) Clamps applied on infundibulopelvic and ovarian ligament

approach can limit lysis of adhesion and inspection of peritoneal surface for signs of malignancy.

Laparotomy

Women with a greater potential for malignancy are best managed by laparotomy, as it provides a large surgical field enough for oophorectomy or cyst enucleation without tumor rupture or spill and for surgical staging if malignancy is found. Frozen section is helpful in identifying the type and malignant potential of the tumors. As adequate sampling of a large ovarian neoplasm often is impossible, final opinion and prognosis must be based on analysis of permanent rather than frozen section.

Role of Gynecologic Oncologist

As ovarian cyst frequently are benign and require surgical treatment so they can be managed by general gynecologist. Whenever malignancy is present formal cancer staging should accompany the surgical excision. There are several studies which support that optimal surgical resection and proper staging performed by gynecologic oncologist during the primary operation for ovarian cancer are major factors in long-term survival. The ACOG 2002 has presented guidelines regarding clinical criteria that should prompt referral to a gynecologic oncologist. These are as follows (Table 17.3).

MULTIPLE CHOICE QUESTIONS

1. Which of the following is the likely diagnosis in a 27-year-old obese women presenting with oligomenorrhea, infertility and hirsutism:
   a. PCOS
   b. Endometriosis

Table 17.3: ACOG 2002 guideline clinical criteria for referral to gynecologic oncologist

Premenopausal women (<50 years)
   a. CA 125 > 200 U/ml
   b. Ascites
   c. Evidence of abdominal or distant metastasis by clinical examination or imaging study
   d. Family history of breast or ovarian cancer in a first degree relative

Postmenopausal women (>50 years)
   a. CA 125 > 35 U/ml
   b. Ascites
   c. Nodular or fixed pelvic mass
   d. Evidence of abdominal or distant metastasis by clinical examination or imaging study
   e. Family history of breast or ovarian cancer (in a first degree relative)

   c. Turner's syndrome
   d. PID
   Ans. a

2. The following hormone is increased in PCOS:
   a. FSH
   b. LH
   c. TSH
   d. 17-OH progesterone
   Ans. b

3. A 28-year female is suspected to have PCOD, sample for testing LH and FSH are best taken on the following days of menstrual cycle:
   a. 1-4
   b. 8-10
   c. 13-15
   d. 24-36
   Ans. a

4. What causes torsion of ovarian tumor:
   a. Trauma
   b. Uterine contraction
   c. Physical movement
   d. All of the above
   Ans. a
5. True regarding benign cystic teratoma:
   a. Rarely undergo torsion
   b. Metastasis is common
   c. 10% are bilateral and malignant
   d. Contains Call-Exner bodies
   Ans. c
6. Complications of benign ovarian tumors are all *except*:
   a. Torsion
   b. Bleeding
   c. Pseudomyxoma peritonei
   d. Metastasis
   Ans. d
7. A 30-year-old female presents to the emergency with complaint of sudden severe abdominal pain, an abdominal mass palpable on examination most likely diagnosis is:
   a. Torsion of subserous fibroid
   b. Twisted ovarian cyst
   c. Rupture of ectopic pregnancy
   d. Rupture of ovarian cyst
   Ans. b
8. The first step in the management of hirsutism due to Stein-Leventhal syndrome is:
   a. OCP
   b. HMG
   c. Spironolactone
   d. Bromocriptine
   Ans. a
9. Tumor marker most helpful in follow-up of a case of epithelial carcinoma of ovary is:
   a. CA 125
   b. Serum alpha fetoprotein
   c. Serum human chorionic gonadotropin
   d. Human placental lactogen
   Ans. a
10. Which is not true of dermoid cyst of ovary:
    a. Commonly more than 10 cm
    b. Has sebaceous material
    c. Bilateral in 30%
    d. Lined by epithelial cells
    Ans. a, c

18. Gynecological Infection and STD

*Great opportunities to help others seldom come,
but small ones surround us every day.*

GENERAL CONSIDERATION

The female genital tract is vulnerable to acquire infection from the external environment because of its anatomical location. At the same time the defense mechanism is so protective that the organisms are not allowed access to the genital tract despite its anatomical vulnerability.

Defense Mechanisms of Genital Tract

Vulva

a. Closure of introitus by apposition of labia protects entry of pathogens.
b. Secretion of the apocrine glands which is rich in undecylenic acid that is fungicidal.

Vagina

a. Vagina is closed by apposition of its anterior and posterior walls.
b. Well-developed and mature stratified squamus epithelium.
c. Vaginal acidity and vaginal flora—The pH level of normal vagina is lower than 4.5 which is maintained by the production of lactic acid. Estrogen stimulated vaginal epithelial cells are rich in glycogen. Vaginal epithelial cells breakdown glycogen and monosaccharide which can then be converted by the cells themselves and lactobacilli to lactic acid. **Lactobacilli (also called *Doderlein bacilli*)** are aerobic gram variable rod-shaped bacteria (Figs 18.1A and B). The vagina also contains gram negative bacteria as well anaerobes. Vaginitis is caused by alteration in normal flora like bacterial vaginosis, candidiasis or by an outside organism like Trichomoniasis.

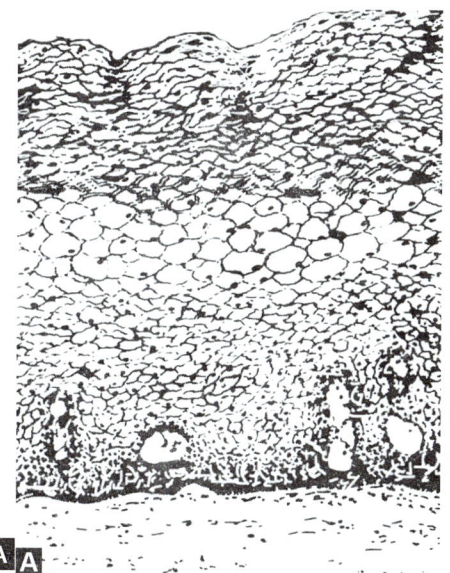
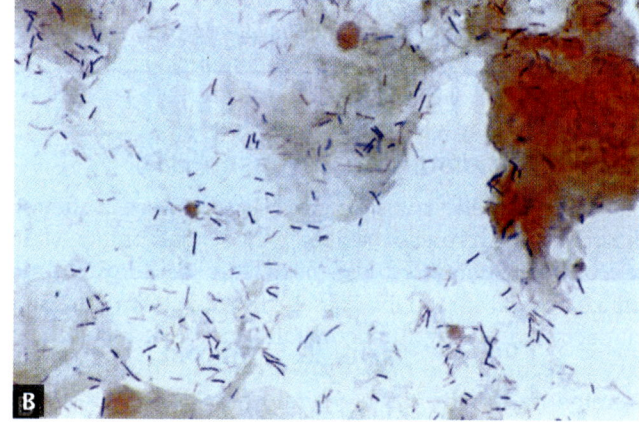

Figs 18.1A and B: Natural barrier to infection: (A) Well developed stratified squamous epithelium and vaginal cells rich in glycogen; (B) Presence of lactobacilli (gram positive rods)

Cervix

Functional closure of the cervix is affected by mucus which is also supposed to be bacteriolytic.

Uterus

Periodic shedding of surface endometrium during menstruation tends to eliminate any infection.

Variations in the Efficiency of Defense Mechanism

a. *Age variation:* The defenses are imperfect during **childhood** and after the **menopause** when, (i) The vagina has thin and vulnerable epithelium, (ii) Its content of glycogen and *Doderlein bacilli* is low and the vaginal acidity is reduced, (iii) The endometrium is poorly developed and does not undergo cyclical shedding.
b. *Menstrual cycle:* During menstruation the cervical plug is absent and vaginal acidity is lowered by the alkaline menstrual discharge. So infection may ascend to upper genital tract.
c. *During puerperium:* In reproductive age group the genital tract defense are weakened during and immediately after miscarriage or delivery because—
   i. There is raw placental site
   ii. There are often breaks in epithelial lining of the cervix and vagina
   iii. The tissues are bruised and devitalized
   iv. The vulva, vagina and cervix are wide open
   v. The discharge of liquor and lochia are alkaline so there is reduced vaginal acidity
   vi. Degenerating blood clots and fragments of decidua can become a focus for infection
   vii. Patient's general resistance is lowered by pregnancy and possibly nutritional deficiency especially in developing countries.

Sexually Transmitted Disease (STD)

The term sexually transmitted disease is used to denote disorders which spread principally by sexual contact. Many sexually transmitted diseases can be acquired by transplacental spread, by passage through birth canal and via lactation during the neonatal period like Hepatitis B, HIV infection. The organisms involved are peculiarly adapted to growth in the genital tract and are present in body secretion or blood. There is rising trend of STDs because of following reasons:

i. Social changes: There has been vast change in last decade in society. There is trend for late marriages, more travels for education and employment, more chances of having multiple sex partners due to change in social values. At the same time there is still lack of sex education and inadequate practice of safer sex. All factors contribute to increasing incidence of sexually transmitted disease.
ii. There is increased used of oral contraceptive pills and intrauterine contraceptive device which cannot prevent STDs.
iii. Development of antibiotic resistance.
iv. Inclusion of more diseases like herpes simplex virus type 1 and 2, cytomegalovirus in sexually transmitted infections.
v. Increased detection due to more awareness as well the diagnostic methods.

Physicians have a critical role in prevention and treatment of STD. The clinician's role is four-fold:

i. To understand the microbiology of STD in order to appropriately diagnose and treat patients.
ii. To alleviate symptoms and prevent future sequelae like infertility, PID.
iii. To prevent transmission to others including health professionals.
iv. For above physician has to do patient education and counseling.

As the future continues to bring advancement in therapy, the physician must be able to adapt to these changes. Pre-exposure vaccination will be trend of future therapy. **In present times prevention through life style and behavioral modification is the primary weapon against the spread of STDs.** Table 18.1 summarized commonly found sexually transmitted infections.

VAGINITIS

Vaginitis is a clinical syndrome characterized by vaginal discharge, vulvar irritation or malodorous discharge. This can be divided into two entities—(a) Infective vaginitis, (b) Atrophic vaginitis. The leading causes of symptomatic vaginal discharge are—(a) Trichomoniasis, (b) Bacterial vaginosis, (c) Candidiasis.

Bacterial Vaginosis

Bacterial vaginosis has previously been referred to as a non-specific vaginitis or *Gardnerella vaginitis*. This common and complex clinical syndrome reflects abnormal vaginal flora.

It is alteration of normal vaginal bacterial flora that results in loss of hydrogen peroxide producing lactobacilli and an overgrowth of predominantly anaerobic bacteria like *Gardnerella vaginalis, Ureoplasma urealyticum, Mobiluncus* species and *Mycoplasma hominis*.

Whether an altered ecosystem leads to lactobacilli disappearance or whether its disappearance results in the changes observed with bacterial vaginosis is unknown.

Risk Factors

Bacterial vaginosis is not considered by Centers for Disease Control and Prevention (CDC) consensus group to be a sexually transmitted disease and it is seen in women without previous sexual experience.

Table 18.1: Types of common STDs

Curable		Incurable	Super infection
Mostly bacterial	Protozoal	Viral	
Ulcerative	Non-ulcerative		
Syphilis	Gonorrhea	HIV/AIDS	Bacterial vaginosis
Chancroid	Chlamydial infection	Hepatitis B	Candidial infection
Herpes	Trichomoniasis	Human papilloma virus	
Lymphogranuloma venereum			
Granuloma inguinale			

It has been postulated that repeated alkalinization of the vagina which occurs with frequent sexual intercourse or douche plays a role. There is increased risk of acquiring STD in women with bacterial vaginosis.

Once normal hydrogen peroxide producing lactobacilli disappear, it is difficult to reestablish normal vaginal flora and recurrence of bacterial vaginosis is common.

Sequelae of Bacterial Vaginosis

Numerous studies have shown an association of bacterial vaginosis with significant adverse sequelae. Women with bacterial vaginosis are at increased **risk for pelvic inflammatory disease, postabortal PID, postoperative cuff infection after hysterectomy and abnormal cervical cytology**. In women with bacterial vaginosis who are undergoing surgical abortion or hysterectomy, preoperative treatment with metronidazole eliminates this risk.

Diagnosis

Office based testing is required to diagnose bacterial vaginosis. It is diagnosed on the basis of following findings:
a. A non-irritating, malodorous vaginal discharge is characteristic but may not always be present.
b. On examination there is thin white gray discharge. Vagina is usually not erythematous and cervical examination reveals no abnormalities.
c. The pH of these vaginal secretion is higher than 4.5 (usually 4.7 to 5.7).
d. Microscopy of the vaginal secretion reveals an **increased number of clue cell** and leukocytes are conspicuously absent. In advanced cases of bacterial vaginosis, more than 25% of the epithelial cells are **clue cells** (Fig. 18.2). *Clue cells are the most reliable indicator of bacterial vaginosis and were originally described by Gardner and Dukes. These vaginal epithelial cells contain many attached bacteria, which create a poorly defined stippled cellular border.*
e. The addition of KOH to the vaginal secretion releases a fishy amine like odor—**Whiff test**. The odor is frequently evident even without KOH. Similarly, alkalinity of seminal fluid and blood are responsible for odor complaints after intercourse and with menstruation. **The finding of both clue cells and positive Whiff test, is pathognomonic even in asymptomatic patients**.

Treatment

Ideally treatment of bacterial vaginosis should inhibit anaerobes but not vaginal lactobacilli. Specific therapy for bacterial vaginosis has been neglected in part because of the rather innocuous symptoms reported. Therapy is required in following situations:
a. For symptomatic women
b. Pregnant women, who are at high risk for preterm labor may benefit from treatment
c. Treatment is recommended for low risk group during pregnancy if patients are infected and symptomatic
d. Asymptomatic carrier before pelvic or abdominal surgery

Guidelines of Treatment Issued by CDC

1. *Metronidazole:* An antibiotic with excellent activity against anaerobes but poor activity against lactobacilli is the drug of choice for the treatment of bacterial vaginosis.

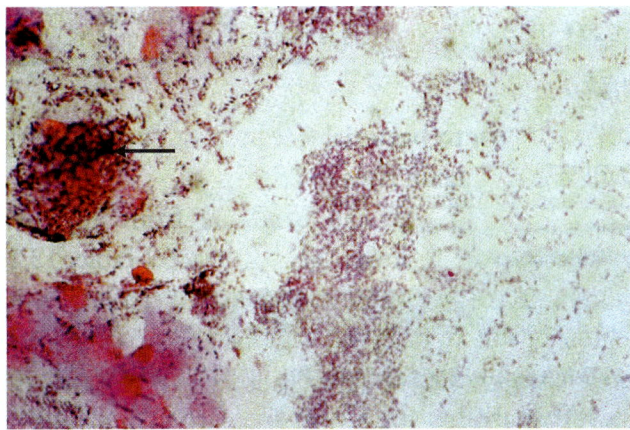

Fig. 18.2: Clue cell seen in bacterial vaginosis with decrease in number of lactobacilli

A dose of 500 mg *metronidazole administered orally twice a day* for 7 days should be used. Patient should be advised to avoid using alcohol during treatment and 24 hours thereafter. *Metronidazole gel 0.75%, one applicator* (5 gm) intravaginally once or twice daily for 5 days, may also be prescribed. It has cure rate of 75 to 84%.

2. *Clindamycin:* Clindamycin in the following regimen is also effective in treatment of bacterial vaginosis:
    i. Clindamycin cream 2% one applicator full (5 gm) intravaginally at bed time for 7 days.
    ii. Clindamycin 300 mg orally twice daily for 7 days.
    iii. Clindamycin ovules 100 mg, intravaginally once at bed time for 3 days.
    iv. Clindamycin bioadhesive cream 2%, 100 mg intravaginally in a single dose.

Treatment of male sexual partner has not been shown to improve therapeutic response and therefore is not recommended.

Vulvovaginal Candidiasis

It is estimated that approximately 75% of women will experience an episode of vulvovaginal candidiasis during their life time. Nearly 45% of women will experience two or more episodes.

Candida albicans is responsible for 85 to 90% of vaginal yeast infection. Other species of candida as *C. glabrata, C. tropicalis* can cause vulvovaginal symptom and may be resistant to therapy.

Candida are dimorphic fungi exist as blastospores which cause transmission and colonize asymptomatically. Myelie result from blastospore germination which enhance colonization and tissue invasion. There can be extracellular toxin or enzyme which causes extensive areas of pruritis and inflammation. There can be role of individual hypersensitivity phenomena which cause chronic, recurrent candidiasis in some patients. Patient having symptomatic candidiasis have higher concentration of these microorganism ($>10^4$ ml) compared with asymptomatic patient ($<10^3$/ml).

Risk Factor

Risk factor that predispose the women to development of symptomatic VVC are:
(a) Antibiotic use,
(b) Pregnancy,
(c) Diabetes.

Diagnosis

Symptoms: **Vulvar itching associated with thick vaginal discharge resembling cottage cheese are usually presenting symptom.** There may be burning sensation following urination, particularly if there is excoriation of the skin from scratching. Widespread involvement of the skin adjacent to the labia may suggest an underlying systemic illness such as diabetes.

Signs
i. Examination can reveal erythema and edema of labia and vulvar skin. Vagina may be erythematous with an adherent whitish discharge. The cervix appears normal.
ii. Diagnosis is based on demonstration of:
    a. Candidal myelia in wet saline preparation (Fig. 18.3).
    b. Normal vaginal pH (pH $\leq$ 4.5). When vaginal secretions are mixed with 10% KOH solution, there is no fishy odor (**Whiff test is negative**) and pseudohyphae (myelia form) of candida are seen.
iii. Gold standard for diagnosis is **culture positive vaginal yeast culture**.

A presumptive diagnosis can be made in the absence of fungal elements confirmed by microscopy if the pH and results of the saline preparation evaluation are normal, but the patient has increased erythema of vulva and vagina on clinical examination. A fungal culture is recommended to confirm the diagnosis.

Treatment

Treatment is reserved only for symptomatic patients. It is helpful to categorize women with VVC as having either uncomplicated or complicated disease.

Classification of vulvovaginal candidiasis (The CDC vulvovaginal candidiasis classification 2006):
a. *Uncomplicated*
    a. Sporadic or infrequent
    b. Mild to moderate symptom
    c. Immunocompetent women
b. *Complicated*
    a. Recurrent symptoms
    b. Severe symptoms
    c. Non-albicans candidal infection
    d. Immunocompromised, e.g. diabetes

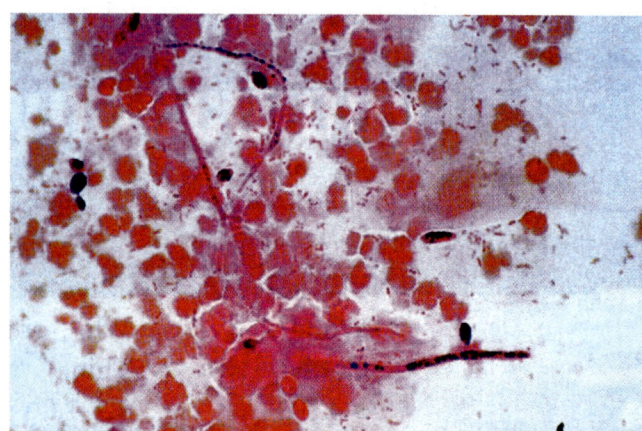

Fig. 18.3: Candidiasis—Gram-positive spores and pseudohyphae seen in wet saline preparation

Treatment of Uncomplicated VVC

1. Topically applied Azole drugs are economically available treatment for VVC and more effective. Nystatin, Miconazole, Clotrimazole, Tioconazole, Terconazole, Butoconazole, can be given for 3–7 days in form of vaginal tablet or cream form.

    There is trend to shorten the therapy to 1–3 days. These short course formulations have higher concentration of the antifungal agent causing an inhibitory concentration in the vagina that persists for several days.

2. Oral antifungal agent: Fluconazole—Is used as a single 150 mg dose. It has equal efficacy to topical Azole in mild to moderate VVC. Patient should be counseled that their symptoms will persist for 2–3 days so they will not expect additional treatment.

Treatment of Complicated VVC

i. Underlying metabolic disorder like diabetes should be well-controlled, and complicating medicines like antibiotics should be discontinued if possible.
ii. Non-absorbent undergarments and douches should be avoided.
iii. Fluconazole 150 mg should be repeated 72 hours after the first dose.
iv. More prolonged topical Azole drugs should be given lasing for 10–14 days.
v. Adjuvant treatment with a weak topical steroid such as 10% hydrocortisone cream may be applied in relieving some of external irritation symptoms.

Recurrent Vulvovaginal Candidiasis

Chronic or recurrent infection is defined when *woman has 4 or more episodes of candidal infection* in a year. Its incidence is 5% of the population. It results from **insufficient duration of therapy, recontamination and/or resistant strains**. These women experience persistent irritative symptoms of the vestibule and vulva. Burning replaces itching as the prominent symptom in patient with recurrent vulvovaginal 'Candidiasis'. **Diagnosis should be confirmed by direct microscopy of the vaginal secretion and by fungal culture.**

Treatment of Recurrent Vulvovaginal Candidiasis

i. High dose estrogen or oral contraceptive use may precipitate infection and therefore should be discontinued.
ii. Treatment consists of introducing a remission of chronic symptoms with Flucanazole (150 mg) every 3 days for 3 doses. After that patient should be maintained on a suppression dose of Flucanazole 150 mg weekly for 6 months. Success of this segment is 90%. But in 57% of women recurrence occurs and they should be given full suppressive therapy again.
iii. *Ketoconazole 100 mg orally each day for 6 month, Itraconazole 100 mg* orally daily for 6 months are equally effective.
iv. Treatment of the male partner may be considered in cases of symptomatic balanitis.
v. Fluconazole and Ketazole are effective against C Tropicalis and *C. Glabrata*, which are resistant to topical Imidazoles.
vi. **Chemicals and dyes:** For non-albicans infection, a 600 mg boric acid gelatin capsule intravaginally daily for 2 weeks has been found successful. 1% gentian violet is an aniline dye, that when painted over vaginal surface once per week is effective against *C. albicans* and *Candida glabrata*. Medications used in treatment of VVC are summarized in (Table 18.2).

During pregnancy: During pregnancy VVC may be more difficult to treat. The azoles have not been well-studied and they should be avoided until second trimester or 1 tablet of Nystatin 100,000 units may be administered vaginally at night for 2 weeks during the first trimester.

Trichomonas Vaginitis

Trichomonas vaginitis is caused by sexually transmitted, flagellated protozoa—*Trichomonas vaginalis*. It is the most prevalent non-viral STD, more commonly diagnosed in women because most men are asymptomatic. The transmission rate is high.

The *Trichomonas vaginalis* exist only in trophozoite form. *It is larger than polymorphonuclear leukocyte but smaller than mature epithelial cells*. It is an anaerobe that has the ability to generate hydrogen to combine with oxygen to create an anaerobic environment. It often accompanies bacterial vaginosis; the incidence of coexistent bacterial vaginosis can be as high as 60%.

The parasite is usually a marker of high risk sexual behavior and co-infection with other STD is also common. Vertical transmission to child during birth is possible and may persist for a year.

Diagnosis

Symptoms

Between 10-50% of women are asymptomatic. Local immune factor and inoculum size influence the appearance of symptoms. **A persistent vaginal discharge is the principal symptom, with or without secondary vulvar pruritis**. The discharge is profuse, extremely frothy and greenish and at times fowl smelling.

On Examination

pH of the vaginal secretion is usually higher than 5.0 and vaginal epithelium and cervix shows generalized vaginal

Table 18.2: Medications used in the treatment of vulvovaginal candidiasis
Butoconazole 2% cream, 1 applicator vaginally, for 3-5 days.
Clotrimazole 1% cream, 1 applicator (5 g) vaginally, for 7 days (14 days if chronic)
Clotrimazole 100 mg tablet, vaginally, for 7 days
Clotrimazole 100 mg tablet, 2 tablets vaginally, for 3 days
Clotrimazole 500 mg tablet, vaginally, for one dose
Miconazole 2% cream, 1 applicator vaginally, for 7 days
Miconazole 100 mg suppository, vaginally, for 7 days
Miconazole 200 mg suppository, vaginally, for 3 days
Tioconazole 2% cream, 1 applicator vaginally, for 3 days
Tioconazole 6.5% cream, 1 applicator vaginally, for one dose
Tioconazole 0.4% cream, 1 applicator vaginally, for 7 days
Tioconazole 0.8% cream, 1 applicator vaginally, for 3 days
Tioconazole 80 mg suppository, vaginally, for 3 days
Boric acid 600 mg gelatin capsule, vaginally at night, for 2 weeks or nightly for 1 week then 2 times per week for 3 weeks
Ketoconazole 200 mg, orally 2 times per day for 5 days
Itraconazole 200 mg, orally 2 times per day for 1 day
Fluconazole 150 mg tablet, orally, for 1 day

erythema with multiple small patechia so called *strawberry spots*. On **wet saline mount microscopy,** there is an increase in poly morphonuclear cells and characteristic motile flagellate in 50 – 70% of culture confirmed cases (Fig. 18.4). It is highly specific but sensitivity is 60 – 70%. Clue cells and positive Whiff test indicates co-existent bacterial vaginosis. Culture is gold standard and provides 95% sensitivity and 100% specificity but is impractical because special media (Diamond media) is required and only few laboratories are equipped.

Nucleic Acid Amplification Tests (NAAT) for Trichomonal DNA are sensitive and specific, but not widely available. Alternatively the OSUM Trichomonas rapid test is an immunochromatographic assay which has 88% sensitivity and 99% specificity. It is available for office use and results are available in 10 minutes.

Trichomonads may also be noted on Pap smear screening and sensitivity is approximately 60%.

Treatment

Metronidazole is drug of choice for treatment of vaginal Trichomoniasis. CDC (2006) recommended treatment is:
a. Primary therapy: Metronidazole single 1 gm dose orally or Tinidazole single 2 gm dose orally.
b. Alternatively: Metronidazole 500 mg orally twice a day for 7 days. It has cure rate of 95%. Patients should abstain from alcohol during use of metronidazole for 24 hours after and for 72 hours after Tinidazole as it may induce disulfiran like reaction. The sexual partner should also be treated with advice of abstinence or barrier contraception.
c. Patients, who do not respond to initial therapy, should be treated again with metronidazole 500 mg twice daily for 7 days. If treatment is not effective, the patient should be treated with a single 2 gm dose of metronidazole once daily for 5 days or Tinidazole 2 gm in a single dose for 5 days.

Inflammatory Vaginitis

Desquamative inflammatory vaginitis is a clinical syndrome characterized by diffuse oxidative vaginitis, epithelial cells exfoliation and profuse purulent vaginal discharge. Etiology is unknown, gram staining reveals *absence of lactobacilli* and their replacement with *gram-positive cocci usually streptococcus*.

Symptoms

Women have complaints of purulent vaginal discharge, vulvovaginal burning or irritation and dyspareunia.

On Examination

Vaginal and vulvar erythema and associated vulvovaginal ecchymotic spots can be seen. Vaginal pH is usually higher than 4.5.

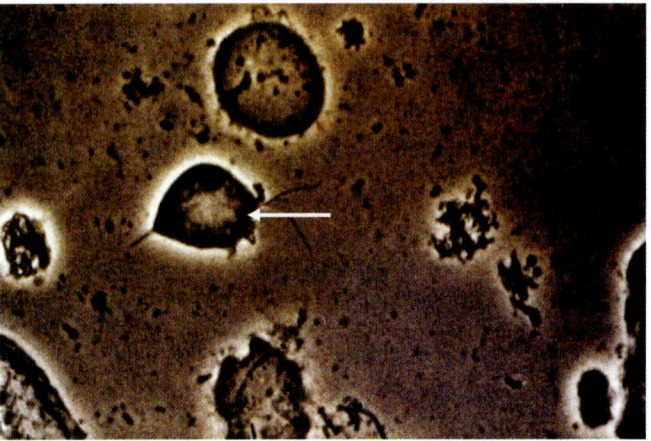

Fig. 18.4: Trichomoniasis—Flagellated trichomonas vaginalis in center

Treatment

Initial therapy is 2% Clindamycin cream, one application full 5 gm intravaginally once daily for 7 days. Relapse is common (30%) who should be treated with intravaginal 2% Clindamycin cream for 2 weeks. If relapse occurs in postmenopausal age group, supplementary hormonal therapy should be considered.

Atrophic Vaginitis

Atrophic vaginitis is inflammatory vaginitis which may be accompanied by an increased purulent vaginal discharge in estrogen deficient states in postmenopausal period either natural or secondary to surgical removal of ovaries or some times in prepubertal age and lactation period.

The pH of the vagina is abnormally high and the normal acidogenic flora of the vagina may be replaced by mixed flora. The vaginal epithelium is thinned and more susceptible to infection and trauma.

Diagnosis

Patients complain of vaginal dryness, spotting, presence of serosanguinous or watery discharge and dyspareunia or even post coital bleeding resulting from atrophy of vaginal and vulvar epithelium.

On Examination

The vaginal mucosa is thin with few or absent vaginal folds. pH of vagina is 5.0–7.0. The wet mount shows small, rounded parabasal epithelial cells and an increased number of polymorphonuclear cells.

Treatment

Atrophic vaginitis is treated with topical estrogen vaginal cream; use of 1 gm of conjugated estrogen cream intravaginally each day for 1-2 weeks generally provides relief. Systemic estrogen therapy should be considered to prevent recurrence of atrophic vaginitis.

Approximately, one third of the vaginal estrogen is systemically absorbed; therefore this treatment may be contraindicated in women with a history of breast or endometrial cancer. The estradiol vaginal ring which is changed every 90 days may provide a more preferred route of administration for some women.

Foreign Bodies

Foreign bodies may cause vaginal discharge and infection in preadolescent girls. Children may require vaginal examination under anesthesia to identify or to rule out a foreign body or tumors in high vaginal vault. In adult forgotten tampon or contraceptive device may cause a malodorous discharge.

Diagnosis

Diagnosis can be made by pelvic examination. Ulcerative lesions, particularly associated with tampon use are typically located in the vaginal fornices and have rolled irregular edges with a red granulation base.

Treatment

Treatment involves removal of the foreign body. Dryness and or ulceration secondary to tampon is transient and heal spontaneously. Rarely antibiotics are required for ulceration or cellulitis of the vulva or vagina.

Cervical Mucorrhea or Vaginal Epithelial Discharge

a. Cervicitis due to cervical polyps or cervical or vaginal cancer can cause a mucopurulent discharge and bleeding.
b. Excessive cervical ectropion may cause excessive discharge of cervical mucus from normal endocervical cells.
c. Vaginal adenosis may cause clear mucoid type discharge, with no associated symptoms.
d. Excessive desquamation of the vaginal epithelium may produce a diffuse grey white pasty vaginal discharge, which may be confused with candidiasis.

Diagnosis

Diagnosis is confirmed by perspeculum examination which will reveal ectropion, or cervical polyp vaginal pH is normal.

On Microscopy

There is normal bacterial flora, mature vaginal squamous cells and no increase in number of leukocytes.

Treatment

a. Reassure if ectropion or normal pelvic examinations.
b. At times, cryosurgery is required.

Parasitic Infection

Less common cause of vaginitis is parasitic infection with pinworms (*Enterobius vermicularis*) and with *Entomoeba histolytica*. Pinworm infection is usually seen in children. Source of infection is fecal contamination at the introitus. Child complains of severe pruritis of perineal area. Diagnosis can be confirmed by microscopic detection of double walled ova. Treatment is deworming.

Toxic Shock Syndrome

Toxic shock syndrome is the most serious complication of improper use of vaginal tampon. The syndrome has been associated with use of high absorbant tampons or at times diaphragm and associated staphylococcal vaginal infection.

Symptoms

Symptoms consist of high grade fever (> 38.9°C, 102°F) and severe constitutional symptoms like sore throat, myalgia, vomiting and diarrhea. There are skin rashes and may be superficial desquamation of the palms and soles. Progressive hypotension may occur and proceed to shock level within 48 hours. Multisystem organ failure may occur, including renal and cardiac dysfunction. *Incidence is 1 in 100000 among females and any menstruating women presenting with sudden onset of febrile illness should be evaluated for toxic shock syndrome.*

Treatment

a. Appropriate supportive measures for correction of hypovolemia and hypotension with I/V fluid and Dopamine infusion is done.
b. The tampon to be removed, culture is sent, vagina is cleansed to decrease organ inoculum.
c. Lactamase resistant penicillin (Cloxacillin, Methicillin) or Vancomycin (if patient is allergic to penicillin) is administered for 10-14 days. Mortality following toxic shock syndrome is 6-10%.

Cervicitis

The cervix is made up of two different types of epithelial cells-squamous epithelium and glandular epithelium. The etocervical epithelium can become inflamed by the same microoraganism that are responsible for vaginitis. Thus, the ectocervical squamous epithelium is an extension of and is continuous with vaginal epithelium. Trichomonas, candida and herpes simplex virus can cause inflammation of the ectocervix.

N. gonorrhoeae and *Chlamydia trachomatis* infect only the glandular epithelium. The infection may be localized or spread upwards to involve the fallopian tube and or parametrium.

Diagnosis

Diagnosis of cervicitis is based on the finding of a purulent endocervical discharge, greenish yellow in color. Cervix is tender on touch or movement, cervix is edematous and congested.

On microscopy of mucopus and gram staining reveal the presence of an increased number of neutrophils (>30 per high power field). Endocervical swab should be taken for bacteriological identification and sensitivity. Test for both gonorrhea and chlamydia using nucleic acid amplification test should be performed. However, the microbial etiology of endocervicitis is unknown in about 50% of cases in which neither Gonococci or Chlamydia is detected.

Sequelae

Acute cervicitis may resolute completely in untreated or incompletely treated cases. The infection may spread to involve the adjacent structure or may become chronic.

Treatment

Treatment of cervicitis consists of an antibiotic regimen recommended for the treatment of uncomplicated lower genital tract infection with both Chlamydia and Gonorrhea. It is imperative that all sexual partners be treated with a similar antibiotic regimen to minimize the bacterial resistance.

Cervicitis is commonly associated with bacterial vaginosis, which if not treated, simultaneously may lead to significant persistence of the symptoms and signs of cervicitis.

Chronic Cervicitis

Chronic cervicitis is one of the commonest lesions found in gynecologic outpatient. It may follow an acute attack or may be chronic from the beginning. The infection usually occurs following child birth or spontaneous or induced abortion by the pyogenic organism like *Staphylococcus, Streptococcus* or *E. coli. Chlamydia trachomatis* is more and more implicated and Gonorrhea is very uncommon.

Pathology

The mucosa and deeper tissues are congested, fibrosed and infiltrated with leukocytes and plasma cells. The glands are hypertrophied with increased secretory activity. There may be associated Nebothian follicles or ectropion.

Clinical Features

Symptoms

In chronic cervicitis leucorrhea may be the chief symptoms. Though it may not be as profuse as acute cervicitis; the discharge may cause vulvar irritation. The discharge may be frankly purulent or thick tenacious, turbid mucus. There can be history of contact bleeding. Lower abdominal pain, lumbosacral backache, dysmenorrhea or dyspareunia may occur occasionally due to associated parametritis.

Infertility may be due to inflammatory changes that result in acidic and hostile cervical mucus to sperm. Urinary frequency, urgency and dysuria may be seen in association with chronic cervicitis.

On Examination

On inspection there may be only abnormal vaginal discharge. There may be fibrosis or stenosis of cervix.

Patulousness of deeply lacerated external os often exposes the endocervical canal, which may bleed when wiped with a cotton applicator.

Investigations

Bacteriological studies to confirm and find the pathogen should be done by *smears on cervical discharge, gram staining and culture and sensitivity*. For Gonorrhea and Chlamydia new technique of nucleic acid amplification methods as polymerase chain reaction (PCR), transcription mediated amplification (TMA) and strand displacement amplification (SDA) are being used recently. The benefit of these techniques is high sensitivity (82–100%) and specificity.

Patient with gonorrhea or chlamydia are at risk for infection with other sexually transmitted diseases. Counseling and testing should be offered for syphilis, hepatitis B and HIV.

Differential Diagnosis

a. **Non-infective cervicitis:** It is most commonly due to effects of endogenous or exogenous hormones. Bimanual examination should be performed to distinguish the signs and symptoms of pelvic tenderness, induration and mass formation.
b. **Early neoplastic process:** Cervicitis must be distinguished from early neoplastic process. This is difficult at times because inflammatory condition may alter the epithelial cells to produce atypia on cytologic examination. Colposcopy, cervical cytology and histological examination by endocervical curettage and biopsy should be performed to distinguish chronic cervicitis from developing cancer of the cervix.
c. **Lesions:** Lesion of syphilis, chancroid and chronic granulomatous ulceration of tuberculosis and granuloma inguinale should be considered and excluded with specific investigation.

Treatment

It is not necessary to treat an asymptomatic patient with chronic cervicitis, who does not test positive for sexually transmitted disease. Antibiotics are of no benefit except in gonococci or proved cases of chlamydial infection.

Surgical Procedures

Surgical procedures may be useful for treatment of symptomatic chronic cervicitis or in the absence of an infectious pathogens or evidence of dysplasia. **Cryosurgery, electrocauterization, and laser therapy** can be used. But the disadvantages are high risk for recurrence and risk for cervical injury.

Pathogens Causing Suppurative Cervicitis

Neisseria Gonorrhoeae

N. gonorrhoeae is a gram-negative diplococcus that forms oxidase positive colonies and ferments glucose. The columnar and transitional epithelium of the genitourinary tract is the principal site of invasion.

Risk Factors

Risk factors are—age less than 25 years, the presence of other STDs, a history of previous gonococcal infection, new or multiple sex partners, lack of barrier protection, drug use and commercial sex worker. Screening for women having no risk factor is not recommended.

Symptoms

Symptomatic gonorrhea may present as vaginitis or cervicitis. Those with cervicitis present with odorless, nonirritating and white to yellow discharge. Gonorrhea can also infect the Bartholin's gland and Skene's gland, the urethra and ascend into the endometrium and fallopian tube to cause upper reproductive tract infection.

Diagnosis

A presumptive diagnosis of gonorrhea can be made based on examination of the stained smear. Confirmation requires positive identification on selective media—Thayer-Martin or Transgrow. Nucleic Acid Amplification Test (NAATs) from endocervical swab, liquid Papanicolaou (Pap specimen), vaginal swab and urine specimen are available.

Complication

The major complication in the female is salpingitis and consequent tubal scarring, infertility and increased risk for ectopic gestation.

Prevention

Gonorrhea is a reportable disease that can be controlled only by detecting the asymptomatic carrier and treating her and sexual partner. It is important to instruct patient to abstain for 7 days after therapy is initiated. All high risk population should be screened by routine culture. Re-examination 3 weeks after treatment is mandatory to rule out reinfection or failure of therapy. Barrier contraception will protect against gonorrhea.

Treatment

Recommendation for single dose therapy of uncomplicated cervical, urethral or rectal infection by CDC is as follows:

Ceftriaxone 125 mg I/M + Doxycycline 100 mg orally twice a day for 7 days or Azithromycin is 1 gm orally.

Or Cefixime 400 mg orally + Doxycycline/Azithromycin.

Or Ciprofloxacin 500 mg orally.

Or Ofloxacin 400 mg orally or Levofloxacin 250 mg orally + treatment for Chlamydia infection if not excluded.

Quinolone resistant *N. gonorrhoeae* is common in parts of Asia and Pacific. So quinolones are no longer recommended for treatment of Gonorrhea acquired in Asia and Pacific.

Alternative Regimen

a. Spectinomycin 2 gm I/M once followed by Doxycycline or Azithromycin as above.
b. Ceftizoxime 0.5 gm, or Cefotaxime 0.5 gm or Cefoxitin 2 gm I/M + Doxycycline or Azithromycin as above.
c. Gatifloxacin 400 mg, Norfloxacin 800 mg or Lomefloxacin 400 mg orally once in nonpregnant, non-lactating patients, over 17 years old.

Treatment in Pregnancy

Pregnant women should not be treated with quinolones or tetracycline. They should be treated with recommended or alternative cephalosporin. If cephalosporins are not tolerated, spectinomycin 2 gm I/M should be given along with treatment for diagnosed or presumptive *C. trachomatis*.

Chlamydial Infection

The spectrum of genital infections caused by serotypes of *C. trachomatis* has only recently become appreciated. Chlamydia is obligate intracellular microorganism that has a cell wall similar to that of gram negative bacteria. They are classified as bacteria and contain both DNA and RNA (Fig. 18.5). They divide by binary fission but like viruses they grow intracellularly. They can be grown only by tissue culture.

With the exception of *L. serotypes*, *chlamydia* attach only to columnar epithelial cells without deep tissue invasion. So the clinical infection may not be apparent. *Chlamydia trachomatis* infections are associated with many adverse sequele due to chronic inflammatory changes as well as fibrosis. The proposed mechanism for the pathogenesis of Chlamydial disease is an immune mediated response.

Risk Factors

Following factors may be predictive of women with greater likelihood of acquiring *C. trachomatis*:
a. Resumption of sexual activity younger than 20 years have Chlamydial infection rates 2–3 times higher than rates of older women.
b. Lower socioeconomic status.
c. Multiple sexual partner.

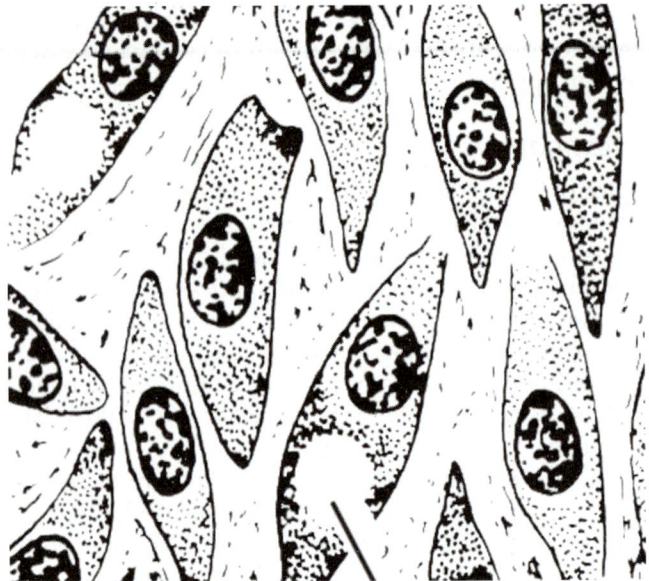

Fig. 18.5: Chlamydia trachomatis

Diagnosis of Chlamydia Infection

Symptoms and Signs

As chlamydia causes columnar epithelial infection, presenting symptoms are mucopurulent discharge, or endocervical secretion. Not uncommonly women are asymptomatic. Urethritis and dysuria may be present.

Diagnosis

a. Microscopic inspection of secretion following a saline preparation typically reveals 20 or more leukocytes per high power field.
b. More specifically culture, NAAT and ELISA are available for endocervical secretions. Cell culture is the detection method of greatest specificity but cost can be prohibitive.

Complications

a. Adverse sequelae of salpingitis, specifically infertility due to tubal obstruction and ectopic pregnancy are the most dire complication of this infection.
b. Pregnant women with cervical chlamydial infection can transmit infection to their newborns. Up to 50% of infant born to such mother can have inclusion conjunctivitis.
c. In 10% of infant, there can be indolent chlamydial pneumonitis at 2–3 months of age and also cause otitis media in neonate.
d. Chlamydia can cause significantly increased fetal and perinatal wastage by abortion, premature delivery, or stillbirth. There is increasing evidence that chlamydial infection in pregnancy is a risk marker for premature delivery and postpartum infection. Women at greatest risk are those with recent chlamydial infection detected by anti-chlamydial IgM. It is hypothesized that

asymptomatic cervicitis predisposes to mild amnionitis, which activates phospholipase A2 to release prostaglandin, which cause onset of premature uterine contraction. Chlamydial infection is associated with higher rates of early postpartum endometritis as well as delayed infection from chlamydia that often presents several weeks postpartum.

Treatment

Recommended treatment is as follows (CDC recommendation 2006):

Primary Treatment

Azithromycin 1 gm orally once or Doxycycline 100 mg orally twice a day for 7 days

Alternative Regimen

Erythromycin base 500 mg orally 4 times a day for 7 days
 Or erythromycin ethylsuccinate 800 mg orally 4 times a day for 7 days
 Or Ofloxacilin 300 mg orally twice a day for 7 days
 Or Levofloxacin 500 mg orally daily for 7 days
 Following treatment, retesting is not recommended if symptoms resolve. To prevent further infection abstinence is recommended, until a woman and her partner are asymptomatic.

Key points in principle for diagnosis and treatment and prevention of PID
 i. Consider the diagnosis in all sexually active women of reproductive age, who present with lower abdominal pain.
 ii. Rule out pregnancy.
 iii. Err on the side of over diagnosis to help to prevent the sequelae of PID.
 iv. Immediate treatment with recommended regimen as soon as possible once the diagnosis is established.
 v. Reassess the patient in 48-72 hours if oral treatment is chosen to ensure response.
 vi. Refer and directly treat all sexual partners.
 vii. Screen for symptomatic gonorrhea and chlamydia in sexually active men and women.
 viii. Encourage barrier methods and spermicidal to help prevent infection.
 ix. When PID is diagnosed, recommend testing for other STDs such as syphilis, HIV, hepatitis B.

GENITAL ULCER DISEASE

Ulceration defines complete loss of the epidermis covering with invasion into the underlying dermis, whereas **erosion** describes partial loss of the epidermis without dermal penetration. They are distinguished by clinical examination. Biopsies are generally not helpful but may be if taken from the edge of a new lesion. Significantly, biopsy is mandatory if carcinoma is suspected.

Genital herpes, **syphilis** and **chancroid** are the most **common ulcerative** lesion, followed by uncommonly found **Lymphogranuloma venereum** or **Granuloma inguinale** (Figs 18.6A to C). Essentially all are sexually transmitted and are associated with increased risk for HIV.

Herpes Simplex

Genital herpes is the most prevalent genital ulcer disease and is a chronic viral infection. The virus enters sensory nerve endings and undergoes retrograde axonal transport to the dorsal root ganglion, where the virus develops life long latency. Spontaneous reactivation by various events results in antegrade transport of virus particles of protein to the surface. Here virus is shed with or without lesion formation. It is postulated that immune mechanism control latency and reactivation.

There are two types of Herpes simplex virus—HSV-1, and HSV-2. Type 1 HSV is the most frequent cause of oral lesion. Type 2 HSV is found more typically with genital lesions. Type 1 and Type 2 both can cause genital herpes.

Symptoms

Patient's symptoms at initial presentation will depend on primarily on whether or not a patient during the current episode has antibody from previous exposure. If a patient has no antibody, the attack rate in an exposed person approaches 70%. There are three stages of lesion:
a. Vesicle with or without pustule formation, which last about a week—painful red, vesicle appear on clitoris, labia, vestibule, vagina, perineum and cervix.
b. Ulceration—vesicle progresses into multiple shallow ulcers.
c. Crusting—vesicle heal up spontaneously by crusting.
 Vesicles predictably shed during the vesicle and ulcerative phase. In this period, the women may have other signs of viremia such as a low grade fever, malaise and myalgia. The most common complaint of HSV infection is pain. Primary herpes out break is typically more severe and lasts longer (12–21 days). Recurrent outbreaks typically last 2–5 days and the symptoms are usually milder. The frequency of HSV recurrence is quite variable. Some women experience a single outbreak and others have recurrences many times a year.

The pain of initial herpes outbreak can be so severe that narcotics, topical anesthetic and even hospitalization may be necessary. Women can have urinary retention, requiring bladder catheterization as urine is extremely irritating to the ulcers.

Diagnosis

The gold standard for diagnosis is tissue culture. It has high specificity but sensitivity is low. PCR testing is 1.5

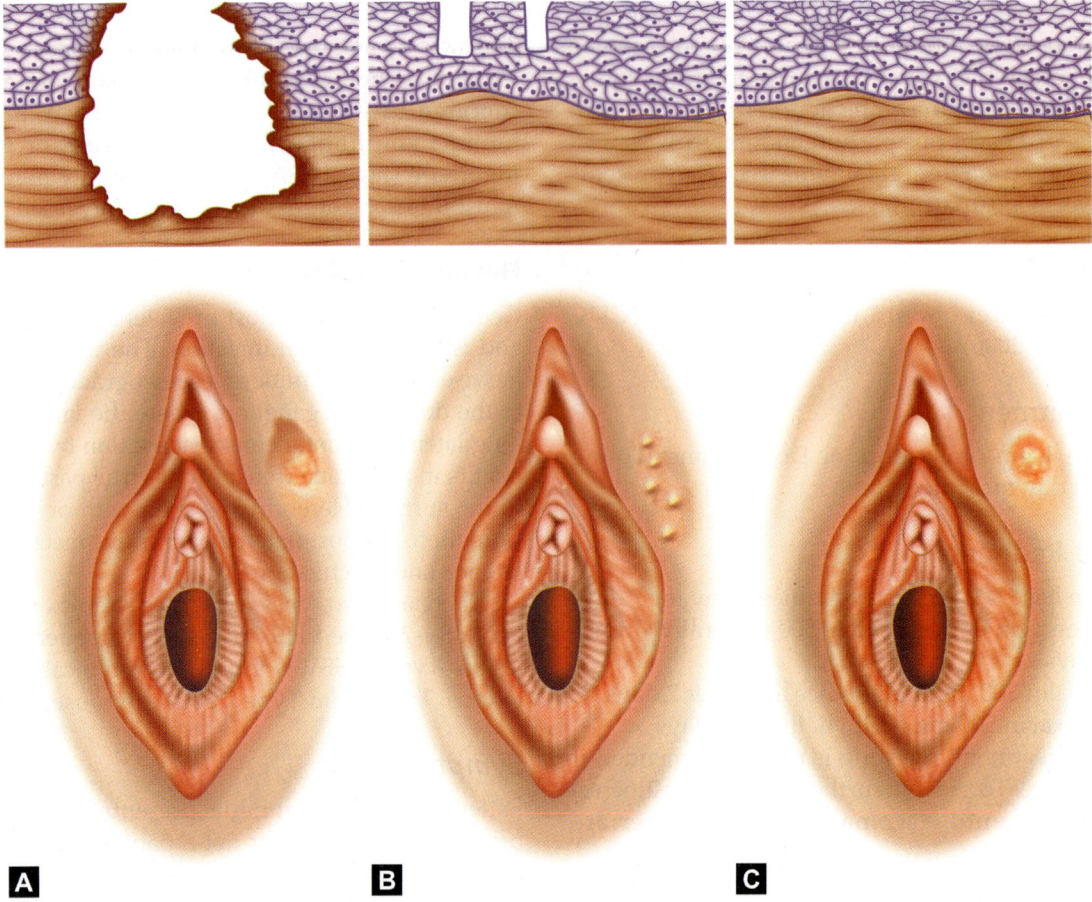

Figs 18.6A to C: Genital ulcer: (A) Chancroid—irregular margin and undermine edge; (B) Syphilis—smooth and indurated border; (C) Herpes—superficial and inflamed

to 4 times more sensitive and is now increasingly being used. The Elisa or Immunofluorescent method antibodies to HSV-1 and HSV-2 can be detected which have a specificity of 96%.

Although these tests may be used to confirm herpes simplex infection, treatment and additional STD screening may be initiated in clinically obvious cases following physical examination alone.

Treatment

Although HSV cannot be cured, the symptoms and duration of both initial and secondary outbreaks can be reduced with antiviral treatment.

Antiviral Treatment

CDC recommended antiviral regimens are listed in Table 18.3. It includes Acyclovir, Valaciclovir, and Famiciclovir. Initial treatment is for 7 days, treatment of recurrence is for 3 days.

Supportive Treatment

Analgesia with NSAIDS drug or mild narcotic such as acetaminophen with codeine may be prescribed. In addition topical anesthetic as lidocaine ointment may provide relief. Local care to prevent secondary bacterial infection is important. Patient education is mandatory and counseling should include natural disease history, its sexual transmission, method to reduce transmission and natural consequences.

Treatment for Recurrent HSV Outbreaks

If episode recurs at interval of 2–3 months, a woman may select daily suppressive therapy, which reduces recurrences by 70-80%. Suppressive therapy may eliminate recurrences and decreases sexual transmission of virus by approximately 50% and Sequelae of HSV infection.

In Pregnancy

There can be transmission to newborn. If woman has an active herpes outbreak or prodroma at the time of vaginal delivery, neonatal infection can be a serious problem. So if woman has a prodroma or active lesion at the time of labor, she should be delivered by cesarean section. At 36 weeks of gestation age, in a woman with history of HSV infection, suppressive therapy can be given. HSV-2 virus infection may be a risk factor for cervical cancer.

Table 18.3: Recommended oral medication regimens for treatment of genital herpes, simplex infection
First clinical episode of genital herpes: Acyclovir 400 mg three times daily for 7–10 days Or Acyclovir 200 mg five times daily for 7–10 days Or Famiciclovir 250 mg three times daily for 7–10 days or Acyclovir 1 g twice daily for 7–10 days
Episodic therapy for recurrent disease: Acyclovir 400 mg three times daily for 5 days or Acyclovir 800 mg twice daily for 5 days Or Acyclovir 800 mg three times daily for 2 days Or Famciclovir 125 mg twice daily for 5 days Or Famciclovir 1 g twice daily for 1 day Or Valaciclovir 500 mg twice daily for 3 days Or Valaciclovir 1 g once daily for 5 days
Oral suppressive therapy options: Acyclovir 400 mg twice daily Or Famciclovir 250 mg twice daily Or Valacicolovir 0.5 to 1 g once daily

Infectivity of Genital Herpes

Although the latent virus is always present in an infected individual's body, spread is by direct contact with virus at the site of an outbreak. Therefore, the virus can only spread when a woman has a secondary outbreak or in the days just prior to the eruption of an ulcer. During the **pre-eruptive period** the patient typically experiences a prodrome of tingling or burning in the effected region and mild systemic symptoms. When a woman has no active lesion and not experiencing a prodrome, she is generally not infective. **Once ulcers are completely healed, they are no longer infective.**

Chancroid

Chancroid is caused by non-motile, non-spore forming, facultative gram negative bacillus—*Hemophilus ducreyi*. Incubation period is 3–10 days, and host access requires a break in the skin or mucous membranes. Chancroid does not cause a systemic reaction and no prodromal syndrome precedes the appearance of infection.

Symptoms

The disease presents as a vesicopustule on the pudendum, vagina or cervix. Later it degenerates into a saucer shaped ragged ulcer circumscribed by an inflammatory wheal. Ulcer base is red and granular in contrast to syphilitic chancre which are typically soft. Lesions are frequently covered with purulent maternal and if secondarily infected, a foul odor will result.

In 50% of patient there is unilateral or bilateral tender inguinal lymphadenopathy. If large and fluctuant, they are termed **buboes**. They may occasionally suppurate and form fistula.

Diagnosis

The most common imitating this presentation is syphilis and genital herpes. Figure 18.6 differentiates characteristics of 3 types of ulcer. Presumptive diagnosis can be made with identification of Gram negative nonmotile rods on a Gram stain of lesion content.

Definitive diagnosis requires *H. ducreyi* growth on special culture media but sensitivity is 80% for obtaining specimen. Superficial pus or crusting should be removed with sterile, saline soaked gauze.

Treatment

Local treatment: Good personal hygiene is important. The early lesion should be cleansed with mild soaps.
Antibiotic treatment: The CDC (2006) recommended regimen is as follows:

    Azithromycin 1 gm orally
    Or Ceftriaxone 250 mg I/M

Or Ciprofloxacin 500 mg orally twice a day in nonpregnant; over 17 years of age and nonlactating women for 3 days.
Or Erythromycin base 500 mg orally 3 times a day for 7 days.

Successful treatment will result in symptomatic improvement within 3 days and objective improvement within 1 week. Lymphadenopathy resolves more slowly, and if fluctuant, incision and drainage may be warranted. Those with coexistent HIV infection may require longer therapy courses and treatment failures are more common.

Granuloma Inguinale (Donovanosis)

It is genital ulcerative disease, caused by intracellular gram negative capsulated bacterium **(Klebsiella Granulomatis)**. The disease is only mildly infective, requires repeated exposure and has long incubation period of weeks to months.

Symptoms

It presents as painless inflammatory nodules which progresses to highly vascular beefy red ulcers that bleeds easily on contact. If ulcer is secondarily infected, they may become painful. Ulcer heals by fibrosis which can result in scarring resembling keloids. Lymph nodes are usually uninvolved but sometimes become enlarged and new lesion may appear along these lymphatic drainage channel.

Diagnosis

Diagnosis is confirmed by identification of Donovan bodies in microscopic evaluation after Wright Giemsa staining.

Treatment

CDC (2006) recommended regimens are:
Doxycycline 100 mg twice a day for minimum of 21 days and until lesions are completely healed.
Or Azithromycin 1 gm orally once a week as above.
Or Ciprofloxacin 750 mg orally twice a day as above.
Or Trimethoprim–Sulfamethoxazole DS orally twice daily as above.

Lymphogranuloma Venereum (LGV)

The causative agent is serotypes L_1, L_2 or L_3 of *Chlamydia trachomatis*. It is more common in tropical and subtropical region. Transmission is via sexual contact. Men are more frequently affected than women. The incubation period is 2–21 days.

Symptoms

The primary lesion is a small painless papule, vesicle or ulcer on fourchette, labia or cervix. The secondary stage is characterized by enlargement of the inguinal glands to form a painful mass which tends to suppurate and form sinuses.

Diagnosis

LGV can be diagnosed by clinical evaluation, exclusion of other etiology and possible Chlamydial testing. Additionally lymph node specimen obtained by swab for cultured for *C. trachomatis* or tested by immune fluorescence or PCR.

Treatment

The 2006 CDC regimen is Doxycycline 100 mg orally twice daily for 21 days or erythromycin base 500 mg orally four times daily for 21 days. It is recommended to diagnose and treat sexual contacts.

Syphilis

Syphilis is a sexually transmitted infection, caused by the spirochete—*Treponema pallidum*, which is a slender spiral shaped organism with tapered ends. Women at higher risk are from low socioeconomic status, adolescent, early onset of sexual activity and multiple sex partners.

Symptoms

The primary lesion is macular which soon becomes papular and ulcerates to form a primary chancre. *Primary chancre* is an indurated painless ulcer with a dull red base. Primary stage lasts for 3–8 weeks if untreated and ulcer spontaneously heals.

In *secondary syphilis*, it develops 6 week to 6 months after primary chancre. It is associated with maculopapular skin rashes. These rashes actively shed spirochetes in warm moist body areas like vulva. This rash may produce broad, pink or grey white highly infectious plaques.

Syphilis is a systemic infection, so there can be fever, malaise. Kidney, liver, joints and central nervous system (CNS) may be involved. In *late syphilis* vulvar lesion termed Gummas appear as squamous lesion or subcutaneous nodule that sometimes ulcerate.

In *tertiary syphilis* this phase may appear up to 20 years after latency, in which cardiovascular, CNS and musculoskeletal involvement may become apparent. However, cardiovascular and neurosyphilis are half as common in females as in males.

Diagnosis

Early syphilis is diagnosed primarily by **dark field examination or direct fluorescent antibody testing of lesion exudates**. In absence of this positive diagnosis, presumptive diagnosis may be reached with serologic non-treponemal test—(a) VDRL (Venereal disease research laboratory), (b) Rapid plasma reagin. Treponemal specific tests are—(a) FTA-ABS fluorescent treponemal antibody absorption, (b) *Treponema pallidum* particle agglutination.

Following treatment sequential non-treponemal test should be preferred. A 4-fold titer decrease is required to define a clinically significant decline.

Treatment

CDC (2006) recommended regimens for syphilis are as follows:
Primary, secondary, early latent (< 1 year) syphilis:
Benzathine Penicillin G 2.4 million units I/M once.
Alternatively—oral regimen in penicillin allergic non-pregnant women.
Doxycycline 100 mg orally twice daily for two weeks
Or Tetracycline 800 mg orally 4 times daily for 2 weeks
Late latent, tertiary and cardiovascular syphilis:
Benzathine Penicillin G 2.4 million unit I/M weekly 3 doses.
Alternative regimen in penicillin allergic, non-pregnant women—Doxycycline 100 mg orally twice daily for 4 weeks.

As with other STDs, all patients treated for syphilis should be tested for other STDs. Patients with evidence of neurologic or cardiac involvement should be treated by an infectious disease specialist.

After initial treatment women should be seen at 6 months interval for clinical evaluation as well as serologic retesting.

Pathogens Causing Mass Lesions

External genital warts are manifestation of **Human Papilloma Virus (HPV)** infection. The non-pathogenic *HPV type 6 and 11 are usually responsible for external genital warts*. Incubation period ranges from 3 weeks to 8 months.

Genital warts display differing morphologies and appearance ranging from flat papule to the classic verrucous exophytic lesion termed **Condyloma acuminata**. Involved tissues vary and external genital warts may develop at sites in the lower reproductive tract, urethra, anus or mouth.

Diagnosis

Warts are typically diagnosed by clinical inspection and biopsy is not required unless coexisting neoplasm is suspected. Similarly HPV serotyping is not required for routine diagnosis (Fig. 18.7).

Treatment

Condyloma acuminata may remain unchanged or spontaneously resolve and the effect of treatment on future viral transmission is unclear. The goal of treatment is removal of the warts; it is not possible to eradicate the viral infection. Treatment is most successful in patient with small warts that have been presented for less than 1 year. Following are treatment options with efficiency percent:
a. Trichloroacetic acid—80-90%
b. Podophyllin—10-25%
c. Cryotherapy—63-88%
d. Imiquimod (5%) cream—33-72%
e. Podofilox (o.5%)—45-88%
f. Electrodessication or cautery—94%
g. Laser—43-93%
h. Interferon—44-61%

Selection of a specific treatment regimen depends on the anatomic site, size, and number of warts as well as expense, efficacy, convenience and potential adverse effect. Recurrence more often results from reactivation of sub-clinical infection than reinfection by a sex partner. So thorough examination of sexual contact is not absolutely necessary, yet many of sexual contact may have external genital warts and may benefit from therapy and counseling concerning transmission of warts.

Molluscum Contagiosum

It is a DNA virus that is transmitted by intimate contact. The host response to viral invasion is papular with central umbilication, giving a characteristic appearance. Lesions may be single or multiple and is commonly seen on the vulva, vagina, thighs and or buttocks.

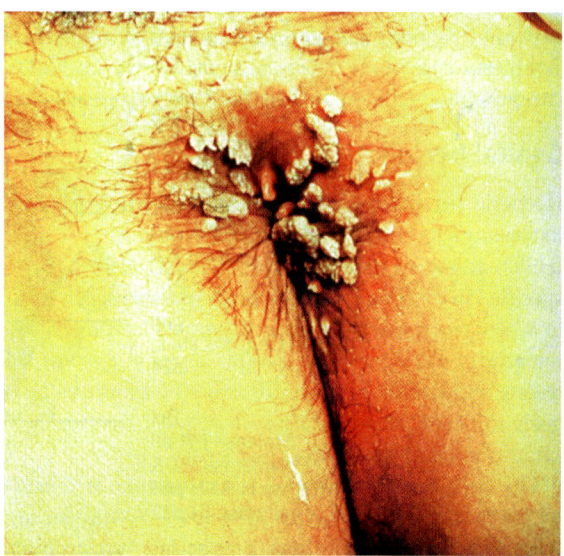

Fig. 18.7: Genital warts caused by HPV

Diagnosis

They are typically diagnosed by visual inspection alone. However, material from lesion can be sent for Giemsa, Gram or Wright staining. **Molluscum bodies-large intracytoplasmic structures are diagnostic**.

Treatment

Most lesions, spontaneously regress over 6 -12 months. If removal is preferred, lesion may be treated by Cryotherapy, Electrosurgical needle coagulation. Alternatively, topical application of agents used in the treatment of genital warts may also be applied effectively to treat molluscum contagiosum.

HUMAN IMMUNODEFICIENCY VIRUS INFECTION

Human immunodeficiency virus was discovered in 1983 by Barre Sinoussi and Colleagues. Human immunodeficiency virus is a **retrovirus** (having double standard RNA) (Fig. 18.8). The virus gains entry into the cells through CD4 receptor on the surface of T cells by the fusion, transcribes genomic RNA into DNA by **reverse transcriptase**. By **Integrase** enzyme it integrates in cell nucleus and transcripts and translates HIV mRNA polyprotein. **Protease** enzymes process virus assembly. Virus remains as provirus until the life of cell. It replicates within the host cell at the expense of host cell resources. When cell death occurs, the HIV viral load is released in large numbers. HIV cells show preference for human T cells where it can lie dormant for many years (Fig. 18.9).

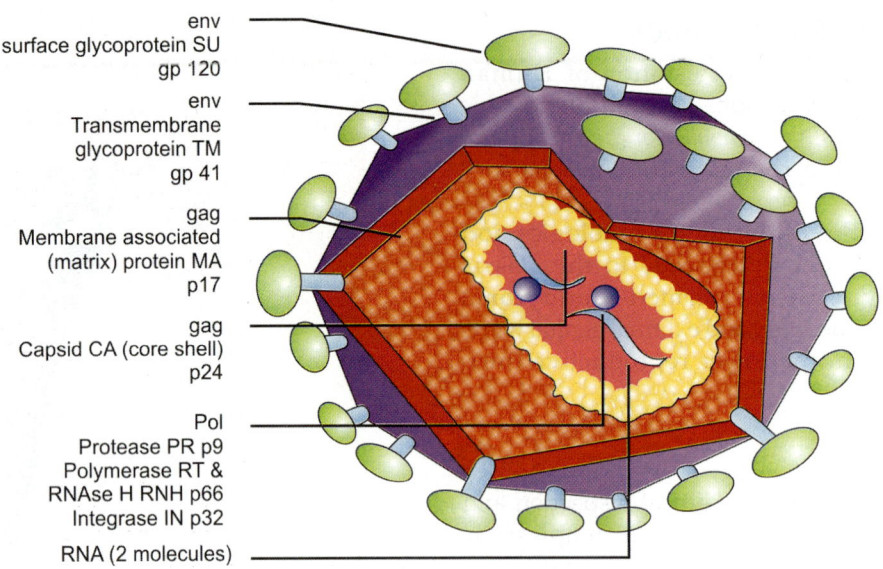

Fig. 18.8: Structure of HIV

Natural History of Disease

Acute HIV Infection

After infection the person may remain asymptomatic or manifests symptoms within 3–6 weeks after initial exposure to HIV virus. Patients may have non-specific **'flu like'** symptoms at this time including fever, fatigue, pharyngitis, swollen lymph nodes and rash. In the period, virus reproduces unopposed by the immune system, causing an initial high viral load.

Window Period

The virus spreads to lymph node. At this time immune system does not begin producing HIV antibodies for several weeks. So the standard testing will be negative but at the same time high amount of virus in the bloodstream makes the patient highly infectious.

Clinical Latency

This period follows acute infections and lasts for 6–10 years. Initially the immune system is able to partially control the level of HIV in the patient's blood. But there is slow but steady decline of immune system.

Full Blown AIDS

With decline of CD4 cell count, the body is no longer able to fight certain diseases and symptoms of AIDS complex begin to manifest like unexplained fever, rashes, weight loss, fatigue, and diarrhea. AIDS define the presence of opportunistic infection like tuberculosis, recurrent oral, vaginal candidiasis, mycobacterial infection, recurrent varicella/herpes zoster, Kaposi's sarcoma and cervical cancer. Natural history of HIV infection is summarized in Figure 18.10.

Epidemiology and Mode of Transmission

About 40–50% of all HIV infected persons are women. In India 5.2 million persons are supposed to be HIV infected in India. Out of which 86% are infected through heterosexual contact. Other modes of transmission are through blood transfusion (2%) and blood product, through I/V drugs needle sharing (2.4%). Maternal to child transmission (vertical or perinatal) accounts for 3.6% of infection.

Route of Transmission

i. **Sexual transmission**
   a. Heterosexual
   b. Homosexual
ii. **Blood contact**
   a. Blood transfusion
   b. I/V drug use
   c. Occupational exposure like needle stick, splash, cut
iii. **Mother to child**
   a. In utero
   b. During delivery
   c. Breastfeeding

Socioeconomic factors like low literacy level, ignorance of mode of transmission, gender disparity, poverty, migration due to various reasons, unprotected commercial sex or casual sex with multiple partners, poverty, and stigmas leading to poor communication and marginalization of infected persons are responsible for spread of HIV/AIDS.

CHAPTER – 18 ♦ Gynecological Infection and STD

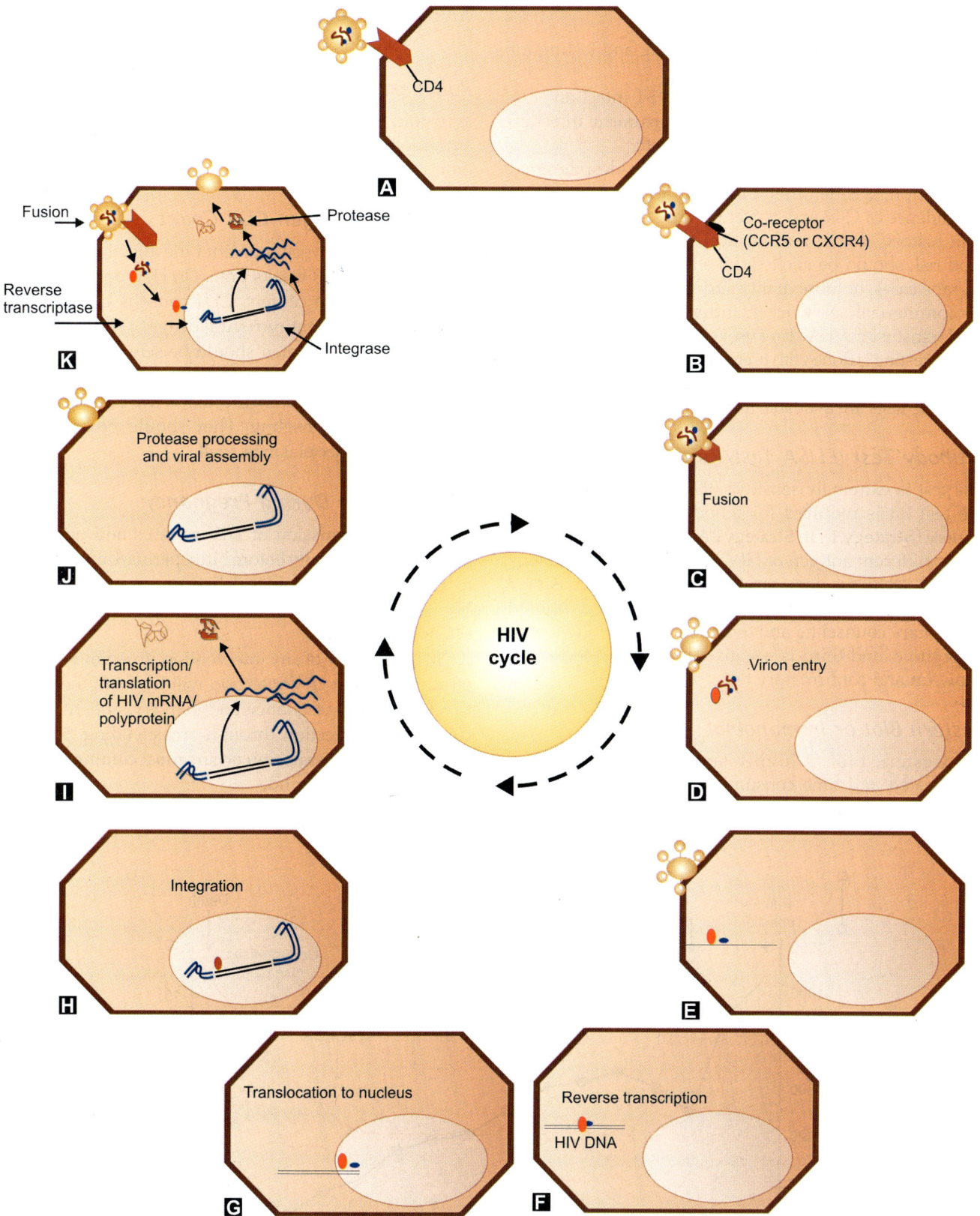

Fig. 18.9: Life cycle of HIV

Diagnosis

The physician should consider counseling and testing for HIV by following symptoms:
a. Individuals with reproductive tract/ST infection.
b. Individuals with symptoms of opportunistic infection like recurrent candidiasis, diarrhea, etc.
c. Individuals with persistent weight loss despite good nutrition. Besides this, in female there is increased incidence of CIN and cancer cervix.

In history, sexual risk, vertical transmission risk and blood risk should be elicited. Like history of commercial sex, rape cases, homosexuality and vulnerable population like commercial sex worker, individuals with multiple blood transfusions, I/V drug user or history of needle prick.

HIV testing is done with pretest counseling and informed consent (NACO Protocol) and proper post test counseling. Following tests are available for diagnosis of HIV.

Antibody Test (ELISA Test/Rapid Test)

Elisa test is extremely sensitive (99.5%) but less specific. One test kit is required for blood bank and screening purpose (**Strategy 1**). In **Strategy 2A** (surveillance) two kits having different antigen of HIV virus is used. In **Strategy 2B and 3**, testing is done serially on same sample using 3 kits, having 3 different antigens. Strategy 2 and 3 is offered at voluntary counseling and treatment centers. If two tests are positive, and third is negative, patient is referred for follow-up and confirmatory test.

Western Blot or Immunoblot

The western blot is highly specific but expensive, complicated and time consuming. It is reactive when a critical pattern of specific antibodies is detected against the three main gene products of HIV.

Polymerase Chain Reaction (PCR)

It is gold standard for diagnosis of HIV. Viral DNA is amplified following isolation of the virus from peripheral mononuclear cells.

Viral 1-24 Antigen CD4 Count

It can be detected very soon after the infection and usually disappears in 8–10 weeks time. On HIV positive persons, and at specialized centers, CD4 count is done to decide about the need of antiretroviral drugs.

HIV positive women should be screened for TB, STI. They should be offered vaccination against hepatitis B, pneumococcal, and influenza with behavioral and psychological counseling. They should be screened for intraepithelial neoplasm as well.

HIV Infection During Pregnancy

Maternal transmission of HIV to fetus and neonate can occur transplacentally before birth, peripartum by exposure to blood and bodily fluid at delivery or postpartum through breastfeeding. Hence all pregnant women should be offered HIV testing.

In the absence of any intervention, an estimated 15–30% of mothers with HIV infection will transmit the infection to fetus during pregnancy and delivery, and 10–20% will transmit the infection through breastfeeding. **50–70% of vertical HIV transmission occurs most commonly during the intrapartum period.**

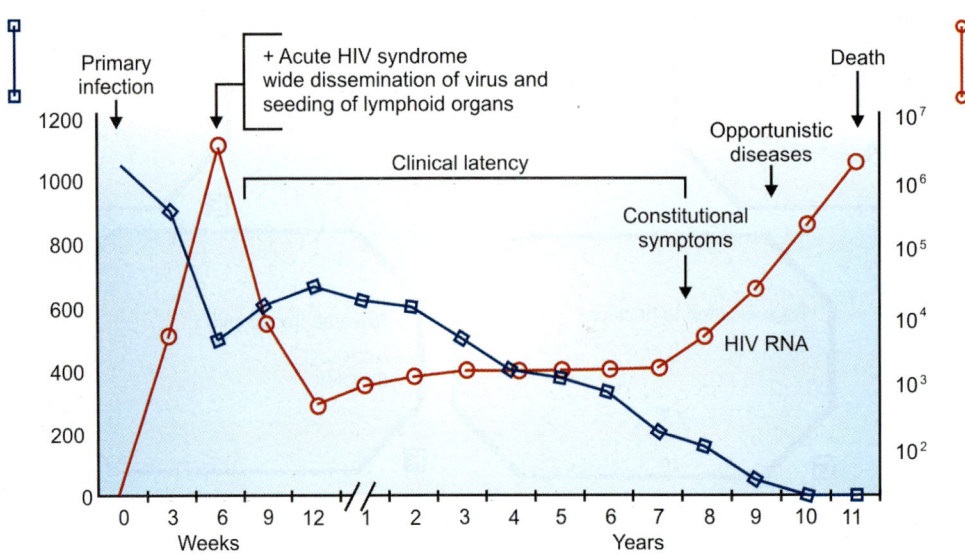

Fig. 18.10: Natural history of HIV infection

Testing protocol for HIV in adults and children more than 18 months old is summarized in Flow chart 18.1, and in children less than 18 months in Flow chart 18.2.

Perinatal Care and Guidelines of Delivery in HIV Positive Women

Perinatal care must be individualized. Patient should be referred to support system ideally in antenatal period. Screening for other STD and HIV related infection should be done. At a minimum a tuberculin skin test with control, chest radiography, cytomegalovirus and toxoplasmosis baseline serological test should be done.

CD4 lymphocyte count should be monitored in each trimester. 3 drug ARV drug for 3 months after 14–28 weeks gestation is best means of preventing vertical transmission. Elective cesarean section and avoidance of breastfeeding further reduces the risk of vertical transmission from 15–30% to less than 1%. In developing countries it may not be affordable and sustainable. In low resource setting vaginal delivery with all standard work precaution like not rupturing amniotic membrane, minimum tissue trauma. Breast and breastfeeding can be considered in developing countries. But *NO mixed feeding is advocated.*

Postpartum care should entail a continuation of blood and bodily fluid precautions. Family planning and safer sex counseling to be continued in postpartum period with consideration given to tubal ligation, if there is no desire for childbearing in future.

Treatment

Decisions regarding initiation of ARV therapy should be guided by monitoring the laboratory parameters of HIV, RNA (Viral load) and CD4 cell count as well as the clinical condition of the patient. The following groups of ARV drugs are available:

Nucleoside Reverse Transcriptase Inhibitor

a. Zidovudine
b. Didanosine
c. Stavidine, Lamivudine

Non-nucleoside Reverse Transcriptase Inhibitor

a. Nevirapine
b. Efavirenz
c. Protease inhibitor
d. Saquinavir
e. Ritonavir
f. Indinavir
g. Nelfinavir

The ARV drug should be offered in women with – (a) Fewer than 350 CD4 T cells (b) Plasma HIV RNA level > 1000 copies/ml.

Flow chart 18.1: Testing protocol of HIV in adults and children more than 18 months

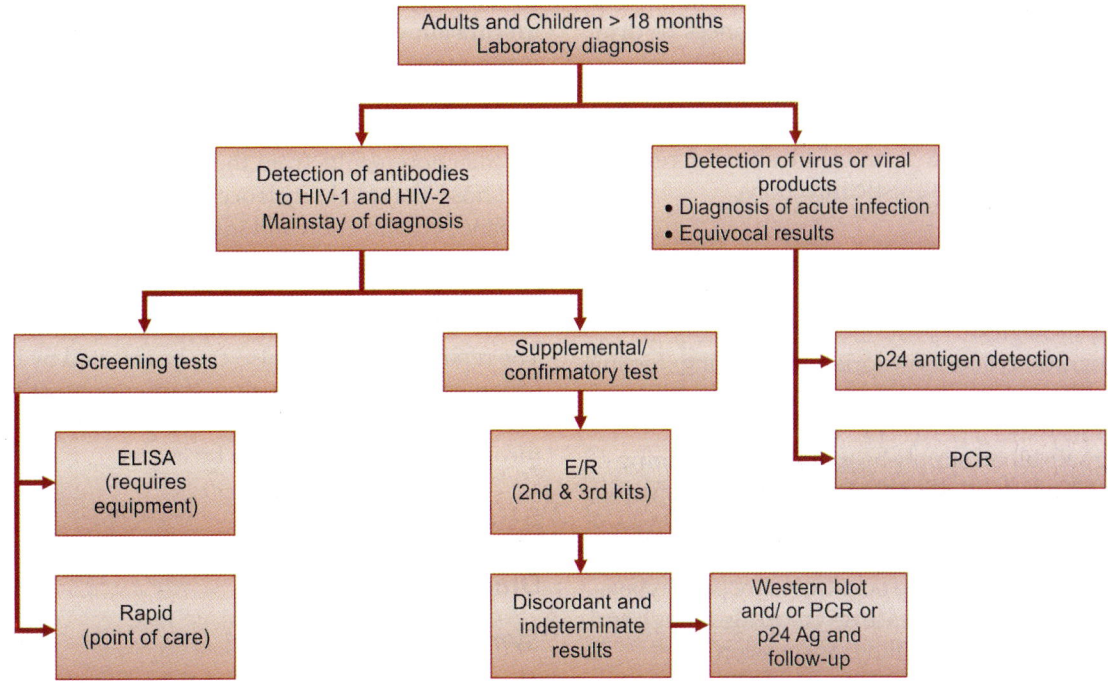

Flow chart 18.2: Testing protocol of HIV in children less than 18 months

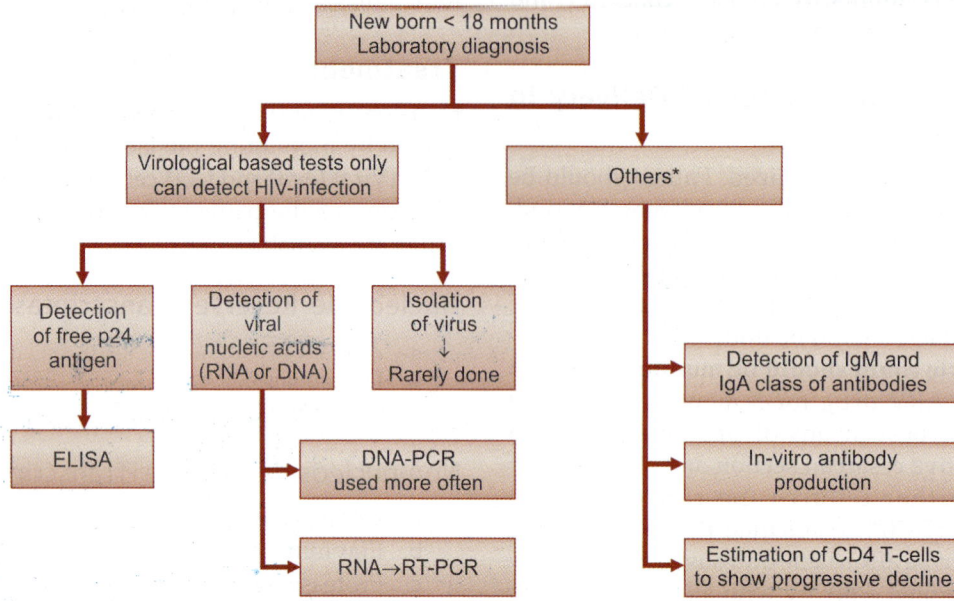

* Tests listed under others are not commonly used for diagnosis

Usually three different ARV drugs are given to reduce the chances of drug resistance. Dual nucleoside regimen with protease inhibitor or NNRI provides a better endurable clinical benefit.

For women diagnosed in labor Nevirapine 200 mg orally in labor cuts transmission significantly but there is 50% chance of developing drug resistance. NVP and AZT 300 mg/ZDV plus lamivudine (3TC) 150 mg orally twice daily for 3–7 days after delivery reduce chances of drug resistance to 10%.

ARV (NVP drop—2 mg/kg) should be offered to newborn within 72 hours of delivery. In addition patients with less than 200 CD4 T cells/µl should receive prophylaxis against opportunistic infections.

Prevention

The HIV epidemic within the community can be prevented by following strategies:
a. Risk recognition, and appropriate counseling, testing and referral.
b. STI management.
c. Ensuring safe blood supply by mandatory screening of donated blood, only rational use of blood transfusion, discouraging professional blood donation.
d. Educating hospital personnel on standard work precaution and appropriate post-exposure prophylaxis.
e. Routine timely HIV testing in pregnancy and prevention of mother to child transmission.
f. Voluntary and confidential counseling, testing promotion and referral.

URINARY TRACT INFECTION (UTI)

Symptomatic urinary tract infections are among the most common bacterial infection.

Pathogenesis

Because of pelvic anatomy, women have more chance of developing UTI than men. The **short length of the female urethra** allows easier access by bacteria to the bladder. The **warm moist vulva and rectum** contribute to contamination due to close proximity. Sexual activity increases bladder inoculation.

Infection results from the interaction between bacteria and host. Bacterial virulence is more common, when they enhance colonization and invasion of the lower and upper urinary tract. Once within the bladder, bacteria may ascend within the ureter, enhanced by vesicourethral reflux into the renal pelvis and cause upper urinary tract infection. The renal parenchyma also can be infected by blood borne organism especially during staphylococcal bacteremia. Mycobacterium tuberculosis gives access to the kidney through this route and also by ascent.

ACUTE CYSTITIS

Diagnosis

Symptoms and Signs

The women with acute cystitis have an abrupt onset of multiple severe UTI symptoms which include dysuria, frequency and urgency associated with suprapubic or low back pain. On physical examination there can be suprapubic tenderness. The current recommendation is that most patients can be treated with a short course of antibiotics without urine analysis or urine culture.

Treatment

High concentration of trimethoprim and fluoroquinolones can eradicate *E. coli*, while minimally altering normal anaerobic and microaerophilic vaginal flora. **Nitrofurantoin 100 mg orally twice a day for 7 days** or **fluoroquinolones (ciprofloxacin 250 mg orally twice a day for 3 days)** are the optimal choice for empirical 3 days therapy for uncomplicated cystitis. Usually empirical therapy can be started and no visit or culture is necessary unless symptoms persist or recur.

Recurrent Cystitis

Fifty percent of women who suffer an uncomplicated acute bacterial cystitis will have another infection within a year. Out of these 5% have recurring symptoms.

Diagnosis

1. **Urine culture and sensitivity:** For recurrent cystitis urinalysis and culture are mandatory. Urine collection should be mid stream, in a sterilized container and should be promptly plated for culture within 2 hours. Urine culture is the gold standard for identifying the cause of UTI and susceptibility testing of that pathogen to variety of antibiotics.

   Significant bacteriuria is most commonly defined as $\geq 10^5$ (colony forming unit)/ml of urine. If urine is collected by catheterization or suprapubic aspirate, colony count $\geq 10^2$ CFU/ml are diagnostic.

   As final urine culture reports are usually available for 48 hours, the empirical treatment is initially begun but modified later on after culture results.

2. **Microscopy:** Microscopy of urine specimen allows identification of both pyuria and bacteriuria. For identification of leukocyte, a specimen should be examined expeditiously because leukocytes deteriorate quickly in urine.

3. **Leukocyte esterase:** This test measures esterase enzyme found in urinary leukocyte. This has high negative predictable value, but it can be false positive if urine specimen has been contaminated with vaginal or colonic bacteria.

4. **Nitrites:** Bacteria metabolically produce nitrites from nitrates. It identifies mainly family of enterobacteria but not the gram positive pathogens. In addition it ideally requires the first morning urine specimen, because more than 4 hours are required for bacteria to convert nitrates to nitrites.

Treatment

Patient may be treated by one of these strategies:
a. Continuous prophylaxis
b. Postcoital prophylaxis
c. Therapy initiated by the patient when symptoms are first noted, and followed thereafter according to urine culture report.

In postmenopausal women having frequent reinfection, hormonal therapy or topical applied estrogen cream along with antimicrobial prophylaxis is helpful in treatment.

ACUTE PYELONEPHRITIS

Diagnosis

The clinical spectrum of acute uncomplicated pyelonephritis may be:
a. Mild—No nausea, vomiting, normal to slightly increased leukocyte count and normal to low grade fever
b. Severe—Vomiting, dehydration, evidence of sepsis, high leukocyte count and fever. Other symptoms are varying degree of flank pain and tenderness to percussion over kidney region. Urine culture should be obtained in all women.

Treatment

In absence of nausea and vomiting and severe illness, outpatient oral therapy can be given for 10–14 days (Table 18.4).

Symptoms usually subside within 48-72 hours. If fever and flank pain persist after 72 hours of therapy, ultrasound or CAT should be considered to rule out a perinephric or internal abscess or urethral obstruction. A follow-up culture should be obtained 2 weeks after the completion of therapy.

Table 18.4: Treatment protocol for mild acute pyelonephritis

Trimethoprim - Sulfamethoxazol 160-800 mg every 12 hours
Outpatient treatment: Quinolone - Ofloxacin 200-300 mg every 12 hours.

Inpatient treatment is indicated for severely ill patients. It includes—Ceftriaxone (1-2 gm daily) Ampicillin (1 gm every 6 hour) Gentamicin or Azithromycin (1gm every 8-12 hours)

MULTIPLE CHOICE QUESTIONS

1. A 35-year-old female presented to gynecologist with complaint of profuse vaginal discharge. The diagnosis of bacterial vaginosis is made upon all the following findings except:
   a. Abundance of gram variable coccobacilli
   b. Absence of lactobacilli
   c. Abundance of polymorph
   d. Presence of clue cells

   Ans. c

2. True about *Trichomonas vaginalis*:
   a. Flagellated parasite
   b. Fungal infection
   c. Pruritis
   d. Sexually transmitted

   Ans. a, c, d

3. Which of the following is best drug of choice for treatment of bacterial vaginosis in pregnancy?
   a. Clindamycin
   b. Metronidazole
   c. Erythromycins
   d. Kanamycin

   Ans. b

4. Which of the following condition is most likely to be associated with vaginal pH<4?
   a. Atrophic vaginitis
   b. Candidal vaginitis
   c. Trichomonas
   d. Gardnerella

   Ans. b

5. Gardnerella vaginalis infection is diagnosed by all except:
   a. pH < 4.5
   b. Fishy odor
   c. Clue cells
   d. Positive Whiff test

   Ans. a

6. Chlamydial infection is best treated by:
   a. Azithromycin + contact tracing
   b. Doxycycline + Metronidazole
   c. Fluconazole + Doxycycline
   d. Metronidazole

   Ans. a

7. Which of the following is not sexually transmitted disease?
   a. Echinococcus
   b. Candida
   c. Molluscum contagiosum
   d. Group β streptococcus

   Ans. a

8. Asymptomatic carrier of gonococcal infection in female is commonly seen in:
   a. Endocervix
   b. Vagina
   c. Urethra
   d. Fornix

   Ans. a

9. Herpes simplex type II cause:
   a. Herpes labials
   b. Common in homosexual
   c. Carcinoma cervix
   d. All

   Ans. a, c

10. Which of the following does Chlamydia trachomatis commonly cause?
    a. Malignancy
    b. Amenorrhea
    c. Postcoital bleeding
    d. Infertility

    Ans. d

19 Pelvic Inflammatory Disease

When you stop learning, stop listening, stop looking and asking questions – Then it's time to die.

Introduction

The term pelvic inflammatory disease describes a spectrum of infection and inflammation involving the upper genital tract (endometrium, fallopian tubes and ovaries) as well as the surrounding peritoneum in varying degrees depending on the severity of the disease. In more severe cases, the infection can spread along the upper peritoneum to the liver capsule, causing perihepatic adhesions. So called Fitz–Hugh–Curtis syndrome.

Etiopathogenesis

Pelvic inflammatory disease comprises usually sequelae of cervical infection with sexually transmitted organism, chiefly *Neisseria gonorrhoeae and Chlamydia trachomatis*. Cervical infection with these organisms breaks down cervical barriers to ascending infection. It allows endogenous superinfection of the upper genital tract by aerobic as well anaerobic organism normally inhabiting the lower genital tract (Fig. 19.1).

In addition, though less commonly *instrumentation of the cervix* and uterus during surgical procedures (such as surgical abortion, dilatation and curettage, hysteroscopy, endometrial and cervical biopsy, insertion of intrauterine device and intrauterine insemination) can cause autoinoculation of the endometrium with endogenous bacteria and lead to pelvic inflammatory disease.

In general the onset of PID caused by *Neisseria gonorrhoeae* is more acute and severe than that caused by *Chlamydia*. The *gonococci* can cause a direct inflammatory response in the human endocervix, endometrium and fallopian tube and is one of the true pathogens of human fallopian tube epithelial cells.

In contrast many cases of PID caused by *Chlamydia* are silent and are only diagnosed in retrospect, when the patient presents with infertility caused by tubal adhesions. It is supposed that **with intracellular *Chlamydia trachomatis*, cell mediated immune mechanism is responsible for resulting tissue injury**. Tubal destruction in women with repeated asymptomatic *Chlamydia* may be the result of a delayed hyperimmune response.

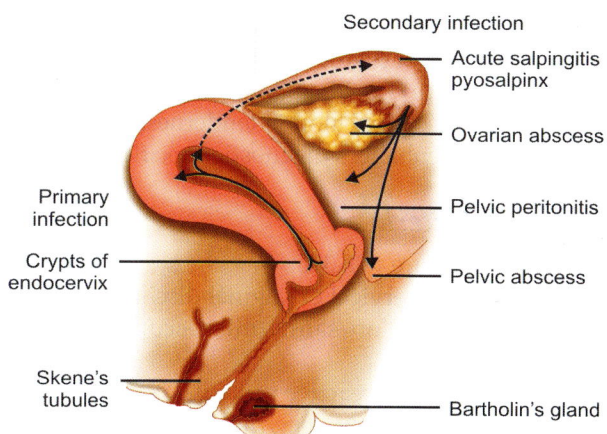

Fig. 19.1: Diagrammatic representation of various sites of pelvic inflammatory disease

Women with **pulmonary tuberculosis** can develop salpingitis and endometritis. Infection is usually blood borne but direct ascent can also be mode of spread. Beside this the fallopian tubes can also be infected by direct extension from inflammatory gastrointestinal disease, especially ruptured abscess, i.e. appendiceal or diverticular.

Diagnosis

Clinical Presentation

Traditionally the diagnosis of PID has been based on a triad of symptoms and signs including *pelvic pain, cervical motion and adnexal tenderness and presence of fever*. It is now recognized that many women with PID exhibit subtle or mild symptoms. So PID can be segregated into 'Silent PID' and a PID.

Silent Pelvic Inflammatory Disease

It is presumed that silent PID results from multiple or continuous low grade infection in asymptomatic women. Silent PID is not a clinical diagnosis but is an ultimate diagnosis when women present with tubal factor infertility, who lack a history of upper genital tract infection. Many of these patients have antibodies to *Chlamydia trachomatis* and or *N. gonorrhoeae* on laparoscopy or laparotomy. These patients may have evidence of prior tubal infection such as adhesion or fallopian tube may be grossly normal. But on salpingoscopy or histopathology there are flattened mucosal fold, extensive dilatation and secretory epithelial cells degeneration.*

Acute Pelvic Inflammatory Disease

The most recent recommended **diagnostic criteria** presented by the CDC (2006) are for sexually active women at risk for STD, who have pelvic or lower abdominal pain, and other etiologies for this are not possible.

Minimum Criteria

(i) Sexually active or history of recent instrumentation of cervix or uterus, (ii) Lower abdominal pain, (iii) Adnexal tenderness, (iv) Cervical motion tenderness. One or more of the following enhances diagnostic specificity.

Additional Criteria

i. Oral temperature >38.3°C.
ii. Mucopurulent cervical or vaginal discharge.
iii. Abundant WBC on saline microscopy of cervical secretion.
iv. Elevated ESR or C reactive protein (CRP).
v. Presence of cervical *N. gonorrhoeae* or *C. trachomatis*.

Elaborate Criteria

i. USG documenting tubo-ovarian abscess.
ii. Laparoscopy visually confirming salpingitis.

Symptoms and Physical Findings

Presenting symptoms will be lower abdominal and or pelvic pain, yellow vaginal discharge, menorrhagia, fever, chills, anorexia, nausea, vomiting, diarrhea, dysmenorrhea, dyspareunia, and dysuria. Yet there is no single symptom or symptoms associated with a physical finding that is specific for this diagnosis. So always other possible sources of pelvic pain should be ruled out.

On Physical Examination

Fever and mild to severe tachycardia are frequently found. **Abdominal examination** shows varying degree of bilateral lower abdominal tenderness and possible rebound and or guarding in more severe cases. Right upper quadrant tenderness will be found with accompanying Fitz-Hugh-Curtis syndrome. On **pelvic examination**, the classic sign of PID is **Chandelier's sign** – that is cervical motion tenderness, which describes severe tenderness and accompanying reaction by the patient on movement of cervix. Palpation of uterus and adnexa also elicits tenderness and frequently an adequate examination may be limited by guarding. Tubo-ovarian abscess if present can be palpated either as unilateral adnexal mass or a mass in the cul-de-sac.

On Speculum Examination

Mucopurulent discharge may be originating from the cervix. In advanced cases, this sign may have resolved since as endogenous superinfection advances, inciting organism (e.g. *Neisseria* and *Chlamydia*) are frequently eliminated.

Laboratory Findings

White Blood Cell (WBC) count is elevated, and ESR and CRP are also raised, though the latter are not usually obtained in the clinical setting. Cervical culture for causative organism is frequently positive, DNA based testing can be done if available. Culdocentesis generally is productive of reaction fluid (cloudy peritoneal fluid) that when stained reveals leukocytes with or without gonococci or other organism. Culture and sensitivity testing of organism from culdocentesis sampling may be done.

Radiological Findings

X-ray examination may show sign of illness but it is not specific. If air is seen under the diaphragm, it indicates ruptured tubo-ovarian or pelvic abscess and demands immediate laparotomy in addition to combination of antimicrobial therapy.

Ultrasound

TVS has increased the diagnostic accuracy of PID. Markers for acute and chronic PID can be differentiated. **Incomplete septation of the tubal wall (Cog wheel sign)** is a marker for acute disease and a **thin wall (beaded string)** indicates chronic disease. Thickening is noted in the pelvic areas during the inflammatory process.

Ultrasound diagnosis is approximately 90% accurate compared with laparoscopy, and it is noninvasive, cheap and easily available. Ultrasonography is very valuable in following the progression or regression of an abscess, after it has been diagnosed. The borders of an abscess confirm to the surrounding pelvic structure and as such do not give a well-defined borders noted in an ovarian cyst (Fig. 19.2).

---

* Intrauterine contraceptive device and PID: Most studies suggest that IUD itself does not cause pelvic infection. Though some association has been noted in prior IUD users and Chlamydial infection and future tubal infertility. So it supports the theory that not the IUD but STD exposure is cause of PID and subsequent tubal damage. If IUD is in place and diagnosis of PID is made along with antimicrobial therapy, IUD should be removed.

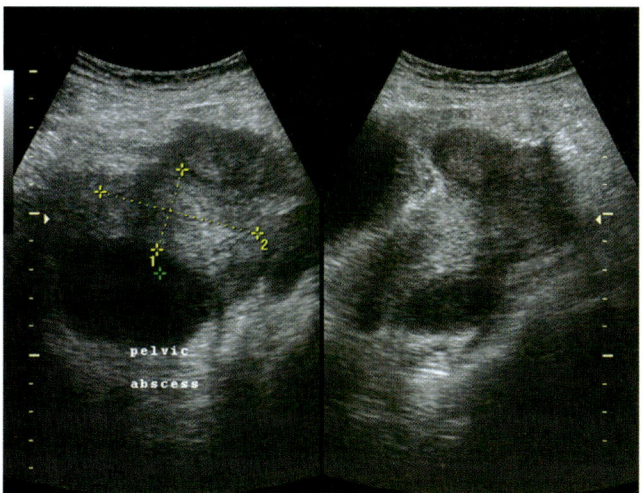

Fig. 19.2: Ultrasound image showing pelvic abscess

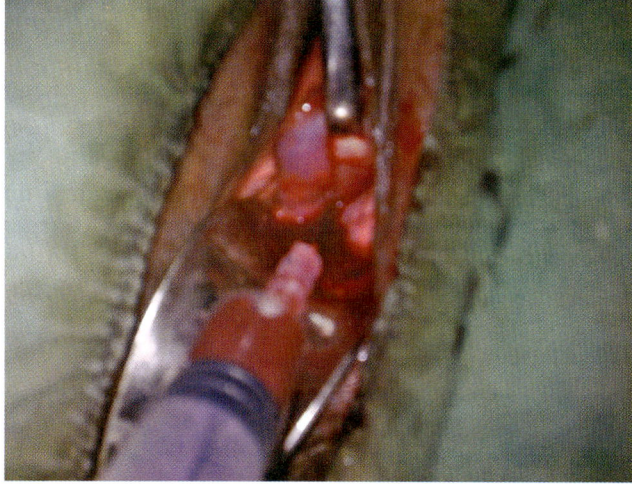

Fig. 19.3: Procedure of culdocentesis

Laparoscopy

Laparoscopy is considered to be the gold standard for the diagnosis of PID as it allows direct culture of the cul-de-sac and endosalpinx. However, it may not detect infection limited to the endometrium (Endometritis) or mild salpingitis. Tubal serosal hyperemia, tubal wall edema and purulent exudates from the fimbrial ends of the fallopian tubes and pooling in the cul-de-sac confirm laparoscopic diagnosis.

But laparoscopy is an operative procedure, it is used infrequently to make the diagnosis of PID, and clinical diagnosis of PID had a positive predictive value of 65–90% when compared with laparoscopy.

Culdocentesis

It is tapping of cul-de-sac which may be helpful in the diagnosis of suspected pelvic infection. Other conditions like ectopic pregnancy, which may simulate infection, can be ruled out by this simple procedure. It is indicated whenever peritoneal material is needed for diagnosis.

In this procedure pouch of Douglas is punctured with a long spinal needle to obtain a sample of the contents of the peritoneal cavity after vaginal membrane preparation with povidine iodine or similar agents. Contraindication of culdocentesis is a cul de sac mass or a fixed retroverted uterus (Fig. 19.3).

Differential Diagnosis

Acute salpingitis must be differentiated from: (a) Acute appendicitis, (b) Ectopic pregnancy, (c) Ruptured corpus luteal cyst with hemorrhage, (d) Diverticulitis, (e) Infected septic abortion, (f) Torsion of adnexal mass, (g) Degenerated leiomyoma, (h) Endometritis, (i) Acute urinary infection, (j) Bowel pathology like ulcerative colitis.

To differentiate

i. Urine or serum human chronic gonadotropins (hCG) to rule out early pregnancy complication like septic abortion or ectopic pregnancy.
ii. Cervical Gram stain or wet preparation of cervical discharge to see WBC and gram-negative diplococci.
iii. A history of anorexia preceding onset of periumbilical pain that eventually localizes to the right lower quadrant is more indicative of appendicitis than PID.
iv. Lower abdominal pain in woman, who is not sexually active, is unlikely to be PID.
v. Ultrasound can differentiate from early pregnancy and other adnexal mass.

Potential Long-term Complications of PID

i. **Infertility secondary to tubal and ovarian adhesion.** There is 20% incidence of infertility with one episode of PID. Risk of infertility is proportionately increased with each additional episode of PID.
ii. **Chronic pelvic pain** is noted in 20% of women with history of PID.
iii. Tubo-ovarian abscess.
iv. Increased risk of ectopic pregnancy.
v. Potential transmission of STD to other sexual partner.
vi. After rupture of tubo-ovarian abscess there can be serious morbidity as well mortality.

Epidemiology and Risk Factors and Prevention of PID

Despite better understanding of etiopathogenesis, improved diagnostic tool and availability of wide ranges of antimicrobial, PID is still a health hazard both in developed and developing countries. Incidence varies from 1 to 2% per year among sexually active women. Out of which 85% are spontaneous and 15% following operative procedure like D and C, insertion of IUD or hysterosalpingography.

Pelvic inflammatory disease is more common in younger women and teens, in lower socioeconomic status, and having high risk sexual behavior, among IUD users, and in women with a history of prior episode of PID. Teenagers have low hormonal and cell mediated immune response to genital tract infection. Besides this teenagers have wide area of cervical epithelium which allow colonization of *Chlamydia trachomatis* and *N. gonorrhoeae*.

Prevention

Barrier contraceptives prevent PID and other STDs as well. Oral contraceptive pills have been associated with lower risk of recurrence of PID because of thick cervical mucus plug and decreased menstrual blood loss. Abstinence in teenagers, sexual monogamy plays preventive role in PID in society.

Early diagnosis and full treatment of minimally symptomatic disease (cervicitis, urethritis) also prevents pelvic inflammatory disease. Aggressive screening of at risk population for STDs particularly *Gonorrhea* and *Chlamydia* will prevent development of PID in general population. Treatment of sexual partner will reduce the incidence of PID.

Treatment

Principle of treatment is that therapy regimen must provide empirical, broad spectrum coverage of likely pathogens including *N. gonorrhoeae, C. trachomatis*, gram-negative facultative bacteria, anaerobes, and streptococci. It is important to note that negative culture does not preclude upper reproductive tract disease and empirical therapy should be given as soon as a presumptive diagnosis is made. The primary goal of therapy is to eradicate bacteria, relieve symptoms, and prevent sequelae.

Outpatient Therapy–Criteria for Outpatient Care

The outpatient therapy for acute PID may be undertaken if:
i. Temperature is less than 39°C or 102.2°F.
ii. Lower abdominal findings are minimal.
iii. The patient is not toxic.
iv. The patient can take oral medication.

Outpatient Treatment Regimen

i. IUD removal if present.
ii. Analgesic and rest.
iii. Antibiotic: Recommended requirement by CDC are:
  a. Ofloxacin 400 mg twice daily or levofloxacin 500 mg orally once daily for 14 days + Clindamycin 450 mg orally 4 times a days or metronidazole 500 mg orally twice a day.
  b. Cefoxitin 2 gm with probenecid 1 gm x 1 dose orally concurrently or ceftriaxone 250 mg I/m x 1 dose, followed by Doxycycline 100 mg orally twice daily for 14 days with or without metronidazole 500 mg twice daily.

If response to therapy is not observed after 72 hours, the patient should be admitted for inpatient therapy. All male sexual partners of women treated for acute PID should be examined for STD and promptly treated with a regimen effective against uncomplicated gonococci or *chlamydia*.

Inpatient Regimen

Clindamycin 900 mg I/V every 8 hours + Gentamicin loading dose I/V or I/m (2 mg/kg body weight) followed by a maintenance dose = 1.5 mg/kg every 8 hours.

Alternative Parenteral Regimen

Levofloxacin 500 mg I/V once daily, with or without metronidazole 500 mg I/V every 8 hours or Ofloxacin 400 mg every 12 hours, with or without metronidazole 500 mg as above or Ampicillin / Sulbactam 3 gm I/V every 6 hours + Doxycycline 100 mg orally or I/V as above.

Hospitalized patients can be considered for discharge when:
i. Their fever has lyzed (<99.5°F for more than 24 hours).
ii. WBC count is normal.
iii. Rebound tenderness is absent.
iv. Repeat examination shows marked amelioration of pelvic organ tenderness.

Tubo-ovarian Abscess

An end stage process of acute PID, tubo-ovarian abscess diagnosed when a patient with PID has a pelvic mass that is palpable during bimanual examination. The condition reflects an agglutination of pelvic organs (tube, ovary, bowel) forming a palpable complex (Fig. 19.4).

Treatment

Abscess is treated with an antibiotic regimen administered in hospital. 75% of women with TO abscess respond to parenteral antimicrobial therapy alone. Failure of medical therapy suggests the need for drainage of abscess, which requires surgical exploration.

GENITAL TRACT TUBERCULOSIS

The incidence of genital tract tuberculosis varies widely with the social status of patient and her environment. In developing countries the incidence is approximately 10% in gynecology outpatient department. While in infertility clinic genital tuberculosis is as high as 5-10%. With prevalence of HIV infection, incidence of genital tuberculosis is also rising. The overall incidence of pelvic

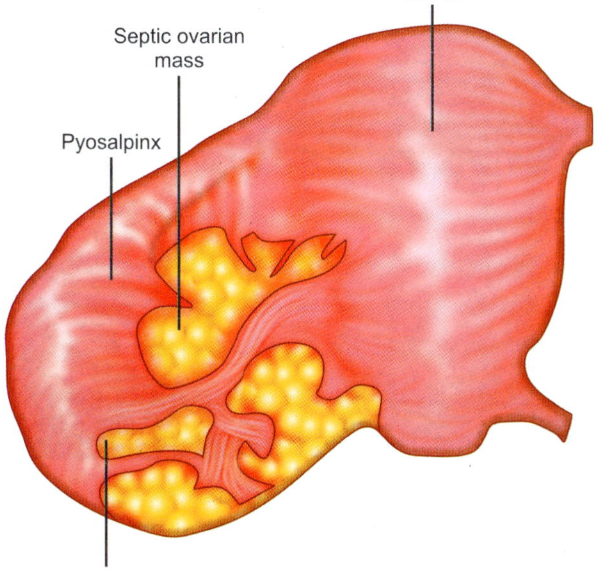

Chapter - 19 ♦ Pelvic Inflammatory Disease

Fig. 19.4: Tubo-ovarian abscess

Pathology of Pelvic Organs

Fallopian Tube

It is the most common site of infection in more than 90% of cases. Both the tubes are affected simultaneously. The initial site of infection is in the submucosal layer (Interstitial salpingitis) of the ampullary part of the tube. Variation of tuberculous salpingitis has been noted on laparotomy and laparoscopy. Increasing use of laparoscope has helped in diagnosing genital tuberculosis.

Tubercular Endosalpingitis

The infection may spread medially along the wall causing destruction of the muscles, which are replaced by fibrous tissues. The wall is thickened, sometimes calcified. There may be sequestration of fallopian tube giving characteristic beading appearance on HSG.

Where the mucosa is involved, it gets swollen and destroyed. The fimbrial ends are everted, pouting and may remain patent. This elongated and distended distal tube with the patent abdominal ostium gives the appearance of **'Tobacco Pouch'**. Occlusion of ostium can also occur due to adhesions.

There may be periodic spill of tubal exudates into the peritoneal cavity, causing frequent exacerbation with flare up of fever and abdominal pain. This flare up can follow hysterosalpingography. If both ends of fallopian tube are sealed by fibrosis, there is collection of cheesy material in the lumen and caseation in the wall of fallopian tube, causing **'Pyosalpinx'**.

There can be dense adhesion around such tuberculous pyosalpinges and present as abdominal lump – **Tubercular tubo-ovarian mass**. Though the content of tuberculous pyosalpinx may be sterile, pyosalpinges are particularly liable to recurrent attack of secondary bacterial infection which may present as acute or recurrent PID.

Occasionally, endosalpinx reveal a hyperplastic edematous pattern or granulomatous lesions which lead to occurrence of ectopic pregnancy (Fig. 19.5).

Tubercular Exosalpingitis

It is usually caused by direct extension of tuberculosis from adjacent organs. The peritoneum surface can be studded with miliary tuberculosis. There can be **frozen pelvis**, when plastic or adhesive type of peritonitis results in a dense inextricable mass of intestinal adhesion to such a degree that surgeon is not able to reach uterus or the adnexa. Any attempt to separate the adhesion in frozen pelvis may result in intestinal trauma and fistula formation.

Interstitial Tuberculous Salpingitis

In this the tube is thickened and indistinguishable from other pelvic inflammatory lesions.

tuberculosis in patients with pulmonary tuberculosis is approximately 5%. Prepubertal tuberculosis rarely results in genital tract infection.

Pathogenesis

The causative organism is *Mycobacterium tuberculosis* of human type. Very rarely the *bovine type* may affect the vulva. Genital tuberculosis is almost always secondary to primary infection elsewhere in the extragenital sites, such as lungs (50%), lymph nodes, urinary tracts, bones and joints.

The fallopian tubes are invariably the primary site of pelvic tuberculosis from where secondary spread occurs to other genital organs.

Mode of Spread

Blood stream: It is the most common method of spread accounting for almost 90% of genital tract tuberculosis. If the postprimary hematogenous spread coincides with the growth spurt of the pelvic vessels and the genital organs, the tubes in particular are likely to be effected. The infection remains dormant for a variable period of time until clinical manifestations appear.

Lymphatic or direct: The pelvic organs are involved directly or by lymphatics from the infected organs as peritoneum, blood or mesenteric nodes.

Ascending: Though rare and difficult to prove, sexual transmission from a male with urogenital tuberculosis is possible causing vulvar, vaginal or cervical lesion.

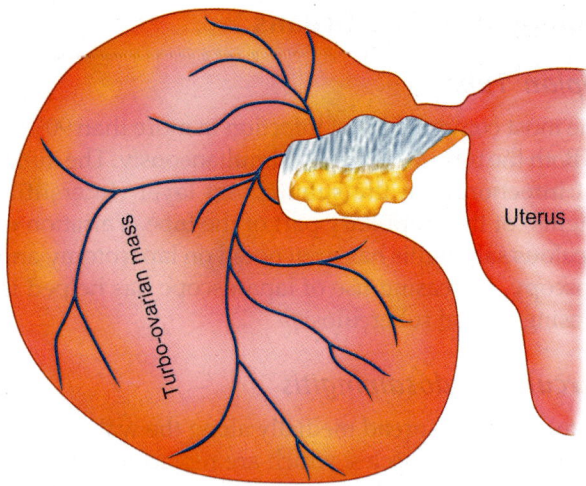

Fig. 19.5: Tubercular tubo-ovarian mass

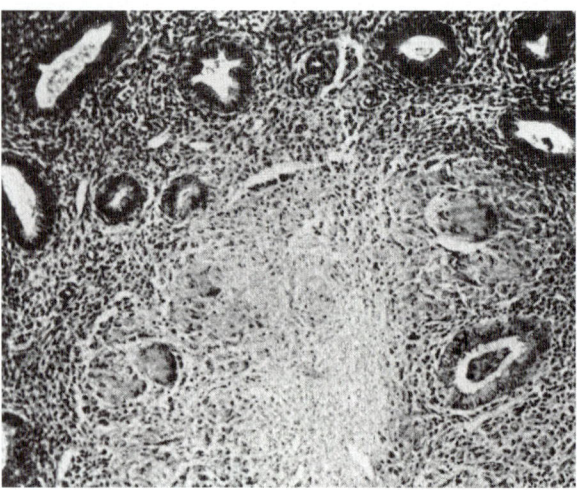

Fig. 19.6: Microscopic picture of tubercular endometritis showing giant cells in the stroma

Uterus

The endometrium is involved in 60% of cases. The infection can be from fallopian tube either by lymphatics or by direct spread through continuity. *Cornual ends are commonly affected due to their dual blood supply and anatomical proximity to tube*. The tubercle is situated in the basal layer of endometrium, which come to surface only premenstrually. So the *endometrial tissue for diagnosis of tuberculosis by microscopy, culture or PCR should be taken premenstrually*.

After the endometrium is shed at each menstruation, reinfection occurs from basal layer or from the fallopian tubes. Endometrial ulceration may lead to adhesion or synechiae formation so called **Asherman's syndrome**, which causes infertility, secondary amenorrhea and recurrent pregnancy loss. Rarely the infection spreads to the myometrium (2.5%) and if caseation occurs, it can result in pyometra, especially in postmenopausal women.

Ovaries

In 30% of cases ovaries are infected. The manifestations on laparoscopy or laparotomy are surface tubercles, adhesions, thickening of the capsule or even caseating abscess in the substance of ovary.

Cervix

In 5-15% of genital tuberculosis cervix is affected. Cervix can be ulcerative or nodular. Both may bleed to touch. Biopsy is essential to rule out carcinoma.

Vulva and Vagina

It is rare (less than 1%). The lesion may be ulcerative with undermined edges. Diagnosis can be made only by histology.

Pelvic Peritoneum

Pelvic peritoneum is involved in about 40-50% of cases. It can be of two types:
a. **Wet:** In wet variety there is ascites with straw colored fluid in peritoneal cavity. The parietal and visceral peritoneum is covered with numerous small tubercles.
b. **Dry:** In dry variety there is dense adhesions with bowel loops. On healing of wet variety there is adhesion formation.

Microscopic Appearance of Lesion

Microscopic picture of the lesion is typical *granuloma consists of infiltration of multinucleated giant cells surrounding a central area of caseation necrosis* (Fig. 19.6).

Diagnosis

Symptoms and Signs

About 10% of women with genital tuberculosis are **asymptomatic**. The only complaint may be **infertility** either primary or secondary due to tubal blockage, uterine synechiae and associated ovulatory dysfunction. In India 10% of infertile women have genital tuberculosis. The patient may also present with menstrual abnormality. In 50% of women menstrual function is normal. Patient may present as menorrhagia or irregular bleeding in early phase of disease due to ovarian involvement, pelvic congestion or endometrial involvement. Adolescent can present as **puberty menorrhagia** and rarely elderly women as **postmenopausal bleeding**. In later phase oligomenorrhea, hypomenorrhea and amenorrhea is more common and it can be the only presenting complaint. It is due to suppression of ovarian function or endometrial synechiae formation.

Chronic pelvic pain, dysmenorrhea can be present in 20-30% of cases. It is often associated with presence of tubo-ovarian mass and may be flared up by tubal patency test and secondary bacterial infection. Chronic pelvic pain is commonly associated with low grade fever, asthenia and weight loss.

Tuberculous peritonitis can present as gross ascites with fluid containing more than 3 gm of protein per 100 ml of peritoneal fluid which is characteristic of tuberculous peritonitis. Cervical or vaginal tuberculosis present as persistent vaginal discharge, not responding to conventional therapy and postcoital bleeding.

Pelvic tuberculosis is many times encountered in the course of gynecologic operations performed for other reasons. The distinguishing features of tuberculosis from other chronic PID are:
i. Extremely dense adhesions without plane of cleavage.
ii. Segmental dilatation of the fallopian tubes.
iii. Lack of occlusion of the tubes at the ostia.

General health is usually unaffected, sometimes there may be constitutional symptoms like weakness, low grade fever, anorexia, anemia, and night sweats. Abdominal findings may be negative or may feel doughy due to matted intestines. Tubercular encysted localized ascites may mimic an ovarian cyst.

Bimanual Pelvic Examination

Pelvic findings may be negative in 50% of cases. There may be thickened adnexa felt through fornices. At times there may be pelvic adnexal mass of varying sizes with restricted mobility.

Laboratory Findings

a. The best direct method of diagnosis in suspected case of genital tuberculosis is detection of acid fast bacteria by Ziehl-Neelsen stain followed by culture on L-Z (Lowenstein-Jenson) media, guinea pig inoculation and nucleic acid amplification.

The specimen can be taken from:
i. Menstrual blood
ii. Endometrial biopsy in premenstrual period
ii. Peritoneal biopsy if there is ascites
iv. Raised sedimentation rate, peripheral blood eosinophilia is suggestive.
v. Mantoux test: Strongly positive Mantoux test are additional evidence of tubercular infection. A negative test excludes tuberculosis.

X-ray Findings

Chest X-ray Film

A chest X-ray film should be taken in any patient with proved or suspected tuberculosis of other organs or tissue for evidence of healed or active pulmonary lesion.

Hysterosalpingography

In a proved case HSG is contraindicated for risk of reactivation of the lesion. HSG done as a routine workup in the investigation of infertility may reveal following picture:
1. Vascular or lymphatic extravasation of dye.
2. A rigid non-peristaltic pipe like tube called lead pipe appearance.
3. Beaded appearance of tube due to variation in filling density.
4. Tobacco Pouch appearance with blocked fimbrial ends.
5. Distal tube obstruction.
6. Bilateral cornual blockage.
7. Coiling of tubes or calcified shadows at places.
8. Tubal diverticula.
9. Irregular outline of uterus or **honey comb** appearance due to uterine synechiae.

Imaging

Abdominal and pelvic ultrasound, CT, and MRI is helpful in case of tuboadnexal mass or and ascites. But it cannot confirm the diagnosis.

Laparoscopy

On laparoscopy one can usually inspect tubercles in the pelvic organs and various characteristic of fallopian tube typical of tuberculosis. At the same time biopsy may be taken from peritoneal tubercles and fluid can be aspirated for cultures. For developing countries the physician should have high degree of suspicion for genital tract tuberculosis in cases of unexplained infertility, amenorrhea, chronic PID and tuboadnexal mass. Thorough investigation should be done to confirm or exclude genital tract tuberculosis (Fig. 19.7).

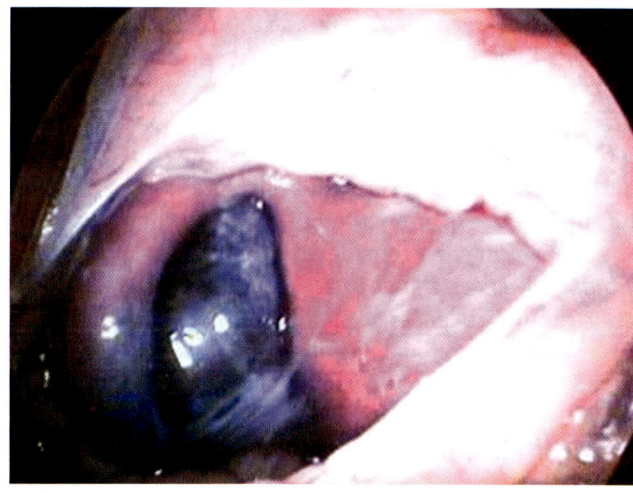

Fig. 19.7: Tuboadnexal mass as seen in laparoscopy suggestive of tuberculosis

Table 19.1: Antituberculous chemotherapy for initial treatment				
Drugs	Dosage	Action	Toxicity	Precaution
Isoniazid	5-10 mg/kg OD Max. 300 mg	Bactericidal	Hepatotoxic Peripheral neuropathy Hypersensitivity	Check liver function • Combine Pyridoxin (50 mg) daily
Rifampicin	10 mg/kg OD Max. 600 mg	Bactericidal	Hepatotoxic Fever Purpuric rash orange urine	• Liver enzyme monitoring • Oral contraceptive to be avoided
Pyrazinamide	20-25 mg/kg Max 2 gm	Bactericidal	Hepatitis Hyperuricemia GIT upset Arthralgia	• Monitor liver enzyme
Ethambutol	15-20 mg/kg OD Max. 2.5 gm	Bacteriostatic	Visual disturbance Optic neuritis Loss of visual acuity	• Ophthalmic examination prior to therapy

Differential Diagnosis

It should be differentiated from:
a. Pyogenic tubo-ovarian mass
b. Pelvic endometriosis
c. Adherent ovarian cyst
d. Chronic ectopic pregnancy
e. Chronic mycotic infection

Treatment

Medical Measures

Antitubercular chemotherapy is treatment of choice. To prevent the emergence of drug resistant strains, the **initial** therapy of tuberculous infection should include 4 drugs – **Isoniazid, Rifampicin, Pyrazinamide and Ethambutol.** Ethambutol is essential to those who have been treated previously or are immunocompromised (HIV positive individual).

Continuation phase: Treatment is continued with two drugs Isoniazid and Rifampicin for a period of 4 months. *The standard drug regimen is continued during pregnancy and lactation (Table 19.1).*

After completion of treatment, diagnostic endometrial curettage is to be done. If there is histological bacteriological evidence of infection, the treatment must be continued further. If these examinations are negative, the endometrium is examined at interval of six months.

A patient may be considered cured if *at least two reports including histological and bacteriological examination become negative.* 90-95% of patient respond well to therapy. In patients not responding to initial antituberculous chemotherapy the second line drugs has to be given (Table 19.2).

Surgical Measures

The primary mode of treatment for pelvic tuberculosis is medical therapy. Indications of surgical intervention are:

Table 19.2: Genital tract tuberculosis—Chemotherapeutic drug used in resistant cases of genital tuberculosis		
Drugs	Dosage	Side effects
1. Capreomycin	15-30 mg/kg I/M	• Auditory • Vestibular renal toxicity
2. Kanamycin	15-30 mg/kg I/M	As above
3. Ethionamides	15-30 mg/kg I/M	Hepatitis hypersensitivity
4. Para-amino-salicylic acid	150 mg/kg	Hepatitis
5. Cycloserine	15-20 mg (1 gm max)	Psychosis convulsion

a. Pelvic mass not responsive to medical therapy.
b. Resistant or reactivated pyosalpinx, pyometra or ovarian abscess.
c. Persistent menstrual irregularities.
d. Persistent pelvic pain.

It is mandatory that medical therapy should be attempted for 12-18 months prior to evaluation for surgery. Before and after surgery antitubercular treatment should be continued.

Types of Surgery

In selected cases isolated *excision of tubo-ovarian mass, drainage of pyometra and fistula repair* is done. In young patient if tubercular tubo-ovarian mass is accidentally discovered during laparotomy, only biopsy should be taken and medical therapy should be given.

In women who have no fertility desire, total hysterectomy with bilateral salpingo-oophorectomy should be done in cases of chronic pelvic pain, pelvic masses, unresponsive menstrual abnormality and unresponsive cervical tuberculosis in cover of full antitubercular drug treatment.

Prognosis

The prognosis for life and health is excellent, if chemotherapy is instituted promptly. Prognosis for fertility is unfavorable. Pregnancy is uncommon (5-10%) and chances of ectopic pregnancy are approximately 40%. Abortion and preterm labor is also common.

ART can be of help in genital tuberculosis, but success rate of ART procedure is lower in these patients due to implantation defects.

POSTOPERATIVE INFECTION

Surgical Site Infection (SSI) Classification

CDC has recommended classification of surgical site infection in two categories:
a. Incisional space—i. Superficial, ii. Deep
b. Organ space

Vaginal cuff infections are considered in the superficial incisional class and parametritis is classified as a deep incisional class. In contrast pelvic infection as adnexal infection, pelvic abscess or infected pelvic hematoma falls into category of organ/space infection.

Diagnosis

The most frequent definition for *febrile morbidity* is an oral temperature of ≥ 38°C on two or more occasions, four or more hours apart and 24 or more hours following surgery.

It is commonly seen after hysterectomy (30–40%), usually is not associated with other signs of infection and *does not require antimicrobial therapy*. A remote non-surgical site may also serve as a cause of fever like I/V site phlebitis, urinary tract infection so women developing febrile morbidity should be thoroughly examined at surgical as well non surgical site.

Pain

Operative site pain following surgery is normal. Patients who develop an operative site infection report increasing pain in SSI area and increasing tenderness is present on physical examination. For most patients with pelvic infection there is deep lower abdominal or pelvic pain. Common site of infection requiring antimicrobial therapy are parametrium and vaginal surgical margin. Less commonly there can be pelvic abscess and infected pelvic hematoma.

Signs

Abdominal palpation is an integral part of SSI diagnosis in gynecology. Mild tenderness is expected after surgery and decreases quickly. Women, who develop pelvic cellulitis or cuff cellulitis, will have increasing tenderness at gentle depression of the lower abdominal wall. Over the infected area tenderness may be bilateral but usually more marked on one side. Peritoneal signs are not present.

In absence of increasing lower abdominal pain and tenderness, bimanual examination is not necessary. But if there is fever with new onset pain and tenderness, gentle bimanual examination is required to identify the infection site and to exclude or diagnose a mass. If patient is too tender, vaginal sonography can be added. Bowel function is usually not altered by soft tissue cellulitis but may be with pelvic abscess or infected pelvic hematoma.

Investigations

a. *Laboratory finding:* Serial complete blood count usually demonstrates leukocytosis and occasionally concealed hemorrhage can be detected. Urinalysis can be of help to exclude or confirm urinary tract infection as a sole or added reason for febrile morbidity. Usually pelvic infection following hysterectomy is polymicrobial and it is difficult to identify true pathogen by culture. So surgeon should not wait for culture results before starting empiric broad spectrum antibiotic therapy. However, if initial therapy is partially effective or unsuccessful then a culture will more predictably identify pathogens. Since, therapy will have eradicated other species the antibiotic regimen then can be changed according to culture result.
b. *X-ray finding:* Chest films are unrevealing in most cases but can be useful if pulmonary complications are suspected.
c. *Ultrasonography:* USG can be helpful if hematoma or tubo-ovarian mass is suspected.

Specific Postoperative Infections

a. Vaginal cuff cellulitis
b. Adnexal infection
c. Ovarian abscess or infected pelvic hematoma
d. Pelvic abscess
e. Abdominal site infection

Within two days following hysterectomy the surgical margin of the vagina appears hyperemic and edematous and there is almost always purulent or seropurulent exudate regardless of patient's clinical condition. For this there is no need to antimicrobial therapy.

Only few women who require therapy are those who usually present after hospital discharge with mild but increasing new onset lower abdominal pain and have a yellowish vaginal discharge. There is more than normal tenderness of vaginal cuff.

Oral antimicrobial therapy with a single broad spectrum antibiotic is appropriate. A patient should be reevaluated to assess therapeutic efficacy.

Pelvic Cellulitis

It is most common infection and develops when inflammatory process spreads into the parametrial regions resulting in lower abdominal pain, regional tenderness and temperature elevation (Fig. 19.5).

Adnexal Infection

This is also common infection and present as pelvic cellulitis. But the area of tenderness is at the adnexal area. This may develop after tubal ligation or other adnexal surgery as ectopic pregnancy.

Ovarian Abscess, Infected Pelvic Hematoma

A rare but life-threatening complication following primarily vaginal hysterectomy is ovarian abscess. In this the ovaries are in close proximity to vaginal surgical margin. There is physiological cuff cellulitis but when ovulation occurs, bacteria in area gain access to ovulation site and corpus luteum. Patients usually present after 10 days of surgery with acute unilateral abdominal pain which becomes generalized later on.

Exploratory laparotomy is necessary immediately with pre- and postoperative antibiotic, evacuation of the abscess and removal of the affected ovary and adjacent fallopian tube. Tubo-ovarian abscess on the other hand can be managed medically with intravenous antimicrobials and surgery is not required unless rupture follows. Antimicrobial therapy should be continued until a woman has been afebrile for 48-72 hours.

Pelvic Abscess

Pelvic abscess not involving an adnexal structure is uncommon but can occur if there is no preoperative prophylactic antibiotic and open vaginal cuff technique is used. Signs and symptoms of pelvic abscess are more central and a mass is noted centrally after 7-10 days of surgery. In order admission with combination intravenous antibiotic is necessary until a woman has been afebrile for 48-72 hours. Sometimes, opening of vaginal surgical margins is required to allow drainage witch aids in treatment.

Abdominal Incision Infection

Risk factors for abdominal incision infections are – **obesity, occlusive dressings, excessive use of electro-surgical coagulation, passive drains, and inflammation in skin at time of surgery**. Erythema and heat are first physical signs. There may be hematoma or serous discharge from wound.

Treatment

Drainage and local care are usually the basis of successful therapy. Wet to dry dressings stimulate fibroblastic proliferation and development of healthy granulation tissue. Several solutions can be used with mechanical debridement of wound margins if necessary. At this stage secondary closure can be considered.

If there is soft tissue cellulitis adjacent to the incision, antibiotic therapy is required (Table 19.3).

Table 19.3: Recommended empirical antibiotic regimen for postsurgical infection

Regimen	Dosage
Single agent intravenous	
Cephalosporin	
Cefoxitin	2 g every 6 hours
Cefoxetan	2 g every 12 hours
Cefotaxime	1-2 g every 8 hours
Penicillin with or without β-lactamase inhibitor	
Piperacillin	4 g every 6 hours
Piperacillin/tazobactam	3.375 g every 6 hours
Ampicillin/sulbactam	3 g every 6 hours
Ticarcillin/clavulanate	3.1 g every 4 to 6 hours
Carbapenems	
Imipenem/cilastatin	500 mg every 8 hours
Meropenem	500 mg every 8 hours
Ertapenem	1 g once daily
Combination agent intravenous	
Metronidazole	Loading dose 15 mg/kg, maintenance dose 7.5 mg/kg very 6 hours
Ampicillin	2 g every 6 hours
Gentamicin	3-5 mg/kg once daily
Clindamicin	900 mg every 8 hours
Gentamicin	900 mg every 8 hours
Gentamicin with or without Ampicillin	900 mg every 8 hours
Oral agents	
Amoxicillin/clavulanate	875 mg twice daily
Levofloxacin	500 mg once daily
Clindamycin	300 mg every 6 hours
Metronidazole	500 mg every 6 hours

Prevention of SSI

Following measures may be helpful to prevent SSI:
i. Preoperative insertion of antibacterial vaginal cream or suppositories especially if cervicitis, bacterial vaginosis is present.
ii. Preparation of vagina with povidone iodine just prior to surgery.
iii. Meticulous attention to hemostasis at operation and gentle handling of tissues. Use of large strangulating hemostatic suture material should be avoided. Non-reactive suture material should be used.
iv. If hemostasis is less than desirable, suction drainage of that area should be accomplished.
v. Preoperative antibiotic prophylaxis has been shown to reduce pelvic infectious morbidity following vaginal and abdominal hysterectomy.
vi. Severe and more advanced infection may be prevented by early diagnosis, drainage and prompt treatment of mild infections.

Chapter - 19 ♦ Pelvic Inflammatory Disease

MULTIPLE CHOICE QUESTIONS

1. Most common cause of tubal block in India is:
   a. Gonorrhoea
   b. *Chlamydia*
   c. Tuberculosis
   d. Bacterial vaginosis

   Ans. c

2. TB endometritis is caused by:
   a. Hematogenous spread
   b. Lymphatic spread
   c. Retrograde spread
   d. Direct spread

   Ans. a

3. Tuberculosis of female genital tract is most common in age group:
   a. Below 10 years
   b. 10-20 years
   c. 20-30 years
   d. Above 60 years

   Ans. c

4. The most common site of genital tuberculosis in women is:
   a. Tubes
   b. Uterus
   c. Cervix
   d. Vagina

   Ans. a

5. The mot common complication of pregnancy after complete treatment of genital tuberculosis is:
   a. Abortion
   b. Ectopic pregnancy
   c. Malpresentation
   d. IUD

   Ans. b

6. The symptoms of pelvic tuberculosis can be:
   a. Foul smelling vaginal discharge
   b. Amenorrhea
   c. Infertility
   d. Dysmenorrhea

   Ans. b,c

7. The most sensitive method for detecting cervical *Chlamydia trachomatis* infection is:
   a. Direct fluorescent antibody test
   b. Enzyme immunoassay
   c. PCR
   d. Culture on irradiated MC ConKey cells

   Ans. c

20 Infertility

May be God created desert, so that man could appreciate the date trees.

General Consideration

The inability to conceive after 1 year of unprotected intercourse of reasonable frequency is termed infertility. It can be subdivided into *Primary infertility* that is there is no prior pregnancy and *Secondary infertility* which refers to infertility which follow at least one prior conception. Conversely *Fecundability* is expressed as the likelihood of conception per month of exposure. It is about 0.2 or 20% in normally fertile couple. This figure is particularly important in trying to understand the success rate for treatment modalities offered to infertility couple.

Fecundity is the probability of achieving a live birth in one menstrual cycle. Fertility as well infertility of a women or couple is best perceived as fecundability. *Sterility* applies an intrinsic inability to achieve pregnancy whereas *infertility* implies a decrease in the ability to conceive and synonymous with sub fertility.

Epidemiology

Approximately 85–90% of healthy young couples conceive within a year therefore 10–15% of couples are affected with infertility. Although the prevalence of infertility is believed to have remained relatively stable during the past 40 years, demand for infertility evaluation and treatment has increased considerably.

Timing for Infertility Evaluation

It is generally agreed that an infertility evaluation should be considered in any couple that has failed to conceive in 1 year. Of note even without treatment approximately half of women will conceive in the second year of attempting. There are some clinical situations when evaluation should be considered sooner for, e.g. history of anovulatory women, diagnosed PCOS in adolescence, history of pelvic inflammatory disease. Furthermore as fecundability is highly age related, so in women older than 35, evaluation should be performed after 6 months.

Etiology of Infertility

Conception requires a complex sequence of events which includes ovulation, ovum pickup by a fallopian tube, fertilization, transport of fertilized ovum into the uterus and implantation into a receptive uterine cavity. With male infertility, sperms of adequate number and quality must be deposited at the cervix near the time of ovulation. *Understanding of these critical events guides the clinician for stepwise evaluation.*

Overall etiology for infertility can be found in 80% of cases with an even distribution of male and female factors, including couples with multiple factors. Male factor is the only cause of infertility in 20% of infertile couples but it may be a contributing factor in as many as 30–40% of cases. Ovulatory dysfunction (20%), tubal/peritoneal factor (20%), cervical factors (5-15%) comprise majority of female factor infertility (Fig. 20.1). In 15-20% the etiology can not be found and diagnosis of unexplained infertility is made. Causes of infertility are summarized in Table 20.1.

The success rate of treatment for infertility depends on a variety of factors, which includes cause of infertility, women's age, duration of infertility, and treatment modality.

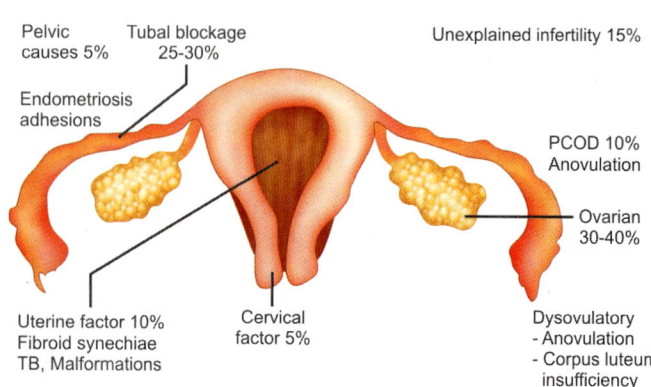

Fig. 20.1: Female factors of infertility

CHAPTER -20 ♦ Infertility

Table 20.1: Causes of Infertility

Male factor
- *Endocrine disorders*
  - Hypothalamic dysfunction (Kallmann's syndrome)
  - Pituitary failure (tumor, radiation, surgery)
  - Hyperprolactinemia (drug, tumor)
  - Exogenous androgens
  - Thyroid disorders
  - Adrenal hyperplasia
- *Anatomic disorders*
  - Congenital absence of vas deferens
  - Obstruction of vas deferens
  - Congenital abnormalities of ejaculatory system
- *Abnormal spermatogenesis*
  - Chromosomal abnormalities
  - Mumps orchitis
  - Cryptorchidism
  - Chemical or radiation exposure
- *Abnormal motility*
  - Absent cilia (Kartagener's syndrome)
  - Varicocele
  - Antibody formation
- *Sexual dysfunction*
  - Retrograde ejaculation
  - Impotence
  - Decrease libido

Ovulatory factor
- *Central defects*
  - Chronic hyperandrogenemic anovulation
  - Hyperprolactinemia (drug, tumor, empty sella)
  - Hypothalamic insufficiency
  - Pituitary insufficiency (trauma, tumor, congenital)
- *Peripheral defects*
  - Gonadal dysgenesis
  - Premature ovarian failure
  - Ovarian tumor
  - Ovarian resistance
- *Metabolic disease*
  - Thyroid disease
  - Liver disease
  - Renal disease
  - Obesity
  - Androgen excess, adrenal or neoplastic

Pelvic factor
- *Infection*
  - Appendicitis
  - Pelvic inflammatory disease
  - Uterine adhesions (Asherman's syndrome)
- *Endometriosis*
- *Structural abnormalities*
  - Diethylstilbestrol (DES) exposure
  - Failure of normal fusion of the reproductive tract
  - Myoma

Cervical factor
- *Congenital*
  - DES exposure
  - Mullerian duct abnormality
- *Acquired*
  - Surgical treatment
  - Infection

Not uncommonly, infertility treatment does not actually make the difference between conceiving and not conceiving but allows for conception in more immediate feature.

Psychological Aspects

Infertility poses an emotional crisis for a couple and diagnosis of infertility is a question on self-image, sexuality and relationship. The couple may progress through stages of denial, anger, grief and resolution. Recognition of these stages may assist the practitioner in providing appropriate support and counseling or referral for the additional therapy.

GUIDING PRINCIPLES IN THE EVALUATION OF INFERTILITY

From the beginning, the evaluation of infertility focuses on the couple and not on one or other partner. In management following four basic aims should be kept in mind:

a. To identify the specific cause or causes of infertility and correct that causes whenever possible. With proper evaluation and treatment, the majority of women will conceive.
b. To provide accurate information and to dispel misinformation commonly acquired from friends and mass media.
c. To provide emotional support and resolve psychological stress.
d. To guide the couple for advanced technique as on ART, use of donor gametes or adoption, in whom standard form of treatment do not achieve success. Counseling must be an ongoing process. Regular consultations to review and critique results and to outline recommendation for further evaluation and treatment are necessary to ensure that all of the couple's medical, emotional and financial needs and concerns are effectively addressed in a timely fashion.

New Patient Assessment

The initial clinical assessment should begin with a thorough history of both the partners. Table 20.2 outlines the facts to be noted for female and male. The history will guide the physical examination beyond general evaluation. For example, a bimanual examination is done to detect adnexal mass in patients having history of PID. Rectovaginal examination is done to detect endometriotic nodularity if there is history of severe dyspareunia. Laboratory, radiological and further test assess factors for fertility that is sperm, oocyte, transport and implantation.

EVALUATION OF MALE FACTORS

Physiology of Spermatogenesis

During evaluation of male infertility patient, it is critical to understand the basics of male reproductive physiology.

Table 20.2: Medical history for male and female factor infertility
Female
In utero diethylstilbestrol (DES) exposure
History of pubertal development
Present menstrual characteristic (length, duration, molimina)
Contraceptive history
Prior pregnancies, outcomes
Previous surgeries, especially pelvic
Prior infection
History of abnormal Papanicolaou (Pap) smear, treatment
Drugs and medications
General health (diet, weight stability, exercise patterns, review of systems)
Male
Congenital abnormalities
Undescended testes
Prior paternity
Frequency of intercourse
Exposure to toxins
Previous surgery
Previous infections, treatment
Drugs and medications
General health (diet, exercise, review of systems)
Decreased frequency of shaving

Testes are analogs to ovary. Testes have two functions: (a) Generation of mature germ cells (sperm), (b) production of male hormones testosterone.

The seminiferous tubules are composed of *germ cells called Spermatogonia and Sertoli cells*. Tight junction between the Sertoli cells form a diffusion barrier known as blood testis barrier (similar to blood-brain barrier) that protects the germ cells from antigen, antibodies and environmental toxins. In between seminiferous tubules Leydig cells are located called interstitial cells, which are responsible for steroid hormone testosterone production (Fig. 20.2A).

Spermatogenesis

In testis there are stem cells that allow ongoing production of mature germ cells throughout a male's life. In a fertile male, approximately 100-200 million sperms are produced each day. As spermatogenesis begins, the diploid (46 chromosomes) spermatogonia grow to become primary spermatocytes, each of which gives rise to 2 spermatids during the second meiotic divisions. After that each spermatid gradually matures to become mature spermatozoa. Approximately half of all potential sperm production is lost during meiosis (Fig. 20.2B).

Production of sperm requires approximately 70 days in completing. An additional 12 to 21 days is needed for sperm to be transported into the epididymis, where they further mature and develop motility. *It is significant to note that due to this prolonged developmental period the result of semen analysis* reflect the event over the past 3 months not a single point in time. To fertilize an oocyte, human sperm must undergo a process known as *capacitation*. Capacitation results in sperm hyperactivation (i.e. extreme increase in movement) as well as the ability of sperm to release acrosomal contents which allow penetration of the Zona Pellucida.

Normal spermatogenesis depends on gene on 'Y' chromosome. Spermatogenesis is directed by genes on the 'Y' chromosomes with important contribution by autosomal genes so genetic abnormalities also adversely effect this process.

Hormonal LH from the anterior pituitary gland stimulates production of testosterone by Leydig cells. FSH increase LH receptors on the Leydig cells and increased

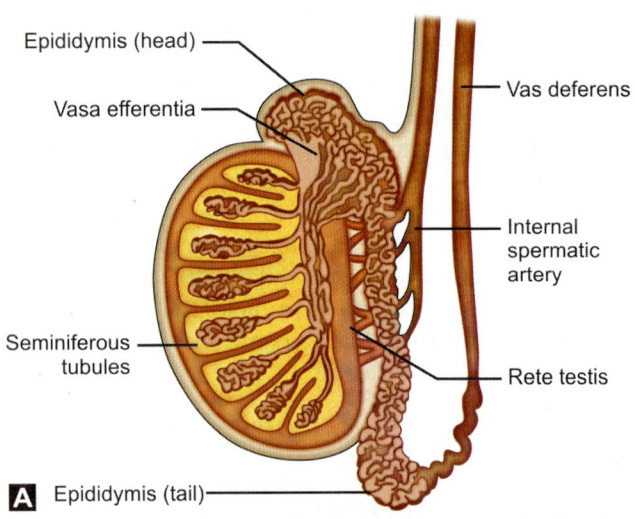

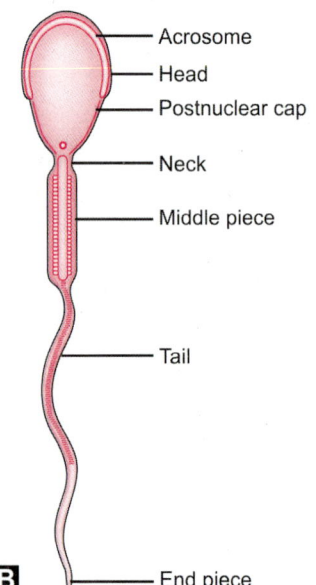

Figs 20.2A and B: (A) Normal anatomy of testis; (B) Normal sperm

production of androgen binding protein. Androgen binding protein binds testosterone in seminiferous tubules.

Testicular volume often reflects spermatogenesis and normal volume is between 15 and 25 ml. The majority of this volume is provided by seminiferous tubules and so decreased testicular volume is a strong indication of abnormal spermatogenesis. Beside this though advancing male age have an impact on fertility, it is probably insignificant compared with the change in women.

Semen Analysis

Semen analysis is a core test in evaluation of male fertility status. For this test man is asked to refrain from ejaculation for 2–3 days and specimen should be received in the lab within 1 hour of collection. The semen undergoes liquefaction, due to conjugative action from the liquid contributing via prostrate gland. Liquefaction normally takes 5-20 minutes and allows more accurate evaluation of the sperm contained in seminal fluid.

Ideally two semen sample repeated by at least one month should be analyzed. The reference values for the semen analysis are shown in Table 20.3.

The semen parameters in normal fertile males vary significantly and the first response to any abnormal results should be to wait an interval of at least one month and repeat the test. If the semen analysis reveals abnormal or borderline parameters, the history should be reviewed for any proximate cause of an abnormality. One should keep in mind that the cycles of spermatogenesis takes about 74 days. A male with less than 5 million sperm per ml warrants an endocrinologic evaluation including FSH, LH and testosterone or a Karyotype in selective cases. The patients should be referred to an urologist with a special interest and infertility specialist.

DNA Assays

Several tests, including sperm chromatin structure assay (SCSA), comet, and terminal DVTP nick end labeling (TUNEL) have been developed to quantify the damage to DNA or chromatin. But these assays are not in wide clinical use.

Other Tests

More detailed assessment of sperm function may include **postcoital test, antibody studies, sperm penetration test**. Such assessments are designed to investigate more subtle problems or abnormalities not revealed by routine semen analysis. Though they can be helpful in some cases, the sensitivity of these assays is still uncertain, and varies with particular laboratory, where the test is performed.

Postcoital Test

Cervical mucus is a heterogeneous secretion containing more than 90% water. It has intrinsic properties as stretchability (spinnbarkeit), ferning and thin watery consistency. It facilitates reservoir for the sperm. Functional sperm must interact normally with the egg and surrounding cells in the uterine tube. It is estimated that less than 1000 sperm will be found in the environment of the oocyte. The initial interaction of sperm and female genital tract can be determined by postcoital examination of the cervical mucus **(Sim-Hunner test)**.

The purpose of postcoital test is to determine the number of active spermatozoa in the cervical mucus and length of sperm survival (in hours) after intercourse. The test should be performed as close to ovulation as possible. Cervical mucus is aspirated with syringe within 6–8 hours of after coitus and checked under the microscope for number and motility of sperm. **If there is less than 10 motile sperm per high power field, it is considered abnormal**. It has limited use in infertility workup and its value has not been proven.

Sperm Penetration Assay

These assays compare the ability of sperm to penetrate the zona free hamster egg. The value of this test is controversial.

Sperm Antibodies

Sperm possess antigen and semen may contain antibodies which includes sperm agglutinating, sperm immobilizing or cytotoxic antibodies. These antibodies can be measured in semen or in serum. *The immunobead test mostly used and considered positive when only 20% or more of motile spermatozoa have immunobead binding.* However, the test is considered to be clinically significant when 50% of sperm are coated with immunobeads.

Hormonal Evaluation of the Male

Hormonal testing in the male is analogous to endocrine testing in an anovulatory female. **It is only recommended if sperm concentration is less than 10 million/ml**.

Table 20.3: Analysis—Normal reference values

Character	Normal reference values
Volume	1.5-5.0 ml
pH	>7.2
Viscosity	<3 (scale 0-4)
Sperm concentration	>20 million/ml
Total sperm number	>40 million/ejaculate
Percent motility	>50%
Forward progression	>2 scale (0-4)
Normal morphology	>50% normal
	>30% normal
	>14% normal
Round cells	<5 million/ml
Sperm agglutination	<2 scale (0-3)

It includes serum FSH and testosterone level. *Elevated FSH and low testosterone level gives evidence of testicular failure.* Low FSH and low testosterone level are consistent with hypothalamic dysfunction as Kallmann's syndrome.

Beside this *elevated serum prolactin level and thyroid dysfunction* impact spermatogenesis and are the most likely endocrinopathies to be detected.

Genetic Testing

Genetic abnormalities are relatively common causes of abnormal semen characteristic. *Approximately 15% of azoospermic men and 5% of severely oligospermic men will have an abnormal karyotype.*

As they can have implication for health of patient or their offspring, karyotyping testing should be obtained on all azoospermic and severely oligospermic men ranging from 3–10 million sperm per ml. *Klinefelter's syndrome has 47 'XXY' finding, observed in 1 in 500 men of general population and accounts for 1–2% of male infertility.* Classically they are tall, undervirilized and have gynecomastia and small firm testes.

Microdeletion of 'Y' chromosome - approximately 15% of men with severe oligospermia or azoospermia will have small deletion in 'Y' chromosome called azoospermia factor region. Obstructive azoospermia may be due to **Congenital Bilateral absence of the vas deferens (CBAVD).** Approximately 70–85% of men with **CBAVD** will be found to have mutation in CFTR gene.

Conventionally essentially all men with clinical cystic fibrosis will have CBAVD. Testicular function in these men is usually normal and adequate sperm may be obtained by epididymal aspiration to achieve pregnancy through IVF.

Careful genetic counseling and testing the female partner for carrier status is critical in these situations.

Testicular Biopsy

Evaluation of a severely oligospermic or azoospermic male may include either open or percutaneous testicular biopsy to determine whether viable sperms are present in seminiferous tubules. The biopsy specimen can be cryopreserved for further extraction of sperm during an IVF cycle. Thus the testicular biopsy can have diagnostic, prognostic and therapeutic value.

History and Physical Examination of Male Partner

The male partner should be questioned regarding pubertal development and sexual dysfunction – erectile as well ejaculatory. STD or frequent genital urinary infection should be asked as they can result in obstruction of vas deferens. History of mumps, cryptorchidism, testicular torsion or testicular trauma may suggest the presence of abnormal spermatogenesis. Medical history of Varicocele, hypertension, diabetes mellitus and neurologic disorders may be associated with erectile dysfunction, or retrograde ejaculation. Smoking, tobacco, alcohol, illicit drugs, environmental toxin and various medications like cimatidine, erythromycin, tetracycline and spironolactone can adversely affect semen parameter. Increasing use of anabolic steroids also decreases sperm production by suppressing the production of intratesticular testosterone. Though the effect of many medication are irreversible, anabolic steroid abuse may lead to lasting or even permanent damage to testicular function.

Examination of Male Patient

Gynecologist at minimum should understand the primary focus of the examination. One should see for secondary sexual character as beard growth, axillary and pubic hair. *Gynecomastia may suggest Klinefelter's syndrome.* **Testicular length should be at least 4 cm**. Small testes are unlikely to be producing normal sperm count. Epididymis should be soft and non tender to exclude chronic infection. Epididymic fullness suggests obstruction of vas deferens. The pampiniform plexuses of veins should be palpated. Congenital bilateral absence of vas deferens is associated with mutation in the gene responsible for cystic fibrosis.

EVALUATION OF FEMALE FACTOR

History

a. *Gynecological history:* Gynecological history should be complete regarding menstrual history, prior contraceptive use, coital frequency and duration of infertility. History suggestive of endometriosis, PID, previous pregnancy, complication should be elicited.
b. *Medical history:* One should elicit symptoms of hyperprolactinemia, thyroid disorder, androgen excess, prior chemotherapy, pelvic radiation.
c. *Surgical history:* Surgical history should focus on pelvic and abdominal surgery for ruptured appendix or ovarian tumor which gives clue to cause of infertility.
d. *Medication:* NSAID may adversely effect ovulation. Use of herbal remedies should be discouraged.
e. *Social:* Lifestyle, eating habits, exposure to toxin, smoking, tobacco, and drug and alcohol consumption should be noted, which have the adverse effect on fertility as well infertility management. Body mass Indices ≥ 25 or <17, is related to abnormalities in GnRH and gonadotropins secretion.

Examination of Female Patient

Vital signs, height and weight should be recorded. Hirsutism, alopecia, acne indicates hyperandrogenism. Acanthosis nigricans indicate insulin resistance. Thyroid abnormalities should be noted. Pelvic examination is particularly informative. **Large uterus may reflect leiomyomas whereas fixed uterus raises the doubt of endometriosis or prior pelvic infection.** All women should have a normal PAP smear test on preceding treatment.

Evaluation for Specific Causes of Infertility

Infertility evaluation can be simplified with confirmation of: (a) Ovulation, (b) Tubal and pelvic factor, (c) Cervical factor.

Ovulatory factor

Ovulatory dysfunction is responsible for approximately 20–25% infertility cases and 40% of female factors infertility. Regular menstrual cycle, with Mittel Schmerz moniliminal symptoms and mild dysmenorrhea suggest ovulatory cycles. Signs and symptoms of systemic disease particularly thyroid disorders, hyperandrogenism may effect ovulation. The extensive exercise, weight gain or weight loss and complaints of hot flushes suggest endocrine or ovulatory dysfunction. Confirmation of ovulation can be done in following ways:

a. *Basal body temperature:* Progesterone has a central thermogenic effect and elevates basal body temperature by an average of 0.8°C during the luteal phase. Basal body temperature should be taken shortly after awakening in the morning. Biphasic monthly temperature pattern is confirmatory evidence of ovulation but the absence of a biphasic pattern may be seen in ovulatory cycles.

b. *Pelvic ultrasonography:* It gives evidence for ovulation. In the follicular phase, the developing follicles can be monitored to maturation and subsequent rupture. *The disappearance of follicle and free fluid in the cul-de-sac document ovulation* (Figs 20.3A and B).

c. *Ovulation predictive kits:* Ovulation occurs 24-36 hours after the onset of the LH surge and 10–24 hours after the peak of the LH surge. The patient can use commercially available urinary LH kit for detection of LH surge and predicting ovulation. The kits can be used to timed intercourse or intrauterine insemination.

d. *Serum progesterone:* Ovulation can also be tested by measurement of mid luteal phase serum progesterone level. Value above 4–6 ng/ml is highly correlated with ovulation and subsequent progesterone production by the corpus luteum.

e. *Endometrial biopsy:* The endometrial biopsy near the end of luteal phase shows secretory endometrium in luteal phase. Generally biopsy is performed 2–3 days before expected onset of menstrual cycle and histological finding should be within 1–2 days determined by morphology of glands and stroma. *Discrepancy in histological and menstrual dating is termed an out of phase biopsy.* Luteal phase defect is a histologic diagnosis made when the endometrium lag 3 days or more behind the expected pattern at the time of endometrial biopsy. But this test has intraobserver and interobserver variability and there is real risk of disrupting a normal conception, if couple has not been advised abstinence in that cycle.*

f. *Cervical mucus:* Within 48 hours of ovulation, the cervical mucus changes under the influence of progesterone to become thicker, tacky and cellular, with loss of crystalline fern pattern on drying.

Female Ageing and Ovulatory Dysfunction

Ovarian Reserve

Ovarian reserve should be evaluated in women older then 35 year of age who are seeking infertility treatment. **Day 2 evaluation of the level of FSH and estradiol** in the early follicular phase may provide helpful guidelines.

Mild elevation in either FSH or estradiol may precede overt ovulatory dysfunction but still indicates a poor prognosis for successful pregnancy. **High level of FSH indicates poor ovarian reserve.**

Paradoxically despite overall depletion of ovarian follicles, estrogen level in older women will be elevated early in cycle due to increased stimulation of ovarian steroidogenesis by elevated gonadotropin.

Anti Müllerian Hormone(AMH): AMH is a member of transforming growth factor beta (TGF-β)family, produced by granulosa cells. The highest level of AMH is present in granulosa cells of secondary, preantral and small antral follicles up to 6 mm. Thus, serum AMH strongly

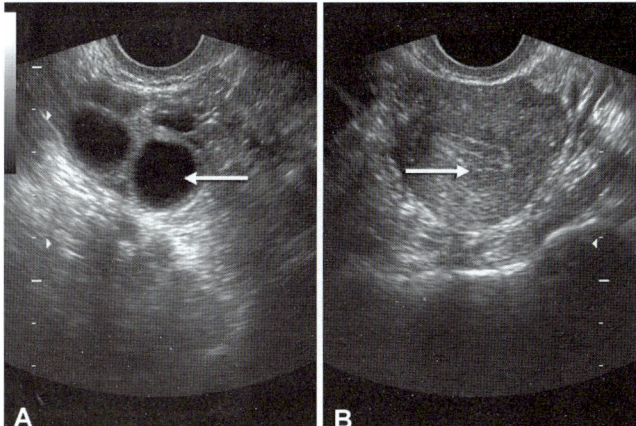

Figs 20.3A and B: Ultrasound image showing: (A) Follicular development; (B) Triple layer proliferative endometrium

---

* It is interesting to note that impressive advances are being made in our understanding of timing of protein expression in endometrial gland and stroma. In the future EB may again become part of infertility evaluation, if expression pattern of protein prove to be predictive of endometrial receptivity.

correlates with age and becomes undetectable at menopause. Serum AMH strongly correlates with number of antral follicles. The major advantage over other markers of ovarian reserve (FSH and estradiol) are that it is cycle independent, so blood sampling for AMH can be done at any period of cycle.

Clomiphene Citrate Challenge Test (CCCT)

It is believed to be more sensitive indicator of ovarian reserve than measurement of stimulated hormone level. *Clomiphene citrate is a nonsteroidal estrogen receptor modulator.* It acts by blocking the negative feedback inhibition of endogenous estrogen on FSH secretion.

In test, a woman takes 100 mg of clomiphene citrate orally on cycle day 5 to 9 (counted from day 1st - 1st day of menstrual cycle). Estradiol and FSH level are compared on day 3rd and 10th. **Elevated FSH at either time point is indication of diminished ovarian reserve.**

CCCT should be considered in women with prior history of ovarian surgery or chemotherapy or irradiation, history of smoking, age greater than 35 years, with family history of early menopause, and poor responders to gonadotropins.

Ultrasound

Transvaginal sonography to assess ovarian volume and antral follicle count in early follicular phase is simple, informative, cheap and noninvasive test. Less than 10 antral follicles predict poor response to gonadotropin stimulation.

Interpretation of Test of Ovarian Reserve

If there are abnormal results in any of the above methods; it indicates poor prognosis for achieving pregnancy. In older women donor oocyte IVF or adoption should be advised. Borderline results in younger women may suggest a need for a more intensive approach.

Tubal and Pelvic Factor Evaluation

The pelvic factor includes abnormalities of the uterus, fallopian tubes, ovarian and adjacent pelvic structures. History and physical examination as described above yields clues to possible tubal and pelvic factor.

There are following approaches for evaluation of pelvic anatomy:

Hysterosalpingography (HSG)

HSG is a fluoroscopic study performed by instilling radio opaque dye into uterine cavity through a catheter to determine the contour of the endometrial cavity and patency of the fallopian tubes (Figs 20.4A and B). Sensitivity and specificity of an HSG are approximately 65% and 85% respectively.

It can be done in outpatient setting with minimal analgesic. The test is performed in early follicular phase. A water bubble or oil soluble dye can be selected. Water soluble dye causes fewer cramps and gives ideal visualization of tubal mucosa while oil soluble dye obscures the details of tubal anatomy. There is evidence of fertility enhancing effect of HSG using oil base dye.

HSG can detect congenital malformation of the uterus, submucous leiomyoma, intrauterine synechiae (Asherman's syndrome), intrauterine polyp, salpingitis isthmic nodosa and proximal or distal tubal occlusion. Acute pelvic infection and allergy to iodine or radio contrast dye are contraindication of HSG. Short-term antibiotic (Doxycycline) before and after procedure is advised. Possible complications are pain and development of acute salpingitis (1-3%).

Sonohysterogram

In this procedure ultrasound scan is done after saline is infused into endometrial cavity during the follicular phase by pediatric Foley's catheter. Endometrial cavity, water fall

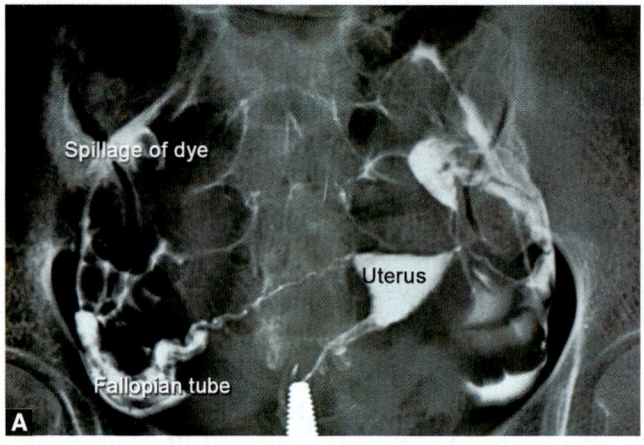

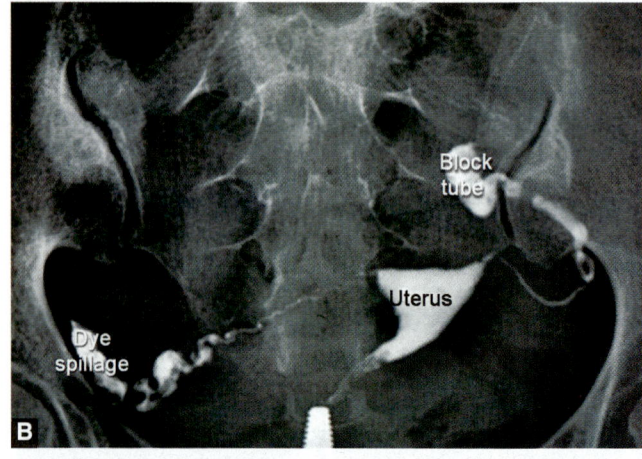

Figs 20.4A and B: HSG showing: (A) Normal uterus and bilateral tubal spillage; (B) HSG showing one tube block

sign from fallopian tube, collection of fluid in pelvis (**Sion test**) and any adnexal mass in pelvis is observed to assess pelvic factors. The procedure has sensitivity of 75% and specificity over 90%.

Laparoscopy with Chemopertubation

It is the gold standard for evaluation of tubal and pelvic factors. When it is performed in conjunction with hysteroscopy, information on uterine contour can be observed simultaneously. Laparoscopy allows endoscopic visualization of internal pelvic anatomy thereby *assesses the pelvis for peritubal or periovarian adhesions, endometriosis, and external structure of the uterus* (Figs 20.5A to C).

For chemopertubation a dilute dye–either methylene blue or indigocarmine is injected through hysterosalpingography cannula and tubal spill is evaluated through laparoscope (Fig. 20.5A).

Another advantage of laparoscopy is that it is not only diagnostic but surgical treatment can be done in same sitting as adhesiolysis, or lysis or ablation of endometriosis, or cystectomy. The necessity of laparoscopy in an infertility workup is controversial. In 1/3rd of patients, pelvic pathology may exist with normal HSG and ultrasound but some believe that a stepwise empiric approach is desirable considering cost and inherent risk of anesthetic and surgery in the procedure (Figs 20.5B and C).

Hysteroscopy

Endoscopic evaluation of the uterine cavity is the primary method for defining intrauterine abnormalities. It can be performed either in office setting, or can be combined with laparoscopy (Fig. 20.6).

Cervical Factor

The cervical glands secrete mucus that is normally thick and impervious to sperm and ascending infection. High estrogen level at midcycle changes the characteristic of cervical mucus and it becomes thin and stretchy. Estrogen primed cervical mucus filters out nonsperm component of semen and forms channels that help direct sperm into the uterus. Midcycle mucus acts as a sperm reservoir, allowing ongoing release during the next 24–72 hours and extending the potential time for fertilization.

Cervical factor for infertility may be indicated by history of abnormal Pap smear test, Postcoital bleeding, Cryotherapy, Conization. This major evaluation is done by pelvic speculum and bimanual examination and properly timed postcoital test. The value of routine cervical culture is controversial.

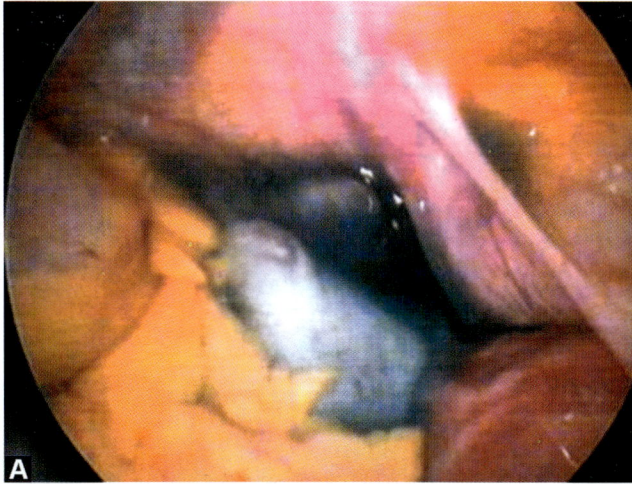
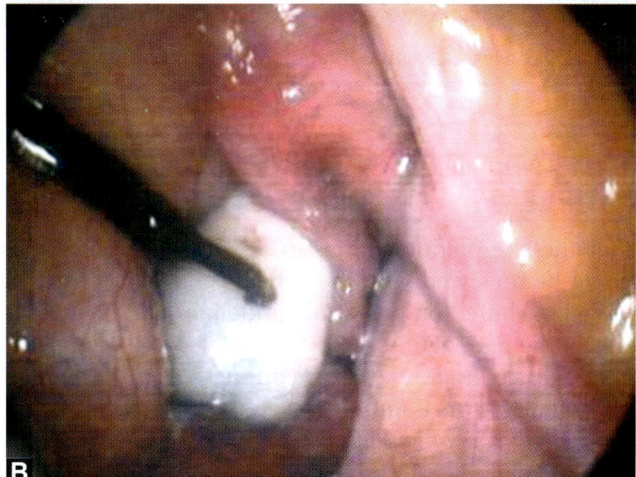
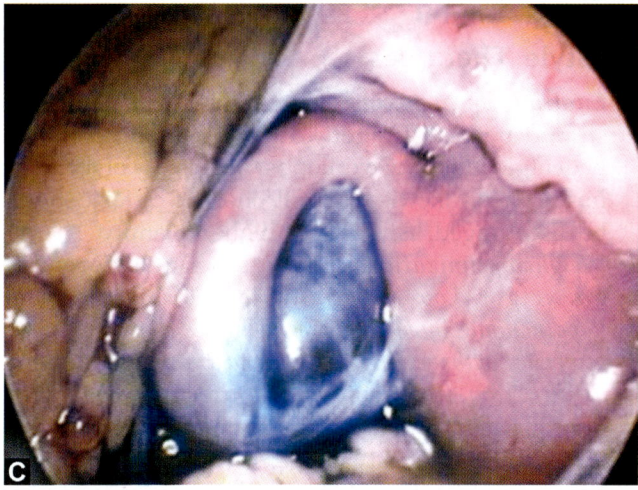

Figs 20.5A to C: (A) Laparoscopy showing patent fallopian tube, methylene dye spilling from fimbrial part of fallopian tube; (B) Laparoscopic ovarian diathermy for polycystic ovaries; (C) Tuboadnexal mass as visualized in laparoscopy

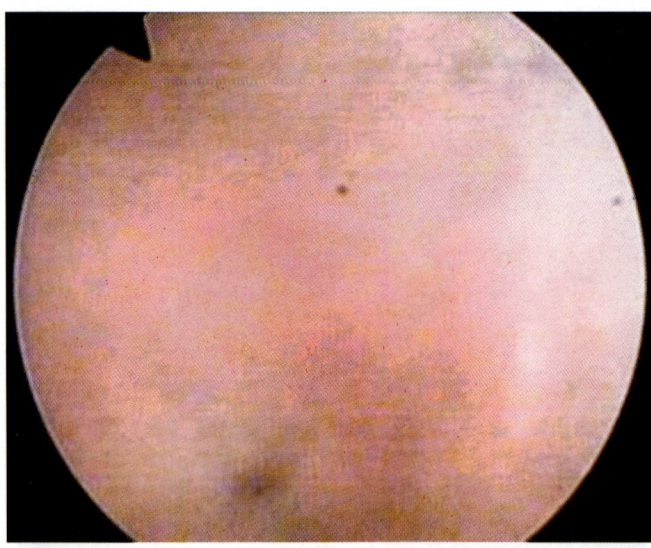

Fig. 20.6: Hysteroscopic image showing smooth normal uterine surface with tubal ostia

TREATMENT PLAN FOR INFERTILE COUPLE

After the completion of diagnostic workup, the finding should be reviewed with the patients and treatment plan is finalized based on physician guidelines and choice and need of the patients.

In approximately 20% of couple, a combination of suboptimal factors is found, and *multiple therapies may need to be instigated simultaneously or sequentially.* For the couple with unexplained infertility either an empiric approach or the additional tests should be discussed.

Lifestyle Therapies

a. *Environmental toxins:* Smoking and use of tobacco should be discouraged for both male and female patients in infertility workup as well history of recurrent miscarriage. Likewise use of alcohol and caffeine should be discouraged, especially in higher quantity.

b. *Weight optimization:* Ovarian function is dependent on weight. *Low body fat content is associated with hypothalamic hypogonadism, while central body fat is associated with insulin resistance and contributes to ovarian dysfunction.* So achieving a normal BMI with appropriate diet and exercise regimen is an important adjuvant for infertility management.

c. *Stress management:* Stress has been implicated in reproductive failure. Infertile couple should be screened for evidence of anxiety and depression. Usually pharmacologic management is not needed but a mind body approach that combines psychological counseling and meditation may help the couple. Advice of cultivating hobby and doing creative pursuit also helps in relieving anxiety.

Correction of an Identified Cause

Male Infertility

The initial evaluation by sperm analysis and hormone assay gives guideline about treatment options (Flow chart 20.1).

a. **In obstruction defect:** Surgical reanastomosis can be done in selected case. *Sperm can be retrieved through Microsurgical Epididymal Sperm Aspiration or Testicular Sperm Aspiration for Intracytoplasmic Sperm Injection.*

b. **Retrograde ejaculation:** Can be treated with alpha sympathomimetic or urine can be centrifuged to collect sperm for IUI.

c. **Primary hypogonadism:** Patient should have a Karyotype as Klinefelter's syndrome (47 XXY) is the most common etiology.

d. **Secondary hypogonadism:** It may be result of pituitary lesion like prolactinoma or hypothalamic etiology as Kallmann's syndrome. Most prolactinoma respond to medical management either with Bromocriptine, or Caberlin. In hypogonadotropic hypogonadism, pulsatile gonadotropin releasing hormone (GnRH) administration with a pump or FSH replacement, restores – testosterone and sperm production.

e. **Varicocele:** It is a dilatation of scrotal veins in the pampiniform plexus. Infertility is a questionable indication for correction of subclinical Varicocele detected by USG or venography.

f. **Mild to moderate oligospermia:** Along with lifestyle modification, *intrauterine insemination* can be offered. In this procedure semen is prepared by washing and culturing to select for highly motile sperm, concentrate sperm and remove seminal fluid. The prepared sperm is then inserted transcervically via a flexible catheter near the anticipated time of ovulation. Intrauterine insemination can be performed with or without super ovulation and is appropriate therapy for treatment of cervical factors, mild and moderate male factors and unexplained infertility.

g. **Severe oligospermia:** ICSI is used in conjunction with IVF for treatment of severe oligospermia that is less than 2 million motile sperm. In this procedure, a sperm is individually injected into each oocyte. Sperm can be taken from normal semen sample or retrieved by microsurgical epididymal sperm aspiration (MESA) or Testicular sperm aspiration (TESA).

h. **Donor sperm:** When male infertility is not amenable to therapy, donor sperm for insemination or IVF offers an opportunity for pregnancy. Donor sperm is taken from accredited semen banks with well informed consent from both partners. All Measures of semen selection like blood group, skin color, eye color, etc. are considered while selecting the sample size. The procedure has good results. Only frozen sample from accredited semen bank can be used to minimize the risk of transmission of infective disease.

Flow chart 20.1: Diagnostic guideline in male factor infertility

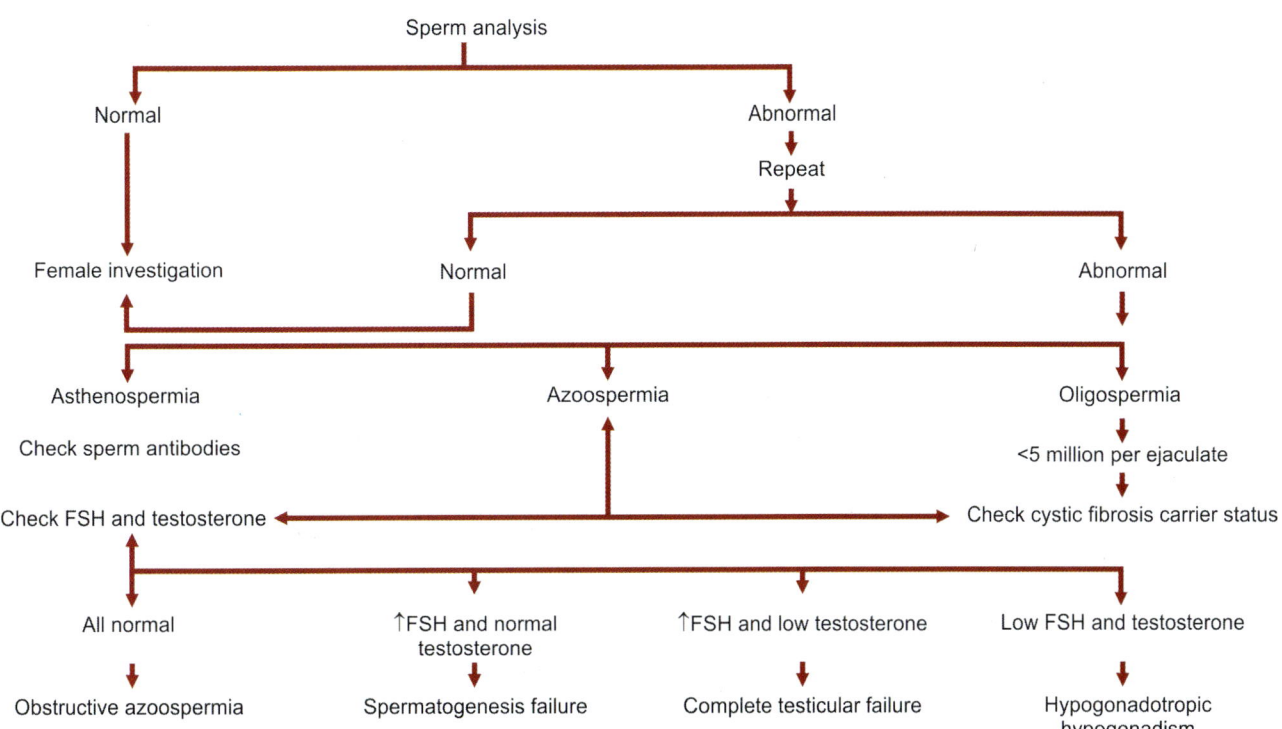

FEMALE FACTOR INFERTILITY

Causes of anovulation are summarized in Box 20.1.

Box 20.1: Causes of anovulation

Primary anovulation	Secondary anovulation
1. Hypothyroidism	1. Polycystic ovarian syndrome
2. Hypothalamic dysfunction	2. Hypo-or Hyperthyroidism
3. Weight related issues	3. Adrenal enzyme disorder
4. Dysgenetic gonads	4. Hyperprolactinemia
	5. Stress
	6. Pregnancy
	7. Premature ovarian failure
	8. Hypothalamic causes

Ovulatory Factor

The modality of treatment and success of specific ovulatory disorder is determined by the age of patient and etiology of anovulation. A stepwise approach *from least to most invasive as well expansive* is desired. It is usually started with clomiphene citrate and progress to ovulation induction with gonadotropins and in last IVF. If premature ovaries failure or early menopause is the cause, the option is oocyte or embryo donation.

a. **Clomiphene citrate:** It blocks the feedback inhibition of estradiol on the hypothalamus and pituitary leading to an increase in endogenous FSH. Dosage is orally started on 3rd or 5th day after the onset of spontaneous or progestin induced menstruation. It is advisable to do sonography to exclude signs of significant spontaneous follicular maturation or residual follicular cyst. Treatment begins with a single 50 mg tablet daily for 5 days. Dosage is increased by 50 mg in subsequent cycles until ovulation is induced. Effective dose of CC ranges from 50 to 250 mg/daily. Alternatively half of patient will ovulate at 50 mg/day and another 25% at 100 mg/day. USG and hormone monitoring of follicular development is an option and desired which gives more information and better control of the cycle. In general, women failing to ovulate with 100–150 mg/day or failing to conceive should be considered for alternative treatments.
Side effects are hot flushes, emotional liability, bloating and visual changes. Usually side effects are mild and disappear on discontinuation of the drug. The incidence of twin gestation is 8% and triplet or higher order multiple pregnancy (HOMP) is less than 1%.

b. **Insulin sensitizing agents:** Hyperinsulinemia plays a pivotal pathogenic role in development of PCOS. So it is reasonable to assume that intervention which reduces circulating insulin level in women with PCOS may restore normal reproductive endocrine function. In addition to weight loss, diet change and exercise, *insulin sensitizing agents* has been developed which may be helpful in induction of ovulation. *Biguanide, Metformin 500 mg orally twice or thrice a day* with or without CC may increase ovulation and pregnancy rate in selected and carefully monitored cases.

c. **Gonadotropins:** In patients when there is no response to clomiphene is termed as **clomiphene resistance.** If there is no pregnancy termed as **clomiphene failure.**

These cases have pituitary insufficiency or hypothalamic insufficiency and should undergo ovulation induction with gonadotropins.

Gonadotropins preparations vary in term of their source – *urinary or recombinant*, and presence or absence of LH activity. Human menopausal gonadotropins (HMG) consists of FSH and LH isolated from urine of postmenopausal women to various levels of purification. Recombinant (FSH and LH) contains purely FSH and LH respectively. Recombinant gonadotropins are administered by subcutaneous route and urinary gonadotropins are given by I/m injection. Overall evidence indicates that efficacy is similar in two preparations.

There are increased risk of side effect as ovarian hyperstimulation syndrome (OHSS), and multiple gestations. Intensive monitoring of number and maturity of follicles with ultrasound and estradiol level is required. Mimicking the effect of the LH surge, **human chorionic gonadotropins (hCG) is used to trigger ovulation**. Gonadotropins are usually used in conjunction with intrauterine insemination to increase pregnancy rate and should be done in supervision of expert persons. Patients with hypogonadotropic amenorrhea have higher success rate than PCOS. With perseverance, cumulative pregnancy rate of 45–90% can be achieved over 3–4 cycles with gonadotropins treatment. But even with careful monitoring there is 25% risk of multiple gestation.

d. *Aromatase inhibitor:* **Aromatase inhibitor effectively inhibit a cytochrome P-450 hemoprotein that catalyzes the rate limiting step in estrogen production**. They are orally administered, easy to use and relatively inexpensive. Letrozole is most widely used, given 2.5–5 mg orally daily for 5 days from 5th day of cycle. Compared with CC, its use is associated with a thicker endometrium and higher pregnancy rates. Relative higher risk of fetal congenital anomaly with Letrozole is controversial.

e. *Ovarian drilling:* Laparoscopic ovarian drilling (LOD) electrosurgical coagulation, laser vaporization or harmonic scalpel may be used to create multiple perforations in the ovarian surface and stroma. It may result in temporarily higher rate of spontaneous ovulation, conception and improved ovulation induction with medications. **Principle is that LOD may destroy ovarian androgen producing tissues and reduce peripheral conversion of androgens to estrogens**. Risk of ovarian drilling is postoperative adhesion, risk of laparoscopic surgery and possibility of premature ovarian failure. As surgery is more invasive, ovarian drilling is generally not offered prior to consideration of medical therapies (see Fig. 20.5B).

f. *Correction of diminished ovarian reserve:* Ovarian dysfunction may result from diminished ovarian reserve due to ageing or ovarian failure due to disease or surgical treatment. If basal 2-3 day level FSH is above 15 IU/L, it predicts the poor response to medical ovulation inductions and option of donor egg should be given to these patients.

g. *Thyroid disorder and hyperprolactinemia:* Both can lead to ovulatory dysfunction. Primary hypothyroidism leads to elevated thyroid stimulating hormone (TSH) levels which is a secretogogue of prolactin. Elevated prolactin level inhibits GnRH secretion causing oligomenorrhea or amenorrhea. If elevated prolactin level is in absence of hypothyroidism or history of drug induced hyperprolactinemia, imaging studies should be performed to identify micro- or macroadenoma of the pituitary gland. Hypothyroidism should be treated with thyroxin supplement and hyperthyroidism with antithyroid drugs. Dopamine agonist is the primary treatment of hyperprolactinemia, which can lead to normalization of cycle. If hyperprolactinemia is not associated with pituitary lesions or if a lesions is less than 10 mm (microadenoma), the dopamine agonist therapy is stopped during pregnancy.

The Pelvic Factors

Tubal factors: Tubal occlusion can results from: (i) Congenital abnormality, (ii) Infection, (iii) Iatrogenic. Following gynecological operative procedures, (iv) idiopathic. *Proximal* tubal occlusion describes obstruction proximal to fimbria and may develop at tubal ostium, isthmus or ampulla. *Distal tubal occlusion* describes obstruction at the tubal fimbria and typically results from prior pelvic infection and may be associated with concomitant adnexal adhesion.

Treatment

Tubal surgery is most likely to be successful if the tubal mucosa has not undergone significant damage. If the tubal mucosa has been obstructed by tubal disease, IVF is probably the best approach. In addition if the tubal damage has resulted in the formation of a hydrosalpinx, there is evidence that removal of tube improves IVF outcomes. Following procedures can be tried for tubal disease according to level of obstruction:

a. *Proximal tubal obstruction:* Hysteroscopic directed tubal cannulation has been tried in proximal tubal occlusion, which should be performed with concurrent laparoscopy. *Surgical segmental resection and reanastomosis* can be performed in proximal obstruction caused by disease or previous sterilization operation, via minilaparotomy or laparoscopy.

b. ***Distal tubal obstruction:*** Neosalpingostomy can be performed via mini laparotomy or laparoscopy. However, risk of ectopic pregnancy is 50%, which should be explained to the patients. **However, hydrosalpinges that is dilated more than 3 cm in diameter, associated with significant adnexal adhesion or that display an obviously attenuated endoscopic vision gives a poor prognosis**. These tubes are best treated by salpingectomy and should be recommended *in vitro* fertilization.

Correction of Uterine Factors

a. **Fibroid:** The role of fibroid in infertility is inconclusive. However, *myomectomy is reserved in cases who have repeated implantation failure with distortion of endometrial cavity, causing recurrent abortion.*
b. **Endometrial polyps:** If polyp is identified, hysteroscopic polypectomy should be done in all infertile women, which shows higher conception rate following procedure.
c. **Intrauterine adhesions:** Hysteroscopic adhesion treatment may range from simple lysis of small bands to excessive adhesiolysis of dense intrauterine adhesions, using scissors, electrosurgical cutting or laser energy. In women with severe Asherman's syndrome, not amenable to reconstructive surgery, gestational carrier surrogacy is valuable option.
d. **Congenital uterine anomalies:** Congenital uterine anomalies like bicornuate uterus, uterine septum are associated with pregnancy loss but generally not associated with infertility. However, uterine anomalies may be associated with severe endometriosis which can impair fertility. Treatment is usually reserved only for women who have experienced pregnancy loss presumably due to uterine anomaly. **Uterus septum can be resected via hysteroscope**. Treatment of bicornuate uterus is usually not recommended. For selected patients metroplasty can be considered.

Treatment of Peritoneal Disease

a. **Endometriosis:** Laparoscopic resection or ablation of moderate or advanced endometriosis enhances fecundity in infertile women for period immediately following surgery. Resection of mild endometriosis at time of diagnostic laparoscopy can also improve pregnancy rate.
b. **Adhesions:** Pelvic adhesion may result from endometriosis, prior surgery or pelvic infection. Adhesion may impair fertility by distorting adnexal anatomy and interfering with gamete and embryo transport even in the absence of tubal disease. **Surgical lysis** may restore pelvic anatomy in some cases, but there is always risk of recurrence.

Correction of Cervical Factors

Inadequate cervical mucus caused by chronic cervicitis and inflammatory changes deserves treatment. Alternatively in decreased cervical mucus volume, exogenous estrogen and use of mucolytic expectorant guaifenesin can be tried but its efficiency is not confirmed. IUI with washed sperm should be considered in cervical abnormalities, which can result in 20–30% of pregnancy rate per cycle in each of the first 3 cycles.

Unexplained Infertility

A diagnosis of unexplained or idiopathic infertility is assigned to couples with normal results of a standard infertility workup. The main treatment option can be: (a) Expectant observation, with lifestyle changes like timed intercourse, (b) Ovarian stimulation with or without IUI, (c) IVF.

The rationale for treatment with superovulation in women with documented ovulation, is that by increasing the number of oocytes available, the likelihood of pregnancy is increased. When fundamental defect in fertilization or embryo transfer to uterus is cause of idiopathic infertility, IVF may play a role in treatment. For many, the hardest course to contemplate is no therapy at all.

ASSISTED REPRODUCTIVE TECHNOLOGY

Assisted reproductive technology describes clinical and laboratory techniques used to achieve pregnancy in infertile couples. **In principle IUI meets this definition. By convention; ART procedures are those that at some point require extraction and isolation of oocyte**. These are:

a. *In vitro fertilization:* During IVF, mature oocytes from stimulated ovaries are retrieved transvaginally under USG guidance. Sperm and ova are then combined *in vitro* to prompt fertilization. If fertilization is successful, viable embryos are transferred transcervically into the endometrial cavity (Figs 20.7A to C).
b. *Intracytoplasmic sperm injection:* It is most applicable to male factor infertility. In micromanipulative technique, cumulus cells surrounding the ova are emzymatically digested and single sperm is directly injected through the zona pellucida and oocyte cell membrane (Fig. 20.8).
c. *Gestational carrier surrogacy:* In this, a fertilized egg is placed into the uterus of surrogate, rather than into the intended mother. Indications are: (i) Uncorrectable uterus factors, (ii) Pregnancy would pose significant health risk to woman, (iii) Repeated unexplained miscarriage. Gestational carrier surrogacy has legal and psychological issues. In most states, a surrogate is the legal parent and therefore adoption must be completed after birth, to give the intended mother her parental rights.

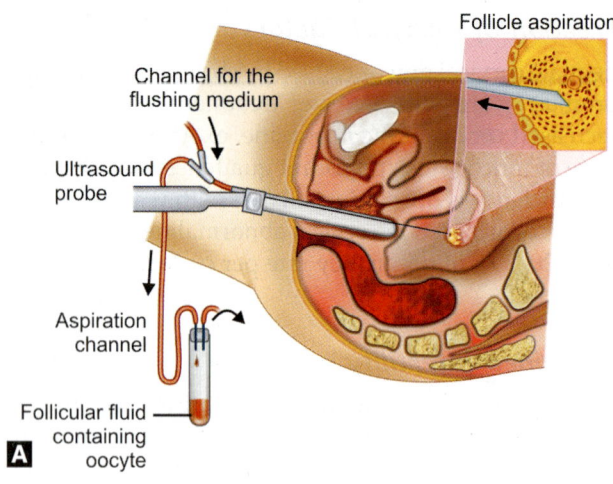

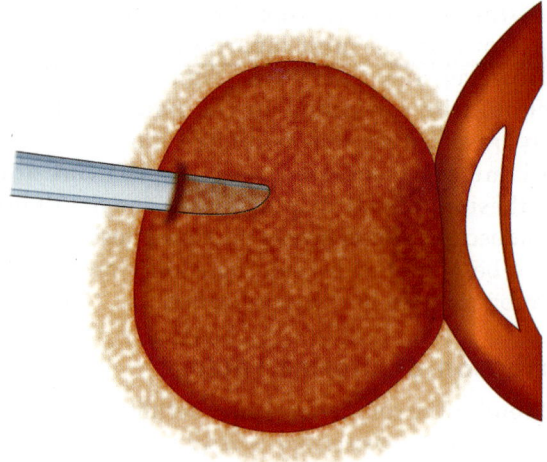

Fig. 20.8: Intracytoplasmic sperm injection

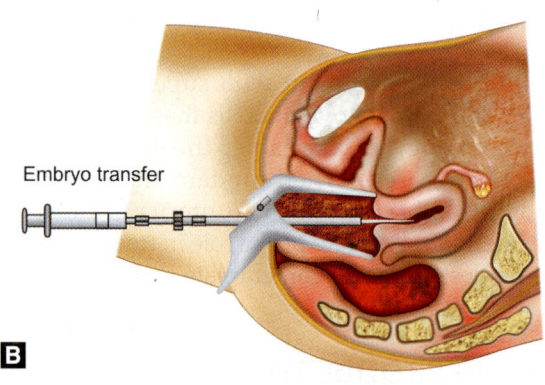

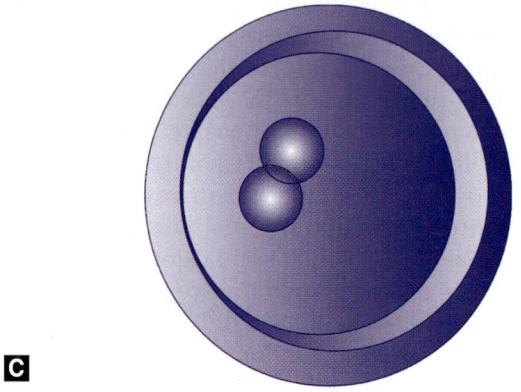

Figs 20.7A to C: IVF technique: (A) Follicle pickup; (B) Embryo transfer; (C) Fertilized embryo

d. *Egg donation:* Egg donation is employed in cases of: (i) Infertility with ovarian failures or diminished ovarian reserve, (ii) When offspring would be at risk for maternally transmitted genetic disease.

e. *Gamete intrafallopian transfer:* It is similar to IVF but in this egg and sperm are placed via catheter through the fimbria and deposited directly into fallopian tube via laparoscopy. Now IVF has largely replaced GIFT.

f. *Zygote intrafallopian transfer:* It is also variety of IVF when embryo transfer is done into fallopian tube at laparoscopy.

g. *Embryo cryopreservation:* In IVF many eggs are retrieved to have ultimately one to three healthy embryos for transfer. This frequency leads to extraembryos. Successful freezing and thawing of embryo has been proved so these extraembryos can be freezed with cryopreservation which can be used in next cycle, without the need for ovarian stimulation and egg retrieval.

h. *Oocyte cryopreservation:* It is still suboptimal and experimental.

i. *In vitro maturation: In vitro* culture of immature oocytes is still experimental.

j. *Preimplantation genetic diagnosis:* In this technique 1 or 2 cell from a developing embryo is removed at 6-8 cell stage to screen for single gene defect, chromosomal disorders.

Success of Assisted Reproductive Technique

Approximately 25% of couples going through an IVF cycle have a live born child. 5% have a miscarriage or ectopic pregnancy. IVF pregnancy abortion rates are similar to spontaneous conception.

Complications of ART

Ovarian hyperstimulation syndrome (OHSS): OHSS is an infrequent but potentially severe complication of IVF. **It is most commonly seen in young women with very high estradiol concentration and many intermediate sized follicles.** OHSS usually presents 1 week after oocyte retrieval. It is characterized by ascites, weight gain and intravascular volume depletion. In severe cases prerenal azotemia, hemoconcentration and hypercoagulable state can be present. **Treatment with aggressive hydration is indicated**. Paracentesis early in course of OHSS can be done and replaced as needed.

Multiple gestation: Multiple gestation is the most common.

Ectopic and heterotopic pregnancy: Patient who undergo ART procedure are at twice at the risk for having an ectopic pregnancy as the general population.

Preterm birth, low birth infant: Risk is independent of maternal age and number of fetuses.

Congenital abnormalities: There is no increased risk of congenital anomalies in children born through IVF as compared to spontaneous conception. There may be minimally increased risk of chromosomal abnormalities and birth defects among children with Intracytoplasmic sperm injection, where a single sperm is directly inserted into an egg's cytoplasm. Currently available data suggest that there are no difference between the psychomotor developments of preschool children conceived by IVF and naturally conceived children.

Cost: It is a quite expensive procedure.

Causes of Failure of IVF

Following may be the causes of failure to conceive through IVF:

a. **Less than optimal ovarian stimulation**, which can be because of diminished ovarian reserve, advanced maternal age or via inappropriately stimulation medication dosing/regimen.
b. Poor fertilization.
c. **Poor embryo quality**, more common with advanced maternal age.
d. **Poor technique of oocyte retrieval or embryo transfer**.
e. **Inadequate uterine receptivity**.

Couple can opt for repeated IVF in case of failure. In general IVF success rate do not fall significantly for couples who have failed one or two prior cycle. Most couples do not attempt more than three IVF cycle.

MULTIPLE CHOICE QUESTIONS

1. A lady with infertility and bilateral tubal block comes for treatment. Best method of management is:
   a. Laparoscopy and hysteroscopy
   b. Hydrotubation
   c. IVF
   d. Tuboplasty
   Ans. a
2. PESA/MESA is helpful in:
   a. Pre-testicular azoospermia
   b. Testicular azoospermia
   c. Post testicular azoospermia
   d. Asthenospermia
   Ans. c
3. Increased FSH level in azoospermic male indicates:
   a. Testicular atrophy
   b. Hypothalamic failure
   c. Cryptorchidism
   d. Hypospadias
   Ans. a
4. Drug used for ovulation induction:
   a. Clomiphene citrate
   b. Danazol
   c. Cyproterone acetate
   d. Tamoxifen
   Ans. a
5. Time of ovulation is detected by:
   a. Urine LH
   b. Urine FSH
   c. Urine HCG
   d. Serum estradiol
   e. BBT
   Ans. a, e
6. Sonosalpingography is done for:
   a. Measuring basal body temperature
   b. To detect pregnancy
   c. Testing tubal potency
   d. Determining anovulatory cycle
   Ans. c
7. Ferning pattern of drying cervical mucus suggests the action of:
   a. Estrogen
   b. Progesterone
   c. Prolactin
   d. 17 ketosteroid
   Ans. a
8. Side effect of clomiphene citrate includes all *except*:
   a. Multiple pregnancy
   b. Increased risk of ovarian cancer
   c. Multiple polycystic ovary
   d. Teratogenic effect on offspring
   Ans. d
9. Which is not ART technique?
   a. GIFT
   b. ZIFT
   c. IVF & ET
   d. Artificial insemination
   Ans. d
10. Most common indication for IVF is an abnormality in:
    a. Uterus
    b. Fallopian tube
    c. Anovulation
    d. Azoospermia
    Ans. b

21. Hirsutism

*This time like all times is very good one,
if we but know what to do with it.*

GENERAL CONSIDERATION

Hirsutism is excessive facial and body hair caused by excess androgen production. It is usually associated with anovulatory ovaries and loss of cyclic menstrual function. There are three types of body hairs:

a. *Lanugo hair follicles:* Lightly pigmented thin in diameter found in neonates.
b. *Vellous hairs follicles:* Fine non pigmented, hairs found in most body regains in adults.
c. *Terminal hair follicles:* Which are pigmented coarse hairs found in scalp, axillae and pubic area of adult men and women and face and chest of men. The hair follicle has three phases in its growth cycle: (a) *Anagen—growth phase*, (b) *Catagen—involution*—hair stops growing and moves up in the follicle, (c) *Telogen—resting phase*—prior to hair loss.

Physiology of Androgen

Androgens are steroid that simulate the development of male secondary sexual characteristic and so promote the growth of sexual hair. The major androgens are: (a) Testosterone, (b) Dihydrotestosterone, (c) Androstenedione, (d) Dehydroepiandrosterone (DHEA and DHEAS).

The production rate of testosterone in the normal female is 0.2-0.3 mg/day. Approximately 50% of testosterone is derived from peripheral conversion of androstenedione whereas the adrenal gland and ovary contributes approximately equal amount (25%) to the circulating level of testosterone. Dehydroepiandrosterone sulfate (DHEAS) arise almost exclusively from the adrenal glands whereas 90% of dehydroepiandrosterone (DHA) is from the adrenal.

About 80% of circulating testosterone is bound to a betaglobulin known as sex steroid hormone binding globulin (SHBG). In women about 19% is loosely bound to albumin, leaving about 1% unbound. *Androgenicity is dependent mainly on the unbound fraction and partially on the fraction associated with albumin.* DHA, DHEAS and androstenedione are not significantly protein bound and routine immunoassay reflect their biologically available hormone activity. Routine assay of testosterone measure total testosterone concentration bound and unbound (Flow chart 21.1).

SHBG production in the liver is decreased by androgens. Hence, the binding capacity in men is lower then in normal women and 2-3% of testosterone circulation is in the free, active form in men. SHBG is decreased by insulin and increased by estrogen and thyroid hormone. Therefore, binding capacity is increased in women with hyperthyroidism, in pregnancy and by estrogen containing medicines. In hirsute women, the SHBG level is depressed by the excess androgens and the percent free and active testosterone as well the metabolic clearance rate of testosterone is elevated. The total testosterone concentration therefore can be in the normal range in women who is hirsute. Though there is little clinical need for a specific assay fore the free testosterone. Because the very presence of hirsutism or masculinization indicates increased androgen effects.

In hirsute women only 25% of the circulating testosterone arise from peripheral conversion and mostly is due to ovarian secretion of testosterone and androstenedione. *The most common causes of hirsutism in women are anovulation and excessive androgen production by the ovaries.*

Flow chart 21.1: Testosterone production and metabolism

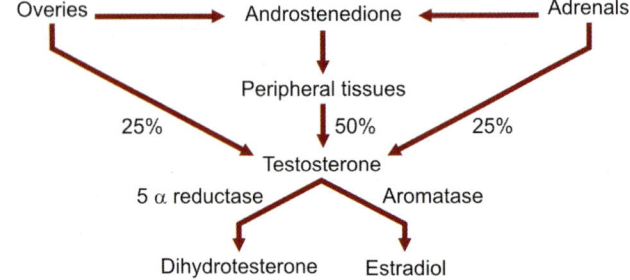

Chapter - 21 ♦ Hirsutism

Causes of Hirsutism

1. *Ovarian non-neoplastic causes:*
   a. Polycystic ovary syndrome,
   b. Stromal hyperplasia,
   c. Stromal hyperthecosis,
   d. Hyperandrogenism, insulin resistance, acanthosis nigricans.
2. *Ovarian neoplastic cause:*
   a. Sertoli-Leydig cell tumor, germ cell tumor, Gynandroblastoma, Hilus cell tumor.
3. *Pregnancy related cancer:*
   a. Theca lutein cyst, luteoma of pregnancy.
4. *Adrenal causes:* Congenital adrenal hyperplasia (CAH), adrenal tumors, Cushing's syndrome and hyperprolactinemia.
5. *Iatrogenic cause:* Methyltestosterone, danazol, Anabolic steroid, 19 norethisterone, idiopathic.
6. *Idiopathic.*

Diagnosis and Clinical Finding

Appropriate questioning allows one to rule out any history of drug ingestion that might cause excessive hair growth to determine the speed of onset of symptoms and to correlate the timing of symptoms of age and puberty (Fig. 21.1). *Anabolic steroid, danazol and testosterone drug have androgenic activity. An abrupt onset of hirsutism is more likely to be associated with androgen producing tumors or exogenous hormone use.*

Special enquiries are made into patient's menstrual history and early or late onset of hirsutism. Knowledge of a family history of hirsutism or of abnormal menstrual cycle may also be informative. A physical examination should be performed to differentiate hypertrichosis from hirsutism and to evaluate for acanthosis nigricans or additional signs of virilization such as clitoromegaly, male pattern balding, deepening voices or decrease breast contour. *Ferriman and Gallwey scoring system is a standardized grading system for scoring hirsutism depending on body site. Less than 8 is normal, greater than 15 is severe.*

Laboratory Findings

Screening Test

a. **Testosterone:** A serum testosterone level less than 200 ng/dl will rule out almost all of the testosterone secreting neoplasm. A total testosterone level higher than 200 ng/dl should be considered evidence of an ovarian tumor until proven otherwise. A normal testosterone level in presence of hirsutism indicates androgens effects, because of decreased level of SHBG.
b. **DHEAS:** A normal or slightly elevated DHEAS level excludes significant adrenal pathology. A DHEAS>700-800 µg/dl can be caused by adrenal tumors.
c. **17 α hydroxyprogesterone (17 OHP):** It is the single most accurate diagnostic test for congenital adrenal hyperplasia due to 21 hydroxylase deficiency. It should be measured immediately upon awakening in the morning. Normal levels are less than 200 ng/dl. Level ranging between 200 and 400 ng/dl warrant further evaluations. **Levels > 400 ng/dl are virtually diagnostic of 21 hydroxylase deficiency.**
d. If alopecia is present, a TSH screen for thyroid function is indicated.
e. A clinician should always consider the possibility of hyperinsulinemia and emphasize preventive health intervention.
f. The single dose overnight dexamethasone test is used to screen for Cushing's syndrome. If the results are abnormal, it should be confirmed by measuring the 24 hours urinary free cortisol.

Treatment

Almost all patients presenting with hirsutism represent excess androgen production in association with steady state of persistent anovulation. Treatment is directed towards interruption of steady state. In those patients who wish to become pregnant, ovulation can be induced. In patients who do not want to become pregnant, the steady state can be interrupted by suppression of ovarian steroidogenesis by utilizing the potent inhibitory action of progestational agents on LH secretion.

Combined Oral Contraceptive Pills

They increase SHBG by estrogen component and decrease ovarian androgen production from ovary.

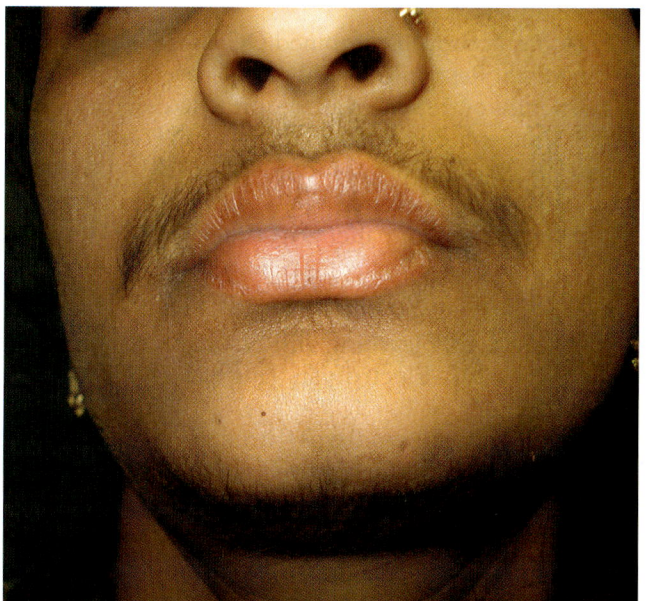

Fig. 21.1: 19-year-old girl with PCO and hair growth

Cyproterone Acetate

It is a potent progestational agent that both inhibits gonadotropins secretion and blocks androgen action by binding to the androgen receptors. It is available as estrogen progestin contraceptive agents called *Diane (2 mg cyproterone acetate and 50 mg ethinyl estradiol)*.

Spironolactone

It is an *aldosterone antagonistic diuretic*. It inhibits ovarian and adrenal biosynthesis of androgens, competing for the androgen receptors in the hair follicle and directly inhibiting 5 α reductase activity. The effect in hirsutism is dose related and better effect is seen with a dose of 200 mg daily. The dose can be gradually lowered to 25-50 mg daily.

Dexamethasone

Dexamethasone suppression of endogenous ACTH secretion is used in women who have an adrenal enzyme deficiency. The 0.5 mg Dexamethasone is given nightly.

Flutamide

(Eulexin) is a nonsteroidal antiandrogen at the receptor level. It has severe toxic effect on liver so a low dose is recommended. A dose of 250 mg daily have a marked beneficial effect on hirsutism within 6 months. Liver enzyme should be monitored meticulously and treatment should be combined with contraceptive method. Because if woman conceives, blockage of androgen receptor in a male fetus can interfere with normal male development.

Finasteride

It inhibits 5 α reductase activity; this blocks conversion of testosterone into dihydrotestosterone. A dose of 5 mg per day decreases hirsutism without side effects. A smaller dose of 1 mg is available for men for treatment of hair loss in men. After extended therapy (6 months to a year) there is little clinical difference in the efficacy of the major drugs used to treat hirsutism.

Vaniqua (Eflornithine Hydrochloride)

13.9% Eflornithine hydrochloride cream inhibits ornithine decarboxylase, an enzyme in the hair dermal papilla that is essential for hair growth. Local application to facial hair will slow overall growth and make hair softer. The cream may make acne worse by obstructing pilosebaceous glands. This treatment is recommended only for treatment complaining of facial hair in specific circumstances as slight increase in hair on the upper lip that occurs after menopause.

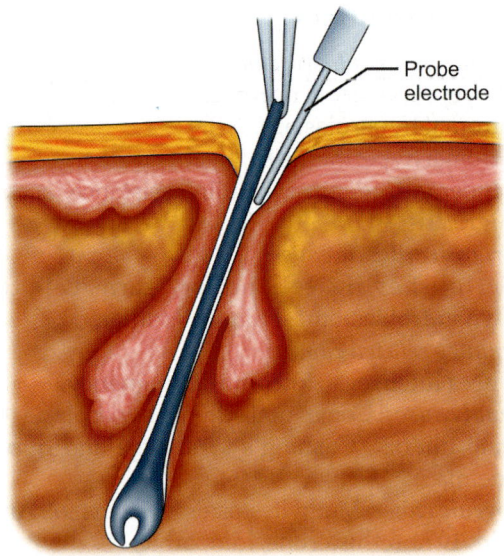

Fig. 21.2: Electrolysis for hirsutism

GnRH Agonist

Because ovarian androgen production is LH dependent, suppression of the pituitary with chronic GnRH agonist treatment improves hirsutism. But results of GnRH agonist treatment are inconsistent and treatment is complicated and expansive. So GnRH agonist should be reserved for severe case of ovarian hyperandrogenism, which is usually due to significant hyperthecosis and marked hyperinsulinemia.

FDA has approved combined OC and Vaniqua cream for hirsutism. Response of drug is relatively slow and at least 6 months of treatment are required to demonstrate an impact. If patients do not respond well to oral contraceptive, antiandrogen should be added, preferably (in order) spironolactone or finasteride. The addition of GnRH agonist should be reserved for patients resistant to initial therapy.

Adjuvant Therapy for Hirsutism

(i) Weight loss, (ii) Bleaching, (iii) Waxing, (iv) Depilation, (v) Shaving, (vi) Electrolysis (Fig. 21.2), (vii) Laser, (viii) Plucking.

Shaving is recommended as it does not increase the rate of growth and there is less risk of folliculitis and scaring.

22 Menopause

A comfortable old age is the reward of well spent youth.

MENOPAUSE

Menopause is defined as the permanent cessation of menstruation resulting from the loss of follicular activity. Natural menopause is defined as 12 months of amenorrhea without another pathologic cause. The average age of menopause is 51 years. *Menopause before age 40 is called premature ovarian failure.*

Perimenopause or Menopausal Transition

It refers to the period prior to menopause and first year after menopause. The average age when perimenopause starts is 47 years and it lasts on average 4 years.

Climacteric

It is the phase during the aging of women marking the transition from the reproductive to the nonreproductive state. Postmenopause refers to the phase of life that comes after the menopause.

Endocrinology and Etiopathogenesis of Menopause

Menopause is due to gradual diminishing of ovarian follicles. There is more rapid depletion of ovarian follicles which starts in late 30's and early 40's and continues until a point when menopausal ovary is virtually devoid of follicles. This process of atresia of nondominant cohort of follicles is largely independent of menstrual cycling. It is the prime event that leads to final loss of ovarian activity and menopause.

It cause decline in level of inhibin, which is a polypeptide hormone synthesized and secreted by granulosa cells. It causes negative feedback on FSH so there is increased FSH production from the pituitary, which accelerates the follicular phase of menstrual cycle and cause high basal estradiol and menstrual irregularity. **So the transitional phase of menstrual irregularity is not one of marked estrogen deficiency.** Occasionally estradiol level will rise to 2-3 times higher than is normally seen, which may be followed by corpus luteum formation, usually with limited progesterone secretion. Thus in premenopausal period, episode of follicular maturation and vaginal bleeding are widely spaced. Premenopausal woman may be exposed to persistent estrogen stimulation of the endometrium in the absence of regular cyclic progesterone secretion.

After menopause granulosa cell gradually lose their ability to produce estradiol, and FSH level rise and androgen level decline by 50%. But the greater decline of estradiol favors a high androgen to estrogen ratio leading to signs of hirsutism and alopecia in some women. *Estrogen production after menopause is principally estrone production by aromatization of androstenedione in adipose tissues.*

Physical Changes Associated with Menopause

Reproductive Tract

As estrogen function is major growth factor of the female reproductive tract, there are substantial changes in the appearance of all the reproductive organs. There is varying degree of atrophic change in vaginal epithelium and reduction of secretion of cervical mucus. Atrophy of uterus is also seen with atrophy of both endometrium and myometrium. This shrinkage can be beneficial to women who enter the climacteric with uterus myomas. Fallopian tube and ovaries also decrease in size postmenopausally—small size of ovaries makes them difficult to palpate during pelvic examination. **Thus, the palpable ovary in a postmenopausal woman must be viewed with suspicion and the presence of an ovarian neoplasm must be considered.** The supporting structure of the reproductive organs suffers loss of tone as estrogen level decline. Postmenopausal estrogen deficiency may lead to symptomatic progressive pelvic relaxation.

Urinary Tract

Estrogen plays an important role in maintaining epithelium of bladder and urethra. In menopause there are atrophic change in these organs which may give rise to atrophic cystitis with complaint of urinary urgency, frequency, incontinence and dysuria. There is tendency to formation of urethral caruncle with resultant dysuria, meatal tenderness and occasionally hematuria. There are more chances of recurrent UID.

CLINICAL CONDITION ASSOCIATED WITH MENOPAUSE

Menstrual Disturbance

Menses may be irregular in more than one half of all women during menopausal transition. **In all women, regardless of menopausal states, the etiology of abnormal bleeding should be determined.** Anovulation is the most common cause of erratic bleeding during the transition. But endometrial hyperplasia, estrogen sensitive neoplasm such as endometrial polyp, uterine leiomyomas and pregnancy should always be considered.

Evaluation of Abnormal Bleeding in Menopause

a. *Sonography:* Transvaginal sonographic measurement of endometrial thickness can be used in postmenopausal women to guide need of biopsy. *Endometrial biopsy is not required, if the endometrial thickness is less than 5 mm but biopsy is suggested if there is a clinical history of a long-term unopposed estrogen exposure.*
b. *Endometrial biopsy:* It is gold standard to assess premalignant and malignant lesions.
c. *Hysteroscopy:* It allows evaluation of focal intrauterine lesions and targeted biopsy of specific lesion as submucous leiomyoma, endometrial polyp or focal area of endometrial hyperplasia or endometrial cancer.

Central Thermoregulation Change

Vasomotor symptoms may be described as hot flushes. Hot flushes and night sweats are the most common medical complaint of women during menopausal transition (75%).

Hot flush is sudden sensation of warmth often accompanied by a flushed sensation of the upper body and face, typically lasting 1–5 minutes. Exact cause is unknown but it is supposed to be due to alteration on the hypothalamic thermoregulatory center due to fluctuation in steroid and peptide hormone levels.

Sleep dysfunction and fatigue: Sleep disruption is a common complaint of women with hot flushes. Disturbed sleep can lead to fatigue, irritability, depressive symptoms, cognitive dysfunction and impairment in daily functioning.

Treatment

Estrogens are the principal medication used to relieve hot flushes. Estrogen blocks both the perceived symptoms and the physiological change by enhancing hypothalamic opioid activity in postmenopausal women. In women who cannot take estrogen, progesterone also blocks hot flushes partially. Clonidine, selective serotonin reuptake (SSRIS), has been tried for hot flushes.

Osteopenia and Osteoporosis

WHO define *osteopenia* as Bone Mineral Density (BMD) that is >1.0 to <2.5 standard deviation (SD) below the young adult mean (called a T score). *Osteoporosis is ≥ 2.5 S.D below the young adult mean.* A Z score is the BMD of the patients compared to her own range. *Z score >1 S.D below the mean is abnormal.* **BMD is best assessed by a dual energy X-ray absorptiometry.** Biochemical markers of bone remodeling include serum markers of bone formation that is osteocalcium, bone specific alkaline phosphatase, precollagen extension peptide. Urinary markers of bone resorption are: hydroxyproline, hydroxylase, N-telopeptides. *In general bone markers increase with increasing bone turnover.*

Types and Causes of Osteoporosis

Primary osteoporosis (Type 1): It refers to bone loss associated with aging and postmenopausal estrogen deficiency. With estrogen deficiency estrogen's regulatory effect on bone resorption is lost, so bone resorption is accelerated and is usually not balanced by compensatory bone formation, which is most rapid in early post-menopausal years.

Other causes of Type 1 osteoporosis are advancing age, excessive smoking, alcohol consumption, poor nutrition (lack of calcium and vitamin D_3, protein). Sedentary life-styles, slender body build and hereditary factors as race.

Secondary osteoporosis (Type II): **If osteoporosis is caused by other disease or medication, it is termed secondary osteoporosis.** Endocrine abnormalities like thyroid, parathyroid, diabetes, hypogonadism, and gastrointestinal abnormalities as malabsorption, anorexia, medications as GnRH agonist, anticonvulsant, glucocorticoid, and methotrexate can cause secondary osteoporosis.

Prevention and Treatment for Osteoporosis

a. All individuals at risk for or who have been diagnosed with osteoporosis should be advised to consume

adequate calcium (minimum of 1200 mg elemental calcium per day) and vitamin D (400–800 IU/day).
b. Lifestyle modification, cessation of tobacco, alcohol, and participation in regular weightbearing exercise should be encouraged.
c. Pharmacologic therapy should be strongly considered in women with BMD score below 1.5 with one or more risk factor. Current therapy available are as follows:
    i. Bisphosphonates.
    ii. Calcium.
    iii. Estrogen with or without progesterone.
    iv. Parathyroid hormone.
    v. Raloxifene.

Bisphosphonates

They are potent antiresorption agents and also cause osteoblast to produce substance that inhibits osteoclast. They increase bone mineral density at the spine, wrist, and hip in a dose dependent manner and decrease the risk of vertebral fracture by 30-35% and nonvertebral facture as well.

Dosages

i. **Alendronate** 5 mg daily or 35 mg weakly for prevention. For treatment of established osteoporosis is 10 mg daily or 70 mg weekly.
ii. **Risedronate** 5 mg daily or 35 mg weekly.
iii. **Ibandronate** 2.5 mg daily and monthly dose is 150 mg.

Administrative Caution

As the intestinal absorption of bisphosphonate is poor so medicine should be *taken with lot of water, empty stomach and nothing should be taken by mouth for after oral dosing, women must remain upright for 30, 60 minutes*. Risks are gastric and esophageal ulceration and rarely osteonecrosis of the jaw.

Calcitonin

Calcitonin is a peptide hormone that inhibits osteoclastic activity and therefore inhibits bone resorption.

Dosage and Administration

Calcitonin 100 IU is given S/C daily or alternative days. The intranasal dose is 200 IU daily, but it may cause rhinitis.

ESTROGEN

Until recently estrogen was the mainstay of therapy for prevention and treatment of postmenopausal osteoporosis. Though osteoporosis is FDA approved indication for estrogen therapy, it is best used in women who should otherwise use estrogen/hormone therapy for management of menopausal symptoms, or in women who cannot tolerate alternate antiresorptive therapies. Estrogen decreases the risk of hip fracture by 25–50%, of vertebral fracture by 50%.

Dosage and Administration

0.3-0.62 mg of conjugated estrogens, 0.5 – 1 mg micronized estradiol, 0.25-0.05 mg of transdermal estradiol. The lower dose (0.3 mg conjugated equine estrogen) is not as effective as higher doses but do prevent bone loss. For best results therapy should begin soon after the menopause.

Parathyroid Hormones (PTHs)

It has been approved by the FDA for treatment of established osteoporosis or who are at high-risk for fracture. Despite its potential deleterious effect on bone, intermittent administration of recombinant PTH stimulates bone formation. *It should be used only in high risk patients because of its high cost and need for daily injection and possible risk for osteosarcoma.*

Selective Estrogen Receptors Modulator

They are nonhormonal agents that bind to estrogen receptors and may exhibit either estrogen agonist or antagonist activity.

Dosage and Administration

Raloxifene 60 mg daily for 2 years is associated with 1–2% increase in lumbar spine and hip bone density.

Tibolone: Its effect on bone is comparable to estrogen but use regarding long-term therapy is currently being evaluated.

Phytoestrogens: They are plant derived compound that have weak estrogen like effects. Role is still inconclusive.

Sexual Dysfunction

The determinants of sexual behavior are complex and interrelated. It is believed to be regulated by three general components: (a) Individual's motivation called desire or libido, (b) Endocrine competence, (c) Sociocultural belief. The hypoestrogenic state can lead to atrophy of internal genitalia. There can be dyspareunia due to vaginal atrophy.

Treatment

Genitalia atrophy responds to estrogen therapy. Role of androgen therapy in female sexual dysfunction is under research. A variety of water soluble vaginal lubricants are available. Alternatively a polycarbophil based gel offers a more sustained correction of vaginal dryness.

Common Clinical Conditions of Menopause and Postmenopausal Women

Cardiovascular Disease

Cardiovascular disease including coronary heart disease, congestive heart failure and stroke are the leading cause of death in both men and women. Most of cardiovascular disease develops from atherosclerotic changes in the major blood vessels. Age alone is a significant predictor of CVD risk in men and women. Other risk factors are same for men and women and they are family history of cardiovascular disease, hypertension, smoking, diabetes mellitus, obesity, and abnormal cholesterol/lipoprotein profile.

Before menopause women have a much lower risk for cardiovascular events compared with men for their age.

Though reasons for protection from CVD in premenopausal women are complex, but estrogen induced greater high density lipoprotein (HDL) is the main cause. After menopause this benefits disappear overtime and there is 2–6 fold higher incidence of CVD in postmenopausal women compared with premenopausal women.

Preventive measures in perimenopausal period can significantly improve quality of life in postmenopausal period. Walking, vigorous exercise prevents cardiovascular events while sedentary lifestyles, central adiposity are risk factor for cardiovascular events.

Weight Gain

Weight gain is a common complaint among postmenopausal women because with ageing a woman's metabolism is slowed down reducing her caloric requirement. That's why eating and exercise habits to be altered in this period. Weight gain in menopausal period is associated with fat deposition in abdomen, which increases the likelihood of developing insulin resistance and subsequent diabetes mellitus and heart disease. **Noncontraceptive HRT, has been shown to have either no effect or if any to decrease slightly the rate of age related increase.**

Skin and Hair Changes

Skin changes like hyperpigmentation, wrinkles are caused in part from skin ageing, which results from the synergetic effects of intrinsic ageing and photo ageing. In addition hormonal ageing of skin causes—reduced thickness due to reduced collagen content, a decrease in sebaceous gland secretion, a loss of elasticity, and epidermal changes. **Estrogen should not be prescribed to improve the appearance of skin, though it has been shown to restore collagen content of skin.** Impact of hormone therapy on skin ageing is difficult to differentiate from the effect of intrinsic ageing, photo ageing and other environmental insults.

After the menopause there is variable loss of pubic and axillary hair. Often there is loss of lanugo hairs on the upper lip, chin and cheeks together with increased growth of coarse terminal hair. A slight mustache may become noticeable, occasionally there is slight balding. All of these changes may be partly as result of reduced level of estrogen in the face of fairly well maintained levels of testosterone.

Other Changes

Dental problem may develop with waning estrogen level in menopause. There can be decreased saliva, increased incidence of cavity, tooth loss. At menopause withdrawal of estrogen and progesterone leads to a relative reduction in breast proliferation. Memory may decrease with advancing age, but the risk factor for decreased cerebral perfusion are transient ischemic attack (TIA), hyperlipidemia, hypertension, smoking, excess alcohol consumption, male gender or postmenopausal age group.

Absence of Estrogen

Psychological and cognitive symptoms may develop during menopausal transition and include depression, mood changes, poor concentration and impaired memory. It is important to remember that menopausal transition is a complex sociocultural as well hormonal event. Psychosocial factors also contribute to mood and cognitive symptoms. During this phase as other factor cause additional emotional stress at this age like dealing with teenagers, onset of any major illness, caring for aging patient, death of family member or divorce, carrier change or retirement.

PATIENT EVALUATION FOR MENOPAUSE

Clinical aim of the menopause transition evaluation is to optimize a woman's health and well-being during and after this transition. This is a time for detailed health evaluation, identifying and presenting risk factor for cardiovascular risk factors, osteoporosis, and certain cancers.

Diagnosis

The diagnosis of menopause can usually be made with documentation of age appropriate symptoms and signs. A patient should undergo thorough examination of constitution (BMI), cognitive, psychological function, skin, breast examination and pelvic examination, which can reveal about changes related to menopause. Differential diagnosis of various menopausal symptoms is summarized in Table 22.1.

Table 22.1: Differential diagnosis of menopausal symptoms

Vasomotor symptoms:
- Hyperthyroidism
- Pheochromocytoma
- Febrile illness
- Anxiety and psychological symptoms

Vaginal dryness, dyspareunia:
- Yeast infection
- Bacterial vaginosis
- Poor vaginal lubrication
- Pelvic pathology
- Marital disharmony

Primary osteoporosis:
- Osteomalacia
- Primary and secondary hyperparathyroidism
- Hyperthyroidism or excess thyroid replacement
- Excess corticoid therapy
- Increased calcium excretion

Abnormal uterine bleeding:
- Anovulation
- Endometrial cancer
- Cervical cancer
- Endometrial hyperplasia
- Endometrial polyp
- Uterine fibroid
- Hormonal treatment
- Urogenital atrophy

Lab Testing

FSH and estrogen level sometime can be done to assess ovarian failure, especially in case of premature ovarian failure or women seeking treatment for infertility. **A FSH level greater than 40 m IU/ml has been used to document ovarian failure associated with menopause.**

Estrogen level may be normal, elevated or low depending on the stage of menopausal transition. After menopause estrogen level are extremely low. Estrogen level can be evaluated by some clinician to assess women's response to hormone replacement therapy. *Usually serum estradiol level of 50–100 pg/ml is desired while woman is on hormone replacement therapy.*

Estrogen maturation index: It is an inexpensive mean to evaluate hormonal influence in women. In a PAP smears test index report is read from left to right and refers to the percentage of parabasal intermediate and superficial squamous cells, which appear on smears. Total sum of all 3 values equal 100%. So 0:30:70 reflects 0% parabasal cell, 30% intermediate cells, and 70% superficial cells. A shift to left indicates increase in parabasal cell that denotes low estrogen level. In the same way a shift to right indicates increase in superficial or intermediate cells, which is associated with higher estrogen level.

MANAGEMENT OF MENOPAUSE

Prevention

Nothing can prevent the physiological menopause and nothing can be done to postpone its onset or slow its progress. Preservation of ovaries while doing hysterectomy for other reasons can prevent symptoms and signs of artificial menopause for a certain period.

Hormone Replacement Therapy

Every woman with menopausal symptoms deserves an adequate explanation of the physiological events she is experiencing, so as to dispel has fears and address symptoms as hot flushes and sleep disturbance. Reassurance should be emphasized. Hormone replacement with estrogen (and a progestin if uterus is present, has been tried in menopause to replace ovarian hormone with a view to relieve menopausal symptoms like hot flushes, urogenital atrophy and gain long-term benefit of estrogen hormone like prevention of osteoporosis. But studies have shown contradictory results.

Some studies have shown a 70–80% improvement in vasomotor symptoms and urogenital atrophy and a 2–5% increase in BMD with a 25–50% decrease risk of vertebral and hip fracture. Other studies have suggested a 20% decrease in risk of colorectal cancer, possibility decreased risk of Alzheimer's disease, 25% reduction in risk of tooth loss while observational studies have pointed to cardio-protective benefit of hormone replacement therapy. Randomized controlled trial have not substantiated this effect. In 2002, a large randomized prospective and controlled study of hormone therapy in menopausal women showed an elevation of cardiac and stroke risk, elevation of thromboembolic event and elevation of breast cancer risk in treated women as compared to non-treated women. While both risk and benefit were small in quantity for any women, the conclusion was that *long-term risk exceeded benefit for HT use in healthy postmenopausal women and that for most women HT should be reserved for treatment of menopausal symptoms for as short duration as possible.*

HRT Preparation and Use

Current indication for HRT are: (a) Relief of menopausal symptoms like hot flushes, vaginal atrophy, (b) Prevention of osteoporosis in only for women who are otherwise taking

HRT for menopause symptoms, or who cannot take antiresorptive therapy for osteoporosis.

For Hot Flushes

A standard dose of estrogen as 0.3–0.625 mg of conjugated equine estrogen, 0.025 mg transdermal estradiol or 0.5 mg oral estradiol should be given daily. Additional formulation containing estradiol, synthetic estrogen and progesterone are also available.

Atrophic Vaginitis

For this vaginal preparation are preferred over systemic estrogens. These preparations are available in the form of creams (conjugated equine estrogen or estradiol 0.25–2 gm giving night by for 2 weeks followed by twice weekly), tablet 25 mg estradiol nightly for 2 weeks followed by twice weekly) and rings (estradiol releasing rings, which remain in place for 3 months).

Though with tablets, rings and lowest dose cream, endometrial proliferation is rare, but if there is use of higher dose or presence of vaginal bleeding, or there are other risk factors, **periodic endometrial biopsy and ultrasound assessment for endometrial thickness is necessary**. Progestins may be necessary to prevent endometrial proliferation in some case.

Progestin Estrogen Therapy

The role of progestin in HRT is to reduce the risk of endometrial hyperplasia with subsequent endometrial cancer which occurs with estrogen only therapy in women who have not had a hysterectomy as there is a 4–8 fold increased risk without progestin.

a. *The combined continuous administration of estrogen plus progestin* is the most common mode of administration today. This regimen promotes endometrial atrophy and results in amenorrhea in 70-90% of women who use continuous therapy for more than one year.
b. Another option is to administer a progestin such as medroxyprogesterone acetate at a dosage of 5-10 mg/day for 12–14 days each month. In this 80-90% of women will experience some vaginal bleeding towards the end of the month.
c. An alternative is to prescribe a lower dosage 2.5 mg continuously. It is important to note that progestin administration can be associated with other uncomfortable side effects including fatigue, depression, breast tenderness, bloating, headaches, or menstrual cramps. Safety of progestin regarding breast cancer has not been established in WHO trial. *Endometrial sampling and ultrasound for endometrial thickness is necessary for the estrogen progestin therapy.*

Contraindication to Estrogen Replacement Therapy

They are as follows:
a. Undiagnosed abnormal vaginal bleeding.
b. Known, suspected or history of cancer of the breast.
c. Known or suspected estrogen dependent neoplasm.
d. Active deep vein thrombosis, pulmonary embolism, or history of these conditions.
e. Arterial thromboembolic disease (MI, Stroke).
f. Liver dysfunction or disease.

Estrogen may have undesirable effects on some patients with *pre-existing seizures, hypertension, fibrocystic disease of the breast, uterine leiomyoma, diabetes mellitus, migraine, headache, chronic thrombophlebitis and gallbladder disease.*

Complications and Risk of HRT

Before discussing the management of estrogen replacement, it is necessary to review the complication and above contraindication to HRT. They play an important role in ultimate decision taken by physician as well patient regarding treatment.

a. **Endometrial cancer:** There is 2–8 fold overall risk of endometrial cancer on estrogen therapy. High dose and prolonged treatment increase the risk.
b. **Breast cancer:** There has been still no conclusive evidence of relationship between HRT and breast cancer. Reanalysis of these studies have found that ever users of HT have a relative risk of breast cancer of 1.14 and current users for 5 or more years have a relative risk of 1.35. The addition of progestin does not appear to decrease risk and even may increase risk. Finally risk does not vary in strata of history of breast cancer or with benign breast disease. It must be remembered that all women are at risk for breast cancer. So the instruction for breast self-examination, a careful breast assessment and routine screening mammography should be a part of the medical care of all older women.
c. **Thromboembolic disease:** Venous thromboembolic disease has been found to be increased with use of HRT. Transdermal estrogen use is associated with lower risk of VTE.
d. **Cardiovascular disease:** The effect of estrogen on cardiovascular disease is unclear. Estrogen has been shown to decrease LDL and total cholesterol while raising HDL and triglycerides. It also decreases lipoprotein, fibrinogen and plasminogen activator inhibitor type 1. Many observational studies have shown a 30-50% decrease in coronary heart disease in estrogen users. A recent RCT found no benefit of HRT over 6.8 years of study. The women's health initiated study show a relative hazard for coronary heart disease of 1.2 of (8/10000 women per year more heart events) after 5.2 years of follow-up in treated Vs untreated women.

e. **Stroke:** Several recent studies suggest that hormone therapy is associated with an increased risk of stroke.
f. **Uterine bleeding:** In women taking estrogen only, the incidence of endometrial hyperplasia can be as high as 25% after only one year of therapy. Thus, a pretreatment biopsy and yearly endometrial biopsy are necessary in all women receiving estrogen alone to assess for presence of hyperplasia. Estrogen withdrawal or combined estrogen progesterone therapy may be employed to treat the hyperplasia.
g. **Gallbladder disease:** There is increased incidence of gallbladder disease following ERT. As estrogen can cause increased amount of cholesterol to collect in bile.
h. **Lipid metabolism:** Estrogen replacement decrease LDL cholesterol and increase HDL cholesterol and triglycerides. Transdermal estrogen is probably less likely to raise triglyceride levels and these are preferred in women with an elevation in triglyceride level.
i. **Miscellaneous:** Other side effects can be generalized edema, mastodynia, abdominal bloating, headache, or excessive cervical mucus. Their side effects may be dose related and are managed by lowering the dosage by use of another agent or by discontinuation of the medicine.

Alternative Medicine for Menopause

a. *Selective estrogen receptor modulators (SERMs):* SERMs are a class of drugs that have estrogen like effect in the urogenital system, hypothalamus, thermoregulatory center, cardiovascular system, and bone as well anti estrogenic properties in breast and endometrium, thus prevent estrogen dependent neoplasm. So they are called designer estrogens. Raloxifene is currently approved for the treatment of osteoporosis and is being studied for potential cardioprotective effects. But it does not improve hot flushes or urogenital atrophy.
b. *Clonidine* is an alpha-adrenergic agonist which may be used to reduce the severity and duration of hot flushes.
c. *Phytoestrogens* containing isoflavones are found to lower the incidence of vasomotor symptoms, osteoporosis and cardiovascular disease.
d. *Soy protein* is also found effective to reduce vasomotor symptoms and act like SERMs.

MULTIPLE CHOICE QUESTIONS

1. HRT is used in all of the following, *except*:
   a. Vaginal atrophy
   b. Osteoporosis
   c. Flushing
   d. Coronary heart disease
   Ans. d
2. All of the following appear to decrease hot flushes in menopausal female, *except*:
   a. Androgen
   b. Raloxifene
   c. Isoflavones
   d. Tibolone
   Ans. b
3. Estrogen administration in menopausal female increases:
   a. Gonadotropin secretion
   b. LDL cholesterol
   c. Bone mass
   d. Muscle mass
   Ans. c
4. The investigation of choice in a 55-year-old postmenopausal female who has presented with postmenopausal bleeding is:
   a. PAP smear
   b. Fractional curettage
   c. TVS
   d. CA 125
   Ans. b
5. Postmenopausal women who is overweight, hypertensive and diabetic, presents with bleeding P/v. The most useful investigation in this patient would be:
   a. TVS
   b. Endometrial sampling
   c. Doppler ultrasound of pelvis
   d. CT scan of pelvis
   Ans. b

23 Premalignant and Malignant Disorders of the Uterine Cervix

*As one lamp lights another, it does not grow less.
So nobleness enkindles nobleness.*

GENERAL CONSIDERATION

The term intraepithelial neoplasm refers to squamous epithelial lesions of the lower genital tract, which are considered to be cancer precursors, but lack feature of invasive cancer. Lesions are diagnosed by properly located biopsy and subsequent histologic evaluation. Cervical, vaginal, vulvar and perineal intraepithelial neoplasia (CIN, VaIn, VIN and AIN) demonstrate a disease spectrum ranging from mildly dysplastic cytoplasmic and nuclear changes to severe dysplasia. In intraepithelial neoplasm, as the name suggests, there is no invasion through the basement membrane, which defines invasive cancer.

Grading of CIN of Uterine Cervix

Cervical intraepithelial neoplasia CIN, formally called dysplasia, means disordered growth and development of the epithelial lining of the cervix. Histologically evaluated lesions are characterized by CIN nomenclature. There are various grades of CIN (Fig. 23.1).

LSIL	HSIL	
CIN	CIN II	CIN III
Mild dysplasia	Moderate dysplasia	Severe dysplasia

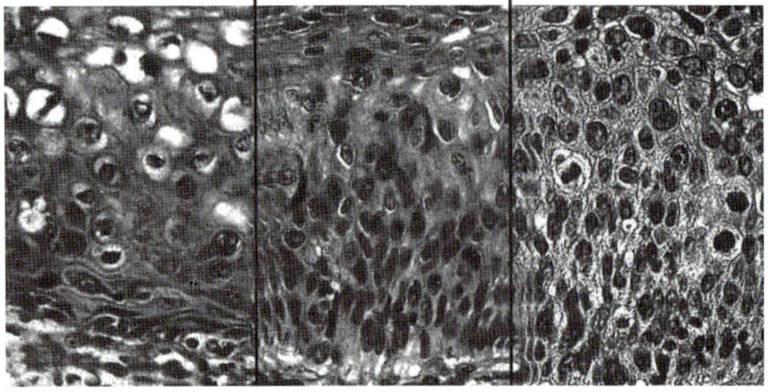

Fig. 23.1: Cytological changes in mild, moderate and severe dysplasia

CIN I (Mild dysplasia): It is defined as disordered growth of the lower third of epithelial lining.

CIN II (Moderate dysplasia): It is abnormal maturation of the lower two third of epithelial lining.

CIN III (Severe dysplasia): It encompasses more than 2/3rd of the epithelial thickness.

Carcinoma in situ: It represents full thickness dysmaturity. In contrast cervical columnar epithelium is only one cell layer thick; it does not demonstrate an analogous neoplastic disease spectrum. Histologic abnormalities are therefore limited to **adenocarcinoma *in situ* (AIS) or adenocarcinoma**.

Bethseda System

Cytologic smears are classified according to Bethseda system (Revised 2001). Briefly atypical squamous cells are divided into **those of undetermined significance (ASC-US)** and those in which a high grade lesions can not be excluded—**ASC-H** (see Table 23.1).

Low-Grade Squamous Intraepithelial Lesions (LSIL)

It encompasses cytological changes consistent with koilocytic atypia or CIN I.

High-Grade Squamous Intraepithelial Lesions (HSIL)

HSIL denotes the cytological finding corresponding to CIN II and CIN III. Bethseda system (2001) has been attempted to reduce confusion in atypical cell category and terms as benign cellular changes or epithelial cell abnormality have been eliminated. Beside this Bethesda system includes Human Papilloma Viruses, cellular changes and CIN I in the same category of low grade squamous intraepithelial neoplasia (LSIL) because they can not be consistently distinguished on the basis of morphology, molecular biology or clinical behavior. Bethseda system has merged CIN II and CIN III because reproducibility in distinguishing them is low, the natural history is same and treatment recommendations are the same.

Pathogenesis of CIN

The cervix is composed of **columnar epithelium**, which lines the endocervical canal and **squamous epithelium**, which covers the exocervix. The point at which they meet is called the *squamous columnar junction (SCJ)*.

Squamous Columnar Junction

It is a dynamic point that changes in response to puberty, pregnancy, menopause and hormonal stimulation. In neonates the SCJ is located in the exocervix. At menarche, the production of estrogen causes the vaginal epithelium to fill with glycogen. Lactobacilli act on the glycogen to lower the pH, stimulating the subcolumnar reserve cells to undergo *metaplasia*. This metaplasia advances from the original SCJ inwards, towards the external os and over the columnar villi. This process establishes an area called the 'Transformation Zone', which extends from the original SCJ to the physiological active SCJ. As the metaplastic epithelium in the transformation zone matures, it begins to produce glycogen and eventually resembles the original squamous epithelium, colposcopically and histologically.

Transformation Zone

The original *squamous epithelium* of the vagina and ectocervix has four layers:
1. **Basal layer:** Single row of immature cells with large nuclei and a small amount of cytoplasm.
2. **Parabasal layer:** It include 2-4 rows of immature cells that have normal mitotic figures and provide the replacement cells for the overlying epithelium.
3. **Intermediate layer:** It is 4-6 rows of cells with larger amount of cytoplasm in a polyhedral shape separated by an intercellular space.
4. **Superficial layer:** It include 5-8 rows of flattened cells with small uniform nucleus and a cytoplasm filled with glycogen. The nuclei become pyknotic and cells detach from the surface called exfoliation. *These exfoliated superficial cells form the basis for Papanicolaou's staining.*

Columnar Epithelium

Columnar epithelium has a single layer of columnar cells with mucus at the top and a round nucleus at the base. This epithelium is composed of numerous ridges, clefts and infolding, and when covered by squamous metaplasia, leads to the appearance of gland openings.

Metaplastic Epithelium

Metaplastic epithelium found at the SCJ begins in the subcolumnar reserve cells. Under stimulation of lower vaginal acidity the reserve cells proliferate, lifting the columnar epithelium. The immature metaplastic cells have large nuclei and a small amount of cytoplasm without glycogen. As the cells mature normally, they produce glycogen, eventually forming the four layers of epithelium. The metaplastic process begins at the tip of columnar villi, which are exposed first to the acid vaginal environment. As the metaplasia replaces the columnar epithelium, the central capillary of the villies regresses and the epithelium flattens out leaving the epithelium with its typical vascular network. As metaplasia proceeds into the cervical clefts, it replaces columnar epithelium and similarly flattens the epithelium, leaving mucus secreting columnar epithelium trapped under the squamous epithelium. Some of these glands open onto the surface, other are completely encased, with mucus collecting in **Nebothian cysts**. Thus glands opening and Nebothian cyst mark the original SCJ and outer edge of the original transformation zone.

In general because of rapid turnover of cells, transformation zone throughout the body are susceptible to carcinogens and carcinogenesis. **The cervix is uniquely susceptible to HPV induced cervical carcinogenesis, when contrasted with the vagina.** Although the vagina has a much greater surface area than the cervix, vaginal cancer is one of the rarest of all malignancies. **Approximately 75 to 80% of all cervical cancers are squamous cell carcinoma, adenocarcinoma account for most of the remaining 25%.**

EPIDEMIOLOGICAL RISK FACTORS FOR CIN

They are same as for cervical cancer and include: (a) Early onset of sexual activity, (b) Multiple sexual partners, (c) High risk sexual partner, (d) HPV infection, lower genital tract neoplasia, (e) History of STD's, (f) Cigarette smoking, (g) HIV infection, (h) AIDS and others form of immunosuppression, (i) Multiparity, (j) Long-term contraceptive use.

Human Papilloma Virus

It is a prime etiologic factor in the development of CIN and cervical cancers. **Analysis of cervical neoplasia lesions shows the presence of HPV in more than 80% of all CIN lesions and in 99.7% of all invasive cervical cancers.** In fact most of the above behavioral and sexual risk factors for cervical neoplasia become statistically insignificant as independent variables after adjusting for HPV infection.

Basic Virology, Life Cycle and Types of HPV

HPV is a non enveloped DNA virus with a protein capsid. It infects epithelial cells exclusively. More than 100 HPV types have now been identified. **Low risk HPV are type 6 and 11**, which cause nearly all genital warts and a minority of subclinical HPV infections. They are rarely oncogenic. **High risk HR-HPV type are 16, 18, 31, 33, 35, 45, and 58**, which account for approximately 95% of cervical cancer world wide. HPV 16, 18, 45 and 31 are most prevalent. Specifically *HPV 16 is the dominant cancer related HPV*, accounting for 40-70% of invasive squamous cells cervical cancer world wide. *HPV 18* is thought to play a dominant role in the development of rapid transit cervical cancers. These cancer develop within 1-3 years of negative cervical cytology, are more likely to be adeno or adenosquamous and develop in younger women.

Transmission

Transmission of genital HPV usually requires sexual contact with genital skin, mucous membrane or body fluid of partner with either warts or subclinical infection. It is one of the most common STD. Vertical transmission from mother to infant is rare.

Outcome of HPV Infection

Genital HPV infection can be latent or expressed. Expressions may be productive with formation of new viruses or neoplastic causing preinvasive disease or malignancy. In cancerous lesions, the circular HPV genome integrates linearly at random locations into a host chromosome. Unrestrained transcription of E_6 and E_7 oncogenes follows. Oncoproteins interfere with the function and accelerate degradation of p53 and pRB which are key host tumor suppressor proteins. This makes the infected cells vulnerable to malignant transformation by loss of cell cycle control, cellular proliferation and accumulation of DNA mutations (Flow chart 23.1).

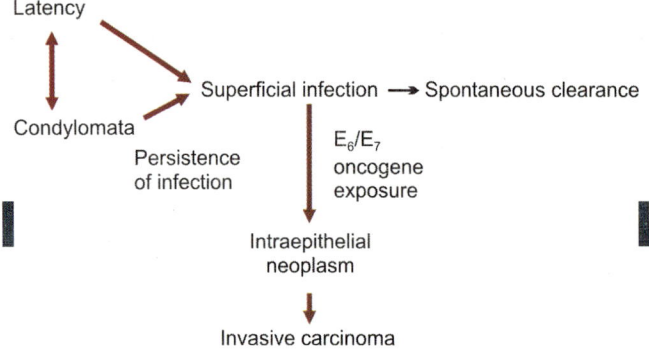

Flow chart 23.1: Outcome of genital HPV infection

The natural history of genital HPV infection, spontaneous resolution is most common outcome and neoplasm is least common manifestation developing over years as a result of persistent infection.

Risk Factors

The strongest risk factors for genital HPV infection are early age of sexual activity and number of life time and recent sexual partners.

Diagnosis of Infection

Infection with HPV is suspected by the appearance of clinical lesions and result of cytology, histology and colposcopy but all are subjective and often inaccurate. In addition serology is unreliable. **A definitive diagnosis can be made only by the direct detection of HPV DNA by PCR, or by Hybrid Capture (HC) technique.** Clinical HPV testing by HC can be done on collection of cervical cells using a small brush device or in conjunction with liquid based cytology. If a typical wart in young women is found or if high grade cervical neoplasia or invasive cancer is identified by cytology or histology then HPV infection is assumed and confirmation by HPV testing is not necessary. *Routine testing for HPV is not* currently indicated outside of cervical cancer screening and triage or surveillance of abnormal cytology.

Treatment

Most HPV infections are transient and warts have a spontaneous regression rate of 60-70%. **The only indication to treat HPV related lower genital tract diseases are the presence of neoplasia or symptomatic warts that cause physical discomfort or psychological distress.**

Prevention

1. *Behavioral intervention:* Sexual abstinence, delaying coitarche and limiting the number of sexual partners are the most logical strategies to avoid or limit genital HPV infections and its effects.
2. *Barrier contraception.*
3. *Vaccines:* Development of vaccines offers the greatest promise for prevention of HPV infection and perhaps limiting or reversing its sequele in those already infected.

Immunology of HPV

Immune response appears to be a key determinant of HPV epidemiology and oncogenicity. At present it is supposed that local and humoral immunity protects against initial infection. Cell mediated immunity likely plays the larger role in HPV infection persistence as well as progression or regression of benign and neoplastic lesions.

Prophylactic Vaccines

These vaccines elicit humoral antibodies that neutralize HPV before it can infect host cells. Although they do not prevent transient HPV positivity, they do prevent establishment of persistent infection and therefore the development of cervical neoplasia.

Gardacil (Merck and Co Inc) has shown 90-100% protection against genital warts plus vulvar, vaginal and cervical neoplasia in women who are serologically and genital tract PCR negative for HPV types covered, i.e. 6, 11, 16, and 18. Gardacil has received approval for vaccination of girls and women aged 9-26 years. A bivalent HPV 16/18 vaccine—**Cervarix** (GSK) has shown similar efficacy. Vaccine is administered in three intramuscular doses during a 6 months period. Both vaccines are safe and well tolerated. *Testing for HPV is not recommended before vaccination.* It is emphasized that vaccination should be done prior to coitarche, when protection provided is nearly 100%. However a history of previous sexual intercourse or HPV related disease is not a contraindication to vaccine administration because exposure to the HPV type targeted by the vaccine is not certain. The vaccination strategy recommends routine administration of vaccine to girls aged 11-12 years and is allowed for 9-26 years old individual irrespective of their sexual activity.

Cigarette Smoking

Cigarette smoking and HPV infections have synergestic effects on the development of CIN and **cigarette smoking is associated with 2-4 fold increase in relative risk for developing cervical cancer**. Cigarette smoke carcinogens have been found to accumulate locally in the cervical mucous and the cumulated exposure as measured by pack years smoked is related to the risk of developing CIN or carcinoma *in situ*.

Dietary Deficiency

Though data are inconclusive, dietary deficiency of certain vitamins such as A, C, E, beta carotene and folic acid may alter cellular resistance to HPV infection, promoting viral infection persistence and cervical neoplasia.

Combined Oral Contraceptive and Parity

Studies are conflicting and inconclusive of role of COC and Parity in development of CIN.

CLINICAL FINDINGS OF CIN

There are usually no symptoms or signs of CIN and the diagnosis is most often based on biopsy findings, following an abnormal routine cervical cytology smear. Because high grade dysplasia probably is a transitional phase in the pathogenesis of many cervical cancers, **early detection is extremely important**.

Screening Guidelines

Based on the American Cancer Society guidelines, which were last reviewed in 2002, all women, **who have reached 21 years or who are 3 years post-coitarche**, should have a pelvic examination and collection of cytologic smear. Cervical cytology smear should be performed yearly if conventional Pap smear is done and biannually if liquid based cytology is done. After age of 30 years and with three consecutive negative smears, the time interval between cervical cytology smears can be extended to every 3 years. Cervical cytology screening can be discontinued at the age of 70 years if the patient had 3 or more consecutive normal smears in the preceding 10 years. Screening cytology smears may also be discontinued if the patient has undergone a total hysterectomy unless it was done for the treatment of cervical dysplasia or cancer.

Method of Cervical Screening

a. *Conventional Pap collection:* Conventional Pap test smear is a smear of cells made directly from collection device to glass slide at the time of sampling.
b. *Liquid based Pap collection:* In this cells are collected in a liquid transport medium that is subsequently processed to produce an even monolayer of cells on a glass slide. In this most of the cellular sample is retained in suspension and random sampling of cells is transferred to the slide in an even preparation. These processing techniques also allow removal of extraneous material such as blood, providing better visualization of the cells.
c. *Computer screening technologies:* Limitation of conventional technique is that more than half of the material remains on the collection device, which is discarded and thus is lost for microscopic analysis. To preserve morphology details, slides are fixed by emersion in alcohol or sprayed with fixative. Air drying limits the interpretation of the specimen. To reduce the false negative results associated with diagnostic evaluation of Pap slides a number of new approaches have been developed using computer image analysis technology, these technologies are cost effective.

Performing a Pap Test

Preparation

Ideally Pap test should be scheduled to avoid menstruation. Patient should abstain from vaginal intercourse, douching or medical cream. Treatment of cervicitis or vaginitis prior to Pap testing is optimal. However, Pap testing should never be deferred due to unexplained infertility condition or bleeding, as these signs and symptoms may be caused by cervical or other genital tract cancers. Pap screening should be performed in high-risk patients whenever an opportunity arises.

Complete history-taking and pelvic examination is essential to accurate interpretation of Pap. Date of LMP, pregnancy, exogenous hormone use, menopausal status, past history of AUB, IUD, high-risk sexual behavior and immunosuppression are important issues for notification. *Location:* Sampling of TZ is paramount to the sensitivity of the Pap test. Adequate visualization of cervix is essential. Touching the cervix should be avoided prior to Pap smear taking as dysplastic epithelium may be inadvertently removed with minimal trauma. Three types of devices are commonly used to sample the cervix: (a) Spatula, (b) Broom, (c) Endocervical brush (Fig. 23.2A).

A spatula is designed to best fit the cervical contour, straddle the squamous columnar junction and sample the distal endocervical canal. All cervical surface is scraped completing at least one full rotation. Plastic spatula is preferred to wood as cells are more readily released from a plastic surface (Fig. 23.2B).

The endocervical brush is used to collect and release endocervical cells. After spatula sample is obtained, the endocervical brush is inserted into the endocervical canal only until the outermost bristle remains visible. It avoids inadvertent sampling of lower segment cells. To avoid excessive bleeding, the brush is rotated only one quarter to one half turn. If the cervical canal is wide as in parous women, the brush is moved to contact all surface of the entire endocervical canal. Broom device have longer central bristles that are inserted into the endocervical canal.

Evaluation of Cytology Results

A cytology report is a medical consultation that interprets a screening test and is not a diagnosis. So **final diagnosis is determined clinically and often supplemented with histologic evaluation**. Pap test is interpreted as either negative for intraepithelial lesions or malignancy, consistent with one or more epithelial cells abnormalities. As mentioned above in Bethesda III system (2001) potentially premalignant squamous lesions fall into three categories. Table 23.1 summarizes Bethesda system for epithelial cell abnormalities.

Table 23.1: Bethesda system*—epithelial cells abnormalities

Squamous Cell
- Atypical squamous cells (ASC)
- Atypical squamous cells of undetermined significance (ASC-US)
- Atypical squamous cells cannot exclude HSIL (ASC-H)
- Low-grade squamous intraepithelial lesion (LSIL)
- High-grade squamous intraepithelial lesion (HSIL)
- Squamous cell carcinoma

Glandular Cell
- Atypical glandular cells (AGC)
- Endocervical, endometrial or not otherwise specified
- Atypical glandular cells, favor neoplastic
- Endocervical or not otherwise specified
- Endocervical adenocarcinoma *in situ* (AIS)
- Adenocarcinoma

* The Bethseda system includes HPV cellular changes and CIN I in the same category of low-grade squamous intraepithelial neoplasia because they cannot be consistency distinguished on the basis of morphology, molecular biology or clinical behavior. It includes CIN II and CIN III together because reproducibility in distinguishing them is low, the natural history is similar and the treatment recommendations are the same.

A. **Atypical Squamous Cell (ASC)**, which is categorized into:
   i. Atypical squamous cell with undetermined significance (ASCUS).
   ii. ASCH, in which high grade lesions must be excluded.

   ASCUS are cells which are suggestive of but do not fulfill criteria for SIL. There are following options for evaluation of ASCUS:
   a. *HPV DNA testing:* If liquid based cytology (LBC) is used, HPV DNA testing is done from the same sample.
      i. If high-risk HPV DNA type is found, colposcopy is indicated as risk of CINI or 3 is equal to that of LSIL cytology.

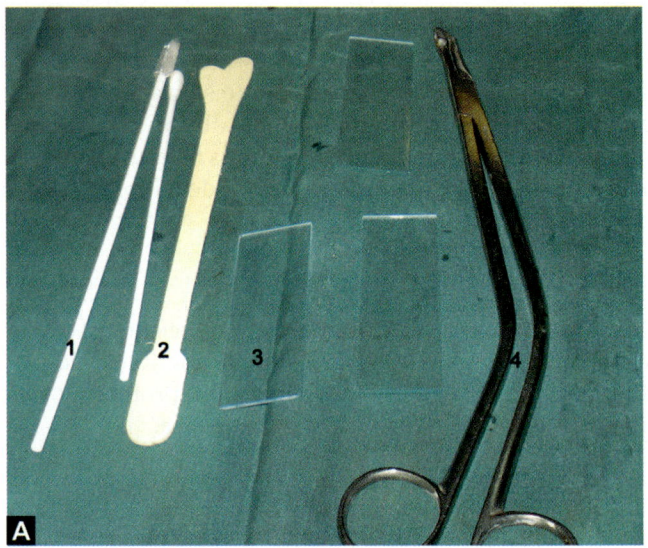

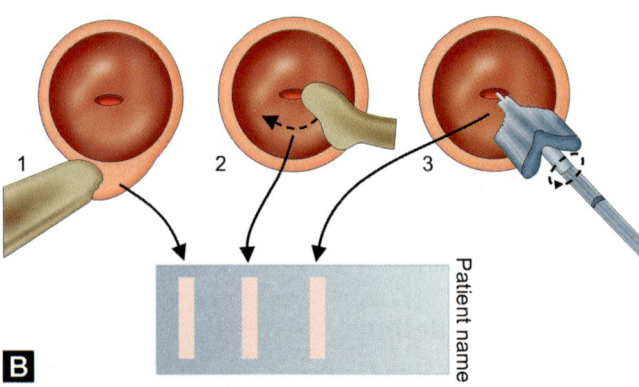

Figs 23.2A and B: (A) Equipment for taking Pap smear and cervical biopsy: (1) Endocervical brush, (2) Ayre's spatula, (3) Slide, (4) Cervical biopsy punch; (B) Method of taking Pap smear: (1) Smear by spatula from posterior fornix, (2) Smear from squamocolumnar junction, (3) Smear from endocervical canal by endocervical brush/broom

ii. If high-risk HPV DNA is absent, a repeat Pap test in 12 months is recommended, or immediate colposcopy in patient who are unlikely to come for follow-up.

B. **ASC-H:** 5-10% of ASC is designated as atypical squamous cells. These are cellular changes, that do not fulfill criteria for HSIL cytology, but for which a high grade lesions cannot be excluded. In these findings colposcopy is indicated for evaluation.

C. **LSIL (Low-grade squamous intraepithelial lesions):** This denotes likely presence of HPV infection or low-grade neoplasia. Colposcopy is indicated for most. In reproductive aged women HPV testing is not useful as in ≈ 80% test will be positive for HPV DNA. In adolescent repeat cytology is recommended, while in postmenopausal women repeat HC HPV testing or repeat cytology at 6 and 12 months is recommended as there is lower rate of positivity in postmenopausal women. **HPV positivity or abnormal repeat cytology is indications for colposcopy (Fig. 23.3A).**

D. **High-grade squamous intraepithelial lesion and (HSIL) glandular abnormalities:** HSIL, all glandular epithelial cells abnormalities and suspicion of carcinoma should be evaluated by *prompt colposcopic evaluation*. HSIL cytology encompasses feature of CIN2 and CIN III (70%) or invasive cancer (1-2%). HPV DNA testing is not useful in the management of HSIL cytology. Alternatively in women aged 21 years and older, diagnostic loop excision can be done. If atypical glandular cells (AGC) cytology is found, squamous neoplasia is the most common diagnosis, but there is also a high-risk of both endocervical and endometrial as well other reproductive tract cancers (Fig. 23.3B). **Therefore in these cases, colposcopic evaluation should include endocervical sampling in nonpregnant patients and endometrial biopsy in women older than 35 years and in younger women if there is a history of abnormal uterine bleeding.** If colposcopy and biopsies are without evidence of neoplasia, management of glandular abnormalities is generally more aggressive than for other abnormalities due to higher risk of occult disease. For initial management of epithelial cells abnormalities refer Flow chart 23.2.

Nonneoplastic Findings

The finding of *Trichomonas vaginalis*, candida species, herpes simplex virus or flora consistent with bacterial vaginosis may be reported. Other non-neoplastic findings may be reactive changes associated with inflammation or repair, radiation, posthysterectomy benign glandular cells. All of these should be managed accordingly.

If benign appearing endometrial cells are found, no evaluation is needed in asymptomatic premenopausal women, **but in postmenopausal women, and those with**

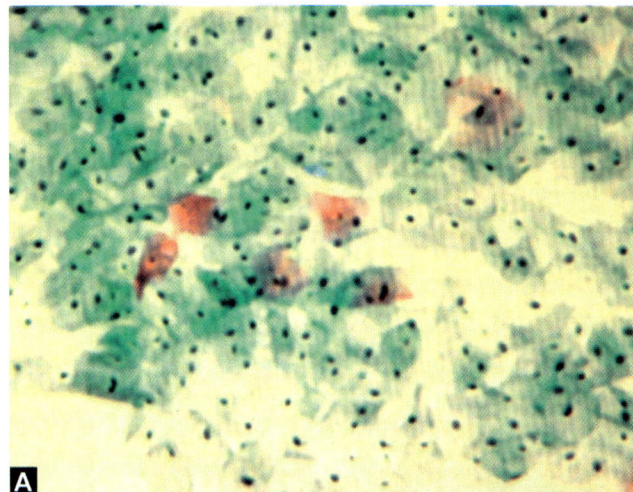

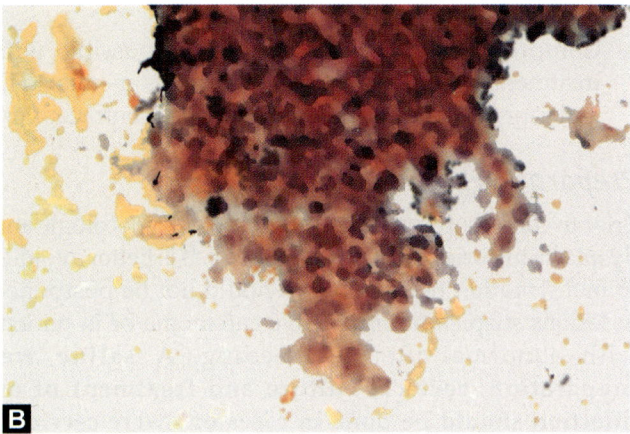

Figs 23.3A and B: Cytology of LSIL and HSIL: (A) LSIL (mild dysplasia); (B) HSIL (severe dysplasia)

abnormal uterine bleeding (AUB) or presence of other risk factors for endometrial disease should undergo further evaluation of the endometrium.

Repeat Cervical Cytology

Prior to performing a repeat smear for ASCUS, patient should be evaluated and treated for potential underlying condition that might cause an atypical smear as antimicrobials for infections or hormones for atrophic vaginitis. Cervical cytology smear should be repeated every 6 months until there are two consecutive normal smears. A 2nd abnormal smear should be evaluated by colposcopy.

COLPOSCOPY

Colposcopy is an outpatient procedure. It is simple, quick and well-accepted. *Colposcopy allows examination of the lower genital tract and anus with microscope to further evaluate abnormal Pap smear test and visible epithelial abnormalities.* Colposcopic examination of cervix is the clinical standard in the evaluation of patients with abnormal cervical cytology.

Colposcope

The colposcope consist of a stereoscopic viewing system with magnification setting ranging from 3–40 fold attached to a free movable stand. A high intensity halogen light provides illumination, use of a green (red free) light filter emphasized contrast by causing the color red to appear black, which aids the examination of vascular pattern (Fig. 23.4).

Advantages of Colposcopy

a. It involves the clinician in diagnosis and management.
b. It permits on the spot assessment of the case.
c. It can easily distinguish between high-grade and low-grade lesion.
d. Therapy can be given under colposcopic guidance by LLETZ or CO_2 or laser.
e. Comprehensive health care become possible with treatment and counseling for condition as anemia, STD, and reproductive tract infection as well contraception.

Preparation

Prior to colposcopy, medical records, past gynecologic and dysplasia histories should be reviewed. It is better avoided in menstruation period, but it should not be postponed in lesions suspicion for invasive carcinoma or in patient with abnormal uterine bleeding. **A saline wet preparation, cervical culture and treatment of an infection should be done in cases of severe cervicitis before performing biopsy or endocervical curettage.** A Pap test at the time of colposcopy is of questionable value and should be individualized according to finding and previous records.

Solutions

Following solutions are used sequentially:

1. **Normal saline**: Saline washing removes cervical mucus and allows vascular and surface feature of lesions to be initially assessed.
2. **Acetic acid**: 3-5% acetic acid is a mucolytic agent that reversibly clumps nuclear chromatin causing lesions to assume various shades of white depending on the degree of abnormal chromatin density. *Epithelium that turns white after application of 3-5% acetic acid is called Acetowhite epithelium, which is characteristic of neoplastic lesion or dysplastic cells* (Figs 23.5A and B).
3. **Lugol's solution**: Lugol iodine solution stains mature squamous epithelial cells in mahogany color due to high glycogen content. Dysplastic cells have lower glycogen content and fail to fully stain and appear faintly yellow. It is useful when abnormal tissue can not be found using acetic acid alone and better defines the limits of transformation zone (Fig. 23.5D).

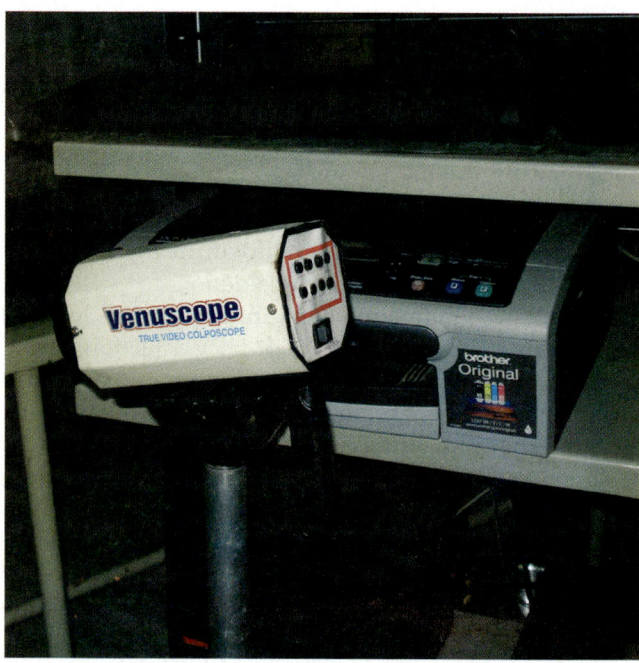

Fig. 23.4: Video colposcope

Colposcopic Grading

A *satisfactory colposcopy* is one where the squamous columnar junction and the full extent of abnormal epithelium are visible. An examination is *unsatisfactory* when the extent of lesion is not seen as when lesion extends into the endocervix and obscured by inflammation or atrophy.

Pattern of colposcopic findings are summarized in Table 23.2.

Table 23.2: Pattern of colposcopic findings

A. Normal colposcopic epithelium
   a. Original squamous epithelium
   b. Columnar epithelium
   c. Transformation zone
B. Abnormal colposcopic finding
   a. Atypical transformation zone
      i. Mosaic
      ii. Punctation
      iii. Acetowhite epithelium
      iv. Hyperkeratosis
      v. Atypical vessels irregular branching on the surface.
   b. Invasive cancer
C. Miscellaneous colposcopic findings
   a. Inflammatory changes
   b. Atrophic changes
   c. Erosion
   d. Condyloma

Patterns of the abnormal ectocervical epithelium containing CIN I are described as *acetowhite, mosaic and punctated*. **Leukoplakia** is white plaque before application of acetic acid. Leukoplakia is caused by a layer of keratin on the surface of the epithelium. Immature squamous epithelial cells have the potential to develop into keratin producing cells or glycogen producing cells. In vagina and the cervix normal differentiation is towards glycogen. *Keratin* production is abnormal in cervicovaginal mucosa and *leukoplakia* is caused by *HPV, keratinizing CIN, keratinizing carcinoma, chronic trauma, from foreign body, or radiotherapy.* Currently the most common reasons for leukoplakia are HPV infection and such area should undergo biopsy to rule out keratinizing carcinoma.

Punctation

Dilated capillaries terminating on the surface appear from the ends as a collection of dots and are referred to as punctation. **When these vessels are seen in a well demarcated area of acetowhite epithelium, they indicate abnormal epithelium.** The punctate vessels are formed as the metaplastic epithelium migrates over the columnar villi. Normally the capillary regresses but in CIN capillary persists and appear more prominent (Fig. 23.5C).

Mosaic

Terminal capillaries surrounding roughly circular or polygonal shaped blocks of acetowhite epithelium crowded together are called mosaics.

These mosaic patterns arise from coalescence of many terminal punctate vessels or from the vessels that surround the cervical gland opening. **Mosaicism tends to be associated with high-grade lesions and CIN II and CIN III.**

Atypical Vascular Pattern

It is characteristic of invasive cervical cancer. **This includes looped vessels, branching vessels and reticular vessels.** Intense acetowhite changes, nonuniform or fused papillae,

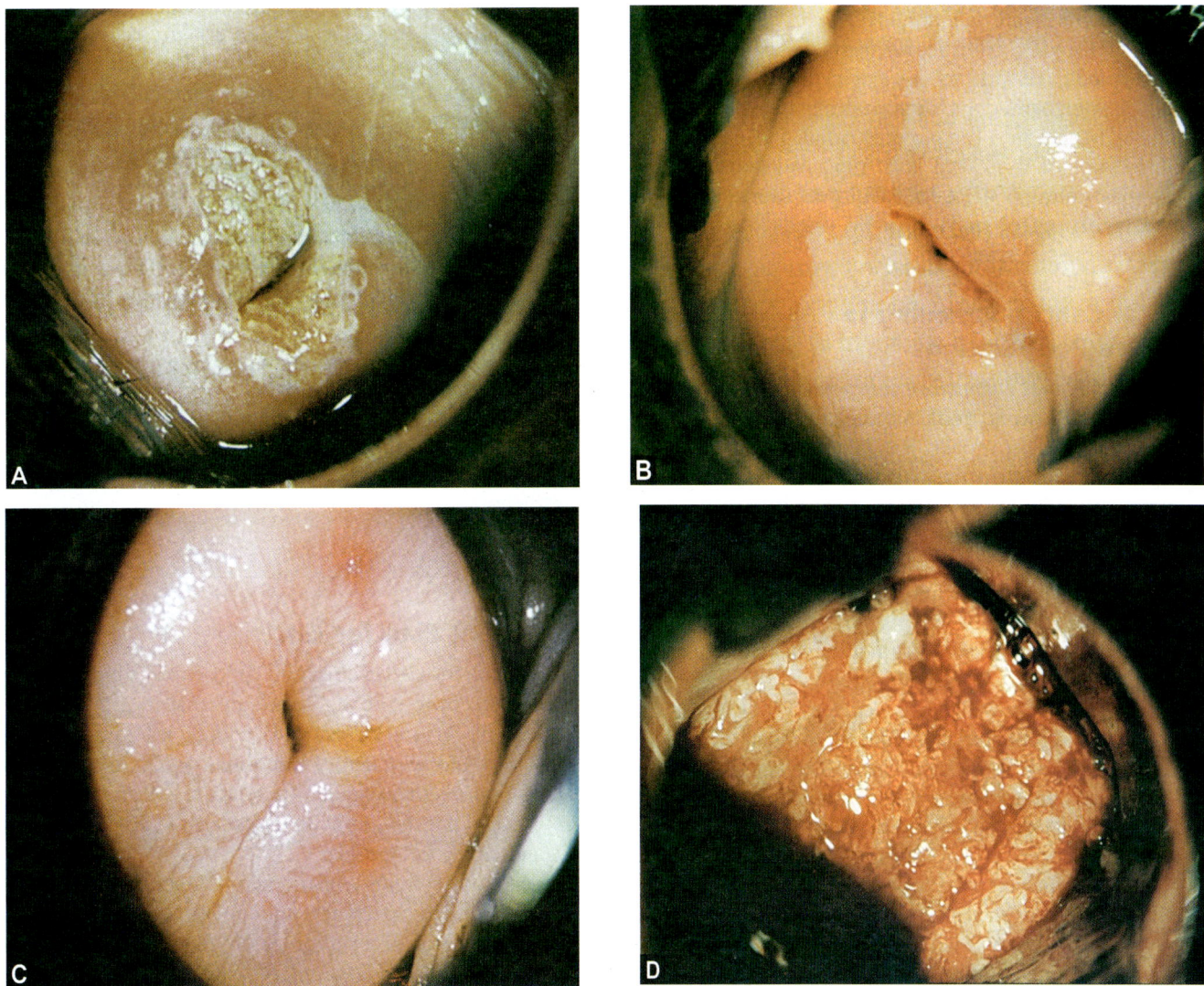

Figs 23.5A to D: Colposcopic findings: (A and B) Acetowhite areas after application of acetic acid; (C) Linear vascular pattern; (D) Negative stain of abnormal area after application of Lugol's iodine

large crypt openings with excessive mucus production and abnormal blood vessels suggest the presence of *adenocarcinoma in situ*. International colposcopic terminology is summarized in Table 23.2.

Biopsy

Colposcopy *directed biopsy* of most abnormal and suspicious areas is taken. If lesion is large or multifocal, multiple biopsies may be necessary to assure complete sample of the affected tissue. Generally biopsy does not require an anesthetic.

Endocervical curettage is used to evaluate tissue within the endocervical canal, not visualized by colposcopy. Normal ECC provides an added degree of assurance that a neoplastic endocervical lesion is not present. It is indicated when:
a. Unsatisfactory colposcopy, common in postmenopausal women.
b. Atypical glandular cells on Pap smear.
c. Ablative treatment is planned.
d. Conization for adenocarcinoma *in situ* has been performed.

ECC is performed by introducing an endocervical currettege 1-2 cm into the cervical canal. Full length and circumference of the canal is firmly curetted, carefully avoiding sampling of ectocervix or lower uterus segment. Alternatively cytobrush may be used to obtain an endocervical tissue specimen.

Cervical Cancer Screening in Resource Poor Settings

a. *Unaided visual inspection with naked eye:* It can be done by paramedical workers. It is the WHO recommended approach for down staging of cancer cervix in developing countries. Sensitivity and specificity is low (40%, 60% respectively).
b. *Visual inspection with acetic acid (VIA):* It consists of unmagnified evaluation of the cervix TZ after application of 3 to 5% dilute acetic acid for visual signs of a high-grade CIN lesions. The test is considered positive if clear and well defined acetowhite areas are detected near SCJ.
c. *Visual inspection with magnification (VIM):* It employs a lower power magnification device to inspect the cervix after treating it with acetic acid. The sensitivity and specificity of above techniques ranges from 49 to 98%. As VIA and colposcopy are based on the same visual technique, precancerous lesions missed by VIA are likely to be missed by colposcopy.
d. *Self-collected samples for detection of human papilloma virus:* Women are said to self-collect samples by inserting a swab in the vagina up to the vault and rotating in the vagina vaults. Swab then is placed in transport media, and collected for further testing for HPV DNA. Self-collection has sensitivity of 74% and specificity of 84%. The lower sensitivity may be acceptable if women who otherwise would not be screened are encouraged to participate.
e. *Cervicography:* A photograph of the cervix is examined for atypical lesions. It has sensitivity comparable to Pap smear but specificity is lower.

MANAGEMENT OF HISTOLOGIC CIN

Understanding the natural history of various degree of CIN is central to the appropriate clinical management of these patients (Table 23.3). In addition the degree of dysplasia, other factors are also considered like patient's age, inciting HPV type, patient's immune competence and smoking habits. Majority of CIN I lesion will spontaneously regress without treatment. However, **9-16% of patient with untreated CIN I are diagnosed with CIN II / CIN III over a 2 years follow-up**. Overall spontaneous regression rates of CIN I is 60%. In young women it is up to 91%. So **it is generally reasonable to expectantly follow the compliant patient with CIN I with repeat cervical cytology at 6 months interval, and HPV test at 12 months interval**. For high risk patient, immediate treatment might be appropriate, as up to 40% of high-risk patients may have persistent or progressive disease that will eventually require therapy. All CIN II and III lesions require treatment. **Treatment is recommended as CIN II progress to carcinoma *in situ* (CIS) in 20% of cases and to invasion in 5%**.

Table 23.3: Natural history of CIN: Spontaneous regression, persistence and progression of CIN

	CIN I	CIN II	CIN III
Regression to normal	60%	40%	30%
Persistence	30%	35%	48%
Progressive to CIN III	10%	20%	
Progressive to cancer	<1%	5%	22%

Treatment Plan for CIN

Ideally both the pathologist and coposcopist should review the colposcopic findings and the results of cytologic assessment, cervical biopsy and endocervical sample before deciding therapy. Current treatment of CIN is limited to local ablations or excisional procedure. *Medical treatment using topical agents is only investigational and not recognized as standard clinical practice.*

Selection of treatment modality depends on multiple factors including patient's age, parity, desire for future fertility, size and severity of lesion, contour of the cervix, prior treatment for CIN and coexisting medical condition as immunocompromised status.

Ablation Therapy

It is appropriate if:
a. There is no evidence of microinvasion or invasive cancer on any of investigation.
b. The lesion is located on the ectocervix and can be seen entirely.
c. There is no involvement of the endocervix with high-grade dysplasia as determined by colposcopy ECC.

Cryotherapy

In cryotherapy a refrigerant gas usually nitrous oxide, through flexible tubing is passed to a metal probe which freezes tissue on contact. Cryonecrosis is achieved by crystallizing intracellular water (Fig. 23.6).

Method

The cryoprobe is positioned on the ectocervix, where it must cover the entire lesion and refrigerating gas is passed until blanching of the cervix extends at least 7 mm beyond the probe in all direction. Introduction of two cycle freeze, thaw, and freeze techniques has improved the efficacy.

Indications

a. CIN grade I / II.
b. Small lesion.
c. Ectocervical location only.
d. Negative endocervical sample.
e. No endocervical gland involvement on biopsy.

Advantage

Easy to learn, low cost, easily available and low complication rate.

Side Effects

There is mild uterine cramping and copious watery vaginal discharge for several weeks. Besides follow-up colposcopic examination can be unsatisfactory because of inability to visualize SCJ.

CO_2 Laser Ablation

Treatment with light amplification by stimulated emission of radiation (Laser) is delivered using colposcopic guidance with a micromanipulator. Laser vaporizes tissue to a depth of 5-7 mm but because of high cost of equipment as well need for special training, this modality has fallen out of favor.

Excision Treatment

Indications

A. *Diagnostic excisional procedure is must if:*
 a. Lesion suspicious for invasive cancer and adenocarcinoma *in situ* of cervix.

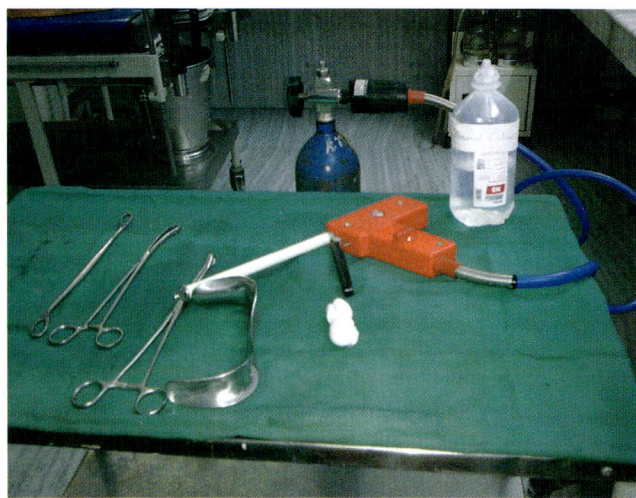

Fig. 23.6: Equipment for cryosurgery attached to source of liquid nitrogen

 b. Patient with unsatisfactory colposcopy.
 c. Histologic CIN.
 d. Unexplained high-grade or recurrent AGC cytology.
 e. Cytologic Vs Biopsy discordance, when histologic results are significantly less severe.

B. **Excision treatment modalities:** Excision is recommended if there is post treat recurrence of high-grade CIN to allow complete histologic evaluation of the specimen.

 a. **Loop electrosurgical excision procedure (LEEP):** This is procedure of choice for treating CIN II and CIN III because of its ease of use, low cost, and provision of tissue for histologic evaluation.
 Method: In this a small thin wire on an insulated handle attached to an electrosurgical generator is used. Electric current is passed and this instrument simultaneously cut and coagulates tissues under direct colposcopic visualization. It can be performed under local anesthesia. The size and shape of tissue excision can be customized by varying loop type and the sequential order in which loop are used. This helps in conserving cervical stroma volume. Fulguration with a roller ball electrode can be added to achieve complete hemostasis. An insulated speculum to prevent conduction of electricity, a grounding pad and a vacuum to remove the smoke are necessary.
 Complication: Complication are minimal. There can be bleeding, infection and cervical stenosis.
 Selection of patients: Those at highest risk for invasive cancer, CIN Grade III, discordance between cytology, biopsy and colposcopy results, patients older than 35 with CIN III, high-grade large lesions, and biopsies showing AIS.

 b. **Cold knife conization:** In this method entire cervical transformation zone including the cervical lesions is excised by scalpel (Fig. 23.7). It is performed under general or regional anesthetic in operation theater. The shape and size of cone excised can be individualized. For example, a wide shallow cone can be obtained for a young patients, where SCJ is on ectocervix. In older patients deeper cone is preferred.

Complications: (a) Bleeding, (b) Infection, (c) Cervical stenosis, (d) Cervical incompetence, (e) Removal of greater than 10 mm depth of cervical tissue is an independent risk factor for preterm labor, (f) Cervical stenosis: It may require dilation for evaluation of recurrence and facilitating progressive labor.

Advantage: It gives a specimen devoid of any thermal artifact, which may complicate the histologic diagnosis. It is particularly important with suspected microinvasive carcinoma and adenocarcinoma *in situ*.

c. **CO_2 laser conization**: It has disadvantage of high cost, need of special training and thermal compromise of margins. But advantages are less blood loss and precise cone size and shape tailoring.

Follow-up

Post-treatment after ablation or excision, additional patient surveillance is required.
a. Patient with excision margin negative for CIN or who have undergone an ablation procedure might be followed with cytology testing alone or with colposcopy every 6 months until two negative evaluations are obtained before returning to routine screening. Alternatively HPV DNA testing may be done between 6-12 months post-treatment and colposcopy performed for persistent HPV infection as this is a sensitive marker of disease persistence. Cytology screening should be continued for at least 20 years thereafter.
b. Patient with positive for CIN II & III or positive ECC, repeat cytology and ECS is done 4-6 months later, but repeat excision is also acceptable.

See and Treat Options

The current cervical cancer screening programs practiced in high resource setting include at least three visits: (a) Screening, (b) Triage of equivocal result, colposcopy with directed biopsy, (c) Treatment, (d) Post-treatment follow-up.

In resource poor setting, screening and treatment in a single visit or providing treatment a short time after screening has been tried. Women who were HPV positive or who had a positive VIA test were assigned randomly to cryotherapy or to delayed treatment. At 6-12 months, high-grade CIN was found to be significantly lower in see and treat group. This can be considered in resource poor setting and women with poor compliance or unreachable population like women living in far off village, hills area.

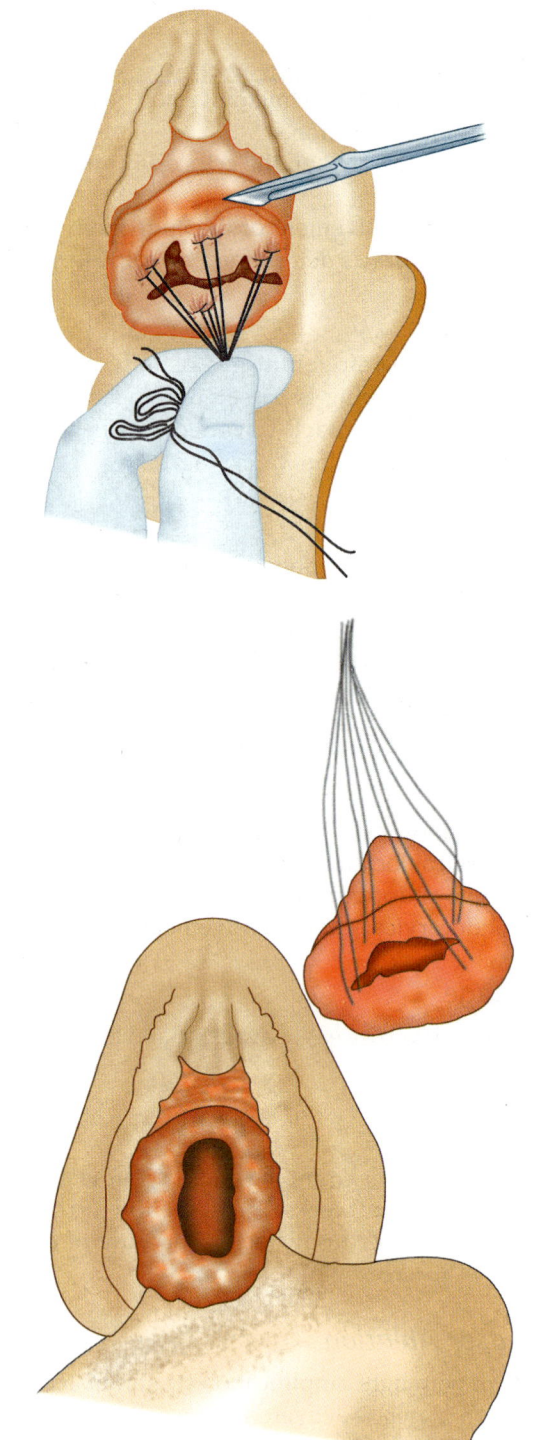

Fig. 23.7: Conization of cervix for the treatment of CIN

Hysterectomy

Hysterectomy is considered too radical for treatment of CIN. It can be considered in following situations:
a. Microinvasive carcinoma.
b. CIN III at margin of cone specimen.

c. AIS where future fertility is not decided.
d. Poor compliance with follow-up.
e. High-grade CIN with completed child bearing and repeat cervical excision is technically not feasible.
f. There are other gynecologic problems requiring hysterectomy as fibroid, prolapse, endometriosis and PID.

Although hysterectomy provides the lowest recurrence rate of CIN, invasive cancer must always be excluded beforehand. Even with negative cervical margin, hysterectomy performed for CIN is not completely protective. Patients particularly immunosuppressed are at risk for recurrent disease and require postoperative interval cytologic screening of the vaginal cuff. Treatment for CIN has been summarized in Flow chart 23.2.

Special Situation

Pregnancy

Pregnant women should routinely undergo cervical cytology screening at first prenatal visit. Colposcopy can be performed for same indication as in non pregnant patient. **But biopsies should be limited and ECC is not performed because of potential risk for infection and abortion.** Colposcopy is challenging as physiological changes of pregnancy produce changes in the cervical epithelium, which mimic those of dysplasia. Patient should be carefully followed up if CIN is discovered and treatment is usually deferred till postpartum period, because of high rate of regression in that period. Conization is only indicated if early invasive disease is suspected.

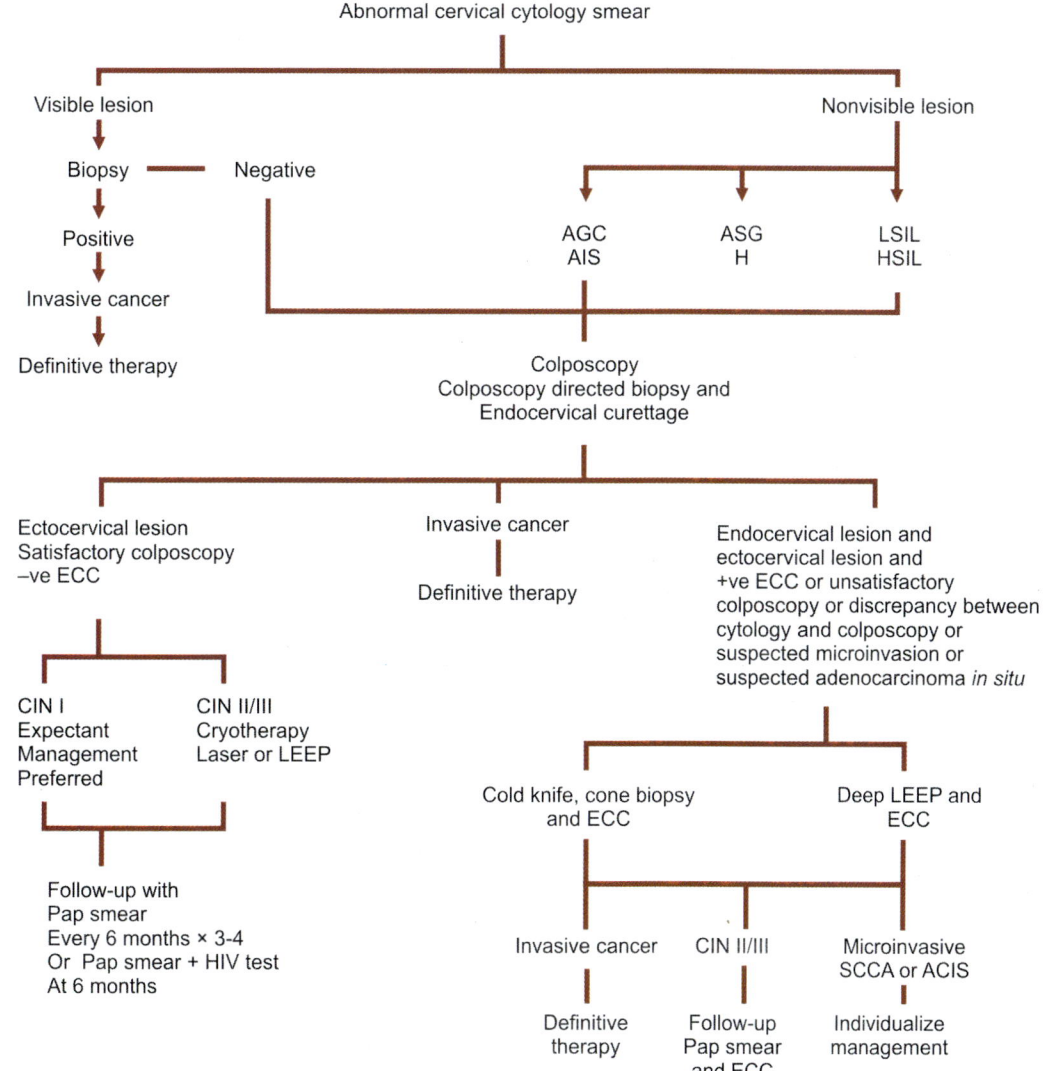

Flow chart 23.2: Plan for management of the abnormal cytology smear with visible or nonvisible cervical lesion

HIV Infection

Management of CIN in the HIV infected patient presents a great challenge. In HIV patient, risk of recurrent CIN is high more so in patients with low CD4 cell count. Use of highly active antiretroviral therapy (HAART) appears to reduce the risk of recurrent or progressive cervical neoplasia.

CANCER OF THE CERVIX

International and Indian Trends in Cervical Cancer

Worldwide cervical cancer is common and ranks second among all malignancies for women. Developing countries contributes 83% of reported cases annually. The highest incidence is seen in Sub-Saharan Africa and Central America, India, Pakistan and most of the African countries where incidence ranges between 20-30/100,000. Most of the developed world, China and Middle East have a low incidence of less than 10 per 100,000.

Developed countries have significantly lower cervical cancer rates and add only 3.6% of new cancers. This incidence disparity highlights the success achieved by organized screening program. Data demonstrates that apart from screening, probably education has an important role in down staging carcinoma of the uterine cervix as noted by markedly reduced rate in Kerala (India). Indian data is mostly collected from Cancer Registry Network, which shows the age adjusted incidence of carcinoma cervix is lowest in Thiruvananthapuram and highest in Chennai. The cervical cancer is developed in general at earlier age than that of other gynecologic malignancies and median age at diagnosis ranges from 40-59 years. In women aged 20-39 years, cervical cancer is the second leading cause of cancer deaths. It also shows that cancer breast was the most common followed by cancer of the cervix (ICMR 2004). In female cancers relative proportion of cancer breast varied between 21-24%, whereas that of cancer cervix was between 14 and 24%.

So the major factors affecting the prevalence of carcinoma cervix in a population are socioeconomic condition, education, sexual behavior and degree of effective mass screening.

Etiology and Epidemiology

The major epidemiological risk factors for cervical cancer are the same as those for CIN. These are:
a. Young age at first intercourse (< 16 years).
b. Multiple sexual partners.
c. Cigarette smoking.
d. Race.
e. High parity.
f. Lower socioeconomic states.

The relationship to oral contraception use has been debated. According to some studies use of oral contraceptive may increase the incidence of adenocarcinoma, but this hypothesis has not been consistently supported.

The initiating event in cervical dysplasia and carcinogenesis is infection with HPV. **HPV infection has been detected in up to 99% of women with squamous cervical carcinoma. HPV 16 is the most prevalent HPV type in squamous cell carcinoma and HPV 18 is most prevalent in adenocarcinoma**. Most recently cervical cancer has been associated with autoimmune deficiency with increased incidence seen in patients after organ transplant and in those with HIV/AIDS disease. In fact CDC has described cervical cancer as an AIDS defining illness in patients infected with HIV.

Pathogenesis and Natural History

Squamous cell carcinoma of the cervix typically arises at the squamocolumnar junction (SCJ), from a pre-existing CIN, which in most cases follow infections with HPV. HPV is epitheliotropic. Once the epithelium is acutely infected with HPV, one of these clinical scenarios can result:

a. **Asymptomatic latent infection:** Most women can readily clear this virus.
b. **CIN:** Women with persistent infection may develop preinvasive *dysplastic cervical disease*. In this HPV undergoes vegetative replication but not integration into the genome.
c. **Neoplastic transformation:** Progression from dysplasia to invasive cancer requires several years, though wide variation also occurs. The molecular alterations involved with cervical carcinogenesis are complex and not fully understood. Carcinogenesis is suspected to result from the interactive effects between environmental insults, host immunity and somatic cell genomic variations. Oncogenic HPV serotype can integrate into human genome, which allows malignant transformation. This causes upregulation of the viral oncogenes E_6 and E_7. E_6 and E_7 oncoprotein impair proliferation inhibition by blocking the function of the p53 and retinoblastoma tumor suppressor pathways.

Tumor Spread

The pattern of local growth may be **exophytic** if a cancer arises from the ectocervix or may be **endophytic** if arises from the endocervical canal.

A. **Lymphatic spread:** Early stromal invasion (Stage IA_1) up to a depth of 3 mm below the basement membrane is a localized process. Penetration of stroma beyond this point carries an increased risk of lymphatic metastasis. The pattern of tumor spread typically follows cervical lymphatic drainage. **These channels principally drain into the peracervical and parametrial lymph nodes,** which passes into obturator lymph nodes and then into the internal, external and common iliac lymph nodes (Fig. 23.8).

Lymphatic channels from the posterior fornix course through the rectal pillars and the uterosacral ligaments to the rectal lymph nodes. Squamous cells carcinoma clinically confined to the cervix involves the regional pelvic lymph nodes in 15-20% of cases. When cancer involves the parametrium (Stage IIB), tumor cells can be found in the pelvic lymph nodes in 30-40% and in peraaortic nodes in 15-30% of cases. The more advanced the local disease, the greater the likelihood of distant metastasis (Fig. 23.9).

B. **Lymphovascular space involvement:** As tumors involves deeper into the stroma, it enters blood capillaries and lymphatic channels so called **lymphovascular space involvement (LVSI)**. This type of invasive growth is not included in clinical staging of cervical cancer. But its presence is considered a poor prognostic factor.

C. **Local tumor extension:** The growth spreads directly to the adjacent structures, to the vagina, and to the body of the uterus. With extension through the perametria to the side walls, ureteral blockage frequently develops. The bladder may be invaded through vesicouterine ligaments. The rectum is invaded infrequently as it is anatomically separated from the cervix by the posterior cul-de-sac.

D. **Blood borne metastasis:** Blood borne metastasis is late and usually by veins rather than arteries. **Lung, ovaries, liver and bone are the most frequently affected organs**. Thus ovarian involvement is rare occurring in 0.5% of squamous cell carcinoma and 1.7% of adenocarcinoma.

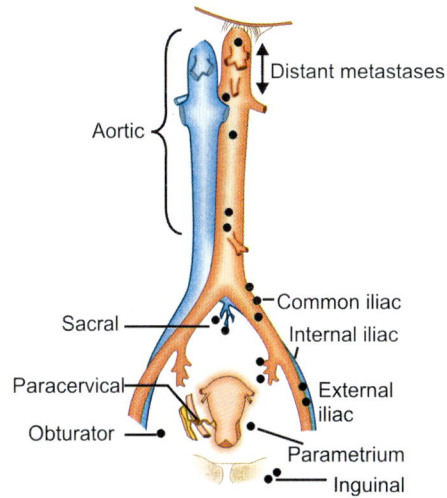

Fig. 23.8: Diagrammatic representation of lymphatic drainage of cervix

Course of Disease

When cancer of the cervix is untreated or fails to respond to treatment, death occurs in 95% of patients within 2 years after the onset of symptoms. **Death can occur from uremia, pulmonary embolism, or hemorrhage from direct extension of tumor into blood vessel.** There can be life-threatening sepsis from complications of pyelonephritis or vesicovaginal and rectovaginal fistula. Large bowel obstruction from direct extension of tumor into rectosigmoid can be the terminal event. Pain from perineural extension is a significant management problem of advanced disease.

Squamous Cell Carcinoma

Squamous cell carcinoma comprises 85% of all cervical cancers, and arises from ectocervix. Histologically variant of squamous cell carcinoma include: (a) Large cell keratinizing, (b) Large cell nonkeratinizing, (c) Small cell types (Fig. 23.10A).

Verrucuous Carcinoma

It is rare subtype associated with HPV6 of well differentiated squamous carcinoma. It is a slow growing, locally invasive neoplasm. Histologically this tumor is composed of well-differentiated squamous cells with frond like papillae and little apparent stromal invasion but it is potentially lethal.

Adenocarcinoma

Adenocarcinoma comprises 10-15% of all cervical cancers and arises from the endocervical mucus producing glandular cells (Fig. 23.10B). They are as follows in order of frequency:
a. Mucinous endocervical adenocarcinoma.
b. Endometrioid adenocarcinoma.
c. Minimal deviation adenocarcinoma.

Mixed Cervical Carcinoma

It is rare and histologically classified as: (a) Adenosquamous, (b) Adenoid cystic, (c) Adenoid basal epithelium, (d) Glassy cell carcinoma.

Neuroendocrine Tumors of the Cervix

These malignancies include large cell and small cell tumors of the cervix. **Large cell neuroendocrine tumors are highly aggressive**. Small cell neuroendocrine tumors resemble small cell carcinoma of lung. Tumor cancer stains positive for neuroendocrine markers. Because of their propensity for early systemic spread, systemic chemotherapy is an integral part of the treatment of neuroendocrine tumors of the cervix.

Other malignant tumors: Rarely the cervix may be the site of sarcoma and malignant lymphomas.

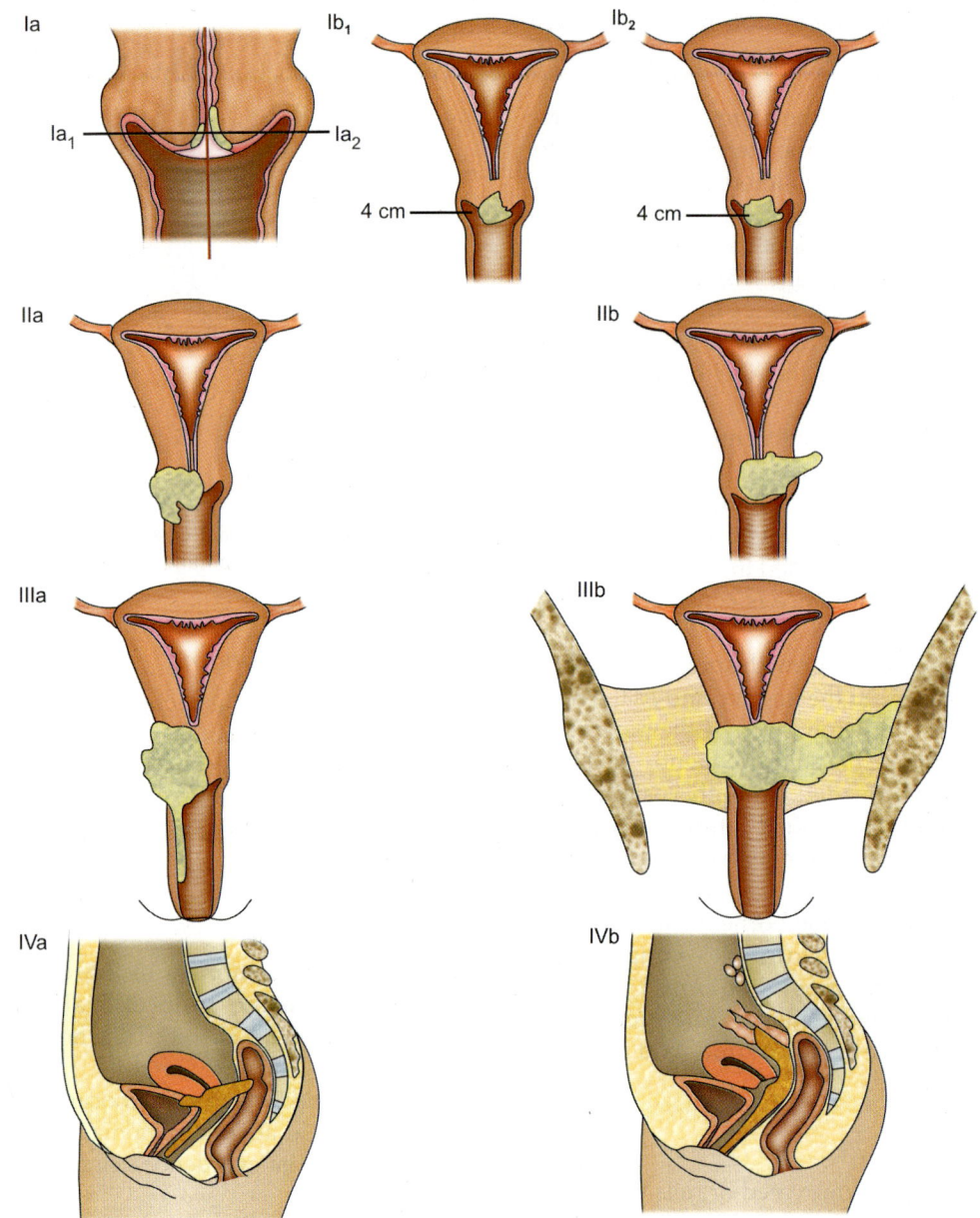

Fig. 23.9: FIGO staging of cancer cervix

Diagnosis of Carcinoma Cervix

Symptoms

A good proportion of women diagnosed with cervical cancer can be asymptomatic. Abnormal vaginal bleeding is the most common symptom of invasive cancer and may take the form of a blood stained leucorrheal discharge, scanty spotting or frank bleeding. A history or complaint of postcoital bleeding can be the presenting symptom. As malignancy advances, bleeding typically intensify and occasionally women may present with profuse hemorrhage from a tumor bed.

Vaginal discharge, which can be sanguinous or purulent, offensive and nonpruritic, is frequently present.

Pelvic pain is often unilateral and radiate to hip or thigh. It is manifestation of advanced disease, caused by involvement of uterosacral ligament and sacral plexus. With ureteral obstruction there can be hydronephrosis and uremia. With bladder involvement, there may be hematuria or symptoms of vesicovaginal or rectovaginal fistula.

Physical Examination

Patient can have normal general physical examination finding. In late stage, patient can be anemic, with weight

Chapter -23 ♦ Premalignant and Malignant Disorders of the Uterine Cervix

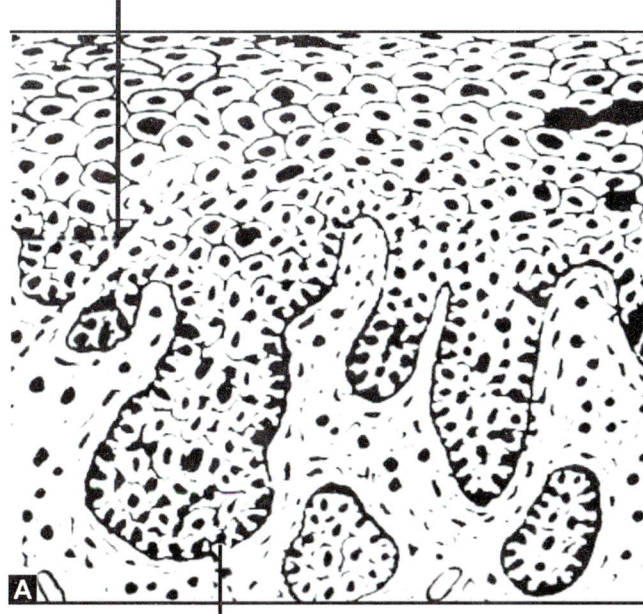

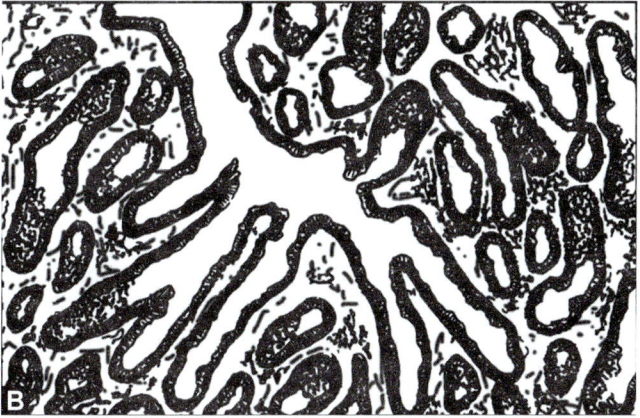

Figs 23.10A and B: Histological picture: (A) Squamous cell carcinoma; (B) Adenocarcinoma

loss. *On perspeculum examination*, cervix may appear grossly normal if cancer is microinvasive. Visible disease can be varied—it may appear as exophytic or endophytic growth, as a polypoid mass, papillary tissue or barrel shaped cervix, as a cervical ulceration or granular mass or as necrotic tissue. There can be watery, purulent, or bloody discharge. *On bimanual pelvic examination*, there can be enlarged uterus, due to tumor invasion or presence of hematometra or pyometra. Advanced cervical cancer may have vaginal involvement. Extensive parametrial involvement by the infiltrative process may produce a nodular thickening of the uterosacral and cardinal ligaments with loss of mobility and fixation of the cervix.

Differential Diagnosis

Cervical cancer may resemble appearance of difficult disease like cervical leiomyoma, cervical polyp, prolapsing uterine sarcoma, vaginitis, cervical erosion, cervicitis, threatened abortion, cervical pregnancy, herpetic ulcer, Condyloma acuminata.

Confirmation of Diagnosis

a. *Cytology:* Because of failure of malignant cells to desquamate and the obscuring effects of inflammatory cells, Pap smears does not always detect cervical cancers. **Pap smear testing has only 55-80% sensitivity for detecting high-grade lesions on any given single test.** So use of Pap smear alone for evaluation of suspicious lesions is discouraged.

b. *Colposcopy:* Colposcopic examination suggesting malignancies: (a) Abnormal blood vessels, (b) Irregular surface contour with loss of surface epithelium, (c) Color tone changes.

c. *Biopsy:* Any suspicious lesions of the cervix should be sampled by adequate biopsy. **Punch biopsy of Schiller positive areas of any ulcerative, granular, nodular or papillary lesions provides the diagnosis in most cases.** Colposcopic directed punch biopsies may permit the diagnosis of frank invasion allowing treatment to be administered without delay.

d. *Conization of cervix:* It may be required: (a) When reports of suspicious or probable exfoliated carcinoma cells are made by the pathologist and visible or palpable lesions of the cervix is not evident, (b) If biopsy reveal carcinoma *in situ*, where invasion cannot be ruled out, (c) In the setting of normal colposcopy and abnormal cytology. Conization of cervix should be performed to determine presence or absence of invasion. **Conization for lesion grossly suggestive of invasive cancer *is not indicated*.** It not only delays the start of appropriate treatment, but also predisposes the patient to serious pelvic infection and bleeding.

e. *Radiological investigation:* (a) Chest X-ray is indicated in all patient with cervical cancer, (b) Intravenous pyelogram (I/VP) or CT urogram should be done to determine signs of ureteral obstructions, like hydroureter and hydronephrosis, (c) MRI, CT Scan, Lymphangiography, PET Scanning, may be done to assess pelvic or pera-aortic lymph node involvement.

Clinical Staging of Cervical Cancer

It is important to estimate the extent of disease not only for prognosis but also for treatment planning. **Staging for cervical cancer is based on clinical examination, preferably done under anesthetic. It includes bimanual pelvic examination, cystoscopy and proctoscopy.** Once assigned, the stage does not change based on progression or intraoperative findings. FIGO 1995 staging system is summarized in Table 23.4.

Table 23.4: FIGO staging of cervical cancer*

Stage	Features
0	Carcinoma *in situ*
	Cervical intraepithelial lesion $(CIN)_3$
1	Carcinoma strictly confined to the cervix (extension to corpus should be disregarded)
1a	Invasion is limited to measured stromal invasion with a maximum depth of 5 mm and no wider than 7 mm
$1a_1$	Measured invasion of stroma no greater than 3 mm in depth
	And no wider than 7 mm
$1a_2$	Measured invasion of stroma greater than 3 mm and no greater than 5 mm in depth and no wider than 7 mm
1b	Clinical lesion confined to the cervix or preclinical lesions greater than 1a
$1b_1$	Clinical lesion no greater than 4 cm in size
$1b_2$	Clinical lesion greater than 4 cm in size
2	Carcinoma extends beyond cervix but has not extended to pelvic wall, it involves vagina, but not as for as the lower third
2a	No obvious parametrial involvement
2b	Obvious parametrial involvement
3	Carcinoma has extended to the pelvic wall, on rectal examination there is no cancer free space between tumor and pelvic wall, tumor involves lower third of vagina, all cases of hydronephrosis or nonfunctioning kidney should be included, unless they are known to be due to another cause
3a	No extension to pelvic wall, but involvement of lower third of vagina
3b	Extension to pelvic wall, or hydronephrosis or non-functioning kidney due to tumor
4	Carcinoma has extended beyond true pelvis or has clinically involved mucosa of bladder or rectum
4a	Spread of growth to adjacent pelvic organs
4b	Spread to distant organs

The staging should include:
a. Examination under anesthesia which should include a combined rectovaginal assessment.
b. Biopsy of suspicious area which should be suitably large to make a definitive diagnosis.
c. Cystoscopy should be considered.
d. Sigmoidoscopy should be considered.
e. Plain X-ray chest.
f. IVP.
g. Other imaging as indicated and according to facilities available—CT and MRI.

TREATMENT

Invasive cancer cervix spreads mainly by direct extension and lymphatic dissemination. Like in any other types of cancer, both primary lesions and potential sites of spread should be evaluated and treated. The therapeutic modalities achieving this goal include primary treatment with—**surgery, radiotherapy, chemotherapy or chemoradiation**. Radiation therapy can be used in all stages of disease; surgery is limited to patients with stage I to II a disease.

Stage IA: The definitive diagnosis of microinvasive squamous cell carcinoma of cervix can only be made by conization. For young women desirous to maintain fertility, only conization is an acceptable treatment, *but only when conization margin are negative, and depth of invasion is up to 3 mm or less*. If women has completed child-bearing, type I hysterectomy (simple hysterectomy, extrafascial hysterectomy) is preferred in which uterus and cervix is removed with excision of parametrium or paracolpium. If there is evidence of lymphovascular invasion, these patients should be treated like stage IA_2 disease. Microinvasive adenocarcinoma presents a management dilemma.

Stage IA_2 to IIA: Patient with early stage cervical cancer may be treated either with: (a) Radical hysterectomy and pelvic lymphadenectomy, (b) Primary radiation with concomitant chemotherapy. The overall 5 years cure rate for surgery and for radiation therapy in operable patients are approximately equal.

Radical Hysterectomy

Surgical Treatment (Stage IA_2 to IIA)

Women with FIGO stage IA_2 to II A cervical cancer may be selected for radical hysterectomy for: (a) Who wish to avoid long-term effect of radiation therapy, (b) Who have contraindication to pelvic radiotherapy, (c) Young patient who desire ovarian preservation and retention of a functional nonirradiated vagina, as radiation causes vaginal stenosis and atrophy.

Following types of radical hysterectomy can be performed:

Modified Radical Hysterectomy (Type II)

It removes the cervix, proximal vagina, and parametrial and peracervical tissues. The ureter is completely dissected from the peracervical tunnel. So that parametrial and peracervical tissue medial to the ureter can be removed. It is suitable for tumors with 3-5 mm depth of invasion and smaller stage IB tumor.

Radical Hysterectomy (Type III)

This operation includes pelvic lymph node dissection along with removal of most of the uterosacral and cardinal ligaments and the upper one-third of vagina. In this the ureters are completely dissected from their beds and the bladder and ureter are mobilized.

Radical Trachelectomy

Radical trachelectomy is a procedure that is gaining popularity as a surgical management options for women with stage IA_2 and IB_1 disease. It can be considered in patients who desire uterus preservation and fertility, tumor less than 2 cm in diameter, and negative lymph node involvement and no lymph vascular space involvement. Trachelectomy can be performed vaginally or abdominally accompanied by pelvic lymphadenectomy and cervical circlage placement. But there is risk of recurrence. If recurrence develops, definitive therapy with surgery or radiation is necessary.

Adjuvant postoperative radiation: Women with localized cervical cancer at **high-risk for recurrence are with positive lymph nodes, positive margin, or microscopic parametrial involvement**. In those patients postoperative adjuvant radiation therapy with concomitant chemotherapy is indicated. Platinum based chemotherapy is superior to adjuvant radiation alone, with an improvement in 4 years progression free interval from 63 to 80%.

Primary Radiation Therapy

For primary radiation of cervical cancer *external beam radiation* is used in combination with *intra cavitary radiation*. External beam radiation is given to shrink the tumor volume and to sterilize the regional lymph nodes. Usually 4500 cGY and 5000 cGY are administered but up to 6000 CGY can be directed to known lymph node deposits. *Brachytherapy* is the second phase and involves insertion of catheter through the cervix into uterus cavity. Radiation is administered directly to the tumor by placing a radiation source (Iridium or Cesium) in the lumen of catheter (Fig. 23.11). Local dose of over 10000 cGY can be given to center of the tumor. Concomitant platinum based chemotherapy has improved the results. It has cure rate of 70% for Ia, 60% for stage II.

Stage IB_2 and Bulky IIA

The management of patients with stage IB_2 and bulky IIA disease is a matter of considerable debate. Proposed management strategies are:
a. Primary radiation therapy with concomitant chemotherapy and option of a subsequent adjuvant extrafascial hysterectomy.
b. Primary radical hysterectomy and therapeutic lymphadenectomy followed by tailored radiation with concomitant chemotherapy when indicated by pathologic finding.
c. Neoadjuvant chemotherapy followed by radial hysterectomy and lymphadenectomy and subsequent chemoradiation, when indicated by pathologic finding.

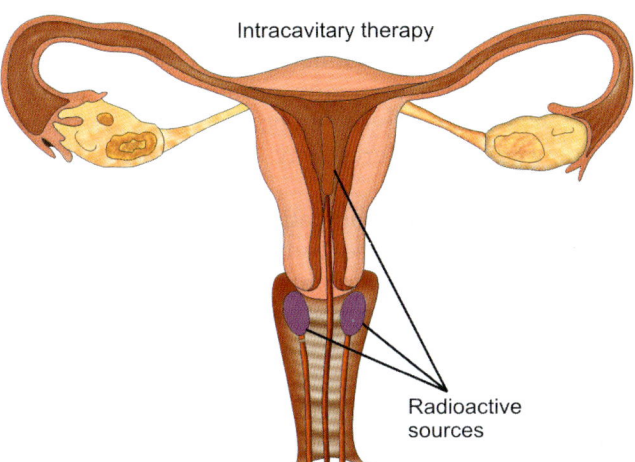

Fig. 23.11: Intracavitary radiotherapy in treatment of cancer cervix

Stage IIb to IVA: Treatment of Locally Advanced Disease

These patients are best treated with primary *radiation (external beam plus brachytherapy) with concomitant chemotherapy*. External beam radiation usually precedes intracavitary radiation, which is one form of brachytherapy. External beam radiation is commonly administered in 25 fractions during 5 weeks. During brachytherapy, to limit bladder and rectal dose, bowel and bladder are packed away from the intracavitary source. During tandem insertion, vaginal packing is done. During staging if pera-aortic nodal metastases are found, then extended field radiation can be added to treat these effected lymph nodes.

Adjuvant Chemoradiation

Concurrent chemotherapy with Cisplatin containing regimen have been associated with best survival rate. Cisplatin is given weekly for 5 weeks and administered concurrently with radiotherapy. Control of symptoms with the least morbidity is of major concern. Radiotherapy has cure rate of 60% for stage II, 45% for stage III and 18% for stage IV.

Treatment of Disseminated Primary (Stage IVB) and Persistent or Recurrent Disease

Patients with stage IVB disease have a poor prognosis and are treated with a goal of palliation. Pelvic radiation is administered to control vaginal bleeding and pain. Systemic chemotherapy is offered to palliate symptoms.

Follow-up surveillance:
a. *Following surgery:* After radical hysterectomy 80% of recurrences are detected within subsequent 2 years.

During surveillance if there is presence of pelvic mass, abnormal pelvic examination, new onset pain and edema in lower extremity prompt, CT scanning of abdomen and pelvis should be done. Pelvic recurrence after radical hysterectomy can be salvaged with radiation therapy.

b. *Following radiotherapy:* Patients are closely monitored to assess their response. Tumors should be expected to regress for up to 3 months after therapy. Pelvic radiological examination should document progressive shrinkage of the cervical mass with thorough manual nodal survey, and yearly chest X-ray. Cervical or vaginal cuff Pap smear should be done every 3 months for 2 years and every 6 months for 3 years. If high-grade lesion or cancer is noted on cervical biopsy, then CT scanning is done to assess disease recurrence is indicated.

Secondary Disease

Secondary disease is defined as either persistent or recurrent cancer. Cervical cancer that has not completely regressed within 3 months of radiotherapy is considered persistent. Disease recurrence is when new lesion develops after completion of primary therapy. There can be following options of treatment for secondary disease:

a. *Pelvic exanteration:* It is one of the most formidable operation of all gynecological operation and requires removal of bladder, rectum, and vagina along with uterus if hysterectomy has not yet been performed. It is followed by the reconstructive phase of the procedure. Exanteration can sometimes be used to palliate severe symptoms as post radiation fistulas or hemorrhage from tumors.
b. *Radiotherapy:* With central or limited peripheral recurrences, curative intent radiation can be given.
c. *Chemotherapy:* Cisplatin is considered the single most active cytotoxic agent in this setting.

Palliative Care

Comprehensive care of a patient with cancer involves in addition to antitumor surgery, radio or chemotherapy, good symptoms relief as well as personal and family support. The palliative care for patients with advanced cervical cancer is challenging and emphasis is on to give comfort, dignity, autonomy of life with personal rehabilitation.

The fowl purulent discharge caused by ulceration of cervix and vagina can be lessened by astringent douches and antimicrobial vaginal cream or suppository. Hemorrhage caused by tissue necrosis can be controlled by packing with gauge impregnated with a hemostatic agent. Severe pain management includes use of long-acting narcotic as morphine or transdermal fentanyl patch with short-acting narcotics for break through pain and nonsteroidal anti-inflammatory agents. Anxiolytics and antidepressant may be of considerable value. In patients with lower back or extremity pain, morphine can be given via peridural catheter. Urinary fistula and bowel obstruction can be managed surgically in a suitable patient. Palliative radiation may be helpful in relief of pain caused by bony metastasis and treatment of recurrent lesions. Palliative chemotherapy is administered only if this treatment does not cause significant decline in patient quality of life.

SPECIAL SITUATION

Carcinoma of Cervical Stump

Early stage cervical cancer detected on a cervical stump (following subtotal (supracervical) hysterectomy for an unrelated conditions) should be treated with *radical trachelectomy and therapeutic lymphadenectomy* in surgically fit patients. Surgery is preferred to chemo and radiotherapy as delivery of adequate radiation dose may be difficult to give in patient with short cervical stump. However, still in advanced disease radiation with concomitant chemotherapy is the preferred treatment modality.

Carcinoma of Cervix During Pregnancy

The incidence of invasive cervical cancer associated with pregnancy is 1.2 in 10,000. A Pap smear should be performed in all pregnant patients at initial prenatal visit. The treatment modality is chosen according to: (a) Stage of CIN/invasive cancer, (b) Duration of pregnancy, (c) Willingness of women to continue or terminate the pregnancy.

Diagnostic Conization in Stage Ia

It can be done in 2nd trimester if patient has *biopsy proven microinvasive* cervical cancer or strong cytologic evidence of invasive cancer, but not detected by colposcopy or biopsy. In 1st trimester conization is associated with high abortion rate (32%), high incidence of hemorrhage and infection. So conization is done only in 2nd trimester.

In stage Ia cervical cancer after conization, definitive treatment can be delayed till fetal maturity. **Classical cesarean is preferred mode of delivery, as vaginal delivery is the significant predictor cause of recurrence**. Patient with 3-5 mm of invasion may also be followed to term or delivered early by cesarean section after establishment of pulmonary maturity. They may be delivered by cesarean birth followed immediately by modified radical hysterectomy and pelvic lymphadenectomy.

Stage Ib

Patient with more than 5 mm invasion should be treated as having frankly invasive carcinoma of cervix. It is unwise

24. Premalignant and Malignant Disorders of the Uterine Corpus

To know and not to do, is not yet to know.

GENERAL CONSIDERATION

Endometrial cancer is the fourth most common cancer in females in world, ranking behind breast, bowel and lung cancer and seventh leading cause of death from cancer in female. In developing world, carcinoma cervix is the most common malignancy. In developed world cancer endometrium is most common malignancies of genital tract. *Endometrial cancer primarily occurs in postmenopausal women and is increasingly virulent with advancing age.* Role of estrogen in the development of most endometrial cancer has clearly been established.

Epidemiology and Risk Factors

Estrogens are implicated as a causative factor in endometrial cancer, because there is a high incidence of this disease in patient with presumed alterations in estrogen metabolism and in those who take exogenous estrogen. **Classically, endometrial cancer affects the obese, nulliparous, infertile, hypertensive and diabetic women,** but it can occur in absence of all these factors.

Obesity risk of endometrial cancer is 3 fold, who are 21-50 pounds overweight and 10 fold, for those more than 50 pounds overweight.

A *nulliparous* patient is *twice* as likely to develop the disease as a woman with one child, and 3 times as likely as a woman with 5 or more children.

Diabetes mellitus is associated with an almost *three* times greater risk for the cancer, independent for weight and age.

Menopause later than age 52 years, have more than twice the risk for developing endometrial cancer.

Patients with *anovulatory cycles* have high risk for endometrial carcinoma due to prolonged period of estrogenic stimulation of the endometrium without the opposing effects of progesterone.

Menopausal estrogen therapy without progestin increases the risk of endometrial cancer 4-8 times. Use of antiestrogen Tamoxifen for treatment of breast cancer is associated with 2-3 fold increased risk for the development of endometrial cancer.

Women with hereditary *nonpolyposis colorectal cancer syndrome (HNPCC),* a cancer susceptibility syndrome with germ line mutation in mismatch repair genes – MLH 1, MSH 2, and MSH 6 have a 40 to 60% life time risk for endometrial as well colon cancers. For this group, routine screening for endometrial cancer is recommended.

Variants of Endometrial Cancer

There appears to be two different pathogenesis for endometrial cancer:

Type I: It accounts for 75 to 85% of cases, occur in younger, perimenopausal women with history of exposure to either exogenous or endogenous estrogen. These are estrogen dependent, better differentiated and have more favorable prognosis. *They are associated with mutation in the PTEN tumors suppressive gene and K-ras oncogene.*

Type II: Endometrial carcinoma occur in women with no source of estrogen stimulation of the endometrium. These estrogen independent tumors tend to occur in postmenopausal, thin women and are present disproportionately in African and Asian women. *These tumors are more often associated with p53 mutations.*

Endometrial Cancer Screening

Currently there is no good screening tool for asymptomatic patient for endometrial cancer. Routine Pap smear is inadequate, and endometrial cytologic assessment is too insensitive and nonspecific. Screening of high risk individual can at best detect only one half of all cases of endometrial cancer. Screening in higher risk cases like women on hormone replacement therapy, women with hereditary nonpolyposis colorectal cancer is only justified, which can be done by office endometrial biopsy and transvaginal ultrasound to measure the thickness of endometrial strips complex.

ENDOMETRIAL HYPERPLASIA

Endometrial hyperplasia represents a spectrum of morphologic and biologic alteration of the endometrial glands and stroma, ranging from an exaggerated physiologic state to carcinoma *in situ*. Usually it occurs as a result of prolonged estrogen stimulation in the absence of progestin influence.

Classification

The classification system used by WHO and International Society of Gynecological Pathologist designates four types with varying malignant potential (Box 24.1).

Box 24.1: WHO classification of endometrial hyperplasia

Types	Progressing to cancer
Simple hyperplasia	1%
Complex hyperplasia	3%
Simple atypical hyperplasia	8%
Complex atypical hyperplasia	29%

Hyperplasia is classified as simple or complex based on the absence or presence of architectural abnormalities such as glandular complexity and crowding. **Atypia** is diagnosed if cells demonstrate cytological (nuclear) atypia. Only atypical endometrial hyperplasia is clearly associated with the subsequent development of adenocarcinoma.

Endometrial Intraepithelial Neoplasia (EIN)

This classification has been introduced recently. EIN is used to describe all endometrium delineated as premalignant by a combination of 3 features: (a) Glandular volume, (b) Architectural complexity, (c) Cytological abnormality.

Clinical Features

Two-third of women with endometrial hyperplasia present with postmenopausal bleeding. However, any type of abnormal uterine bleeding should warrant prompt diagnostic evaluation. Occasionally adnexal mass may be palpable, which is usually benign ovarian cyst but some times coexisting granulosa cell tumor.

Diagnosis

Transvaginal sonography of endometrial thickness and endometrial biopsy is mainstay of diagnosis.

Treatment

Management of women with endometrial hyperplasia depends mainly on the patient's age and presence or absence of cytologic atypia. However, nonsurgical therapy is inherently risky due to the inconsistency of diagnosis and uncertainty in predicting the natural history of individual lesions.

Nonatypical Endometrial Hyperplasia

a. *Premenopausal women:* They can be given 3-6 months course of low dose progestin therapy in following forms:
   i. Cyclic medroxyprogesterone acetate (MPA) (provera) orally for 12-14 days each month at a dose of 10-20 daily.
   ii. Combined OC pills.
   iii. Progesterone containing intrauterine devices.
   Patient is kept under surveillance with transvaginal sonography. Endometrial biopsy is done during surveillance biopsy. If no residual hyperplastic endometrium is found during surveillance biopsy, then patient is continued on progestins and monitored until menopause. *Repeat biopsy should be done after 2-6 weeks of hormonal withdrawal.*
b. *Postmenopausal women:* Simple hyperplasia often are followed without therapy. Complex hyperplasia without atypia is treated with low dose cyclic medroxyprogesterone acetate, continuous 2.5 mg/day. In older women office endometrial biopsy is performed annually to surveile these women. Overall 90% of non atypical hyperplasia regresses with progestin therapy. Patient with persistent disease should be given higher dose regimen 40-100 mg orally medroxyprogesterone acetate or megestrol acetate 160 mg daily. *Hysterectomy should be reconsidered for lesion refractory to medical management.*

Atypical Endometrial Hyperplasia

Hysterectomy is the best treatment for women at any age with atypical endometrial hyperplasia because the risk of concurrent subclinical invasive disease is high. Premenopausal women who strongly wish to preserve fertility are the main exception. High dose progestin therapy may be most appropriate for highly motivated patients. Serial endometrial biopsy should be repeated after every 3 months until the response is documented otherwise hysterectomy should be recommended.

ENDOMETRIAL CANCER

Diagnosis

Symptoms and Signs

Endometrial carcinoma most commonly occurs in women in the sixth and seventh decades of life. **About 90% of women with endometrial carcinoma have abnormal uterine bleeding, most common presentation is**

postmenopausal bleeding, 10% of patients may present with vaginal discharge. Occasionally patients with cervical stenosis may have a pyometra or hematometra. In more advanced disease, women may experience pelvic pressure or discomfort indicative of uterine enlargement or extra-uterine disease spread. Less than 5% of women diagnosed with endometrial cancer are asymptomatic and detected as the results of abnormal Pap smear, on pelvic sonography or CT scan for an unrelated reason.

Physical examination is usually normal, *though obesity and hypertension are commonly associated constitutional factors.* **Abdominal examination** is usually normal, except in very advanced cases when ascites or hepatic or omental metastasis may be palpable. On **gynecological examination**—the vaginal introitus and suburethral area, as well as the entire vagina and cervix should be carefully inspected and palpated. Atrophic vaginitis is frequently identified in these elderly women but postmenopausal bleeding should never be associated to atrophy without a histologic sampling of endometrium to rule out endometrium carcinoma.

Bimanual and rectovaginal examination of the uterus in the early stages of the disease will be normal unless hematometra or pyometra is present. It should be performed specifically to evaluate the uterus for size and mobility, the adnexa for masses, the parametria for induration and the cul-de-sac for nodularity.

Investigations

a. *Papanicolaou test:* The Pap smear has not been a sensitive tool to diagnose endometrial cancer and *50% of women with endometrial cancer will have normal findings.* Presence of benign endometrial cells is considered normal in premenopausal women, but in postmenopausal women it is associated with 3-5% risk of endometrial carcinoma. So endometrial biopsy should be considered with this finding.

b. *Endometrial biopsy:* Office endometrial biopsy is the accepted first step in evaluating a patient with abnormal uterine bleeding or suspected endometrial pathology with diagnostic accuracy of 90 to 98%. Pipllae, Novak curette and vibra aspirator are available, which are narrow plastic cannula. They can often be used without a tenaculum and causes less uterine cramping (Figs 24.1A and B). Complications are rare. Endocervical curettage may also be performed at the time of endometrial biopsy, if cervical pathology is suspected.

c. *Fractional curettage:* Dilatation and fractional curettage, (D&C) is the definitive procedure for diagnosis of endometrial carcinoma. It should be performed under anesthetic for thorough and more accurate pelvic examination. It is carried out by careful and complete curettage of the endocervical canal followed by dilatation of the canal and circumferential

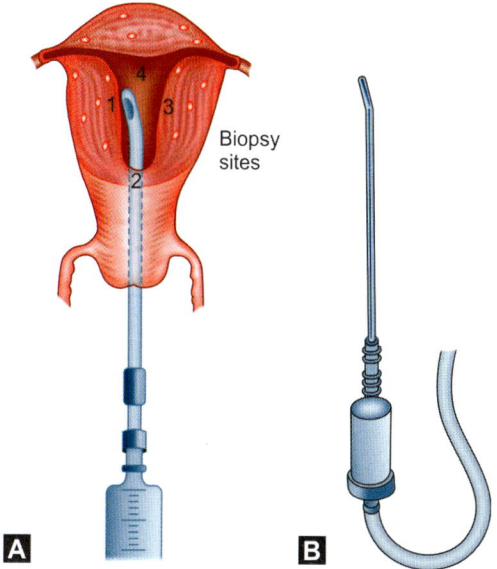

Figs 24.1A and B: (A) Technique of endometrial biopsy with novak curette; (B) Vabra aspirator

curettage of the endometrial cavity. When obvious cancer is present with the first pass of the curette, the procedure should be terminated as long as sufficient tissue for analysis has been obtained from the endocervix and endometrium. Perforation is a common complication and can be avoided by gentle surgical technique and limitation of the procedure to the extent necessary for accurate diagnosis and staging. D&C is never considered curative and should not be performed vigorously.

d. *Hysteroscopy:* Office hysteroscopy has proved less helpful in diagnosing hyperplasia. However, it can increase diagnostic accuracy in case of localized hyperplasia or polyp but hysteroscopy can promote the transtubal spread of tumor cells into the peritoneal cavity.

e. *Pelvic ultrasonography:* Transvaginal ultrasonography is a useful adjunct to endometrial biopsy for evaluating AUB. The *finding of an endometrial thickness greater than 4 mm, a polypoid endometrial mass or collection of fluid within the uterus requires further evaluation.*

f. *Imaging studies:* In general, for women with well differentiated type 1 endometrioid tumors chest radiograph is the only required preoperative imaging study. CT scan or MRI imaging is usually not necessary.

g. *Estrogen and progesterone receptor arrays:* Estrogen and progesterone receptor assays if available, helps in planning adjuvant or subsequent hormone therapy. *In general, patients with tumors positive for one or two receptors have longer survival than patients with receptor negative tumors.* Moreover, patients with receptor positive tissues might be candidate for hormone based therapy of recurrent tumor disease.

Pathology

Histologic Classification of Endometrial Carcinoma

WHO histologic classification of endometrial carcinoma is shown in Box 24.2.

Box 24.2: WHO histological classification of endometrial carcinoma

---
Endometrioid carcinoma (75-80%)
a. Variant with squamous differentiation
b. Villoglandular variant
c. Secretory variant
d. Ciliated cell variant
Mucinous carcinoma (1-2%)
Serous carcinoma (5-10%) – Uterine papillary serous carcinoma (UPSC)
Clear cell carcinoma
Squamous cell carcinoma (75%)
Mixed cell carcinoma
Undifferentiated carcinoma (1-2%)

The vast majority of endometrial carcinomas are endometrioid in histology (75-80%). Papillary serous tumors comprise less than 10% of endometrial carcinomas, display early intraperitoneal spread and are very aggressive cancer. Clear cell carcinoma are rare (only about 4%) but are also a more aggressive subtype (Figs 24.2A to C). Common metastatic tumors to the endometrium include *breast, ovary, stomach, colon and pancreas*. Approximately 3% of endometrial cancers are sarcomas such as malignant mixed Müllerian tumors and endometrial stromal tumor.

Histologic Grading

The FIGO grading system for endometrial carcinoma is most widely used.

Grade 1: 5% or less of the tumor shows a solid growth pattern.

Grade 2: 6 to 50% of the tumor shows a solid growth pattern.

Grade 3: More than 50% of the tumor shows a solid growth pattern.

The presence of notable nuclear atypia that is inappropriate for the architectural grade increase the tumor grade by one.

Mode of Spread

Direct Extension

Endometrial cancer spreads most commonly by direct extension to the adjacent organs such as by invasion through the myometrium to the serosa of the uterus and to the cervix. Tumor situated in lower uterine segment tends to involve the cervix early, whereas those in the upper corpus tend to extend on the fallopian tube or serosa.

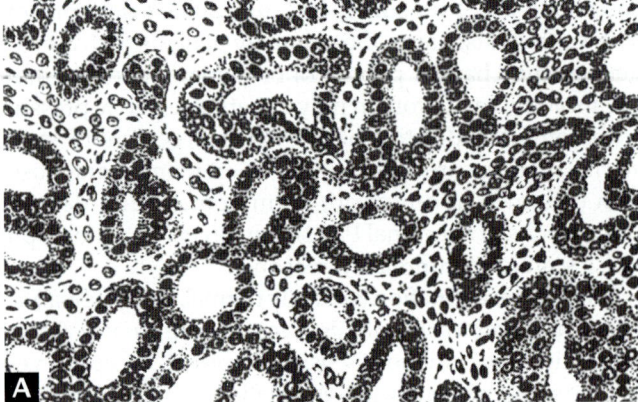
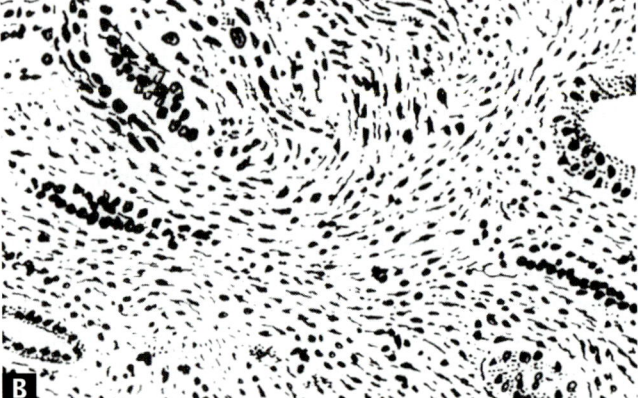
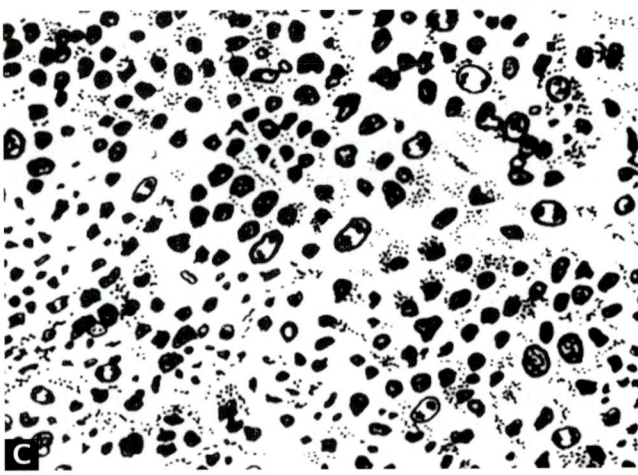

Figs 24.2A to C: Histological picture: (A) Adenoacanthoma; (B) Adenosquamous carcinoma; (C) Clear cell carcinoma

Advanced regional growth may lead to direct invasion of adjacent pelvic structure, including the bladder, large bowel, vagina and broad ligament.

Lymphatic Spread

Metastasis to the pelvic and para-aortic nodal chains can occur if tumor penetrates the myometrium. The lymphatic network draining the uterus is complex and patients can have metastasis to any single nodal group as well combination of groups. This haphazard pattern is in contrast to cervical cancer in which lymphatic spread usually follows a stepwise progression from pelvic to para-aortic or scalene nodal group.

Hematogenous Dissemination

Most common blood spread of cancer is to lungs followed by liver, brain, bone and other sites. Deep myometrial invasion is the strongest predictor of the spread.

Retrograde Transtubal Transport

Exfoliated endometrial cancer can reach peritoneal cavity by retrograde fallopian tube transport.

Staging of Endometrial Cancer

Clinical Staging

As to 1971 FIGO system, clinical staging should be performed in patients who are deemed not to be surgical candidates because of their poor clinical medical conditions or the spread of their disease (Table 24.1):

Table 24.1: FIGO clinical staging of endometrial carcinoma

Stage	Characteristic
I	Confined to corpus
Ia G_{123}*	Uterine cavity < 8 cm
Ib G_{123}	Uterine cavity > 8 cm
II	Involves the corpus and cervix but has not extended outside to uterus
III	Extends outside the uterus, but not outside the true pelvis
IV	Extends outside the true pelvis or obviously involves the mucosa of the bladder or rectum
IVa	Spread to adjacent organs
IVb	Spread to distant organs

* $Gr_{1,2,3}$ according to FIGO histological grading

Surgical Staging

Most patients with endometrial cancer should undergo surgical staging based on the 1988 FIGO system (Table 24.2). *At a minimum, the surgical procedure should include sampling of peritoneal fluid for cytologic evaluation, exploration of the abdomen and pelvis with biopsy or excision of any extrauterine lesions suggestive of metastatic cancer, extrafascial hysterectomy, and bilateral salpingo-oophorectomy.* The uterine specimen should be opened and tumor size, depth of myometrial involvement and cervical extension assessed.

Treatment

The majority of endometrial cancer cases are diagnosed at an early stage and can be treated with high cure rates. **The most important treatment modality is surgery with total simple or radical hysterectomy, bilateral salpingo-oophorectomy and staging, including pelvic and para-aortic lymphadenectomy.** To manage a patient optimally it is imperative to carefully review the histopathologic description of the preoperative biopsy findings. For example, papillary serous features suggest the possibility of intraperitoneal disease in the upper abdomen, so the vertical incision is most appropriate for proper exploration. Traditionally laparotomy has been the standard approach, but laparoscopic surgical staging is being used increasingly nowadays for endometrial cancer in cases where clinically cancer appears to be confined to the uterus.

Table 24.2: FIGO surgical staging for endometrial carcinoma (1981)

Stage	Grade	Finding
Ia	1,2,3	Tumor limited to endometrium
Ib	1,2,3	Tumor involves less than 50% of the myometrium
Ic	1,2,3	Tumor invasion to 75% of myometrium
IIa	1,2,3	Endocervical glandular involvement
IIb	1,2,3	Cervical stromal invasion
IIIa	1,2,3	Tumor involves serosa and/or adnexa/or positive peritoneal cytology
IIIb	1,2,3	Vaginal metastasis
IIIc	1,2,3	Metastasis to pelvic and/or para-aortic lymph nodes
IVa	1,2,3	Tumor invasion of bladder and/or bowel mucosa
IVb	1,2,3	Distant metastasis, including intra-abdominal and/or inguinal lymph nodes

Surveillance

Most surgically treated patients should be followed by pelvic examination every 3-4 months for the first two years and twice yearly for 3 years, before returning to annual visits. Pap smears are not mandatory part of follow-up as they are not cost-effective and fail to identify vaginal recurrence in majority of cases. Women with advanced disease requiring postoperative radiation or chemotherapy or both require more aggressive monitoring. Serum CA-125 may be valuable especially in uterine papillary serous carcinoma (UPSC). CT scanning or MRI may sometimes be indicated for recurrence.

Adjuvant Therapy: Chemotherapy

TAP chemotherapy – Paclitoxil (Taxon), Daxorubicin (Adriamycin) and Cisplatin is adjuvant treatment of choice for advance endometrial cancer. A less toxic alternative is combination of paclitoxil and carboplatin. In practice, cytotoxic chemotherapy is frequently combined with radiotherapy in patients with advanced endometrial cancer.

Radiation

Primary Therapy

Primary radiation is considered only in rare instances, when a patient is an exceptionally poor surgical candidate. Intracavitary brachytherapy with or without external beam pelvic radiation is the typical method.

Adjuvant Therapy

a. *Stage I:* It is controversial. It is claimed to reduce incidence of vaginal vault recurrence stage 1, but cost and toxicity should be balanced against evidence that it does not improve survival or reduce distant metastasis. However, in women with *stage Ic grade 3 endometrial adenocarcinoma* postoperative *external beam pelvic radiotherapy is recommended.*
b. *Stage II:* Usually external beam pelvic radiation or brachytherapy both can be given but currently there is no standard approach and in most patients treatment is individualized based on coexisting risk factors.
c. *Stage III:* In these tumor directed postoperative external beam radiation is indicated with or without chemotherapy.
d. *Stage IV:* In this stage role of radiotherapy is generally palliative. As intraperitoneal metastasis most often lie outside directed radiation field so chemotherapy is preferred.

Hormonal Therapy

Primary: Endometrial cancer is hormone responsive. In a few exceptional circumstances progestin is used for primary treatment. In situations when clinical stage I disease and grade I adenocarcinoma with a poor surgical candidate, intrauterine progestational device may be useful but should be used only with great caution.

Adjuvant: Tamoxifen with progestin shows high response rate in women with advanced disease with low toxicity. However, this combination is used most commonly for recurrent disease.

Prognostic Indicators

Stage of disease at time of diagnosis is the most significant prognostic factor in patients with endometrial cancer; younger women have a better prognosis than older. Some histologic types like UPSC or clear cell adenocarcinoma carry a worse prognosis. Table I summarize the factor associated with poor prognosis (Box 24.3).

Box 24.3: Poor prognostic variable in endometrial cancer

1. Advanced surgical stage
2. Older age
3. Histologic type: UPSC or clear cell carcinoma
4. Advanced tumor grade
5. Presence of myometrial invasion
6. Presence of lymphovascular space invasion
7. Peritoneal cytology positive for cancer cells positive
8. Increased tumor size
9. High tumor expression level of ER and PR

Survival Rate

The overall survival rate for patients with endometrial cancer is about 60-70%. However, patients with early stage disease fare much better than those with late stage disease (Box 24.4).

Box 24.4: Survival rate of various FIGO stages

FIGO Stage	Survival %
IA	91
IB	91
IC	85
IIA	83
IIB	66
IIIA	50
IIIB	50
IIIC	57
IVA	25
IVB	20

UTERINE SARCOMA

Malignant tumors of uterus are broadly divided into 3 main types: (a) Carcinoma, (b) Sarcoma, (c) Carcinosarcoma.

Sarcoma and carcinosarcoma are mesodermally derived, highly malignant tumors and account for 2 to 6% of uterine malignancies.

Histogenesis and Classification

Uterine sarcoma can be separated into 4 major categories:
1. **Leiomyosarcoma** (Tumors of the uterine smooth muscles).
2. **Endometrial stromal sarcoma (ESS)** (Pure homologous endometrial sarcoma)
   a. High grade (Fig. 24.3)
   b. Low grade (endolymphatic stromal myosis).
3. **Malignant mixed mesodermal tumor (MMMT)** (Mixed epithelial/stromal tumors).

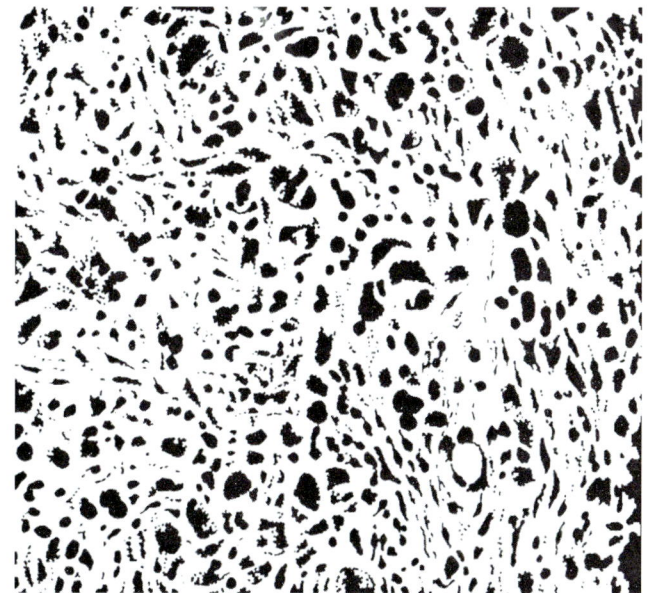

Fig. 24.3: Histopathological picture of endometrial stromal sarcoma

a. Homologous carcinosarcoma
b. Heterologous carcinosarcoma
4. Adenocarcinoma: (Mixed epithelial/stromal tumors)
   a. Homologous
   b. Heterologous

Several of identifiable risk factors for uterine sarcoma are same as that observed in endometrial carcinoma. However, the morphologic diversity of uterine sarcoma suggests a variety of potential pathways. *Leiomyosarcoma have monoclonal origin*, although commonly believed to arise from benign leiomyoma. Usually they appear to develop denovo as solitary lesions. In *endometrial stromal tumor* there are heterogeneous chromosomal aberrations. A loss of tumors suppressor gene function is suspected. In general MMMT (Malignant Mixed Müllerian tumors) are also monoclonal neoplasm. So both carcinoma and sarcoma components are thought to arise from a common epithelial progenitor cells.

Diagnosis, Symptoms and Signs

Abnormal uterine bleeding is the most common presenting symptoms for all histologic types of uterine sarcoma. Other complaints are pelvic discomfort, constipation, urinary frequency and presence of growing mass low in the pelvis. On examination there can be grape like structure of Sarcoma Botryoidis protruding from the cervix. Uterus is enlarged, soft and globular. If cancer has invaded adjacent structure, fixation or asymmetry of parametria may be evident.

Investigations

a. *Laboratory findings:* It should include complete blood count, liver and renal function studies. CA 125 may be a somewhat useful marker of disease response.
b. *Endometrial sampling:* Sensitivity of an office endometrial biopsy to detect uterine sarcoma is lower than that of endometrial carcinoma.
c. *Imaging studies:* Chest radiograph may show metastatic coin lesions. If routine *X-ray is negative, a chest CT scan* should be considered, because uterine sarcoma commonly metastasizes to the lungs. *Pelvic ultrasound* may confirm the presence of pelvic mass or helps to differentiate an adnexal from a uterine mass. Though as a diagnostic tool USG is far less helpful. *CT scan of abdomen and pelvis* should be performed routinely because of two reasons – first sarcoma often violate normal soft tissue planes in the pelvis and unresectable tumors can be identified preoperatively and extrauterine metastasis may be visualized. *MRI* is useful for distinguishing uterine sarcoma from a benign myoma. *Positron emission tomography (PET)* scanning is used most effectively for disease monitoring of the completion of treatment.

Mode of Spread

Uterine sarcoma fall into two categories of malignant behavior: (a) Leiomyosarcoma, high grade undifferentiated sarcoma, and MMMTS are consistently characterized by an aggressive growth pattern, and early lymphatic and hematogenous dissemination, (b) Endometrial stromal sarcoma and adenosarcomas have an indolent growth pattern with lung disease free interval. However, all of these tumors grow by direct extension to some extent. Leiomyosarcoma spread mainly by blood and lung metastasis is particularly common. With MMMT half of patients with clinical stage 1 tumors will have nodal metastasis.

Staging

There are no specific staging systems for uterine sarcomas due to their rarity. Currently FIGO surgical staging system for endometrial cancer to stage uterine sarcoma is used (Box 24.5).

Box. 24.5: FIGO staging of uterine sarcoma

Stage	Description
I	Sarcoma confined to uterus
II	Sarcoma involving both the corpus and cervix
III	Sarcoma extended outside the uterus but not outside the true pelvis
IV	Sarcoma extended outside the true pelvis or has involved the mucosa of the bladder or rectum

Treatment

Surgery

Surgery is the cornerstone of the treatment plan and should be the central focus. In general abdominal approach is preferred because of the typical features of parametrial extension and tumors metastasis. During laparotomy, surgical staging should be revised as in endometrial cancer with uterine leiomyosarcoma. All patients should undergo a hysterectomy. Lymph node dissection should be reserved for patients with clinically suspicious nodes. Endometrial stromal tumors and adenosarcoma also are best treated by hysterectomy. A more radical procedure may be required to encompass local disease for uterine MMMT. Hysterectomy and bilateral salpingo-oophorectomy are mandatory. Lymph node metastasis develops in 15-20% of patients with clinical stage I disease, so retroperitoneal nodes should be sampled. Extended surgical staging with infracolic omentectomy and random peritoneal biopsy is advisable.

Adjuvant Therapy

Radiation

As the primary modality, radiation has produced dismal results. In conjunction with surgery, pelvic irradiation or brachytherapy with or without chemotherapy for surgical stages I and II leiomyosarcoma, MMMT and high grade undifferentiated sarcoma is still supported to reduce recurrence.

Chemotherapy

Adjuvant progestin or Tamoxifen therapy is recommended for ESS. For receptor negative tumor Doxorubicin based chemotherapy is used.

Emergency Measures

Hemorrhage from uterine sarcoma can be severe and requires prompt attention. In acute hemorrhage blood volume should be replaced promptly by packed red blood crystalloid solution, volume expanders, and fresh frozen plasma. Emergency D & C should be used only to obtain tissue for analysis. Vigorous curettage is likely to aggravate profuse bleeding. High dose bolus radiation is more reliable and safe method of controlling bleeding. A dose of 400-500 CGy administered daily to the whole pelvis over 2-3 days usually control acute hemorrhage. If this is not successful, emergency embolization or ligation of the hypogastric arteries sometimes controls hemorrhage, if hysterectomy is not indicated or technically feasible.

Surveillance

Surgically treated stage I patients should have a physical examination every 3 months for the first 2 years and than at 6-12 months interval thereafter. Pap test is largely irrelevant and CA-125 levels are usually not helpful. A chest radiograph should be performed every 3-6 months for 2 years and then annually. In many cases intermittent CT scanning or MR imaging may be indicated.

Prognosis

In general, uterine sarcoma has a poor prognosis. **FIGO staging and tumor histology is the most important predictor of clinical outcome.** Leiomyosarcoma have the worst prognosis, followed by MMMT and high grade undifferentiated sarcoma.

MULTIPLE CHOICE QUESTIONS

1. The risk of endometrial carcinoma is highest with the following histological pattern of endometrial hyperplasia:
   a. Simple hyperplasia without atypia
   b. Simple hyperplasia with atypia
   c. Complex hyperplasia without atypia
   d. Complex hyperplasia with atypia
   Ans. d

2. The risk of complex hyperplasia of endometrium with atypia progressing to malignancy in a postmenopausal women is:
   a. 3%
   b. 8%
   c. 15%
   d. 88%
   Ans. d

3. The most malignant endometrial carcinoma is:
   a. Adenocarcinoma
   b. Adenoacanthoma
   c. Mixed adenosquamous
   d. Clear cell carcinoma
   Ans. d

4. In endometrial carcinoma, lymph node spread is not to:
   a. Para-aortic
   b. Inguinal
   c. Inferior mesenteric
   d. Presacral
   Ans. c

5. Most common histology of carcinoma of endometrium is:
   a. Squamous cell
   b. Clear cell
   c. Adenocarcinoma
   d. Anaplastic carcinoma
   Ans. c

6. At laparotomy for endometrial cancer the growth was found invading inner half of myometrium, right ovary and upper part of vagina. What is the staging?
   a. IIb
   b. IIIa
   c. IIIb
   d. IVa
   Ans. c

Chapter -24 ♦ Premalignant and Malignant Disorders of the Uterine Corpus

7. Indications for radiotherapy in carcinoma endometrium include all, *except*:
   a. Pelvic node involvement
   b. Deep myometrial involvement
   c. Enlarged uterine cavity
   d. Poor differentiation
   Ans. c

8. What is choice of treatment for a 55-year female with simple hyperplasia of endometrium with atypia?
   a. Simple hysterectomy
   b. Medroxyprogesterone acetate
   c. Levonorgesterol
   d. IUCD
   Ans. a

9. Long-term tamoxifen therapy may cause:
   a. Endometrium cancer
   b. Ovary cancer
   c. Cervix cancer
   d. Vagina cancer
   Ans. a

10. Investigation of choice in a 55-year-old postmenopausal women who has presented with postmenopausal bleeding:
    a. Pap smear
    b. Fractional curettage
    c. Transvaginal ultrasound
    d. CA-125 estimation
    Ans. b

11. Which of the following direct lymph node dissection in endometrial carcinoma:
    a. Penetration into half of myometrium
    b. Clear cell carcinoma
    c. Fundal involvement
    d. Peritoneal metastasis
    Ans. a,b,c

12. A 45-year-old woman has negative Pap smear with +ve endocervical curettage. Next step in the management will be:
    a. Colposcopy
    b. Vaginal hysterectomy
    c. Conization
    d. Wertheim's hysterectomy
    Ans. d

13. Indication of adjuvant radiotherapy in cancer endometrium is/are:
    a. Cervical involvement
    b. Lymph node involvement
    c. Carcinoma *in situ*
    d. Papillary serous tumor
    Ans. a,b,c

25 Premalignant and Malignant Disorders of Ovaries and Fallopian Tubes

A room without books is like a body without soul.

GENERAL CONSIDERATION

Ovarian cancer accounts for 3-4% of cancer in women. 23% of gynecological cancers are ovarian in origin but ovarian cancer is responsible for more than half of gynecological cancer death. In general ovarian cancer is a disease of postmenopausal women; highest incidence is at age 65-74. The lifetime risk of developing ovarian cancer is approximately 1.4% and lifetime risk of dying from ovarian cancer is almost 0.5%. Ovarian cancer is a diverse term describing several different histologies. Each type has a different natural history, *70% of ovarian cancer are epithelial in origin. 15% are germ cells, 10% are sex cord/ stromal cells and 5% are metastatic tumors of the ovary.*

Etiology and Risk Factors

a. *Family history:* Family history of breast or ovarian cancer is most important risk factor. Approximately 5-10% of patients have an inherited genetic predisposition.
b. *Incessant ovulation:* For other 90-95%, **most risk factors are related to a pattern of uninterrupted ovulatory cycles during the reproductive years**. Ovarian cancer has been associated with low parity and infertility. On the other hand protective factors are multiparty, use of oral contraception and history of breastfeeding. Theoretically, it is supposed that surface epithelium undergoes repetitive disruption and repair, which lead to a higher probability of spontaneous mutation that can unmask germ line mutations or otherwise lead to the oncogenic phenotype. Likewise early menarche and late menopause also have been associated with an increased risk of ovarian cancer.
c. *Diet:* Diet high in saturated animal fats seem to confer an increased risk by unknown mechanism.
d. *Tubal ligation and hysterectomy:* Have been associated with a substantial reduction in the risk of developing ovarian cancer. It is postulated that any gynecologic procedure that precludes irritants from reaching the ovaries via ascending lower genital tract might exert a similar protective effect. As women who regularly use perineal talc have an increased risk.
e. *Genetic risk:* Approximately 90% of ovarian cancer are sporadic in which familial or hereditary patterns account for 5 to 10% of all malignancies.

   Hereditary ovarian cancer: Most hereditary ovarian cancer is associated with mutations in the BRCA1 gene, located on chromosome 17. A small proportion of inherited disease is associated with mutations in BRCA2 gene, located on chromosome 13. It is now believed that site specific hereditary ovarian cancer and hereditary breast ovarian cancer syndrome represent a continuous of mutations with different degree of penetrance within a given family. In addition there is higher than expected risk of ovarian and endometrial cancer in the Lynch II syndrome, which is also known as **HNPCC syndrome** – *hereditary nonpolyposis colorectal cancer syndrome*. The mutations are inherited in an autosomal dominant fashion so a full pedigree analysis must be carefully evaluated. *Hereditary ovarian cancer in general occurs in women approximately 10 years younger than those with nonhereditary tumors.*

Prevention of Ovarian Cancer

Ovarian cancer screening: Still there is no proof that routine screening with serum markers, sonography or pelvic examination decrease mortality. Thus, for women at average risk routine screening is not recommended. *In high risk women* screening strategies are directed to BRCA1 or BRCA2 mutation carriers, in women with a strong family history of breast and ovarian cancer. Beside this cancer antigen CA-125 measurement and transvaginal sonography have been tested only with marginal success. Still in BRCA1 or BRCA2 mutation carriers, who do not wish to undergo prophylactic surgery, a combination of thorough pelvic examination, transvaginal sonographic evaluation and CA-125 blood testing should be offered.

Physical examination: **For near future the only recommendation for prevention of ovarian cancer in asymptomatic women is annual pelvic examination.** There is no additional technique that has proved to be effective in routine screening.

Chemoprevention: Oral contraceptive pills use is associated with 50% decreased risk of developing ovarian cancer. However, there is a short-term increased risk of developing breast cancer that should be considered in counseling.

Prophylactic surgery: **In BRCA1 or BRCA2 mutation carrier prophylactic bilateral salpingo-oophorectomy should be recommended on completion of childbearing or at age 35 years (AICOG 1999).** This procedure is 90% effective in preventing epithelial ovarian cancer. But it is not 100% protection as there can be occasional peritoneal carcinoma even after surgery. In HNPCC syndrome hysterectomy is mandatory when performing prophylactic bilateral salpingo-oophorectomy because of coexisting endometrial cancer risk. These patients should also undergo periodic screening mammography, colonoscopy and endometrial biopsy if not hysterectomized.

Histopathology

Ovarian cancer can be divided into three major categories based on the cell of origin.

Histopathologic Categories of Ovarian Cancer (Table 25.1)

1. Epithelial
2. Germ cell
3. Sex cord and stromal
4. Neoplasm metastatic to the ovary: Breast colon, stomach, endometrium lymphoma.

Epithelial Neoplasm

Epithelial neoplasm accounts for more than 60% of all ovarian neoplasm and for more than 90% of malignant ovarian tumor (Table 25.2).

Table 25.1: Major histological categories of ovarian cancer

Epithelial: Serous mucinous, endometrioid clear cell, transitional cell (Brenner) undifferentiated
Germ cell: Dysgerminoma, endodermal sinus tumor, teratoma, embryonal carcinoma, choriocarcinoma, gonadoblastoma, mixed germ cell, polyembryoma
Sex cord and stromal: Granulosa cell tumor, fibroma, thecoma, Sertoli-Leydig cell, gynandroblastoma
Neoplasm metastasis to the ovary: Breast, colon, stomach, endometrium, lymphoma

Table 25.2: Histologic classification of epithelial tumor

Histologic type	Cellular type
Serous: Benign, borderline, malignant	Endosalpingeal
Mucinous: Benign, borderline, malignant	Endocervical
Endometrioid Benign, borderline, malignant	Endometrial
Clear cell, Mesonephroid: Benign, borderline, Mullerian	Malignant
Brenner: Benign, borderline, malignant	Transitional
Mixed epithelial: Benign, borderline, malignant	Mixed
Undifferentiated	Anaplastic
Unclassified	Mesothelium

Serous Tumor

Serous tumors develop by invagination of the surface ovarian epithelium and named because they secrete serous fluid and form **psammoma bodies**. Approximately 10% of all ovarian serous tumors are in category of *borderline tumor or tumor of low malignant potential* and 50% of these occur before age of 40 years. Ten percent of these borderline serous ovarian tumors have *extraovarian implants* which can be invasive or non-invasive. In *malignant serous carcinoma* stromal invasion is present. In these the grade of tumor should be identified—well differentiated, moderately differentiated or poorly differentiated. Laminated calcified Psammoma bodies are found in 80% of serous carcinoma.

Mucinous Tumors

They represent 8 to 10% of epithelial ovarian tumors. These tumors have loculi secreting epithelium, which resemble those of endocervix, gastric polyposis or intestine. They are notable for the large size and can fill the entire abdominal cavity. Bilateral tumors occur in 8-10% of carriers. In 95-98%, mucinous lesions are intraovarian. It is *histologically indistinguishable* from metastatic carcinoma of the gastrointestinal tract.

Pseudomyxoma peritonei is a clinical term used to describe the finding of abundant mucoid or gelatinous material in the pelvis and abdominal cavity surrounded by fibrous tissue. It is most commonly secondary to a well differentiated appendiceal carcinoma, though reported to occur rarely with cystadenocarcinoma of the ovary and mucocele of appendix. Histologically, it is benign in appearance but pseudomyxoma peritonei has a protracted and potentially morbid course causing bowel obstruction with a mortality rate of 50%.

Endometrioid Neoplasm

They constitute 6 to 8% of epithelial tumors which shows an adenomastoid pattern resembling endometrial carcinoma. It is bilateral in 30-50% of cases. Rarely this arises in foci of endometriosis. Borderline (low malignant potential) and malignant are defined based on degree of differentiation in glandular architecture. **As many as 30% of patient with endometrioid carcinoma of the ovary have a synchronous, endometrial carcinoma of the uterus.** Identification of multifocal disease is important, because patients with distant metastasis from the uterus to ovaries have a 30-40% 5 years survival rate, while those with synchronous multifocal disease have a 75 to 80% 5 years survival rate.

Clear Cell Carcinoma (Mesonephroid Tumors)

Clear cell carcinoma of the ovary are biologically aggressive and can be associated with hypocalcemia and hyperpyrexia. The external surface is smooth and bosselated histologically– two cell types may be present **clear cell and hobnail cells**.

Transitional Cell (Brenner) Carcinoma

It accounts for less than 1% of epithelial cancer. It is comprised of cells that resemble low grade transitional cell carcinoma of the urinary bladder. Patients typically presents with advanced stage disease and exhibit a poorer prognosis.

Undifferentiated Carcinoma

They are less than 10% of epithelial neoplasm and characterized by absence of any distinguishing microscopic feature to be placed in any histologic category.

Nonepithelial Ovarian Cancers

Nonepithelial ovarian cancer accounts for about 10% of all ovarian cancers.

Germ cell neoplasm: Germ cell tumors are derived from the primordial germ cells of the ovary. Although 20 to 25% of all benign and malignant ovarian neoplasm are of germ cell origin, out of which only about 3% of these tumors are malignant.

Dysgerminoma

It is most common malignant germ cell tumors, (30% of all germ cell tumors). It is female *counterpart of Seminoma in the male*. It is unilateral in 85-90% of cases. It is a solid tumor which may contain areas of softening due to degenerative changes. *Histologically*, it mimics the pattern seen in primitive grade with nest of germ cells appearing as large rounded cells with central nucleus. A lymphocytic infiltrate is considered a favorable prognostic indicator.

Endodermal Sinus Tumor

Yolk sac tumors are third most common germ cell neoplasm. It is bilateral in 100% of cases and one of the most rapidly growing neoplasms. Patient commonly presents with acute abdomen. The lesion on *gross appearance* is friable, focally necrotic. *Microscopically*, it is composed of primitive epithelial cells mimicking primitive gut or liver. The pathognomonic finding is *Schiller Duval* bodies which is a single papillae lined by tumor cells with central blood vessels. This commonly produces *a-fetoprotein,* which as a serum marker is useful in following the response to therapy.

Immature Teratoma

They are second most common germ cell malignancy and the *malignant counterpart of the mature cystic teratoma or dermoid*. Malignant teratomas are found most commonly in patients younger than 20 years. They are bilateral in less than 50% of cases. The serum AFP is usually elevated in patients with an immature teratoma. Microscopically they reveal a disordered collection of tissues derived from the three germ layers, with at least some of the component having an immature embryonic appearance. Immature teratoma can be graded from 1 to 3 based on the amount of immature neural tissue they contain. Tumor grade is correlated with prognosis.

Mature Teratoma — Dermoid

They are common ovarian neoplasm found in women aged 20-30 years. They are most common neoplasm diagnosed during pregnancy. Less than 1% of all teratoma are malignant.

Embryonic Carcinoma

It is rare, found at near age of 15 years. The neoplasm has highly aggressive growth pattern with early extensive spread. *Histologically*, they consist of solid sheets of large polygonal cells, with pale eosinophilic cytoplasm. Serum hCG and serum AFP levels are usually elevated. Estrogen can be produced by these tumors and may serve as a serum marker.

Choriocarcinoma

It is rare germ cell tumor, not related to pregnancy. Primary choriocarcinoma of ovary is associated with somewhat lower elevation of hCG. It can cause precocious puberty, uterine bleeding or amenorrhea. Microscopically neoplasm is composed of cytotrophoblast.

Gonadoblastoma

It is rare neoplasm composed of nest of germ cells and sex cord derivative surrounded by connective tissue stroma. They usually occur in second decade of life. Gonadoblastoma are found in patients with abnormal gonadal development in the presence of Y chromosome.

Mixed Germ Cell Tumors

They are approximately 10% of germ cell neoplasm. As implied by the name, these neoplasms contain two or more germ cell element.

Polyembryoma

Polyembryoma of the ovary is an extremely rare tumor, most commonly seen in perimenarchal girls with signs of pseudopuberty. The tumor secretes AFP and hCG, is composed of embryoid bodies, and mimics the structure of the true somatic layers of early embryonic differentiation.

Sex Cord Stromal Tumors of the Ovary

They account for 5-8% of all ovarian malignancies. This group is derived from sex cords and the ovarian stroma or mesenchyme. The tumors usually are composed of various combination of elements, including the female cells (i.e. granulosa and theca cells), and male cells (Sertoli and Leydig cells).

Granulosa Stromal Cell Tumors

They include granulosa cell tumor, thecoma and fibroma. Granulosa cell tumors, which secrete estrogen, are rare in women of all age, and 50% occur in prepubertal girls. They are bilateral in only 2% of cases. It is low grade malignancy. *Histologically* granulosa cells which exhibit characteristic grooved coffee bean nucleus, can exhibit microfollicular, trabecular, insular or solid growth pattern. In most common variety, granulosa cells shows a tendency to arrange themselves in a cluster or rosettes around a central cavity, so there is resemblance to primordial follicle, i.e. **Call-Exner bodies**. **Thecoma** are associated with hyperestrogenism. This is commonly benign and consists of lipid laden stromal cells.

Sertoli-Leydig Tumors

They are rare, most frequently seen in the third and fourth decades of life. The tumors typically produce androgens and clinical virilization is noted in 70 to 85% of patients. Microscopically both Sertoli and Leydig cells are present.

Neoplasm Metastatic to the Ovaries

Cancer metastasizing to the ovary accounts for 5-6% of all ovarian malignancies. Most common sites are female genital tract, breast or the gastrointestinal tract. Microscopically, the origin of an ovarian metastasis might be difficult to determine. Gastrointestinal carcinoma metastatic to the ovary resembles a primary mucinous adenocarcinoma of the ovary in which characteristic **signet ring cells** are seen. Signet ring cells are identified by large locules lined by tall columnar mucin secreting epithelial cells, which are separated by fibrous trabeculae. Likewise in metastatic breast carcinoma the histologic appearance of the ovary may be different when compared to the primary breast tumor. **Krukenberg tumor** represents carcinoma of the stomach, metastatic to the ovary. However, the eponym is commonly used to denote any gastrointestinal carcinoma metastatic to the ovary. **Immunohistochemistry** is commonly used to facilitate the characterization of ovarian tumor. The ovarian tumor is expected to stain positive for cytokeratin (CKT) and negative for CK 20, while a metastatic lesion from a primary mucinous adenocarcinoma of the colon is likely to show the reverse pattern of (CKT negative, CK 20 positive).

DIAGNOSIS OF OVARIAN CANCER

Symptom

More than 80% of patients with ovarian cancer are diagnosed after menopause. The median age at diagnosis is about 62 years. Ovarian cancer typically develops as an insidous disease with few warning signs or symptoms. A history of nonspecific gastrointestinal complaints like nausea, dyspepsia and altered bowel habit is particularly common. Urinary urgency, pelvic pain, constipation and back pain may be noted. Occasionally patient may present with nausea, vomiting and partial bowel obstruction if carcinomatosis is widespread. Unfortunately in many women clinician attribute these symptoms to menopause, aging, dietary changes, psychological or functional bowel problem. As a result there is delay in diagnostic investigation.

Menstrual abnormalities may be noted in 15% of reproductive age patients with ovarian neoplasm or as postmenopausal bleeding. The cause of bleeding may be the presence of synchronous endometrial carcinoma or as a result of metastatic disease to lower genital tract or in hormone producing germ cell tumor. Granulosa theca cell tumors are classically estrogen producing tumors that present with abnormal vaginal bleeding. In advanced stage disease patient most often have symptoms related to the presence of ascites, omental or bowel metastasis.

Physical Examination

The most important sign of ovarian cancer is the presence of pelvic mass in physical examination. The presence of flank fullness and shifting dullness implies the presence of ascites or a large pelvic abdominal mass. Together with these signs, tympanic percussion noted over the lateral abdomen is consistent with a large mass that displaces the bowel to the periphery. A central tympanic percussion note is suggestive of ascites. Recent eversion of umbilicus in patients with abdominal distention may result from an increase on intra-abdominal pressure secondary to ascites.

Box 25.1: Differentiating feature between benign and malignant ovarian tumor on clinical examination

Benign	Malignant
Mobile	Fixed
Cystic	Solid and firm
Unilateral	Bilateral
Smooth	Nodular

Pelvic Examination

A pelvic or pelvic abdominal mass is palpable in most patients with ovarian cancer. A careful and thorough pelvic examination provides many helpful clues regarding the etiology of pelvic mass. Differentiating feature between benign and malignant tumor on clinical examination is summarized in Box 25.1.

Unilateral cystic masses in reproductive age women are benign in up to 95% of cases. These masses particularly when less than 6-8 cm in size are followed through next two menstrual cycles as they may represent functional cyst and spontaneously resolve. An enlarging mass or one that is associated with pain warrants prompt investigation. *Fixed, bilateral, firm nodular masses are suggestive of malignancy. To aid surgical planning a rectovaginal examination should also be performed.* Chest auscultation is important because patients with malignant pleural effusion may not be overtly symptomatic. Palpation of peripheral nodes should be done.

Differential Diagnosis

Ovarian neoplasm must be differentiated from benign neoplasm and functional cyst of the ovary. A range of benign condition like *pelvic inflammation disease, endometriosis and pedunculated uterus leiomyomas can simulate ovarian cancer.* Nongynecologic causes of pelvic tumors such as *inflammatory bowel disease* or *neoplastic colonic mass* must be excluded. A *pelvic kidney can simulate ovarian cancer.*

Investigation

a. **Lab evaluation:** A routine *complete blood count and metabolic panel* should be obtained. In 20-25% of patients there can be thrombocytosis (Platelet count $> 400 \times 10^{9L}$) probably caused by release of cytokines induced by ovarian malignant cells. Hyponatremia ranging between 125 – 135 mEq/lit, is another common finding because of tumor secretion of a vasopressin like substance.
b. **The serum hCG level** should be measured in any female in whom pregnancy is a possibility. **Serum AFP and lactate dehydrogenase (LDH)** should be measured in young girls and adolescent who present with adnexal masses because of the greater likelihood of malignant germ cell tumor.
c. **Serum CA-125** is integral to management of epithelial ovarian cancer. For a postmenopausal patient with an adnexal mass and a very high serum CA-125 level (>200 U/ml), *there is a 96% positive predictive value for malignancy.* For premenopausal patient, the specificity of test is less because CA-125 level tends to be elevated in common benign condition.
d. Paracentesis is not advocated as a routine procedure for patients with ascites, but diagnostic thoracocentesis for cytology is recommended in pleural effusion for staging purpose.

Imaging

Ultrasound

Ultrasound is the most common radiographic test to evaluate adnexal masses. Transabdominal examination requires a full bladder as an acoustic window for optimal visualization of the adnexa. A transvaginal examination does not have this requirement, but may not be useful for the assessment of large adnexal masses. Ultrasonographic characteristic of benign compared to malignant ovarian masses are mentioned in Table 25.3.

In patients with advanced disease, sonography is less helpful. The pelvic sonogram may be particularly difficult to interpret when a large mass encompasses the uterus, adnexa and surrounding structure. Ascites if present is easily detected but, abdominal sonography has limited use (Figs 25.1A to 25.2C).

CT/MRI

The main advantage of CT scanning is in treatment planning of women with advanced ovarian cancer. Preoperatively it may detect disease in the liver, retroperitoneal, omentum or elsewhere in the abdomen and thus guides cytoreduction. But CT scanning is not superior to USG in differentiating benign mass from malignant tumor and not particularly reliable in detecting intraperitoneal disease smaller than 1-2 cm in diameter.

Table 25.3: Ultrasonic differentiating features between benign and malignant ovarian neoplasm

Benign	Malignant
1. Simple cyst <10 cm in size	Solid or echogenic
2. Septation <3 mm in thickness	Multiple septation >2-3 mm in size
3. Unilateral	Bilateral
4. Calcification especially teeth	Not seen
5. Gravity dependent layering of cysts contents	
6. No papillary projection	Papillary projection
7. Doppler flow = no neovascularization	Neovascularization

Chapter -25 ♦ Premalignant and Malignant Disorders of Ovaries and Fallopian Tubes

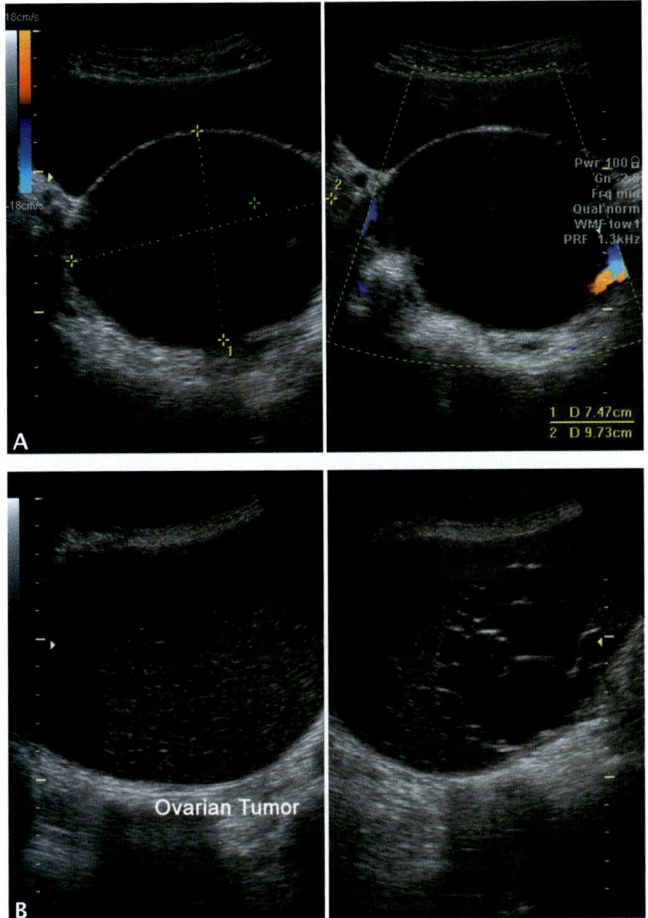

Figs 25.1A and B: (A) Ultrasound image of simple benign ovarian cyst; (B) Ultrasound image of solid ovarian tumor with variegated echogenicity which should raise the doubt of malignancy

In general other radiologic studies as MRI imaging, bone scan, and positron emission tomography (PET) usually gives little valuable information preoperatively.

Radiography

Every *patient with suspected ovarian cancer should have chest radiography* to detect pulmonary effusion or infrequently pulmonary metastasis. Rarely a barium enema is helpful clinically in excluding diverticular disease or colon cancer or in identifying involvement of the rectosigmoid by ovarian cancer. Diagnosis of an ovarian cancer requires an exploratory laparotomy.

Mode of Spread

Ovarian epithelial cancers spread primarily by exfoliation of cells into the peritoneal cavity, by lymphatic dissemination and by hematogenous spread.

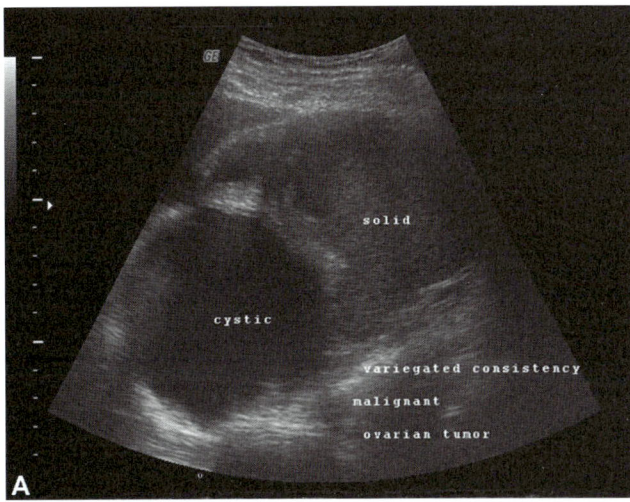

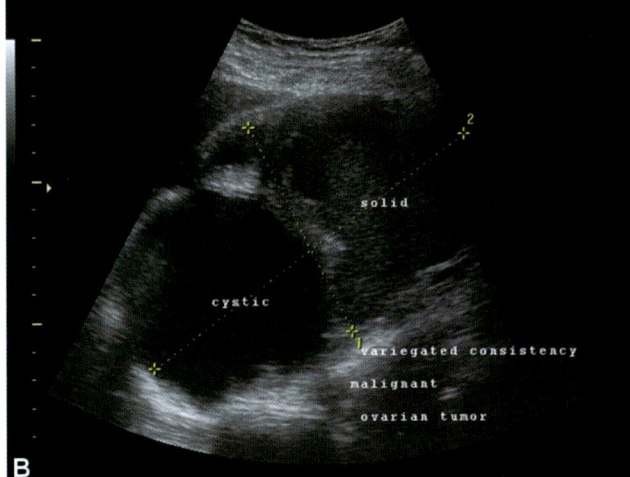

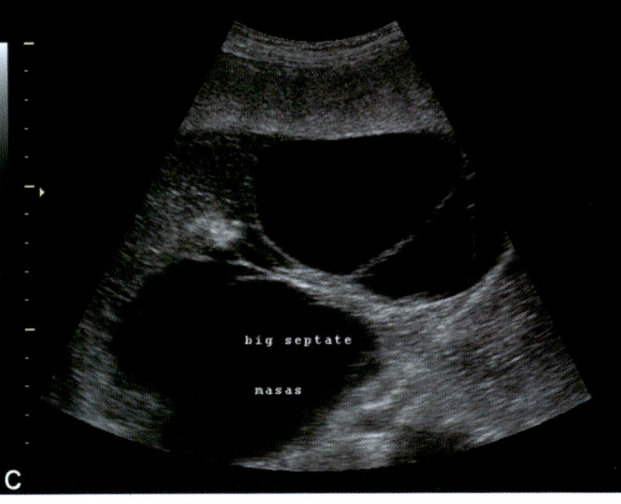

Figs 25.2A to C: Ultrasound images showing malignant ovarian cyst

Transcoelomic

The most common and earliest mode of dissemination of ovarian epithelial cancer is by exfoliation of cells that implant along the surface of the peritoneal cavity. The cells tend to follow the circulatory path of the peritoneal fluid. The fluid tends to move with the forces of respiration from the pelvis, up the paracolic gutters, especially on the right along the intestinal mesenteries to the right hemidiaphragm. So the metastases are typically seen on the posterior cul-de-sac, paracolic gutters, right hemidiaphragm and liver capsule, the peritoneal surface of the intestines and their mesenteries and omentum. **A unique characteristic of ovarian cancer is that metastatic tumors usually do not infiltrate visceral organs but exist as a surface implants** (As a result aggressive, debulking is possible with reasonable morbidity). **Omentum is the most frequent location because of its marked vascularity.**

Lymphatic Dissemination

It is the other primary mode of spread. Malignant cells may spread via channels that follow the ovarian blood supply along the infundibulopelvic ligament to pelvic obturator, internal iliac and external iliac and para-aortic lymph nodes. Infrequently metastasis may follow round ligaments to the inguinal nodes and through retroperitoneal spread to supraclavicular lymph nodes. **About 80% of patients with stage III have positive pelvic lymph nodes.**

Hematogenous Spread

It is uncommon. Metastasis to the liver or lung, brain or kidneys is observed in patients with recurrent disease, not at initial diagnosis.

Direct Extension

Direct extension of a progressively enlarging ovarian cancer may result in confluent tumor involvement of pelvic peritoneum and other structure like uterus, rectosigmoid colon and fallopian tubes.

Staging of Ovarian Neoplasm

Ovarian cancer is staged surgically based on typical pattern of spread. FIGO surgical staging system for ovarian cancer is listed in Table 25.4. It is important as subsequent treatment will be determined by the stage of disease. Whenever ovarian cancer is considered or likely diagnosis, a gynecologic oncologist trained to address both the surgical and medical needs of the patients should be consulted. Intraoperative differentiation of benign and malignant masses and procedures in the surgical staging of ovarian cancer are summarized in Tables 25.5 and 25.6, respectively.

Table 25.4: FIGO surgical staging system for ovarian cancer

Stage	Surgical pathologic findings
IA	Growth limited to one ovary
IB	Growth limited to both ovary
IC	Tumor limited to one or both ovaries, but with disease on the surface of one or both ovaries, or with capsule(s) ruptured, or with malignant ascites or positive peritoneal washing
IIA	Extension and or metastases to the uterus and/or tubes
IIB	Extension to other pelvic tissues
IIC	Tumor limited to genital tract or other pelvic tissue, but with disease on the surface of one or both ovaries, or with capsule(s) ruptured; or with malignant ascites or positive peritoneal washing
IIIA	Tumor grossly limited to the true pelvis with negative nodes but with histologically confirmed microscopic seeding of abdominal peritoneal surface
IIIB	Abdominal implants less than 2 cm in diameter with negative nodes
IIIC	Abdominal implants at least 2 cm in diameter and/ or positive pelvic, para-aortic, or inguinal nodes
IV	Distant metastases, including malignant pleural effusion or parenchymal liver metastases

Table 25.5: Intraoperative differentiation of benign and malignant ovarian neoplasm

Benign	Malignant
a. Simple cyst	Multiloculated with solid areas
b. Unilateral	Bilateral
c. No adhesion	Adhesions
d. No ascites	Ascites
e. Smooth surface	Area of hemorrhage, necrosis
f. Intact capsule	Papillary excrescences

Table 25.6: Procedures in the surgical staging of ovarian cancer

a. Sample of ascites or peritoneal washing from the paracolic gutter, and pelvic and subdiaphragmatic surface for cytology
b. Complete abdominal exploration
c. Intact removal of tumor
d. Hysterectomy
e. Infracolic omentectomy
f. Biopsies of the abdominal peritoneal implant
g. Pelvic and para-aortic lymph node biopsies
h. Cytoreductive surgery to remove all visible disease

MANAGEMENT OF EPITHELIAL OVARIAN CANCER

Stage I

After a comprehensive staging laparotomy only a minority of women will have local disease (FIGO stage I).

The primary surgical treatment for stage I epithelial ovarian cancer is surgical and patient should undergo total abdominal hysterectomy, bilateral salpingo-oophorectomy and surgical staging.*

Adjuvant Chemotherapy

In general patients with stage IA or IB, grade 3 epithelial ovarian cancer and all patients with stage IC and II tumors should be treated with 3-6 cycles of carboplatin and paclitaxel chemotherapy. Despite adjuvant chemotherapy, more than 20% of women with early stage disease develop recurrence within 5 years suggesting need of better treatment strategies.

Surveillance

After completion of treatment, early stage ovarian cancer may be followed every 2-4 months for the first 2 years, then twice yearly for 3 years and then annually with complete physical pelvic examination and serial CA-125 determination.

Management of Advanced Ovarian Cancer

In stages III and IV, the multimodality therapy is particularly important to achieve the most successful outcome. ***Surgical cytoreduction or debulking*** is performed to remove the primary tumor as well as the associated metastatic disease. The operation typically includes the performance of the total abdominal hysterectomy and bilateral salpingo-oophorectomy with complete omentectomy and resection of any metastatic lesion from the peritoneal surface or from the intestines.

The advantages of debulking is the:
a. Removal of bulky tumor mass may reduce the volume of ascites.
b. Improve appetite and nutritional status and facilitate the patient's ability to tolerate subsequent chemotherapy.
c. Beside this bulky tumor removes poorly vascularized areas which are exposed to suboptimal concentration of chemotherapeutic agent and more likely to be relative resistant to treatment.
d. After cytoreductive surgery there is smaller residual mass with a relatively higher growth fraction so require fewer cycles of chemotherapy.
e. The removal of necrotic masses improve drug delivery to remaining well vascularized cells.
f. Removal of bulky disease potentially enhances the immune system.

Since, goal of cytoreductive surgery is maximal resection of ovarian cancer and all metastatic disease, laparoscopic surgery has virtually no role.

Interval cytoreductive surgery:

In some patients, who are medically too compromised, interval cytoreduction can be offered after 3-4 courses of chemotherapy.

Chemotherapy

Advanced ovarian cancer is considered to be relatively sensitive to cytotoxic agents. Though duration of survival has increased with recent advances in chemotherapy, only fewer than 20% will be cured.

a. *Intravenous chemotherapy:* The preferred regimen in patients with advanced disease is nowadays *six courses of Paclitaxel and carboplatin combination.*
b. *Intraperitoneal chemotherapy:* Intraperitoneal *Paclitaxel* and *Cisplatin* has been under trial, and initial results are promising.

Complication of Chemotherapy

Combination of chemotherapy makes an impact on the patient day-to-day activities and can be associated with a variety of potentially life-threatening side effects. Table 25.7 lists the common side effects of commonly used drugs. *Nausea, vomiting and alopecia* are anticipated side effects. New antiemetics are more effective. *Myelosuppression* is another common side effect and complete blood counts are always monitored between cycles of therapy. Synthetic erythropoietin and colony stimulating factor can be administered to lessen the severity and duration of anemia and granulocytopenia.

Management of Patients in Remission

In most women with advanced ovarian cancer, the combination of surgery and platinum based chemotherapy will result in clinical remission. However, up to 80% will relapse eventually and die from disease progression.

Table 25.7: Toxicity of commonly used chemotherapeutic drugs	
Drug	Toxicity
Cisplatin	Nephro, neuro, ototoxicity
Carboplatin	Thrombocytopenia, neutropenia
Cyclophosphamide	Hemorrhagic cystitis, pulmonary fibrosis
Paclitaxel	Myelosuppression
Altretamine	Peripheral neuropathy
Etoposide	Myelosuppression
Bleomycin	Pulmonary fibrosis
Doxorubicin	Cardiac toxicity
Vincristine	Neuropathy
Ifosfamide	Hemorrhagic cystitis, central neurotoxicity

---

* Fertility sparing surgery in early stage ovarian cancer – Since, 10% of epithelial ovarian cancer develop in women younger than 40 years of age, uterus and contralateral ovary can be preserved in women with stage Ia, grade 1-2 disease in selected patients. The condition of women has to be carefully monitored with routine pelvic examination and serum CA 125 levels. Generally the other ovary and the uterus are removed at the completion of childbearing.

Surveillance

Patients should be followed regularly with pelvic examination and CA-125 determination. In advanced cases, imaging studies may be indicated more frequently.

Second Look Surgery

It is usually done in the setting of an investigational protocol. The main indication is to assess the completion of response and to resect residual tumor. A laparotomy is performed to obtain multiple specimens from peritoneal surface and suspicious areas. **Second look laparoscopy is an acceptable, less morbid alternative for selected patients**. However, the additional morbidity and cost must be weighed against the expected benefit for an individual patient.

Management of Germ Cell Neoplasm

In contrast to epithelial ovarian neoplasm, most germ cell neoplasm are at early stage at the time of diagnosis. For young women with germ cell neoplasm of the ovary, removal of involved adnexa with preservation of the normal appearing contralateral adnexa and uterus is generally advocated. In view of low incidence of bilaterality, biopsy of the contralateral ovary is not recommended because of risk of peritoneal and periovarian adhesion. Complete surgical staging of germ cell neoplasm is the same as for epithelial ovarian neoplasm and should be performed in all cases. Certain characteristic unique to germ cell neoplasm make an impact on their surgical management. Dysgerminoma of the ovary has the propensity to metastasize to the pelvic and para-aortic lymph nodes in the absence of other evidence of metastatic disease. *Dysgerminoma have the best prognosis of all malignant ovarian germ cell tumors variant. Endodermal sinus tumor of the ovary is the most rapidly growing neoplasm known to occur at any site. All patients are treated with chemotherapy regardless of the stage. Individuals with stages II-IV disease have a survival rate of less than 10%.*

Immature teratoma of the ovary may present with numerous peritoneal implants consistent with metastatic disease. These lesions must be biopsied. However, two-third of immature teratoma are stage I at diagnosis and have a 5 years survival rate of 95%. Patient with stages II-IV disease have a 70-80% 5 years survival rate and unilateral salpingo-oophorectomy is the standard treatment.

Chemotherapy of Germ Cell Neoplasm

Dysgerminoma is the most radiation sensitive neoplasm identified. But Cisplatin regimen has been administered with excellent results. *The significant advantage of chemotherapy is the potential to preserve future reproductive potential compared to radiation therapy.* For adjuvant therapy treatment with bleomycin, etoposide and cisplatin (BEP) is recommended.

Management of Malignant Sex Cord Tumors

Surgery: Surgical resection is the mainstay of treatment for patients with an ovarian SCST. The aims of surgery are to establish a definitive tissue diagnosis, determine the extent of disease by appropriate ovarian cancer staging procedures and remove all grossly visible disease. Staging laparotomy or laparoscopy is essential to determine the extent of disease and the need for adjuvant therapy in most individuals with potential malignant SCST subtypes.

Hysterectomy with bilateral salpingo-oophorectomy is performed for those who have completed childbearing. Unilateral salpingo-oophorectomy with preservation of uterus may be appropriate in the absence of obvious disease spread to other organs, if patient is young and willing for retaining fertility. Endometrial biopsy must be done in women with granulosa cell tumor because many of these patients have coexistent hyperplasia or adenocarcinoma that may effect the decision for hysterectomy.

Chemotherapy in SCST

In general SCST display less sensitivity to chemotherapy than other ovarian malignancies but most common at high risk for disease progression. SCST can be treated successfully with adjuvant Cisplatin based chemotherapy. Malignant stage I ovarian SCST may require adjuvant chemotherapy if there are high suspicion of recurrence. Stages II-IV disease warrants postoperative treatment. Five days BEP – bleomycin, etoposide and cisplatin regimen is the most widely used first line chemotherapy combination, given in 3 courses every 3 weeks in incompletely resected disease.

Radiotherapy

It has a very limited role and only reserved for palliation of local symptoms. Chemotherapy is primary mode of adjuvant treatment because of better tolerance, accessibility and ease of administration.

Surveillance

In general women with stage I ovarian SCST have an excellent prognosis following surgery. Surveillance includes a general, physical, pelvic examination, serum marker testing and imaging tests as clinically indicated.

Prognosis

The prognosis for patients with ovarian cancer is primarily related to stage of disease and histological types. **The 5 years survival rate for patient with stage I epithelial ovarian cancer is 76 to 93% depending upon tumor grade, 60 to 74% for stage II, 23 to 41% for stage III, 5 to 11% for**

stage IV disease. In general patients with well differentiated diploid neoplasm with an S phase fraction of less than 8-10% do better than patients who have poorly differentiated, aneuploid, rapidly proliferating (high S phase fraction) neoplasm.

In general germ cell tumors are associated with better 5 years survival rate than epithelial ovarian neoplasm. Patient with dysgerminoma have a 5 years survival rate of 95%, immature teratoma have 70-80%. Epithelial ovarian neoplasms of low malignancy potential are characterized by 5 years survival rate of 95%, reflecting their protracted and indolent course.

MALIGNANT NEOPLASM OF FALLOPIAN TUBE

Primary carcinoma of fallopian tube is the least common cancer, accounting for approximately 0.3% of all cancers of the female genital tract. **In histologic features and behaviors fallopian tube carcinoma is similar to epithelial ovarian cancer so evaluation and treatment are the same**. Secondary neoplasm of the fallopian tube can occur from other primary sites like ovaries, endometrium, gastrointestinal tract or breast.

Clinical Features

They are seen most frequently in fifth and sixth decade of life. Women having germline mutation in BRCA1 and BRCA2 are at substantially higher risk for developing fallopian tube carcinoma, so prophylactic surgery in these women should include a complete removal of both tubes along the ovaries.

Symptoms and Sign

The classical triad of symptoms are:
a. Prominent watery vaginal discharge (Hydrops, tubal profluens)
b. Pelvic pain
c. Pelvic mass

Vaginal discharge or bleeding is the most common symptom reported in 50% of cases with fallopian tube carcinoma. On *examination* a pelvic mass is present in about 60% of patients, and ascites may be present if advanced diseases exist.

Mode of Spread

They spread like epithelial ovarian malignancies, principally by transcoelomic exfoliation of cells and lymphatic channels.

Staging

It is surgically staged (Table 25.8).

Table 25.8: Modified FIGO staging of fallopian tube cancer (Based on Operative Findings before Debulking and Pathologic Findings)

Stage	Features
0	Carcinoma in situ* (limited to tubal mucosa)**
I	Growth is limited to the fallopian tubes
Ia	Growth is limited to one tube with extension into the submucosa*** and/or muscularis but not penetrating the serosal surface; no ascites.
Ib	Growth is limited to both tubes with extension into the submucosa*** and/or muscularis but not penetrating the serosal surface; no ascites.
Ic	Tumor either stage Ia or Ib but with tumor extension through or onto the tubal serosa; or with ascites present containing malignant cells or with positive peritoneal washings.
II	Growth involving one or both fallopian tubes with pelvic extension.
IIa	Extension and/or metastasis to the uterus and/or ovaries.
IIb	Extension to other pelvic tissues.
IIc	Tumor either stage IIa or IIb but with tumor extension through or onto the tubal serosa; or with ascites present containing malignant cells or with positive peritoneal washings.
III	Tumor involves one or both fallopian tubes with peritoneal implants outside of the pelvis and/or positive retroperitoneal or inguinal nodes. Superficial liver metastases equals stage III. Tumor appears limited to the true pelvis but with histologically proven malignant extension to the small bowel or omentum.
IIIa	Tumor is grossly limited to the true pelvis with negative nodes but with histologically confirmed microscopic seeding of abdominal peritoneal surfaces.
IIIb	Tumor involving one or both tubes with histologically confirmed implants of abdominal peritoneal surfaces; none exceeding 2 cm in diameter, lymph nodes are negative.
IIIc	Abdominal implants greater than 2 cm in diameter and/or positive retroperitoneal or inguinal nodes.
IV	Growth involving one or both fallopian tubes with distant metastases. If pleural effusion is present, there must be positive cytology to be stage IV. Parenchymal liver metastases equals stage IV.

* The staging system does not distinguish between microscopic foci or replacement of tubal epithelium by malignant epithelium and grossly evident masses in the tubal lumen that do not penetrate the wall beyond the epithelium. The former have not been reported to spread beyond the tube, whereas the latter can extend beyond the tube, recur, and the fatal.
** The mucosa presumably refers to the epithelium because involvement of the lamina propria component of the mucosa requires staging of the tumor as Ia.
*** Because the fallopian tube has no *submucosa*, this designation presumably refers to the lamina propria.

Histology

Ninety-five percent are papillary carcinoma. In 40-50% it is bilateral. **Grossly the affected tube is fusiform or sausage shaped and resembles pyosalpinx or tubo-ovarian inflammatory disease.**

Treatment

It is same as epithelial ovarian cancer. **Exploratory laparotomy is necessary to remove the primary tumor, to stage the disease and to resect metastasis.** After surgery the most frequently employed treatment is carboplatin, and paclitaxel chemotherapy.

Prognosis

Prognosis depends on stage of disease. Overall 5 years survival rate is approximately 56%.

MULTIPLE CHOICE QUESTIONS

1. All of the following are known risk factors for the development of ovarian carcinoma, *except*:
    a. Family history of ovarian carcinoma
    b. Use of oral pills
    c. Use of clomiphene
    d. BRCA1 positive individual
    Ans. b
2. The most common germ cell tumor of the ovary is:
    a. Choriocarcinoma
    b. Dysgerminoma
    c. Embryonal cell tumor
    d. Malignant teratoma
    Ans. b
3. In case of dysgerminoma of ovary following tumor marker is increased:
    a. Serum hCG
    b. Serum CA-125
    c. AFP
    d. LDH
    Ans. c
4. Call-Exner bodies are seen in:
    a. Dysgerminoma
    b. The carcinoma cell tumor
    c. Granulosa cell tumor
    d. Polyembryoma
    Ans. c
5. Which are seen in endodermal sinus tumor:
    a. Schiller-Dual bodies
    b. Reed-Sternberg cells
    c. Reinke's crystals
    d. Russell bodies
    Ans. a
6. Which of the following is correct regarding granulosa cell tumor of ovary:
    a. Common in puberty
    b. Associated with cancer endometrium
    c. Malignant change occur rarely
    d. It is bilateral
    Ans. b
7. Feature of dysgerminoma are:
    a. Unilateral
    b. Postmenopausal
    c. Virilizing
    d. Cut section gritty
    Ans. a
8. A 20-year-old girl presents with history of rapidly developing hirsutism and amenorrhea with change in voice. To establish a diagnosis you would like to proceed with which of following test:
    a. 170 H progesterone
    b. DHEA
    c. Testosterone
    d. LH FSH estimation
    Ans. c
9. CA-125 is a specific marker of:
    a. Choriocarcinoma
    b. Teratoma
    c. Epithelial cell carcinoma of ovary
    d. Seminoma
    Ans. c
10. A lady with Ca ovary in follow-up with raised CA-125 level, next step will be:
    a. CT
    b. PET
    c. MRI
    d. Clinical examination and serial follow-up of CA-125
    Ans. b
11. A 25-year-old married nullipara undergoes laparoscopic cystectomy for ovarian cyst which on histopathologic reveals ovarian serous cystadenocarcinoma. What would be nest management?
    a. Serial CA-125 measurement and follow-up
    b. Hysterectomy and bilateral salpingo-oophorectomy
    c. Hysterectomy + Radiotherapy
    d. Radiotherapy
    Ans. a
12. All are components of Meigs' syndrome, *except*:
    a. Pleural effusion
    b. Ovarian tumor
    c. Ascites
    d. Pericardial effusion
    Ans. d
13. What is the stage of ovarian cancer with superficial liver metastasis with bilateral ovarian mass:
    a. Stage I
    b. Stage II
    c. Stage III
    d. Stage IV
    Ans. c
14. The following tumor commonly metastasis to ovary, *except*:
    a. Malignant melanoma
    b. Stomach
    c. Esophagus
    d. Lymphoma
    Ans. a

Chapter -25 ♦ Premalignant and Malignant Disorders of Ovaries and Fallopian Tubes

15. A 55-year-old female patient has carcinoma of ovary with bilateral involvement with ascites fluid in the abdomen. The stage is:
    a. II
    b. III
    c. IV
    d. IC
    Ans. d
16. A 30-year-old female presents to the emergency with complaint of sudden severe abdominal pain, an abdominal mass on examination, most likely diagnosis is:
    a. Torsion of subserous fibroid
    b. Twisted ovarian cyst
    c. Rupture of ectopic pregnancy
    d. Rupture of ovarian cyst
    Ans. b
17. A 12-year-old female is admitted as a patient of dysgerminoma of right ovary 4 × 5 cm in size with intact capsule. Best treatment will be:
    a. Ovarian cystectomy
    b. Oophorectomy on the involved side
    c. Bilateral oophorectomy
    d. Hysterectomy with bilateral salpingo-oophorectomy
    Ans. b
18. The following are long-term complication of PCOS, *except*:
    a. Diabetes mellitus type II
    b. Cardiovascular disease
    c. None
    d. Ovarian cancer
    Ans. c
19. Which of the following ovarian tumor is prone to undergo torsion during pregnancy:
    a. Serous cystadenoma
    b. Mucinous cystadenoma
    c. Dermoid cyst
    d. Theca lutein cyst
    Ans. c

26 Premalignant and Malignant Disorders of the Vulva and Vagina

Mind like muscle is developed by use.

GENERAL CONSIDERATION

The vulvar skin is one component of the anogenital epithelium, extending from the distal vagina to the perineum and perianal skin. The lower genital tract epithelium is of common cloacogenic origin. Neoplasia of the vulvar skin is often associated with multiple foci of dysplasia in the lower genital tract.

VULVAR INTRAEPITHELIAL NEOPLASIA (VIN)

Premalignant lesions of the vulva occur in both premenopausal and postmenopausal women with the median age being approximately 40 years.

Diagnosis

Symptoms and Signs

The most common presenting symptom is **pruritis**, which is seen in more than 60% of VIN. Burning pain, soreness, discharge, urination discomfort, persistent ulcer, different color and texture of skin, lump or wart like growth are other presenting symptoms. On careful **inspection**, the vulvar lesion may be typically white and hyperkeratotic, or gray, pink or brown. In 1-2% of young women it is found with cervical dysplasia and they have **multifocal** vulvar, vaginal and perianal area dysplasia as **these surfaces arise from a cloacogenic origin**.

Investigations

Colposcopy and biopsy of any suspicious lesion should be performed and is the gold standard for diagnosis. An abnormal vascular pattern is most frequently associated with a severe degree of dysplasia, carcinoma *in situ*, or early invasive disease. Adequate biopsy can be taken by using a local anesthetic and biopsy punch up to 6 mm diameter. If lesions are close to clitoris, a general anesthetic is required. Careful documentation and mapping of vulvar area biopsy helps in management.

Pathology

International Society for the Study of Vulvar Disease (ISSVD) has adopted a standard of reporting vulvar dysplastic lesion. The degree of loss of epithelial cell maturation in a given lesion defines the grade of VIN.

VIN I: Immature cells occur in the lower one-third of epithelium.

VIN II: Intermediate between VIN I and VIN III.

VIN III: Complete loss of cellular maturation in the full thickness of epithelium. In new modified terminology VIN I have been eliminated and VIN II and III categories are combined. It is as follows:
a. **VIN (Usual type):** Warty, Basaloid (Mixed, formerly VIN II, VIN III, Vulvar CIS, carcinoma *in situ*).
b. **VIN (Differentiated type):** 2-10% of former VIN III lesion, older postmenopausal women, oncogenic HPV infection uncommon.
c. **VIN (Unclassified type):** Rare pagetoid lesions.
VIN are often multicentric, may be discrete or diffuse, single or multiple, flat or raised. They can be white velvety red or black.

On Microscopy

There is loss of stratification and cellular organization, which is seen in full thickness of the epithelium.

Risk Factors

VIN has been associated with sexually transmitted disease, primary human papilloma virus. **Approximately 80% of VIN lesions are positive for high risk HPV types particularly HPV–16.** Other risk factors are smoking and other genital precancers or cancers.

Natural History and Management

VIN I: The progression of VIN I to VIN III has not been established and modified 2004 ISVVD terminology has eliminated the VIN I category entirely. Lesions reported as VIN I may be reassessed annually and generally resolve without treatment.

VIN II and III: Treatment of VIN II and III is individualized and based on lesion location, size and clinical expertise. Many patients are best treated by excision or ablation.

Excision

Extensive vulvar surgery for VIN is not always necessary, if patient is under close monitoring for disease progression or recurrence. **Wide local excision with a surgical margin that includes at least 5 mm of normal tissue is done.** As disease recurrence is related to surgical margin status, frozen section histology of the specimen margin should be evaluated intraoperatively. Wide local excision may require skin grafting and can be disfiguring. All vulvar surgeries require thorough preoperative counseling.

Ablation Treatment

Laser ablation can be used. It provides better cosmetic result but it does not allow histologic evaluation of a surgical specimen. So presence of invasive carcinoma must be excluded beforehand.

Topical Treatment

Topical treatment is currently under investigation. Five fluorouracil or imiquinod have been tried.

Prognosis and Prevention

It is currently not possible to predict high grade VIN lesion behavior. Regardless of the treatment modality chosen, recurrence is common, especially in patients with multifocal disease and immunocompromised status.

VULVAR CANCER

Incidence and General Consideration

Vulvar cancer is uncommon representing 3 to 5% of malignancies of the female genital tract. The incidence appears to have increased during the last century. However, this may reflect the longer average lifespan of women. **Vulvar cancer is primarily a disease of postmenopausal women with a peak incidence in women ages 60-70 years.**

Etiopathogenesis and Risk Factors

Recent studies suggest two different etiological types of vulvar cancer:
a. **Basaloid or warty type:** It occurs in younger women, which is related to human papilloma virus (HPV) and smoking and commonly associated with vulvar intraepithelial neoplasia (VIN). Epidemiologic risk factor for basaloid or warty type squamous cell carcinoma of the vulva are similar to those for cervical cancer and include a history of multiple lower genital tract neoplasia, immunosuppression and smoking.
b. **Keratinizing type:** This presents mostly in older women, this is more common type. *It is unrelated to smoking or human papilloma virus infection and concurrent VIN.* In keratinizing carcinoma, associated lichen sclerosis or squamous hyperplasia is found in more than 80% of patients yet their causative role is not well defined.

Types of Invasive Vulvar Cancer

Types of invasive vulvar cancer are summarized in Table 26.1.

Mode of Spread

Vulvar cancer spreads by following routes:
1. *Direct extension* to involve adjacent structure such as vagina, urethra and anus.
2. *Lymphatic embolization* to regional inguinal and femoral lymph nodes. Lymphatic flow in the vulva runs anteriorly from the labia towards the mons and then laterally to the ipsilateral groin. The most common site of initial metastasis is to the *superficial inguinal nodes*. From there spread is usually through the fossa ovalis to the *deep femoral nodes*, then proximally to the *iliac chains*. In general lymphatic drainage travel in a step wise fashion from the superficial to deep inguinal nodes and then to pelvic lymph nodes, i.e. iliac and obturator lymph nodes, whereas the term inguinofemoral lymph nodes is usually described for collective deep and superficial inguinal nodes. **Any spread beyond the inguinal lymph nodes is considered distant metastasis.** Lymphatic decussate in the mons central and post fourchette and cross midline, so centrally occurring lesions involving clitoris, anterior labia, mons and perineum have an increased incidence of contralateral groin involvement. There are lymphatics in the anterior introitus and clitoris, which drain under the symphysis directly into the *pelvic lymph channels*, but they are of minimal clinical significance as pelvic metastasis without inguinal pathology is exceedingly rare.

Table 26.1: Types of vulvar cancer	
Types	Incidence (%)
Squamous	92
Melanoma	2-4
Basal cell	2-3
Bartholin's gland (adenocarcinoma, squamous cell, transitional cell, adenoid cystic)	1
Metastatic	1
Verrucuous	<1
Sarcoma	<1
Appendage (e.g. Hidradenocarcinoma)	Rare

3. *Hematogenous spread* to distant sites including lung, liver and bone.
4. *Direct extension* to involve adjacent structure such as the vagina, urethra and anus.

Staging of Vulvar Cancer

Currently the International Federation of Gynecology and Obstetric (FIGO) advocates surgically staging of a women with vulvar cancer (Table 26.2).

Diagnosis

Symptoms

Most patients are asymptomatic at time of diagnosis. If symptoms exist the most common presenting complaint is **itch (45%) or a lump or palpable mass (45%)**. Pain, bleeding, ulceration or dysuria is present in at least 10% of cases. In most patients symptoms are mild and persist for months before medical treatment is sought. Failure of apparently routine infection (like candida) to respond to standard therapy, should raise the suspicion of cancer.

Signs and Examination

A careful inspection of the vulva should be part of every gynecologic examination. On physical examination, vulvar carcinoma is usually raised and may be **fleshy, ulcerated,**

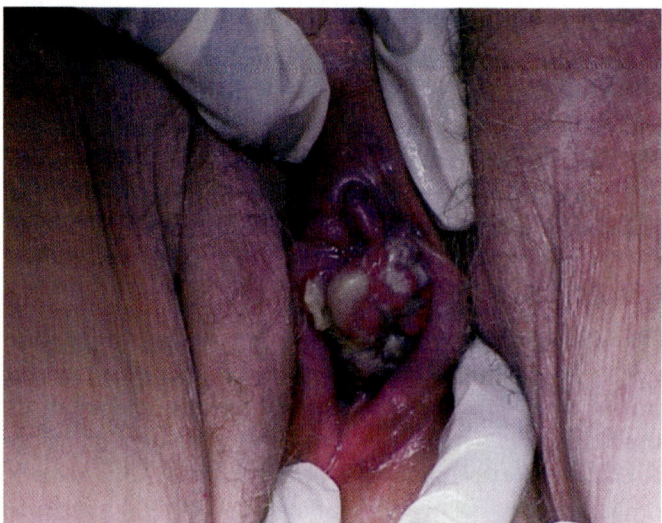

Fig. 26.1: Invasive vulvar carcinoma

leukoplakic or warty in appearance (Fig. 26.1). It may be pigmented, red or white, and tender or painless. It may be clinically indistinct especially in the presence of VIN or vulvar dystrophies. **Thus, any lesion of the vulva warrants a biopsy**. Most squamous carcinoma of the vulva occurs on the labia majora and minora (60%) but the clitoris (15%) and perineum (10%) also may be the primary sites.

In examination a careful assessment of the extent of the lesion including whether it is *unifocal or multifocal* should be done. The *groin lymph nodes* should be evaluated carefully and a complete pelvic examination should be performed. *Colposcopy* of the cervix and vagina should be performed because of common association with other squamous intraepithelial or invasive neoplasm of the lower genital tract.

Investigations

A **wedge biopsy** specimen is required for diagnosis. Women who have a well defined mass can have a direct punch biopsy for pathologic examination. In others **vulvoscopy** is done, and vulva is soaked with 3% acetic acid for 5 minutes, which allows for adequate penetration into keratin layer which aids identification of acetowhite areas and abnormal vascular pattern. Biopsy specimen is obtained with Key's punch forceps which should be approximately 4 mm thick to include surface epithelial lesion and underlying stroma.

Treatment

Surgery is the primary therapy for vulvar cancer. The procedure can be—**(a) Wide local excision, (b) Radical partial vulvectomy, (c) Radical complete vulvectomy.** Lymphadenectomy may accompany these procedures and typically includes excision of the deep and superficial inguinal lymph nodes. Skinning *vulvectomy* refers to

Table 26.2: FIGO staging of invasive cancer of the vulva

Stages	Clinical Pathological Findings
Stage 0 – CIS	Carcinoma *in situ*, intraepithelial carcinoma
Stage 1 – $T_1N_0M_0$	Tumor confined to the vulva and/or perineum, 2 cm or less in greatest dimension No Nodal metastasis
Stage 1A	Lesion 2 cm or less in size confined to the vulva or perineum and with stromal invasion no greater than 1.0 mm^3 (no nodal metastasis)
Stage 1B	Lesion 2 cm or less in size, confined to the vulva or perineum and with stromal invasion greater than 1.0 mm (no nodal metastasis)
Stage 2 – $T_2N_0N_0$	Tumor confined to the vulva and or perineum, more than 2 cm in greatest dimension (no nodal metastasis)
Stage 3 – $T_3N_0M_0$ $T_1N_1M_0 T_2N_1M_0$	Tumor any size with: a. Adjacent spread to the lower urethra and or vagina or the anus and/or
	b. Unilateral regional lymph node metastasis
Stage 4A $T_1N_2M_0$ $T_2N_2M_0$ $T_3N_3M_0$ T_4 any NM_0	Tumor involves any of the following – Upper urethra, bladder, mucosa, rectal mucosa, pelvic bone and/or bilateral regional node metastasis
Stage 4B	Any distant metastasis including pelvic lymph nodes

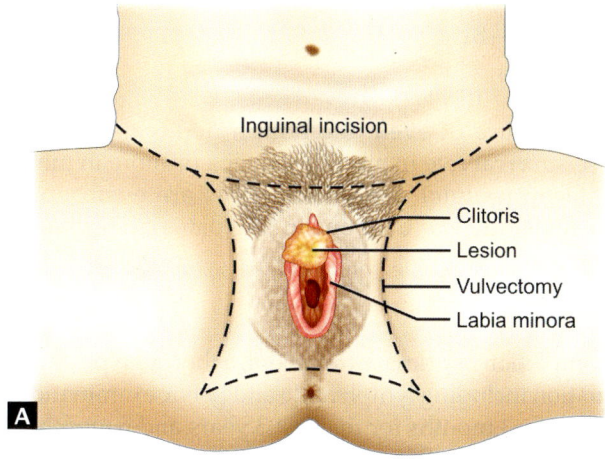
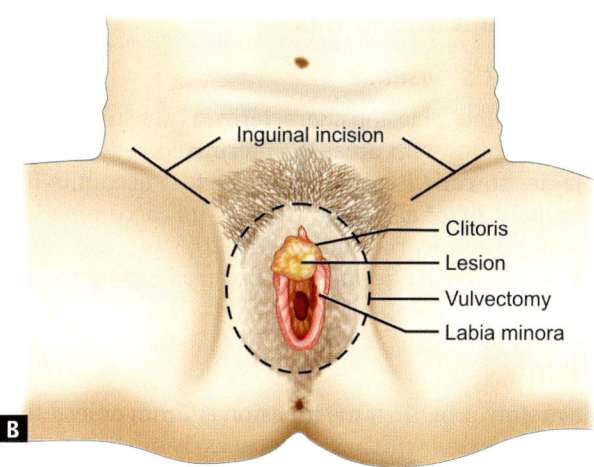
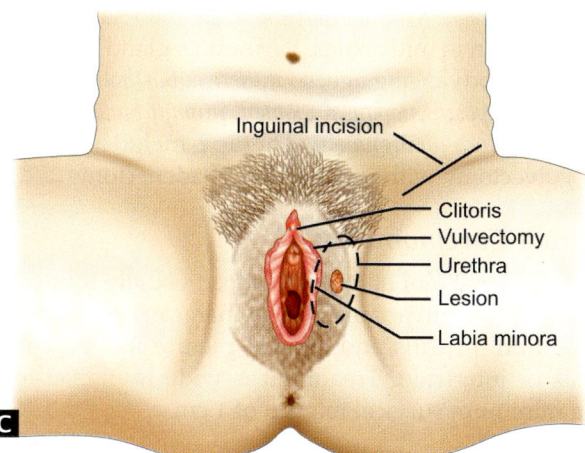

Figs 26.2A to C: Types of vulvectomy used in treatment of vulvar cancer: (A) En bloc radical vulvectomy with bilateral inguinal lymphadenectomy; (B) Radical complete vulvectomy with bilateral inguinal lymphadenectomy; (C) Radical partial vulvectomy with ipsilateral inguinal lymphadenectomy

removal of only skin and superficial subcutaneous tissue. This has no role in invasive vulvar cancer, but may be used in noninvasive disease such as cases with widespread multifocal VIN 3.

Stagewise Choice of Surgical Procedure (Figs 26.2A to C)

a. *Microinvasive tumor:* For curative resection these patients can undergo **wide local excision, also termed simple partial vulvectomy** to obtain 1-2 cm surgical margins around the lesion with dissection done to the superficial fascia of the urogenital diaphragm. Lymphadenectomy is not indicated for these very low risk patients.

b. *Early stage vulvar cancer:* Stage **IB**, II and few stages of III require radical resection of the primary tumor. An enbloc total radical vulvectomy involves excision of vulvar tissue between the labiocrural folds from the perineal body to the superior border of mons pubis. Dissection is up to level of perineal membrane (deep fascia of the urogenital diaphragm). Conceptually the rationale behind radical enbloc 'butterfly' resection is to excise three areas—the vulvar lesion, superficial and the deep inguinal lymph nodes and the lymphatic in between to remove all possible cancer infiltrated tissues. This has high immediate and long-term morbidity and cause severe perineal disfiguration.

c. *Radical partial vulvectomy:* Current modified surgical resection of a primary tumor is termed *radical partial vulvectomy*. In this vulvar lesion with clear surgical margin of 1-2 cm around the tumor is removed down to the perineal membrane, but other healthy tissue is not excised. Inguinal lymphadenectomy is performed using small, separate incisions below and parallel to the inguinal ligament.

d. *Radical complete vulvectomy:* In this entire vulva is removed. The borders of resection are generally the mons pubis superiorly, the perineal body inferiorly, and the labiocrural fold laterally. The clitoris is removed and deep margin is expanded to the perineal membrane. This is rarely used in early stage vulva cancer.

e. *Role of groin dissection and lymphadenectomy:* It is effective treatment to reduce surgical morbidity. The en bloc dissection of the groin nodes in continuity with vulva was replaced by an operation using three separate incisions. This depended on the principle that lymphatic metastases developed initially by embolization. Ipsilateral groin dissection is required for lesions that are unilateral (>1 cm from midline) and that involve >1 mm or are >2 cm in width. If these nodes are negative, the risk for isolated contralateral metastasis is less than 3% overall. If any of the ipsilateral nodes are positive, the contralateral groin must be surgically evaluated. Some doctors advocate pelvic node dissection when groin nodes are positive but evidence indicate that postoperative radiation to the groin and hemipelvis is superior to pelvic lymph node dissection in maintaining local control. Lesion that are <1 cm from the midline require bilateral groin evaluation if dissection is required, because the propensity for contralateral spread is much higher as the midline is approached.

Stages III and IV Cancer

These cancers involve adjacent mucosal structures or inguinal lymph nodes. A few advanced stage vulvar cancers can be treated with primary surgery in the form of a radical partial vulvectomy. But most advanced stage vulvar cancers require resection using some variation of pelvic exanteration and radical vulvectomy.

Role of Chemoradiation

Radiation is used predominantly for locally advanced disease. Due to the geometry of this body region, attaining homogeneous dosing is difficult. Chemotherapy is useful for disease that has metastasized out of the pelvis. In this setting neither surgery nor radiation can address all of the lesions. Response rate to chemotherapy alone are up to 30%, but the duration of response is generally short.

Complications of Treatment

a. Wound breakdown and infection is the most common complication. But with triple incision technique it is usually only a minor problem.
b. Ostitis pubis is rare but can be very serious complication. It requires intensive and prolonged antibiotic therapy.
c. Secondary hemorrhage.
d. Thromboembolic disease is life-threatening complication associated with surgery of malignant disease. It can be presented by combination of preoperative epidural analgesia to ensure good venous return with subcutaneous heparin started 12-24 hours before operation.
e. Chronic leg edema is present in 15% of women.
f. Numbness and paresthesia over anterior thigh.
g. Loss of body image and impaired sexual function.

Prognosis and Survival

Tumor stage especially lymph node involvement, tumor thickness, location on the vulva, lymphatic vascular space involvement and histologic differentiation are all important prognostic factors for women with vulvar cancer. Five years survival rates are as follows:

Stage I — 91%
Stage II — 81%
Stage III — 48%
Stage IV — 15%

The presence of even one lymph nodes metastasis decrease survival rate in all stages by 5% or more in most series. Deep (pelvic) nodal metastasis are even more omnius with only less than one in five patients surviving for five years.

Surveillance

After completion of primary treatment, a thorough physical examination including lymph node and pelvic examination is done every 3 months for the first 3 years and 6 monthly for next 2 years. Vulvoscopy and biopsy are performed if areas of concern are noted.

Other Vulvar Carcinomas

Vulvar Paget's Disease

It is an intraepithelial lesion characterized by a superficial, velvety thickening with areas of intermixed redness and leukoplakia, so called **cake icing effect**. It accounts for approximately 2% of all vulvar tumors. It is accompanied by invasive adenocarcinoma in 10-20% of cases and 20-30% of patient will have or develop an adenocarcinoma at other nonvulvar location.

Treatment

It displays slow growth. If the invasion is 2 mm or less, the lesion can be treated with a wide local excision. If invasive disease is suspected a radical partial vulvectomy is needed.

Bartholin's Gland Adenocarcinoma

It account for 1% of vulvar malignancies and its incidence peeks in women in mid sixties. Bartholin's gland infection decrease with advancing age, so *if there is Bartholin's gland enlargement in postmenopausal women, prompt biopsy should be done to exclude malignancy.* Therapy includes radical partial vulvectomy with inguinal lymphadenectomy.

Basal Cell Carcinoma (BCC)

It is in less than 2% of all vulvar cancer, usually found in elder women. In vulvar area BCC is characterized by poor pigmentation, pruritis and clinical picture like eczema, psoriasis or intertrigo. Treatment is wide local excision using a minimum surgical margin of 1 cm.

Vulvar Sarcoma

It is rare. Tumor typically develops as isolated masses in the labia majora, clitoris or Bartholin's gland. Recommended treatment for most types is primary surgery followed by adjuvant radiation or chemotherapy or both.

CHAPTER -26 ♦ Premalignant and Malignant Disorders of the Vulva and Vagina

PREINVASIVE DISEASE AND CANCER OF THE VAGINA

Incidence

Vaginal cancer is rare, accounting only 1 to 2% of malignant neoplasm of female genital tract. **Approximately 90% of vaginal cancer are squamous and develop slowly from precancerous epithelial changes similar to CIN called vaginal intraepithelial neoplasia (VaIN).**

Risk Factor of VaIN

Though the natural history of VaIN is less understood, the risk factors are thought to be similar as CIN. Cervical or vulvar neoplasia increases the risk for VaIN and vaginal squamous cancer. HPV virus infection can begin its growth in a healing abrasion in the same way as it infects transformation zone in cervix and initiate dysplastic change. The upper third of vagina is vulnerable to development of dysplasia and carcinoma *in situ*, whether or not hysterectomy has been performed previously for intraepithelial neoplasia. So women, who have had a hysterectomy with history of HPV or intraepithelial neoplasia, should continue to have periodic cytologic screening of the vaginal apex. In the same way VaIN and cancer vagina can develop after prior radiation for a pelvic cancer. Condylomatous lesions of the lower genital tract may demonstrate associated dysplasia. So a biopsy should be made of condylomatous growth of vagina prior to treatment.

Diagnosis

Symptoms

Generally all lesions of VaIN are asymptomatic. If present, symptoms may be vaginal bleeding, discharge and odor.

Signs and Investigations

Abnormal cytology is usually the first sign of the disease. Diagnosis is confirmed by **colposcopic examination with directed biopsy**. Because of redundant vaginal tissue, vaginal colposcopy is difficult to perform. A clear plastic speculum may help in visualization of all quadrants of vagina. Tissue in upper 1/3rd of vaginal vault requires proper attention. Technique is similar as in cervical colposcopy. After application of 3-5% acetic acid to the vagina a VaIN may appear as acetowhite epithelium, and may have mosaicism or punctation. Lugol's iodine may also help to identify the border of a lesion.

Treatment

VaIn lesions usually do not require treatment, as lesions typically regress. VaIN II and III can be treated either by excision or ablation.

Excision

Focal lesion should be best removed with local excision. If multifocal disease is present a total vaginectomy may be performed with a split thickness skin graft vaginal reconstruction.

Ablation

a. **Medical ablation:** Persistent VaIN I or II and selected VaIN III lesions may be medically treated using 5% Fluorouracil (5FU). Before medical ablation, possibility of invasive cancer must be excluded.

b. **CO_2 laser ablation:** It is suited for eradication of multifocal lesions and cause less scarring and blood loss than excisional modalities.

Prognosis

VaIN tends to be multifocal with cervical and vulvar involvement in many cases so the patients must be closely monitored every 3-4 months with colposcopic examination of lower genital tract and cytology.

CANCER OF VAGINA

Incidence

Primary vaginal cancer is relatively uncommon, representing only 1-2% of malignant neoplasm of female genital tract. Approximately 85% are squamous cell cancers and remaining in order of frequency are adenocarcinoma, sarcoma and melanomas. Secondary carcinoma of vagina is seen more frequently than primary vaginal cancer. Secondary or metastatic tumors may arise from cervical, endometrium or ovarian cancer, breast cancer, gestational trophoblastic disease, colorectal, urogenital or vulvar cancer.

Risk Factors

There are no causative agents identified for squamous lesions, which constitute 70-80% of all primary vaginal causes. Bacterial infections, trauma with pessary or prolapse and HPV exposure have all been postulated as predisposing factors, but scientific evidence of causation is lacking. **Exposure to synthetic estrogen diethylstilbestrol (DES) *in utero* is associated with increased incidence of adenocarcinoma of the vagina especially clear cell subtypes.** VaIN can be combined as premalignant phase of vaginal invasive cancer, but exact incidence of progression of VaIN to invasive cancer is not known. **Beside this by convention any new vaginal carcinoma developing at least 5 years after cervical cancer should be considered a new primary lesion.**

Screening

Routine screening of all patients for vaginal cancer is inappropriate. If the patients have a history of cervical

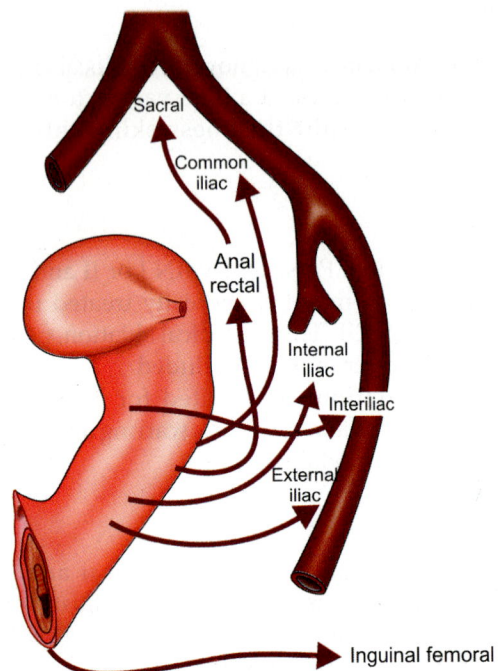

Fig. 26.3: Lymphatic drainage patterns of the vagina

dysplasia or cervical cancer, yearly screening is recommended.

Mode of Spread

Cancer of the vagina most often spread by direct extension into the pelvic soft tissue and adjacent organs. Metastasis to the pelvic and para-aortic lymph nodes may occur in advanced disease (Fig. 26.3). Hematogenous dissemination to lungs, liver or bones may occur as a late phenomenon.

Diagnosis

Age group: Though vaginal cancer has been reported in every decade of life. It is predominantly disease of elder women, with about 70% of patients diagnosed after age of 90. *The notable exceptions are Sarcoma Botryoidis and vaginal endodermal sinus tumor. These rare tumors demonstrate a predilection for infants and children.* Beside this clear cell adenocarcinoma, which arise in conjunction with vaginal adenosis is detected in young women, who had a history of exposure to diethylstilbestrol (DES) *in utero* at average age of 19 years.

Symptoms

Vaginal cancer is often asymptomatic, discovered only in routine vaginal cytologic examination. **Vaginal discharge with or without bleeding is the most common complaint.** Difficulty with voiding or intercourse is also reported due to tendency of the cancer to restrict the normal pliability of the vagina. Often the diagnosis is delayed due to subtlety of the symptoms.

Signs and Investigations

A diagnosis of primary vaginal cancer cannot be established unless metastasis from another source is excluded by thorough pelvic examination, cervical cytologic examination, and endometrial biopsy. Vaginoscopy with colposcope is done as described in VaIN and directed biopsy taken with Tischler biopsy forceps. No other specific lab testing is needed. If extent of cancer expansion is unclear, MRI imaging can be done. Vaginal cancer evaluation should include:

a. Vaginal biopsy
b. Physical examination
c. Endocervical curettage
d. Endometrial biopsy
e. Cystourethroscopy
f. Proctosigmoidoscopy
g. Chest radiograph
h. Abdominal/Pelvic CT scan or MRI.

Staging of Vaginal Cancer

FIGO staging of vaginal cancer is summarized in Box 26.1. It is clinical staging, not surgical (Figs 26.4A to D).

Box 26.1: FIGO staging of vaginal cancer

Stage	Features
0	Carcinoma *in situ*—preinvasive carcinoma
I	Carcinoma limited to the vaginal mucosa
II	Carcinoma involving subvaginal tissue but not extended to the pelvic wall
III	The carcinoma extended to the pelvic wall
IV	Tumor extended beyond the true pelvis, or has invaded bladder or rectal mucosa
IVA	Direct extension into adjacent organs
IVB	Distant metastasis

Treatment

Treatment is individualized based on tumor type, stage, location and size. Stage I and *in situ* lesion can be managed with surgical excision. In some patients radical hysterectomy is performed to obtain adequate margins, when deep invasion is present. External beam radiation to the whole pelvis is given initially to reduce the primary tumor volume and sterilize the regional lymphatics. External beam therapy is followed by intracavitary or interstitial treatment, which allows cytotoxic doses to be delivered directly to the tumor while minimizing damage to surrounding normal tissue. Persistent or recurrent disease can be treated with exenterative procedures if the disease has not spread distantly with reported success rate of 40%.

CHAPTER -26 ♦ Premalignant and Malignant Disorders of the Vulva and Vagina

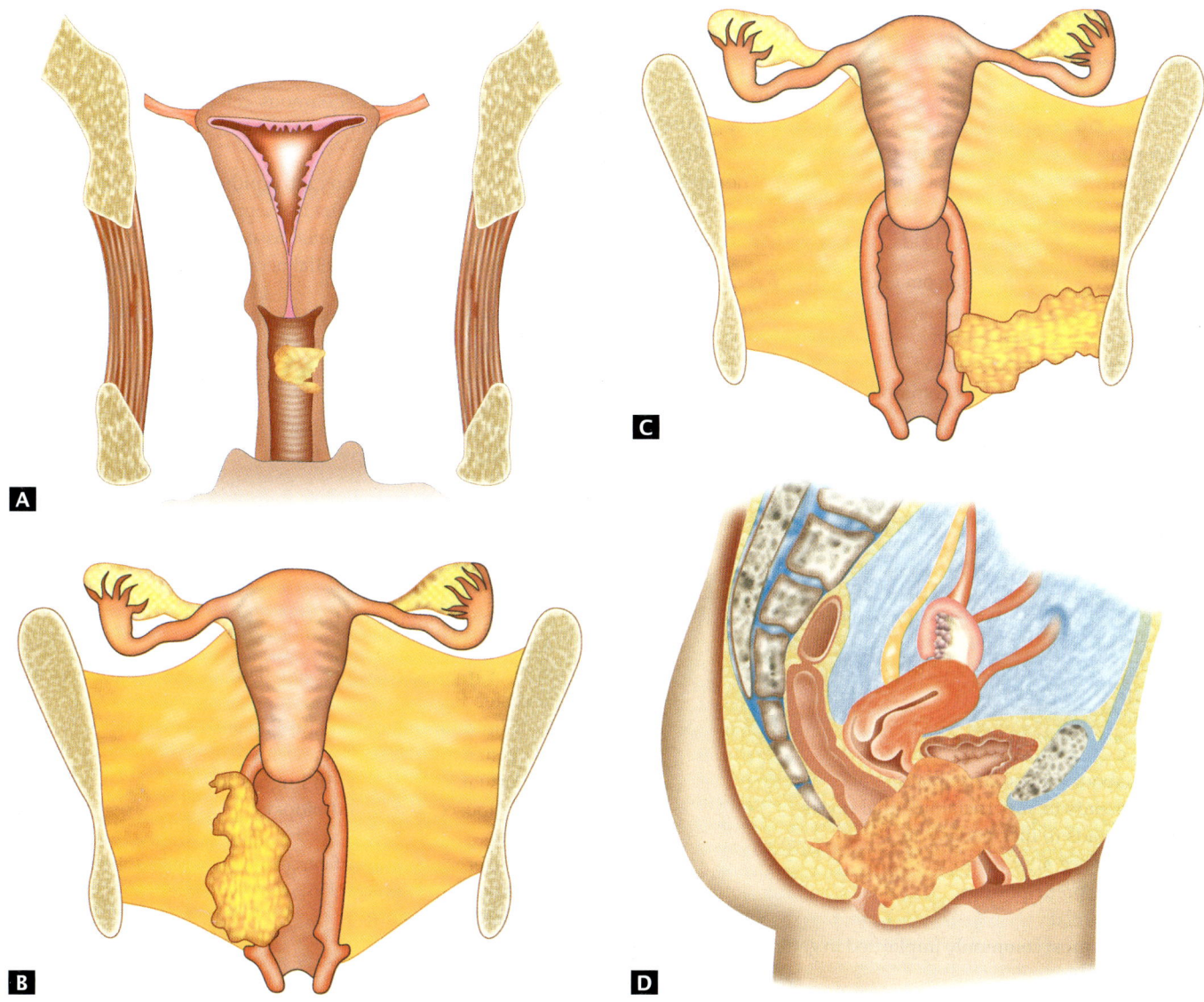

Figs 26.4A to D: FIGO staging of vaginal cancer: (A) Stage I; (B) Stage II; (C) Stage III; (D) Stage IV

Prognosis

Five years survival rate in vaginal cancer is as follows:
Stage I—70%
Stage II—40%
Stage III—30%
Stage IV—15-20%

Verrucuous Carcinoma of Vagina

It is extremely rare variant of squamous cell carcinoma. It presents as a warty and fungating mass. For diagnosis multiple biopsies are done. **Treatment** is surgical resection. They are resistant to radiotherapy and can be transformed into conventional squamous cell carcinoma after radiation. So radiation treatment is contraindicated.

Vaginal Adenosis

It is defined as presence of subepithelial glandular structure lined by mucinous columnar cells. These are residual glands of mullerian origin. Clinically, they appear as red granular spots.

Adenocarcinoma

Usually vaginal adenocarcinoma is a metastatic disease from endometrium. **Treatment** is like squamous cell carcinoma.

Clear Cell Adenocarcinoma

It has been linked to *in utero* exposure to DES treatment is like squamous cell carcinoma.

Embryonal Rhabdomyosarcoma (Sarcoma Botryoides)

It is most common malignancy of vagina in infant and children. This rare tumor develops in girls aged younger than 5 years. It presents as multiple polyp like structure or solitary growth. Treatment is primary chemotherapy.

MULTIPLE CHOICE QUESTIONS

1. All are true regarding sarcoma Botryoidis *except*:
   a. Seen in vagina
   b. Seen in elderly women
   c. It is an adenocarcinoma
   d. Familial incidence is common
   Ans. b, c, d

2. Most common vaginal carcinoma is:
   a. Squamous cell Ca
   b. Adenocarcinoma
   c. Botryoid's tumor
   d. Columnar hyperplasia
   Ans. a

3. Pelvis is involved in a case of vaginal carcinoma of stage:
   a. I
   b. II
   c. III
   d. IV
   Ans. c

4. True about carcinoma vulva is:
   a. Spreads to superficial inguinal nodes
   b. Spreads to iliac nodes
   c. Presence after menopause
   d. Viral predisposition
   Ans. a, b, c, d

5. Which is most commonly implicated in genital (Vulva) warts
   a. HPV 16
   b. HPV 18
   c. HPV 31
   d. HPV 6
   Ans. a

6. Patient diagnosed as squamous cell intraepithelial lesions, which of the following has the highest risk for progression to carcinoma:
   a. Low grade squamous intraepithelial neoplasm
   b. High grade squamous intraepithelial neoplasm
   c. Squamous intraepithelial associated with HPV
   d. Squamous intraepithelial neoplasia associated with HPV
   Ans. d

7. Pyometra is a complication associated with all of the following condition *except*:
   a. Ca vulva
   b. Ca Cx
   c. Carcinoma endometrium
   d. Pelvic radiotherapy
   Ans. a

8. Brachytherapy is used in:
   a. Stage IB Ca cervix
   b. Ovarian cancer
   c. Stage IV Ca vagina
   d. Stage II fallopian tube Ca
   Ans. a

9. A 35-year-old female, presents with postcoital bleeding. The next step is:
   a. Clinical examination and Pap smear
   b. Visual inspection with acetowhite
   c. Visual inspection with Lugol's iodine
   d. Colposcopy directed biopsy
   Ans. a

10. Characteristic feature of carcinoma fallopian tube is:
    a. Watery discharge P/V
    b. Hemorrhage
    c. Pain
    d. Sepsis
    Ans. a

27 Gestational Trophoblastic Diseases

Conscious learning becomes unconscious knowledge.

GENERAL CONSIDERATION

Gestational trophoblastic disease is an abnormal proliferation of placental type tissue resulting from a union of egg and sperm with abnormal DNA content. Histologic finding may include vesicular chorionic villi and proliferative trophoblast. **GTD refers to variety of diseases which include invasive mole, choriocarcinoma, and placental site trophoblastic tumor.** These diseases are characterized by reliable tumor marker – beta hCG and have varying tendencies towards local invasion and spread. **Gestational trophoblastic neoplasia (GTN) refers to the subset of gestational trophoblastic disease that develops malignant sequele.** These tumors require formal staging and typically respond to chemotherapy. Usually, GTN develops after a molar pregnancy but may follow any gestation.

Epidemiology and Risk Factors

The incidence of complete and partial mole is in 1 in 945 and 1 per 695 pregnancies respectively. *Maternal Age—* Women less than 20-year-old appear to have a slightly higher incidence of GTT while women older than 40 years have a 10 fold higher risk of GTD. *Ethnic and racial variation—*The prevalence of GTD is 10 times higher in Asia than in North America and Europe. In Japan incidence of molar pregnancy is 2 per thousand.

Obstetrical History

A history of prior unsuccessful pregnancies increases the risk of gestational trophoblastic disease. Previous spontaneous abortion at least doubles the risk of molar pregnancy and a personal history of gestational trophoblastic disease increase the risk of developing a molar gestation in a subsequent pregnancy by 10 fold. **So women with a prior history of GTD should undergo first trimester sonographic examination in subsequent pregnancies.**

Other Factors

Vitamin A deficiency and low dietary intake of carotene is associated with increased risk of complete mole. In some studies combined oral contraceptive (COC) pills have been associated with an increased risk of GTD.

Pathogenesis

GTD arise in fetal rather than maternal tissue. A complete mole results, when an empty egg lacking maternal DNA is fertilized by a haploid sperm that duplicates its chromosomes or by two haploid sperm simultaneously. **The karyotype of a complete mole is paternally derived 46 XX in 90% of cases, and paternally derived 46 XY in 10% cases. A partial mole is triploid 69 XXY (70%), 69 XXX (27%), or 69 XYY (3%).** It arises when an ovum with an active nucleus is fertilized by a duplicated sperm or two haploid sperm. This explains the occurrence of homozygous conception with a propensity of altered growth (Figs 27.1A and B).

Pathology

Hydatidiform Mole

It is an abnormal pregnancy characterized grossly by multiple grape like vesicles filling and distending the uterus, usually in the absence of intact fetus (Fig. 27.2).

Microscopically: It is identified by 3 classic findings – edema of the villous stroma, avascular villi and nest of proliferating syncytiotrophoblast or cytotrophoblast element surrounding villi (Fig. 27.3). The likelihood of malignant sequele is higher in patients whose trophoblastic cells show increased proliferation and anaplasia.

Invasive Mole

An invasive mole occurs in 20% of patients who have undergone evacuation of a molar pregnancy. It is essentially a hydatidiform mole that invades the myometrium or

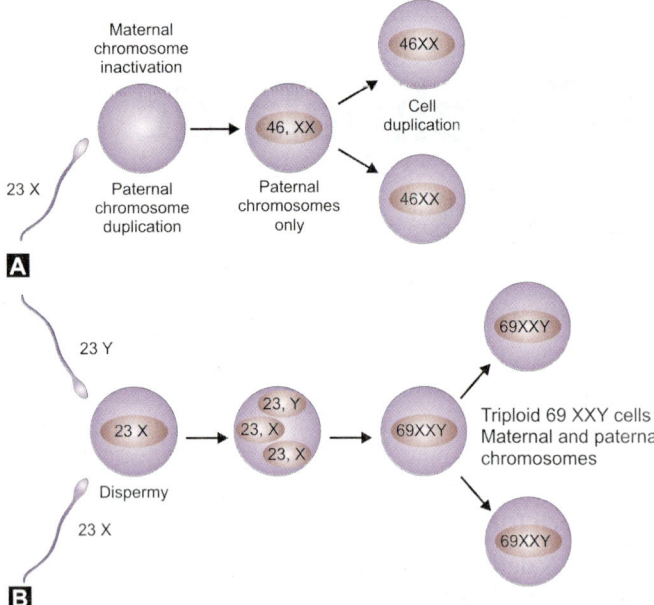

Figs 27.1A and B: Pathogenesis of complete and partial mole: (A) 46 XX complete mole; (B) partial mole formed if two sperm either bearing 23X or 23Y fertilize a 23 X containing egg or a haploid egg is fertilized by diploid 46 XY sperm

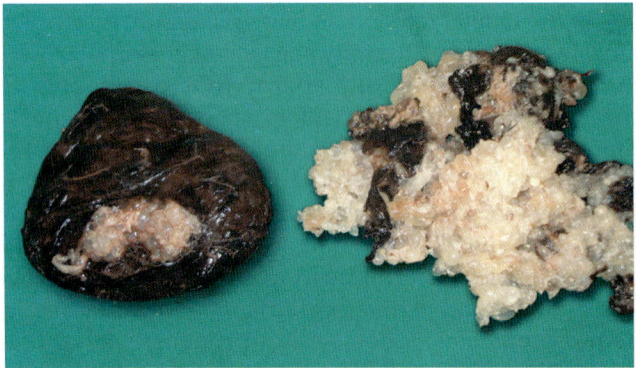

Fig. 27.2: Big vesicular mole showing grape like vesicles

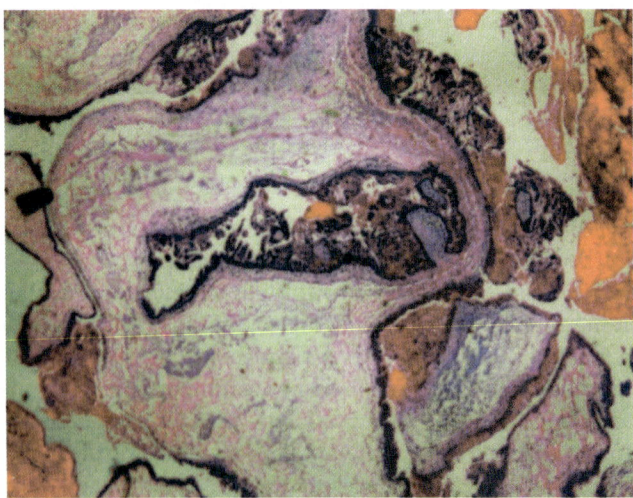

Fig. 27.3: Histology of complete hydatidiform mole showing extensive stromal edema of villi

adjacent structures. It can completely penetrate the myometrium and cause subsequent uterine rupture and hemoperitoneum (Fig. 27.4).

Choriocarcinoma

It is a pure epithelial tumor composed of syncytiotrophoblast and cytotrophoblast cells. It may be associated or follow any type of pregnancy. *Histology* shows sheets or foci of trophoblast on a background of hemorrhage and necrosis but no villi. It is important that curettage specimen must be processed in its entirety, as the specimen may contain only small isolated areas of choriocarcinoma.

Placental Site Trophoblastic Tumors (PSTTs)

It is derived from the intermediate trophoblast of the placental bed with minimal or absent syncytiotrophoblastic tissue. PSTT may occur with any type of pregnancy or present months to years thereafter. *Histologically* local invasion occurs into the myometrium and lymphatics and less commonly into the vasculature.

Clinical Presentations

Patients with complete molar pregnancy are increasingly being diagnosed earlier in pregnancy and treated before they develop the classic clinical signs and symptoms. This is because of changes in clinical practice, as the vaginal ultrasound and beta-hCG is being done in early pregnancy. Following is a description of the classic and current features of complete molar pregnancy:

a. *Vaginal bleeding:* It is the most common presenting symptoms occurring in more than 90% of patients with molar pregnancy. Three fourth of these patients present prior to the end of the first trimester.
b. *Excessive uterine size:* Excessive uterine enlargement relative to gestational age is one of the classic signs of a

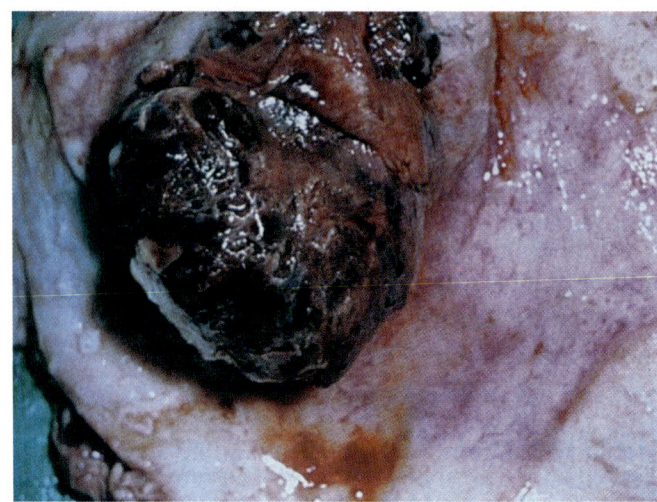

Fig. 27.4: Invasive mole

complete mole present in about half of the patients. It is caused by expansion of endometrial cavity with chorionic tissue and retained blood.

c. *Pre-eclampsia:* Pre-eclampsia was once observed in 27% of patients with a complete hydatidiform mole but now only 1 in 74 patients. Hydatidiform mole should be considered whenever pre-eclampsia develops early in pregnancy.
d. *Hyperemesis gravidarum:* Nausea and vomiting is reported in 14-32% of patients with GTD and 10% of these patients have symptoms severe enough to require hospitalization.
e. *Hyperthyroidism:* Clinically evident hyperthyroidism may be observed in 70% of patients with a complete molar gestation. The women may have tachycardia, warm skin, tremors. Diagnosis can be confirmed by elevated serum level of free thyroxine (T_4) and (T_3). Hyperthyroidism develops almost exclusively in patients with very high hCG levels.
f. *Trophoblastic embolization:* In the past, 2% of patients develop respiratory distress but nowadays it is rare. Respiratory insufficiency may result from trophoblastic embolization and the cardiopulmonary complications of thyroid storm, pre-eclampsia and massive fluid replaced.
g. *Theca lutein cyst:* Prominent theca lutein ovarian cyst (6 cm in diameter) develops in about one-half of patient with a complete mole. They results from high serum hCG levels, which cause ovarian hyperstimulation. Usually, they are detected on ultrasound examination. **After molar evacuation theca lutein cyst normally regress spontaneously within 2-4 months.**

Clinical Presentation of Partial Hydatidiform Mole

Patient with partial hydatidiform mole usually do not have the typical clinical feature characteristic of complete molar pregnancy. In general these patients have the signs and symptoms of incomplete or missed abortion; *partial mole is diagnosed after histologic review of the tissue obtained by curettage.*

Investigations

a. **Ultrasound:** Ultrasound is a reliable and sensitive technique for the diagnosis of complete molar pregnancy. Chorionic villi exhibit diffuse hydropic swelling. Complete mole produce a characteristic vesicular ultrasonographic pattern even in first trimester (Fig. 27.5).
b. **β-hCG estimation:** The principal characteristic of GTT is their capacity to produce β-hCG. Level of β-hCG closely correlates with the number of viable tumor cells. So monitoring of β-hCG level is a necessary tool for the diagnosis, treatment and follow-up of the disease process.

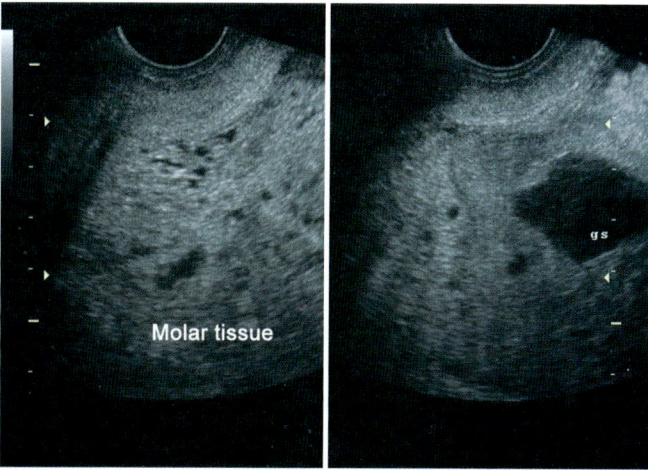

Fig. 27.5: Ultrasound image showing snowstorm appearance of partial mole, at one side empty gestational sac is seen

Differential Diagnosis

Gestational trophoblastic disease must be differentiated from a normal or ectopic pregnancy. USG is useful. Quantitative β-hCG levels improve the accuracy of the diagnosis. Analysis of tissue obtained from a dilatation and curettage for histology and DNA content will prove invaluable.

Treatment

After diagnosis of molar pregnancy, the patient should be evaluated carefully for the presence of associated medical complications like pre-eclampsia, hyperthyroidism, electrolyte imbalance and anemia. After stabilization, method of evacuation of molar tissue can be considered depending on age, desire of fertility, gestational age and associated complications.

A. **Suction curettage:** It is the preferred method of evacuation regardless of uterine size for patients who desire to preserve fertility. It involves the following steps:
   a. *Oxytocin infusion:* This is started before induction and may be continued 24 hours postoperatively. It facilitates uterine evacuation and minimizes the risk of uterine perforation.
   b. *Cervical dilatation:* Usually with dilatation bleeding starts.
   c. *Suction curettage:* The use of largest cannula is strongly advised to facilitate rapid evacuation. If uterus is larger than 14 weeks of gestation, one hand should be placed on top of the fundus and the uterus should be massaged to stimulate uterine contraction and reduce the risk of perforation.
   d. *Sharp curettage:* When suction evacuation is believed to be complete, gentle sharp curettage is performed to remove any residual molar tissue. Because trophoblast cells express Rh factor, patients who are

Rh negative should receive Rh immunoglobulin at the time of evacuation.

B. *Hysterectomy:* Hysterectomy remains an option for good surgical candidates not desirous of future pregnancy and for older women. If theca lutein cyst are encountered at hysterectomy the ovaries should remain intact, because regression to normal size will occur as the hCG titer diminishes. Careful follow-up with β-hCG titer is required even after hysterectomy.

C. *Hysterotomy:* It is no longer a method of choice in typical cases. Current recommendation restricts hysterotomy to cases complicated by hemorrhage.

D. *Prophylactic chemotherapy:* The use of prophylactic chemotherapy at time of molar evacuation is controversial. Studies demonstrate that it prevents metastasis and reduce the incidence and morbidity of local uterine invasion. **Prophylaxis is particularly useful in management of high risk complete molar pregnancy as age > 35 years; history of prior molar pregnancy, trophoblastic hyperplasia or when poor follow-up is anticipated.**

Follow-up

Regardless of the method of termination, close monitoring with raised β-hCG titer is essential for every patient because of the 20-30% incidence of malignant disease. The patients should be monitored with weekly determination of β-hCG until the levels are normal for 3 consecutive weeks followed by monthly determination until levels are normal for 6 consecutive months. On an average, normal beta hCG level is achieved in about 9 weeks. If patient achieves a non-detectable beta-hCG level the risk of developing tumor relapse is very low and may approach zero. After completion of follow-up patients can plan pregnancy.

Contraception

Patients are encouraged to use effective contraception in period of follow-up. IUCD should not be inserted because of possible risk of uterine perforation. Oral contraceptive or barrier methods should be used.

PERSISTENT GESTATIONAL TROPHOBLASTIC TUMOR (GTT)

Gestational trophoblastic tumor refers to invasive or metastatic form of gestational trophoblastic disease. There can be three types:
a. **Invasive or nonmetastatic persistent mole,** characterized by molar tissues invading the uterine myometrium.
b. **Choriocarcinoma,** metastatic malignant tumor.
c. **Placental site trophoblastic tumor,** which is rare and highly aggressive neoplasm.

Only two-third of GTT follows a molar pregnancy. The remaining one-third of cases follows miscarriage, therapeutic abortion or ectopic pregnancy.

Invasive GTT develops in about 15% of patients after evacuation of a complete mole and infrequently after other gestation. The patients may present with:
a. Irregular vaginal bleeding
b. Theca lutein cyst
c. Uterine subinvolution or asymmetric enlargement
d. Persistently elevated serum β-hCG levels.

The trophoblastic tumor may perforate the myo-metrium, causing intraperitoneal bleeding, or erode into uterine vessels, causing vaginal hemorrhage. Bulky necrotic tumor may be foci for infection and may present with purulent vaginal discharge and acute pelvic pain. After molar evacuation, persistent GTT may exhibit the histologic feature of either hydatidiform mole or choriocarcinoma. But after a non molar pregnancy, persistent GTT always has the histologic pattern of choriocarcinoma.

METASTATIC GESTATION TROPHOBLASTIC TUMORS (DISEASE)

Metastatic GTT occurs in about 4% of patients after evacuation of a complete mole but it is seen more often when GTT develops after nonmolar pregnancies. Metastasis is usually associated with choriocarcinoma, which has a tendency towards early vascular invasion with widespread dissemination. As trophoblastic tumors are perfused by fragile vessels, they are frequently hemorrhagic and symptoms of metastasis may result from spontaneous bleeding at metastatic foci.

The common sites of metastasis are:
a. Lung 80%
b. Vagina 30%
c. Pelvis 20%
d. Liver 10%
e. Brain 10%

Lung

At the time of diagnosis **lung involvement is visible by chest radiography in 80% of patients with metastatic GTT.** Patients with pulmonary metastasis can have chest pain, cough, hemoptysis, dyspnea or can be asymptomatic. Chest X-ray can show four principal types of findings.
i. An alveolar or snow storm pattern
ii. Discrete rounded densities
iii. Pleural effusion
iv. An embolic pattern caused by pulmonary arterial occlusion.

Because respiratory symptoms and X-ray findings can be alarming, the patient may be thought to have a primary pulmonary disease. Pulmonary hypertension can develop if there is pulmonary arterial occlusion by trophoblastic emboli.

Vaginal

Vaginal metastasis occurs in 30% of the patients with metastatic tumor. These lesions are usually highly vascular and may bleed vigorously when biopsied. The metastatic deposit in fornices or suburethra may produce irregular bleeding or a purulent discharge.

Hepatic

In 10% of cases with metastatic GTT, there is hepatic metastasis, which usually occurs if there is delay in diagnosis. It can present as epigastric or right upper quadrant pain and rarely may be hemorrhagic causing intraperitoneal bleeding.

Central Nervous System

It is seen in advanced cases, in 10% of patient usually with concurrent pulmonary or vaginal involvement or both. **Patient may present as acute focal neurologic deficits.**

Diagnosis of GTN

Most GTN are diagnosed clinically using hormonal evidence of persistent trophoblastic disease. *Criteria for the diagnosis of GTN are:*
1. Plateau of β-hCG last for four measurements over a period of 3 weeks or longer (day 1, 7, 14 and 21).
2. Rise of β-hCG of 3 weekly consecutive measurement or longer, over a period of 2 weeks or more (day 1, 7 and 14).
3. β-hCG remains elevated for 6 months or more.
4. Histologic diagnosis of choriocarcinoma.

When serologic criteria are met for GTN, a new intrauterine pregnancy should be excluded with ultrasound.

Diagnostic Evaluation

A thorough pretreatment assessment is done to determine the extent of the disease. **The initial evaluation should include a pelvic examination, chest radiograph and abdominal pelvic computed tomography (CT) scan.** If there is pulmonary lesion CT scan of chest and brain should be done. If conventional imaging doest not demonstrate metastatic disease, PET/CT position emission tomography/computed tomography may be useful in the evaluation of occult choriocarcinoma.

Staging

1. Anatomic staging (FIGO) (Table 27.1).
2. Prognostic scoring system (WHO) (Table 27.2).

Anatomic staging (FIGO): It is summarized in Table 27.1.

	Table 27.1: FIGO anatomic staging of GTN
Stage I	Patient have persistently elevated β-hCG level and tumor confined to the uterine corpus.
Stage II	Patient have metastasis to the vagina and pelvis or both
Stage III	Patients have pulmonary metastasis with or without uterine, vaginal or pelvic involvement.
Stage IV	Patients have advanced disease and involvement of the brain, liver, kidney or gastrointestinal tract.

Prognostic scoring system: A prognostic scoring system proposed by the WHO reliably predicts the potential for resistance to chemotherapy. It is as follows:

Table 27.2: Modified WHO prognostic scoring system as adapted by FIGO

Score	0	1	2	4
Age	<40	≥40	–	–
Antecedent pregnancy	Mole	Abortion	Term	–
Interval month from index pregnancy	>4	4 - <7	7 - <13	≥13
Pretreatment serum β-hCG (mIU/ml)	>10^3	10^3 - <10^4	10^4 - <10^5	≥10^5
Largest tumor size including uterus	–	3 - <5 cm	≥5 cm	–
Site of metastasis	Lung	Spleen, kidney	Gastrointestinal	Liver, brain
Number of metastasis	–	1 - 4	5 - 8	>8
Previous failed chemotherapy drug	–	–	1	≥2

Patients with WHO scores of 0-6 are considered to have low risk disease, whereas those with a score of 7 or higher are assigned to the high risk GTN group. The addition of risk scoring to anatomic staging has been shown to best reflect the disease behavior. Women with high risk score are best treated initially with combination chemotherapy. The FIGO classification system has been reported to be a better predictor of disease free interval than the WHO scoring system. Women diagnosed with FIGO Stages I, II, III GTN has a survival rate approaching 100%.

Management of GTN

Surgical Management

Most patients diagnosed with postmolar GTN have persistent tumors confined to the endometrial cavity and are treated primarily with chemotherapy. **Repeat dilatation and curetting has risk of uterine perforation, hemorrhage, infection, uterine adhesion and anesthetic complication.** Though in Europe repeat curettage is part of standard management of postmolar GTN and has been shown to reduce the need and dose of chemotherapeutic agents.

Hysterectomy may play several roles in treatment of GTN. The indication can be as follows:

i. To treat placental site trophoblastic tumor, epithelioid trophoblastic tumor or chemotherapy resistant cases.
ii. Severe intractable vaginal or intra-abdominal bleeding may necessitize as an emergency lifesaving procedure.
iii. Adjuvant hysterectomy decrease the total dose of chemotherapy in low risk GTN. So patients who do not desire future fertility should be counseled about this option.

Chemotherapy

Low-Risk GTN

a. *Methotrexate* is the most common treatment for low risk disease. Methotrexate is a folic acid antagonist that inhibits DNA synthesis by causing an acute intracellular deficiency of folate coenzymes. Ideally the 5 days treatment cycle is given every other week because tumor re-growth becomes significant after treatment gap of 2 weeks or longer. Once negative titer is achieved additional course is administered. The most common side effect is stomatitis. The less common side effects are nausea, vomiting, anorexia, hair thinning, leukopenia, hepatotoxicity and renal toxicity. Routine *Folinic acid* or calcium folinate is commonly administered several hours following methotrexate to replenish folate and minimize side effects.

b. If resistance to methotrexate occurs, manifested either by rising or plateau titer or by development of new metastasis the patient should be given **Dactinomycin**. There is a tendency not to be aggressive in treating these patients, because of low risk designation but failure of drug therapy does occur in approximately 10% of cases and meticulous follow-up with specialist is necessary for good results.

High-Risk GTN

High-risk GTN must be treated with combination chemotherapy such as EMACO (etoposide, methotrexate, actinomycin D, alternating with cyclophosphamide, vincristine (EMF/CO). Chemotherapy is a well tolerated and highly effective regiment for high-risk GTN and should be considered *primary treatment* in most circumstances. Treatment is continued for 2-3 courses beyond an undetectable b-hCG level. Survival is approximately 70%. High risk GTN patients, who have refractory or relapse from EMA/CO chemotherapy, may be treated effectively by replacing the cyclophosphamide and vincristine component with etoposide and cisplatin (EMA/EP). Other alternatives for second or third line therapy include—paclitoxel and alternating etoposide and cisplatin (TE/TP) and cisplatin and bleomycin combined with either vinblastine (VPB) or etoposide (BEP).

Brain Metastasis

Patients with GTN metastatic to the brain usually can be cured with aggressive multimodality therapy that may include chemotherapy, surgery and radiation. In addition, emergency craniotomy may be indicated in selective patients who display rapidly deteriorating signs.

Placental Site Trophoblastic Tumor

PSTT generally is resistant to chemotherapy; hysterectomy is the recommended choice of treatment. Partial uterine resection involving the tumor is possible if the patient desire to retain fertility. Chemotherapy is indicated in case of metastatic disease EP – EMA is preferred regimen over EMA/CO with (cisplatin/etoposide) paclitoxel and topotecan used, when resistance develops. The greatest adverse outcomes are associated with an interval >2 years from antecedent pregnancy to diagnosis.

Post Treatment Surveillance

Patients with Stages I, II, III GTN are monitored with weekly β-hCG measurement until the level is undetectable for 3 weeks followed by monthly titer until the level is undetectable for 12 months. Women with stage IV disease are followed for 24 months because of the greater risk of late relapse. Patients are motivated to use effective contraception in entire surveillance period.

Subsequent Pregnancy Outcome

The majority of pregnancies following treatment for a molar pregnancy or GTT result in normal healthy babies. The risk of a second molar pregnancy is only 10%. A woman who has 2 molar pregnancies has 15-28% chances of having a third. The risk of following three molar pregnancies is nearly 100%. This elevated risk appears to persist even when the women has a different male partner.

Phantom β–hCG

Occasionally, there is mild elevation of serum β-hCG which can lead to misdiagnosis. This phantom β-hCG results from presence in serum of heterophilic antibodies that interfere with the β-hCG immunoassay and cause false positive results. It can be clarified by negative urine pregnancy test and unchanged level of β-hCG in serial dilution.

Secondary Tumors

Etoposide based combination chemotherapy has been associated with increased risk of leukemia, colon cancer, melanoma and breast cancer up to 25 years after treatment for GTN. So etoposide is reserved to only patients resistant to single agent chemotherapy.

Chapter -27 ♦ Gestational Trophoblastic Diseases

MULTIPLE CHOICE QUESTIONS

1. The following conditions are associated with molar pregnancy *except*:
   a. Pregnancy induced hypertension
   b. Thyrotoxicosis
   c. Gestational diabetes
   d. Hyperemesis gravidarum
   Ans. c

2. The current imaging technique of choice for the diagnosis of hydatidiform mole is:
   a. Computed tomography
   b. Ultrasonography
   c. Plain X-ray abdomen
   d. Magnetic resonance imaging
   Ans. b

3. For a multiparous 40-year-old woman having molar pregnancies, the treatment of choice would be:
   a. D and C followed by regular follow-up
   b. Hysterectomy
   c. Hysterotomy and tubectomy
   d. VAT following by radiation
   Ans. b

4. The essential investigation to be included in follow-up of hydatidiform mole is:
   a. Ultrasound abdomen
   b. Chest X-ray
   c. Serum level of hCG
   d. Serum level of TSH
   Ans. c

5. The immediate complication of vesicular mole evacuation is:
   a. Bleeding
   b. Infection
   c. Incomplete evacuation
   d. Sepsis
   Ans. a

6. Chromosome number of hydatidiform mole is:
   a. 46 XX
   b. 45 XO
   c. 46 XY
   d. XXY
   Ans. a

7. The presence of lutein cyst in vesicular mole is due to excess:
   a. FSH
   b. LH
   c. Estrogen
   d. hCG
   Ans. d

8. Choriocarcinoma commonly metastasizes to:
   a. Brain
   b. Lung
   c. Vagina
   d. Ovary
   Ans. a, b

9. The following conditions are associated with molar pregnancy *except*:
   a. PIH
   b. Thyrotoxicosis
   c. Gestational diabetes
   d. Hyperemesis gravidarum
   Ans. c

10. The point of distinction between partial mole to complete mole is:
    a. Partial mole is triploid or tetraploid
    b. Partial mole is more prone to term malignant
    c. Typical of partial mole is cellular atypia
    d. Partial mole shows trophoblastic proliferation with absent villi
    Ans. a

28. Contraception

Give people room to grow and they will stay with you.

INTRODUCTION

The history of contraception is a long one dating to ancient time. However, the voluntary control of fertility is even more important in modern society. Effective control of reproduction is essential to a woman's ability to accomplish her individual goals. From a larger perspective the rapid growth of human population in this century threaten the survival of all. At the same time decision making concerning fertility control is a deeply personal and sensitive issue, often involving religious or philosophical convictions. So, it is important for the medical personnel to approach the subject with particular sensitivity, sympathy, maturity and nonjudgmental behavior.

Contraception in India—Past, Present and Future

Asia accounts for 60% of total world population and India contributes about 16% of world population. India has crossed the 1 billion people mark. While global population has increased nearly during this century from 2 to 6 billion, the population of India has increased nearly 5 times from 238 million (23 crores) to 1 billion in the same period. India's current annual increase in population is 15.5 million.

In 1952, India was the first country in the world to launch a national program, emphasizing family planning to the extent necessary for reducing birth rates to *stabilize the population at a level consistent with the requirement of national economy.*

The first five years plan called for an explicit population policy and considered family planning as a step toward improvement in health of mother and children. The basic strategy in the first plan was to treat family planning as a part of health program and provide 100% funds for it as a centrally sponsored program. Initially family planning program was intended to be promoted through a network of family planning clinics, which was replaced by an extensive education approach in 2nd and 3rd five years plan. Health department operated incentive based, target oriented and time bound program. During 1966–69, family planning program was integrated not only in health system but also specifically made a part of the Maternal and Child Health (MCH) program implemented through the primary health centers in rural areas and urban family planning centers in the town. In 1974-79, the mass sterilization camps were organized and 8.26 million sterilizations done in 1976-77. However there was a lot of criticism and again the policy was reviewed and after 1977 the program was changed from family planning to family welfare. In 6th five years plan the health based time bound target oriented family planning program was revised with reduced emphasis on sterilization and greater emphasis on spacing methods and on child survival program with help of international organization like UNICEF, WHO, universal immunization programs and extended program of immunization. It was continued till 1991. In 1992 the enactment of Panchayat Raj and reservation of 1/3rd of the seats in Panchayat empowered women politically in all decision making issues pertaining to social development including family planning. In 1994, Reproductive and Child Health (RCH) approach to family planning and population stabilization was accepted, which owes its origin to the recommendation of the International Conference on Population and Development (ICPD) in Cairo. ICPD recommended that population policies should be viewed as an integral part of program for women's development, right, reproductive health, poverty alleviation, and sustainable development.

The National Population Policy 2000 (NPP 2000) offers the commitment of Govt. towards voluntary and informed choice for contraceptive methods and consent of citizens while availing of reproductive health care services and continuation of the target free approach in administering family planning services.

Efficacy of Contraception

Contraception efficacy is generally assessed by measuring the number of unplanned pregnancies that occur during specified period of exposure and use of a contraceptive

method. There are two methods for measuring contraceptive efficacy:
a. Pearl index.
b. Life table analysis.

Pearl Index

The pearl index is defined as number of failure per 100 woman years of exposure. The denominator is the total months or cycles of exposure from the onset of method until completion of study.

$$\text{Pregnancy rate per 100 women year} = \frac{\text{Total accidental pregnancy} \times 1200}{\text{Total months of exposure to unintended pregnancy}}$$

With most methods of contraception the failure rate decline with duration of use. The pearl index fails to accurately compare methods at various duration of exposure. This limitation is overcome by using the method of life table analysis.

Life Table Analysis

It is being used more and more nowadays. It calculate failure rate for each month of use. A cumulative failure rate can then compare methods for any specific length of exposure.

METHODS OF CONTRACEPTION

The methods currently available for contraception are:
1. **Natural method:** Abstinence, with drawl and fertility awareness.
2. **Permanent sterilization:** Vasectomy (male), tubal ligation (female).
3. **Barrier method:** Diaphragm, cervical cap, male and female condom.
4. **Spermicidal**
5. **Intrauterine contraceptive devices:** Copper T – 250, 380, levonorgestrel (Mirena).
6. **Hormonal:**
   a. **Oral contraceptive** (OCP's, combination and progestin only).
   b. **Injectable**
      i. Depot medroxyprogesterone acetate (Depo Provera).
      ii. Lunelle (estradiol cypionate and medroxy-progesterone acetate).
   c. **Implant**
      i. Norplant (6 rods of levonorgestrel).
      ii. Vaginal ring (Nuva ring – ethinyl estradiol and etonorgestrel).
      iii. Transdermal patch (Eura – ethinyl estradiol and norgestimate).
   d. **Emergency contraception** (hormonal and copper IUD).

Natural Methods

Coitus Interruptus

It is withdrawal of penis before ejaculation. It has high failure rate from 4/100 women to 27 per 100 women years.

Lactational Amenorrhea

The lactational amenorrhea method is an effective method for breastfeeding women to utilize physiology to space births. *Sucking elevates prolactin levels and reduces gonadotropin releasing hormone (GnRh) from the hypothalamus, reducing leuteinizing hormone (LH) release and thus, inhibiting follicular maturation.* The duration of this suppression is variable and is influenced by the frequency and duration of nursing, length of time since birth and probably by the mother' nutritional status. Even with continued nursing, ovulation eventually returns but is unlikely before 6 months especially if woman is amenorrheic and fully breastfeeding with no supplement food to the infant. *To prevent pregnancy, another method of contraception should be used from 6 months after birth or earlier if menstruation resumes.*

Fertility Awareness Based Methods

It requires avoiding intercourse or use of barrier methods during the fertile period around the time of ovulation. For this proper instruction is critical and complex charting is involved. There can be following methods:

a. **Standard days method:** It is based on self-reported regular monthly cycles of 26 to 32 days during which users avoid unprotected intercourse during cycle from day 8 to 19.
b. **Periodic or rhythmic abstinence:** Human ovum is particularly susceptible to successful fertilization for only 12–24 hours after ovulation and sperm can live up to 6 days in the reproductive tract. This is the basic of fertility awareness methods. It has pregnancy rate from 5-40 per 100 women years. Following methods can be used:
   i. *Calendar rhythm method:* Ovulation most often occurs 14 days after the onset of last menstrual period. So, IPPF (1982) concluded that this method is not considered an effective method of family planning.
   ii. *Temperature rhythm method:* This method relies on a slight increase 0.4 to 1° increase in morning basal body temperature that occur just before ovulation and women practice abstinence from first day of menses through the third day after the increase in temperature—this is not a popular method but with excellent compliance, unwanted pregnancy rate is only about 2% in the first year.
   iii. *Cervical mucus rhythm method (Billing's method):* It depends on awareness of vaginal dryness and

wetness. Abstinence is required from the beginning of menses until 4 days after slippery mucus is identified. This is also not popular but with accurate use the first year failure rate is only about 3%.

iv. **Symptothermal method:** This system combines the use of change in cervical mucus and calendar method and change in basal body temperature to estimate the time of ovulation. The use of home kit to detect luteal hormone increase in the urine on the day prior to ovulation may improve the accuracy of periodic abstinence methods.

Barrier Methods

Barrier methods both the male and female condom provides a physical barrier that prevents sperm and egg interaction. *Diaphragms, caps and sponges use two different mechanisms—a physical barrier as well as a spermicidal chemical.*

Male Condom

Condom or contraceptive sheath is made of latex. They are most widely used barrier contraceptive in the world today.

Advantages

a. It protect against sexually transmitted infection (STI) including Chlamydial Herpes virus, HIV, Gonorrhea, Syphilis and Trichomoniasis.
b. It also protects and prevents premalignant cervical changes, probably by blocking transmission of human papilloma virus.
c. It provides immediate protection without much prior planning.
d. It has easy access.
e. No systemic side effects.

Disadvantages

a. There is need for a high degree of motivation for use.
b. Discomfort with use.
c. It has failure rate of 3-4/100 couple years of exposure.
d. Latex allergy very rare, but could lead to life threatening anaphylaxis in either partner from late condom. Non-latex condom of Polyurethane and Tactylon should be offered to these couples.

Female Condom (Vaginal Pouch)

The female condom is made of the polyurethane material with 2 flexible rings at each side. Open ring remains outside the vagina and closed internal ring is fitted under the symphysis like a diaphragm.

Advantages

a. It is in control of female partner.
b. It offers protection against STD and HIV.

Disadvantages

a. Costly.
b. Overall bulky.
c. Slippage and displacement rate is about 3%.
d. Pregnancy rate is higher than with the male condom.

Vaginal Diaphragm

This diaphragm consist of a circular rubber dome of various diameter supported by circumferential metal spring (Figs 28.1A and B). It can be very effective when used in combination with spermicidal jelly or cream. They are designed to fit in the vaginal cul-de-sac and over the cervix.

Fitting of diaphragm should be performed as follows:
a. A vaginal examination should first be performed.
b. A set of test diaphragm of various sizes is used and correct size diaphragm is inserted and checked by palpation.
c. The patient should practice insertion and should be reexamined to confirm proper position of the device.
d. The diaphragm can be inserted hours before intercourse but if more than 2 hours elapse, additional spermicidal jelly should be placed in the upper vagina. The diaphragm should be left in place for at least 6 hours after intercourse to allow for immobilization of sperm. Because toxic shock syndrome has been described following its use, the diaphragm should not be left in place for longer than 24 hours.

Disadvantages

a. It require fitting by a physician or trained personnel.
b. Necessity for anticipating the need for contraception.
c. Failure may result from improper fitting or displacement.
d. It can not be used with significant pelvic relaxation, short vagina or sharply retroverted or anteverted uterus.
e. Increased risk of urinary tract infection due to pressure of the rim against the urethra and alteration in the composition of the vaginal flora.
f. It has failure rate of 2-6/1000 women years.
g. It provide some protection against STDs.

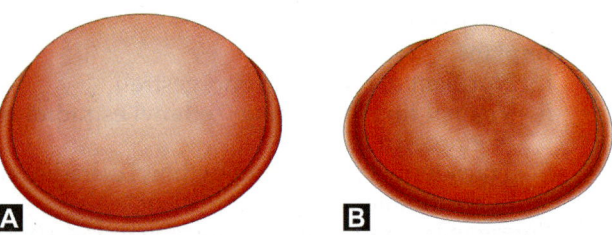

Figs 28.1A and B: Vaginal diaphragms: (A) Coil spring type; (B) Flat spring type

Cervical Cap

The prentif cervical cap is a flexible cup like device made of natural rubber that is fitted around the base of the cervix. It is now no longer available. A new version of cervical cap made of silicone rubber was approved by FDA and marketed under name of Fim Cap. Fim Cap requires a clinician fitting and prescription for use.

Lea's Shield

It is reusable, washable, barrier made of silicone which is placed against the cervix. It safety and efficacy are similar to that of other vaginal barrier method, acceptability is high.

Spermicidal Preparation

Currently available vaginal spermicidal preparation combines a spermicidal chemical either *nonoxynol–9 or Octoxynol* with a base of cream, jelly, aerosol foam, foaming tablet, film, suppository or polyurethane sponge. Nonoxynol–9 is a nonionic surface active detergent that immobilizes sperm. Nonoxynol–9 spermicidal alone appear considerably less effective in preventing pregnancy than condom or diaphragm.

Recent evidence indicates that spermicidal containing nonoxynol–9 are not effective in preventing cervical gonorrhea, chlamydia or HIV infection. In addition frequent use of spermicidal containing nonoxynol –9 without a barrier has been associated with genital lesion, which may be linked to increased risk of HIV transmission.

The Sponge Today

The today sponge is a polyurethane dome shaped device containing nonoxynol–9. It is moistened with water and then inserted high in the vagina to cover the cervix. It combines the advantages of a disposable barrier with spermicides and provides protection for 24 hours.

Intrauterine Device (IUD, IUCDs)

IUCD are made of plastic or metal or a combination of these materials meant for insertion into uterine cavity for contraception.

Mechanism of Action

An intrauterine device causes a foreign body reaction within the uterine cavity, thus altering sperm motility or integrity. It alters tubal fluids thereby interfering with ova and sperm transport and interaction. Finally an IUD alters the uterine linings so that it becomes unfavorable for implantation.

Copper intrauterine device: These IUCDs release free copper and copper salts which have both a biochemical and morphologic impact on the endometrium. It also produce alteration in cervical mucus and endometrial secretions. The copper IUD is associated with an inflammatory response marked by production in endometrium of cytokine peptides known to be cytotoxic. Progestin releasing IUDs add the endometrial action of progestin to the foreign body reaction. The endometrial is decidualized with atrophy of the glands. *The progestin thus inhibits implantation and sperm capacitation and survival. It also thickened the cervical mucus creating a barrier to sperm penetration.* The progestin IUD decreases menstrual blood loss (about 40-50%) and dysmenorrhea.

Various Types of IUDs (Figs 28.2A to F)

a. *Lippe's loop:* It was once most widely used type IUCD. It is made of polyethylene and impregnated with barium sulfate for radio-opacity. It is inserted with *Pushout* method of contraception. In India it is now being replaced by CUTs.
b. *Copper T 200:* This device is made of polypropylene integrated with barium sulfate and carries 12 mg of 0.25 mm diameter copper wire around vertical limb. The tail end bears two polypropylene transcervical threads. Its effective life is 4 years.
c. *Multiload copper 250 and multiload copper 375:* These are copper releasing devices made of polypropylene with 250 sq mm or 375 sq mm of exposed copper in the form of a wire wrapped around the vertical shaft. The arms are flexible plastic serrated fins that hold the device in place without stretching the uterine cavity. These devices are available in preloaded special inserter of the withdrawal type which helps in their insertion high up in the uterus. The inserter has no plunger. **In India**

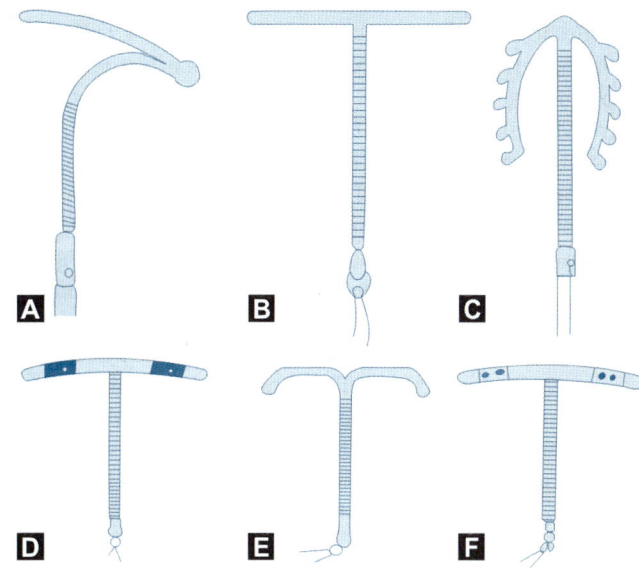

Figs 28.2A to F: Copper releasing IUDs. (A) Copper 7; (B) Copper T 200; (C) Multiload Copper 250; (D) Copper T 380 A, (E) Nova T; (F) Copper T 220 C

multiload- 250 recommended life span of 3 years and multiload copper 375 of 5 years are available. It is available in sterilized packs and can be inserted without prior handling which is a great advantage.

d. *CuT 380 A, CuT 380 Ag and CuT 380s:* They are T-shaped, have 314 square mm copper wire on the vertical stem and two 33 sq. mm copper sleeve on each of the two transverse arms. The wire in the 380 Ag has a silver core. They have specialized inserters of withdrawal type. **The approved life span of the CuT 380 A is 10 years, and CuT 380 Ag is 4 years.** In the USA CuT 380 A is only type of IUD available since 1988.

e. *Nova CuT 200 (Nova 7):* It is modified CuT 200 with a silver core added in the copper wire around the stem, 200 sq. mm of copper is exposed to surface. The inserter is of withdrawal type. The silver core increases its effective life to 5 years.

f. *CuT 220 C:* The device was developed by Population Council and has 7 copper sleeves, two on the transverse arm and 5 on the stem with a total exposed surface of 220 sq. mm. It has an estimated life of 3 years. All the copper devices have two transcervical monofilament nylon threads but some ML Cu 250 and 375 have one nylon thread.

Hormone Releasing IUD

a. *Progestasert (Progesterone IUD):* The device is T-shaped made of ethylene vinyl acetate copolymer impregnated with barium sulfate. The vertical shaft is fitted with a capsule containing 38 mg of progesterone dispensed in silicone oil. It delivers progesterone to the uterus at the rate of 65 µg/day. The progestasert has its own special method of insertion without a plunger but with an armcocker to pull the arm together during insertion and a thread retaining plug. The USFDA approved effective life is only one year. The contraceptive effectiveness of progestasert is similar to that of Cu IUDs. It reduces menstrual blood loss. It is slightly thicker than Cu IUD and insertion is more difficult (Fig. 28.3A).

b. *Levonorgestrel IUD 20 (LNG 20, Levonova, Mirena):* LNG 20 is a longer acting hormone releasing device. It is shaped like the Nova T but with a capsule on the stem. The core of the capsule contains a mixture of silicone rubber and 40-60 mg of levonorgestrel and releases 20 µg of the hormones per day (Fig. 28.3B). The insertion is of the withdrawal type. The contraceptive efficacy is for 5 years. It has a protective effect against ectopic pregnancy, reduces menstrual blood loss, sometime resulting in complete amenorrhea. It is slight difficult in insertion. Removal is not difficult.

Effectiveness

The CuT 380 A and levonorgestrel T have remarkable low pregnancy rates less than 0.2/100 women years. Considering all IUDs together, the actual use failure rate in

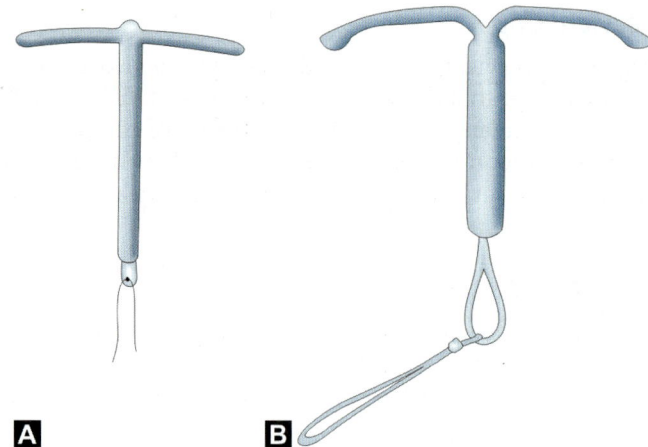

Figs 28.3A and B: Progesterone releasing IUDs: (A) Progestasert; (B) LNG 20

the first year is approximately 3% with a 10% expulsion rate and 15% rate of removal for bleeding and pain. With increasing duration of use and increasing age failure rate decrease as well the removal for pain and bleeding.

Benefits

Modern IUD provides excellent contraception without continued effort by the user. The levonorgestrel device reduces menstrual blood loss and reduced risk of endometrial cancer and improvement in symptoms of endometriosis.

Side Effects and Risk

a. *Infections:* IUD related bacterial infection is now believed to be due to contamination of endometrial cavity at the time of insertion *so the major risk of infection is at the time of insertion and does not increase with long-term use.* There is also a small increased risk of pelvic infection for up to the first 20 days. The problem of infection can be minimized with careful screening and the use of aseptic technique. Doxycycline (500 mg) or Azithromycin 500 mg administered orally one hour prior to insertion can provide protection against insertion associated pelvic infections but prophylactic antibiotics are probably of little benefit for women at low risk for RTI. With long-term use of current devices, pelvic infection rates are comparable to those in oral contraception users. Any infection after 45-60 days should be considered sexually transmitted and appropriately treated. The significance of Actinomyces infection in IUD user is unclear. Some studies have reported 7% of Actinomyces species seen on cytology smears from women using IUDs compared with less than 1% in non-users. In some cases pelvic infection or even pelvic abscess has been reported. ACOG (2005c) recommends that if symptomatic infection develops in women, who harbor actinomyces, then the IUD should be removed and antibiotic therapy should be given.

b. *Cramping and bleeding:* It is common for women to have uterine cramps and some bleeding soon after IUD insertion. It can be minimized by administration of NSAID.
c. *Menstrual problem:* The symptoms most commonly responsible for IUD insertion are increased uterine bleeding and increased menstrual pain. Within 1 year 5-15% of women discontinue IUD use because of these problems. Smaller copper IUDs and progestin IUDs have reduced incidence of pain and bleeding considerably but a careful menstrual history is still important in helping a women for considering and selecting an IUD. Women with menorrhagia or significant dysmenorrhea may not be able to tolerate copper IUDs but may benefit from a progestin IUD. Menorrhagia and cramping associated with IUCD can be effectively treated with NSAIDS. NSAIDS should begin at the onset of menses and be maintained for 3 days.
d. *Uterine perforation:* There can be clinically apparent or silent perforation, which occurs while sounding or during insertion. Perforation occurs at a rate of approximately 1 per 1000 insertions. Uncommonly device may migrate into and through the uterine wall.
e. *Expulsion:* Approximately 5% of patients spon-taneously expel the CuT 380 A within the first year. Younger women than 20 years have a higher incidence than older and it is associated with cramping, vaginal discharge or uterine bleeding. Patient should be continued to request immediate attention if expulsion is suspected. A partially expelled IUDs should be removed and if there is no pregnancy or infection, a new IUD can be inserted immediately.
f. *Ectopic pregnancy:* **If pregnancy occurs in an IUD user it will be ectopic in about 5% of cases.** Because fallopian tubes are less well protected against pregnancy than is the uterus. But compared with women having no contraception, there is 80%-90% reduction in the risk of ectopic with CuT 380 A or levonorgestrel T. *The largest WHO multicentric study includes that IUD users are 50% less likely to have an ectopic pregnancy when compared with women using no contraception.*
g. *Fertility:* Tubal factor infertility is not increased among nulligravid women who have used copper IUDs but exposure to sexually transmitted pathogens such as *Chlamydia trachomatis* does increase risk.
h. *Pregnancy with IUD in situ:* Spontaneous miscarriages occur more frequently (40-50%) among woman who become pregnant with IUDs in place. A woman with IUD in place has amenorrhea, should have a pregnancy test and pelvic examinations. If an intrauterine pregnancy is diagnosed and confirmed and IUD thread is visible, the IUD should be removed as soon as possible to prevent later septic abortion, premature rupture of membrane and premature births. If IUD strings are not visible, then ultrasound examination should be performed to localize the IUD and determine whether expulsion has occurred. If there is IUD in uterus and live pregnancy. There are 3 options for management:
 a. Therapeutic abortion.
 b. Ultrasound guided intrauterine removal of the IUD.
 c. Continuation of the pregnancy with the device left in place.

If patient wishes to continue pregnancy location of the IUD is detected by ultrasound. If the IUD is not in a fundal location ultrasound guided removal using small alligator forceps is advised. If location is fundal IUD should be left in place. If *pregnancy is continued with an IUD* in place the patient must be cautioned for symptoms of (a) *Intrauterine infection* like fever, chills, abdominal cramping or bleeding. At the earliest signs of infections high dose intravenous antibiotic therapy should be given and the pregnancy evacuated promptly (b) *Congenital anomalies*—there is no evidence that exposure of a fetus to medicated IUD is harmful, (c) *Preterm labor and birth* is increased approximately 4-fold when an IUD is left in place during pregnancy.

Clinical Management of IUD

Patient Selection

Patient selected for successful IUD users require attention to menstrual history and risk for STDs. Age and parity are not the clinical factors in selection. **The risk factors for STI are the most important consideration.** Nulliparous and nulligravid women can safely use the IUD if there is monogamous relationship. Patients with menorrhagia should be told about the possibility of increased menstrual bleeding with copper IUDs. Women on anticoagulant are not good candidate for copper IUDs but they might benefit from progestin IUDs.

Medical eligibility criteria for selection and continuation of IUCD are summarized in Table Annexure 1.

There are conditions which can reduce the success of IUCD. Women having abnormalities of uterine anatomy (Bicornuate uterus, cervical stenosis) may not accommodate IUD. Few individuals who have allergy to copper or have Wilson's disease should not use copper IUDs. Immunosuppressed patients should not use IUDs. In patient at risk for endocarditis like rheumatic valvular heart disease should be treated with prophylactic antibiotic at time of insertion and removal. It is to be emphasized that there is no increase in adverse events with copper IUD use in patients with *diabetes mellitus.*

A careful per speculum and bimanual examination is essential prior to selection for IUD insertion and absence of cervical or vaginal infection should be established before insertion. Insertion should be delayed if a mucopurulent discharge of the cervix or a significant vaginitis is present.

Contraindications to use of an IUCD

They are listed in Table 28.1.

Table 28.1: Contraindications to use of an IUCD

General:
1. Pregnancy or suspicion of pregnancy
2. Abnormalities of the uterus resulting in distortion of endometrial cavity
3. Acute PID, or H/o PID unless there has been a subsequent uterine pregnancy
4. Postpartum endometritis or infected abortion in past 3 months
5. Known or suspected uterine or cervical neoplasia or unresolved abnormal cytological smear
6. Genital bleeding of unknown cause
7. Untreated acute cervicitis or vaginitis
8. Couple having multiple sexual partner
9. Immunocompromised conditions like Leukemia, HIV positive, I/V drug abuse

Levonorgestrel IUCD is contraindicated in:
1. Hypersensitivity to any component of this procedure
2. Known or suspected breast cancer
3. Active liver disease or tumor

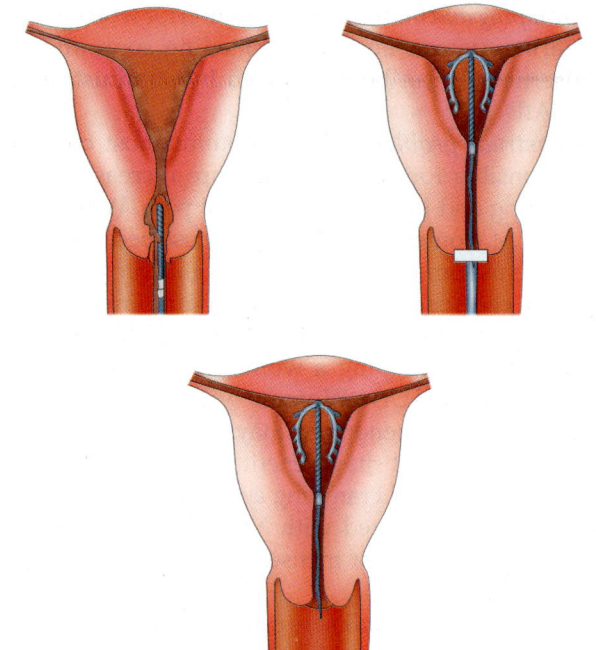

Fig. 28.4: Insertion of multiload Cu IUDs

Timing of Insertion

An IUD can be safely inserted at any time after delivery (postpartum), spontaneous miscarriages, induced abortion and during the menstrual cycle. IUD insertion during post menstrual period has the advantage that there is more open cervical canal so insertion is easy, there is masking of insertion related bleeding and knowledge that women is not pregnant. Beside this there is lower rate of expulsion and termination request if IUCD are inserted postmenstrualy. However, it can be inserted at any point of cycle as long as the patient is not pregnant.

An *'interval'* insertion is defined as insertion in women who are neither postpartum or post abortion or insertion in women 6 weeks after delivery.

Technique of Insertion

a. The cervix is exposed with speculum.
b. Vaginal vault and cervix are cleaned with bactericidal solution as iodine containing solution.
c. The uterine cavity size and direction is noted with a uterine sound.
d. Use of tenaculum is must to prevent perforation. It straighten the angle between the cervical canal and uterine cavity.
e. In withdraw technique the insertion with the device placed inside is introduced through the cervical canal right up to the fundus and after positioning it by the guard, the inserter is withdrawal, keeping the plunger in position. So, IUD is held in place by the plunger and inserter is withdrawn (Fig. 28.4).
f. The excess of the nylon thread beyond 2-3 cm from the external os is cut and instruments are taken off.
g. Levonorgestrel IUD is inserted somewhat differently. The inserter tube is introduced into the uterus until the present sliding flange on the inserter is 1.5-2 cm from the external os of the cervix. The arm of the T device is then released upward into the uterine cavity and the inserter is pushed up under them to elevate the IUD up against the uterine fundus.

Special Situations

a. **Embedded IUD:** If removal is not easily accomplished, direct visualization of IUD with sonography or hysteroscopy can be helpful.
b. **Finding a displaced IUD:** If the thread of IUCD can not be visualized the device may have been expelled or perforated the uterus. In both situation pregnancy can occur. *One should never assume that device has been expelled unless it was seen.* Initially gentle probing of uterine cavity can be done as thread simply may be in the uterine cavity. If tail is not felt, sonography should be done. If IUD can not be visualized with sonography additional X-rays are necessary because IUD can be high and hidden. X-rays should be taken with a uterine sound inserted into utrine cavity. *An extrauterine copper bearing IUD induce an intense local inflammatory reaction and adhesion and laparotomy may be needed to remove them.*

Hormonal Contraception

Hormonal contraception is female sex steroids-synthetic estrogen and synthetic progesterone (progestin) or progestin only. They can be administered in the form of

OCs, patches, implants and injectables. The most widely used hormonal contraceptive is the combination OC.

Mechanism of Action of Oral Contraception Pills

Estrogen component of the pill inhibits ovulation in part by suppression of Follicle Stimulating Hormone (FSH) and Luteinizing Hormone (LH). Progestational agent inhibits ovulation by suppressing LH, it thickens cervical mucus and thus hampers sperm transport and there is Decidualization of endometrium. It has possible effect on secretion and peristaltic movement within the fallopian tube, which gives additional benefit.

Mechanism of Action of Only Progestin Preparation

The mode of action of progestin only contraception are highly dependent on the dose of the compound. With **low level of progestin** in blood, there may be occasional ovulation. At **moderate level of progestin** in blood, normal basal level of FSH and LH are present and some follicle maturation may occur. But as there is no LH surge, ovulation does not occur. At **higher levels of progestin** in the blood, the amount of basal FSH is reduced and there is less follicular activity, less estradiol production and no LH surge.

Transdermal Hormonal Contraception

These patches have combination of ethinyl estradiol and a potent progestin, which provides sustained release of the steroids. It results in relatively constant screen levels which are less than peak level seen with OC's but sufficient to prevent ovulation.

Hormonal Implants

Subdermal implants release levonorgestrel for 3-5 years. With this there is some follicular maturation and estrogen production but LH peak are low and ovulation is often inhibited. In first year of use about 20% of cycles are ovulatory. The low dose progestin makes cervical mucus dry and scant, thus inhibits sperm migration into the upper tract. Progestin causes decidualization of endometrium and effect tubal motility. Progestin decrease nuclear estrogen receptor levels, decrease progesterone receptors and induce activity of the enzyme 17 hydroxysteroid dehydrogenase, which metabolizes natural estradiol. The sustained release offered by contraceptive implants allows for highly effective contraception at relatively low blood level of the hormones.

Steroid Pharmacology

Estrogen Component

Oral contraceptives contain either ethinyl estradiol or mestranol. Addition of an ethinyl group at 17 position of estradiol makes them orally active. Mestranol is the **3 methyl ether of ethinyl estradiol.**

Dose of estrogen component of the pill is of major importance.

Progestin Component

Progestins are synthetic compounds that mimic the effect of natural progesterone but differ from it structurally. The progesterone differ from each other in their affinities for estrogen, androgen and progesterone receptors, their ability to inhibit ovulation and their ability to substitute for progesterone and antagonize estrogen.

Orally active derivation of testosterone was developed in form of ethisterone. In 1951, it was discovered that removal of 19 carbon from ethisterone forms Norethindrone, which was not destroyed by oral intake and changed the major hormonal effect from that of androgen to progestational agent.

Norethinderone family contains – Norethindrone, norethynodrel, norethindrone acetate, ethynodiol diacetate, lynesternol, norgestrel, norgestimate, desogestrel and gestodene. Norgestrel is an equal mixture of two stereoisomer identified as dextronorgestrel, levonorgestrel.

New Progestin

Desogestrel, Gastodene and Norgestimate. They are viewed as more selective than other 19 nor progestin as they have little androgenic effect at doses required to inhibit ovulation. *The decreased androgenicity of new progestin is reflected in increased sex hormone binding globulin and decreased free testosterone concentration to a greater degree than older OC's.* This difference has clinical implication in treatment of acne and hirsutism. Besides they promote favorable lipid changes.

Drospirenone is a progestin that is an analogue of spironolactone. It has antiandrogenic and anti-mineralocorticoid activity and thus effective in treating premenstrual syndrome. Its use should be avoided in women with abnormal renal, adrenal or hepatic function.

New Formulation

The multiphasic preparation alter the dosage of both estrogen and progestin component periodically throughout pill taking schedule. They were developed in an effort to reduce the amount of total progestin per cycle without sacrificing contraceptive efficacy.

Pack is started with low dose of progestin and increasing it later in the contraceptive cycle. It results in reduction in progestin induced metabolic changes and adverse side effects. The estrogen dose may be kept constant or may be increased later in the cycle. Usually estrogen dose is kept between 20-40 μg of ethinyl estradiol. There are certain disadvantages of these formulations– which are confusion due to multicolor pills and increased breakthrough bleeding or spotting.

Drug Interaction

Oral contraceptives interferes with action of some drugs- *Phenytoin (anticonvulsant)* and *Rifampicin (antitubercular)* are believed to increase breakthrough bleeding and reduce efficacy of contraceptive pills especially containing less than 50 μg of ethinyl estradiol. Many antiretroviral drug (used in HIV and other viral infections) decrease contraceptive efficacy so barrier contraception is recommended. *Ampicillin* and *Tetracycline* may reduce efficacy of OC's, vitamin C competes for active sulfate in the intestinal wall and increase the bioavailability of ethinyl estradiol.

Efficacy of hormonal contraception: When used continuously combined OC's have pregnancy rate as low as 2-3 per 1000 women per year. Progestin only OC's are less effective then combination estrogen progestin preparation with best results of 3-4 pregnancies per 100 women years.

Safety of Hormonal Contraception

In general hormonal contraception and OC's have proven to be safe for most women.

Beneficial Effects

Besides providing a very effective method of contraception, the noncontraceptive benefits of OC's are many which should be highlighted to women.

The benefits of OC's can be categorized as:

1. *Fertility related benefit:* OC's by providing effective contraception reduces maternal morbidity and mortality due to pregnancy complication and cause – (i) reduction in ectopic pregnancy (ii) reduction in trophoblastic disease (iii) reduction in pelvic inflammatory disease.
2. *Menstrual benefits:*
   a. Reduction in menorrhagia and dysfunctional uterine bleeding.
   b. OC's are highly effective in relieving dysmenorrhea and premenstrual syndrome.
   c. It makes menopause easier by soothing mood swings, insomnia and hot flushes associated with perimenopausal period.
   d. In OC's user menstrual blood loss is reduced to 50% so they confirm protection against iron deficiency anemia. It is significantly important in developing countries like India where incidence of nutritional iron defficiency anemia and related maternal and child morbidity is high.
3. *Protection against benign disease:*
   a. There is less risk of benign breast disease like fibroadenoma or fibrocystic disease of breast.
   b. OC use protects from functional ovarian cyst. The benefit is ovulation related and applies to only current pill users.
   c. It controls symptoms of endometriosis to a good extent.
   d. Low dose OC helps to reduce risk of develop uterine fibroid.
4. *Protection against malignancies:* OC helps to protect against endometrial cancer, ovarian cancer (by 50%) and colorectal cancer.
5. *Other possible health benefits:*
   a. Low does OC's and newer OC's are effective in treating hyperandrogenic side effects like acne and hirsutism.
   b. It may stabilize or even increase bone density.
   c. It can have protective effect in the development of rheumatoid arthritis.

Possible Adverse Effects

1. *Lipids and lipoprotein:* In general COC's increase serum triglyceride and total cholesterol level. Estrogen decrease concentration of low density lipoprotein, cholesterol and increase high density lipoprotein (HDL) cholesterol. Progestin causes the reverse overall. The clinical impact on lipid is inconsequential for the vast majority of women.
2. *Carbohydrate metabolism:* Oral contraceptive do not increase risk of diabetes even in women with history of gestational diabetes. COC's may be used in women who have diabetes not complicated by associated vascular disease.
3. *Liver disease:* Cholestasis and cholestatic jaundice are uncommon complications of oral contraceptive. If they develop, signs and symptoms clear on stopping of oral contraceptives. There is no reason to withhold COC's in women recovering from viral hepatitis.
4. *Neoplasia:*
   a. **Endometrial and ovarian cancer:** COC's reduce the risk of subsequent endometrial cancer and ovarian cancer. In 2nd and 4th year of use OC's reduces the risk of endometrial cancer by 40%, and 60% respectively. There is 50% and 80% reduction in ovarian cancer risk for women who take OC's for 4 years and 10 years respectively. Benefit continues for at least 15 years from last use.
   b. **Cervical cancer:** There may be a weak association between OC use and squamous cancer of the cervix. But it is unclear that if these associations have a causal basis as COC's users are not protected from exposure to HPV virus and they are more frequently screened cytologicaly for cervical dysplasia. To reduce risk, however women who are not in mutual monogamous relationship should be advised to use barrier methods in addition to hormonal contraception.
   c. **Breast cancer:** By meta-analysis it has been concluded that breast cancer risk is not increased

for current or past users of OC's and did not increase with prolonged or with high estrogen or OC use.
   d. **Liver tumor:** Older contraceptive with larger estrogen doses were linked circumstantially with hepatic focal nodular hyperplasia and benign hepatic adenoma. But *recent large multicentric studies have found no association between use of OC's and subsequent Liver cancer.*
5. *Cardiovascular effects:*
   a. **Thrombosis and embolism:** The absolute risk of thrombosis in OC users taking pills containing 30-35 µg EE is 3 per 10,000 per year, compared with 1 per 10,000 in reproductive aged women not using OC's and 6 per 10,000 in pregnancy. The risk of thrombosis is related to estrogen dose and decreases with low dose EE formulation. Risk is apparent by 4 months after COC's and does not increase further with continued use. Risk is highest during the first year of use.
   b. **Ischemic heart disease:** Ischemic heart disease and stroke were the major causes of death attributed to OC use in the past. It is now known that the principal determinants of risk are advancing age and cigarette smoking. After adjusting for age, illness, smoking, ethinicity and body mass index, *risk for myocardial infarction has not found to be increased by OC users.* ACOG 2000b state that there is no contraindication to COC in nonsmoking women older than 35 years. Smoking is an independent risk factor for myocardial infarction and **smoking and COC's act synergistically to increase this risk especially beyond age of 35.**
   c. **Stroke:** Studies conclude that COC's use by healthy nonsmoking women is not associated with an increased risk of stroke. But smokers taking COC's had 7 times the risk of ischemic (thrombotic) stroke when compared with smokers who do not use COC's. Likewise hypertensive women had 10-fold increased risk if they took COC's but a five-fold risk if they did not. *Women taking COC's who have migraine headache with aura have a two to four-fold increased risk of stroke compared with non users.* So WHO has changed the medical eligibility criteria to exclude women with migraines from taking COC's. It is advisable also to preclude women who have migraine headache without aura from taking these combination contraceptives. For that a progestin only pill, barrier method or an IUD is more appropriate.
   D. **Hypertension:** Current low dose COC's increase the absolute risk of clinically significant hypertension only slightly. ACOG 2005b recommend a thorough evaluation of women who currently have hypertension and control of hypertension before COC use is considered.
6. *Effect on Reproduction:* After discontinuing OC's, return of ovulatory cycle occurs within 3 months. If there is post pill amenorrhea after COC's discontinuation it likely reflects preexisting problem. There is no evidence that COC's are teratogenic with the exception of sex organ development.
7. **Lactation:** There are limited data on the interaction of COC's and lactation. For women who are exclusively breast feeding, progestin only OC's are preferred. Those who are only intermittently breast feeding should use effective contraception within 3 weeks postpartum and can start oral contraceptive as soon as lactation is established.
8. **Weight Gain:** Review of 42 RCT and Cochrane database has concluded that available evidence was insufficient to determine effects of COC on weight but no larger effect was evident.

Other Effects

a. *Cervical leukorrhea:* May develop in response to estrogen component which at times cause pruritis, vaginitis or vulvovaginitis especially caused by candida species.
b. *Hyperpigmentation chloasma:* It is more likely in women who have chloasma during pregnancy. It is much less common in low dose COC's.
c. *Leiomyoma:* Do not increase with COC's.

Contraindications of COC's

It is argued that because pregnancy is usually more dangerous than COC that no contraindication to COC's should be considered absolutes. Pragmatically Box 28.1, list the condition in whom COC's should probably not be prescribed and alternative methods should be encouraged.

Medical eligibility criteria for initiating and continuing use of COC and combined injectable are summarized in Table Annexure II.

Transdermal Hormonal Contraception

The combined contraception patch (ortho Evra) patch has contact surface area of 20 sq. cm. and measures 4.5 sq. cm. It can be applied to the buttock/ upper outer arm/ lower abdomen/ upper torso. It delivers 150 µg norelgestromin (NGMN) and 20 µg ethinyl estradiol (EE) per day. The patch is worn for one week, discarded and replaced with a new one. A patch free week follows three weeks of continuous use. Data suggest that women who weigh 90 kg or more are at increased risk of contraceptive failure. It is an effective alternative hormonal contraceptive for women who do not prefer daily dosing and find a transdermal method acceptable.

Box 28.1: Contraindication for combined oral contraception

1. Thrombophilia or thromboembolic disorder
2. History of deep vein thrombosis or thrombotic disorder
3. Cerebrovascular or coronary artery disease
4. Thermogenic cardiac vasculopathies
5. Migraine with focal neurologic symptoms
6. Current pregnancy
7. Age > 35 years in the setting of smoking more than 20 cigarette per day
8. Hypertension (BP > 160/100mm hg) or with vascular disease
9. Active liver disease (Benign hepatic adenoma, liver cancer, active viral hepatitis, severe cirrhosis)
10. Major surgery with prolonged immobilization or any surgery of the legs
11. Presence or family history of hypercoagulable disease

Transvaginal Administration

An intravaginal hormonal contraceptive ring (**Nuva ring**) is a flexible polymer ring with an outer diameter of 54 mm and inner diameter of 50 mm. Its core contains ethinyl estradiol and the progestin Etonogestrel, which are released at rate of 15 µg and 120 µg per day respectively. The rings are refrigerated and once dispensed their shelf life is 4 months. The ring is initially placed within 5 days of menstrual cycle and removed after 3 weeks of use for 1 week to allow withdrawal bleeding. It is highly effective, ovulation inhibition is complete and failure rate is 0.65 per 100 women year.

Intramuscular Administration

There is only one combination preparation for intramuscular injection—**Lunelle**. This contains 25 mg of medroxy-progesterone acetate plus 5 mg of estradiol cypionate which is given monthly.

Progesterone Contraceptive

Oral progestins: Progestin only pills also known as mini pill contain Norethindrone. It does not reliably inhibit ovulation. It causes alteration in cervical mucus and endometrium. *Because the mucus changes do not persist beyond 24 hours, to be maximally effective it should be taken at the same time every day.* Even a delay of 2-3 hours reduces the contraceptive efficacy for coming 48 hours.

Advantage

Progestin only contraception is ideal for women when estrogen is contraindicated like smokers, migraine headache, hypertension. It is an excellent choice for lactating mothers. In combination with breast feeding. It is virtually 100% effective for up to 6 months and does not impair milk quantity.

Disadvantages

There are more chances of contraceptive failure and relative increased risk of proportion of ectopic pregnancies. They have to be taken at fixed time. There effectiveness is decreased by medication like phenytoin, carbamazepine and Antitubercular drug Rifampicin. Women taking any of these drugs should not use minipills. Unlike COC, minipill does not improve acne, may even worsen in some women.

Injectable Progestin Contraceptives

Depo Provera (DMPA) contains depot medroxy-progesterone acetate 150 mg suspended in aqueous solutions, which is given deep intramuscularly every 3 months. It is highly effective, having pregnancy rates of about 0.3/100 women per year.

Mode of action: In addition to thickening of cervical mucus and alteration of the endometrium the circulating level of the progestin is high enough to effectively block the LH surge and so ovulation does not occur. Suppression of FSH is not as intense as with COC so, follicular growth is maintained sufficiently to produce estrogen level comparable to follicular phase of normal menstrual cycle. Symptoms of estrogen deficiency as vaginal atrophy do not occur.

Advantages

1. It is not associated with compliance problem and not related to coital event.
2. It is highly effective method of contraception comparable or better than COC's.
3. It has no impairment on lactation.
4. It is useful for women who lead disorganized life and who are mentally retarded. It should be considered in patients with seizure disorders.
5. It is indicated in women where estrogens are contraindicated like H/o thromboembolism, smokers or hypertensive.
6. Reduced incidence of anemia due to oligomenorrhea or amenorrhea associated with its use.
7. There is a decreased risk of endometrial cancer comparable with COC's.
8. It has other noncontraceptive benefit like less PID, less endometriosis, fewer uterine fibroids and fewer ectopic pregnancies.

Problem with Depo Provera

a. *Irregular menstrual bleeding:* The principal disadvantage of depot progestin is irregular menstrual bleeding and 25% women discontinue its use because of irregular bleeding. Persistent irregular bleeding can be treated by adding low dose estrogen temporarily like conjugated estrogen 1.25 mg per day for 10-21 days at a

time. Mifepristone 50 mg every 2 weeks can reduce breakthrough bleeding in new users.
b. *Fertility:* There is prolonged anovulation after discontinuation resulting in delayed return of fertility. However, 70% of former users desiring pregnancy conceived within 12 months and 90% conceived within 24 months. Suppressed menstrual function persisting beyond 18 months after the last injection is not due to the drug and deserves evaluation.
c. *Breast cancer:* Studies has not found evidence for an overall increased risk of breast cancer and risk did not increase with duration of use.
d. *Other cancers:* Cervical and hepatic malignancies do not appear to be increased and the risk of ovarian and endometrial cancer is decreased.
e. *Effect of bone density:* Studies conclude that degree of bone loss if any is similar to the benign bone loss associated with lactation and it is regained after discontinuation of drug. However, loss of BMD is more relevant for teenagers because bone density increases most rapidly from age 10-30. There is addition of black box warning to clinician that Injectable contraceptive should be used longer than 2 years only if other methods of birth control are inadequate.
f. *Metabolic effect:* There are no clinically significant changes in carbohydrate metabolism or coagulation factors.

Indications and Contraindications

Indications

Depo Provera should be considered for contraception:
a. If at least 1 year of birth spacing is desired.
b. In lactating mothers.
c. If private, coital independent method is desired.
d. Who are not reliable to take daily pill.
e. Whom estrogen is contraindicated.
f. In sickle cell disease, seizure disorder.

Contraindications

Absolute
1. Pregnancy.
2. Unexplained genital bleeding.
3. Coagulation disorders.
4. Previous sex steroid induced liver adenoma.

Relative
1. Liver disease.
2. Severe cardiovascular disease.
3. Rapid return of fertility desired.
4. Difficulty with injections.
5. Severe depression.

Progestin Implants

In these systems a progestin is delivered by a subdermal implant device which contains the drug and coated with a compound to prevent fibrosis. Currently, there are two preparations:
a. **Norplant (Wyeth):** It has 6 capsules each containing 36 mg crystalline levonorgestrel made of silastic. Its contraceptive efficacy persists for 60 months, after that the system should be removed.
b. **Implanon:** It is a single flexible rod 4 cm long that contains 68 mg of etonogestrel and has an ethylene vinyl acetate copolymer cover.

Advantages
a. Implants are safe, highly effective, continuous method of contraception which require little effort and rapidly reversible.
b. It can be used in lactating women and in women where estrogens are contraindicated.

Disadvantages
a. They cause disruption in bleeding patterns especially in first year of use.
b. They have to be inserted and removed by trained personnel.
c. They do not provide any protection against STI's.

Emergency Contraception

Implantation of the fertilized ovum is believed to occur on the 6th day after fertilization. This interval provides an opportunity to prevent pregnancy even after fertilization occurs. **Emergency contraception may act via interfering with corpus luteum function, thickening of cervical mucus and alteration in tubal transport of sperm, egg or embryo. They do not interrupt already established pregnancy.** Prevention of pregnancy can be accomplished using hormonal agents singly or in combination or IUD's. There are following regimens for emergency contraception.
a. *Yuzpe regimen combination method:* 200 mcg of ethinyl estradiol and 1 mg of levonorgestrel in two divided dose 12 hours apart is given (2 ovral tablet followed by 2 more tablet 12 hours later). Risk of pregnancy is reduced by 74%. Nausea and vomiting is common and an antiemetic should be prescribed. Preven is a prepackaged kit containing instruction for emergency contraception, appropriately dosed estrogen and progestin pill and a pregnancy test kit.
b. *Progestin (Levonorgesterol) only methods:* Levonorgestrel alone 0.7 mg initially followed by another 0.75 mg 12 hours later is more effective than combination method and it is the method of choice for emergency contraception. It has fewer side effects. There is evidence that these dose of levonorgestrel have almost as much efficacy at 3-5 days after coitus, hence women who present after 3 days but before 5 days should not be refused treatment.
c. *Copper intrauterine device:* The IUD is a less frequently used method of emergency contraception. It can be inserted up to 7 days after ovulation to prevent

pregnancy. The failure rate is very low (0.1%). This method has the additional advantages of providing long term contraception.

d. *Mifepristone (RU 486):* The antiprogesterone Mifepristone (RU 486) is also highly effective for postcoital contraception without any significant side effects. A dose of 100 mg is effective for emergency contraception. 200 mg Mifepristone is also highly effective in inducing menstruation when taken on day 27th of menstrual cycle, well beyond the 72-120 hours window. It can be considered for postcoital contraception.

Medical eligibility criteria for use of emergency contraception are described in Table Annexure III.

Special Consideration for Contraception

a. *Adolescent:* Concern about confidentiality and lack of money deter teenagers from seeking and obtaining contraception. Combined oral contraceptives are excellent choice for this age group because they provide effective contraception, increase bone density and can be used to improve acne and regulate menstrual cycle. The only disadvantage is daily requirement of pill taking. *Injectable depot* medroxyprogesterone may be considered as it is use and forget method but disadvantage is menstrual irregularity, loss of bone mass and need for 3 monthly injections.

b. *Barrier method:* Provide protection against STD's but still they are not good choice for adolescent as they require preplanning and motivation for proper use. Barrier method should be considered primarily as backup method and protective method for STD.

c. *Contraception for older than 35 years:* Though fertility begins to decline at about 35-40 years, there is still the risk for unwanted pregnancy and STD's. The choice for them are as follows:
   i. *Combined oral contraceptive:* They are highly effective well tolerated and have many health benefits with normal risk. Healthy, nonsmoking women may use low dose COC until the menopause.
   ii. *Injectable depot medroxyprogesterone acetate:* In women who have contraindication for estrogen, this is highly effective hormonal contraception that can be used. Because of the association with bone loss, this method should be used with caution for longer than 2 years in perimenopausal women.
   iii. *Intrauterine device:* It is a good choice for women with completed family and monogamous relationship.
   iv. *Barrier method:* They can be used either as a primary or adjunct contraceptive. Their effectiveness improves with advancing age.

d. *Women with medical illness:* Women with chronic illness may present special problem that should be considered in the choice of method of contraception. *The illness may make pregnancy more complicated and dangerous for these women, thus, making effective contraception all the more important.* The choice of the most effective and safe method of contraception is dependent on the disease and how it is modified in by pregnancy. For many women an important strategy is to prescribe a progestin only method and to avoid estrogen containing hormonal contraception.

e. *Lactating mothers:* Breastfeeding is important to infant health and to child spacing. Lactating in it self is not a reliable method of family planning. Waiting for first menses involves a risk of pregnancy because ovulation usually antedates menstruation. *Progestin only contraception is preferred choice in most case.* COC's can be started after 6 months if infant is on exclusive breastfeeding and after 3 months or as soon as lactation is established. If infant is on partial breastfeeding IUCD can also be recommended.

Missed Pill

It is estimated that only one-third of women were documented to have missed no pills in first month of use and by third month, about one-third of women missed three or more pills with many episodes. To ensure regular pill taking and to avoid missing pills, the pill should be keyed to a daily event like with dinner or at bed time. Missing a pill can impair the contraceptive efficacy and also cause symptoms like irregular spotting or bleeding. The following advice is usually given in cases of missed pills:

a. If pill is missed by the women she should take the pill as early as possible, when she remembers and next pill is taken at routine time. No back up is required.
b. If women misses two pills in the first two weeks she should take two pills on each of the next two days. It is better to have a backup method for seven days.
c. If two pills are missed in the third week or more than two pills are missed any time. Backup method in form of barrier contraception should be used immediately and for next seven days and a new pack of pills should be started.

STERILIZATION

Female Sterilization

Female sterilization is the surgical procedure used to end a women's ability to become pregnant. The procedure involves ligation with or without resection or blocking of both the fallopian tubes so that egg and sperm can not meet. Female sterilization is the most widely used contraceptive method is the world.

Timing of sterilization: It is now agreed that tubal ligation can be done at any time according to suitability of the patient. However, there are certain factors which govern the timing of procedure to some extent.

Cesarean ligation: Postpartum tubal sterilization at time of cesarean delivery adds no risk other than a slight prolongation of operating time. Cesarean birth poses more risk than vaginal birth and planned sterilization should not influence the decision to perform cesarean delivery.

Puerperal ligation: Advantage of tubal ligation done early in puerperium for those who wishes for sterilization are –
a. Sterilization is technically easier because of easy and ready approach to fallopian tube through small incision. Because in postnatal period uterus remains enlarged and opposed to the anterior abdominal wall for several days after delivery.
b. Minimal hospital stay as postoperative and postpartum period coincides.
c. Women and her family are sensitized to need of contraception. However, if there is a chance of postpartum infection it is better to postpone the operation to a later date.

Interval ligation or sterilization: Interval sterilization is done six weeks after delivery or any time in nonpregnant women. Tubal ligation should be done within 7-10 days of onset of menstruation to avoid early clinically undetectable pregnancy.

Postabortal ligation: Following MTP or D & C, tubal ligation can be done at the same time either vaginally or abdominally.

Preoperative Procedure

Clear comprehensive counseling is essential for women who are considering tubal sterilization. The couple should be explained that the procedure should be considered as a permanent method. There can be rare possibility of failure as well complication related to anesthesia and infection and surgical related complications. The other alternative temporary method of contraception should also be discussed.

Surgical Techniques

Technique of female sterilization basically consists of:
a. Ligation and resection of fallopian tube at minilaparotomy.
b. The application of variety of permanent rings or clips to fallopian tubes usually by laparoscopy.
c. Electrocoagulation of a segment of the fallopian tube usually through a laparoscope.

Pomeroy procedure: In classic Pomeroy procedure a loop of tube is excised after ligating the base of the loop with a single absorbable suture (Figs 28.5A to D).

Modified Pomeroy procedure: It is excision of the mid portion of the tube after ligation of segment with two separate absorbable sutures.

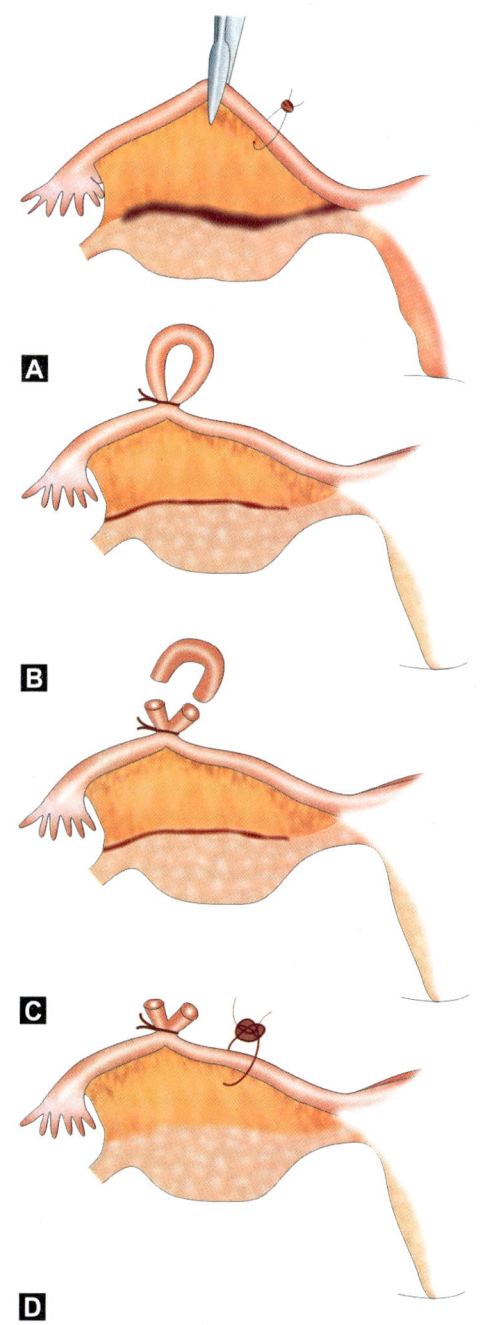

Figs 28.5A to D: Pomeroy method of tubectomy: (A and B) Making of loop; (C) Loop of tube excised and ligated at both ends; (D) Modified Pomeroy method—A silk stitch is applied on medial side

Irving method: In this the tube is cut in between two ligatures and medial stump is burried into a hole made in uterine wall and lateral stump is peritonized (Figs 28.6A to C).

Madlener technique: A loop of tube in the middle third portion is crushed at the base and ligated with non absorbable suture like thread or silk. In practice combination

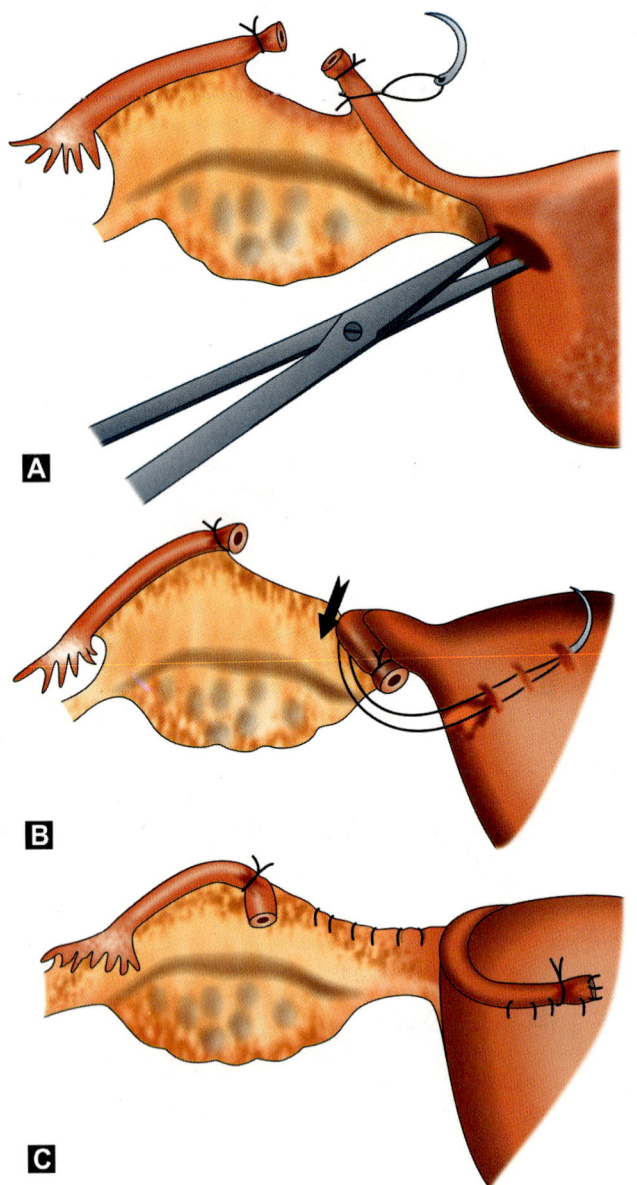

Figs 28.6A to C: Irving method of tubectomy. (A) Tube is cut between two ligature; (B and C) Medial stump is burried in uterine wall

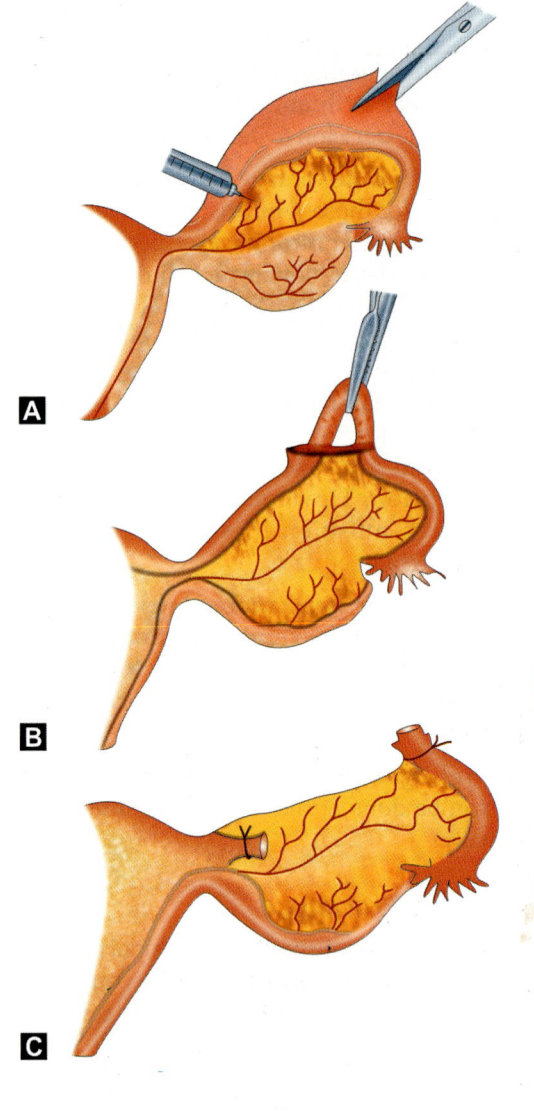

Figs 28.7A to C: Uchida method of tubectomy: (A and B) Tube is pulled out; (C) Two end of tube are ligated and medial stump is burried in mesosalpinx

of Pomeroy and Madlener technique is used when loop of tube is crushed at base in the middle third portion, excised and cut segments are ligated with non absorbable suture.

Uchida technique: In this saline with epinephrine is injected into mesosalpinx which is then cut open. The muscular tube is pulled out. After removing a portion of tube the ends are ligated and medial stump is burried in the mesosalpinx. In Pomeroy and combined method procedure have failure rate of 1-4 per 1000 case; while pregnancy is almost nil after Irving or Uchida method (Figs 28.7A to C).

Laparoscopic Approach

The laparoscopes are thin metal tube of 5 to 10 mm diameter with inbuilt lens with prism which give direct vision of operating field. They have fibro optic light bundle system to transmit cold light from external source directly in to the abdomen (Fig. 28.8). Nowadays laparoscopic method of sterilization can be done in a short time with rapid recovery. It is now use as a method of choice for camp sterilization.

Sterilization is done by any of the three techniques:
a. Bipolar electrical coagulation.

Chapter - 28 ♦ Contraception

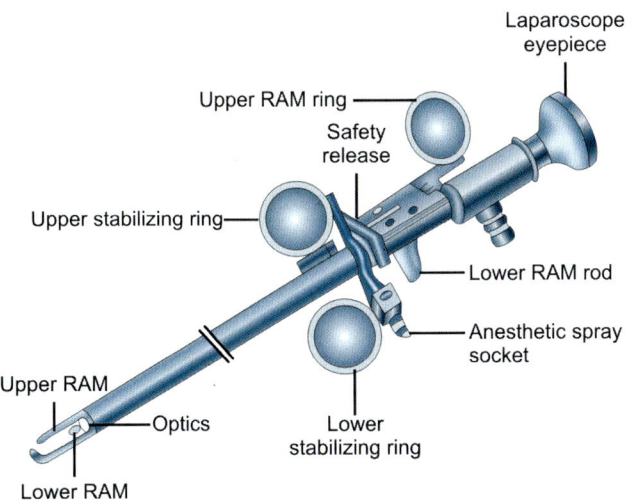

Fig. 28.8: Single puncture operative laparoscope, specially designed for tubectomy

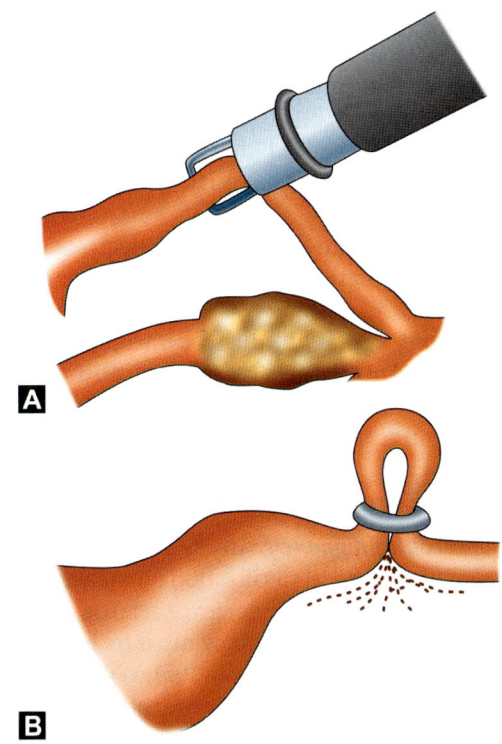

Figs 28.9A and B: Laparoscopic sterilization by silastic bend (Falope ring): (A) Picking of tube by laparoscope; (B) Placement of silastic band on tube

b. Application of a small silastic rubber bend (Falope ring) (Figs 28.9A and B).
c. The plastic and metal Hulka clip or Filschie clip (Fig. 28.10).

Bipolar coagulation can be used with any type of fallopian tube. The fallopian ring and clips can not be applied if the tube is thickened from previous salpingitis. Failure of Falope ring or clips generally results from misapplication and pregnancy if it occurs is usually intrauterine. *After bipolar coagulation pregnancy may result from tuboperitoneal fistula and is ectopic in more than 50% of cases.*

Minilaparotomy: In this a small Suprapubic incision is given 2-4 cm in length. Additional uterine elevator is useful which elevates the uterine fundus and keeps it opposed to the anterior abdominal wall. The fallopian tube is occluded by simple Pomeroy or modified Pomeroy method. **Minilaparotomy is favored approach nowadays because of its safety, simplicity and adaptability to ambulatory or camp approach.** In this no specialized equipment and training is required. However, patient's characteristics as obesity, previous pelvic infection or previous surgery are the principal determinants of complications.

Vaginal approach: Although vaginal techniques are still used for tubal sterilization, high rate of infection and occasional pelvic abscess following vaginal approach have almost abandoned this approach. However, this can be preferred in women who are undergoing pelvic or organ prolapse repair like, Fothergill Manchester operation as an adjacent procedure.

Hysteroscopic approach: Essure is a coil device with polyester fibers. It is placed hysteroscopically within the proximal segments of the fallopian tubes spanning the utero

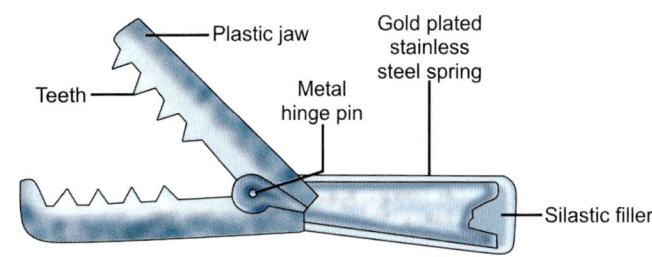

Fig. 28.10: Hulka-Clemens clips

tubal junction. It expands when released, anchoring it self in place. The device stimulates a tissue reaction which is fibrotic and occlusive. After backup contraception for three months hysterosalpingogram is performed to confirm occlusion. The procedure is quick, performed in the outpatient settings often without analgesia. Effective permanent sterilization is achieved in about 85-90% of women.

Risk of Tubal Sterilization

Tubal sterilization is remarkably safe.
1. *Failure rate:* Laparoscopic and minilaparotomy sterilization are not only convenient but almost as

effective as older laparotomy technique. From the CREST study 1.3% of 10,685 tubal sterilization were followed by subsequent pregnancy. The cause of failure can be:
a. Surgical error in 30-50% of cases.
b. An occlusion method failure may be due to fistula formation especially with electrocoagulation procedures.
c. Equipment failure as defective electric current for electrocoagulation.
d. In some cases woman was already pregnant at time of surgery. To avoid this contraception should be continued until day of surgery and a sensitive pregnancy test should be routinely performed on the day of surgery.

Long-term Complications

a. *Risk of ectopic pregnancy:* Any symptoms of pregnancy in a woman after tubal sterilization must be investigated with sensitive urinary serum test for βHCG and ultrasound. **Ectopic pregnancy must be excluded.**
b. *Post tubal ligation syndrome:* In 1951, William in 22 years experience noted increased incidence of menorrhagia and intermenstrual bleeding. But recent CREST and other studies have found no evidence of menstrual abnormalities following 2-5 years of tubal ligation.

Tubal ligation reversal: The tubal sterilization reversal procedures are technically difficult, expensive and not very successful. Success rate depends and varies with the women's age, the amount of remaining tube and used technology. Almost 10% of women undergoing tubal sterilization reversal have an ectopic pregnancy. Reversal can be done by laparoscopy in experienced hands or conventional laparotomy approach. Pregnancy rates are similar with either method. However, no women should undergo tubal sterilization believing that subsequent fertility is guaranteed by either surgery or assisted reproductive techniques.

Male Sterilization—Vasectomy

Vasectomy is excision of a portion of the vas deferens. It is safer, easier, less expansive and has a low failure rate than female sterilization. It is readily accomplished with local anesthetic in an office setting. It does not decrease sexual performance.

Technique

The basic technique is to palpate the vas through the scrotum. Vas is grasped with fingers or a traumatic forceps, then small incision is made over the vas and vas is pulled into the incision. A small segment is removed and a needle electrode is used to coagulate or vas is ligated at cut ends. Improved techniques include the *nonscalpel vasectomy* in which the pointed ends of the forceps are used to puncture the skin over the vas. This small variation reduces the chances of bleeding and avoids the need to suture the incision. Another variation is the **open end vasectomy** in which only the abdominal end of the severed vas is coagulated while the testicular end is left open. This is believed to prevent congestive epididymitis (Figs 28.11A to D).

Follow-up

An important caution after vasectomy is that sterility is not immediate complete. Expulsion of sperm stored in the reproductive tract beyond the interrupted vas deferens takes about three months. Semen analysis should be done to confirm azoospermia. Before azoospermia is documented, another form of contraception must be used.

Failure rate: Failure rate is less than 1%. Cause is failure from unprotected intercourse too soon after ligation, failure to occlude the vas defers or recanalization.

Reversal of male vasectomy: It depends on several factors. Overall success rate is 50%. There is a slightly higher rate following microsurgical reanastomosis.

Long-term effects: Apart from regret other consequences are rare. There is no difference in the incidence of myocardial infarction or stroke as well prostatic or testicular cancer following vasectomy.

Short-term complications: Operative complications include scrotal hematoma, wound infection and epididymitis but serious sequele are rare.

MULTIPLE CHOICE QUESTIONS

1. Which of following is correct for the calculation of Pearl Index?
   a. Number of accidental pregnancies × 1200/Number of patients observed × months of use.
   b. Number of accidental pregnancies × 1200/Number of patients observed × 2400.
   c. Number of patients observed × months of use/Number of accidental pregnancies.
   d. Number of patient observed × 2400/Number of accidental pregnancies × 1200.

   Ans. a

2. Pearl's index indicates:
   a. Malnutrition.
   b. Population.
   c. Contraceptive failures.
   d. LBW.

   Ans. c

3. Spermicidal jelly acts through:
   a. Acrosomal enzyme.
   b. Cervical enzyme alternation.
   c. Glucose uptake inhibition by sperms.
   d. Disruption of cell membrane.

   Ans. d

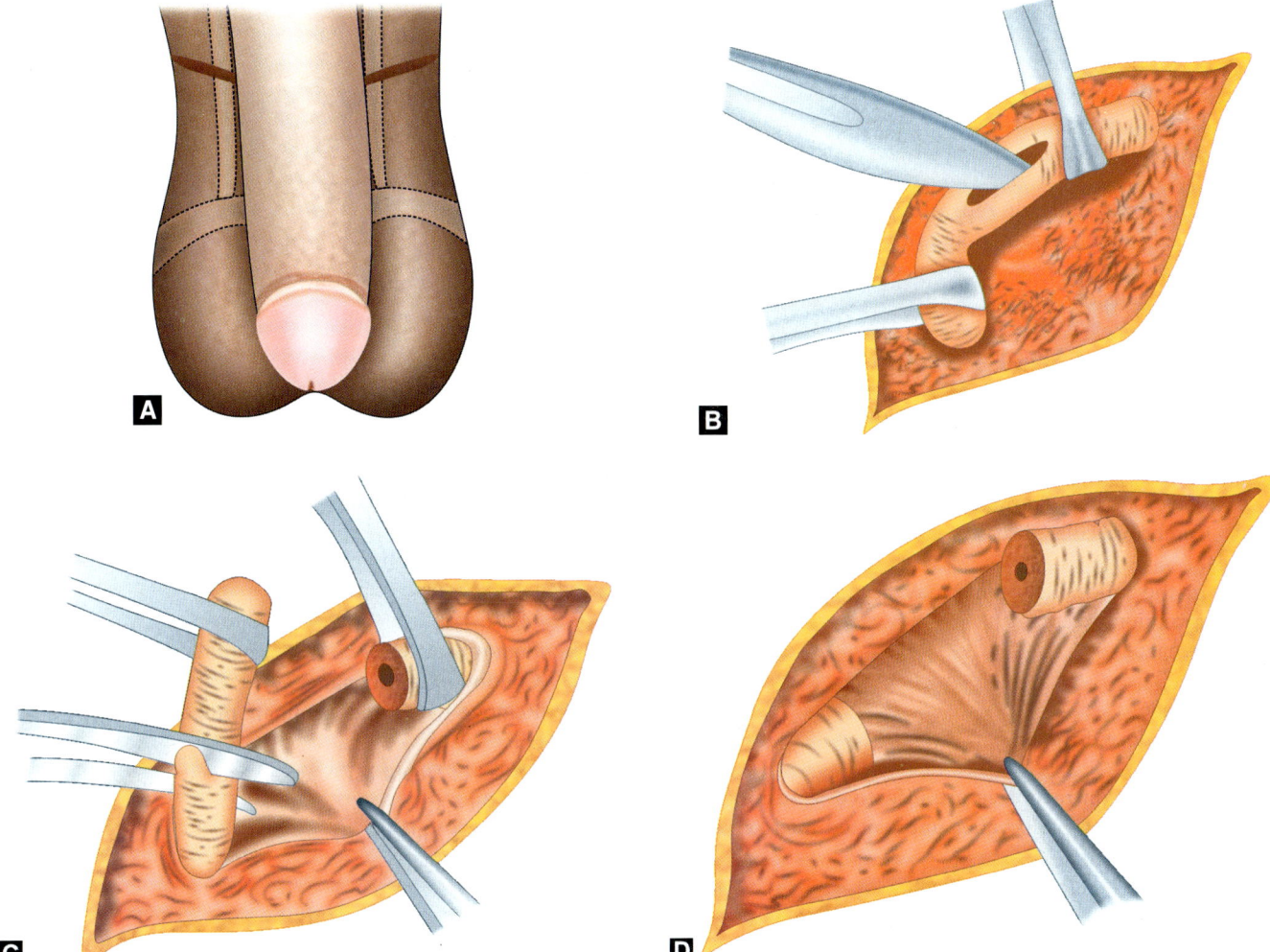

Figs 28.11A to D: Step of vasectomy: (A) Incisions on the skin; (B) The sheath of the vas being cut open; (C) A portion of the vas is being removed; (D) The vas is ligated at cut ends

4. Spermicidal preparations are:
   a. Nonoxynol
   b. Menfegol
   c. Progestasert
   Ans. a, b

5. Among the following which one is the absolute contraindication for combined oral contraceptive pills:
   a. Diabetes mellitus
   b. Migraine
   c. Previous history of thromboembolism
   d. Heart disease
   Ans. c, d

6. Use of oral contraceptive are known to decrease the incidence of all of the following, *except*:
   a. Ectopic pregnancy
   b. Epithelial ovarian malignancy
   c. Hepatic adenoma
   d. Pelvic inflammatory disease
   Ans. c

7. Oral contraceptive pills give protection against following cancers:
   a. Endometrial
   b. Ovary
   c. Cervix
   d. Breast
   Ans. a, b

8. Minimum effective dose of ethinyl estradiol in combined oral pills is:
   a. 20 µg
   b. 35 µg
   c. 50 µg
   d. 75 µg
   Ans. a

9. Oral contraceptive pills efficiency is reduced by simultaneous use of:
   a. Rifampicin
   b. Carbamazepine
   c. Propranolol
   d. Tricyclic antidepressant
   Ans. a

10. Oral contraceptive pills intake causes psychiatric symptoms, and abdominal pain. Diagnosis is:
    a. Acute intermittent porphyria
    b. Systemic lupus
    c. Thrombosis
    d. Anemia
    Ans. a
11. In a young female of reproductive age, an absolute contraindication for prescribing oral contraceptive pills is:
    a. Diabetes
    b. Hypertension
    c. Obesity
    d. Impaired liver function
    Ans. d
12. Oral contraceptive pills are contraindicated in all, *except*:
    a. Smoking 35 years
    b. Coronary occlusion
    c. Polycystic ovarian disease
    d. Cerebrovascular disease
    Ans. c
13. All of the following agents may be used for postcoital contraception except:
    a. Danazol
    b. Cu 7
    c. RU 486
    d. High dose estrogen
    Ans. a
14. Emergency contraceptive are effective if administered within following period after unprotected intercourse:
    a. 24 hours
    b. 48 hours
    c. 72 hours
    d. 120 hours
    Ans. d
15. The progesterone of choice for emergency contraception is:
    a. Norethisterone
    b. Medroxyprogesterone acetate
    c. Levonorgesterol
    d. Desogesterol
    Ans. c
16. Mechanism by which IUCD does not act:
    a. Chronic endometrial inflammation
    b. Increase the motility of tubes
    c. Inducing endometrial atrophy
    d. Inhibition of ovulation
    Ans. d
17. Which of following IUCD have life span for 10 years:
    a. Cu T 380 A
    b. Cu T 200
    c. Nona T
    d. Multi load
    Ans. a
18. Mirena is:
    a. Used in abortion
    b. Antiprogesterone
    c. Progesterone IUCD
    d. Hormonal implant
    Ans. c
19. Composition of NOVA T is:
    a. Copper and silver
    b. Copper only
    c. Copper and aluminum
    d. Copper and selenium
    Ans. a
20. Absolute contraindication of IUCD is:
    a. Endometriosis
    b. Iron deficiency anemia
    c. Dysmenorrhea
    d. Pelvic tuberculosis
    Ans. d
21. A lady with IUCD becomes pregnant with tail of IUCD being seen. Next course of action is:
    a. MTP
    b. Removal of IUCD
    c. Continue the pregnancy
    d. Remove IUCD and terminate pregnancy
    Ans. b
22. Side effect of Depot MPA are all except:
    a. Weight gain
    b. Irregular bleeding
    c. Amenorrhea
    d. Hepatitis
    Ans. d
23. Permanent sterilization is all, *except*:
    a. Electrocoagulation
    b. Vasectomy
    c. Medroxyprogesterone
    d. Tubal ligation
    Ans. c
24. Best prognosis for reversibility is seen in:
    a. Isthimo isthmic type
    b. Isthmic ampullary type
    c. Ampullary interstitial type
    d. Ampullary fimbrial type
    Ans. a
25. Best mode of contraception for a patient with heart disease is:
    a. IUCD
    b. Depo Provera
    c. Barrier method
    d. Oral contraceptive pills
    Ans. c

29. Breast Disease

To be trusted is a greater compliment than to be loved.

INTRODUCTION

The breasts are secondary reproductive glands of ectodermal origin. They are frequently referred to as modified sweat gland. In women breast are the organs of lactation, whereas in men the breast are normally functionless and undeveloped.

Anatomy and Histology

Breast lies on the superior aspect of chest wall. The adult female breast contains glandular and ductal elements. Stroma consists of fibrous tissue that binds the individual lobes together and adipose tissue within and between lobes.

Each breast consists of 12-20 conical lobes. The base of each lobe is close to the ribs and the apex of each lobe is deep to areola and nipple. Each lobe consists of group of lobules. The lobules have several lactiferous ducts which unites to form a major duct that draws the lobe as they goes towards the nipple areolar complex. Each of the major ducts widens to form an ampulla as they travel towards areola and then narrow at its individual opening in the nipple. The lobules are held in place by a meshwork of loose fatty areolar tissue. Approximately 80-85% of the normal breast is adipose tissue. The breast tissues are joined to the overlying skin and subcutaneous tissues by fibrous stroma. In the nonpregnant nonlactating breast, the alveoli are small and tightly packed. During pregnancy the alveoli hypertrophy and their lining cells proliferate in number. During lactation the alveoli cells secretes protein and lipids, which comprise breast milk. The deep surface of the breast lies on the fascia covering the chest muscle. The fascial stroma forms the fascial ligament—coopers ligament which run from breast into the subcutaneous tissues. These bands may be distorted by tumor resulting in pathologic skin dimpling (Fig. 29.1).

Vessels, Lymphatic and Nerves

Blood Vessels

The breast has a rich blood supply from following:
a. Branches from internal thoracic arteries.
b. Small branches from the arterial intercostals arteries.
c. Pectoral branch of the thoracoacromial branch of the axillary artery.
d. External mammary branch of the lateral thoracic artery.
e. External mammary artery.

The medial and lateral arteries tend to arborize in the supra-areolar area, so the arterial supply to the upper half of breast is almost twice that of the lower half (Fig. 29.2).

Veins

Venous returns from the breast closely follows the route of arterial system. Blood return to the superior vena cava via

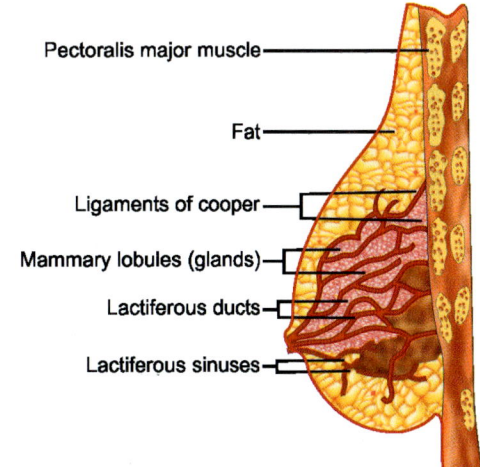

Fig. 29.1: Anatomy of female breast sagittal section of mammary gland

Section -2 ♦ Gynecology

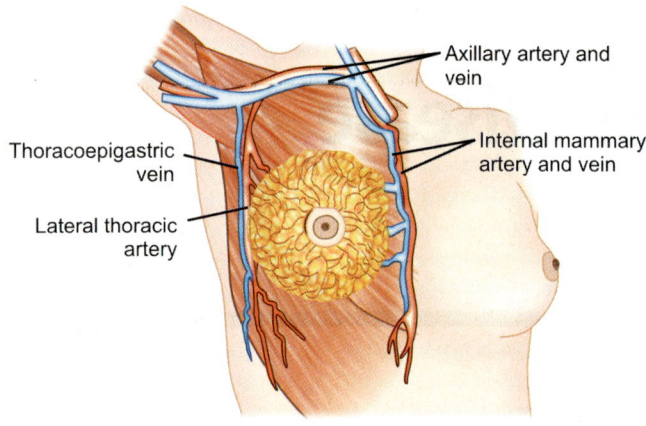

Fig. 29.2: Boold vessels of breast

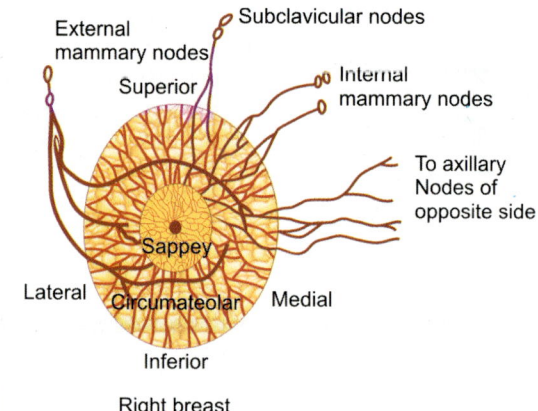

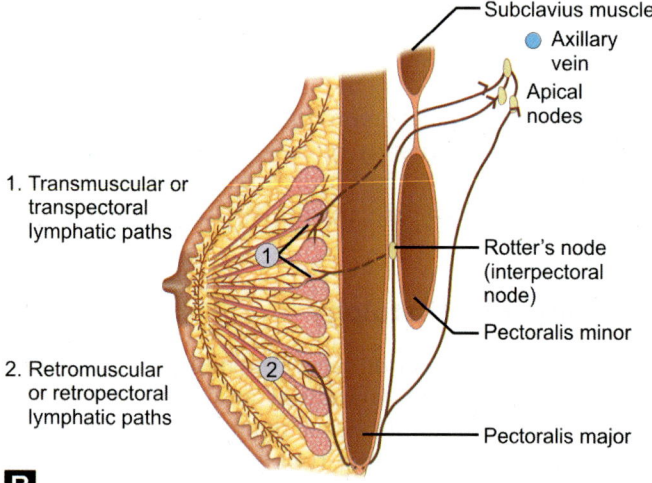

Figs 29.3A and B: Lymphatic drainage of breast: (A) Accessory drainage pathways; (B) Classic axillary drainage pathways

the axillary and internal thoracic veins and through vertebral venous plexuses.

Lymphatics

A thorough knowledge of the lymphatic drainage of the breast is of critical importance to the clinician. It has significant clinical implication in several disease etiologies including breast cancer. Lymphatic drainage can be divided into two main categories:
a. Superficial (including cutaneous) drainage
b. Deep parenchymatous drainage.

Superficial drainage: A large lymphatic plexus exists in the subcutaneous tissues of the breast deep to the nipple areolar complex. This plexus drain the areola and nipple region with cutaneous and subcutaneous tissues close to nipple areolar complex.

Deep parenchymatous drainage: The deep parenchymatous lymph vessels drains the rest of breast and some portion of the skin and subcutaneous tissues of the nipple areolar complex. Small periductal and periacinal lymph vessels collect parenchymal lymph and deliver it to the larger interlobar lymphatics. Once in the deep parenchymatous drainage, the lymph is delivered to the subareolar plexus for efferent transport. The majority of lymphatic drainage from both the retroareolar and deep interlobar lymphatics of the breast travel to the **ipsilateral axillary lymph nodes.** In general the drainage of the breast is to the **anterior axillary or subpectoral nodes**, which are located deep to the lateral borders of the pectoralis major muscle, close to the lateral thoracic artery. From these nodes lymph travel to nodes in close proximity of the axillary vein. The lymph then passes superiorly via the axillary chain of lymph vessels and nodes. Eventually the drainage occurs in the **highest nodes in axilla**. This is the most common pattern of lateral and superior breast lymphatic drainage. Other paths are common particularly when the lateral and superiorly directed channels are obstructed (Figs 29.3A and B).

Nerves Supply

The lateral and anterior cutaneous branches of T4-T6 supply the cutaneous tissues covering the breast.

Benign Breast Condition

Benign breast disorders account for most breast problems. Their lifecycles reflect different reproductive phases in a women's life and associated with unique breast manifestation.

Early Reproductive Period (15-25 Years)

In this age, lobule and stroma formation occurs. The aberration of normal development and involution (ANDI) to disease state results in the formation of fibroadenomas which can be multiple and assume big size.

Mature Reproductive Period (25-40 Years)

Cyclic hormone changes affect glandular tissue and stroma. In this phase ANDI is an exaggeration of these cyclic effects such as cyclic mastalgia and generalized nodularity.

In Age 35-55 Years

There is involution of lobules and ducts or turnover of epithelia. The ANDI associated with lobular involution are macrocyst (lumps) and sclerosing lesion (mammographic abnormalities). Those associated with ductal involution are **duct dilatation (nipple discharge) and periductal fibrosis (nipple retraction) and those with epithelial turnover are mild hyperplasia.**

Fibrocystic Disease of Breast

Fibrocystic change is one of the most common benign lesions of the breast characterized by fibrosis of breast stroma and formation of cysts within the breast.

Symptoms and Signs

Fibrocystic change may produce an asymptomatic mass that is smooth and mobile. Fibrocystic disease is more commonly accompanied by pain or tenderness and sometimes nipple discharge. Pain may coincide with premenstrual phase of the cycle. Fluctuations in size and rapid appearance or disappearance of a breast mass are common. Multiple or bilateral masses appears frequently. Cyclic breast pain is the most common associated symptom of fibrocystic disease.

Clinical Stages

1. Mazoplasia (Mastoplasia)
   a. In early 20's
   b. Breast pain is in upper and outer quadrant
2. Adenosis
   a. In 30's
   b. Pain and tenderness in premenstrual phase, less severe
   c. Multiple small breast nodules from 2 to 10 mm in diameter
3. Cystic
   a. In 40's
   b. Sudden pain with pin point tenderness and discovery of lump
   c. Fluid aspirated is colored dark brown or green

Differential Diagnosis

Pain, fluctuation in size, multiplicity of lesion and bilaterality are most distinguishing feature from carcinoma. If a dominant mass is present, always the diagnosis of cancer should be suspected until it is disproved by cytologic aspiration of cyst or histopathological analysis.

Histological Finding

There are gross and microscopic cyst, papillomatosis, adenosis, fibrosis and ductal epithelial hyperplasia.

Diagnostic Test

a. **Ultrasonography:** Characteristic ultrasound finding are: (i) Mass with thin walls, (ii) Smooth round shape, (iii) Absence of internal echoes, (iv) Posterior acoustic enhancement (Fig. 29.4).
b. **Mammography:** It may be helpful but there are no mammographic signs diagnostic of fibrocystic change.
c. **Biopsy:** Any lesion that is suspicious by mammography or ultrasonography should be biopsied. In following situation the biopsy should be done:
   i. No cyst fluid is obtained
   ii. Fluid is bloody
   iii. Fluid is thick
   iv. Cyst is complex
   v. Intracystic mass
   vi. A mass persist after aspiration
   vii. A persistent mass noted during follow-up

Surgery should be conservative. Women with fibrocystic disease are not at increased risk for breast cancer.

Management

It is normal evolutionary change in breast development and involution and does not require a specific treatment other than a good clinical examination and age appropriate mammography screening.

Following treatment option can be effective:
1. Support
2. Diet reduction in intake of tea, coffee, cold drink, chocolate
3. OC's or supplement progestin—40% of women's symptoms are relived
4. Danazol—drug of choice. In dose of 100-200 mg daily for 4-6 months. It relieves symptom in 90% of patient. Danazol is not given more than 6 months because of side effect.
5. Second option drugs:
   a. Bromocriptine 5 mg daily
   b. Tamoxifen
   c. Alpha linoleic acid with evening primrose oil

Regular self-examination should be advised every month after menstruation and inform the physician if a mass appears.

Mastalgia

Mastalgia is a distressing constellation of symptoms that is classified as cyclic, noncyclic or extramammary. Cyclic mastalgia is related to exaggerated premenstrual symptoms. Noncyclic mastalgia is independent of menstrual cycle. Extramammary pain is perceived to be located in the breast sites but is related to extramammary sites. *Chest wall muscular pain, costal cartilage symptoms, herpes zoster radiculopathies are some of the common cause of extramammary pain. Costochondritis (Tietze's syndrome) is a manifestation of chest wall pain that is frequently interpreted as breast pain.*

Management

Oral contraceptive or HRT can cause mastalgia. If mastalgia is disturbing, withdrawal of hormone can be considered. Various treatments have been used which include analgesic, low dose diuretic, danazol, reduction in caffeine intake. **Women with mastalgia are not at increased risk of breast cancer.**

Fibroadenoma

They are the most common benign tumors of the breast. They are not associated with an increased risk of breast cancer. It most frequently occurs in young women usually with few years after puberty. Multiple tumors in one or both breast are found in 10-15% of patients.

Clinical Presentation

The typical fibroadenoma is round, firm, discrete, relatively mobile, nontender mass, 1-5 cm in diameter. In women older age than 30 years fibrocystic disease and carcinoma of breast should be considered while in young age the diagnosis is not difficult. Cyst can be identified by ultrasound examination and aspiration.

Treatment

a. Careful clinical observation—close follow-up of 2 years can be done in compliant patient as fibroadenoma may involute during surveillance.
b. Excision—large or growing fibroadenoma must be excised.

Cystosarcoma Phyllodes

It is type of fibroadenoma with cellular stroma that tends to grow rapidly. This tumor may reach a large size and if inadequately excised will recur locally. The lesion can be rarely malignant.

Treatment

Local excision of the mass with a margin of surrounding normal breast tissue is done. In malignant cystic sarcoma phyllodes complete removal of tumor with a rim of normal tissue should prevent recurrence. As these tumors tend to be large, simple mastectomy is often necessary to achieve complete control.

Breast Condition Requiring Evaluation

Nipple Discharge

Nipple discharge is a presenting breast symptom in 4.5% of patient seeking evaluation of breast symptoms—in 48% it is spontaneous and in 52% it is provoked. The following characteristic of the discharge should be evaluated by history and physical examination:

a. Nature of discharge—serum, bloody or other
b. Association with or without mass
c. Unilateral or bilateral
d. Single duct or multiple duct discharge
e. Discharge that is spontaneous, persistent or intermittent or must be expressed.
f. Relation to menstruation
g. Premenopausal or postmenopausal
h. Hormonal medication

Diagnosis and Management

Purulent Discharge

Purulent discharge can originate in a subareolar abscess and may require excision of the abscess and related lactiferous sinus.

Chronic unilateral nipple discharge: Unilateral spontaneous serous, bloody or serosanguinous discharge from a single duct is usually caused by intraductal papilloma uncommonly by an intraductal malignancy. **Usually a palpable mass is not present.** The involved duct may be identified by pressures at different sites around the nipple at the margin of the areola. Blood discharge is usually caused by benign papilloma in the duct, but can be suggestive of malignancy.

Bloody discharge is an indication for resection of the involved ducts. Mammography and USG are performed to rule out an associated mass. On occasions ductography may be preformed to identify filling defect system but ductography is not a substitute of excision.

When localization is not possible and no mass is palpable the patient should be re-examined every week for one month. *If unilateral discharge persists even without definite localization or palpable mass, exploration must be considered.* The alternative approach can be careful follow-up at interval of 1-3 months with accompanying mammography.

Treatment

a. The involved duct and if mass if present should be excised. Cytology of discharge may identify malignant cells but negative findings do not rule out cancer which is more likely if woman is older than 50 years.
b. In premenopausal women spontaneous multiple duct discharge, unilateral or bilateral is most marked just before menstruation. It usually is caused by fibrocystic change. The discharge may be green or brownish. Biopsy may be necessary to establish the diagnosis. Usually papillomatosis and ductal ectasia are seen or biopsy.

Milky Discharge (Galactorrhea)

Galactorrhea from multiple ducts in the nonlactating breast reflects increased secretion of pituitary prolactin. An endocrine work-up is usually indicated. Causes of galactorrhea are summarized in Table 29.1.

Table 29.1: Causes of galactorrhea	
Drug Induced	Idiopathic
	Phenothiazine, Reserpine, Methyldopa, Imipramine, oral contraceptive agent, metoclopramide sulpiride
Central nervous system lesion (CNS lesion)	Pituitary tumors, empty sella, hypothalamic tumors, head trauma
Medical condition	Hypothyroidism, chronic renal failure, Cushing's disease, hepatic cirrhosis
Chest wall lesion	Thoracotomy, herpes zoster

Treatment

Treatment is directed to cause like discontinuation of drug treatment of hypothyroidism. If increased prolactin level-bromocriptine is given.

Fat Necrosis of Breast

It is rare but clinically important because it produces a mass often associated with skin or nipple retraction which is indistinguishable from carcinoma. It often presents as confusing clinical finding. Diagnostic imaging studies are insufficient. **As a rule safest course is needle core or excisional biopsy of the entire mass to rule out carcinoma.** Though in untreated case mass associated with fat necrosis usually disappears.

Breast Abscess

Lactational Mastitis

Infection in the breast is usually with lactation period. Lactation mastitis is caused by transmission of bacteria during nursing and hygiene. Common organism is *Staphylococcus aureus*. In mastitis manual pressure, antibiotic, analgesic and continued breastfeeding is recommended. Antibiotic preferred is Oxacillin 500 mg 4 times a day, or Dicloxacillin 250 mg 4 times a day.

Lactational Abscess

If lesion progresses to form a palpable mass with local and systemic signs of infection, the abscess is diagnosed and needs to be drained.

Nonlactational Abscess

It is uncommon, but may develop in young or middle aged women. The current approach to nonlactational abscess is conservative. A suspected abscess should be evaluated with preliminary sonography to detect presence of mass, frank, solitary cavity or multiloculated abscess. Aspiration of pus is done, if present antibiotic therapy is started and reaspiration is done. A single aspiration is sufficient in 50% of cases. Recurrent abscess formation is low (10%). If these infections recur after multiple aspirations, incision and drainage followed by excision of the involved lactiferous ducts or ducts at the base of the nipple may be necessary during a quiescent interval. Usually the cause of reinfection is maxillary sinus (Lactiferous duct fistula). Inflammatory carcinoma is considered if erythema of breast is present. *Patient should not undergo prolonged treatment for an apparent infection unless biopsy has eliminated the possibility of inflammatory carcinoma.*

Subareolar Abscess

Subareolar abscess and fistula of lactiferous ducts secondary to squamous metaplasia can occur. **The definitive treatment for lactiferous duct sinus is excision of the lactiferous duct and drainage of the abscess cavity.**

Malformation of the Breast

Many women are concerned about abnormality of either the size or asymmetry of their breast. Difference in size between two breasts is common. If there is extreme difference, it may be corrected by cosmetic surgery.

Macromastia

Overtly long breast are usually not caused by any endocrine or pathologic abnormalities and these patients can be considered for cosmetic surgery. Less common malformation are amastia, complete absence of one or both breast or presence of accessory nipples and breast tissue along the embryologic milk line.

Evaluation of Breast Mass

Breast Examination

In general breast examination should be methodical and consistent. As breast tumors, particularly cancerous ones are asymptomatic and are discovered only by physical examination or screening mammography. Most of cases of breast cancer present with a palpable breast mass.

Examine the patient in seated and supine position. Ask the patient to flex the pectoralis muscle and open the axilla, which can be done by asking the patient to place the ipsilateral hand behind the head. If mass is discovered—size, contour, consistency and mobility of mass are noted, with attachment to skin or overlying fascia. Careful examination of the axillary and supraclavicular nodes should be the part of examination. Any nipple discharge or rash should be noted. A simple diagram of the breast with finding drawn facilitates subsequent examination.

Self-examination of breast: It increases breast health awareness and promotes early detection of cancer and may improve the survival rates for patient with breast carcinoma.

The following points represent essential component of breast examination:
a. Position
b. Palpation

c. Pads of fingers for palpation
d. Pressure
e. Perimeter
f. Pattern of search
g. Patient education

The women should examine the breast at 7-10 days after menstrual cycle and in postmenopausal women selection of a specific calendar date is helpful way to remember to perform a monthly breast examination. Breast examination should be done in following position:

a. While standing or sitting for minor inspection looking for any asymmetry, skin dimpling or nipple retraction.
b. Elevating her arm over the head or pressing her hands against hips to contract pectoralis and again inspect and palpate.
c. In bending over position.
d. In lying down position. Palpation should be done systemetically for each quadrant with three pressures—light, moderate and deep, covering from clavicle to inframammary fold, and from sternum to latissimus dorsi laterally.

Breast Imaging Mammography

The best method for imaging of the breast is screen film mammography. Slow growing breast cancer can be identified by mammography at least 2 years before the mass reaches a size detectable by palpation. The indications of mammography are:

a. To screen at regular interval of women who are at high risk of developing breast cancer.
b. To evaluate a questionable or ill defined breast mass or other suspicious change in the breast that is detected by clinical breast examination.
c. To establish a baseline breast mammography for follow-up.
d. To reach for occult breast cancer in a patient with metastatic disease in axillary nodes.
e. To screen for unsuspected cancer before cosmetic surgery or biopsy.
f. To monitor breast cancer patients who have been treated with breast conserving surgery and radiation.

Mammographic Abnormalities

They include:
a. Mass (Solid vs cystic).
b. Microcalcification.
c. Asymmetric density.
d. Architectural distortion.
e. Absence of new density.

There are eight morphologic categories of mammographic abnormalities:

a. Calcification distribution.
b. Number of calcification.
c. Description of calcification.
d. Mass margin.
e. Shape of mass.
f. Density of mass.
g. Associated finding.
h. Special cases.

Mammographic abnormalities should be visible on two veiws usually craniocaudal. Mammographic features suggestive of malignancy are:

 i. Irregular or ill defined border.
 ii. Architectural distortion.
 iii. Asymmetric density.
 iv. Skin thickening retraction.
 v. Nipple retraction.

Correlation of Mammographic Findings

Biopsy must be performed on patients with dominant or suspicious mass despite absence of mammographic finding. **Mammography is never a substitute for biopsy as it may not reveal clinical cancer.** Sensitivity of mammography is 75% with specificity of 92.3% depending on patient age, breast density, use of hormone therapy. Mammography is less sensitive in young women with dense breast tumor than in older women who tend to have fatty breast like with small tumors. Particularly those without calcification are more difficult to defect, especially a women with dense breast.

Ultrasonography

It is generally used for focused scanning of questionable finding or for evaluation of a mammography finding. Indications of breast ultrasound examination:
a. Palpable abnormalities.
b. Ambiguous mammography finding.

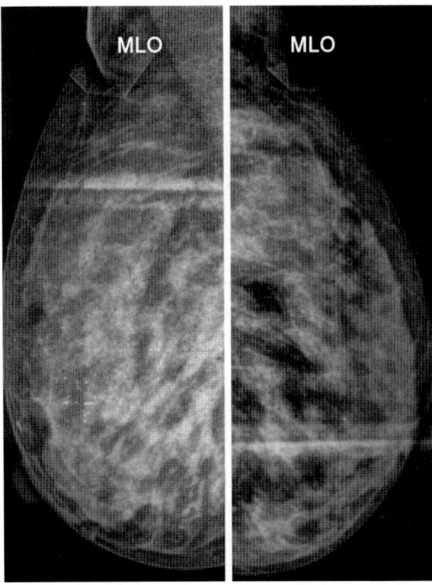

Fig. 29.4: Mammography showing fibroadenosis

c. Mass in women younger than 30 years, lactating or pregnant.
d. Guidance for interventional procedure.
e. Possible role for additional imaging in high-risk individual.

Sensitivity and specificity: Real time ultrasound is 95 to 100% accurate in differentiating solid mass from cysts. However, the finding is of limited clinical value because a dominant mass should be evaluated by biopsy and a cystic mass can be studied by needle aspiration, which is far less expensive than ultrasound.

Magnetic Resonance Imaging

MRI can be used in following specific indication:
a. Stage tumor to rule out multicentric disease.
b. Differentiate postoperative scar from recurrence after breast conserving surgery.
c. Find a lesion seen only in one view of mammography.
d. Evaluate positive axillary nodes in the presence of negative mammography and clinical breast examination results.
e. Rule out silicone implant.
f. Assess focal asymmetry.
g. The future consideration can be: (i) Assessment of BrCa 1 and 2 mutation carrier, (ii) Women with personal history of breast cancer.

Positive Emission Tomography Scanning

It is a diagnostic modality that assesses the metabolic activity of tumor. This technique has been used to identify occult breast lesion with positive axillary lymph nodes.

Fine Needle Aspiration Cytology (FNAC)

In this cell from breast tumors are aspirated with a small, usually 22-gauge needle and examined by pathologist. It is easy, inexpensive with no morbidity and noninvasive. It is rapid to perform and report.

The Triple Test

The triple test results are more powerful than each modality alone. Concordance between fine needle aspiration cytology, physical examination and mammography is foundation of breast evaluation.

Core Needle Biopsy

In this a core of tissue is obtained from palpable lesion using a large cutting needle. It is a reliable diagnostic alternative to surgical excision of suspicious nonpalpable breast lesion.

Open Excisional Biopsy

Open biopsy with local anesthetic as a separate procedure before deciding definitive treatment is the most reliable means of diagnosis. It is required when the result of needle biopsy are non diagnostic or equivocal.

Histologic Analysis

Histological evaluation with hemotoxylin and eosin staining confirms benign or malignant disease.

Ductal Lavage Cytology

Using a microcatheter is new modality used in high-risk women. *The cytologic assessment of a sample obtained by ductal lavage is more sensitive than nipple aspiration.*

BREAST CANCER

General Consideration

Breast cancer accounts for approximately one-third of all cancer in women and is second only to lung cancer as the leading cause of cancer death among women. *Predisposing factors* are age, family history of breast cancer, history of breast cancer in the opposite breast, hormone replacement therapy (HRT) for longer than 10 years, early menarche and/or late menopause, nulliparity and a history of colon or uterine cancer. The Gail model is a computer model that analyze a women's various risk factors to give her an "accurate" individualized risk assessment. There has been a slight increase in the risk of breast cancer with use of HRT. Duration of HRT therapy appears to correlate with risk, so women should be assessed for baseline risk of breast cancer before start of HRT. Women with history of breast cancer have a 50% risk of developing microscopic cancer and 20-25% risk of developing clinically apparent cancer in the contralateral breast which occur at a rate of 1-2%.

Diagnosis

Symptoms

The presenting complaint in approximately 70% of patients with breast cancer is a lump (usually painless) in the breast. Approximately 90% of breast masses are discovered by the patient herself. Less frequent symptoms are—breast pain, nipple discharge, erosion, retraction, enlargement or itching of the nipple, and redness, generalized hardness. Rarely an axillary mass, swelling of the arm, or bone pain from metastasis may be the first symptoms. Approximately 35-50% of women involved in organized screening program have cancer detected by mammography alone.

Signs

Breast cancer most commonly arises in the upper outer quadrant. The standard screening modalities of mammography and physical examination are complementary. *Approximately 10-50% of cancers detected mammographically are not palpable whereas physical examination detects 10 to 20% of cancers not seen radiologically.*

Palpable breast cancer lump usually consist of a nontender, firm or hard lump with poorly delineated margins generally caused by local inflammation. Slight skin or nipple retraction is an important sign as it affects staging. Minimal asymmetry of the breast may be noted. Very small (1-2 mm) erosion of the nipple epithelium may be the only manifestation of the Paget's carcinoma. Watery, serous or bloody discharge from the nipple is an occasional early sign, but is more often associated with benign disease.

The signs of advanced carcinoma are edema, redness, nodularity or ulceration of skin, the presence of large primary tumor (> 5 cm), fixation to the chest wall, enlargement, shrinkage or retraction of the breast, marked axillary lymphadenopathy, distant metastasis, and supraclavicular lymphadenopathy.

Special Clinical form of Breast Carcinoma

a. **Paget's disease:** It refers to eczematous changes around the nipple and is associated with cancer in 99% of cases. An underlying mass is palpable in 60% of patients with Paget's disease. It accounts for approximately 1% of all breast cancer. It is important because it appears innocuous and frequently diagnosed and treated as dermatitis or bacterial infection, leading to unfortunate delay in diagnosis. **Treatment**—total mastectomy and lymph node dissection.

b. **Inflammatory carcinoma:** These patients initially appear to have acute inflammation of the breast with corresponding redness and edema. There can be variable presentation from complete absence of a dominant mass to the presence of either satellite skin nodules or large palpable abnormality. If there is more than one-third of the breast involved with erythema and edema, it should be suspected. Biopsy of involved area including the skin shows metastatic cancer in the subdermal lymphatics. **Treatment** is combination of chemotherapy and radiation therapy. Surgery is not part of initial management. Mastectomy may be indicated for patients who remain free of distant metastatic disease after chemotherapy and radiation.

c. **Breast cancer in pregnancy** (details in obstetric section).

Early Detection and Screening Program

a. **Mammography:** Mammography remains the single test screening procedure for the early detection of breast cancer. Approximately 40% of early malignancies can be detected only by mammography. Another 40% can be detected by palpation. Sensitivity of mammography is 70-90% and specificity is greater than 90%.

b. **Self-examination:** Described.

c. **Genetic testing:** A positive family history of breast cancer is recognized as a risk factor for the subsequent development of breast cancer. With the discovery of two major breast cancer predisposition genes – BrCa (17q21) and BRCA2 (13q1213), there has been increasing interest in genetic testing. Mutations in these two genes are associated with an elevated risk for breast cancer as well as ovarian; colon, prostates and pancreatic cancer. Of all women with breast cancer, approximately 5-10% may have mutation in BRCA1 or BRCA2. **The estimated risk of a patient developing cancer with a BRCA1 and BRCA2 mutation is believed to be between 40% and 85%.** Genetic testing is available and may be considered for member of high risk family.

Diagnostic Evaluation

1. *Mammography:* It is the most reliable means of detecting breast cancer before a mass can be palpated in the breast. Indication and finding are summarized before.
2. *Biopsy technique:* Cytology:
   a. Fine needle biopsy
   b. Open biopsy
   c. Image guided localization biopsy.
3. *Laboratory finding:* A complete blood cell count, liver function test and βhCG in premenopausal patients to diagnose pregnancy should be obtained as part of initial evaluation.
4. *Radiographic findings:*
   a. *Plain X-ray*: PA and lateral chest X-ray may show pulmonary disease involvement and provides radiographic evaluation of the cardiac silhouette.
   b. **CAT scan of brain and liver** is only required for locally advanced disease.
   c. **MRI** is usually not used. In T_0N_1 patient may be helpful in better characterizing the soft tissues of the tumor.
   d. **Radionuclear scanning**: There is no role for this imaging in screening or in routine work-up of the patient. In evaluation of metastatic breast cancer, bone scans using technetium 99 m labeled phosphonates are important tools.

Pathology and Staging

Staging

a. *Clinical staging:* It is based on TNM tumor, node and metastasis system of the international union against cancer. This classification considers tumor size, clinical assessment of axillary nodes and presence or absence of distant metastasis. The breast cancer surgical staging is summarized in Table 29.2.

b. *Histological staging:* It is determined following surgery and along with clinical staging helps in determining prognosis.

Chapter - 29 ♦ Breast Disease

Table 29.2: Breast cancer surgical staging

T Stage		Stage grouping
Tis	In situ	0
T1	≤2 cm	I
T2	>2 cm but ≤ 5 cm	IIA
T3	>5 cm	
T4	Involvement of skin or chest wall or inflammatory cancer	IIB
N Stage		
N0	No lymph node involvement	IIIA
N1	1-3 nodes	
N2	4-9 nodes	
N3	≥10 nodes or any infraclavicular nodes	IIIB
M Stage		
M0	No distant metastases	IIIC
M1	Distant metastases	IV

Table 29.3: Histologic types of breast cancer

Type	Percentage occurrence
Invasive duct (not specified)	8-85%
Medullary	3-6
Colloid (mucinous)	3-6
Tubular	3-6
Papillary	3-6
Invasive lobular	4-10
Noninvasive	15-20
Intraductal	80
Lobular *in situ*	20

Pathologic Types

Numerous pathologic subtypes of breast cancer can be identified histologically. The main types are summarized in Table 29.3. In general breast cancer either arises from the epithelial lining of the large or intermediate sized ducts (**ductal**) or from the epithelium of the terminal ducts of the lobules (**lobular**). The cancer can be invasive or *in situ*. Most breast cancers arise from the intermediate ducts and are **invasive (invasive ductal or infiltrating ducts)** and most histologic types are merely subtypes of invasive ductal cancer with unusual growth patterns (colloid, medullary, scirrhous, etc.). The histologic subtypes have only slight bearing on prognosis, when outcome are compared after accurate staging.

Hormone Receptor Sites

It is advisable to obtain an estrogen receptor assay for every breast cancer at the time of initial diagnosis. The presence or absence of estrogen receptor in the cytoplasm of the tumor cells is of critical importance in managing patients with initial, recurrent and metastatic disease. If tumors have estrogen receptor, up to 60% of patients with metastatic breast cancer will respond to hormonal stimulation. Likewise if tumors have progesterone receptor, 80% of tumors will respond to hormonal manipulation. Receptors probably have no response to chemotherapy.

Treatment

a. *Surgical treatment:* Traditionally the treatment of breast cancer has been surgical, but the type of procedure has remained controversial and highly emotional issue.
   i. *Radical mastectomy:* In this entire breast, the underlying pectoralis muscles and contiguous axillary lymph node in continuity is removed.
   ii. *Extended radical mastectomy:* In this en block internal mammary lymph node are removed, but this did not enhance overall survival rate.
   iii. *Modified radial mastectomy:* In this pectoralis major muscle is preserved. The breast is removed like radical mastectomy but axillary lymph node dissection and skin excision is not extensive. Nowadays modified radical mastectomy has replaced radial mastectomy.
   iv. *Total mastectomy:* In this entire breast, nipple and areolar complex is removed without resection of the underlying muscle or intentional excision of axillary lymph nodes. Low lying lymph node in upper outer portion of breast and low axilla are often excised. It has a local control rate comparable to radical or modified radical mastectomy but has a higher risk of axillary recurrence.
b. *Breast conservation therapy (BCT) with or without radiation therapy:* It involves a surgical procedure as lumpectomy—an excision of tumor mass with a negative surgical margin, an axillary evaluation and postoperative irradiation. Segmental mastectomy, partial mastectomy and quadranectomy are also used in conjunction with radiation and are part of surgical component of BCT. BCT has gained increasing acceptance as a treatment option of stages I and II breast cancer.

Adjuvant Therapy

a. *Postmastectomy radiation therapy:* Recent recommendation of radiation therapy is for women with T3 (>5 cm) primary tumors and 4 or more positive axillary lymph nodes. Postmastectomy radiation therapy has shown to reduce risk of local regional failure by 20% and absolute survival benefit of 10% at 10 years in stages II to III breast cancer.
b. *Chemotherapy:* The goal of adjuvant chemotherapy is to eliminate occult microscopic metastasis that is often responsible for late recurrence. It is a systemic treatment and should not be confused with effort to address local disease. *The current National Institute of Health (NIH) recommends the addition of chemotherapy in women with localized breast cancer >1 cm regardless of nodal, menopausal*

or *hormonal static*. Polychemotherapy (≥ 2 agents) is superior to single agent chemotherapy. 4-6 cycles' often give optimal benefit without subjecting the patient to undue toxicity associated with more prolonged treatment. Cytotoxic chemotherapy with an: (i) Anthracycline based (Doxorubicin A) or (Epirubicin E) regimen is favored, (ii) Traditional regimen of 6 cycle of CMF—Cyclophosphamide, methotrexate and 5 fluorouracil which do not cause alopecia are as good as 4 cycle of AC—Doxorubicin and cyclophosphamide regimen.

The choice of adjuvant chemotherapy is complex. The medical oncologist must consider multiple tumor and patient feature and individualize treatment for breast cancer patients.

c. *Hormone therapy:* There is firmly established role for adjuvant hormonal therapy. The drugs used are tamoxifen and aromatase inhibitor which are used alone or in combination with a cytotoxic regimen.

Tamoxifen: It is an estrogen analog, given a dose of 20 mg/day for 5 years. It reduces the annual risk of recurrence by 50% and annual risk of death by 25% in women with estrogen receptor positive disease regardless of chemotherapy treatment.

Aromatase inhibitor: Anastrozole have been approved for use in the adjuvant treatment of patient with estrogen receptor positive cancers. They act by inhibiting the aromatase enzymes, thus blocking the conversion of androgens into estrogens. These drugs should be used only in postmenopausal patients or premenopausal women who have undergone chemical ovarian suppression or oophorectomy. Compared to tamoxifen the use of AI confers a smaller risk of endometrial cancer, venous thromboembolism events and hot flushes for patients. But AIS have higher risk of musculoskeletal disorder and fracture when compared to tamoxifen.

Follow-up care: After primary treatment, breast cancer patient should be followed for life because of the long insidious natural history of breast cancer. The recommendation are—patient should undergo a physical evaluation every 4 months for the first 2 years, then every 6 months until 5 years and annually for life. **Routine laboratory test** including CBC, chemistry profile and liver function test can be done yearly especially if patient has received chemotherapy.

Prognosis

a. The stage of breast cancer is the single most reliable indicator of prognosis. Patient with disease localized to the breast and no evidence of regional spread after microscopic examination of the lymph nodes have by far the most favorable prognosis.
b. Estrogen and progesterone receptor is an important prognostic variable.
c. Clinical cure rate with most accepted method when cancer is localized to breast with no evidence of regional spread is 75-80%. Patient with small estrogen and progesterone receptor positive tumors and no evidence of axillary spread have 5 years survival rate of nearly 90%.
d. When axillary lymph nodes are involved, the survival rate drops to 50-60% at 5 years and probably to less than 25% at 10 years.
e. In general breast cancer appears to be somewhat more aggressive in younger than in older women which may be related to the fact that relatively few younger women have estrogen receptor positive tumors.

Recurrent and Metastatic Breast Cancer

In these situations following palliative therapy can be given:
a. *Radiotherapy:* It is of use when:
   i. Locally advanced cancer with distant metastasis in order to control ulceration, pain in breast and regional nodes.
   ii. In treatment of certain bone or soft tissue metastasis to control pain or avoid pathologic fracture.
b. *Hormonal therapy:* Tamoxifen is recommended as treatment of choice for hormonal therapy in premenopausal women with advanced breast cancer. In postmenopausal women aromatase inhibitors (AIs) and Tamoxifen are the initial therapy of choice for metastatic breast cancer amenable to endocrine manipulation. Other agent can be gonadotropin releasing hormone agonist as alternative to oophorectomy. Progestin, megestrol acetate and medroxyprogesterone acetate are alternative agents reserved mainly for cases resistant to Tamoxifen. Ovarian ablation by bilateral surgical oophorectomy has been done in past.
c. *Chemotherapy:* Cytotoxic drug is indicated:
   i. If visceral metastasis is present.
   ii. If hormonal treatment is unsuccessful.
   iii. If tumor is estrogen and progesterone receptor negative.
d. *Bisphosphonates therapy:* If bone metastasis is confirmed by plan X-ray, MRI and/or CT scan. The bisphosphonate therapy should be started. It along with other palliative systemic treatment has been shown to reduce bony as well visceral metastasis. It is given intravenously every 3-4 weeks for 2 years or for the duration of other systemic treatment.

Section Three

Obstetrics

30. Preconceptional Counseling, Physiological Changes in Pregnancy and Antenatal Care

A child's mind is like a bank. What you put in, you get back in the years with interest.

PRECONCEPTION COUNSELING

Preconceptional counseling is preventive medicine for obstetrics. Factors that could potentially affect perinatal outcome are identified and women are advised of her risks. If and when possible, a strategy is provided to reduce or eliminate the pathological influences which are detected by her family, medical or obstetrical history or specific testing.

Role of Preconceptional Counseling

a. *Decrease birth defect:* Intervention to reduce birth defects need to be done prior to or at conception to be effective. By the time of the first prenatal visit usually at 6-8 weeks of gestation, organogenesis has started and exposure to teratogen might have already occurred.
b. *Identification, assessment and possible alteration of risk factors:* The risk factors that may influence maternal and fetal outcome during pregnancy can be identified and interviewed during preconceptional counseling. Ideally dosage adjustment or withdrawal of medications especially drugs in class C,D should be done before conception.
c. *Timing of pregnancy in women with special risk factors:* Women having special risk factors should be counseled about timing of pregnancy. Women with chronic medical conditions should try to conceive when their disease is under optimal control. In family history of genetic disorders some couple may want to complete screening for some genetic disorder to determine their risk more precisely and explore the possibility of prenatal diagnosis.
d. Preconceptional counseling is a good occasion to assess and **reinforce folic acid supplementation** and to review the importance of seeking early and regular prenatal care.

Timing and Persons for Preconceptional Counseling

Ideally preconceptional counseling should be discussed with all women of childbearing age, especially if they are considering pregnancy in the next 1-2 years. When women seeks medical advice for contraception or infertility or routine visit for any medical problem, the women should be given preconceptional advice regarding diet, alcohol use, smoking, vitamin intake, exercise and other behaviors.

Preconceptional counseling (PCC) can be performed by family physicians, general obstetrician and gynecologist, geneticist or maternal fetal medicine (MFM) specialist. Basic advice can be given by primary care provider. Counselor should be knowledgeable about relevant medical disease, prior surgery, and reproductive disorders on genetic conditions and should be able to interpret data and recommendation provided by other specialist. If the practitioner is uncomfortable in providing counseling they should refer the women or couple to a counselor with special expertise.

Information Obtained during Preconceptional Counseling

1. *Medical and surgical history* like diabetes, renal disease, hypertension, epilepsy, heart disease, thromboembolism, psychiatric disorders.
2. *Maternal age*—extremes of maternal age has an impact on pregnancy outcome.
3. *Gynecological and reproductive history* with attention to potentially recurrent obstetric complication.
4. *Family history* focused on ethical and social background, congenital anomalies and genetic disorders.
5. *History of medications*.
6. *Social and nutrional assessment:*
    a. *Tobacco use:* The key to prevention of drug related fetal damage is to have the women provide an honest assessment of her usage. Questions should be nonjudgmental. Smoking affects fetal growth in a dose dependent manner. It increases risk for preterm labor, fetal growth restriction and low birth weight as well as attention deficit hyperactivity disorder and behavioral and learning problems in school going age.

Smoking also increases the risk of pregnancy complications related to vascular insufficiency as uteroplacental insufficiency and placental abruption.
   b. *Alcohol* related mental retardation is currently the only mental retardation syndrome, amenable to prevention.
   c. *Environmental exposure*: While every one is exposed to environmental substances, only a few increase pregnancy risk. Pregnant industrial workers may be exposed to heavy metals or chemicals such as organic solvents. Patients living in rural area may be exposed to potentially harmful pesticides or contaminated cold water.
   d. *Diet*: Deficiency of protein, iron and other minerals in diet can be corrected by counseling like advice of increasing cheese, milk product and leafy fresh vegetables. Obesity is associated with a number of maternal complications as hypertension, pre-eclampsia and gestational diabetes. Anorexia and bulimia increase the risk for electrolyte disturbance, cardiac arrhythmias.
   e. *Exercise*: There is no data to suggest that exercise is deleterious during pregnancy. But the women should be cautioned about balance problem.
   f. *Domestic violence*.
7. *Physical examination including pelvic examinations.*
8. *Laboratory tests in preconceptional counseling*:
   a. Hematocrit for iron deficiency anemia, and lowered mean corpuscular volume as a screen for hemoglobinopathies should be done.
   b. *Rubella titer:* Immunization if nonimmune in pregnant state.
   c. Screening of HIV with appropriate pre- and post-test counseling and treatment.
   d. Screening for other sexually transmitted disease like syphilis, hepatitis B.
   e. Screening for specific genetic disorders according to the family history and ethnic origin.
   f. Routine preventive health care like Pap smear, cholesterol screening and immunization.

Genetic Disease

The 2-3% incidence of serious birth defects found at delivery in the general population has remained unchanged for decades. **Of all malformations 15-20% are thought to be genetic, 8-10% are a result of environmental factors or maternal disease (i.e. diabetic) and the remaining 65% are of unknown etiology.**

As advances are made in the treatment of other obstetrical and newborn complications, genetics will play a proportionately larger role in neonatal morbidity and mortality. The preferable strategy is:
1. **Primary prevention:** Avoidance of causal factors which is becoming possible for more congenital disease as their etiologies are discovered.
2. **Secondary prevention:** Identifying and terminating affected pregnancies is an alternative strategy for single gene disorders and other nonpreventable defects.
3. **Tertiary prevention:** Surgical correction of structural defect but it is not possible for most genetic disorders. The benefits of preconceptional counseling usually are measured by comparing the incidence of new cases before and after the initiation of a counseling program.

Primary Protection

Some following congenital conditions are clearly benefited from counseling.
a. **Neural tube defect:** The incidence of neural tube defect is 1-2 per 1000 live births and they are next only to cardiac anomalies in overall fetal malformations. Some NTDs are associated with a specific mutation in the methylene tetrahydrofolate reductase gene. The adverse effect of which is largely overcome by periconceptional folic acid supplementation. **The CDC recommends that women who had a previous NTD affected pregnancy should take 4 mg of folic acid per day beginning at least 1 month prior to conception and continuing throughout the first trimester.** Risk factors for NTD other than a previous NTD affected pregnancy include maternal diabetes (Pregestational), maternal intake of valproic acid or carbamazepine and history of NTD in patient or close relative. Still there is no evidence to support periconceptional high dose folic acid (4 mg/ or 4000 µg) but they should definitely take at least 0.4 mg of folic acid daily and consideration can be given to increasing their daily periconceptional folic acid intake to 4 mg. The potential risk of the higher dose of folic acid include masking the hematological signs of vitamin B_{12} deficiency (Pernicious anemia) without preventing its irreversible neurologic effects. In women with no history of an NTD affected pregnancy, supplementation with a multivitamins containing 0.4 mg (400 µg) folic acid will prevent at least 50% of NTDs, when taken before conception and continued throughout the first trimester. Since more that 50% of pregnancies are unplanned, **all women of childbearing age should consume 0.4 mg (400 µg) of folic acid daily.** Additional intake of food rich in folate can raise the average intake, but naturally occurring folate is less readily absorbed then synthetic folic acid in supplements or fortified food. Besides this it is important to remember that folic acid supplements are the only method of folic acid supplementation that has been tested and shown to decrease the primary and secondary incidence of NTD. The most of multivitamin, over the counter preparation, contain 0.4-0.8 mg folic acid. *These multivitamins preparations should not be used to increase folic acid intake up to 1 mg or more, since they contain other vitamins that could have adverse effects when taken in large quantities such as vitamin 'A'.*

b. **Phenylketonuria (PKU):** PKU is an inborn error of phenylalanine metabolism. It is an example of a disease in which the fetus is not at risk to inherit the disease but may be damaged by the effects of maternal genetic disease. With preconceptional counseling and adherence of phenylalanine restricted diet before pregnancy the incidence of fetal malformation caused by high blood phenylalanine is dramatically reduced.
c. **Tay-Sachs disease:** This disease is a severe autosomal recessive neurodegenerative disorder that leads to death in childhood. The identification of carrier through genetic testing, provision of prenatal testing has helped in reducing incidence of Tay-Sachs disease to great extent.
d. **Thalassemias:** These disorders of globin chain synthesis are the most common single gene disorders worldwide. Primary and secondary prevention can reduce the incidence of new cases by at least 80%.

Vitamin 'A' and Pregnancy

Vitamin 'A' is an essential vitamin with requirement in pregnancy of 5000 IU. An average balanced diet supplies 7000-8000 IU/day so additional supplementation is usually not needed. Daily vitamin A intake > 25000 IU/day as with diet rich in liver and cod oil as well as supplemental vitamin A intake increase the risk of birth defects. So **vitamin A intake supplementation in pregnancy is not recommended and may have harmful effects. Therefore, it should be discontinued.**

Maternal Medical Condition

a. **Pregestational diabetes:** It is associated with an increased risk of birth defects (cardiac defects and neural tube defects are the most frequent). Risk is further increased if glycemic control is suboptimal. Ideally optimal blood sugar control, assessed by glycosylated hemoglobin can be achieved before conception. In diabetic women overall health status is evaluated including blood pressure, renal, cardiac or retinal evaluation, which is useful in counseling patients about both impact of pregnancy on her disease and risk of fetal and pregnancy related complication due to her diabetes.
b. **Epilepsy and seizure disorders:** Women with epilepsy are 2-3 times more likely to have infants with structural anomalies than unaffected women. It is thought to be due to anticonvulsant medicines. **Preconceptional counseling usually includes recommendation to switch to monotherapy with the least teratogenic medications. Besides this epileptic women are advised to take supplemental folic acid.**
c. **Hypertension:** Assessment of cardiac and renal function are probably best gauge for complications during pregnancy. Current medications should be assessed and angiotensin converting enzyme inhibitors should be avoided.
d. **Connective tissue disorder:** In disorders like systemic lupus erythematosus, current renal function, hypertension and pericardial/pleural involvement is evaluated to assess risk of pregnancy to underlying disease as well as potential for pregnancy complications. Women positive for antibodies like anticardiolipin antibody, lupus anticoagulant but no history of thrombosis, adverse pregnancy outcome or previous child with congenital heart block, there is no evidence that treatment affects outcome of pregnancy.

Risk Associated with Advanced Maternal Age > 35 Years

a. Fertility decreases as the maternal age advances.
b. Chromosomal anomalies increase with advancing maternal age and this increase is mainly due to an increase in trisomies (The most frequent being Trisomy 21 or Down syndrome) due to an increase in non-disjunction associated with maternal age.
c. The spontaneous abortion rate is increased with maternal age, mainly secondary to the increase in chromosomal anomalies.
d. Other birth defects (Nonchromosomal) are not increased with maternal age.
e. Maternal complication such as pre-eclampsia, gestation diabetes and placenta previa are more frequent in women ages 35 or older. It may be age related or due to predisposing medical conditions.
f. The cesarean section rate is increased in older women.

Cardiac Evaluation

Women with following conditions should receive a cardiac assessment (e.g. electrocardiogram, echocardiogram) prior to conception:
a. Pregestational diabetes.
b. Chronic hypertension (longer than 10 years, or over age 40).
c. Congenital heart disease.
d. Signs and symptoms suggestive of cardiac disease.

Absolute Contraindication of Pregnancy

Risk has to be individualized for every patient but cardiac conditions associated with marked maternal mortality (50% or more) include *Eisenmenger syndrome, primary pulmonary hypertension, Marfan's syndrome with marked dilation of aortic root, complicated coarctation of the aorta, uncorrected tetralogy of Fallot and dilated cardiomyopathy.*

PHYSIOLOGICAL CHANGES DURING PREGNANCY: GENERAL CONSIDERATION

During pregnancy there are progressive and many anatomical, physiological and biomechanical changes not only in the genital organs but to all system of the body. These changes begin from after fertilization and continue throughout gestation. Most of these changes occur as adaptation in response to physiological stimuli provided by the fetus. It is also significant to note that these changes are almost completely reversed after delivery and lactation.

A basic knowledge of these adaptations is critical for understanding normal laboratory measurements, knowing the drugs likely to require dose adjustment, and recognizing women who are predisposed to medical complications during pregnancy.

Cardiovascular System

Anatomical Changes

With uterine enlargement and diaphragmatic elevation, the heart rotates on its long axis in a left upward displacement. As a result of these changes, the apical beat (point of maximum intensity) shifts laterally. Overall the heart size is increased by 12%, resulting from both an increase in myocardial mass and intracardiac volume ($\approx$ 80 ml). All heart sounds are louder and first sound is splitted. A systolic ejection murmur is normal and a diastolic murmur is heard occasionally.

The ECG may show low voltage QRS complexes, flattening or inversion of the T wave and depression of the ST segment. Atrial or ventricular extrasystoles are common.

Cardiac output rises from 7 liters/min at 8-11 weeks to 9 liter/min at 36-39 weeks. The rise is caused by an increased stroke volume (64-71 ml) and an increase in heart rate (8 beat/min by 8 weeks, 16 beats/min by term). Myocardial contractility is increased. The arteriovenous oxygen difference is reduced in early pregnancy (33 ml/liter) but returns to nonpregnant values at term (45 ml/liter) (Fig. 30.1).

Cardiac output is lowest in sitting or supine positions and highest in the right or left lateral or knee chest position. *Cardiac output returns to prelabor values by one hour following delivery and to the prepregnant level by another 4 weeks of time.*

Multiple gestations have even more profound effects on the maternal cardiovascular system. In twin pregnancies, cardiac output is about 20% greater than for singletons because of greater stroke volume (15%) and heart rate (3.5%).

Blood Pressure

Systolic blood pressure does not change in pregnancy, diastolic pressure is reduced in the first-two trimester and returns to nonpregnant level at term. The combination of increased cardiac output and decreased diastolic blood pressure indicates that peripheral resistance is reduced. This is caused by the placenta, which acts as an arteriovenous shunt together with peripheral vasodilatation and factors such as estrogen and progesterone and increased endothelial synthesis of prostaglandin and prostacyclin. Blood pressure is lower when the women is lying down (supine or on her side) than when she is sitting. Both blood pressure and cardiac output are reduced during epidural analgesia.

Venous pressure progressively increases in the lower extremities but not in the arms, particularly when patient is supine or sitting. The increase is due to mechanical obstruction by the uterus and its contents and to the high pressure of venous outflow from the uterus, also possibly from the pressure of the fetal presenting part on the common iliac veins. The femoral venous pressure is raised from 8-10 cm of water during pregnancy in lying down position and to about 80-100 cm of water in standing position. This explains the fact that physiological edema of pregnancy subsides by rest alone.

The rise in venous pressure, together will fall of colloid osmotic pressure in the blood, explains the leg edema (which occurs in 40% of pregnant women), varicose veins, piles and deep vein thrombosis.

Blood Flow in the Individual Organs

Uterine blood flow increases during pregnancy, reaching volumes around 700 ml/min at term. Blood flow also increases in other organs, the target changes being in the kidneys (up to 400 ml/min) and the skin (up to 500 ml/min), the hands show the most striking increase. As with cardiac output, most of the rise in extrauterine sites occurs during first 10 weeks of pregnancy.

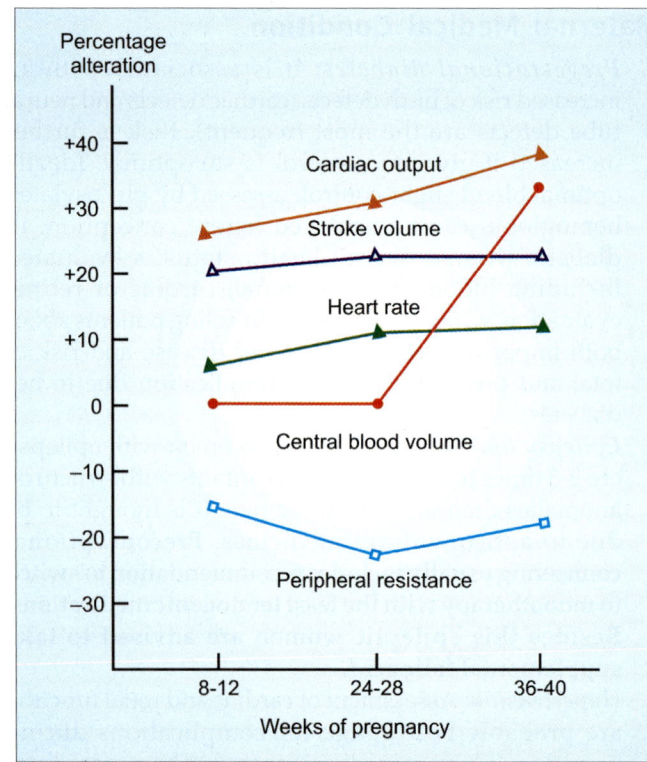

Fig. 30.1: Cardiovascular changes in pregnancy (% alteration over nonpregnant level occurring in pregnancy)

Blood Volume and Composition

Plasma volume increases during pregnancy, reaching a plateau at 32-34 weeks. The increase is 1250 ml in a first pregnancy and 1500 ml in subsequent pregnancies (non-pregnant volume 2600 ml).

Red cell mass increases by 240 ml (400 ml for those given iron, nonpregnant mass > 1400 ml). Increased red cell production is probably stimulated by a three fold rise in erythropoietin level and is associated with an increase in the proportion of fetal hemoglobin (HbF). Changes in cellular composition of blood are shown in Table 30.1.

Table 30.1: Changes in cellular composition of blood

Component	Changes
Total white cell count	Increase
Neutrophil	Increase
Lymphocyte	No change
Eosinophil	Fall sharply during labor and delivery
Platelet	Decrease
Red cell count	Decrease
Hematocrit (Packed cell volume)	Decrease
Hemoglobin concentration	Decrease (acceptable minimum 11 gm/dl)
Mean cell hemoglobin concentration	No changes
Mean cell volume	Small increase
Red cell fragility	Increase
ESR	Increase

Red Blood Cells

The red cell mass expands by about 33% or by approximately 450 ml of erythrocytes for the average pregnant women. The increase is greater with iron supplementation. The greater increase in plasma volume accounts for physiological anemia of pregnancy. For example, maternal hemoglobin is average 10.9 ± 08 S D gm/dl in the second trimester and 12.4 ± 1.0 gm/dl at term.

White Blood Cell

The total blood leukocyte count increases during normal pregnancy from prepregnancy level from 5000 to 12000/μl. Reduced polymorphonuclear leukocyte adherence has been reported in the third trimester. These changes may predispose pregnant women to infection.

Placenta

Some studies have reported decreased production of platelet (thrombocytopenia) during pregnancy that is accompanied by progressive platelet consumption. Platelet count falls below 1,50,000/μl in 6% of gravidas in third trimester. This pregnancy associated thrombocytopenia, which appears to be caused by increased peripheral consumption, resolves with delivery *and is of no pathological significance*. Level of prostacyclin a platelet aggregation inhibitor, and thromboxane A2—an inducer of platelet aggregation and vasoconstrictor, increase during pregnancy.

Clotting Factors

Circulatory level of several coagulation factors increase in pregnancy. Fibrinogen factor I and factor VIII level increase markedly whereas factors VII, IX, X and XII increase to a lesser extent. Plasma fibrinogen concentration begins to increase from nonpregnant level (1.5-4.5 gm/lit) during the third month of pregnancy and progressively rise by nearly two fold by late pregnancy (4-6.5 gm/lit). The high estrogen level of pregnancy may be involved in the increased fibrinogen synthesis by liver.

Plasma level of factors VII, VIII, IX, X and XII together with fibrin degradation products increase during pregnancy. Factor IX and antithrombin III level decrease. Fibrinolytic activity is depressed during pregnancy through a poorly understood mechanism. Plasminogen concentration increases concomitantly with fibrinogen but there is still a net procoagulant effect of pregnancy. Understanding physiologic alteration of coagulation and fibrinolytic system is critical for management of some of the more serious pregnancy disorders including hemorrhage and thromboembolic disorders.

Iron

The enhanced erythropoiesis of pregnancy increases utilization of iron which can reach 6-7 mg/day in the latter half of pregnancy. Many women begin pregnancy in an iron deficient state, making them vulnerable to iron deficiency anemia. So the supplemental iron is commonly given to pregnant women.

Placenta actively transports iron from the mother to fetus, the fetus is generally not anemic even when mother is severely iron deficient.

Pulmonary System Adaptation in Pregnancy

During pregnancy, the diaphragm rises 4 cm, the transverse diameters of the chest increases by 2 cm and subcostal angle increases from 68 to 103°. Overall there is an increase in ventilation attributed to a greater depth of breathing but not an increase in rate. The prime stimulus to this is the increase in circulating progesterone levels.

Oxygen consumption increases during pregnancy from 250 to 300 ml/min. Because this 20% increase is less then 50% for alveolar ventilation, there is an effective hyperventilation. Both alveolar and arteriolar PCO_2 are reduced (35-40 mm Hg in nonpregnant, 30 mm Hg in pregnancy). This in turn, leads to increased renal bicarbonate excretion and a reduction in plasma bicarbonate and sodium and hence in osmolality. Arterial pH is unchanged. Arterial PCO_2 shows a small increase. Maternal hyperventilation may be protective in that it prevents the fetus from being exposed to high CO_2 tensions, which might adversely effect the development of respiratory control and other critical regulatory mechanism.

Renal System

Anatomical Changes

During pregnancy, the length of kidney increases by 1-1.5 cm, with a proportional increase in weight. The calyces and pelvis are dilated in pregnancy with the volume of renal pelvis increased up to 6 fold compared to nonpregnant volume of 10 ml. The ureters are dilated above the brim of the bony pelvis, with more prominent effect on the right.

The ureters become elongated, wider and become more curved. The entire dilated collecting system may contain up to 200 ml of urine, which predispose to ascending urinary infection. Several factors likely to contribute to the hydronephrosis and hydroureter of pregnancy:
a. Pregnancy hormones, e.g. progesterone.
b. Enlargement of the ovarian vein complex in the infundibulopelvic ligament may compress the ureter at the brim of bony pelvis.
c. Hyperplasia of smooth muscle in distal 1/3rd of the ureter may cause reduction in luminal size, leading to dilatation in the upper 2/3rd.
d. The sigmoid colon and dextrorotation of the uterus likely reduce compression (and dilatation) of left ureter relative to the right.

Renal Function

Renal blood flow (effective renal plasma flow) increases 70-80% by mid pregnancy, during the third trimester it decreases but is still 50-60% above nonpregnancy level. Glomerular filtration increases by 30-50% during pregnancy, beginning in the first-two weeks of pregnancy. As a result plasma level of creatinine and urea fall. The upper limit of normal in late pregnancy is 70 μm mol/ml and 4.5 m mol/liter respectively. Clearance of uric acid is also increased, but this is balanced by increased tubular reabsorption, and in late pregnancy the plasma level is similar to those in the nonpregnant state.

Renal excretion of a variety of material during pregnancy is increased owing to an increase in filtered load, which is greater than tubular reabsorptive capacity. Such material include—glucose and other sugar, water soluble vitamins, serum protein (including albumin and transferrin) and amino acid.

Cumulative water retention in pregnancy is 7.5 liter and this is accompanied by 900 m mol sodium. The increase in filtered load of sodium (from 20,000 m mol/day to 30,000 m mol/day) is balanced by greater tubular reabsorption. This pattern is influenced by a variety of hormones, most notably the sodium retaining steroid aldosterone and deoxycorticosterone (DOC), both of which increase during pregnancy. The increased aldosterone, results at least in part from the elevated plasma concentration of renin. Angiotensin I and II are also substantially increased and pregnant women are highly resistant to the pressure effect of infused angiotensin II. The uterus and amniotic fluid contain high level of renin like maternal.

Renal acid base regulation (bicarbonate absorption and acid H^+) excretion is unchanged during pregnancy. There is slight retention of potassium (total 350 mEq). Although plasma osmolality is reduced by 10 mosmol, vasopressin level is normal, presumably owing to resetting of osmoreceptors. The ability to excrete a water load is subject to marked postural effect, being greater in the lateral recumbent position than in either the supine or upright position. This may be the result of compression of renal veins by the gravid uterus. Thus, measurement of urinary function must take into account of maternal posture. Collection period should be at least 12-24 hours as there is large urinary dead space. Similarly the creatinine clearance is higher at night in contrast to the nonpregnant state.

Urinary Bladder

As the uterus enlarges, the urinary bladder is displaced upward and flattened in the anterior posterior diameters. One of the earliest symptoms of pregnancy is increased urinary frequency which may be related to pregnancy hormones. In later gestation mechanical effect of the enlarged uterus may contribute to increased frequency. Bladder vascularity increases and muscle tone decreases which increase bladder capacity up to 1500 ml.

Gastrointestinal System

Anatomical Changes

As the uterus grows, the stomach is pushed upward and the large and small bowel extend into more posterolateral regions. The appendix is displaced superiorly in the right flank area. These organs return to their normal position in the early puerperium.

Oral cavity: The gum may become hypertrophic and hyperemic and bleed easily, which may be caused by increased systemic estrogen. Pregnancy per se does not predispose to tooth decay or to mobilization of bone calcium.

Esophagus and stomach: Reduced competence of the lower esophageal sphincter may lead to reflux esophagitis. Gastric secretion of both acid and peptide enzymes is reduced in mid pregnancy. Pregnancy is associated with greater production of gastrin which increases stomach volume and acidity of gastric secretion. Gastric tone and motility are also reduced, especially during labor, and the emptying time increased from 50 to 100 minutes.

Intestines: Both the small and large intestines have reduced motility during 2nd and 3rd trimester, whereas 1st trimester and postpartum transit times are similar. The slow transit time of food through the gastrointestinal tract potentially enhances water absorption, predisposing to constipation. However, diet and cultural expectation may be more important factors in this disorder.

Gallbladder: Gallbladder motility and emptying rate is reduced in pregnancy. Bile stasis of pregnancy increases the risk for cholesterol gallstone formation, although the chemical composition of bile is not appreciably altered.

Liver: Liver morphology does not change in normal pregnancy. Plasma albumin level is reduced to a greater extent than the slight decrease in plasma globulin. This fall in the albumin/globulin, ratio mimics liver disease in non-pregnant individuals.

Serum alkaline phosphatase activity can double as the result of alkaline phosphate isoenzyme produced by the placenta.

Skin

Hyperpigmentation

Hyperpigmentation is one of the well recognized changes of pregnancy, which is manifested in linea nigra and chloasma. Chloasma is exacerbated by sun exposure, develops in 70% of pregnancies and is characterized by an uneven darkening of the skin in the centrofascial malar area. This hyperpigmentation is because of the elevated concentration of melanocytic stimulating hormone and or estrogen progesterone effect on the skin.

Striae gravidarum: It consists of bands or lines of thickened, hyperemic skin. These stretch marks begin to appear in the second trimester on the abdomen, breast, thighs and buttocks. Decreased collagen adhesiveness and increased ground substance formation are characteristically seen in this skin condition. There is probably a genetic predisposition. And there is no effective preventive or therapeutic treatment.

Other cutaneous changes are:
a. Spider angioma
b. Palmer erythema
c. Cutis marmorata—mottled appearance of skin secondary to vasomotor instability
d. Development or worsening of varicosity in nearly 40% of pregnancy as compression of *vena cava* by gravid uterus increases venous pressure in lower extremities, which dilates veins in the legs, anus (hemorrhoids) and vulva.
e. Nail becomes brittle and can show horizontal grooves (Beau's lines).
f. Thickening of hair during pregnancy is caused by an increased number of follicles in anagen (growth phase) which ends 1-5 months postpartum, with the onset of the telogen (resting phase) which results in excessive shedding and thinning of hair. Normal hair growth returns within 12 months.

Metabolic Changes

Maternal Weight Gain During Pregnancy

Maternal weight gain average 0.35 kg/weak in early pregnancy, 0.45 kg/weak in mid pregnancy and 0.35 kg/weak in late pregnancy. The average total weight gain is 12.5 kg. The contributions to this weight gain from identified sources are shown in Table 30.2.

Table 30.2: Contribution of different organs in maternal weight gain

Tissues/Fluid	Gain (gm)
Fetus	3400
Placenta	650
Amniotic fluid	800
Uterus	970
Mammary glands	400
Blood	1250
Extracellular extravascular fluid	1700
Fat	3500

Carbohydrate Metabolism

Normal pregnancy is characterized by mild fasting hypoglycemia. After an oral glucose meal there is both prolonged hyperglycemia and hyperinsulinemia in pregnant women with a greater suppression of glucagon. This mechanism is likely to ensure a sustained or maintained postprandial supply of glucose to the fetus. In pregnancy action of insulin is blunted, this unmask latent diabetes and aggravates existing diabetes.

Protein

The protein accounts for about 1 kg of maternal weight gain which is evenly divided between the mother (uterine contractile protein, breast glandular tissue, plasma protein and hemoglobin) and the fetoplacental unit.

Lipid

There is general increase in plasma lipid levels during pregnancy including triglycerides, cholesterol, phospholipid, nonesterified (i.e. free) fatty acids and lipoproteins. Unlike the situation in adult, fatty acids are not a significant energy source for the fetus. Fetal tissue can synthesize fatty acids, triglycerides and cholesterol. It has been suggested that more fat is stored centrally during mid pregnancy and as fetus extracts more nutrition in the latter months, fat storage decreases.

Water Metabolism

Increased water retention is a normal physiological alteration of pregnancy. At term, the water content of the fetus, placenta and amniotic fluid constitutes about 3.5 liter. Increase in maternal blood volume and size of uterus and breast, amniotic fluid added to another 3.0 liter of water. So the minimum amount of extra water retained in pregnancy is about 6.5 liter, which explains presence of pitting edema of ankle and leg in a substantial proportion of normal pregnant women.

Acid-base Equilibrium

Maternal ventilation increases during pregnancy which causes a respiratory alkalosis by lowering the PCO_2 of blood. There is a moderate reduction in plasma bicarbonate from 26 to about 22 m mol/liter which partially compensates for this. Consequently there is only a minimal increase in blood pH.

Vitamins

There are rise in plasma concentration of carotenoids (Provitamins A) and tocopherol (Vitamin E) and reduction in retinol (Vitamin A), ascorbic acid (Vitamin C), folate, vitamin B_{12}, vitamin B_6, biotin, Thiamine (Vitamin B_1), Riboflavin and nicotinic acid. These fats soluble vitamins are increased while increased renal excretion causes a fall in level of water soluble vitamins. Fetal levels of water soluble vitamins are generally higher than maternal levels.

Calcium

Approximately 30 gm of calcium is incorporated into the fetus by term; mostly in the second half of pregnancy. This is associated with reduction in maternal plasma total calcium and magnesium, while ionized calcium and phosphate are unchanged. Absorption of dietary calcium is associated with an increase in 1,25, dihydroxycholecalciferol (calcitriol) and parathormone. There is a reduction in maternal bone density during pregnancy especially in 3rd trimester. Extra requirement of calcium and vitamin D can be met by a normal diet, although majority of women in India require calcium and vitamin D supplement, because of various socioeconomic factors. Fetal plasma concentration of calcium and phosphate are greater than maternal plasma concentration because of active placental support.

Musculoskeletal System

Progressive lordosis is a characteristic feature of normal pregnancy. It compensates for anterior position of the enlarging uterus, the lordosis shifts the center of gravity back over the lower extremities. There is increased mobility of the sacroiliac, sacrococcygeal and pubic joints during pregnancy, presumably due to hormonal changes. This mobility contributes to alteration of maternal posture and discomfort in lower portion of back.

During late pregnancy, occasionally there is aching, numbness and weakness in upper extremities. This possibly is from the marked lordosis with anterior neck flexion and slumping of the shoulder girdle, which in turn produce traction on the ulnar and median nerve. Similarly paresthesia and sensory loss over the anterolateral aspect of thigh may occur, which is due to compression of the lateral cutaneous nerve of the thigh.

Genital Tract Changes in Pregnancy

Uterus

During pregnancy the uterus is transformed into a relatively thin walled muscular organ of sufficient capacity to accommodate the fetus, placenta and amniotic fluid. By the end of 12 weeks, the uterus has become too large to remain totally within the pelvis. As the uterus continues to enlarge, it contacts the anterior abdominal wall, displaces the intestines laterally and superiorly, and continues to rise, ultimately reaching almost to the liver (Figs 30.2A to D).

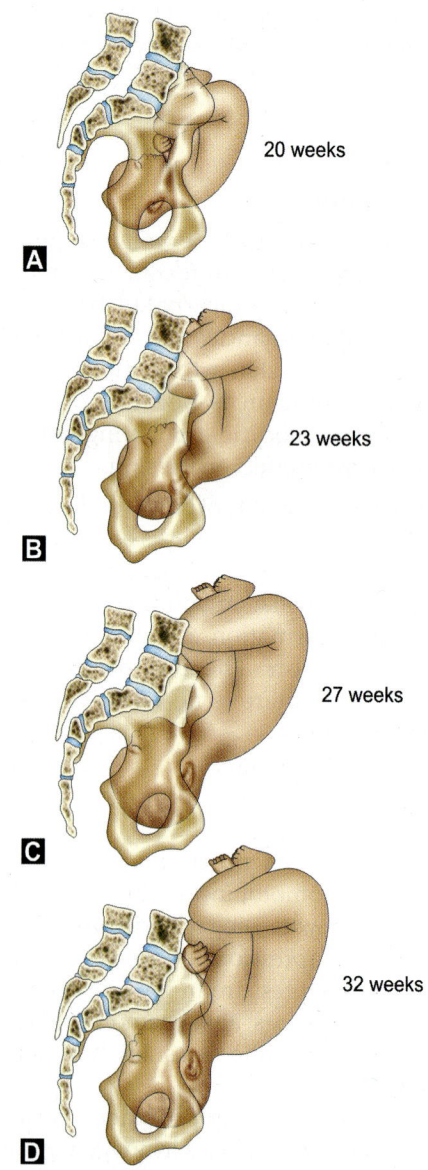

Figs 30.2A to D: Enlargement of uterus in normal pregnancy

There is dextrorotation of uterus, likely to be caused by the rectosigmoid. At term the uterus weighs 900-1000 gm and measures 35 cm in length as compared to 50 gm weight and 7.5 cm length in nonpregnant state. From the first trimester around the uterus undergoes irregular contraction, which is normally painless. Such contractions appear unpredictably and sporadically and are usually non-rhythmic (Braxton Hicks contractions). During the last weeks or two of gestation, the contractions may be more frequent and regular, accounting for so called false labor.

Placental perfusion is dependent upon uterine blood flow through uterine and ovarian arteries. There is a progressive increase in uteroplacental blood flow during pregnancy ranging from 450-600 ml/minute.

Cervix: During pregnancy, there is pronounced softening of the cervix and the cervical glands undergo marked proliferation. Soon after conception, there is thick mucus obstructing the cervical canal. It is expelled at onset of labor, resulting in a bloody show.

Ovaries: There is persistence and growth of the corpus luteum, which reaches its maximum at 8th week, when it measures about 2.5 cm and become cystic. Regression occurs following decline in the secretion of hCG from the placenta. Colloid degeneration occurs at 12th week which later becomes calcified at term.

Estrogen and progesterone secreted by the corpus luteum maintain the environment for the growing ovum, before placenta assumes its function. The hormones not only control the formation and maintenance of decidua of pregnancy, but also inhibit ripening of the follicle. Thus, both the ovarian and uterine cycle of the normal menstruation remain suspended.

PRENATAL CARE

Prenatal care as we know it today is a relatively new concept in medicine, which was introduced largely by social reformers and nurses. It is an example of preventive health care at its best. It originated in Boston in the first decade of the 20th century. Before that time a pregnant patient only used to visit any physician either only for confirmation of pregnancy or at time of delivery. The nurses of the instructive Nursing Association in Boston, thinking that they might contribute to the health of pregnant mothers, began making house calls in all mothers registered for delivery at hospital. These visits were so successful that the principle behind them was gradually accepted by physician and our present system of prenatal care which stress on prevention, evolved.

Pregnancy is a normal physiologic event that is complicated by pathologic process dangerous to the health of the mother and fetus in only 5-20% of cases. The aims of prenatal care is to:

a. Define the health status of the mother and fetus.
b. Determine the gestational age of fetus.
c. Prevent, identify, and or ameliorate maternal or fetal abnormalities that adversely effect pregnancy outcome including socioeconomic, emotional, medical and obstetric factors.
d. Educate the patient about pregnancy, labor, delivery and parenting as well about ways she can improve her overall health.
e. Promote adequate psychosocial support from family.

So prenatal care is a continuum from the preconceptional period through the first postpartum year.

Initial Visit (First Prenatal Visit)

First prenatal visit is an important visit, when the following measures are carried out:

a. Risk assessment to include genetic, medical, obstetrical and psychosocial factors.
b. Estimated due date.
c. General physical examination.
d. Laboratory test includes hematocrit, urinalysis, urine culture, blood group, Rh, syphilis screen, Pap smear, HbSAg testing, HIV testing with pre- and post-test counseling.
e. Patient education about daily activity, diet, avoidance of alcohol and tobacco.

Prenatal Records

Use of standardized prenatal record greatly facilitates antepartum and intrapartum management. There are several definitions pertinent to establishment of an accurate prenatal record.

a. *Primipara:* **A women who has been delivered only once of fetus or fetuses, who reached viability.** So completion of any pregnancy beyond the stage of abortion bestows parity upon the mother.
b. *Multipara:* A women who has completed two or more pregnancies to viability. It is the number of pregnancies reaching viability and not the number of fetus delivered that determines parity. Parity is not greater if a single fetus, twins or quadruplets were delivered, nor lower if the fetus or fetuses were stillborn.
c. *Nulligravida:* A women who is not now and never has been pregnant.
d. *Gravida:* A women who is or has been pregnant, irrespective of the pregnancy outcome with the establishment of the first pregnancy, she becomes a primigravida and with successive pregnancies a multigravida.
e. *Nullipara:* A women who has never completed a pregnancy beyond an abortion. She may or may not have been pregnant or have had a spontaneous or elective abortion.
f. *Parturient:* A women in labor.
g. *Puerpera:* Women who has just given birth.

Good record keeping is important during pregnancy and formats can be framed which show:
a. Compel the obtaining of information, examinations and diagnostic test at appropriate times.
b. Allow easy recognition of significant risk factors and problems.
c. Detail management plans.

It is important to document all recognized problems legibly both for ease of giving care at future encounters and for medicolegal reasons.

Determination of Gestational Age

The duration of pregnancy calculated from the first day of the last normal menstrual period is 280 days or 40 weeks. It is possible to estimate the expected date of delivery by adding 7 days to the date of the first day of the last normal menstrual period and counting back 3 months **(Naegele rule)**. Frequently however variation in the cycle and the timing of ovulation, use of oral contraception on the month preceding the LMP, and appearance of menstrual like bleeding during early pregnancy renders the calculation of expected date of delivery inaccurate.

In these situations other parameters confirming or indicting a different expected date of course and delivery can be used:
a. Date of positive urine (about 4-5 weeks after the LMP) or serum (8-10th postconceptional days) pregnancy test.
b. Uterine size during the first half of pregnancy.
c. Time of quickening (16-20 weeks).
d. Time of listening of first heard fetal heart sounds with electronic Doppler equipment (10-12 weeks) and non-electronic fetoscope (18-20 weeks).
e. Ultrasound using the crown rump length in the first trimester (error of 7 days) and the fetal biometry in late first trimester and second trimester that includes— biparietal diameter, femur length, head and abdominal circumferences, and other measures (with an error of 7-10 days). Ultrasonic estimates of gestational age are much less accurate in the third trimester.

Historical Information

a. *Medical:* Many chronic medical conditions have an effect on pregnancy outcome, conversely pregnancy usually has a distinct effect on the course of the condition itself.
b. *Surgical:* In particular any prior surgical or anesthetic complications and need for transfusions should be noted.
c. *Obstetric and gynecologic:* Some events in the patient's obstetric history often recur in subsequent pregnancies like fetal and neonatal deaths, low birth weight infants, preterm deliveries, intrauterine growth restriction, fetal macrosomia (over 4 kg at birth) birth defects, abruptio placenta, pre-eclampsia or hypertension and postpartum hemorrhage. A history of recent infertility treatment, pelvic inflammatory disease or ectopic pregnancy is significant for identifying early pregnancy compli-cations such as tubal pregnancy or multiple gestations. A history of past sexually transmitted disease should also be taken.
d. *Family history:* Enquiring of inherited disease is important because with time progressively more of these conditions are becoming amenable to prenatal; diagnosis. History of congenital malformations, neural tube defects, cerebral palsy and mental retardation should be enquired. History of blood dyscrasias like hemophilia, thalassemia, cystic fibrosis and muscular dystrophy should be elevated.
e. *Social:* Psychosocial background and lifestyle are also important as they frequently affect pregnancy and neonatal outcome. Questions about smoking, use of alcohol and illicit drugs, use of prescription and over the counter medications, employment and type of occupation and the existence of problems at home such as domestic violence should be asked.

Physical Examination at First Visit

a. *General physical examination:* A general physical examination of all prenatal patients should be performed. This examination may be first or only one over a several year period for many women, and thus it is important for health maintenance. Recording blood pressure and weight, listening to heart and lungs, and palpating the breast and abdomen for any abnormalities are the principal components.
b. *Obstetrical examination:* The fundal height is measured in centimeter from the symphysis pubis to the top of the uterus. Serial measurements over the course of pregnancy provide an excellent assessment of the fetal growth with a rough approximation between centimeters and weeks gestation from 18 to 34 weeks in a patient with normal bodily habits (e.g. 18 cm symphysiofundal distance in 18 weeks gestation). Fetal heart tones should be auscultated. Fetal presentation, fetal parts and estimated fetal weight are determined during the last trimester. Lastly uterine contraction can be easily palpated during a routine examination and if frequent and remote from term may point to the possibility of preterm labor.
c. *Pelvic examination:* It can detect abnormalities of the vulva, vagina, cervix, uterus and adnexa. In early pregnancy size of gravid uterus in weeks is estimated and cervical length is assessed. A Pap smear should be taken. Culture for sexually transmitted infection and wet preparation for any vaginal discharge can be taken. In late pregnancy clinical pelvimetry is done to determine pelvic adequacy in primigravida. In multiparous who have experienced a previous abnormal labor or difficult delivery, anomalies of the vagina and perineum including pelvic organ prolapse is noted.

Laboratory Investigation

Prenatal laboratory test at initial visit in low risk patients are:

Initial Visit

a. Blood hematocrit
b. Urinalysis, screen for bacteriuria
c. Blood group and Rh type
d. Antibody screen
e. Serological test for syphilis
f. Rubella titer
g. Hepatitis B surface antigen
h. HIV antibody with pretest and post-test counseling
i. Pap smear.

Subsequent Visit

a. Blood hematocrit is repeated at 28, 36 weeks.
b. Antibody screening test (Rh negative patients at 28 weeks).
c. Urine dipstick test (at each visit for urinary protein and sugar).

Laboratory test for special indications:

a. ***Gestational diabetes:*** For women at risk for gestational diabetes, screening is recommended between 24-28 weeks.
b. ***Group β streptococcal:*** Eradication of this organism during labor decreases early onset neonatal sepsis. One recommendation is to perform cervical rectal screening culture at 35-37 weeks and to offer intrapartum treatment with penicillin if the culture is positive.
c. ***Screening for genetic disease:*** This screening can be offered based on family history or the ethnic or social background of the couple like test for thalassemia, sickle cell anemia.
d. ***Triple marker test:*** At 15-20 weeks in high risk cases as maternal age more than 35 years, history of previous neural tube defects in women or family.
e. ***Gonorrhea culture, Chlamydia PCR:*** Can be done in high-risk patient with bad obstetrical history.

Subsequent Prenatal Visit

Traditionally the timing of subsequent prenatal examinations is scheduled at interval of 4 weeks until 28 weeks and then every 2 weeks until 36 weeks and weekly thereafter. However, fewer visits are acceptable in uncomplicated pregnancies. Conversely women with complicated pregnancies often require return visits at 1-2 weeks interval.

At each revisit a brief interval history is obtained to uncover any new problems as well as to provide follow-up on existing ones. Every patient should be asked about pain, uterine contraction or cramping, pelvic pressure, bleeding, discharge, dysuria, gastrointestinal problems, presence and number of fetal movement and emergence of any new or other problem since last visit. Patients with medical conditions or known complications should be reviewed with treatment given by physician of other specialties. Women desiring sterilization should be counseled well ahead of delivery.

At each revisit the patient blood pressure and weight is recorded. The gravid uterus is examined by measuring fundal height; fetal position is determined by Leopold's maneuvers in last trimester. Fetal growth and weight is assessed and fetal heart sounds are auscultated. Other examinations including vaginal are done as indicated by the patient's interval history of problems.

Maternal Weight

Maternal weight gain during pregnancy influences birth weight of the infant. Women with a weight before pregnancy of 50 kg are at increased risk for preterm labor. Additionally there is a high risk for a low birth weight infant among under weight women, who gain weight poorly and for a macrosomic baby in over weight patients or those gaining excessively. The rate of weight gain from 8 to 20 weeks is about 0.7 lb/week while after 20 weeks weight gain should be about 1lb/week (Table 30.3).

Table 30.3: Recommended total weight gain ranges for pregnant women in singleton pregnancies

Prepregnancy BMI	Recommended Ponds	Total gain kg
Low (BMI <19.8)	28-40	12.5-18
Normal (BMI 19.8-26)	25-35	11.5-16
High (BMI > 26-29)	15-25	>-11.5
Obese (BMI > 29)	> 15	> 7

Women gaining weight poorly or excessively as the pregnancy progress need further investigation. Cause of poor weight gain may be excessive nausea, vomiting, esophageal reflux, which often responds to medical therapy. Poor eating habit or history of smoking requires counseling. Excessive weight gain often points to lack of physical activity or increased consumption of high caloric foods. It is important to emphasize that initially overweight patients should be allowed some weight gain and no attempt should be made at weight reduction until postpartum. **If there is a sudden spurt of weight gain (> 2 lb/ week or 6 lb/ month) it suggests fluid retention and should alert the caregiver for possibility of pre-eclampsia.** Most of the women lose almost all of their weight gain by 6 months postpartum. But some who gain excessively retain some of this weight, which potentially contributes to lifelong excess weight problem.

Nutrition in Pregnancy

The mother's nutrition from the moment of conception is an important factor in the development of the infant's metabolic pathways and future well-being. The pregnant women should be encouraged to eat a balanced diet and should be made aware of special needs for iron, folic acid, calcium and zinc. *The average women weighing 58 kg have a normal dietary intake of 2300 K Cal/day. An additional 500 K Cal/day is needed during pregnancy and an additional 500 K Cal/day is needed during lactation (Table 30.4).*

Nutritional Requirement

a. **Protein:** Protein needs in the second half of pregnancy are 1 gm per kg plus 20 gm/day (approximately 80 gm/day for the average women). Protein intake is essential for embryonic development.
b. **Calcium:** Calcium intake should be increased to 1.5 gm/day in the last trimester and during lactation. If calcium intake is inadequate, fetal needs will be met through demineralization of the maternal bone system.
c. **Iron:** To avoid iron deficiency anemia, supplementation of 30 mg/day of elemental iron is recommended during second and third trimester. If iron deficiency anemia is diagnosed, the therapeutic doses of elemental iron are prescribed in range of 60-120 mg/day.
d. **Vitamins and prenatal minerals:** Till now only routine folate supplementation (0.4 mg/day) is recommended to prevent neural tube defect. Iron supplementation is recommended during pregnancy, when requirement could not be made by diet alone. Nutrient that can potentially exert toxic effects are iron, zinc, selenium and vitamins A, B, C and D. **Vitamin and mineral intake more than twice the recommended daily dietary allowances should be avoided during pregnancy. Routine multivitamin supplementation is not recommended until the maternal diet is deficient.**

Common Complaint and Maternal Concerns During Prenatal Visits

Nausea and Vomiting in Pregnancy (NVP)

These are common complaints during the first half of pregnancy. Erroneously called morning sickness, symptoms usually commence between the first and second missed menstrual period and continue till about 14-16 weeks. The genesis of pregnancy induced nausea and vomiting is not clear. High level of serum hCG have been implicated in causing nausea. This is likely a surrogate for increasing estrogen levels which are known to cause such symptoms.

The mainstay of treatment is symptomatic therapy with close attention to fluid balance. Frequent small meals and avoidance of aggravating food souces are important. If these simple measures fail, antiemetic such as metoclopramide (Reglan), phenothiazines and ondanserton (Zofran) are effective and appear to be safe in pregnancy. Vitamin B_6 and methylprednisolone has also been reported to be effective in controlling severe hyperemesis.

Table 30.4: Recommended daily intake of various nutrient in pregnancy

Protein	50 g	*
Thiamin	1.0 mg	*
Riboflavin	1.5 mg	*
Niacin	14-16 mg niacin equivalents	*
Vitamin B_6	1.0-1.5 mg	*
Total folate	400 µg	**
Vitamin B_{12}	3.0 µg	*
Vitamin C	60 mg	*
Zinc	16 mg	*
Iron	32-36 mg	***
Iodine	150 µg	*
Magnesium	300 µg	*
Calcium	1100 mg	*
Phosphorus	1200 mg	*
Selenium	80 µg	*
Vitamin A	750 IU retinal equivalents	
Vitamin E	7.0 IU α-tocopherol equivalents	
Sodium	920-2300 mg	
Potassium	1950-5460 mg	

* Indicates an increased requirement compared to nonpregnant female 19-54 years
** Daily requirement is doubled to 400 µg daily
RDI = 200 µg in a nonpregnant female 19-54 years
*** RDI is expressed as a range to account for differences in bioavailability in foods. RDI is for second and third trimesters.

Heart Burn

This is one of the most common complaints of pregnant women. It is caused by reflux of gastric contents into the lower esophagus resulting from the upward displacement and compression of the stomach by the uterus combined with relaxation of the lower esophageal sphincter. In most patients symptoms are relieved by a regimen of more frequent but smaller meals and avoidance of bending over or lying flat. Antacid preparation may provide symptomatic relief.

Pica

There has been popular notion for the alleged cravings (Pica) of pregnant women for strange food and even nonfood as ice (pagophagia), starch (amylophegia) or clay (geophagia). But scientific observations suggest that Pica is more legend than reality.

Pityalism

Excessive salivation (sialism, ptyalism) is an infrequent but troublesome complaint of pregnant women. Most cases are unexplained.

Bowel Habits

Constipation is common because of reduced gastrointestinal motility and compression of the lower bowel by the uterus and the fetus. Bleeding and painful fissures may develop in the edematous and hyperemic rectal mucosa. There is more frequency of hemorrhoids. Taking sufficient quantities of fluid and high roughage diet and reasonable amount of daily exercise relieves the symptoms. Sometimes stool softening agents can be prescribed.

Care of Teeth

Examination of the teeth should be included in the prenatal examinations and good dental hygiene is encouraged. Dental carries is not aggravated by pregnancy. Likewise pregnancy is not a contraindication to dental treatment.

Backache

Low back pain to some extent is reported in half of the pregnant women. Back pain can be reduced by having women squat rather bend over when reaching down and by using back support with a pillow when sitting down. However, severe backache should not be attributed simply to pregnancy until a thorough orthopedic examination has been conducted.

Varicosities

These engorged and enlarged veins generally result from congenital predisposition and are exaggerated by prolonged standing, pregnancy and advancing age. Varicose vein becomes more prominent as pregnancy advances as weight increases and if length of time spent upright is prolonged. *The treatment is generally limited to periodic rest with elevation of the legs, elastic stockings or both.*

Exercise

In general it is not necessary for the pregnant women to limit exercise, if she does not become excessively fatigued or risk injury.

Employment

Law in most of the nations prohibits employers from excluding women from job categories on the basis that they are or might become pregnant. However, any occupation that subjects the pregnant women to severe physical strain should be avoided.

Travel

Travel by healthy women has no harmful effects on the pregnancy. Travel in properly pressurized aircraft also poses no unusual risk.

Coitus

If there is risk of abortion or preterm labor, coitus should be avoided. In general in last 4 weeks abstinence should be preferred.

Fatigue

Early in pregnancy most women complain of fatigue and desire for excessive period of sleep. The condition usually remits spontaneously by the 4th month of pregnancy. Persistent fatigue may be sign of nutritional anemia, infection, cardiac problem and should be thoroughly evaluated.

Leukorrhea

In pregnancy there is usually increased vaginal discharge which is caused by increased mucus formation by cervical glands in response to hyperestrogenism. However, in women with history of preterm labor, reproductive tract infection, the complaint should be evaluated by proper perspeculum examination, smear and relevant investigation.

Smoking, Caffeine and Alcohol

Smoking and alcohol should be avoided in pregnancy, because of multiple effects on maternal and fetal health.

Medications

With exception of any drug that exerts a systemic effect in the mother will cross the placenta to reach the embryo and fetus. All physicians should develop the habit of confirming the likelihood of pregnancy before prescribing any drug for women.

Maternal Immunization During Pregnancy

Current recommendations for immunization during pregnancy are summarized in Table 30.5.

DIAGNOSIS OF PREGNANCY

The diagnosis of pregnancy is usually made on the basis of a history of amenorrhea and a positive pregnancy test. Sometimes it may be crucial to diagnose pregnancy before the first missed menstrual period to prevent exposure of fetus to X-ray or teratogenic drugs, to manage ectopic or nonviable pregnancies and to provide better health care for the mother.

The manifestation of pregnancy can be classified into three groups:
(a) Presumptive, (b) Probable, (c) Positive

Presumptive Manifestation

Symptoms

a. *Amenorrhea:* Cessation of menstrual bleeding is caused by increasing estrogen and progesterone levels produced by the corpus luteum. Thus, amenorrhea is a fairly reliable symptom of pregnancy in healthy reproductive aged women who have regular menstrual cycles. Spotting

Table 30.5: Recommendation for immunization during pregnancy	
Live virus vaccine	Inactivated bacterial vaccine
Measles contraindicated	Pneumococcal—same as nonpregnant
Mumps contraindicated	Meningococcus—same as nonpregnant
Varicella zoster contraindicated	Hemophiliac— same as nonpregnant
Live bacterial vaccine:	Cholera—risk vs benefits
Typhoid (Ty 1 a1) Risk Vs Benefit	*Toxoid:*
Poliomyelitis—no longer recommended	Tetanus—Diphtheria—same as nonpregnant
Yellow fever—only in high-risk area	
Inactivated virus vaccine:	
Influenza—after first trimester request	
Rabies—same as nonpregnant	
Hepatitis A and B—same as nonpregnant	
Enhanced poliomyelitis risk of exposure	
Japanese encephalitis—weigh risk vs benefits	
Hyperimmunoglobulin:	
Hepatitis B: Postexposure prophylaxis along with hepatitis B vaccine initially then vaccine alone 1 and 6 months	
Rabies: Postexposure prophylaxis	
Tetanus: Postexposure prophylaxis	
Varicella: Consider for postexposure within 96 hours	
Pooled immune serum globulin:	
Hepatitis A: Postexposure prophylaxis	
Measles: Postexposure prophylaxis	

caused by bleeding at implantation site may occur from the time of implantation until 29-35 days after the LMP in many women. Conversely delayed menses without pregnancy may be caused by other factors such as emotional tension, chronic disease, opioid and dopaminergic medication, endocrine disorders and certain genitourinary tumors.

b. *Nausea and vomiting:* This common symptom occurs in approximately 50% of pregnancies and is most marked at 2-12 weeks gestation.
c. *Breast changes:* In first pregnancy breast changes are quite characteristic. There is mastodynia or breast tenderness. There is enlargement of circumlacteal sebaceous glands of the areola (Montgomery's tubercles) at 6-8 weeks gestation. Colostrum secretion may begin after 16 weeks gestation. In nullipara these signs are less obvious.
d. *Quickening:* The first perception of fetal movement occurs at 18-20 weeks in primigravida and or 14-16 weeks in multigravida, which is termed quickening.
e. *Urinary tract:* There is slight increase in urinary frequency because of increased bladder circulation and pressure from the enlarging uterus. Urinary tract infection must always be ruled out because pregnant women are more likely than nonpregnant women to have significant bacteriuria which may at times be asymptomatic. Asymptomatic bacteriuria should be treated preferably in accordance with urine culture and sensitivity report because this can lead to pyelonephritis, which is associated with miscarriage, preterm birth and intrauterine fetal demise.

Signs of Pregnancy

1. *Increased basal body temperature:* There is persistent elevation of basal body temperature over a 3 weeks period.
2. *Skin changes:* There is *chloasma* (a darkening of the skin over the forehead, bridge of the nose, or cheekbones). Chloasma usually occurs after 16 weeks gestation and is intensified by exposure to sunlight. **Linea nigrae** is darkening of lower midline of the abdomen from umbilicus to the pubis. These changes are caused by stimulation of melanophores induced by increase in melanocyte stimulating hormone. Stretch marks or striae of breast and abdomen are caused by adrenocorticosteroid response induced separation of collagen.

Probable Manifestation

a. Symptoms are as presumptive ones.
b. **Signs:**

CHAPTER -30 ♦ Preconceptional Counseling, Physiological Changes in Pregnancy and Antenatal Care

Pelvic organs: Following signs are elicitible due to changes in pelvic organs by experienced physician:

i. *Chadwick's sign:* It is bluish discoloration of vagina and cervix caused by congestion of the pelvic vasculature.
ii. *Changes in cervical mucus:* There is an increase in vaginal discharge due to hormonal stimulation. Cervical mucus if spread on glass slide and allowed to dry no longer forms a fernlike pattern but has a granular appearance.
iii. *Hegar's sign:* This is widening of softened area of isthmus, resulting in compressibility of the isthmus on bimanual examination and can be elicited in 2/3rd of cases between 6-10 weeks.
iv. Bone and pelvic ligaments are relaxed, which is most pronounced at pubic symphysis.
v. *Palmer's sign:* At 4-8 weeks regular and rhythmic uterine contraction can be elicited on bimanual examination.
vi. *Osiander sign:* There is increased pulsation felt through lateral fornices at 8 weeks.
vii. *Goodell's sign:* Softening of cervix around 6 weeks.
viii. *Abdominal enlargement:* There is progressive abdominal enlargement from 7-28 weeks. At 16-22 weeks growth may appear more rapid, as the uterus rises out of pelvis and into the abdomen.
ix. *Uterine contraction:* The pregnant uterus is soft and elastic in consistency. On bimanual examination during early pregnancy, it is felt to undergo regular painless rhythmic contraction (Palmer's sign). As the pregnancy progresses the interval between the contractions become longer. *Braxton Hicks contractions* are painless uterine contractions which are felt as tightening during the third trimester. These contractions usually disappear with walking or exercise, whereas in true labor contraction becomes more intense.

Positive Manifestation

The above mentioned signs and symptoms of pregnancy are often reliable but none is diagnostic. A positive diagnosis must be made on objective findings. These are as follows:

a. *Detection of fetal heart tones:* It is possible to detect fetal heart tone as early as 10-12 weeks by hand held Doppler and by stethoscope by 20 weeks of gestation.
b. *Palpation of fetal parts:* After 22 weeks the fetal outline can be palpated through the maternal abdominal wall.
c. *Ultrasound examination of fetus:* Sonography is one of the most useful technical aids in diagnosing and monitoring pregnancy.

Pregnancy Test

Detection of βhCG in maternal blood or urine provides the basis for endocrine test of pregnancy. This hormone is a glycoprotein with high carbohydrate content. It is a heterodimer composed of two dissimilar subunits – α and β which are noncovalently linked. The alpha subunit is similar to those of LH, FSH and TSH. hCG prevents involution of the corpus luteum, the principal site of progesterone formation during the first 6 weeks. It can be detected by following test:

1. *Urine pregnancy test:* This is the most common method used to confirm pregnancy, which use antibodies identifying the β subunit of hCG. Test is quick, affordable, reliable and fast tool to diagnose pregnancy in OPD. The urine pregnancy test is qualitative—positive or negative based on color change with the level of hCG detection ranging between 5-50 mIU/ml, depending on the kit used.
2. *Home pregnancy test:* hCG is detected in a first voided morning urine sample, because the accuracy of the home pregnancy test depends on technique and interpretation, it should always be repeated in the office.
3. *Serum pregnancy test:* hCG can be detected in the serum as early as a week after conception. The serum pregnancy test can be quantitative or qualitative with a very low threshold level of 2-4 mIU/ml depending on the technique. *The serum pregnancy test is a reliable method to diagnose an early pregnancy especially in women with recurrent early pregnancy failure, in follow-up of assisted reproductive technology technique, threatened abortion, ectopic pregnancy.*

PRENATAL DIAGNOSIS

The incidence of major abnormalities discovered at birth is 2-3%. Prenatal diagnosis is the science of identifying these structural or functional abnormalities in the developing fetus with prenatal diagnosis. Prenatal diagnosis hope to alter the severity of congenital disease by offering an ever expanding choice of fetal treatment or surveillance as well as optimal delivery in some situation or consideration of pregnancy termination in others. It is important to remember that most such infants are delivered of mothers with no known risk factor for a fetal malformation. The general public believes that most birth defect occur because of exposure during pregnancy to teratogenic drugs, chemicals, X-ray or viruses. However, the available scientific data reveal that **of all birth defects only 2% are due to exposure to these teratogens. Ninety-eight percent occur secondary to random mutations, the expression of lethal genes in the parents, autosomal or multifactorial genetic expression, and aneuploidy and so on.** This tremendous public confusion has substantially increased the difficult challenge obstetrician face when a malformed baby is delivered. Therefore, the obstetrician has an increased responsibility to detect fetal anomalies in those gravidas at risk.

Diagnostic evaluation typically involves 3 major categories:
1. Fetuses at high-risk for a genetic or congenital disorder.
2. Fetuses at unknown risk for congenital abnormalities.

3. Fetuses discovered ultrasonographically to have structural or developmental abnormalities.

Indication of Prenatal Diagnosis

In following conditions prenatal diagnosis should be offered:

Mothers at risk for having a congenital abnormal fetus with any of the following:
a. Chromosomal abnormality
b. Genetic disease
c. Neural tube defects
d. Congenital malformation

Mothers with:
a. Teratogen exposure
b. Abnormal maternal serum screening test
c. Abnormal ultrasound examination
d. Family history of chromosomal/congenital abnormalities
e. Exposure to infections
f. Others:
   i. History of prior neonatal death
   ii. Hemoglobinopathies
   iii. Tay-Sachs disease
   iv. Cystic fibrosis
   v. Fragile X-syndrome.

Fetus at high-risk for genetic or congenital disorder:
a. Maternal age of 35 years or older
b. Previous child with a chromosomal abnormality
c. Chromosomal abnormality in either parent, including balanced translocation, aneuploidy or mosaicism
d. Chromosomal abnormality in a close family member
e. Abnormal fetus in ultrasound scan
f. Abnormal maternal serum screening test/abnormal triple screen (α-Fetoprotein AFP) estriol ($4E_3$) β hCG.
g. Prior child with neural tube defects.

Principle of Genetic Disorders and Sex Chromosome Anomalies

Single Gene Defect

Single gene defect yield a specific abnormality and are classified as follows in decreasing frequency as: (a) Dominant, (b) Recessive, (c) X-linked

Types of inheritance: It can be: (a) Autosomal dominant, (b) Autosomal recessive, (c) X-linked recessive

Autosomal dominant: In this it is assumed that a mutation has occurred in 1 gene of an allelic pair and that the presence of this new gene produces enough of changed protein to give a different phenotypic effect. The characteristic of autosomal dominant inheritance:
a. The trait appears with equal frequency in both sexes.
b. For inheritance to take place at least 1 parent must have the trait unless a new mutation has just occurred.
c. When a homozygous individual is mated to a normal individual, all offspring will carry the trait. When a heterozygous individual is mated to a normal individual 50% of the offspring. The examples of autosomal dominant conditions and traits are:
   i. Achondroplasia
   ii. Accoustic neuroma
   iii. Color blindness yellow blue
   iv. Mitral valve prolapse
   v. Several form of deafness
   vi. Muscular dystrophy
   vii. Intestinal polyposis, Keloid formation

Autosomal recessive: In this type of inheritance the mutant gene will not be capable of producing a new characteristic. In the heterozygous state in this circumstance under customary environmental condition, i.e. with 50% of the genetic material producing the new protein; the phenotypic effect will not be different from that of the normal trait. When the environment is manipulated the recessive trait occasionally becomes dominant. The characteristic of this form of inheritance is as follows:
a. The characteristic will occur with equal frequency in both sexes.
b. For the characteristic to be present, both parents must be carrier of the recessive trait.
c. If both parents are homozygous for the recessive trait all offspring will have it.
d. If both parents are heterozygous for the recessive trait 25% of the offspring will have it.
e. In pedigree showing frequent occurrence of individuals with rare recessive characteristics, consanguinity is often present for, e.g. albenism, total color blindness, cystic fibrosis, Wilson's disease.

X-linked recessive: This condition occurs when a gene on the X chromosome undergoes mutation and the new protein formed as a result of this mutation is incapable of producing a change in phenotype characteristic in the heterozygous state. As the male has only one X chromosome the presence of this mutant will allow for expression should it occur in the male. The following are characteristics of this form of inheritance:
a. The condition occurs more commonly in male than in female.
b. If both parents are normal and an affected male is produced, its must be assumed that the mother is a carrier of a trait.
c. If the father is affected and an affected male is produced, the mother must be at least heterozygous for the trait.
d. A female with a trait may be produced in 1 or 2 ways:
   i. She may inherit a recessive gene from both her mother and her father, if the father is affected and mother is heterozygous.
   ii. She may inherit a recessive gene from one of her parents and may express the recessive characteristics as a

function of the **Lyon hypothesis**. It assumes that all female are mosaics for their functioning X chromosomes. In this it is assumed that at about the time of implantation each cell in the developing female embryo selects one X chromosome as its functioning X and that all progeny cells thereafter use this X chromosome as their functioning X chromosome. The other X chromosome becomes inactive. Because this selection is done on a random basis, it is conceivable that some females will be produced who will be using primarily the X chromosomes bearing the recessive gene. Thus a genotypically heterozygous individual may demonstrate a recessive characteristic phenotypically on this basis. Egs are complete and incomplete androgen insensitivity syndrome, red green color blindness, and diabetes insipidus.

X-linked dominant: In this situation the mutation will produce a protein that when present in the heterozygous state is sufficient to cause a change in characteristic. The following are characteristic of this type of inheritance:
a. The characteristic occurs with the same frequency in males and females.
b. An affected male mated to a normal female will produce the characteristics in 50% of the offspring.
c. An affected homozygous female mated to a normal male will produce the affected characteristic in all offspring.
d. A heterozygous female mated to a normal male will produce the characteristic in 50% of the offspring.
e. Occasional heterozygous females may not show the dominant trait on the basis of Lyon hypothesis, e.g. orofacial digital syndrome, hyperammonemia.

Polygenic Inheritance

Polygenic inheritance is defined as the inheritance of a single phenotypic feature as a result of the effects of many genes. Most physical features in humans are determined by polygenic inheritance. Many common malformations are determined in this way also. For example, cleft palate with or without cleft lip, club foot, anencephaly, meningomyelocele, dislocation of the hip, and pyloric stenosis. Each occurs with an approximate incidence of 0.5-2/1000. These anomalies are present in siblings of affected infants, when both parents are normal at a rate of 2-5%. They are also found more commonly among relatives than in general population. The increase in incidence is not environmentally induced because the frequency of such abnormalities in monozygotic twin is 4-8 times higher than that of dizygotic twins and siblings. *The higher incidence in monozygotic twin is called concordance. Sex* also plays a role in polygenic inheritance, for example, cleft lip occurs in 6% of the offspring of women with cleft lip as opposed to 2.8% of offspring of men with cleft lip.

Many racial variations in disease are believed to be transmitted by polygenic inheritance, which makes a social background—a determinant of how prone an individual will be to a particular defect. Environment also plays a role in polygenic inheritance because seasonal variations alter some defects and their occurrence rate from country-to-country in similar populations.

Epigenetics

Epigenetics is the regulation of gene expression not encoded in the nucleotide sequence of the gene. Gene expression can either be turned on and off by DNA methylation or histone modification (Methylation, acetylation, phosphorylation or ADP—ribosylation). Epigenetic can subsequently be inherited by its descendents.

Genomic Imprinting

Genomic imprinting is an epigenetic process by which male and female genomes are definitely expressed. The imprinting mark on genes is either by DNA methylation or histone modification. The imprinting patterns are different according to paternal origin of the genes. Genomic imprints are erased in primordial germ cells and re-established again during gemetogenesis. **The imprinting process is completed by the time of round spermatid formation in males and at ovulation of metaphase II oocytes in females.** The imprinted gene survives the global waves of DNA methylation and remethylation during early embryonic development. In normal children the set of chromosome is derived from the father and other from the mother. If both sets of chromosomes are from only one parent, the imprinted genes expression will be unbalanced, e.g. in Prader-Willi syndrome both 15q/3 regions are from the father and in Angelman syndrome both 15q/3 regions are from the mother.

Cytogenetics

Chromosomes

The chromatin of human nucleus is arranged in 46 chromosomes (22 pairs of autosomes and one pair of sex chromosomes XX or XY). Each chromosome contains a double helix of deoxyribonucleic acid. The autosomes are grouped according to size. Group 'A' being the largest and group 'G' is the smallest. When the centromere is centrally placed, the chromosome is *metacentric*. If it is off the center the chromosome is *submetacentric*, and if it is near the end of one arm it is *acrocentric*. The chromosome adjacent to centromere consists largely of genetically inert heterochromatin which remains densely coiled during interphase (euchromatin only becomes coiled during mitosis or meiosis).

Chromosomes which are not metacentric have long arm and short arms. Chromosomes are similar in size and shape may be distinguished by means of banding techniques with dyes such as **quinacrine (Q banding) and Giemsa**

(G binding). G and Q banding technique stains the same adenine—thymine rich portions of chromosomes and a reverse technique (R banding) stains guanine—cytosine rich areas. Banding pattern shows genetic polymorphism.

In the female (XX) one of the X chromosome exists in a tightly coiled form and after staining with basic dyes can be seen as the **sex chromatin or barr body**. As according to Lyon hypothesis only the terminal portion of the arm of this chromosome remains active. Inactivation of one of the X chromosome is controlled by a specific inactivation site in the X chromosome. Thus the female carrier of an X-linked defficiency will have 50% of the normal amount of different substance, e.g. a carrier of hemophilia will have about 50% of the normal level of factor VIII. The short stature of patients with Turner's syndrome is due to loss of a gene in the short arm (p) arm of X and genes in the long (q) arm are critical for ovarian development.

The Y chromosome is less than half the size of the X chromosome and can be identified by brilliant fluorescence of the outer two-third of the long arm (q) after aquamarine staining. The genes for testicular formation (testis determining factor TDF) are situated in the short arm.

The Cell Cycle

The cell cycle is divided into phase G_0-G_1-S-G_2-M. S is the phase of nucleic acid synthesis and DNA replication and M is the phase of mitosis once the cell has moved from quiescence G_0 to G_1, there are 3 possibilities:
1. Progression to mitosis and division
2. Arrest in G_1
3. Cell death

The cell death is the process of apoptosis which differs from necrosis in that there is no loss of membrane integrity or inflammatory reactions. The apoptotic cell is removed by adjacent cells or macrophages.

Mitosis and Meiosis

Mitosis

During S phase of the cell cycle, the 2 DNA strands of a chromosome separate. Each strand then acts as a template for the formation of a complementary strand; the resulting double strand is thus identical with parental DNA.
a. *Prophase:* The duplicated chromatin condenses into well defined chromosomes joined at the centromere and the centrioles and their associated microtubules from the mitotic spindle.
b. *Metaphase:* In this the chromosomes assemble at the mid point of the spindle called metaphase plate. *In this phase the chromosomes can be visualized by karyotyping and identified by banding.*
c. *Anaphase:* In anaphase the new sets of chromosomes separate to opposing poles of the nucleus guided by mitotic spindle.
d. *Telophase:* The nuclear reforms in the telophase.

Cytokinesis: The cytoplasmic contents are divided.

Meiosis

Meiosis occurs only in germ cells in the ovary and testis and involves two successive divisions:

Ist Stage

Each of the 46 chromosomes duplicates into two chromatids, which remains attached at the centromere. They assemble side to side in homologous pairs except for the X and Y chromosomes in the male, which assemble end to end. Cross linkage and recombination at chiasmata leads to an interchange of DNA. This does not occur between the X and Y chromosome which overlap end to end, but do not pair side by side. The short arm of X chromosome is involved in this partial coupling. The long arm sometimes loops back to reach the other end of the Y chromosomes. The X and Y chromosome occupy a separate site on the meiotic spindle, the sex chromosome vesicle. The prophase stage of 1st meiotic division is summarized: (a) Leptotene, (b) Zygotene (c) Pachytene, (d) Diptotene, (e) Diakinesis (Fig. 30.3).

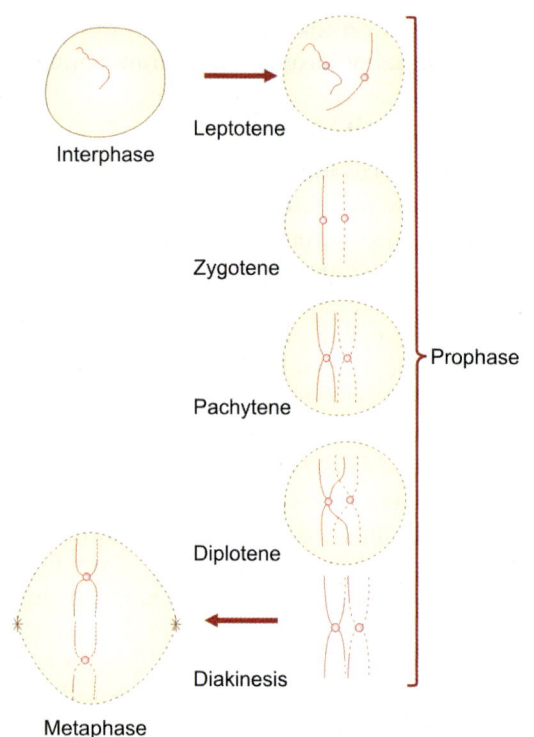

Fig. 30.3: First Stage of meiosis

IInd Meiotic Division

In second meiotic division there is no replication of DNA. In the testis the result of meiosis is the formation of 4 spermatids from germ cells. **Each spermatid has one chromosome from pair (haploid). In the ovary only one oocyte is formed from the two meiotic divisions. The excess genetic maternal is extruded as two polar bodies**—one at the first meiotic division (containing 23 paired strands of DNA) and one at the second meiotic division (containing 23 single strands of DNA). *The process of meiosis in the oocyte is arrested at the diplotene stage around time of birth and resumed just prior to time of ovulation.*

In the oocyte both X chromosomes are active, whereas in sperm the single X chromosome is inactive. In the extraembryonic tissues including the placenta of an XX embryo, it is always paternally inherited X chromosome which is inactivated.

CHROMOSOMAL ABNORMALITIES

Trisomy

It is the presence of an extra chromosome and these are most common type of chromosomal abnormality. Most Trisomies are lethal causing failures of implantation or early abortion. The three most common surviving autosomal trisomies are—**Trisomies 21 (Down syndrome), 13 (Patau syndrome) and 18 (Edward's syndrome).** Even in these cases most affected embryos are aborted, e.g. only 20% of Down's embryo attain viability. **The best known Trisomy of sex chromosome is XXY —Klinefelter's syndrome**.

Monosomy

Only one monosomy, where one of the chromosomes is absent, occurs. **This is called Turner's syndrome (XO), where one of the X chromosomes is missing.** This is the most common abnormality at conception.

Mechanism for Formation of a Trisomy

Nondysjunction

It is the most common cause of chromosomal abnormality. It is a failure of the relevant chromosomes to separate at meiosis, usually during the first phase. After fertilization the zygotes has either an extra chromosome (e.g. XXY) or a missing chromosome (e.g. XO). Nondysjunction takes place in the mother. This becomes more common with advancing maternal age. Nondysjunction in the father is not related to paternal age. In 80% of cases of Turner's syndrome the meiotic error arises in the father. Aneuploid ova and sperm are common and loss of chromosome is more common than an additional chromosome in the secondary oocytes. Some of these are the result not of nondysjunction, but of anaphase lag, where a chromosome is excluded from a new cell during division. 10% of sperm and nearly 50% of secondary oocytes are aneuploid.

Mosaic

It is an individual with cells of different chromosome constitution arising from the same zygote. **This may be due to nondysjunction during early divisions or anaphase lag.** In anaphase lag the chromosome is delayed during its return down the nuclear spindles and does not reach the cell before the nuclear membrane closes. This gives rise to a mosaicism with a normal and an abnormal cell line.

Chimera

In this also there are cells of separate constitution, but **two cell lines result from too zygote lineage, e.g. fertilization of both the polar body and the ovum, which subsequently fuse** or fertilization of two ova, which then fuse. The rare XX/XY from of gonadal dysgenesis occurs in this way.

Translocation

It is transfer of a segment of one chromosome to another. The outcome is two morphologically new chromosomes. If the total chromosomal complement is unchanged this is harmless and described as *balanced*. Such an individual is however a carrier. When a break occurs in two chromosomes and the chromosome material is exchanged between the two, the translocation is said to be reciprocal. If the breakage occurs at the centromere of two acrocentric chromosomes, the tiny short arm fragments are lost and the long arms join together. This is known as *Robertsonian translocation or centric fusion* (Fig. 30.4).

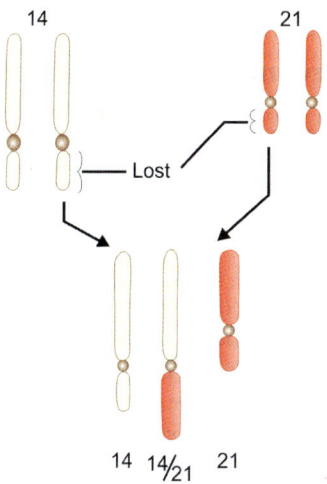

Fig. 30.4: Robertsonian translocation

Deletion

If a break in chromosome takes place and the fragment is lost; deletion has occurred. If the deletion is such that the cell cannot survive, the condition may be lethal. If a break takes place at either end of a chromosome and the chromosome heals by having the two ends fuse together, a ring chromosome is formed. Examples of these have been seen clinically in all of the chromosomes of the karyotype and generally they exhibit a variety of phenotypic abnormalities.

Isochromosomes

At times chromosome will divide by a horizontal rather than longitudinal split of the centromere. So one daughter cell receives both long arms and other both short arms of the chromosome. Such chromosomes are referred to as an isochromosome and individual is essentially trisomic for 1 arm and monosomic for the other arm of the chromosome.

Inversion

It is occurrence of two breaks within the chromosomes and rotation of the center fragments at 180 degrees. So the realignment allows for a change in morphology of the chromosome although the original number of genes is preserved.

APPLIED GENETICS

Currently the most common use for applied genetics in obstetrics and gynecology is in prenatal counseling, screening and diagnosis. Prenatal diagnosis first came into use in 1977 with the discovery of direct relationship of serum alpha fetoproteins and incidence of neural tube defects. Nowadays we can screen not only for NTDs but also for Trisomy 21 and Trisomy 18. In addition cystic fibrosis, sickle cell and Hutington's disease as well many inborn errors of metabolism and other genetic disorders can now be identified prenatal.

Prenatal Screening and Diagnostic Test

The distinction between screening and diagnosis is often blurred in common usage. *Screening test* is performed in all women in order to identify a subset of patients who are at high-risk of disorder. They do not confer any risk to pregnancy and performed for disorders with a relatively high prevalence for which there is an accurate prenatal diagnostic test. **Diagnostic test** can be, on the other hands are carried out on pregnancies that have been identified as high-risk by a prior screening test. They are usually invasive and carry a small risk of miscarriage. So the risk of being affected by the conditions should be severe enough to warrant consideration for a diagnostic test. Difference between prenatal screening and diagnostic test are summarized in Table 30.6.

Table 30.6: Difference between prenatal screening and diagnostic test

	Screening	Diagnostic test
Population tested	All women	Women at high-risk
Purpose of test	Select a high-risk group	To diagnose abnormalities
Usual method of testing	Maternal history Maternal biochemistry Maternal virology ultrasound	Ultrasound Amniocentesis Chorion villous Sampling Cordocentesis
Prerequisite of test	Diagnostic test available	Patient aware potential risk
Risk of test	Anxiety of a screen Positive result	Small risk of miscarriage

The aim of prenatal diagnosis is related to identification of fetal abnormality so that:

a. Parents can be reassessed by reducing the likelihood of undiagnosed fetal abnormality.
b. Maximum information can be given to parents if there is any abnormality detected and assist them in decision-making.
c. If parents decide to continue with pregnancy, patient should be mentally prepared.
d. Allow appropriate perinatal management and intrauterine treatment.
e. Enable parents at risk of inherited conditions to have healthy children by diagnosis of abnormality and termination of affected fetus.

The incidence and classification of common congenital abnormalities are summarized in Table 30.7.

Techniques Used in Prenatal Diagnosis

a. Maternal serum screening/multiple marker screen
b. Ultrasound
c. Chorionic villus sampling

Table 30.7: Classification of congenital abnormalities

Congenital abnormalities	Example	Incidence per 1000 birth
Structure	Congenital heart disease	4-6
	Neural tube defect	2-6
	Cleft lip/palate	1-2
	Talipes equinovarus	1
Chromosomal	Trisomy 21 (Down syndrome)	1.5
	Monosomy (Turner's syndrome)	0.3
	Other Trisomies 13,18	0.3
Genetic	Cystic fibrosis	0.5
	Sickle cell disease	Depends on ethnicity
Miscellaneous	Viral infection	0.2

d. Amniocentesis
e. Magnetic resonance imaging (MRI)
f. Percutaneous umbilical blood sampling
g. Ultrasound-guided tissue biopsy.

Multiple Marker Screen

These test use biochemical markers in the maternal serum to calculate the risk for a birth defect and chromosomal anomaly. The most common abnormalities for which risk can be calculated are NTD, Trisomy 21, Trisomy 18 and Trisomy 13.

In the multiple marker screen serum, α fetoprotein, hCG, unconjugated estriol (μE_3) and inhibin A are used. AFP was the first fetal biochemical analog found to have altered serum concentration in the mother of a fetus with Down syndrome. AFP is produced by the yolk sac first, then fetal gastrointestinal tract and fetal liver. **The AFP level and maternal age can be used to calculate a risk for Down syndrome. The AFP is about 20% lower in the serum of mother of fetus with a Down syndrome. hCG produced by the placenta is about twice as high in the serum of a woman with a fetus with Down syndrome. E_3 is 25% lower than normal.** It is produced by the fetal adrenal gland, fetal liver and placenta. The three values are combined and a specific risk for an individual pregnancy is given. Inhibin A is low in Trisomy 21 and 18. In calculation of multiple marker test the other information which should be considered are: (a) Maternal age, (b) Gestational age, (c) Race, (d) Diabetes mellitus, (e) Maternal weight.

Ultrasound

For pregnancies at risk of a malformation or a genetic disorder based on family history, results of MSAFP screening, exposure to teratogen or infections or maternal conditions, detailed target scanning of fetus is indicated. **Fetal echocardiography** is done to determine fetal congenital heart defect and indicated (i) When a first degree relative (Sibling or parent) has a cardiac defect, (ii) The fetus has a chromosomal abnormality, (iii) Malformation or suspected cardiac defect detected by ultrasonography, (iv) The fetus is at risk for a genetic disorder associated with a cardiac defect, (v) The mother has insulin dependent diabetes, (vi) The mother uses a medications associated with a cardiac defects. The RCOG (UK) has recommended a two stage scan program for screening for structural abnormalities: **An initial scan at booking (11-14 weeks) and further scan at or around 20 weeks.**

A detailed anatomic ultrasound scan of fetus can detect anatomic congenital anomalies and also there are ultrasound genetics markers, which give clue to chromosomal abnormalities and help in selecting the fetus for further evaluation. Some of genetic markers for trisomy are:
a. Small for date fetus
b. Short femur
c. Echogenic bowl
d. Heart malformation
e. Thickened nuchal fold.

Chorionic Villus Sampling (CVS)

CVS is a procedure in which placental tissue is obtained between 10 and 12 weeks for cytogenetic studies. The primary advantage of CVS is that results are available earlier in pregnancy which decreases parental anxiety when results are normal. At the same time it allows earlier and safer method of pregnancy termination, when they are abnormal. CVS is generally performed at 10-13 weeks. Placental villi are obtained through transabdominal or transcervical access to the placenta. The complications are slightly higher miscarriage rate of 1-5% and an association with distal limb defect. An amniotic fluid AFP cannot be done simultaneously. **Maternal serum AFP and fetal anatomic ultrasound survey are recommended at around 16 weeks and at 18-20 weeks, respectively.**

Genetic Amniocentesis

It is a technique in which amniotic fluid is removed from around the fetus. Amniocentesis is generally carried out at 15-17 weeks of gestation with the risk of procedure related losses of 1 in 200-3000. **Early amniocentesis is done before 16 weeks**. The pregnancy loss rate following early amniocentesis is 2.5% and other complication is *fetal club foot (Talipes)*. Beside this there is significantly higher cell culture failure. So many countries do not recommend amniocentesis before 15 weeks.

In this under ultrasound guidance, a 20-22-gauge special needle is passed into amniotic sac, avoiding the placenta, umbilical cord and fetus. The initial aspirate of 1-2 ml of fluid is discarded to decrease the chance of maternal cell contamination. Approximately 20 ml of fluid is collected for analysis and needle is removed. The puncture site is observed for bleeding and fetal heart rate is monitored. **The fluid or the cells suspended in the fluid can be used for specific metabolic tests, recombinant DNA technique or obtaining a karyotype (chromosomes).**

Percutaneous Umbilical Cord Blood Sampling (PUBS)

Ultrasound-guided aspiration of a fetal blood sample can be obtained generally from 18 weeks gestation onwards. Sampling can be done from the umbilical cord and fetal intrahepatic vein. The fetus may need to be immobilized via medication.

Advantage and Disadvantage of PUBS

Advantage of PUBS are access to the entire spectrum of diagnostic studies afforded by a peripheral blood sample, including karyotype in 48 hours and hematologic infections, immunologic and acid-base assessment and for treatment of such condition as fetal arrhythmia, Hydrops fetalis. Disadvantages are 3-5/100 fetal loss rate depending on circumstances.

Laboratory Analysis of Invasive Diagnostic Test

a. *Cytogenetic analysis:* Cells obtained from invasive diagnostic tests are cultured until enough cells in mitosis are available to make a cytogenetic diagnosis. The more rapidly the tissue divides, the quicker the results are available. Hence, the time taken for diagnosis for amniocentesis is 2-3 weeks, for CVS 1-2 weeks and cordocentesis is 24-48 hours. *The use of FISH* (Florence *in situ* hybridization) can facilitate rapid results with amniocentesis. The FISH technique detects and localizes specific DNA sequence directly in interphase or metaphase, so cell culture is not required. It allows the rapid prenatal diagnosis of major aneuploidies for chromosome 13, 18, 21 and XY in 24-28 hours.

b. *DNA analysis*: Fetal DNA obtained from invasive test can be used for DNA probe (sickle cell disease and cystic fibrosis), PCR for fragile X syndrome.

c. *Biochemical and enzymatic analysis:* When DNA analysis is not possible, biochemical or enzymatic assays can be performed for specific disease like congenital adrenal hyperplasia and mucopolysaccharidosis.

Preimplantation Genetic Diagnosis (PGD)

PGD for prenatal diagnosis involves participation in an *in vitro* fertilization program and is currently available for a limited number of genetic conditions. The basis for PGD is as—**early in human gestation, when the vast majority of cells are destined for trophoblastic development, a single cell at the 8 cell stage or a dozen cells at the blastocyst stage can be removed without subsequent damage to the fetus.** These cells provide sufficient DNA for PCR directed molecular analysis of inherited disease or fluorescent *in situ* hybridization for aneuploidy (FISH).

Fetal Cells in Maternal Circulation

Acquisition of fetal DNA without invasive studies has been an area of research for several decades. Attempts are underway to identify the most sufficient means of isolating the fewer cells from the overwhelming number of maternal cells. Once isolated, fetal cells provide information about the fetus through PCR and molecular studies as fluorescent *in situ* hybridization for aneuploidy.

First trimester screening: It is an option that involves multiple serum screening and an early ultrasound.

MULTIPLE CHOICE QUESTIONS

1. Appropriate method for antenatal diagnosis of genetic disorders includes all of the following, *except:*
   a. Fetal blood
   b. Amniotic fluid
   c. Chorionic villi
   d. Maternal urine
   Ans. d

2. The risk of mongolism in a mother at the age of 20 years is 1:3000. What would be the ratio when she is 45-year-old:
   a. 1:6000
   b. 1:3000
   c. 1:1040
   d. 1:50
   Ans. d

3. AFP is raised in all, *except:*
   a. Polycystic kidney
   b. Trisomy
   c. IUD
   d. Esophageal atresia
   Ans. b

4. In which of the following condition would maternal serum AFP values be highest:
   a. Down syndrome
   b. Omphalocele
   c. Gastroschisis
   d. Spina bifida occulta
   Ans. c

5. The one measurement of fetal maturity that is not affected by a bloody tap during amniocentesis:
   a. L/S ratio
   b. Phosphatidylglycerol
   c. AFP
   d. Bilirubin measured by optical density at 450
   Ans. d

6. CVS done before 10 weeks may results in:
   a. Fetal loss
   b. Fetomaternal hemorrhage
   c. Oromandibular limb defect
   d. Sufficient material not obtained
   Ans. c

7. Mr and Mrs X has a 2-month-old baby suffering with Down syndrome. Karyotype of Mrs X shows a translocation variety of Down syndrome. Which of the following investigation you will advice before next pregnancy:
   a. Triple test
   b. AFP
   c. Karyotyping of father
   d. β-hCG
   Ans. c

8. Amniotic fluid contains acetyl cholinesterase enzymes, what is the diagnosis:
   a. Open spina bifida
   b. Gastroschisis
   c. Omphalocele
   d. Osteogenesis imperfecta
   Ans. a

Chapter -30 ♦ Preconceptional Counseling, Physiological Changes in Pregnancy and Antenatal Care

9. Which of the following test on maternal serum is most useful in distinguishing between open neural tube defect and ventral wall defects in a fetus?
   a. Carcinoembryonic antigen
   b. Sphingomyelin
   c. Alpha fetoprotein
   d. Pseudocholinesterase
   Ans. d
10. Which of the following fetus on second trimester ultrasound is not a marker of Down syndrome?
    a. Single umbilical artery
    b. Choroid plexus cyst
    c. Diaphragmatic hernia
    d. Duodenal atresia
    Ans. b
11. DNA analysis of chorionic villi/amniocentesis is not likely to detect:
    a. Tay-Sachs disease
    b. Hemophilia A
    c. Sickle cell disease
    d. Duchenne muscular dystrophy
    Ans. a
12. Earliest detectable congenital malformation by USG is:
    a. Anencephaly
    b. Spina bifida
    c. Meningocele
    d. Cystic hygroma
    Ans. a
13. What is the finding seen earliest on USG?
    a. Yolk sac
    b. Fetal heart
    c. Chorion
    d. Placenta
    Ans. a
14. At what level of β-hCG is that normal pregnancy can be earliest detected by TVS:
    a. 500 IU/ml
    b. 1000 IU/ml
    c. 1500 IU/ml
    d. 2000 IU/ml
    Ans. b
15. The best time to do chorionic villous sampling is:
    a. Between 6-8 weeks
    b. Between 7-9 weeks
    c. Between 9-11 weeks
    d. Between 11-13 weeks
    Ans. d
16. Which of the following is not diagnosed by chorionic villus biopsy:
    a. Neural tube defect
    b. Down syndrome
    c. Phenylketonuria
    d. Sickle cell anemia
    Ans. a
17. Which of the following is not done for maternal diagnosis of Down syndrome?
    a. Amniotic fluid volume estimation
    b. Alpha fetoprotein estimation
    c. Cordocentesis
    d. Chronic villus biopsy
    Ans. a
18. Nuchal translucency at 14 weeks is suggestive of:
    a. Down syndrome
    b. Esophageal atresia
    c. Trisomy 18
    d. Foregut duplication cyst
    Ans. a
19. Which of the following is not an indication for antiphospholipid antibody test:
    a. Three or more than one first trimester pregnancy loss
    b. Unexplained cerebrovascular accidents
    c. Early onset severe pre-eclampsia
    d. Gestational diabetes
    Ans. d
20. Most useful investigation in the first trimester to identify risk of fetal malformation in a diabetic mother is:
    a. Glycosylated hemoglobin
    b. Ultrasound
    c. MSAFP
    d. Amniocentesis
    Ans. a
21. Which one of the following is not a sign of early pregnancy:
    a. Goodell's sign
    b. Hegar's sign
    c. Cullen's sign
    d. Palmer's sign
    Ans. c
22. Hegar's sign of pregnancy is:
    a. Uterine contraction
    b. Bluish discoloration of vagina;
    c. Softening of isthmus
    d. Quickening
    Ans. c
23. Pregnancy is confirmed by:
    a. Morning sickness
    b. Fetal heart activity
    c. Fetal sac in USG
    d. Fetal movement by examiner
    Ans. b, c, d
24. Use of folic acid to prevent congenital anomalies should be best initiated:
    a. During first trimester of pregnancy
    b. During second trimester of pregnancy
    c. During third trimester of pregnancy
    d. Before conception
    Ans. d
25. Cardiac activity of fetus by transabdominal scan is seen earliest at what gestational age:
    a. 5th week
    b. 6th week
    c. 8th week
    d. 9th week
    Ans. c
26. Folic acid supplementation reduces the risk of:
    a. Neural tube defect
    b. Toxemias of pregnancy

c. Down syndrome
d. Placenta previa
Ans. a

27. Hegar's signs can be elicited by:
    a. 8 weeks
    b. 10 weeks
    c. 12 weeks
    d. 15 weeks
    Ans. a

28. Braxton Hicks contractions:
    a. Is a positive feedback system
    b. Is another term for labor contraction
    c. Occurs during most of the months of pregnancy
    d. Result in hypoxia if the fetus
    Ans. c

29. Calcium requirement per day during the third trimester of pregnancy:
    a. 20 mg
    b. 100 mg
    c. 750 mg
    d. 1000 mg
    Ans. d

30. Daily caloric needs in pregnancy is about:
    a. 1000 Kcal
    b. 1500 Kcal
    c. 2500 Kcal
    d. 3500 Kcal
    Ans. c

31. Which is the proper time to do pelvic assessment in primigravida:
    a. 32 weeks
    b. 34 weeks
    c. 36 weeks
    d. 40 weeks
    Ans. d

32. Quickening can be felt at ... weeks.
    a. 14 weeks
    b. 15 weeks
    c. 16 weeks
    d. 19 weeks
    Ans. c

33. Increased demand of following occurs in pregnancy, *except*:
    a. Folic acid
    b. Iron
    c. Vitamin B_{12}
    d. Zinc
    Ans. c

34. Term delivery implies that the gestational age of the fetus calculated from the time of onset of last menstrual period in:
    a. 40 weeks
    b. 42 weeks
    c. 38 weeks
    d. 260 days
    Ans. a

35. Dietary supplement alone cannot compensate the increased requirement of which nutrition in pregnant woman:
    a. Iron
    b. Iodine
    c. Magnesium
    d. Calcium
    Ans. a

31. First Trimester Vaginal Bleeding

*If something comes to life in other because of you,
then you have made an approach to immorality.*

INTRODUCTION

Two out of 10 pregnant women have vaginal bleeding in the first trimester; of these 50% will go on to have normal pregnancies, while the other 50% will have a pregnancy loss. **The presence of vaginal bleeding, abdominal pain, fever or passage of tissues requires immediate evaluation.** It is important to make the diagnosis because ectopic pregnancy is a life-threatening situation while vaginal bleeding in a viable pregnancy can be associated with subsequent adverse pregnancy outcome.

Differential Diagnosis of First Trimester Vaginal Bleeding

1. Early pregnancy failure – spontaneous, missed abortion, or induced abortion.
2. Molar pregnancy.
3. Viable intrauterine pregnancy.
4. Ectopic pregnancy.
5. Gynecological cause, e.g. vaginal trauma, cervical lesions, cervical neoplasia, vaginal / vulvar varicosities.

Evaluation of the Pregnant Patient with Vaginal Bleeding

In these patients a systematic examination in the following order should be performed:
1. Obtain vital signs.
2. Obtain a menstrual history; confirm pregnancy, gynecological history and history of a coagulation disorder.
3. Perform a physical examination to assess uterus size, adnexal masses, and evaluate for peritoneal signs.
4. Use diagnostic aid like urine pregnancy test. If possibility of molar pregnancy or ectopic pregnancy, quantitative serum hCG and ultrasound evaluation.

Careful history taking, proper physical and pelvic examination and guided investigation are useful in diagnosing the cause of 1st trimester vaginal bleeding.

ABORTIONS

Definition

Abortion is spontaneous or induced termination of pregnancy before age of viability, which is usually considered prior to 20 weeks gestation or less than 500 gm birth weight. *Spontaneous abortion* is delivery of all or any part of the products of conception with or without a fetus weighing less than 500 gm.

Threatened Abortion

Threatened abortion is bleeding of intrauterine origin occurring before the 20th completed weeks with or without uterine contraction, without dilatation of cervix and without expulsion of the products of conception (Fig. 31.1A).

Complete Abortion

It is the expulsion of all of the products of conception before the 20th completed weeks of gestation.

Incomplete Abortion

It is the expulsion of some but not all of the products of conception.

Inevitable Abortion

It refers to bleeding of intrauterine origin before the 20th completed weeks with dilatation of the cervix without expulsion of the products of conception.

Missed Abortion

The embryo or fetus dies but the products of conception are retained in uterus (Fig. 31.1B).

Septic Abortion

Infection of the uterus and sometimes surrounding structure occur.

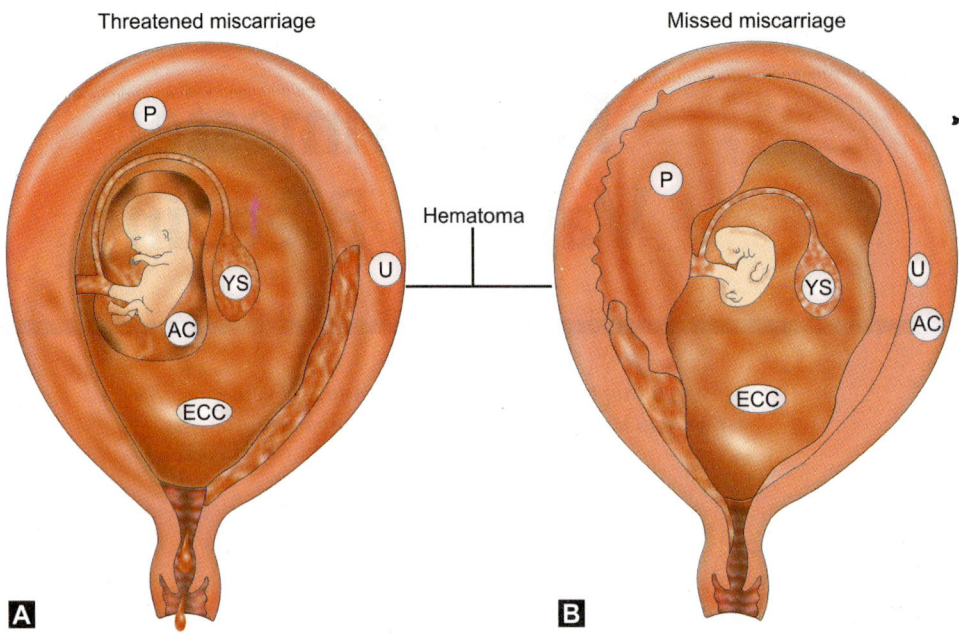

Figs 31.1A and B: (A) Threatened abortion; (B) Missed abortion. (P—Placenta, U—Uterus, AC—Amniotic cavity, YS—Yolk sac, ECC — Extracoelomic cavity)

Incidence of Abortion

The true incidence of spontaneous abortion is unknown. At least 12-15% of clinically recognized pregnancies terminate in fetal loss, 60% of chemically evident pregnancies end in spontaneous abortion, 80% of spontaneous abortion occur prior to 12 weeks gestation.

Etiology of Abortion

Causes of spontaneous abortion are summarized in Table 31.1.

Morphologic and Genetic Abnormalities

Overall genetic abnormalities account for 50-70% of spontaneous abortions, fetal chromosomal abnormalities account for 50-70% of first trimester abortions and 30% of second trimester abortions but only 3% of stillbirths. *It is to be emphasized that incidence of a chromosomally abnormal abortion markedly increases after a maternal age of 35 years.*

Autosomal trisomy is the most frequently identified chromosomal abnormality associated with first trimester abortions. Trisomies 13,16,18,21 and 22 are the most common of these. Monosomy (X) 45 X is the next most common chromosomal abnormality. Triploidy is often associated with hydropic placental degeneration. The remaining half of early abortions has normal chromosomal complements; of these 20% have other genetic abnormalities. Mendelian or polygenic factors resulting in anatomic defects may play a role.

Table 31.1: Causes of spontaneous abortion

Causes	Pathology
Genetic cause	a. Trisomy b. Polyploidy/aneuploidy c. Translocation
Environmental cause	a. Uterine—Congenital uterine anomalies, leiomyoma, Intrauterine adhesion or synechia b. Cervical—Incompetent cervix c. Endocrine— 　i. Inadequate luteal phase 　ii. Untreated thyroid disorder 　iii. Uncontrolled diabetes mellitus 　iv. Hyper secretion of LH d. Immunologic 　i. Autoimmunity: antiphospholipid syndrome, SLE 　ii. Alloimmunity e. Infections: *Toxoplasma, Chlamydia, Mycoplasma hominis, herpes simplex, Treponema pallidum, Neisseria gonorrhoeae* f. Toxins: Alcohol, caffeine, smoking, anesthetic gases, high dose radiation, medication (Methotrexate, Misoprostol) g. Trauma

Environmental Factors

Uterine Factors

1. **Congenital anomalies** that reduce or distort the size of uterine cavity such as unicornuate, bicornuate or septate uterus carry a 25-50% risk of miscarriage.

2. **Acquired anomalies** like submucous myomas or intramural myomas have been associated with spontaneous abortion.
3. **Previous scarring of the uterine cavity** following D and C (Asherman's syndrome), myomectomy or unification procedures have been implicated in spontaneous miscarriage. Anatomic or functional incompetence of uterine cervix causes second trimester or early third trimester abortions.
4. **Endocrine disorders:** Insufficient progesterone secretion by the corpus luteum or placenta has been associated with an increased incidence of abortion. Women with subclinical hypothyroidism and with thyroid auto-antibodies may be at increased risk of miscarriage. Spontaneous abortion and major congenital malformation are increased in women with insulin dependent diabetes. The risk is related to degree of metabolic control.
5. **Immunological abnormalities:** Two primary pathophysiological models for immune related spontaneous abortion are: (a) Autoimmune (immunity against self), (b) Alloimmune theory (immunity against another person). Up to 15% of women with recurrent pregnancy loss have autoimmune factors. The best established autoimmune disorder associated with spontaneous abortion is the **antiphospholipid antibody syndrome**. Antiphoshpholipid antibodies are acquired antibodies targeted against phospholipid, which can be of IgG, IgA or Igm isotype and are most commonly detected by testing for **Lupus Anticoagulant (LAC) and anticardio-lipin antibody (ACA)**. Blood group incompatibility due to ABO, RH Keil or other antigen has been associated with spontaneous abortion. Similar maternal and paternal human leukocyte antigen (HLA) status may enhance the possibility of abortion by causing insufficient maternal immunologic recognition of the fetus.
6. **Infections:** Herpes simplex, HIV, maternal syphilitic seroactivity, and vaginal colonization with group B streptococci has been associated with increased risk of spontaneous abortion.
7. **Toxins:** Smoking has been associated with an increased risk for euploid abortion. Alcohol use during the first 8 weeks of pregnancy may result in both spontaneous abortion and fetal malformation. Radiation, antineoplastic drugs, anesthetic gases have been shown to be embryotoxic.
8. **Trauma:** Direct trauma in accident or indirect trauma such as surgical removal of an ovary containing the corpus luteum of pregnancy may result in spontaneous abortions. There is no conclusive evidence that nutritional deficiency and emotional disturbances causes spontaneous abortion.

Pathology

In spontaneous abortion hemorrhage into the decidua basalis often occurs, necrosis and inflammation appear in the area of implantation. The pregnancy becomes partially or entirely detached. Uterine contraction and dilatation of the cervix results in expulsion of most or all of the products of conception.

Clinical Findings

Threatened Abortion

It is a clinical entity when the pregnancy is so far intact but there is an obvious risk to its continuation. The presenting symptom is that of bleeding, which usually precedes the onset of pain. If predominant symptom is pain followed by bleeding, the possibility of an ectopic pregnancy must be excluded. The amount of bleeding is variable but usually never heavy. On *vaginal examination* the uterus is soft and corresponds to the period of gestation and the internal os is closed. **Ultrasound** confirms the diagnosis of intact and viable pregnancy. **β-hCG** levels are normal for gestational age.

Inevitable Abortion

Abdominal or back pain and bleeding with an open cervix indicate impending abortion. Abortion or rupture of membrane is noted.

Incomplete Abortion

An inevitable abortion will proceed to discharge the products of conception outside the uterine cavity either partially in incomplete abortion.

Complete Abortion

Complete abortion is identified by passage of the entire conceptus. Slight bleeding may continue for a short-time, although pain usually ceases after pregnancy has traversed the cervix.

Missed Abortion

Missed abortion implies that the pregnancy has been retained following death of the fetus. Why the pregnancy is not expelled is not known, it is possible that normal progestogen production by the placenta continues while estrogen level fall, which may reduce uterine contractility.

Blighted Ovum

Blighted ovum or anembryonic pregnancy represents a failed development of the embryo so that only a gestational sac with or without a yolk soc is present. Various types of abortions are diagrammatically represented in Figure 31.2.

Investigation

1. *Complete blood count:* If significant bleeding has occurred, the patient will be anemic. Both the leukocyte

SECTION -3 ♦ Obstetrics

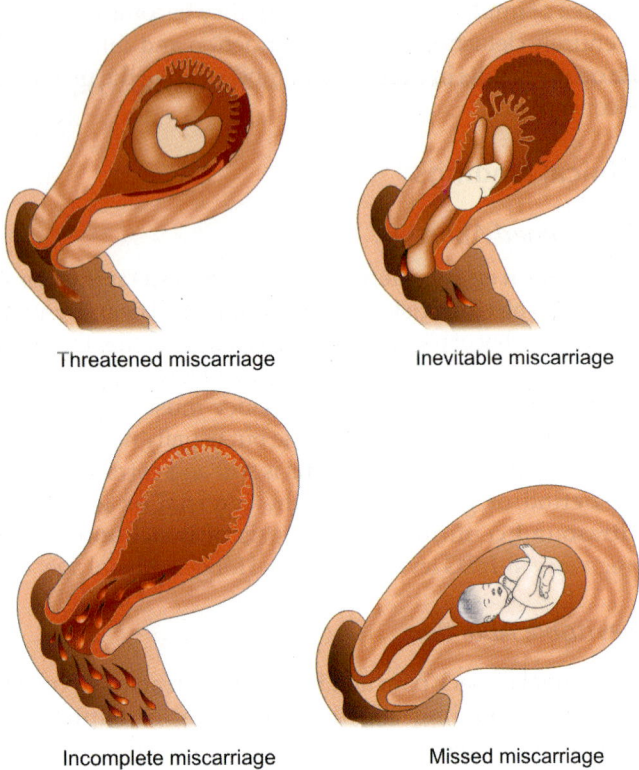

Fig. 31.2: Various types of miscarriages

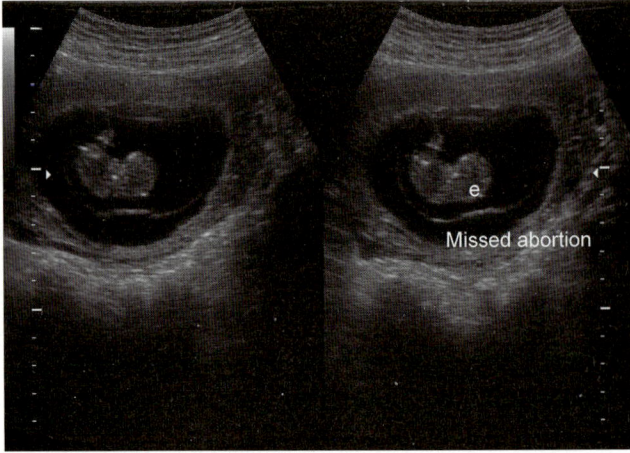

Fig. 31.3: Ultrasound image of missed abortion (embryo shows growth lag and absent cardiac activity)

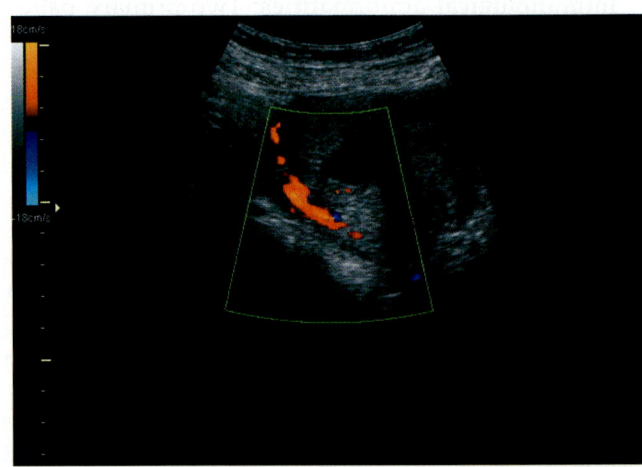

Fig. 31.4: Ultrasound image of blighted ovum (empty gestational sac without embryo)

count and sedimentation rate may be elevated even without the presence of infection.

2. *Pregnancy test:* Falling or abnormally rising plasma levels of β–human chronic gonadotropin (hCG) are diagnostic of an abnormal pregnancy, either a blighted ovum, spontaneous abortion or ectopic pregnancy. Higher levels of β-hCG are found in vesicular mole.

3. *Ultrasonography:* Ultrasonography is quick and useful in diagnosing intrauterine pregnancy and excluding an ectopic pregnancy. Ultrasound is useful in determining which pregnancies are viable and which are most likely to miscarry. The USG findings in different types of abortions are as follows:
   a. *Threatened abortion:* There is a normal gestational sac and viable embryo. However, a large or irregular sac or eccentric fetal pole, presence of a large retrochorionic bleed, and or a slow fetal heart rate (<85 bpm) carry a poor prognosis.
   b. *Incomplete abortion:* The gestational sac is deflated and irregular, echogenic tissue shadows representing placental tissue is seen in the uterine cavity.
   c. *Complete abortion:* The endometrium appear closely apposed with no visible products of conception.
   d. *Missed abortion:* An embryo or fetus without cardiac activity is seen (Fig. 31.3).
   e. *Blighted ovum:* An abnormal gestational sac without a yolk sac or embryo is consistent with blighted ovum (Fig. 31.4).

Complications of Abortion

a. Severe or persistent hemorrhage during or following abortion may cause anemia and sometimes may be life-threatening due to hypovolemia.
b. Sepsis usually develops in neglected care or induced abortion in unsafe place and hands.
c. Intrauterine synechiae, infertility and infection involving adnexa and uterus are late complication of abortion.

Management

Threatened Abortion

a. Bed rest and pelvic rest is recommended until bleeding stops.
b. Hormone therapy with intramuscular progestational agent or micronized progesterone, oral or vaginal is widely used, but evidence of its efficacy is lacking.

c. Ixosuprine is not effective at this period of gestation and may do more harm than good, as it is a vasodilator and can potentially increase bleeding.

Ultrasonography should be repeated after one to two weeks to ensure fetal viability. A per speculum examination is advised if bleeding continues, to rule out any lesion in lower genital tract. Usually the prognosis for pregnancy continuation is good but the pregnancy continues at a greater risk than normal. Premature labor, intrauterine fetal death and antepartum hemorrhage are about 3 times more common. Patient is kept under clinical surveillance including weekly ultrasound examination until patient symptoms are cured and fetal viability and growth is confirmed on ultrasound.

Complete abortion: No further intervention is necessary. The patient is observed for further bleeding. Diagnosis of complete abortion can be confirmed by ultrasound, which reveals empty uterus.

Incomplete abortion: I/V hydration is given and evacuation of uterus by suction curettage should be done. Determination of blood group and Rh typing and blood for cross matching should be done.

Missed abortion: Surgical evacuation using suction curettage is the standard method of treatment for missed abortion in first trimester. Medical methods for termination of pregnancy by using Mifepristone and Misoprostol can be used. If abortion has occurred after the first trimester or if a dead fetus is retained in uterus for more than 4-6 weeks, hospitalization is needed. Prostaglandins, oxytocin is given to felicitate contraction of the uterus, limiting blood loss and aids expulsion of blood clot and products of conception. Suction curettage or D & C is necessary if products of conception are retained or if significant bleeding persist. In these cases there is a potential danger of serious coagulation defect and in those cases, beside other treatment; replacement of blood components is needed as indicated by laboratory test.

Rh Sensitization In Abortion

Rhesus antigen has been found on fetal red cells as early as the 38th day of pregnancy. **It is recommended that 50 µg of polyclonal anti D gamma globulin should be administered after spontaneous or induced abortion before 12 weeks within 72 hours of abortion. In the case of medical abortion, Anti D can be administered along with the first dose of mifepristone.** After 12 weeks of gestation, a full dose of Anti D (300 µg) should be administered.

RECURRENT PREGNANCY LOSS (RPL)

Recurrent abortion in its broadest definition is defined as 2 or 3 more consecutive pregnancy loss before 20 weeks of gestation each with a fetus weighing less than 500 gm.

Incidence of RPL

Repeated spontaneous abortions are likely to be chance phenomena in the majority of cases. Approximately 1-2% of women have recurrent pregnancy loss.

Causes and Evaluation

Generally a complete evaluation is recommended after 3 consecutive losses. However, it depends on the patient's age and level of concern. An identifiable cause is found in 50-60% of cases.

Causes of Recurrent Pregnancy Loss

a. Genetic factors.
b. Anatomic abnormalities of the uterine like bicornuate uterus, septate uterus, cervical incompetence.
c. Endocrine disorders – uncontrolled diabetes, thyroid dysfunction, luteal phase deficiency.
d. Autoimmune disorder – antiphospholipid syndrome, lupus anticoagulant.
e. Alloimmune disorder.
f. Environmental cause – alcohol, tobacco, anesthetic agent.
g. Infections – *Ureoplasma urealyticum, Mycoplasma hominis.*
h. Thrombophilia.

Work-up should include:
a. **Karyotype** of both parents and or products of conception to rule out genetic factors.
b. **Lab tests to rule out endocrine factors**: TSH, serum glucose, prolactin, luteal phase assessment by progesterone level and endometrial biopsy.
c. **Ultrasound or hysterosalpingogram, and or hysteroscopy** to rule out uterine abnormalities.

Treatment

Treatment depends on the cause identified:
a. *Genetic error:* Artificial insemination by donor, embryo transfer, prenatal testing, preimplantation diagnosis.
b. *Anatomic abnormalities:* Uterine operation, hysteroscopic resection of septum, myomectomy, cervical circlage operation, reconstruction of cervical issues.
c. *Hormonal abnormalities:* Thyroid replacement, progesterone or clomiphene citrate, diabetic diet and or insulin as indicated.
d. *Infection:* Appropriate antibiotic.
e. *Acute immune disease:* Low dose aspirin and heparin.
f. *Exogenous agent:* Discourage smoking, alcohol and drugs.
g. *Immunological factor:* Treatment is under investigation.

Prognosis

After two consecutive miscarriages the chance of livebirth is about 70-75%. After three consecutive losses with a previous livebirth, the chances of a subsequent livebirth are

70%. After three consecutive losses without a previous live birth the chance of live birth is 50-65%. Details are in Appendix-4.

SEPTIC ABORTION

Causes

Infection may occur with missed miscarriage and with incomplete miscarriage, especially which result from inexpert mechanical interference or from inadequate surgical evacuation in the first trimester. Causative organisms are usually *E. coli*, streptococci, (hemolytic, nonhemolytic and anaerobic), *Staphylococcus aureus* and *Cl. welchii*.

Symptoms and Signs

Symptoms are fever, malodorous vaginal discharge, pelvic and abdominal pain. On examination there can be cervical motion tenderness, signs of peritonitis and sepsis. Trauma to cervix or upper vagina may be recognized.

Investigations

A complete blood count, urinalysis, endometrial cultures, blood culture, chest X-ray and abdominal X-ray to rule out uterine perforation should be obtained. Ultrasound is helpful in detecting retained products of conception, presence of pelvic masses and pelvic abscess.

Treatment

Hospitalization is done. Intravenous antibiotic therapy is given with selection of antibiotics for both aerobic and anaerobic coverage. Under antibiotic coverage D & C is done to remove retained products of conception. In rare cases if infection does not respond to treatment, a hysterectomy may be necessary.

INDUCED ABORTION

Induced abortion is the medical or surgical termination of pregnancy before the time of fetal viability. There are many countries where induced abortion or termination of pregnancy is still not legalized. In India the abortion was legalized by Medical Termination of Pregnancy Act of 1971, and has been enforced in year April 1972. The provisions of the act have been revised in 1975.

Medical Termination of pregnancy

In the present day form, the provision of the MTP act are as follows:
1. *Indications of MTP*
   a. When the continuation of pregnancy would involve serious risk of life or grave injury to the physical and mental health of the pregnant women.
   b. There is substantial risk of the child being born with serious physical and mental abnormalities so as to be handicapped in life–eugenic consideration.
   c. Social: When the pregnancy is caused by rape both in case of major and minor girl and in mentally handicapped women.
   d. Pregnancy caused as a result of failure of contraceptive.
2. *Qualification of MTP provider:* The MTP act also mentions the qualification required of a registered medical practitioner, who is eligible to perform an MTP. These are as follows:
   a. A registered medical practitioner, who has assisted in at least 25 MTP operations in a recognized MTP training center and holds a certificate.
   b. A person who has undergone residency training in obstetric and gynecology for at least 6 months.
   c. Any person holding a diploma or postgraduate degree in obstetrics and gynecology.
3. *Place for MTP:* The MTP act specifies that an MTP can only be performed in hospitals established and maintained by the government or places approved by the government.
4. *Consent:* Pregnancy can be terminated only after obtaining the written prior consent of the women (husband consent not necessary). In case of minor or mentally retarded individual the written consent of parent or the legal guardian is necessary before undertaking an MTP.
5. For performing a first trimester (up to 12 weeks) MTP the opinion of one medical practitioner suffices, however for undertaking a second trimester MTP (12-20 weeks) the opinion of two medical practitioner are required.
6. The abortion has to be performed in confidence and to be reported to the Director of Health Services of the state in prescribed form.

In India about 2.0% of pregnancies are terminated. Almost 80-85% of these are first trimester pregnancies and 15-20% is second trimester pregnancies.

Methods of Termination of Pregnancies

First Trimester MTP

1. **Medical Methods:** Women with first trimester pregnancies less than 49 days from their first day of the last menstrual period may be eligible for medical abortion. Following medical methods are available:
   a. *Mifepristone (RU – 486) and Misoprostol:* Mifepristone (RU-486) acts as a progesterone receptor antagonist, which block the effect of natural progesterone. It is given 200–600 mg dose on day 1. On day 3 Misoprostol (PGE) is given 400–800 µg orally or vaginally which helps in expulsion of products of conception. Abortion occurs spontaneously usually within 5 days of commencement

of therapy. The patient is called for examination after 10-14 days. If there is persistent bleeding or profuse bleeding or there is any doubt ultrasonography is recommended. Success of method is 95% and 2% patient require curettage for completion of abortion and chance of continuation of pregnancy is about 1%. **Mifepristone should not be used in women > 35 years of age, in smokers and in women on long term corticosteroid treatment for medical disorders.**

b. *Methotrexate and Misoprostol:* Methotrexate blocks Dihydrofolate reductase, an enzyme involved in producing thymidine during DNA synthesis. Thus it inhibits synctialization of the cytotrophoblast, which prevents implantation. Methotrexate 50 mg/m² IM before 56 days of gestation followed by 7 days later Misoprostol 800 µg vaginally is highly effective. Misoprostol may be repeated after 24 hours if it fails. This regimen is less expensive, has similar success rate to that of methotrexate/ misoprostol, but it takes longer time up to 4 weeks for the abortion to occur.

c. *Tamoxifen and Misoprostol:* Oral tamoxifen 20 mg weekly for 4 days followed by misoprostol 800 µg vaginally results in complete abortion in 92% of cases in gestational age less than 63 days.

d. *Misoprostol alone:* 800 µg vaginally repeated for up to 3 doses. Regimen for medical method of termination are summarized in Box 31.1.

Side effects in medical methods of abortion are: (a) Bleeding and pain, (b) Nausea (12-47%), (c) Vomiting (9-45%), (d) Diarrhea (7-67%), (e) Warmth or chills (14-89%), (f) Headache (12-27%), (g) Dizziness and fatigue.

Complication of medical abortion: Complication in medical abortion are hemorrhage requiring emergency dilatation and curettage (<1%), post abortal endometritis (0.09-0.5%), incomplete abortion (5%) (Box 31.1).

Surgical Methods

These methods are simple, one time, effective, well evaluated and safe in expert hands. The techniques are as follows:

Box 31.1: Regimen for medical method of termination of early pregnancy

Mifepristone/Misoprostol
Mifepristone—100-600 mg orally followed by
Misoprostol 200-600 mg orally or 800 mg vaginally, multiple doses over 6-72 hr.
Methotrexate 50 mg/m³ I/m or orally followed by
Misoprostol 800 mg vaginally in 3-7 days
Misoprostol 800 virginally repeated for up to 3 dose

1. **Menstrual regulation:** In this, content of endometrial cavity are aspirated using a 5-7 mm polyethylene cannula attached to a Kerman's 50 ml plastic syringe in which vacuum of 675 mm can be created prior to the procedure. This menstrual regulation syringe has a thumb operated pressure control valve, a position tacking handle or arm catcher which helps to hold in place a self-retaining plunger and locking device which prevent the withdrawal of piston from the syringe incorporated into it. This MR syringe can be used to evacuate intrauterine pregnancy of less than 42 days duration.
   Complication of MR syringe method can be:
   a. Failure of MTP and continuation of pregnancy,
   b. Infection,
   c. Bleeding,
   d. Uterine perforation,
   e. Cervical trauma,
   f. Missed ectopic pregnancy,
   g. Drug allergy.

2. **Manual vacuum aspiration:** In this method a wide bore Karman's polyethylene cannula is used along with plastic syringe with reusable aspirator. Products of conception are evacuated by manually generated vacuum. It has proved very useful in developing countries or low resource setting, where electrical supply or electrically operated suction machine is not available.

3. **Suction evacuation and/or curettage:** First trimester MTPs can be safely and successfully done by suction evacuation. It is usually followed by curettage. Procedure is done under local anesthetic paracervical block with sedation or under general anesthetic. The cervix is dilated slowly using gradually increasing number of Hegar's dilators. Size of Hegar's dilator/sialistic dilator should correspond to duration of pregnancy in weeks, which is followed by insertion of plastic Kerman cannula or metal cannula attached to electrically power suction machine (Figs 31.5A and B). It is very safe and effective method of first trimester pregnancy termination. The advantage of suction over surgical curettage are that suction curettage empties the uterus more rapidly, minimize blood loss and reduces the likelihood of perforation of the uterus.
   Complication of suction curettage are less than 1% for infection, 2% excessive bleeding, less than 1% for uterine perforation. The risk of major complications as persistent fever, excessive hemorrhage, perforation ranges 0.2 to 0.6%. Prior knowledge of the size and position of the uterus and volume of content is mandatory for safe suction curettage.

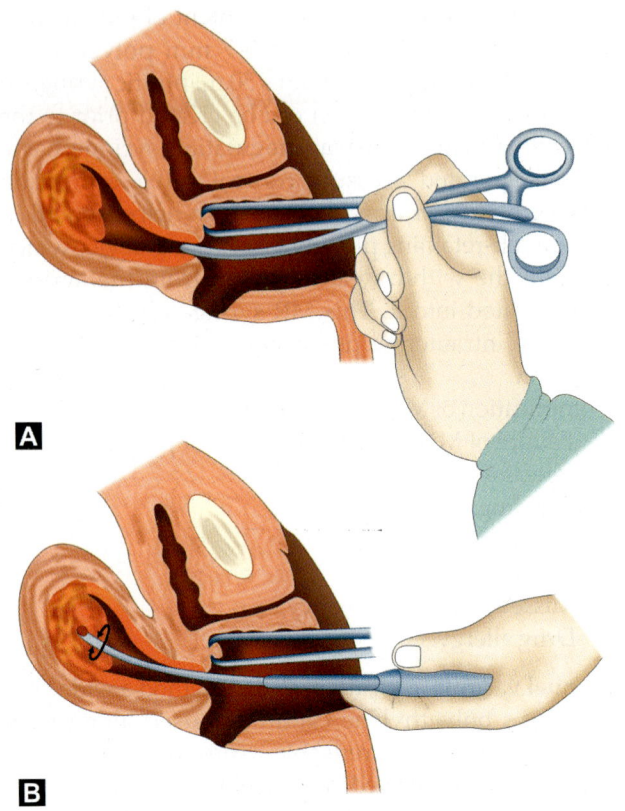

Figs 31.5A and B: Technique of first trimester suction evacuation: (A) Anterior lip of cervix is held with volsellum and internal os is dilated; (B) Products of conception is taken out by suction evacuation

Table 31.2: Medical vs surgical abortion	
Medical abortion	Surgical abortion
Usually avoid operative procedure	Involves operative procedure
Usually avoids anesthesia	Allows use of sedation and anesthesia
Requires two or more visit	One step procedure
Take days to week to complete	Completed in predictable period
Confined to 49-56 days of gestation	Can be used in later gestation
High success rate 95%	High success rate 99%
Requires follow-up to ensure complete abortions	Usually not required

Surgical Curettage/Dilatation and Curettage

1. *Rapid method:* In absence of suction curettage equipment, standard dilatation and curettage can be performed as a method of first trimester medical termination of pregnancy. The blood loss, duration of procedure and likelihood of the damage to uterus and cervix are more as compared to suction curettage. Risk of uterine synechiae or Asherman's syndrome is also increased.
2. *Slow method:* Slow dilation of the cervix can be achieved by inserting Lasminaria tents (Hygroscopic osmotic dilators) into the cervical canal (Synthetic dilators like Dilapan, Lamicol). This is followed by evacuation of uterus after 12 hours. Vaginal misoprostol (PGE1) 400 µg 3 hours before surgery is equally effective. This has an advantage of less chance of cervical injury. But the drawbacks are need of hospitalization and more chance of sepsis.

Advantages and disadvantage of medical verses surgical abortion are summarized in Table 31.2.

Second Trimester Termination (13-20 Weeks)

The second trimester MTP accounts for about 15-20% of all MTP's. Second trimester carry a five fold higher morbidity. So attempts should be made to encourage women to seek MTP early in pregnancy rather than face the consequence of mid trimester termination.

Method of Termination of Pregnancy Between 13-15 Weeks of Gestation

Surgical Methods

1. *Dilatation and evacuation:* It is less commonly done. The procedure should be done in following stages:
   a. Preoperative cervical softening using $PGF_{2\alpha}$ or PGE_2 gel, misoprostol vaginal tablet or laminaria tent.
   b. Oxytocin infusion to enhance uterine tone and facilitate evacuation.
   c. Administration of paracervical local anesthetic block with adequate sedation.
   d. Cervical dilatation sufficient to allow insertion of large sized cannula fallowed by suction evacuation of products of conception by electrically powered suction machine. If procedure is performed under ultrasound guidance it enhances safety and efficacy.
2. *Aspirotomy:* In this under local paracervical block and oxytocin infusion cervix is dilated. Membranes are ruptured and liquor amni is aspirated. Fetal parts are removed with help of specially designed aspirotomy forceps. Decidua and membrane are removed with help of suction cannula. The procedure can be performed under ultrasound guidance. It is a one step procedure but operation is gruesome and most surgeons prefer alternative procedure.

Medical Methods—Induction of Labor

Extra-amniotic installation of 0.1% Ethacridine Lactate: Ethacridine lactate 0.1% in dose of 10 ml/week of gestation but not exceeding a total dose of 150 ml is instilled via Foley's catheter. Foley's catheter is introduced transcervically for about 10 cm above the internal os between membrane and myometrium. After instilling the drug, bulb of Foley's catheter is inflated with 10 ml saline and catheter is clamped. After interval of 6-8 hours the Foley's catheter is removed. The average induction abortion interval ranges from 24-36 hours. Augmentation by oxytocin infusion after 24 hours of instillation helps in reducing the induction abortion interval and enhances success rate.

Likewise 1.0 ml $PGF_{2\alpha}$ diluted in 1 extra-amniotic space at time of removal of Foley's catheter results in marked shortening of the induction abortion interval to less than 24 hours. It acts by stimulating uterine motility, adversely influencing fetal placental complex and initiate the process of expulsion of products of conception.

Extra-amniotic 20% hypertonic saline administration: This method has been given up because of risk of serious complications like hypernatremia, consumptive coagulapathy.

Prostaglandin: Prostaglandin and their analogs are very much effective and used extensively for midtrimester abortion. The commonly used drugs are:

a. **Intramuscular:** (i) **15 methyl $PGF_{2\alpha}$** (Carboprost Tromethamine) 250 µg I/m every 3 hours for a maximum of 10 injections. (ii) **Sulprostone** (PGE_2 Analo) 500 µg administered intramuscularly at every 8 hours.
b. **Vaginal:** (i) PGE_2 analog (Misoprostol) 200 µg every 12 hours. PGE_2 (Dinoprostone) suppository 20 mg every 3 hours.

Misoprostol has fewer side effects like nausea, vomiting, diarrhea, low grade fever, bronchospasm, allergy and risk of hypertonus.

Methods of Terminating Pregnancy Between 16-20 Weeks of Gestation

a. ***Intra-amniotic instillation of abortifacient drugs:*** Intra-amniotic 20% hypertonic saline, ethacridine lactate, hyperosmotic urea, along with Prostaglandin can be instilled via intra-amniotic route.

Procedure: Preliminary amniocentesis is done by a 15 cm, 18-gauge needles. To be sure that needle is in the amniotic cavity, clear amniotic fluid should come out. After that a fine polythene tube is passed through the needle into amniotic sac, needle is withdrawn and polythene tube is connected with the drip set containing the required amount of hypertonic saline/urea/ethacridine lactate. The amount is calculated as number of weeks of gestation multiplied by 10 ml and is infused slowly at rate of 10 ml/minutes.

Though the method is effective in 90-95% of cases with induction abortion interval of 32-36 hours. These methods have now fallen out of favor because of risk of grave complications like hypernatremia, consumptive coagulopathy and renal failure.

b. ***Extra-amniotic administration*** of ethacridine lactate, prostaglandin can be done.
c. ***Prostaglandin*** by parenteral, vaginal, intra-amniotic and extra-amniotic route can be used. Prostaglandins are now preferably used.
d. ***Hysterotomy:*** The hysterotomy is currently reserved only for special circumstances such as the failure to complete a mid trimester abortion due to cervical stenosis or the management of other complications. Hysterotomy have high rate of morbidity as compared to other methods and should not be used as a primary method. It should also considered if women wants permanent sterilization (tubal ligation) at the same time.

Follow-up of patients after induced abortion: Follow-up care after all procedure must be ensured:

a. After abortion by all methods, human Anti D (Rh immunoglobulin) should be administered promptly if the patient is Rh negative.
b. The patient should take her temperature and report fever or unusual bleeding at once.
c. Follow-up care should include pelvic examinations to rule out endometritis and parametritis, salpingitis, failure of ovulation, or continued uterine growth.
d. Finally effective contraception should be made available according to patient's need and desires. *As ovulation is resumed as early as two weeks after an abortion, so contraception should be initiated soon after abortion.*

Complications Following Mid Trimester MTP

The complications of MTPs are 3-5 times higher in mid trimester pregnancy termination as compared to first trimester MTP. Complications can be as follows:

Immediate

a. **Trauma** to the cervix and uterus leading to hemorrhage and shock.
b. **Hemorrhage** and shock due to trauma, incomplete abortion, atonic uterus or rarely coagulation failure.
c. **Thrombosis and embolism**.
d. Postabortal triad of pain, bleeding and low grade fever due to retained clots or products. If needed repeat evacuation is to be done under antibiotic cover.
e. **Related to method** employed: Like hypernatremia, pulmonary edema, DIC, renal failure in *hyperosmotic saline*, nausea, vomiting, diarrhea, hypertonus, cervicouterine injury with use of prostaglandins.
f. **Uterine perforation:** This is the one of the serious and common complications of MTP. Recognition of uterus perforation is important. It is suspected *if suction curette has gone in for a greater depth without resistance. Sudden unexpected bleeding, appearance of omentum, mesenteric fat or intestine in the cannula or ovum forceps, or patient if under local anesthetic complain of diffuse abdominal pain.* Treatment depends upon extent of perforation,

gestational age, amount of bleeding and desire for future childbearing.

For a suspected small perforation, procedure is stopped; patient is kept under observation for vital, any sign of peritonitis, hemorrhage. If there is no further evidence of infection, hemorrhage or peritonitis, no further treatment is needed. Otherwise the patient should be shifted to OT. Laparoscopy can be carried out to visualize the extent of damage. Pelvis, gut is observed. A small rent can be repaired laparoscopically and medical termination of pregnancy is completed under laparoscopic vision. If there is damage to intestines, presence of gut content or active bleeding, immediate laparotomy is needed. Repair of uterus and gut is done. Sterilization can be performed at the same time, if no further childbearing is desired. If there is a wide rent in the uterus or broad ligament hematoma following uterine artery tear, hysterectomy may be required.

g. **Postabortal hematometra:** This usually develops within 12 hours of suction evacuation. The patient complains of pain, uterus is enlarged and boggy. Diagnosis can be confirmed by ultrasound. Prostaglandin analog can help to expel the clot. Sometimes a repeat evacuation is required.

Remote Complications

Though in expert hands and safe place in first trimester abortion there are no serious long-term sequele. Vacuum aspiration does not increase the subsequent incidence of abortion or preterm labor. But there can be following remote complications:
a. Chronic pelvic inflammatory disease.
b. Infertility as a consequence of infection.
c. Scar endometriosis (1%).
d. Multiple sharp curettage may increase the chance of uterine synechiae, various grades of Asherman's syndrome, or placenta previa.
e. Usually risks of ectopic pregnancies are not increased, except in women with pre-existing chlamydial infection or in those who develop postabortal infection.

Mortality and Cause of Death

Unsafe abortion still account for 8.9% of all maternal death in India. In strictly medical terms nearly all abortion death are avoidable. The chief causes of death are sepsis, hemorrhage and shock. Following severe shock and hemorrhage, there may be anemia and uremia. So there is sharp decrease in mortality, when there is access to antibiotic and blood transfusion.

ECTOPIC PREGNANCY

The fertilized ovum (blastocyst) normally implants in the endometrial lining of the uterine cavity. **If fertilized ovum implants in an area other than the endometrial lining of the uterus, it is termed as ectopic pregnancy.**

Incidence

The incidence of ectopic pregnancy has increased from 4.5 in 1000 in 1970 to 19.7 in 1000 in 1992. This may be due to higher incidence of fallopian tube inflammation, an increase in IUCD and tubal sterilization as well ovulation induction and tubal surgery, ART techniques. Ectopic pregnancy is a significant cause of maternal morbidity and mortality. However, development of sensitive βhCG assay along with increasing use of ultrasound and laparoscopy has helped in earlier diagnosis of ectopic pregnancy and decrease in both maternal morbidity and mortality.

Classification

Ectopic pregnancy can be classified as follows:
1. **Tubal (>95%)** – It includes:
    a. Ampullary (55%).
    b. Isthmic (25%).
    c. Fimbrial (17%).
    d. Interstitial (2%).
2. **Other sites (<5%):**
    a. Cervical.
    b. Ovarian.
    c. Abdominal: Primary abdominal pregnancy have been reported, but most abdominal pregnancies are secondary abdominal, from tubal abortion or rupture with subsequent implantation in the bowel, omentum, or mesentery.
    d. Intraligamentous.
4. **Heterotopic pregnancy:** An ectopic pregnancy occurs in combination with an intrauterine pregnancy in 1 in 15000–40000 spontaneous pregnancies and in up to 1% of patients undergoing *In vitro* Fertilization.
5. **Bilateral ectopic:** Very rare.

Various sites of ectopic pregnancy have been shown in Figure 31.6.

Etiology

Tubal Damage

The destruction of the normal tubal anatomy remains the major cause of ectopic pregnancy. Tubal damage can result from inflammation, infection and surgery.
1. **Inflammation and infection** may cause damage without complete tubal obstruction. *After one episode of PID the ratio of ectopic pregnancy to intrauterine pregnancy is increased by 6 folds. Chlamydia* is important pathogen causing tubal damage and subsequent tubal pregnancy. If *Chlamydia trachomatis* antibody titer is higher than 1:64, the chances of ectopic pregnancy is 3 fold increased.
2. **Contraceptive use:** *Inert and copper containing IUCD* prevent both intrauterine and extrauterine pregnancies. But if women conceive with IUCD in place, there are 0.4–0.8 times higher chance of tubal pregnancy.
Hormonal contraceptive: The risk of ectopic pregnancy with combined oral contraceptive is 0.5-4%. Past use of

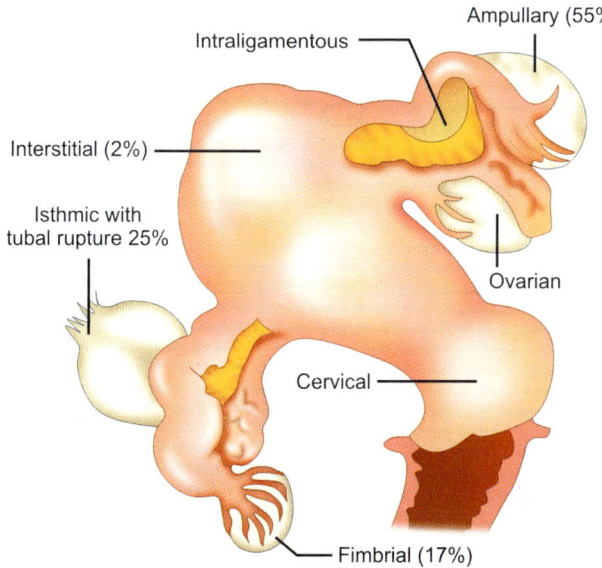

Fig. 31.6: Diagram showing different sites of ectopic pregnancy

oral contraceptive does not increase the subsequent risk of ectopic pregnancy. Progesterone only pills and subdermal implants protect against intrauterine and ectopic pregnancy, when compared with no contraceptive but if pregnancy does occur there is 4 to 10% chance of ectopic pregnancy with the mini pill and up to 30% with subdermal implants. Barrier contraception protects against both intrauterine and ectopic pregnancy.

3. **Tubal sterilization:** If pregnancy occurs following sterilization, there is 15–50% chance of being ectopic. The risk is highest in first two years after sterilization and with technique of laparoscopic fulguration without tubal resection.
4. **Tubal surgery:** Tubal reconstructive surgery is associated with increased risk for ectopic pregnancy, either due to surgical procedure or from the underlying problem. Sterilization reversal also increases risk for ectopic pregnancy.
5. **Prior abdominal surgery:** Role of abdominal surgery in ectopic pregnancy is unclear.
6. **Others:**
   a. *Previous ectopic pregnancy:* There is 10-15% chance of repeat ectopic pregnancy.
   b. *Abortion*: There is no increase in ectopic pregnancy with spontaneous abortion or uncomplicated elective abortion. In unsafe abortion the risk of ectopic pregnancy is increased 10 fold, because of secondary postoperative infection and improperly performed procedures.
   c. *Infertility:* There is a significant increase of ectopic pregnancy in nulliparous women undergoing infertility treatment. Hormonal alteration caused by clomiphene citrate and gonadotropins ovulation induction cycle may predispose tubal implantation. Tubal factor infertility is associated with further increased risk of ectopic pregnancy of 17%.
   d. *Salpingitis isthmic nodosa (SIN):* It is noninflammatory pathologic condition of the tube in which tubal epithelium extends into myosalpinx and forms a true diverticulum. This can be predisposing factor for ectopic pregnancy.
   e. *Exposure to diethylstilbestrol:* Women exposed to DES *in utero*, who subsequently conceive are at increased risk of ectopic pregnancy.
   f. *Smoking:* Cigarette smoking is associated with a more than two fold increased risk for tubal pregnancy.
   g. *Zygote abnormalities:* It is reported that abnormal pre-embryos are more likely to result in abnormal or ectopic implantation.
   h. *Ovarian factors:* Fertilization of an unextruded ovum, transmigration of the ovum into the contralateral tube with subsequent delayed and faulty implantation can result in ectopic pregnancy.

Pathogenesis of Tubal Pregnancy

The fertilized ovum may lodge in any portion of tube giving rise to ampullary, isthmic and interstitial tubal pregnancies. Because tube lacks a submucosal layer, the fertilized ovum promptly burrows through the epithelium and zygote lies within the muscular wall. At the periphery of zygote is a capsule of rapidly proliferating trophoblast which invades and erodes the subjacent muscularis. Maternal blood vessels are opened and blood pours into the space lying within the trophoblast.

Tubal Mole

Repeated small hemorrhages occur in choriodecidual space, which separate the chorionic villi from its attachments. The tubal mole can: (a) Be completely **absorbed**, (b) Can be expelled through tubal ostium as **tubal abortion** with a variable amount of internal hemorrhage. The encysted blood which is collected in the pouch of Douglas is called *Pelvic Hematocele.*

Tubal Abortion

Tubal abortion is common in ampullary tubal pregnancy. Choriodecidual hemorrhage occurs around the ovum, which gets detached and is expelled into the tubal lumen. If this is complete, tubal peristalsis may expel the ovum through the abdominal ostium resulting in **complete abortion**. If abortion is incomplete, part of the products of gestation remain attached to the endosalpinx and bleeding continues. The blood may collect in the pouch of Douglas to form a **pelvic hematocele.**

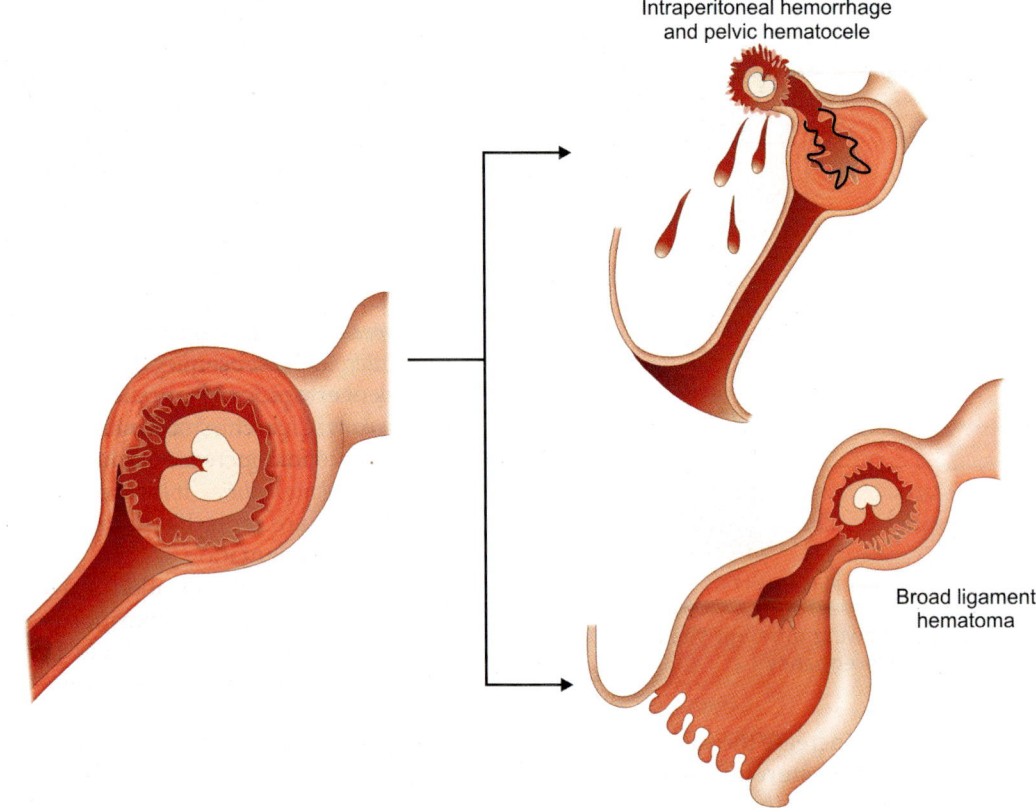

Fig. 31.7: Sequelae of tubal rupture

Tubal Rupture

Tubal rupture is common in isthmic and interstitial implantation. In isthmic portion tubal wall is narrow and less distensible, so the wall is easily eroded by the chorionic villi and patient comes in an acute presentation with shock and hemoperitoneum. *Isthmic rupture usually occurs at 6-8 week, the ampullary one at 8-12 weeks and the interstitial ectopic pregnancy at about 4 month (Fig. 31.7).*

Abdominal Pregnancy

If only the fetus is extruded at the time of tubal rupture the effect on the pregnancy will vary depending on the extent of injury sustained by the placenta. The fetus dies if the placenta is damaged appreciably. But if the greater portion of the placenta remains attached to fallopian tube wall and the periphery of placenta grows beyond the fallopian tube and implants on the surrounding structure like omentum, intestines and adjacent structures, fetus may survive.

Criteria for diagnosing primary abdominal pregnancy are defined as **Studiford's criteria**. They are:
a. Both the tubes and ovaries are normal without evidence of recent pregnancy.
b. Absence of utero peritoneal fistula.
c. Presence of a pregnancy related exclusively to the peritoneal surface and young enough to eliminate the possibility of secondary implantation following primary nidation in the tube.

Broad Ligament Pregnancy

If tubal rupture occurs towards the mesosalpinx the gestational contents may be extruded into a space formed between the folds of the broad ligament and then become an intraligamentous or broad ligament pregnancy (Fig. 31.7).

Ovarian Pregnancy

Spiegelberg's criteria for identification of an ovarian pregnancy is:
a. The tube including fimbria ovarica must be intact.
b. The gestational sac must occupy normal ovarian position.
c. The sac must be connected to the uterus by utero ovarian ligament.
d. Ovarian tissue must be identified histologically in the wall of gestational sac.

Interstitial Pregnancy

Implantation within the tubal segment that penetrates the uterine wall results in an interstitial or cornual pregnancy. It account for about 3% of all tubal gestation. Tubal rupture may not occur up to 16 weeks. As the implantation site is located between the ovarian and uterine arteries, there is severe hemorrhage.

Heterotopic Ectopic Pregnancy

It defines a uterine pregnancy coexisting with a second pregnancy in an extrauterine location. Usually most heterotopic ectopic pregnancies are tubal and uterine, they are seen with ovarian, cervical and other pregnancies. The natural incidence of heterotopic ectopic pregnancy is approximately 1/30,000 pregnancy. With increasing use of ART, its incidence has increased to 1 to 7,000 overall. It should be considered if:
a. Conception is achieved by assisted reproductive technology.
b. Persistent or rising hCG level after dilatation and curettage for an induced or spontaneous abortion.
c. Uterine size larger than menstrual dates.
d. Sonographic evidence of uterine and extrauterine pregnancy.

Cesarean Scar Pregnancy

Implantation of an otherwise normal pregnancy into a prior cesarean delivery uterine scar is called cesarean scar pregnancy. Its reported incidence is about 1:2000 pregnancies. Its clinical presentation is pain and bleeding. In 40% of cases women are asymptomatic and diagnosis is made during routine sonographic examination.

Histologic Characteristics

Chorionic villi usually found in the lumen are pathognomic findings of tubal pregnancy. Gross or microscopic evidence of an embryo is seen in two third of cases. Hemoperitoneum is nearly always present but is confined to the cul-de-sac unless tubal rupture has occurred.

Change in the Uterus

Under the influence of estrogen, progesterone and chorionic gonadotropin, there is varying amount of enlargement of the uterus with increased vascularity. The decidua develops all the characteristic of intrauterine pregnancy except that it contains no evidence of chorionic villi. After tubal abortion or rupture when ovum is dead, decidua is disintegrated and comes out piecemeal or in a single piece as a decidual cast. **Arias-Sella** reaction is characterized by localized hyperplasia of endometrial glands that are hypersecretory. *Arias-Sella reaction is a nonspecific finding that can be seen in patients with intrauterine pregnancies.*

Clinical Features

There are no specific symptoms or signs pathognomonic for ectopic pregnancy. Early diagnosis is important so high index of suspicion should be maintained whenever any pregnant woman in the first trimester presents with bleeding and or abdominal pain. 15-20% of ectopic gestation will present as surgical emergencies.

History

Patient with ectopic pregnancy generally have an abnormal menstrual pattern or the perception of a spontaneous pregnancy loss. Careful history taking should be taken for menstrual pattern, previous pregnancy and history of infertility, use of contraceptive, risk factor assessment and current symptoms.

Symptoms

The classic symptom triad of ectopic pregnancy is *pain, amenorrhea* and *vaginal bleeding*.
a. **Pain:** Pain is the most common presenting symptom. Pain may be unilateral or bilateral and may occur in upper or lower abdomen. The pain may be dull, sharp or cramping and either continuous or intermittent. When there is tubal rupture the patient may experience transient relief of the pain, as stretching of the tubal serosa ceases. The shoulder pain or subdiaphragmatic pain can be due to intra-abdominal hemorrhage.
b. **Bleeding:** Abnormal uterine bleeding, usually spotting occurs in roughly 75% of cases and represents decidual sloughing. A decidual cast is passed in 5-10% of ectopic pregnancies and may be mistaken for products of conception.
c. **Amenorrhea:** Secondary amenorrhea is variable. Approximately half of woman with ectopic pregnancies have some spotting at the time of their expected menstruation and thus do not realize that they are pregnant.
d. **Syncope:** If there is dizziness, light headedness and or syncope, it represents advanced stages of intra-abdominal bleeding and present in one third to one half of the cases.

Signs

a. *Tenderness:* Diffuse or localized abdominal tenderness is present in over 80% of ectopic pregnancies. Adnexal tenderness and cervical motion tenderness is present in over 75% of cases.
b. *Adnexal mass:* A unilateral adnexal mass may be palpable in up to 50% of cases but the mass varies markedly in size, consistency and tenderness. Occassionaly a mass in pouch of Douglas is present. The patient's discomfort may preclude an adequate examination and one should be cautious not to cause iatrogenic tubal rupture by overzealous assessment.
c. *Uterine changes:* The uterus may undergo typical changes of pregnancy including softening and a slight increase in size. The uterus may be pushed to one side by an ectopic mass.

d. *Hemodynamic instability:* Before rupture vital signs are generally normal. Early response to rupture may range from no change in vital signs to a slight rise in blood pressure or a vasovagal response with bradycardia and hypotension. Blood pressure will fall and pulse rise only if bleeding continues and hypovolemia develop.

Laboratory Findings

a. *Hematocrit:* After hemorrhage, depleted blood volume is restored towards normal by hemodilution over the course of a day or longer. Therefore, hemoglobin or hematocrit readings may at first show only a slight reduction.

b. *Urinary pregnancy test:* Ectopic pregnancy cannot be diagnosed by a positive pregnancy test alone. The key issue is to demonstrate that whether the woman is pregnant. Current test using Enzyme Linked Immunoabsorbent Assays (ELISA) are sensitive to 10-50 mIU/ml of β-hCG and are positive in 95% of ectopic pregnancies.

c. *Serum β-hCG assays:* β-hCG is a glycoprotein produced by trophoblastic tissues, can be measured in the serum within 8-12 days after fertilization. Two reference standards are used by various labs. The first is the International Reference Preparation (IRP) which is identical to the third international standard of the World Health Organization (WHO). The second is the Second International Standard (SIS) which approximates one half the value of IRP. The IRP is most commonly used. During the first 6-7 weeks the serum hCG level approximately doubles every 48 hours in 90% of viable intrauterine pregnancies. A subnormal rise <66% is seen in 85% of nonviable pregnancies and rise of <20% is almost 100% predictive of a non viable pregnancy. **Two third of ectopic pregnancies have abnormally rising values whereas the remaining third show a normal progression.**

Special Examination

1. **Ultrasound**
    i. *Abdominal sonography:* Identification of pregnancy in the fallopian tube is difficult using abdominal sonography. On abdominal ultrasound, if there is absence of uterine pregnancy with a positive pregnancy test, fluid in the cul-de-sac and an abnormal pelvic mass, it indicates the ectopic pregnancy. But it is important to remember that intrauterine pregnancy is usually not recognized using abdominal ultrasound until 5-6 menstrual weeks or serum β-hCG concentration greater than 6000 mIU/ml, and presence of blood clot *in utero* may be reported in uterine pregnancy. In the same way corpus luteal cyst and matted loop may look like ectopic adnexal mass.
    ii. *Vaginal sonography:* Vaginal sonography can detect uterine pregnancy as early as 1 week after missed menstruation when serum β-hCG level is approximately 1000-1500 mIU/ml. **An empty uterus with a serum β-hCG concentration of 1500 mIU/ml or higher is extremely accurate in identifying an ectopic pregnancy.** A normal intrauterine sac appears regular and well defined on ultrasound. It has been described as a **double ring**, which represents the decidual lining and amniotic sac. In ectopic pregnancy, ultrasound may reveal only a thickened decidualized endometrium. With more advanced ectopic decidual sloughing with resultant intracavitary fluid or blood may create a *pseudo-gestational sac*. The presence of adnexal mass with an empty uterus raises the suspicion for an ectopic pregnancy, especially if the β-hCG titers are above discriminatory zones (Fig. 31.8). Specific findings with endovaginal probes for *ectopic pregnancy include tubal ring (1-3 cm mass with 2-4 mm concentric echogenic rim surrounding a hypoechoic center) in 68% of tubal pregnancies*. If rupture has occurred, a dilated fallopian tube with fluid in the cul-de-sac may be visualized. The most likely alternative diagnosis to an adnexal mass in early pregnancy is a corpus luteum cyst, which can rupture and bleed thus mimic ectopic pregnancy.
    iii. *Color and pulsed Doppler ultrasound:* This technique consist of identifying a uterine or extrauterine site of vascular color in a characteristic shape, the so called '**Ring of Fire**' pattern and a high velocity, low impedence flow pattern that is seen with placental perfusion. If this pattern is seen outside the uterine cavity, the diagnosis of ectopic pregnancy is made.
2. **Serum progesterone:** A value exceeding 25 ng/ml, excludes ectopic pregnancy with 97.5% sensitivity. Values less than 5 ng/ml suggest that fetus embryo is

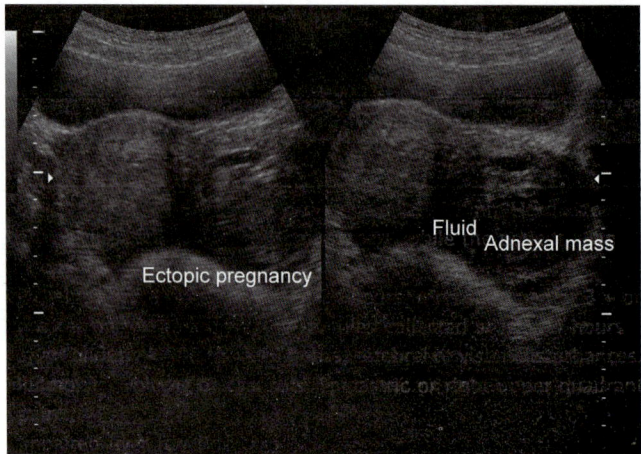

Fig. 31.8: Ultrasound image of ectopic pregnancy showing adnexal mass and free fluid in pouch of Douglas

dead but do not indicate its location. Progesterone level between 5 and 25 ng/ml are inconclusive.

3. **Laparoscopy:** The need for laparoscopy in the diagnosis of ectopic pregnancy has declined with the increasing use of ultrasound. It is used in limited situations, when a definitive diagnosis is difficult to make. If unruptured ectopic pregnancy is diagnosed by laparoscopy, definitive surgical treatment can also be performed at the same time. Despite the low morbidity and quick recovery time laparoscopy is associated with risk and high cost.

4. **D and C:** It may confirm or exclude intrauterine pregnancy in the case of undesired or nonviable pregnancy. On histological examination if chorionic villi are recovered, the diagnosis of an intrauterine pregnancy is confirmed. On the other hand, if only decidua is obtained on D and C, ectopic pregnancy is highly likely.

5. **Culdocentesis:** It is the transvaginal passage of a needle into the posterior cul-de-sac in order to determine whether free blood is present in the abdomen. With the advent of accurate serum hCG values and endovaginal probe ultrasound, culdocentesis is now usually not required. The nonclotting blood obtained via culdocentesis in ectopic pregnancy results from lysis of blood that has clotted previously.

6. **Magnetic resonance imaging:** MRI is a useful adjunct to ultrasound in cases where an unusual ectopic laceration is suspected. An accurate diagnosis of ectopic pregnancy at cervix, cesarean scar or interstitial pregnancy urges conservative intervention with methotrexate (MTX) in order to avoid the potentially catastrophic hemorrhage associated with surgical management of these sites.

Management

Ectopic pregnancy can be treated either medically or surgically. Both methods are effective and the choice depends on the clinical circumstances, the site of ectopic pregnancy and available resources.

Expectant Management

Many ectopic pregnancies resolve spontaneously and with βhCG and endovaginal sonography ectopic pregnancy is diagnosed early. In asymptomatic compliant patient or under hospital observation, patient sometimes can be managed expectantly if bhCG titer are low (<200 mIU/ml) or decreasing and the risk of rupture is low.

Medical Management

Methotrexate: Methotrexate a Folinic acid antagonist has been shown to destroy proliferating trophoblast and may be effective in the medical management of small, unruptured ectopic pregnancies in asymptomatic women.

Criteria for Patient selection for Medical Management
a. No intrauterine gestational sac or fluid collection is detected by transvaginal ultrasonography, the hCG level is greater than 2000 mIU/ml, the hCG level is rising and an ectopic pregnancy mass of 4.0 cm or less without cardiac activity or 3.5 cm or less with cardiac acting is visualized.
b. β-hCG level is persistent after salpingostomy or salpingotomy.

Dosage
Single dose of methotrexate 50 mg/m² I/m is given and patient is followed up by measuring β-hCG level at day 4 and 7. If fall in βhCG level is ≥15%, methotrexate injection is repeated weekly until β-hCG level is < 15 mIU/ml. But if difference is less than 15%, Methotrexate injection is repeated and started as new day 1. If on 7th day fetal cardiac activity is present, Methotrexate dose is repeated and started as new day 1. **If β-hCG levels are not decreasing or fetal cardiac activity persists after 3 dose of methotrexate surgical treatment should be done.**

Variable Dose

Methotrexate 1-mg/kg IM is given on day 1, 3, 5, 7 until βhCG decreases ≥ 15% in 48 hours, or 4 dose methotrexate are given. After that weekly β-hCG is estimated until value is less than 5.0 mIU/ml. Leukovorin 0.1 mg/kg/M is given on day 2, 4, 6, 8. Along with follow-up β-hCG level, a complete blood count, serum creatinine and serum asparatate transaminase are also obtained for comparison with baseline values.

Exclusion criteria for methotrexate therapy:
1. Noncompliant patient.
2. Women who completed childbearing.
3. Peptic ulcer disease.
4. Immunodeficiency.
5. Pulmonary disease.
6. Liver disease.
7. Renal disease.
8. Blood dyscrasias.
9. Hemodynamic instability.
10. Free fluid in the cul-de-sac with pelvic pain.
11. Sensitivity to methotrexate.

Indication for Surgical Intervention

Persistent and worsening pain in conjunction with a hemoperitoneum on ultrasound and or hemodynamic instability mandates immediate surgical intervention.

Efficacy of Treatment

Median success rate is 85% (65-95%) in carefully selected patients. It has also been reported to be successful in treating interstitial, abdominal and cervical pregnancies, which have substantial surgical risk. Tubal patency after methotrexate treatment approaches 80%.

Risk of Methotrexate Treatment

The traditional complications are stomatitis, dermatitis, pleuritis and altered liver function.

Other medical treatment:
i. Actinomycin – D is a more potent chemotherapeutic agent than MTX. It has been used successfully in treating a limited number of ectopic pregnancies, especially in advanced gestation (hCG level>10000 mIU/ml) in which methotrexate has a high failure rate.
ii. **Potassium chloride, KCl injected into the fetal heart** in advanced ectopic pregnancy has been reported to induce asystole and may have a role in treating heterotopic pregnancy.
iii. **Mifepristone (RU 486):** It is an anti progestin used for pregnancy terminations. Recent data suggest that 600 mg Mifepristone with methotrexate injection, the success rate of medical treatment can approach 97%.

Anti D Immunoglobin

If the woman is Rh –ve but not yet sensitized to D-Antigen then Anti D immunoglobulin should be administered.

Surgical Treatment

Once the surgical treatment was mainstay for ectopic pregnancy, now is reserved for patients with contraindication to medical management. The extent of surgery depends on the sequence of damage to the uterus and adnexa. Tubal surgery for ectopic pregnancy is considered *conservative* when there is tubal salvage by procedure of salpingostomy, salpingotomy and fimbrial expression of the ectopic pregnancy. *Radical surgery* is defined when salpingectomy is required. Preservation of ovary should be attempted if feasible.

Salpingostomy

Linear salpingostomy is currently the procedure of choice, when the patient has an unruptured ectopic pregnancy and wishes to retain her potential for future fertility. A small incision is made into the tube on its antimesenteric border and products of conception are removed. Incision can be made with needle tip cautery, laser, scalpel or scissor, by laparoscopy or laparotomy. Linear incisions is allowed to heal by secondary intention which minimize the recurrent ectopic as compared to salpingotomy. Both methods yield similar subsequent pregnancy rates of 40-90%.

Milking the pregnancy out of distal end of the tube is tempting but has been associated with persistent trophoblast and need for re-exploration as well increased risk of ectopic pregnancy.

Segmental Resection with Anastomosis

With an isthmic ectopic pregnancy, **segmental resection with anastomosis** is typically recommended. In isthmic part of fallopian tube muscularis is well developed, forcing the pregnancy to grow in lumen. More conservative treatment such as salpingostomy or salpingotomy would likely cause scarring of lumen. Beside this tubal fistula may result if the tube is allowed to heal by secondary intention.

Plucking Out

With fimbrial pregnancy, products of conception are often visible at the most distal end of the tube, which may be plucked out.

Salpingectomy

Tubal resection can be performed through laparoscopy or via laparotomy, for ruptured as well unruptured ectopic pregnancies (Figs 31.9A and B).

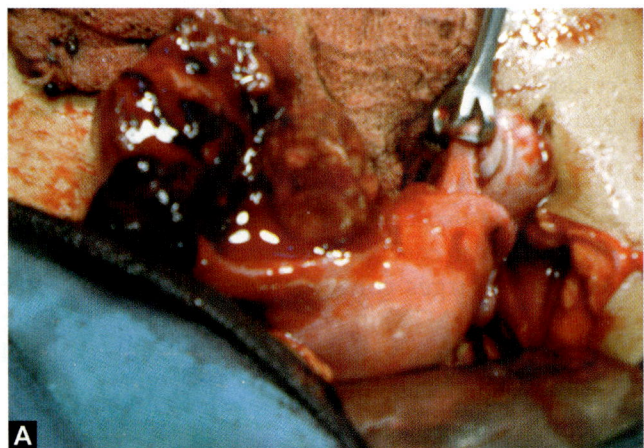

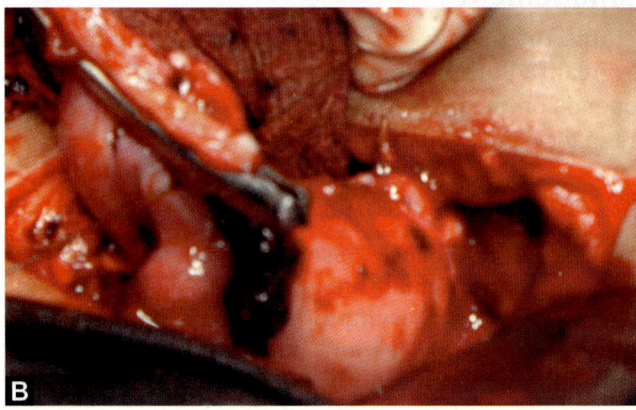

Figs 31.9A and B: (A) Ectopic pregnancy in fallopian tube; (B) Salpingectomy being done

Interstitial and Cervical Pregnancy

These pose a high surgical risk with the potential for massive intra-abdominal bleeding. Most cases are managed with a cornual wedge resection, uterine reconstruction and sometimes salpingectomy on the affected side. If there is extensive tissue damage or if the patient is unstable, a hysterectomy may be needed. Cervical ectopics may also be associated with massive vaginal bleeding with potential for hysterectomy. In both situations medical management should be strongly considered.

Other management modes can be:

Circlage

Hemorrhage associated with cervical pregnancy can be managed successfully by placing a heavy silk ligature around the cervix. It effectively ligates the bilateral descending cervical branches of the uterine artery at a level above the pregnancy to control bleeding.

Curettage and Tympanode

Some author has reported success with suction curettage immediately followed by insertion of Foley's catheter into the cervical canal.

Arterial Embolization

Medical management: Methotrexate can be given systemically or injected directly into the gestational sac with or without potassium chloride to induce fetal death.

Ovarian Pregnancy

It requires oophorectomy and routine salpingectomy on the affected side.

Abdominal Ectopic

Surgery involves delivery of the fetus with ligation of umbilical cord close to the placenta. The placenta is usually left in place to avoid hemorrhage following removal.

Laparoscopy vs Laparotomy

Salpingostomy, salpingectomy or segmental resection can be accomplished by laparoscopy or laparotomy. The approaches used depend on the hemodynamic stability of the patient, size and location of ectopic mass and surgeon's expertise. *Laparotomy* is indicated in: (a) Hemodynamically unstable patient, (b) Ruptured ectopic with presence of large blood clot, (c) Cornual and interstitial pregnancy, (d) Ovarian and abdominal pregnancy.

Laparoscopy has advantage over laparotomy in management of ectopic pregnancy in term of short hospital stay and rapid recovery, less blood loss and equivalent pregnancy, tubal pregnancy rates.

Emergency Treatment

Immediate surgery is needed when the diagnosis of ectopic pregnancy with hemorrhage is made. Blood products should be available because transfusion is often necessary. There is no place for conservative therapy in hemodynamically unstable patients.

Reproductive Outcome

Pregnancy rates are similar in patients treated by either laparoscopy or laparotomy. Tubal patency on the ipsilateral side after conservative laparoscopic management is about 84%.

MULTIPLE CHOICE QUESTIONS

1. Abortion is defined as expulsion of fetus less than …gm:
   a. 500
   b. 800
   c. 900
   d. 1000
   Ans. a
2. MTP act does not protect act of termination of pregnancy after … weeks:
   a. 20
   b. 24
   c. 28
   d. 30
   Ans. a
3. Most common cause of abortion is:
   a. Ovofetal factor
   b. Maternal hypoxia
   c. Uterine fibroid
   d. Cervical incompetence
   Ans. a
4. According to MTP act 2nd, doctors opinion is required when pregnancy is:
   a. 10 weeks
   b. 6 weeks
   c. >12 weeks
   d. >20 weeks
   Ans. c
5. Recurrent spontaneous abortion is seen in all, *except*:
   a. TORCH agent
   b. Uterine pathology
   c. Herpes
   d. None
   Ans. d
6. Cervical incompetence is characterized by:
   a. 1st trimester abortion
   b. 2nd trimester abortion
   c. Premature rupture of membrane
   d. Circlage operation done
   Ans. b, c, d

7. In cervical incompetence encirclage operation done are:
   a. McDonald operation
   b. Purandare operation
   c. Abdominal sling operation
   d. Shirodkar operation
   Ans. a, d
8. The best method for inducing mid trimester abortion is:
   a. Injection of hypertonic saline
   b. Ethacridine
   c. Prostaglandin
   d. D & C
   Ans. c
9. The most common prostaglandin used for termination of pregnancy in 2nd trimester is:
   a. PGE_1
   b. PGI_2
   c. PGA_2
   d. 15 methyl PGF_2
   Ans. a
10. For recurrent spontaneous abortion, following investigation is unwanted:
    a. Hysteroscopy
    b. Testing antiphospholipid antibody
    c. Testing for TORCH infection
    d. Thyroid function test
    Ans. c
11. The most common chromosomal abnormality in early spontaneous abortion is:
    a. Monosomy
    b. Autosomal trisomy
    c. Triploidy
    d. Tetraploidy
    Ans. b
12. Which of the following cannot be used for MTP in a patient with bronchial asthma:
    a. Prostaglandin
    b. Oxytocin
    c. NTT
    d. Ethacridine
    Ans. a
13. Which one of the following causes the greatest risk of ectopic pregnancy?
    a. Pelvic inflammatory disease
    b. IUCD use
    c. Previous ectopic pregnancy
    d. Previous MTP
    Ans. a
14. What is the treatment of choice of unruptured tubal pregnancy with serum βhCG titer < 2000 IU/ml?
    a. Single dose of methotrexate
    b. Variable dose of methotrexate
    c. Expectant management
    d. Laparoscopic salpingostomy
    Ans. a
15. The following drug is not helpful in treatment of ectopic pregnancy:
    a. Methotrexate.
    b. Misoprostol
    c. Actinomycin D
    d. RU 486
    Ans. b
16. In which of the following conditions medical treatment of ectopic pregnancy is contraindicated?
    a. Sac size 3 cm
    b. Blood in the pelvis < 70 ml
    c. Presence of fetal cardiac activity
    d. Previous ectopic pregnancy
    Ans. b
17. Increased incidence of ectopic pregnancy is seen with:
    a. Copper T
    b. OCP's
    c. Progestastert.
    d. Barrier contraceptive
    Ans. c
18. Most constant symptom present in undisturbed ectopic is:
    a. Pain in lower abdomen
    b. Bleeding P/v
    c. Amenorrhea
    d. Hypotension
    Ans. a
19. The expelled products in ectopic pregnancy originate from:
    a. Decidua basalis
    b. Decidua vera
    c. Decidua capsularis
    d. Chorionic villi
    Ans. b
20. Unruptured tubal ectopic pregnancy is best diagnosed by:
    a. Ultrasonography
    b. Laparotomy
    c. Estimation of hCG
    d. Aspiration through posterior fornix
    Ans. a
21. Best modality for diagnosing unruptured tubal pregnancy:
    a. Abdominal USG
    b. Transvaginal USG
    c. X-ray abdomen
    d. CT scan
    Ans. b
22. Arias Stella reaction is not seen in:
    a. Ovarian pregnancy
    b. Molar pregnancy
    c. Interstitial pregnancy
    d. Salpingitis isthmic nodosa
    Ans. d

32 Late Pregnancy Complications

The great end of life is not knowledge but action.

PRETERM LABOR

Definition

Preterm labor is strictly defined as frequent uterine contractions with or without pain in the face of progressive cervical dilatation or effacement, occurring after the 20th week up to 37 weeks of gestation. ACOG (1997) has proposed the following criteria to document preterm labor between 20 and 37 weeks of gestation:
a. Contraction occurring at a frequency of 4 in 20 minutes or 8 in 60 minutes, plus progressive change in the cervix.
b. Cervical dilatation greater than 1 cm.
c. Cervical effacement of 80% or greater.

Incidence

Preterm labor occurs in 5-15% of all pregnancies. The incidence varies with the population studied. Preterm delivery is responsible for more than 50% of all cases of perinatal morbidity and mortality. Out of major reasons for increase in incidence of preterm labor is the increase in the number of multiple pregnancies, particular higher order pregnancies, use of fertility drugs and assisted reproduction. Beside this higher antepartum surveillance and early intervention in high-risk pregnancies has reduced still birth but increased preterm birth.

Risk Factors Associated with Preterm Labor

Numerous factors have been attributed to result in preterm labor but often no cause is found and the condition remains an enigma.

Epidemiological Factors

a. *Maternal age*—Pregnancy at extreme of age like advanced maternal age and maternal age less than 20 years.
b. *Smoking or tobacco*—Smoking and tobacco consumption is directly related to a higher incidence of both preterm labor and intrauterine growth restriction. It is a significant independent factor for preterm labor.
c. *Low socioeconomic status*—It is associated with poor nutrition, the inadequate antenatal care and strenuous work which all result in increased incidence of preterm labor.
d. *Nutrition and body mass index*—Women with low body mass index and poor maternal weight gain in pregnancy are at increased risk.

Psychosocial Factors

Anxiety related factors like stress, depression, negative life events, domestic violence, very hard work is found to be associated with increased incidence of preterm labor.

Obstetrical Factors

a. **History**
   i. Previous induced abortion—Two or more first trimester abortion or one second trimester abortion.
   ii. History of previous preterm delivery.
   iii. Short interpregnancy interval.
   iv. History of urinary tract infection or asymptomatic bacteriuria.
   v. History of previous cervical surgery.
b. **Complications in present pregnancy**
   i. *Uterine anomalies* as malformation of uterus, cervical incompetence.
   ii. *Pregnancy complications* as pre-eclampsia, antepartum hemorrhage, premature rupture of membrane, polyhydramnios.
   iii. *Medical and surgical illness* in pregnancy
      1. Acute fever, acute pyelonephritis, diarrhea, acute appendicitis, toxoplasmosis, abdominal surgery.
      2. Chronic disease like hypertension, nephritis, diabetes, decompensated heart lesion, severe anemia.

iv. *Genital tract infections* as bacterial vaginosis, hemolytic streptococcus, bacterioides, chlamydia, mycoplasma.

Fetal Risk Factor

Multiple pregnancies, congenital malformation in fetus and intrauterine death.

Placental Factors

Placenta previa, abruption, placental infarction is associated with preterm labor.

Iatrogenic

Elective induction of labor in certain high risk situations like hypertensive disorders in pregnancy, Rh incompatibility.

Idiopathic

In majority of cases no cause can be found. Premature effacement of the cervix with hyper irritable uterus and early engagement of head are often associated. In the absence of any high risk factors it is presumed that there is premature activation of the system involved in initiating labor at term. Genetic factors like single gene polymorphism of cytokines in both mother and fetus may be responsible for initiation of preterm labor. Polymorphism involving tumor necrosis factors—Alpha 308, Interleukin 11-1B and 11-6 has been most consistently associated with spontaneous preterm labor and preterm birth.

Pathogenesis

Preterm labor may either be physiological process that has occurred prematurely or a pathological process following in abnormal stimulus like infection. Progesterone withdrawl can play a role in initiation of labor. Infection, intrauterine bleeding induces an intra-amniotic inflammatory response which activates number of cytokines in amniotic fluid, which in turn trigger preterm contraction.

Prediction of Preterm Labor

The first step in prevention of preterm labor is early identification of women at risk. The following test has been tried to predict preterm labor.

Risk Scoring System

A number of scoring system have been proposed combining various risk factors like demographic, social and economic status, past obstetric history has been devised. But the overall positive predictive value of scoring system is low 20-30% and clinical utility is low.

Fetal Fibronectin

Fetal fibronectin (fFN) is an extracellular glycoprotein secreted by the chorionic tissue at the maternal fetal surface. It acts as biological glue which binds the blastocyst to the endometrium. fFN can be normally present in cervicovaginal secretion up to 20–22 weeks of gestation. Around 22 weeks the chorion fuses completely with the underlying decidua. This prevents fibronectin to leak into the vaginal secretion any further until at term a few weeks before labor when the cervix dilates or the membrane rupture. Thus, presence of fFN between 24 and 37 weeks can provide an important marker of preterm labor. The test is more accurate in predicting spontaneous preterm birth within 7-10 days in women with symptoms of threatened preterm labor. Swab is taken from the ectocervix or posterior vaginal fornix and an enzyme linked immunoabsorbent assay (ELISA) with an FDC–6 monoclonal antibody is used to detect fetal fibronectin. A cut off value of 50 ng/ml is usually considered positive. A negative fFN indicates a very low risk of preterm delivery.

Cervical Length Assessment

Cervical incompetence is defined as cervical changes in absence of uterine contraction. Initially it was considered as a congenital or acquired mechanical or anatomical defect. But now it is considered that there can be functional insufficiency of varying degree caused by inflammatory response with upregulation of cytokines and prostaglandins, which result in premature cervical softening and effacement. It can result in premature myometrial contractions.

Method of Assessment of Cervical Length

a. *Digital:* As shortening of cervix precedes internal os changes, digital detection of cervical change can be too late in predicting preterm labor. But if cervix is dilated more than 2 cm, it can better detect digitally as compared to ultrasound.

b. *Transabdominal ultrasound:* It is less useful because full bladder in transabdominal ultrasound can observe internal os dilatation or may produce false elongation of the cervix.

c. *Transvaginal ultrasound:* It is better than transabdominal ultrasound because cervix is close to transvaginal probe and there is no need of full bladder. The normal length of cervix is distributed along a bell shaped curve with mean of 3.5 cm at 20-28 weeks of gestation. The women with progressively shorter cervix had increased rate of preterm delivery.

d. *Funneling:* Internal os diameter ≥ 5 mm is also an independent risk factor for preterm delivery. When fFN and transvaginal ultrasonic assessment of cervical length is combined, the predictive value for preterm labor is increased (Fig. 32.1).*

---

* In normal patients internal os apppers T shaped on translabial ultrasound. In early effacement internal os appears Y shaped while in late effacement it looks like U or V shape.

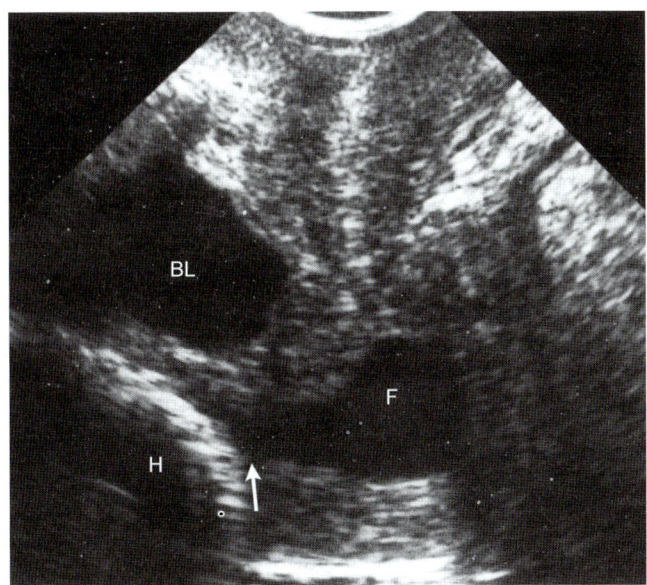

Fig. 32.1: Ultrasound image showing prolapse membrane in shape of funnel (F)

Ambulatory Uterine Monitoring

The home uterine activity monitoring has been tried to decrease preterm deliveries but it has not been found to be useful predictor for preterm labor.

Salivary Estriol

It has not been found beneficial.

Other

Elevated cytokine level in vaginal secretion is found but tests are not yet standardized and currently not recommended.

Prevention of Preterm Labor

In many cases there are no preventive factors. Though the following measures may help in:

Antenatal Care

Intervention like increased prenatal visit, patient education, nutritional counseling, social and psychological support have shown variable effect on rate of preterm delivery.

Cervical Circlage

Women with proven cervical incompetence are candidates for cervical circlage. Cervical circlage should be performed in the absence of uterine contraction. It has proven to be beneficial in selected cases. There are two common transvaginal cervical circlage techniques—**McDonald cervical circlage** is simple purse string suture using No. 4 silk or nylon or Mersilene tape. Five or six deep bites are taken and tied anteriorly. **In Shirodkar operation** vaginal mucosa is dissected away from the cervix before placing the suture. Cervical circlage should be placed at 13-16 weeks of pregnancy. But it can be performed up to 23 weeks of pregnancy. It is not normally done after gestational age of fetal viability. *Contraindications* to cervical circlage are presence of uterine contraction, ruptured fetal membranes, intrauterine infection, fetal growth restriction, and fetal anomalies. ***Risk of cervical circlage***—Procedure related risks are anesthetic risk, maternal soft tissue injury, bleeding, infection, rupture of fetal membrane and abortion. Late complication can be cervical laceration, fistula formation and increased incidence of cesarean section. Cervical circlage should be removed at 37-38 weeks of gestation, before onset of labor to reduce the risk of cervical injury and uterine rupture.

Bed Rest and Hydration

It is widely used but their utility in prevention of preterm labor is not established.

Antibiotics

Bacterial vaginosis—It is a polymicrobial overgrowth of predominantly anaerobic bacteria and is found to be associated with 1.5–3 times increased risk of spontaneous preterm birth. In high risk group treatment of bacterial vaginosis with oral Clindamycin and metronidazole reduce risk of abortion and preterm labor. Currently screening and treatment for lower genital tract infection by Trichomonas, chlamydia in prevention of preterm labor is not recommended.

Progesterone

Progesterone for prevention has been used with variable efficacy in prevention of preterm labor.

Diagnosis and Evaluation of Patient with Possible Preterm Labor

1. **Baseline history:** A detailed history should be elicited for pregnancy complications, gestational age, symptoms of premature rupture of membrane, sign and symptoms of any infection, e.g. (cystitis, pyelonephritis or chorioamnionitis), hydration status and risk factors for preterm labor and cardiac history.
2. **Symptoms and signs:**
   a. *Uterine contraction*—Regular uterine contraction at frequent intervals is documented by palpation or cardiotocography. In possible preterm labor it is generally more than two in one half hour.
   b. *Dilatation and effacement of cervix*—Documented cervical change in dilatation or effacement of at least 1 cm or a cervix that is well effaced and dilated at-least 2 cm is considered diagnostic.

c. *Vaginal bleeding*—Patients may present with bloody show. If there is significant bleeding, patient should be evaluated for abruptio placenta or placenta previa.
3. *Evaluation:*
   a. *Gestational age*—Gestational age must be between 20 and 37 weeks estimated gestational age (EGA), which should be calculated based upon patient's last menstrual period or previous sonographic estimation.
   b. *Fetal weight*—It should be estimated by ultrasound examination.
   c. *Presenting part*—The presenting part must be noted because abnormal presentation is more common in earlier stages of gestation.
   d. *Fetal monitoring*—To assess fetal well-being.
4. *Laboratory studies:*
   a. Complete blood count for leukocytosis and hematocrit.
   b. Urinalysis to assess degree of hydration and infection.
   c. Cervical culture for group B streptococcus. A wet mount should be performed to look for signs of bacterial vaginosis.
   d. Fetal fibronectin (fFN) enzyme immunoassay kits have been approved by FDA, as a mean to assess risk of preterm labor. A negative test is effective at ruling out imminent labor. A positive test is however less sensitive.
   e. *Amniocentesis*—It may be useful in some cases to ascertain.
      i. Fetal lung maturity – When estimated gestational age is uncertain, the size of fetus is in conflict with estimated gestational age like too small or too large or the fetus is more than 34 weeks, amniotic fluid lecithen/sphingomyelin ratio can be done to assess lung maturity.
      ii. To confirm chorioamnionitis—Amniotic fluid is tested for Gram's stain, bacterial culture, glucose level, cell count and if available—Interleukin level.

Treatment of Preterm Labor

Decisions regarding management of preterm labor are made based on evaluation of fetal gestational age, estimated weight of fetus and presence of contraindication to suppress preterm labor.

Followings are contraindication to suppress preterm labor:
1. *Maternal factors*
   a. Severe hypertensive disease
   b. Pulmonary or cardiac disease
   c. Advanced cervical dilatation (>4 cm)
   d. Maternal hemorrhage like abruptio placenta, placenta previa
2. *Fetal factors*
   a. Fetal death or lethal anomaly
   b. Fetal distress
   c. Intrauterine infection
   d. Therapy adversely effecting two fetus
   e. Estimated fetal weight >2500 gm
   f. Erythroblastosis fetalis
   g. Severe IUGR

If the patient is not having any contraindication the management can be one of the two categories—(a) Expectant management, (b) Intervention

A. **Bed rest and hydration:** In threatened preterm labor bed rest should be instituted. Hydration can be supplemented though of inconclusive benefit. At the same time risk of preterm labor can be assessed using fetal Fibronectin level and transvaginal scanning of cervix. Decision about further treatment of preterm labor with tocolysis and administration of corticosteroids can be based upon result of further evaluation.

B. **Corticosteroids:** The administration of corticosteroids to accelerate fetal lung maturity is now the standard care for all women at risk of preterm delivery between 24-34 weeks of estimated gestationalage. Steroids reduce the incidence of respiratory distress syndrome by 30-40%, reduction in intraventricular hemorrhage by 60% and decrease in necrotizing enterocolitis by 65%. There is also a significant reduction of overall mortality in preterm neonates who have received antenatal steroids. Steroids can be given according to two protocols:
   1. Betamethasone 12 mg I/M every 24 hours for a total of 2 doses
   2. Dexamethasone 6 mg I/M every 12 hours for a total of 4 doses

The maximum benefit of antenatal corticosteroids are seen 24 hours after administration, peak at 48 hours and continued for 7 days. If therapy for preterm labor is successful and pregnancy is continued beyond one week, there appears to be no added advantage with repeat dose of corticosteroids. In fact multiple courses may be associated with growth abnormalities and delayed psychomotor development in infant.

C. **Tocolysis:** If the patient is high risk for preterm labor and continue to have uterine contraction with short cervix and positive fFN level, tocolytic therapy to treat preterm labor can be initiated. Aims of tocolytic therapy are as follows:
   a. **Short-term**—(i) To continue pregnancy for 48 hours after steroid administration to achieve maximum benefit of steroids, (ii) To inhibit uterine contraction while patient is being shifted to higher center with NICU facility.
   b. **Long-term** goal is to continue pregnancy beyond 34-36 weeks after which fetal morbidity and mortality is dramatically reduced.

Various Tocolytic Agents

a. *β adrenergic agonist:* They activate β adrenergic receptors and thus increase adenylcyclase with a concomitant increase in intracellular cyclic adenosine monophosphate

(CAMP) which reduces intracellular calcium and thus sensitivity of myosin actin contractile unit to calcium.
b. *Magnesium sulphate:* It competes for calcium entry into muscle cells or calcium storage in muscle cell endoreticulum.
c. *Calcium channel blockers:* They interfere with influx of calcium into cells through voltage mediated channels.
d. *Prostaglandin synthetase inhibitors:* They prevent formation of prostaglandins from arachidonic acid.

Contraindications of Tocolysis

Contraindication include all contraindication to inhibit preterm labor with additional complications are—(a) Known intolerance to tocolytic, (b) Pulmonary hypertension.
Dosage and administration of tocolytics:
a. *Oral tocolytic agent:* Terbutaline 5 mg every 4-6 hours. Ritodrine 10-20 mg every 4-6 hours
b. *Calcium channel blockers:* Nifedipine and verapamil. Nifedipine as 40 mg loading dose over 40 minutes followed by 10 – 30 mg every 3-6 hours.
c. *Prostaglandin synthetase inhibitors:* Indomethacin and Ibuprofen in standard dose. Their use appears to be complicated by oligohydramnios and possible premature closure of the ductus arteriosus.

Parenteral Tocolytic Agents

Intravenous β agonists: Ritodrine and Terbutaline have been used as tocolytic agent. *Terbutaline* is used as infusion in dose of 10-15 µg/minute started at a low rate of 2.5 µg/M and increased in incremental doses every 10 minutes to achieve tocolysis. Subcutaneous Terbutaline sulphate 0.25 mg (250 µg) subcutaneously every 3-4 hours, *Ritodrine* infusion gives 50 µg/minute, increased every 20 minute to a maximum of 350 µg/minute. *Magnesium sulphate* is given in 4-6 gm bolus every 20 minutes and then continued at 2-4 gm/hours to cessation of contractions.

Side-effects of Tocolytics

a. *Use of I/V Beta-agonist* may be complicated by hypotension, pulmonary edema, cardiac arrythmia, chest pain, tachycardia, myocardial ischemia, hypergylycemia, glucose intolerance and hypokalemia. Twin gestations are at greater risk of pulmonary edema secondary to tocolysis. Fetus can have tachycardia, hyperglycemia, hypoglycemia and ileus.
b. *Magnesium sulphate infusion* may be complicated by hypotension, flushing, lethargy, hyporeflexia, pulmonary edema and respiratory and cardiac depression. Neonatal suppression may also occur.
c. *Calcium channel blockers* can causes flushing, headache and maternal hypotension. The concomitant use of magnesium sulphate and calcium channel blockers should be avoided because of increased risk of respiratory depression.
d. *Indomethacin* may cause maternal gastric irritation and prolongation of bleeding time. Indomethacin may also cause decreased fetal renal perfusion and oligo hydramnios as well as premature closure of the ductus arteriosus.

Follow-up of Patient with Tocolytics

a. *For patient on I/V Beta-agonist:* It is necessary initially to evaluate the hematocrit, potassium and glucose. Each patient should be examined for history of cardiac ischemia, valvular lesions, congestive heart failure and arrythmias or previous intolerance to β agonist. So a careful **cardiac and pulmonary examination** should be performed along with routine physical examination. These patients should be followed with **serial potassium and glucose** every 6-24 hours. Frequent physical examination and close **monitoring of urine output** is important for evidence of volume overload or pulmonary edema. **Oral and parenteral fluid** should be limited to not more than 100-125 cc/hours to decrease the risk of pulmonary edema. If there is complaint of chest pain, infusion is to be stopped and ECG should be done.
b. *Patient on magnesium sulphate:* Should be followed up with serial blood pressure and examined for **deep tendon reflexes, alertness and urine output**. Fluid intake should be strictly limited. Serial magnesium and calcium levels may be followed to assess adequacy of infusion. 5-8 mg/dl is considered therapeutic while respiratory depression may occur at >10 mg/dl. As magnesium sulphate is renaly excreted, so renal function and adequate urine output must be assumed. If there is evidence of cardiac or respiratory depression, infusion must be stopped and one ampoule of 10% calcium gluconate is given to competitively inhibit the elevated magnesium concentration.

Newer Tocolytics

a. *Atosiban:* Oxytocin antagonist have been evaluated as tocolytics. In initial trials Atosiban was found to have comparable efficacy and fewer side-effects.
b. *No donors:* Nitric oxide is a potent endogenous hormone causing smooth muscle relaxation. Nitroglycerine, a nitric oxide donor has been used for the treatment of preterm labor. The initial report does not recommend use of nitroglycerine for clinical practice.
c. *Progesterone:* Progesterone therapy is reported to be of same benefit to women with a documented history of previous preterm labor. Further studies are needed to optimal preparation dosage and route of administration.

Antibiotics

Antibiotic therapy as a treatment of preterm labor has shown no benefit in delaying pregnancy. Patient with preterm labor should be started on antibiotics for prevention of neonatal GBS infection if the patient's GBS status is positive or not known. Penicillin or Ampicillin is used as a first line agent. If patient is allergic to penicillin, Cefazolin, Clindamycin, erythromycin or Vancomycin can be used. If there is inhibition of uterine contraction and there is no sign of imminent delivery, GBS prophylaxis can be discontinued.

Conduct of Labor and Delivery

Premature infants less than 34 weeks should be delivered in a **hospital equipped for neonatal intensive care** whenever possible. The preterm fetus should be monitored closely for sign of hypoxia during labor, preferably by continuous electronic fetal monitoring. Digital vaginal examination should be kept to minimum. There is **no benefit of episiotomy or forceps application** and only resorted when indicated. **Ventouse is contraindicated** in preterm delivery due to soft skull of the baby. Neonatalogist must attend the delivery of preterm infant. There is no evidence for a benefit of routine delivery by cesarean section where presentation is cephalic. However, hypoxia is a major risk factor for the development of periventricular leukomalacia and therefore there should be a relatively low threshold for delivery by cesarean section in the presence of abnormal fetal heart rate pattern. However, premature breech infants weighing less than 2000 gm are generally delivered by cesarean section. If cesarean section is indicated it is important to ascertain that the uterine incision is adequate for extraction of the fetus without delay or unnecessary trauma. If a premature birth occurs after the unsuccessful use of parenteral tocolytic agents, the potential adverse effects of drug on neonate like hypotension, hypoglycemia, hypocalcemia, and ileus must be kept in mind.

Cord pH and Blood Gases

Apgar scores are often low in low birth weight babies. These findings do not indicate asphyxia or compromised status but reflects the immaturity of the physiologic systems. *So it is crucial to obtain cord pH and blood gas measurement for preterm infant to document the status at birth.*

Role of Surfactant in Outcome of Premature Infants

Administered neonatally, synthetic surfactant has been shown to reduce neonatal morbidity and mortality. It has been used as rescue treatment in markedly premature infants (<1000 gm), as prophylactic measure in extremely premature infants and as a rescue treatment in larger infants (<2000 gm).

Prognosis

Excellent neonatal care in the delivery room and NICU will do much to ensure a good prognosis for the preterm infants. Lower birth weight babies have a lesser chance of survival and greater chance of permanent sequele in direct relationship to size.

PRETERM PREMATURE RUPTURE OF MEMBRANE (PPROM)

Preterm premature rupture of the membrane (PPROM) is a term used to denote spontaneous rupture of fetal membrane before the onset of labor (premature) and prior to term (preterm). If there is rupture of membrane for > 24 hours before delivery it is termed prolonged rupture of membrane.

Pathophysiology and Risk Factors

Spontaneous membrane rupture occurs physiologically at term either before or after the onset of symptomatic contractions because of progressive weakening of membrane with advancing gestation. When PROM occurs before term, the process of membrane weakening may be accelerated by a number of factors such as stretch, inflammation and local hypoxia. Risk factors from PROM are as follows:

a. Maternal infection, e.g. urinary tract infection, lower genital tract infection and sexually transmitted disease.
b. Intrauterine infection.
c. Cervical incompetence
d. Multiple previous pregnancies
e. Low socioeconomic status and nutritional deficit
f. Smoking
g. History of 2nd trimester of pregnancy loss
h. Family history and previous history of PROM
i. Chronic steroid use

Choriodecidual inflammation and infection lead to a cascade of leukocyte activation and cytokine release resulting in premature cervical ripening and possible membrane rupture.

Incidence of PROM

PROM occurs in 10-15% of all pregnancies including 10% of term pregnancies. PPROM complicates 2-4% of preterm pregnancies.

Diagnosis of PROM

Symptoms—Symptoms are the key to diagnosis. The patient usually reports a sudden gush of fluid or continuous leakage.

Evaluation

1. Digital examination should not be done as even one digital examination can increase the chance of infection

by carrying vaginal organism into the cervix and the uterus.
2. Sterile speculum examination is done. The following are the hallmark finding with PROM:
   a. Pooling—The collection of amniotic fluid in the posterior fornix.
   b. Nitrazine test—A sterile cotton tipped swab should be used to collect fluid from the posterior fornix and it is applied to Nitrazine paper. If there is alkaline amniotic fluid the Nitrazine paper is turned blue.
   c. Ferning—Fluid from the posterior fornix is placed on a slide and allowed to air dry. Amniotic fluid will form a fern like pattern of crystalization.
   d. During the speculum examination the patient's cervix should be visually inspected to determine the degree of dilatation and effacement of cervix and the presenting part.
   e. If vaginal pool is significant the pool can be collected and sent for lung maturity determination, if the gestational age is > 32 weeks.
   f. Cervical secretion can be sent for culture and sensitivity.
   g. *Other methods*—If no free fluid is found on per speculum examination, following test can be done:
      i. A dry pad is placed under the patient's perineum and observed for leakage.
      ii. Observed loss of fluid from cervical os on coughing or Valsalva maneuver.
      iii. Ultrasound examination to detect Oligohydramnios.
      iv. Some times a dilute solution of Evans blue or indigocarmine dye can be injected after performing amniocentesis. At the same time amniotic fluid is sent for bacterial and leukocyte count and culture. After 15-30 minutes, examination of patient perineal pad will reveal blue dye if there is rupture of membrane.
      v. **Immunochromatographic (Amnisure)**—It is new generation test, which detect trace amount of placental microglobulin–1 (PAMG–1). It has 99% sensitivity and 100% specificity. PAMG–1 is a protein produced by the cells of the decidual part of the placenta, which can be detected in amniotic fluid after the rupture of membranes.
      vi. **Physical examination,** once PROM is confirmed a careful physical examination is necessary to search for other signs of infection.

Investigation

i. Complete blood count, urine culture and sensitivity.
ii. Ultrasound examination for fetal weight, presenting part, amniotic fluid estimation and added color Doppler to assess fetal hypoxia.

Complications of PPROM

a. The most common complication of PPROM is *preterm birth*. The latency is the interval between rupture of membrane and onset of labor. It is inversely proportional to the gestational age at which PROM occurs. Majority of patients (80-90%) deliver within 24 to 48 hours.
b. *Chorioamnionitis*: Infection occurs in 15-30% of patient including chorioamnionitis, fetal infection and endometritis. Infections are usually polymicrobial, cultured organism are ureaplasma, Mycoplasma, Gr β hemolytic *streptococcus, peptostreptococci, Gardrenella vaginalis, E. coli, Bacterioides*. Neonatal sepsis account for 3-20% of neonatal deaths and most important predisposing factor is the development of cerebral palsy.
c. *Cord prolapse* especially in nonvertex presentation.
d. *Increased number of cesarean section* because of malpresentation.
e. *Placental abruptio*.
f. *Neonatal morbidity* is due to prematurity, pulmonary hypoplasia. Orthopedic deficits are found with severe, early and prolonged oligohydraminios. Incidence of pulmonary hypoplasia in newborn is directly related to gestational age at birth. The incidence decreases from 50% at 19 weeks to 1% at 31.1 weeks. Neonatal sepsis is another major cause of neonatal morbidity and mortality in PPROM.

Management of PPROM

The management of PPROM depends upon several factors; the most important are gestational age and presence or absence of chorioamnionitis.
1. *Condition that indicate termination of delivery* are symptoms and signs of *chorioamnionitis, non reassuring fetal testing, significant vaginal bleeding, advanced labor and concurrent pregnancy complication like pre-eclampsia.*
2. *Conservative management:* In absence of chorioamnionitis or above conditions a gestational age based conservative management should be considered. It is as follows:
   a. *Term 37 weeks or more:* Term pregnancy (EGA greater than 37 weeks) with PROM in the absence of infection can be managed actively or expectantly. Expectantly management is nonintervention while waiting for the patients to go into spontaneous labor. It is an acceptable initial line of treatment. But if the patient does not go into labor within 6-12 hours after PROM, labor should be induced to minimize the risk of infection. Active management is induction of labor with oxytocin with onset of PROM.
   b. *Preterm 34-36 weeks:* Women with PROM should be managed as a term pregnancy, because there is no evidence that antibiotics, corticosteroids or tocolytics improve the outcome in these patients. Though there

is risk of morbidity at this gestation, the risk of infections and umbilical cord compression outweigh the potential benefit of conservative management. Intrapartum GBS prophylaxis should be given.
  c. *Preterm 32-33 weeks*
     i. If there is indication of delivery as chorioamnionitis, fetal distress, delivery is to be expedited.
     ii. In absence of indication for delivery, following is line of management:
        1. Confirm lung maturity. If fetal lungs are mature, delivery should be expedited as in PROM at 34-36 weeks.
        2. If lungs are immature, steroid prophylaxis should be given followed by delivery at 24-48 hours.
        3. A broad spectrum antibiotic should be administered to reduce maternal and neonatal infection.
        4. Once steroid benefit has been achieved, the patient should be assessed regarding the potential for extended latency (>1 week) before 34 weeks of gestation. During conservative management maternal and fetal assessment is done closely.
  d. *Preterm 23-31 weeks:* Because the risk of neonatal morbidity and mortality resulting from prematurity is very high. These cases are best managed expectantly to prolong pregnancy in absence of evident infection, abruptio, or fetal compromise. During conservative management the following things are considered:
     i. Extended fetal and maternal monitoring for uterine contraction, nonreassuring fetal heart rate pattern.
     ii. Daily clinical assessment for evidence of labor, sign of chorioamnionitis.
     iii. Antenatal corticosteroids for fetal maturation are recommended.
     iv. Broad spectrum antibiotics to be administered I/V 48 hour therapy with Ampicillin (2 gm every 6 hours) and erythromycin 250 mg I/V every 6 hours followed by 5 day oral antibiotic is recommended.
     v. Ultrasound should be performed every 2 weeks to assess fetal growth. It is not necessary to repeat amniotic fluid volume as worsening oligohydramnios is not an indication for delivery.
     vi. Role of tocolytic: The role of tocolytic in PPROM should be limited to 48 hours duration to permit transfer of patient to higher center and administration of steroid and antibiotics.
  e. *Preterm less than 23 weeks:* When PROM occurs prior to the limit of viability, a best gestational age determination should be made based on ultrasound and maternal history. The patients should be counseled with a realistic fetal and neonatal outcome result. Management options are:
     i. Labor induction with high dose oxytocin, intravaginal prostaglandin E2 or oral or vaginal prostaglandin E1—misoprostol.
     ii. Conservative management with strict fetal and maternal monitoring, steroid, antibiotics and strict bed rest and termination of pregnancy if there is any indication for delivery.

Preterm Neonate

The preterm infant is anatomically and functionally immature to handle the extrauterine environment. The preterm infant is small in size with relatively larger head. The sutures are widely separated, bilateral pad of fat is absent, and ear cartilage is deficient. In males the testis are undescended and in females the labia are widely separated. The body systems are functionally immature. The central nervous system is not fully developed leading to decreased physical activity, poor sucking and swallowing and sluggish reflexes (Fig. 32.2). Resuscitation at birth is difficult due to small and stiff lungs.
Preterm neonate can have following problems:
  Respiratory complication
  a. **Inadequate expansion of lungs**.
  b. **Hyaline membrane disease (HMD) or Respiratory distress syndrome (RSD)**—It is due to lack of pulmonary surfactant leading to progressive atelectasis, loss of functional residual capacity. It presents within a few hours after birth with tachypnea, grunting, retraction and cyanosis. The incidence of morbidity due to RDS has been decreasing due to administration of antenatal steroids and surfactant replacement. The main stay of therapy includes adequate ventilation, oxygenation, circulation and temperature control. Exogenous surfactant is administered through endotracheal tube at dose of approximately 100 mg/kg body weight.

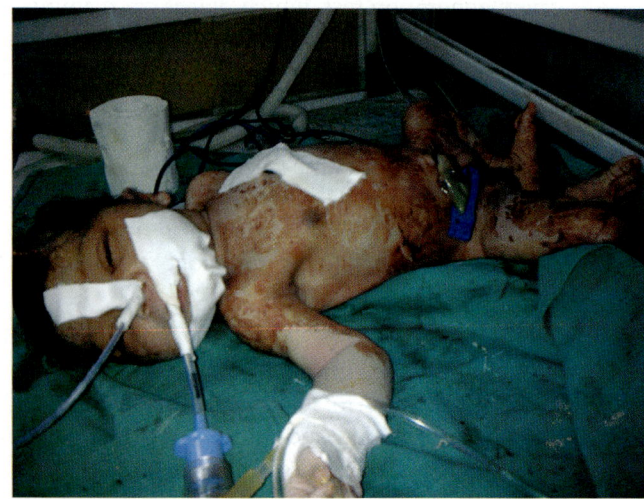

Fig. 32.2: Preterm neonate require intensive care management

c. **Hypoglycemia** occurs due to poor glycogen stores, delay of feeding and birth asphyxia.
d. **Hypothermia** occurs because of lack of subcutaneous fat and large body surface area. So environmental temperature need to be regulated.
e. **Hyperbilirubinemia** requiring phototherapy and sometimes exchange transfusion.
f. **Infection** is a leading cause of death in preterm babies. Low cellular immunity and antibody levels and the prolonged stay in neonatal intensive care units make them vulnerable to infections.
g. **Nutritional defficiency:** Preterm babies are prone to nutritional defficiency, anemia, hypocalcemia, hypoproteinemia, acidosis and hypoxia.
h. **Retinopathy of prematurity**: This is common cause of impaired vision in preterm babies. Incidence is proportional to level of prematurity, level of sickness, duration of oxygen exposure and blood transfusions. In many babies retinopathy of prematurity regresses on its own but it may progress to retinal detachment and blindness. So routine serial screening should be initiated.

Long-Term Prognosis

A higher proportion of preterm babies compared to term babies are affected with neurological disability, low intelligence quotient and visual and hearing impairment.

POST-TERM PREGNANCY

General Consideration

Post-term pregnancy is an inclusive term to describe all patients whose pregnancy extends beyond 41 menstrual weeks (287 days) without regard for accuracy of the assigned gestational age. *Post-term pregnancy* is the term defined to those pregnancies that continue beyond 41 weeks with well established pregnancy dating generally by first or early second trimester ultrasound or known date of conception. *Prolonged pregnancy* is term used for well dated pregnancies that extend beyond 42 completed weeks. This group represents 3-5% of all pregnancies. *Postmaturity syndrome* refers to the dysmature neonatal product of a prolonged gestation.

Cause of Post-term Pregnancy

As the complex mechanism in initiation of labor remains unknown the cause of prolonged pregnancy remains obscure. Certain facts are related with postmaturity—
a. Wrong dates due to inaccurate LMP.
b. Biological variability may be seen in the family.
c. Maternal factors like primiparity, history of post-term delivery in a previous pregnancy are the most significant risk factors for prolonged pregnancy. Sedentary habits and elderly Multipara are related to higher incidence of post-term birth.
d. Fetal factors: Anencephaly which have abnormal fetal hypothalamic pituitary axis (HPA) and adrenal hyperplasia which results in diminished fetal cortisol response.
e. Placental factor: Sulphatase defficiency leading to low estrogen.

Diagnosis

The diagnosis of prolonged pregnancy is made by confirmation of the gestational age by referring to records of early pregnancy test and ultrasound examination and clinical parameters like date of last menstrual period, quickening and detection of fetal heart tone. Routine ultrasound before 24 weeks of pregnancy significantly reduces the rate of induction of labor for post-term pregnancies.

To adequately assess the risk of fetal compromise due to prolonged pregnancy the following protocols should be used for pregnancies beyond 41 weeks gestation—
a. Perform nonstress testing two times weekly.
b. Ultrasonic monitoring should be performed atleast twice weekly to assess amniotic fluid volume and biophysical profile.
c. Daily fetal movement count by mothers.

Risk of Prolonged Pregnancy

a. *Maternal risk:* Maternal risk are related to large fetal size which can result in dysfunctional labor, arrested progress of labor and fetopelvic disproportion. There is increased incidence of operative delivery due to fetal hypoxia and abnormal fetal heart rate pattern during labor.
b. *Fetal risk*
   i. Placental insufficiency is thought to be associated with aging of the placenta and resultant fetal hypoxia.
   ii. There is more chance of Meconium aspiration syndrome.
   iii. Oligohydramnios, which is more common in post-term gestation can lead to cord complications.
   iv. Fetal dysmaturity occurs in 10% of cases. These fetuses tolerate labor poorly and are frequently born with a low Apgar score.
   v. Large fetal size due to prolonged pregnancy can result in birth injury like shoulder dystocia. Complications resulting from prolonged pregnancy result in 2-3 times higher perinatal mortality and morbidity as compared to infants born at 37-42 week. In the survivors there is increase chance of neurologic sequelae.*

---

* Postmaturity syndrome—The postmature infant presents a unique and characteristic appearance feature of postmaturity. These are wrinkled, patchy, peeling skin, a long thin body suggesting wasting and advanced maturity because the infant is open eyed, unusually alert and appears old and worried. Skin wrinkling can be particularly prominent on the palms and soles. The nails are typically long.

Management

Patients with hypertension, pre-eclampsia, growth restriction, pregestational diabetes or multiple gestations should not be permitted to reach postdate. In uncomplicated postdated pregnancies and poorly documented dates, expectant treatment can be done. Twice weekly nonstress test should be done at 41-42 weeks with modified biophysical profile which includes amniotic fluid index. Alternatively traditional biophysical profile or contraction stress test can be utilized. Umbilical artery Doppler assessment does not appear to have a role in post date testing. In well dated post term pregnancies modified biophysical profile (BPP) testing should be done twice weekly from 41 week gestation.

Induction of Labor

Induction of labor should be considered as:
a. Cervix is favorable (Bishop score more than 6) or positive fFN.
b. Antepartum testing non-reassuring.
c. Pregnancy becomes prolonged 42 ± week with good dates and 43 weeks in poorly documented dates. **Cochrane review have reinforced that routine induction of labor at 41 weeks of gestation (with good documentation of date) reduces cesarean section rate and perinatal mortality.**

Method of Induction

Prostaglandins are first choice for induction of labor when cervical ripening is required. Vaginal misoprostol appears to be more effective than prostaglandin or oxytocin. Patient with previous uterine scar with postdatism should be preferably managed by repeat cesarean section.

Intrapartum Management

There should be continuous electronic fetal heart rate monitoring. If there are nonreassuring fetal heart rate patterns or thick meconium, cesarean section should be done. There is more chance of shoulder dystocia and one should have facility for prompt intervention. At delivery there should be availability of neonatal resuscitation team. If amniotic fluid meconium is present, umbilical cord blood gases should be obtained.

INTRAUTERINE FETAL DEATH (IUFD)

WHO define intrauterine fetal death occurring after 20 weeks of gestational age or fetal weight more than 500 gm when gestational age is not known. This is further divided into early IUFD (20-27 weeks) and late (> 28 weeks) fetal death.

Incidence

There is a gradual decline in the incidence of IUFD due to improved preconceptional and antenatal care. It is estimated to be 5-7/1000 birth.

Etiology

The fetal deaths are related to **maternal, placental or fetal complications.** Complication can be in normal course of pregnancy or acute to produce placental insufficiency. In about 25-35% of cases the causes are unknown. Risk factors of IUFD are summarized in Table 32.1.

1. *Maternal factors*
   a. Advanced maternal age
   b. Obesity
   c. Diabetes
   d. Pregnancy induced hypertension
   e. Smoking and tobacco use
   f. Low socioeconomic status
2. *Thrombophilias*—As normal placental circulation is vital for a favorable pregnancy outcome. Thrombophilias—both inherited and acquired causes increased tendency for vascular thrombosis, causes increased pregnancy complication like miscarriage, pre-eclampsia and still birth. The highest risk of still birth was found in women with combined defects as compared to isolated antithrombin III deficiency, protein C and S deficiency. **Antiphospholipid syndrome is an acquired autoimmune condition which is characterized by vascular thrombosis and adverse pregnancy outcome.** It has been found to be associated in 10-15% of fetal death after 20 weeks.

Table 32.1: Risk factor of IUFD
Pregnancy related factors
a. Antepartum hemorrhage due to placental abruptio or placenta previa.
b. Preeclampsia and eclampsia
c. Polyhydramnios
d. Blood group incompatibility
e. Multiple pregnancy
f. Infection
g. Diabetes
h. Nuchal cord
Labor
a. Abruptio placenta
b. Uterine rupture
c. Cord accident (Fig. 32.3)
d. Birth trauma
e. Fetal hypoxia
Newborn
a. Prematurity
b. Chromosomal defect
c. Congenital anamolies
d. Infection
e. Hypoxia
Social demographic variable
a. Advanced maternal age
b. Obesity
c. Backache
d. Socioeconomic status
e. Smoking and tobacco use

Chapter -32 ♦ Late Pregnancy Complications

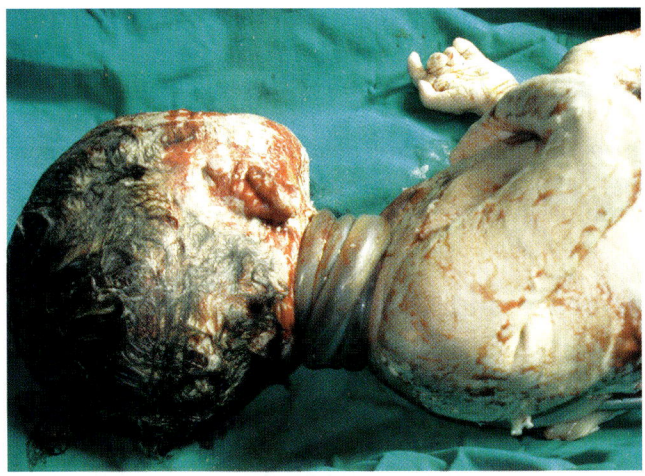

Fig. 32.3: Multiple loops of cord around the neck causing IUFD

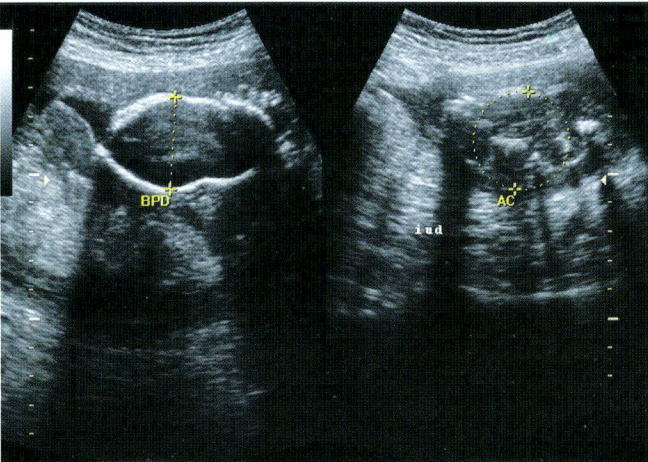

Fig. 32.4: Ultrasound image showing collapsed cranial bone in intrauterine fetal death

3. *Infection:* In utero the viral infection most commonly *Parvovirus B10* and *cytomegalovirus* are implicated in causing still birth. Bacterial infection *Listeria monocytogenes, E. coli*, Gr B streptococcal and *Ureaplasma urealyticum* can cause stillbirth. Syphilis can also cause stillbirth.
4. *Obstetric complication:* IUGR is the most important condition which predispose to IUFD. Placental abruptio, congenital anomalies and chromosomal defect are important cause of intrauterine fetal death.

Diagnosis

Symptoms and Signs

IUFD is clinically suspected when mother reports loss of fetal movement. On examination fundal height is less as compared to gestation age. There is absent fetal heart rate on auscultation.

Investigation and Evaluation

1. **Ultrasound** confirmation of IUFD in all cases should be confirmed with ultrasound. Ultrasound signs are:
   a. Absent cardiac activity during a 10 minute period of careful observation.
   b. Collapsed cranial bones (Fig. 32.4).
   c. Gross oligohydramnios
2. **Plane X-ray abdomen**: Though it is not done not at present for IUFD. However, the radiological signs of IUFD are:
   a. Spalding signs – It is irregular overlapping of the cranial bones. It usually appears 7 days after death.
   b. Hyperflexion of the spine—Ball's sign.
   c. Crowding of the rib shadows.
   d. Appearance of gas shadows in heart and great vessels— Robert's sign. It may appear as early as 12 hours but difficult to interpret.
3. **Hematological** evaluation should include the following–
   a. Blood group and Rh type
   b. VDRL
   c. Postprandial blood sugar
   d. Glycilated hemoglobin
   e. Maternal renal function test
   f. Thyroid profile
   g. TORCH screening
   h. Lupus anticoagulant and anticardiolipin antibodies
   i. Clotting factors estimation
4. **After delivery of baby**
   a. Naked eye examination of placenta and cord with histology.
   b. Postpartum examination of baby sometimes can give clue to etiology of IUFD.
   c. Cytogenetic study by Karyotyping of baby when there is congenital anomaly or IUGR.

Complications of IUFD

a. Psychological upset
b. **Infection:** Infection can occur due to presence of dead tissue. If membranes are ruptured there is more chances of infection especially by gas forming organism like *Cl.Welchi*.
c. **Coagulation disorders:** If dead fetus is retained for more than 4 weeks, there is possibility of silent Disseminated Intravascular Coagulopathy (DIC) caused by gradual absorption of thromboplastin liberated from the dead placenta and decidua into the maternal circulation.
d. **During labor:** There can be uterine inertia, retained placenta and postpartum hemorrhage.

Management

After the diagnosis of IUFD, the diagnosis should be immediately communicated to parents. Spontaneous labor usually ensures within two weeks in 80-90% of cases, but early termination of pregnancy is favored to avoid the complication of DIC and infection due to retained dead fetus and availability of good induction agents like prostaglandin.

Induction of Labor

Various method of induction of labor are available. Induction in IUFD differs from other situations that:
a. There is no need to take account of fetal well being.
b. Induction is required over a wide range of gestational age.

Before starting induction, blood sample must be obtained for hemoglobin level, prothrombin time and partial thromboplastin time. Blood should be sent for grouping and cross matching.

Method of Induction

a. *Oxytocin infusion*—20 unit of oxytocin in 500 ml of ringer lactate solution at rate of 30 drop/minute is started and can be increased to 40 units in 500 ml.
b. *Prostaglandin gel*—Vaginal administration of prostaglandin (PGE2) gel is very good method of induction when cervix is not favorable.
c. *Misoprostol (PGE1)*—50 µg misoprostol, vaginal or sublingually is effective method. Prostaglandin gel or misoprostol can be supplemented with oxytocin infusion.
d. *Foley's catheter insertion in uterus with extra amniotic infusion of normal saline/ Ethacridine lactate.*

Course of labor is monitored. Individualized care, emotional support and adequate pain relief should be looked after in management of labor.

Indications of Cesarean Section

Indications of cesarean section are limited and only for other obstetric indication like major degree of placenta previa, previous cesarean section and malpresentation or repeated failed induction of labor. *Active management of 3rd stage* is indicated as chance of retained placenta and postpartum hemorrhage is high.

ISOIMMUNIZATION AND OTHER BLOOD GROUP INCOMPATIBILITY

General Consideration

A fetus receives half of its genetic component from its mother and half of its father. So fetus may have different blood group than its mother. Same blood group may act as antigen in individual not possessing those blood groups. The antigen is on red blood cells. If enough fetal cells cross into maternal blood, antibodies are produced in mother. If these maternal antibodies cross the placenta they can enter into fetal circulation and destroy the fetal erythrocytes which cause hemolytic anemia in fetus. Hemolytic anemia leads to fetal responses to meet the challenge of enhanced blood cell breakdown. These changes in the fetus and newborn are called *erythroblastosis fetalis*. Several blood groups are capable of producing fetal risk but Rh group incompatibility constitutes the majority of cases of erythroblastosis fetus.

Incidence and Genetics of Rh Factor

About 15% of Caucasian race are Rh negative. In African American incidence is 7-8%. Approximately 5% of Indian population is Rh negative. The incidence is less than 1% in Chinese and Japanese. The Rh blood group is the most complex blood group. The Rh antigens are grouped in three pairs—**Dd, Cc and Ee.** The major antigen in the group is Rho (D) or Rh factor, which is of particular concern. An individual may be homozygous or heterozygous, for each of these inheriting one set from each parent. The practical implication is that the heterozygous father has 50% chance of passing one Rh negative gene to his offspring so in such case child of an Rh negative mother has a 50% chance of being Rh negative and therefore is unaffected. If father is homozygous all of his children will be Rh positive. In contrast the Rh negative individual is always homozygous.

Pathogenesis

Maternal Rh Isoimmunization—Rh antigens are lipoproteins, which are confined to the red cell membranes. Isoimmunization can occur by two mechanisms:
a. Following incompatible blood transfusions.
b. Following fetomaternal hemorrhage between a mother and incompatible fetus.

Fetomaternal hemorrhage may occur during pregnancy or at delivery with no apparent predisposing factors. Fetal red cells can be detected in maternal blood in 6.7% of women during first trimester, 15.9% in during second trimester and 28.9% during third trimester. Factors which predisposes fetomaternal hemorrhage are—(a) Spontaneous or induced abortion, (b) Amniocentesis, (c) Chorionic Villious sampling, (d) Abdominal trauma, (e) Placenta previa, (f) Abruptio placenta, (g) Fetal death, (h) Multiple pregnancy, (i) Manual removal of placenta, (j) Cesarean section.

Though exact number of Rh positive cells necessary to cause Isoimmunization of the Rh negative pregnant women is not known, but as little as **0.1 ml of Rh positive cells can cause sensitization**. A very important protective factor is that about 30% of Rh negative persons never become sensitized (Nonresponders) when given Rh positive blood. ABO incompatabilty also have a protective effect. The initially maternal immune system in response to Rh sensitization produces low level of immunoglobulins Igm. Within 6 weeks to 6 months IgG antibodies become detectable. IgM is not able to cross placenta but IgG is capable of crossing the placenta and destroying fetal Rh positive cells (Figs 32.5A to E).

Other Blood Group Isoimmunization

Other blood groups that may evoke an immunoglobulin capable of crossing the placenta (called atypical or irregular immunizing antibodies), which may cause severe hemolysis are – (a) Kell, (b) buffy, (c) Kidd, (MNSS and Diagio), (d) Xg, (e) P. They may cause fetal hemolysis, but it is usually less severe. **Isoimmunization by Kell antigen results in fetal anemia through red cell destruction.** It is believed that Kell also causes anemia through erythroid suppression, which makes management more complicated than for Rh isoimmunization. Lewis antibodies Lea and Leb do not cause fetal anemia, because they are Igm antibodies and their structure does not allow them to cross the placenta.

Fetal Effects in Isoimmunization

The passage of maternal anti D antibodies into the fetal circulation and the subsequent destruction of Rh positive fetal erythrocyte is the basic pathogenic mechanism responsible for Rh hemolytic disease of the newborn. It can result in following situations:

a. *Extravascular hemolysis:* The spleen is the major origin of destruction of Rh sensitized RBC. This pattern of splenic destruction of IgG sensitized RBC is called extravascular hemolysis.

b. *Intravascular hemolysis:* When there is very high level of Rh sensitization, intravascular hemolysis can occur.

c. *Fetal anemia and extramedullary hemopoesis:* Fetal hemolysis stimulates extramedullary erythropoietic sites to produce high level of nucleated red cell elements. There may be compensatory placental hyperplasia to increase oxygen transfer. The increased fetal bilirubin is produced which is usually cleared via placenta into the maternal circulation but some reaches amniotic fluid which provides a useful marker of the severity of RBC breakdown.

d. *Severe anemia and erythroblastosis fetalis:* When fetal red blood cells destruction far exceeds production and severe anemia occurs erythroblastosis Fetalis may result. **This is characterized by extramedullary hemopoiesis, heart failure, edema, ascites and pericardiac effusion.** Tissue hypoxia and acidosis may result. Normal hepatic architecture and function may be disturbed by extensive liver erythropoeisis, which may lead to decreased protein production, portal hypertension and ascites. If left untreated, the fetus dies in utero (Figs 32.6A and B).

Neonatal Effects

After birth, bilirubin is no longer cleared across the placenta and the fetus is unable to cope with the excess load of unconjugated bilirubin so there is rapid development of jaundice. **A particular risk for the baby is Kernicterus which is a permanently crippling disorder caused by high level of unconjugated bilirubin crossing the blood brain barrier and damaging the basal ganglion.**

MANAGEMENT IN Rh NEGATIVE PREGNANCY

Management of Unsensitized Rh Negative Pregnancy

1. *Prepregnancy or first prenatal visit:* The ABO and Rh group of all pregnant patients should be determined at the first antenatal visit. If a woman is Rh D negative, it is important to know the Rh status of the partner. If partner is Rh D negative no further investigation is required.

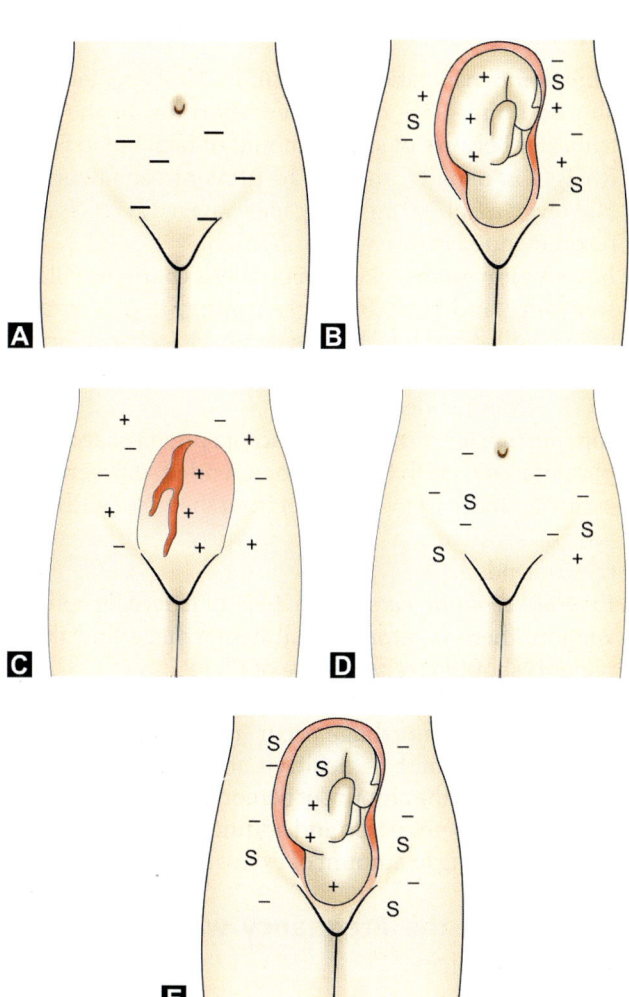

Figs 32.5A to E: (A) Rh –ve women before pregnancy; (B) Pregnancy with Rh +ve fetus; (C) Separation of placenta during delivery; (D) Following delivery Rh isoimmunization and development of Rh antibodies; (E) Next pregnancy with Rh +ve fetus. Maternal antibodies cross the placenta and attach to Rh +ve RBC causing hemolysis

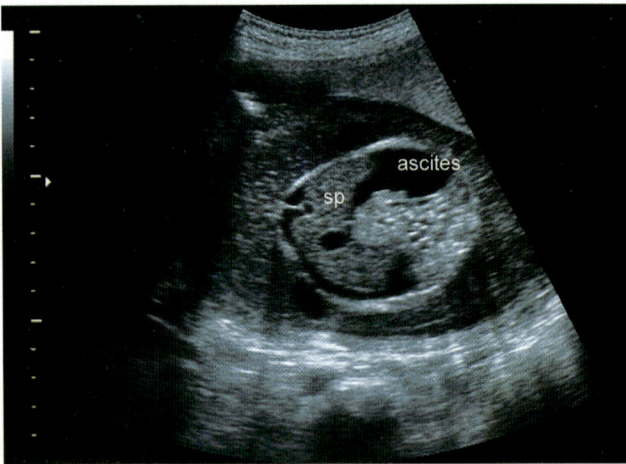

Fig. 32.6A: Fetal ascites

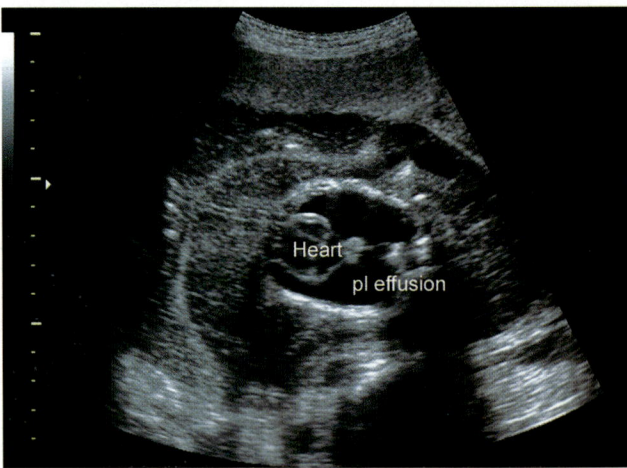

Fig. 32.6B: Fetal pleural and pericardial effusion

If partner is Rh D positive a test for the presence of antibodies should be done in all Rh D negative women irrespective of parity.

2. *Rh antibody estimation at 28 weeks:* Routine antibody testing is done by indirect Coomb's test. In this technique the patient serum is incubated with Rh positive red blood cells. These cells are then washed three times with isotonic saline to remove non adherent human protein and then suspended in antihuman globulin (Coomb's) serum. If the red blood cells are coated with anti D they are agglutinated by the antihuman globulin serum giving a positive test result. The antibody titer is expressed as a reciprocal of the highest dilution of serum that causes agglutination. Critical titer is the antibody level in the maternal serum that signifies that more invasive testing is needed to manage in isoimmunized pregnancy. Critical titer is 1:8 and 1:32 dilution, at which level there is significant risk of Hydrops fetalis. Antibody titer screening is performed at 28 weeks. If it is negative, 300 µg of Rh immunoglobulin is given. If it is positive the patient should be managed as Rh sensitized.

3. *Visit at 35 weeks:* Antibody screening is repeated, if later is negative the patient is kept under observation. If screening is positive the patient is managed as Rh sensitized.

Postpartum

If the infant is Rh positive or D4 positive, 300 µg of Rh immunoglobulin is administered to the mother. If maternal antibody screening is negative Rh IgG should generally be given within 72 hours after delivery. It has been shown to be effective in preventing Rh isoimmunization if given even up to 28 days after delivery. If the antibody screen is positive the patient is managed as if she is Rh sensitized during next pregnancy.

Special Risk Status

a. *Abortion:* Sensitization will occur in 2% of spontaneous abortion and 4-5% of induced abortion. In the first trimester because of small amount of fetal blood 50 µg Rh IgG is usually enough to prevent sensitization. However, a full 300 µg dose can be given. Rh IgG is also recommended in threatened abortion.

b. *Invasive procedure:* Like amniocentesis chorionic villous sampling and cord blood sampling, if placenta is traversed by needle, there is up to 11% chance of Rh isoimmunization. So in unsensitized patient 300 µg Rh IgG is recommended.

c. *Antepartum hemorrhage:* In placenta previa or abruptio placenta, 300 µg Rh IgG is recommended. If pregnancy is carried more than 12 weeks from the time of Rh IgG administration, a repeat prophylactic dose is recommended.

d. *External cephalic version:* In 2-6% of external cephalic version, there is fetomaternal hemorrhage and these patients should receive 300 µg of Rh IgG.

e. *Delivering with fetomaternal hemorrhage:* Extensive fetomaternal hemorrhage occur in 0.4% of patients. If the Antibody titer is positive after 300 µg Rh IgG administration the amount of hemorrhage is quantitated by Kleihaure Bethke test, and additional dose of Rh IgG given according to amount of excess hemorrhage.

Evaluation of the Pregnancy with isoimmunization

Evaluation in these cases is guided by two factors—(a) whether the patient has a history of affected fetus in a previous pregnancy as fetus with severe anemia or hydrops, (b) Maternal antibody titer.

A. *If no history of previous fetus affected by Rh isoimmunization*—Once the antibody screen is positive for isoimmunization. In these patients antibody titer is estimated at 20 weeks gestational age and then every 4 weeks. If antibody titer is below critical level of 1:16/1:32 (according to laboratory norm) there is no indication for further intervention. If antibody titer reaches critical level, **amniocentesis** is performed because fetus is at significant risk for death before 37 weeks. An alternative to serial amniocentesis in patient with abnormal antibody titer is assessment of *blood flow in middle cerebral artery by Doppler*. Ultrasound is performed to identify circle of Willis and blood flow by Doppler is estimated in proximal third of middle cerebral artery. *A value of greater than 1.5 Multiples of Median (MOM) for gestational age is highly suggestive of fetal anemia.* The test can be performed from 18 weeks to 35 weeks at 2 weeks interval but not useful after that due to high false positive rate. Using this method, more invasive diagnostic intervention can be avoided until evidence of severe anemia is reached.

B. *Evaluation in patients with history of a prior fetus effected by Rh isoimmunization*—When there is previously effected fetus that has undergone intrauterine transfusions or an infant who has undergone neonatal transfusion, maternal antibody titers are not helpful in predicting the onset of fetal anemia after the first affected gestation. Once a woman is sensitized to D Rh antigen, there is no role of any amount of anti D. Depending on the history, close surveillance is needed. Atypical antibodies are monitored every 2-4 weeks from booking. If antibodies are at a low level (<10-15 IU/ml), the fetus is unlikely to be affected. If antibodies rise by >15 IU/ml, fetal medicine options must be sought. If facility is available, than heterozygous or homozygous paternal phenotype is checked. If there is heterozygous paternal phenotype, *an amniocentesis is performed at 15 weeks gestation to determine fetal red cell antigen status.* If an antigen negative fetus is found, and paternity is assumed no further testing is warranted. *If fetus is Rh positive, serial MCA Doppler assessment or serial amniocentesis is preformed started at 18 weeks gestation at 15 days interval.*

Amniocentesis: Amniotic fluid is analyzed by **spectrophotometry**. Amniotic fluid contains bilirubin, which is an indirect marker of fetal hemolytic disease. Liley graph is a plot on semilogarithmic paper between the change in optical density at 450 mm (delta OD 450) of the amniotic fluid bilirubin, plotted against gestational age between 27 and 41 weeks. The graph is divided into 3 zones—Zone 1 indicates unaffected zone. Zone 2 is an affected fetus and Zone 3 indicates a fetus that is at risk of intrauterine death. If the fetus is in zone 3 amniocentesis is repeated at 2-3 weeks interval (Fig. 32.7).

MCA Doppler: The alternative of MCA Doppler peak velocity is now also used for fetal assessment.

Other role of ultrasound in fetal evaluation: Ultrasound is used to evaluate fetal heart size, amniotic fluid index and detect edema, pericardial effusion and ascites. Serial ultrasound helps in the progression or reversal of disease.

Management of the Pregnancy with Rh Isoimmunization

Line of management is indicated by amniotic fluid bilirubin spectrophotometry or MCA Doppler.

a. *Mildly effected fetus*—The fetus that falls into zone 1 on Liley's curve (Fig. 32.7) or has normal MCA Doppler is considered to be unaffected or mildly affected. Testing is repeated at every 2-3 weeks and delivery should be near term, after the fetus has achieved pulmonary maturity.

b. *Moderately affected fetus*—The fetus that falls into zone 2 or has MCA Doppler studies nearing 1.5 multiples of the median should be tested more frequently every 1-2 weeks. Delivery may be required prior to term and fetus is delivered as soon as the pulmonary maturity is reached. In some case enhancement of pulmonary maturity by use of corticosteroid may be necessary.

c. *Severely affected fetus*—The severely effected fetus falls into 3 zone on the Liley cases, has MCA Doppler studies >1.5 multiples of the median or has frank evidence of Hydrops like ascites, pleural or pericardial effusion, subcutaneus edema. **In these case cordocentesis with intrauterine blood transfusion is needed to allow a fetus to reach a gestational age at which delivery and neonatal risk are fewer than the risk of *in utero* therapy.**

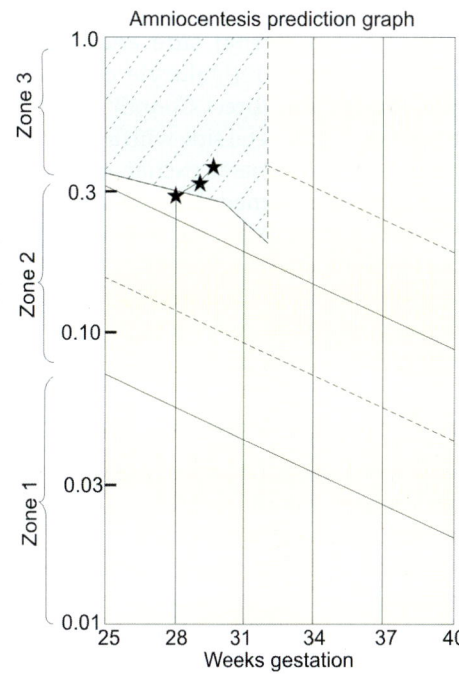

Fig. 32.7: Liley's graph showing zone, 1, 2, 3 in graph plotted on X axis = week in gestation, Y axis = optical density of amniotic fluid δ OD amniotic fluid

Intrauterine transfusion: The procedure is done in conscious sedation with local anesthetic. Prophylactic antibiotic are given. Under ultrasound guidance, a sample of fetal blood is taken from umbilical vein for hematocrit and other values. A small dose of paralytic agent is administered to cause cessation of fetal movement. Once severe anemia is confirmed, the transfusion is performed using *O negative, cytomegalovirus negative, washed, leukocyte depleted irradiated packed red cells.* The volume of red cell is calculated depending on fetal hematocrit values and ultrasound estimated fetal weight. A final sample is taken to measure the fetal hematocrit at the conclusion of the procedure. After the procedure the patient undergoes continuous fetal monitoring until there is resumption of fetal movement. An ultrasound is performed the following day to assess fetal viability.

After transfusion repeat intrauterine transfusion or delivery usually will be necessary as production of fetal blood markedly decreases or ceases. The timing of repeat intrauterine transfusion may be assisted by ultrasonic determination of MCA Doppler studies. Delivery should take place, when the fetus has documented pulmonary maturity.

Mode of Delivery in Rh Negative Women

Vaginal delivery at near term is the goal of management. If for any reason delivery must take prior to 32 weeks gestation, cesarean section is recommended. In other conditions, labor may be induced. Careful fetal heart monitoring is mandatory. Every effort should be made to ensure adequate oxygenation and optimal fetal condition during labor and delivery. After delivery the umbilical cord should be clamped early and should not be milked. The cord blood should be collected from the maternal side and **analyzed for hemoglobin, hematocrit, reticulocyte count, bilirubin, blood group and Rh and direct Coomb's test.*** The cord should be kept long on the fetal side with aseptic precaution in the anticipation of neonatal exchange transfusion. If cesarean delivery is performed, fetomaternal hemorrhage should be minimized by reducing maternal exposure to placental and cord blood. The placenta should be allowed to separate spontaneously. Oxytocin infusion is preferred over methylergometrine or prostaglandin for active management of 3rd stage of labor.

Neonatal Exchange Transfusion

Indications of neonatal exchange transfusion are as follows:
a. Cord bilirubin level is >5 mg/dl.
b. Cord hemoglobin level is <10 gm/dl.
c. Bilirubin level is rising >1 mg/dl per hours despite phototherapy.
d. Hemoglobin level is between 11 and 13 gm/dl, and the bilirubin level is rising over 0.5 mg/dl per hour despite phototherapy.
e. Bilirubin level is approaching 20 mg/dl in the early neonatal period.
f. Progression of anemia despite adequate control of bilirubin by other methods.

Indications of repeat exchange transfusion are same: All infants should be under phototherapy while decision regarding exchange transfusion is being made.

Principle of Neonatal Exchange Transfusion

It removes particularly hemolysed and antibody coated RBCs and unattached antibodies and is replaced by donor RBCs which are lacking in sensitized antigen. Bilirubin is removed from the plasma; extravascular bilirubin will bind to albumin in the exchange blood. Usually within half an hour, after the exchange transfusion bilirubin level return to 60% of pre exchange levels, which shows that bilirubin, is rapidly influxed into the vascular space. *Fresh blood (less than 7 days old), cross matched against mother blood is kept prepared for the neonates.* Exchange transfusion usually involves double the volume of the infant's blood and is known as a *two volume exchange.* This replaces 87% of the infant's blood volume with new blood. After the exchange transfusion, phototherapy is continued and bilirubin levels are measured every 4 hours.

Other treatment for newborn:
a. Phenobarbitone in a dose of 5-8 mg/kg every 24 hours induces microsomal enzymes, increases conjugation and excretion and increases bile flow.
b. High dose intravenous immunoglobulin—500–750 mg/kg over 2-4 hours has been used to reduce bilirubin level.

Anti D Immunoglobulin

D isoimmunization is prevented by administration of high titer anti D antibodies extracted by cold alcohol plasma fractionation and ultra filtration. A standard intramuscular dose provides 300 μg of D—Antibody as determined by radio immunoassay. It is given to Rh negative non-sensitized mother to prevent sensitization after pregnancy related events. A 50 μg dose of anti D immunoglobulin is available for early abortion.

Routine Antepartum Administration of Anti D Immunoglobulin

American College of Obstetrician and Gynecologist (ACOG 1999 b) recommends that one dose of anti D immunoglobulin is given prophylactically to all D negative women at approximately 28 weeks. With such prophylaxis the incidence of D sensitization is 0.07% as compared with 1.8% in women who had not received antenatal prophylactic dose.

It is important to remember that regardless of antepartum administration at 28 weeks, a second dose is required after

---

* Direct Coomb's test—It is used to detect an affected fetus at birth. Cell from cord blood are suspended with the reagent and if the baby is affected (has maternal antibody attached) agglutination with occur.

delivery because the half life of immunoglobulin is only 24 days and protective levels predictably persist for only 6 weeks. Beside, fetal maternal hemorrhage is more likely at delivery. Each 300 μg dose of Anti D immunoglobulin will protect the average sized mother from a fetal hemorrhage of up to 15 ml of D positive red cells or 300 ml of fetal whole blood. The initial 300 μg dose will produce a weakly positive 1:1 to 1:4 indirect Coomb's test in the mother.

When there is more severe fetomaternal hemorrhage, one 300 μg dose of D immunoglobulin may not be sufficient. Recent studies indicate that at least 1% of susceptible mother can have large fetomaternal hemorrhage more than 30 ml without any known risk factor. So it is now recommended that all D negative women should be tested at delivery with the Kleihaur Betke* test and the dosage of anti D immunoglobulin is calculated from the estimated volume of fetomaternal hemorrhage. One 300 μg dose is given for each 30 ml of fetal whole blood to be neutralized. To determine if the dose was adequate after it is given, the indirect comb test is performed. A positive result indicates that there is excess anti D immunoglobulin in maternal serum, which shows that dose was sufficient.

Grandmother Theory

It is recognized that in virtually all pregnancies, small amount of maternal blood enters the fetal circulation, unlike fetus to maternal bleeding, physiologically significant maternal to fetal hemorrhage is uncommon. but rarely the Rh negative fetus is exposed to maternal D antigen and become sensitized. When such female fetus reaches adulthood, she will produce anti D antibodies even before or early in her first pregnancy. This mechanism of isoimmunization is called *Grandmother theory* because the fetus in current pregnancy is jeopardized by antibody initially provoked by its grand mother erythrocytes.

MULTIPLE CHOICE QUESTIONS

1. Risk of preterm delivery is increased if cervical length is:
   a. 2.5 cm
   b. 3.0 cm
   c. 3.5 cm
   d. 4.0 cm
   Ans: a
2. ON TVS which of the following shape of cervix indicates preterm labor:
   a. T
   b. V
   c. U
   d. O
   Ans: c
3. All are used in preterm labor to decrease uterine contraction *except*:
   a. Methyl alcohol
   b. Ritodrine
   c. Magnesium sulphate
   d. Dexamethasone
   Ans: d
4. Which of the following drug may be used to arrest preterm labor?
   a. Aspirin
   b. Alpha methyldopa
   c. Magnesium sulphate
   d. Diaz oxide
   Ans: c, d
5. All are tocolytic *except*:
   a. Ritodrine
   b. Salbutanol
   c. Ixosuprine
   d. Misoprostol
   And: d
6. A 32-year-old female with a history of 2 mid trimester abortion comes with 32 weeks of pregnancy and labor pains with os dilated 2 cm. All are done *except*:
   a. Immediate circlage
   b. Betamethasone
   c. Antibiotics
   d. Tocolytics
   Ans: a
7. Rupture of membrane is said to be premature when it occurs at:
   a. 38 weeks of pregnancy
   b. 32 weeks of pregnancy
   c. Prior to 1st stage of labor
   d. 2nd stage of labor
   Ans: b
8. A woman comes with postdated pregnancy at 42 weeks. The initial evaluation should be:
   a. Induction of labor
   b. Review of previous menstrual history
   c. Cesarean section
   d. USG
   Ans: b
9. Post-term labor is seen in.
   a. Hydramnios
   b. PID
   c. Anencephaly
   d. Multiple pregnancy
   Ans: c
10. Post-term pregnancy is that which continues beyond:
    a. 300 days
    b. 294 days
    c. 280 days
    d. 270 days
    Ans: b

---

* Kleihaure Test – The presence of fetal cells in the mother's circulation can be demonstrated by this test. It depends on the fact that fetal hemoglobin is more resistant than adults to the acid elution. When a blood film is stained following elution, the fetal cells will stand out against the adult ghost cells. It is roughly quantitated by counting the number of fetal cells per 50 low power fields. Five cells per 50 fields indicate– a bleed of 0.5 ml.

11. Which is not a feature of postdated pregnancy:
    a. Cord compression
    b. Fetal distress
    c. IUGR
    d. Polyhydramnios
    Ans: d
12. In post-term pregnancy there is increased risk of all except:
    a. Postpartum hemorrhage
    b. Meconium aspiration syndrome
    c. Intracranial hemorrhage
    d. Placental insufficiency leading to fetal hypoxia
    Ans: a
13. True about intrauterine fetal death is:
    a. Gas bubbles in great vessels
    b. Halo's sign
    c. Overlapping of skull bones
    d. Reduced amniotic fluid volume
    Ans. a, c, d
14. An elderly multiparous woman with IUFD was admitted with strong labor pain. Patient suddenly goes in shock with cyanosis, respiratory disturbances and pulmonary edema. The most likely clinical diagnosis is:
    a. Rupture of uterus
    b. Congestion heart failure
    c. Amniotic fluid embolism
    d. Concealed accidental hemorrhage
    Ans. c
15. following fetal death spontaneous labor will begin within two weeks in:
    a. 25%
    b. 35%
    c. 50%
    d. 75%
    Ans. d
16. One of the following indicates death of fetus in utero:
    a. Spalding sign
    b. Failure of uterus to enlarge
    c. Blood stained discharge
    d. Absence of fetal movement
    Ans. a
17. Which is the most likely complication of IUFD is:
    a. Hypofibrinogenemia
    b. Sterility
    c. Cervical tear
    d. None
    Ans. a
18. In a pregnant woman of 28 weeks gestation IUD is earliest demonstrated X-ray is:
    a. Increased flexion
    b. Overlapping of cranial bones
    c. Spalding's sign
    d. Gas in vessels
    Ans. d
19. The Kleihauer test for detecting the fetal erythrocytes is based on the fact that:
    a. Adult erythrocytes are larger than those of fetus
    b. HbA has higher oxygen affinity than HbF
    c. HbF is more resistant to acid elution than HbA
    d. HbA takes up eosin stain less than HbF
    Ans. c
20. At 28 weeks gestation amniocentesis reveals optical density at 450 of 0.20, which is at the top of 3rd zone of Lilley's curve. The most appropriate management of such a case is:
    a. Immediate delivery
    b. Intrauterine transfusion
    c. Repeat amniocentesis at 1 week
    d. Plasmapharesis
    Ans. c
21. Anti D prophylaxis should be given in all of the following conditions except:
    a. Medical abortion for 63 days of pregnancy
    b. Amniocentesis at 16 weeks
    c. Intrauterine transfusions at 28 weeks
    d. Manual removal of placenta
    Ans. c
22. In Hydrops fetalis, on USG the earliest sign is the development of fetal:
    a. Pericardial effusion
    b. Ascites
    c. Pleural effusion
    d. Skin edema
    Ans. d
23. Anti D immunoglobulin must be given to a mother of 0-ve group with a baby of 0 +ve group within:
    a. At birth
    b. 4 hours
    c. 24 hours
    d. 72 hours
    Ans. d
24. Which does not cause Hydrops fetalis:
    a. Syphilis
    b. Rh isoimmunization
    c. ABO incompatibility
    d. None of the above
    Ans. c
25. Most severely effected child in Rh iso immunization:
    a. Rh -ve mother with Rh +ve in 2nd child
    b. Rh +ve mother with Rh -ve in 2nd child
    c. Rh -ve mother with Rh -ve in 2nd child
    d. Rh +ve mother with Rh +ve in 2nd child
    Ans. a
26. The dose of anti D gamma globulin give after term delivery for a Rh -ve mother and Rh +ve baby is:
    a. 50 µg
    b. 200 µg
    c. 300 µg
    d. All incorrect
    Ans. c

33 Disproportionate Fetal Growth

Education is not filling the bucket but lighting a lamp.

GENERAL CONSIDERATION

Weight at birth was initially considered evidence of prematurity (birth weight <2500 gm) or postmaturity (macrosomia birth weight more than 4500 gm). These criteria have been revised, because it was realized that abnormal growth was reflected in factors other than birth weight. Normal standard such as birth weight, length and head circumference (HC) according to gestation age were developed. Now the following terms are defined:

a. **Large for gestational age:** The infants having birth weight more than 90th percentile are classified as large for gestational age.
b. **Intrauterine growth restriction:** Infants who have birth weight less than the 10th percentile of those born at the same gestational age or two standard deviation below the population mean are considered growth restricted. This defines small for gestational age (SGA) fetus. All SGA fetus may not be necessarily growth restricted, as many of these may be only constitutionally small and not at risk of any adverse outcome. So IUGR term strictly refer to fetus that are small for gestational age and display other signs of chronic hypoxia or failure to thrive. The incidence of this condition is estimated to be approximately 3-5% of pregnancies depending on the population.

INTRAUTERINE GROWTH RESTRICTION

Definition

Currently accepted classification as per birth weight percentile:

a. Very small for gestational age - <3rd percentile
b. Small for gestational age - <10th percentile
c. Appropriate for gestational age - 10th to 90th percentile
d. Large for gestational age - >90th percentile

It does not differentiate between normal small neonate from growth restricted fetus.

Normal Fetal Growth

The control of fetal growth is a complex process affected by multiple variables:

a. **Epidemiologic factors:** Like race, socioeconomic status, maternal height.
b. **Biological factors:** Depend upon *genetic potential* and *substrate supply*. The genetic is derived from both parents, and is mediated through growth factors as insulin like growth factors. Substrate supply is derived from the placenta which is dependent on the uterine and placental vascularity. *Rate of fetal growth is about 5 gm per day at 14-15 weeks of gestation, 10 gm per day at 20 weeks, and 30-35 gm per day at 32-34 weeks, after which growth rate decreases.* Symphysiofundal height-measured from upper border of symphysis pubis to the level of uterine fundus increases by approximately 1 cm per week between 14 and 32 weeks. Abdominal girth increases by 1 inch per week after 30 weeks. So it is about 30 inches at 30 weeks in an average built woman.

Types of Intrauterine Growth Restriction

Clinically three categories of IUGR can be defined depending upon the time of onset and pathologic process:

Type I or Symmetrical or Intrinsic IUGR

It occurs due to growth inhibitions early in pregnancy. The early phase of embryonic and fetal development from 4-20 weeks is characterized by active mitosis and is called the *hyperplastic stage*. If there is any pathology affecting fetal growth at this level, it leads to reduced number of cells in the fetus and overall decreased growth potential.

Incidence and Cause

Symmetrical IUGR accounts for 20-30% of growth restricted fetus. Causes are:

a. Intrauterine infection like herpes simplex, rubella, cytomegalovirus

b. Chromosomal disorders
c. Congenital malformation
d. In unidentified cause, 25% fetus with symmetrical IUGR have chromosomal abnormalities like aneuploidy.

Features of Symmetrical IUGR

All parameters, i.e. head and abdominal circumferences, length and weight are below the 10th percentile for gestational age so these infants have **normal ponderal index** which is – birth weight/height. They have proportionality small brains, liver is frequently affected. Blood flow to the lungs may be decreased, which can cause oligohydramnios and accelerated pulmonary maturity.

Type II or Asymmetrical IUGR

It occurs as a result of restriction of nutrient supply *in utero* that is uteroplacental insufficiency, usually after 28 weeks of gestation.

Incidence and Cause

Asymmetrical IUGR accounts for approximately 70-80% of growth restricted fetus. Causes are usually **maternal disease** like chronic hypertension, renal disease and vasculopathy.

Features of Asymmetrical IUGR

The fetus has near normal total number of cells but the cell size is reduced. There is brain sparing effect so that head growth is normal but abdominal growth is slowed down. Ponderal index is low with low birth weight and abdominal circumference but normal head circumference and fetal length. Cerebral abnormalities may be caused by decreased myelination and altered protein synthesis. Liver size is reduced due to diminished glycogen stores. Renal blood flow is frequently reduced resulting in oligohydramnios. This type of growth restriction can result in chronic hypoxia and fetal death.

Intermediate Type

It is combination of type I and type II. In this causative factor effects fetal growth during the intermediate phase so affect both hyperplasia and hypertrophy.

Incidence and Cause

It is seen in approximately 5-10% of all growth restricted fetus. Chronic hypertension, lupus nephritis and maternal vascular disease, which are severe and have onset in early 2nd trimester result in intermediate IUGR.

Etiology and Risk Factor

IUGR in itself not a disease but manifestation of fetal, maternal and placental disorder that affect fetal growth. The fetal prognosis is largely dependent on the causes. Causes can be enlisted as follows:

A. **Fetal cause:**
   a. Chromosomal disorders like Trisomy 13,18,21, and Autosomic deletion.
   b. Congenital infection like viruses as rubella, cytomegalovirus, varicella, HIV, protozoa like malaria, Toxoplasma.
   c. Structural anomalies.
   d. Genetic cause- inborn error of metabolism like Galactosemia, Phenylketonuria.
   e. Drugs and medications as coumarin, anticonvulsant and antineoplastic agent.

B. **Placental cause:** Like single umbilical artery, abnormal placental implantation, velamentous umbilical cord insertion, bilobed placenta.

C. **Maternal cause:**
   a. Maternal characteristic like age, nulliparity or grand multiparity, history of IUGR.
   b. Maternal disease like hypertension, renal disease, autoimmune disorder, hyperthyroidism, diabetes mellitus.
   c. Smoking, alcohol and drugs.
   d. Thrombophilia.
   e. Nutritional deficiency.

Complications of IUGR

The perinatal mortality and morbidity of IUGR infants is 3-20 times greater than normal infants depending on etiology.

Complications in Antepartum Period

The incidence of stillbirth and oligohydramnios is increased.

Intrapartum

Increased risk of intrapartum complication is due to decrease in placental reserve. There is higher incidence of meconium aspiration, fetal distress and acidosis during labor. There are more cord compression and increased risk of cesarean due to fetal distress.

Neonatal Complications

a. Polycythemia
b. Hypoglycemia
c. Hyperbilirubinemia
d. Hypothermia
e. Apnoeic spells
f. Need for intubations for resuscitation
g. Seizures
h. Sepsis
i. Low Apgar score
j. Neonatal death.

Childhood

a. Increased risk of cerebral palsy (4-6 fold)
b. Impaired cognitive development.

Long-term Risk

Increased risk of coronary heart disease, hypertension, Type II diabetic mellitus, dyslipidemia and stroke in adulthood.

Diagnosis of Fetal Growth Restriction

a. *Identification of high risk patients for developing IUGR:* Identification of high risk patient is based on history and clinical examination. Risk factors like poor maternal nutrition and body mass index at conception, pre-eclampsia and renal disease to be identified.
b. *Calculation of gestational age:* It is of utmost importance for diagnosis of IUGR. Calculation from last menstrual period and ultrasound dating before 21 weeks of pregnancy gives a more accurate estimation of gestational age.
c. *Serial measurement of symphysis fundal height and abdominal girth:* A lag in fundal height of 4 weeks is suggestive of moderate IUGR while a lag of over 6 weeks suggests severe IUGR. Method has low sensitivity (44%) but suspicion on clinical examination warrants additional evaluation.
d. *Sonographic evaluation:* Serial ultrasound examinations are important in documenting growth and excluding anomalies. **Crown rump length is best parameter for early dating of pregnancy.** The biparietal diameter and head circumference are most important in the second trimester. Head circumference is more useful than BPD in establishing gestational age in the third trimester because BPD loses its accuracy secondary to variation in shape.

   Abdominal circumference measurements are less accurate than BPD, HC and femur length but are the most useful measurement for evaluating fetal growth. The fetal abdominal circumference reflects the volume of fetal subcutaneous fat and the size of the liver, which is turn correlates with the degree of fetal nutrition.

   The femur length is not helpful in identification of IUGR, but can identify skeletal dysplasia.
e. *Amniotic fluid index:* Decreased amniotic fluid volume is clinically associated with IUGR and may be the earliest sign detected on ultrasound. But the presence of normal amniotic fluid should not preclude the diagnosis of IUGR.
f. *Placental changes:* Placental changes are not specific of IUGR. Acceleration of placental maturation may occur with IUGR and PIH.
g. *Doppler velocimetry:* It is not useful as a screening technique. Doppler studies are useful once the diagnosis has been made. *It helps to differentiate the IUGR fetus from the constitutionally small baby.*

   i. **Umbilical artery Doppler:** It share the chronologic process of deterioration which is characterized by Increased umbilical artery resistance (↑S:D ratio)
   ↓
   Absent end diastolic velocity
   ↓
   Finally reversal of end diastolic flow
   Fetus with absent or reverse end diastolic flow in umbilical artery is at significant risk of perinatal morbidity and mortality as well adverse long-term outcome. If umbilical artery flow is normal, this group is usually not at risk for adverse perinatal outcome.

   ii. **Middle cerebral artery:** In growth restricted fetus the fetal response to chronic hypoxia is redistribution of blood flow to the tissues most needed as brain, heart and adrenal glands known as brain sparing effect. The cerebral placental ratio (CPR) is the ratio between MCA and umbilical artery pulsatility index (PI), resistance index (RI) or S:D ratio. *A CPR below 1.0-1.1 is considered abnormal. A decreased MCA PI reflects hypoxia induced vasodilatation.*

h. *Other diagnostic test:* They are considered based on maternal history and ultrasound findings. **Karyotype** is indicated with early onset and severe IUGR, especially if there is normal liquor or structural abnormality. An **infectious** etiology occurs in 5-10% of IUGR pregnancies and maternal antibody titer for rubella, cytomegalovirus, varicella, syphilis and *Toxoplasma gondii* should be considered if severe symmetric IUGR is present. Ultrasound feature associated with intrauterine infection are noted which are cerebral ventriculomegaly, nonimmune Hydrops, microscopically intracranial hemorrhage or calcification. The **thrombophilia** disorder should be investigated, if there is 2nd or 3rd trimester fetal demise.

Management of IUGR

Prevention

Though many cases of IUGR are nonpreventable, following intervention have proved effective:

i. Cessation of smoking, alcohol and drugs.
ii. Antimalarial chemoprophylaxis in selected groups.
iii. Balanced protein and energy supplementation especially in adolescent pregnancy and low socioeconomic class.
iv. Avoid contact with individuals with viral infection.
v. Testing for immunity of rubella in nonpregnant population and immunization in nonimmunized women.

vi. Avoidance of X-ray in premenstrual period in reproductive age.
vii. Low dose aspirin and dipyridamole: It is postulated that these drugs may increase prostacyclin production in certain patient and thus prevent idiopathic placental insufficiency.
viii. Maternal oxygen therapy: It has not shown conclusive benefit in management of IUGR.
ix. Preventive measure for maternal disease causing IUGR: Correction of maternal anemia, treatment of hypertension can have a positive effect on birth weight. Intestinal parasite should be appropriately treated preferably before pregnancy. Inflammatory bowel disease should be treated if required but preferable pregnancy should be deferred in active phase.

Treatment

Treatment of IUGR pregnancy presupposes an accurate diagnosis.

A. **Bed rest:** It is often recommended but no evidence shows that it result in improvement in fetal outcome.
B. **Serial antepartum surveillance:** The crux of treatment for IUGR is- serial antenatal testing for biophysical profile, NST and ultrasound with Doppler studies to predict which fetus are at risk for intrauterine fetal demise and may benefit from early delivery. In general when Doppler systolic/diastolic ratio remains within normal limit, the pregnancy can be followed with weekly Doppler evaluation. The biophysical profile NST and amniotic fluid index can be used as an interval test between Doppler examination or twice weekly.
C. **Timing of delivery:** Every IUGR pregnancy must be individually assessed for the optimal time of delivery. A growth restricted fetus should be delivered when it is felt that the risk of fetal death exceeds the risk of neonatal death. This is often difficult to determine but the possible indications of delivery are:
   a. Nonreassuring fetal testing- BPP 4 or below.
   b. Lack of growth in serial biometry.
   c. Significant oligohydramnios beyond 34 weeks.
   d. Strong consideration should be given to delivering even the preterm viable fetus who has severe ductus venosus Doppler changes after a course of steroid. *Expectant management is recommended for small fetus with normal amniotic fluid, antepartum surveillance and normal UA and MCA Doppler velocimetry.*
   e. Role of steroid: Antenatal glucocorticoid administration reduces the incidence of respiratory distress syndrome, intraventricular hemorrhage and death in IUGR fetus less than 1500 gm.
D. **Mode of delivery:** The mode of delivery must be individualized. Fetus with significant IUGR should be preferably delivered in well equipped centers. Continuous electronic fetal heart rate monitoring should be performed during labor in all cases. Vaginal delivery can be allowed as long as there is no obstetrical indication for cesarean section and fetal heart rate is normal. Judicious use of oxytocin for induction or augmentation of labor can be done, when there is no contraindication to vaginal delivery. **Indications of cesarean section are as follows:**
   a. Fetal monitoring shows fetal compromise (Late deceleration, absent variability and progressive moderate to serve deceleration especially if accompanied by acidotic fetal blood pH value should be delivered by cesarean section).
   b. Malpresentation.
   c. Difficult or traumatic vaginal delivery might be expected.
   d. In all cases of IUGR with fetal acidosis, cesarean section should be performed without trial of labor. The signs of fetal acidosis are- *late deceleration, poor biophysical profiles and reversal of end diastolic flow in umbilical artery, abnormal venous Doppler and blood gas analysis showing acidic pH on cordocentesis.*

Prognosis

IUGR pregnancy, *per se* is not considered life-threatening for the mother. However, increased maternal morbidity and mortality may result from an underlying conditions, e.g. hypertension or renal disease. As already mentioned, infants with a low birth weight have a relatively high morbidity and mortality.

LARGE FOR GESTATIONAL AGE AND FETAL MACROSOMIA

Large for gestational age refers to a birth weight equal to or greater than the 90th percentile for gestational age. Fetal macrosomia is growth beyond the certain weight usually 4000 or 4500 gm, regardless of gestational age.

Risk Factors for Development of Macrosomia

Factors which predispose to large for gestational age are as follows:

Maternal Factors

a. *Diabetes:* Gestational and pregestational diabetes. Chemical diabetes is termed with a positive one hour screen with negative 3 hours – (100 gm) glucose tolerance.
b. Prior history of a macrosomic infant.
c. Elevated maternal pregnancy weight – maternal obesity.

d. Excessive weight gain during pregnancy.
e. Multiparity.
f. Ethnicity.

Fetal Factors

a. Male fetus.
b. Gestational age > 40 weeks.
c. Genetic or congenital disorder like **Beck with Weidman's** syndrome – in this there is pancreatic islet cell hyperplasia, Carpenter syndrome or fragile X-syndrome.
d. Constitutionally large fetus.

Diagnosis

Prediction

Identification of risk factor helps in selection of patients for screening. However, clinical measurement like Leopold maneuver and fundal height measurement have reported sensitivity of 10-43%, specifically of 99-99.8% and positive predictive value of 28-53%. With fetal weight exceeding 4500 gm, without maternal diabetes, ultrasound biometry is useful with positive predictive value of 30-44%.

Complications of Macrosomia

There can be following possible maternal and fetal complications:
a. **Maternal:**
   i. Increased risk of operative vaginal delivery.
   ii. Perineal trauma.
   iii. Shoulder dystocia.
   iv. Postpartum hemorrhage.
   v. Increased rate of cesarean section.
b. **Fetal complications:**
   i. Shoulder dystocia.
   ii. Stillbirth.
   iii. Anomalies.
c. **Neonatal complications:**
   i. Birth injury like clavicular fracture.
   ii. Hypoglycemia.
   iii. Hypocalcemia.
   iv. Polycythemia.
   v. Increased rate of cesarean section
   vi. Feeding difficulties
d. **Long-term complications:**
   i. Obesity.
   ii. Type II diabetes.
   iii. Neurological behavioral problem.

Management

Patient with the risk factors for macrosomia should be evaluated for possible fetal macrosomia with an ultrasound estimated fetal size and weight. In gestational diabetes maternal glucose level should be adequately controlled. *A role of induction of labor in high risk pregnancy for reducing the incidence of intrapartum complication is not proved*, though it is in use in clinical practice. Cesarean section reduces risk of birth trauma in fetal macrosomia. But its routine use in all macrosomic fetuses is still not recommended.

In labor management partogram should be carefully followed and careful consideration should be given before performing operative vaginal delivery as there is risk of shoulder dystocia. Vacuum extraction should be avoided if fetal weight greater than 4000 gm. There should be availability of senior obstetrician, neonatologist and anesthetist. Labor should occur in settings where immediate cesarean can be accomplished.

Prognosis

Any women who deliver a large for gestational age baby should be informed that the risk of having another large for gestational age baby is increased by 2.5-4 fold. These women should be screened for previously undiagnosed chemical or insulin independent diabetes. Even if initial screening test is negative they should be carefully followed in any subsequent pregnancy for gestational diabetes mellitus. Obese women should be strongly encouraged to lose weight prior to conception. Women should be encouraged to seek early care in subsequent pregnancy to minimize the possibility of postdatism.

MULTIPLE CHOICE QUESTIONS

1. All are causes of IUGR *except*:
   a. Anemia
   b. PIH
   c. Maternal heart disease
   d. Gestational diabetes

   Ans. d

2. IUGR is seen in:
   a. Rubella
   b. Syphilis
   c. CMV
   d. Chickenpox
   e. HPV

   Ans. a, b, c, d

3. Best parameter for ultrasound evaluation of IUGR is:
   a. Placental membrane
   b. Length of femur
   c. Abdominal circumference
   d. BPD

   Ans. c

4. A pregnant lady with persistent late deceleration with cervical dilatation of 6 cm shifted to OT for surgery, which of the following is not done in management:
   a. Supine position
   b. O_2 inhalation

c. IV fluid
   d. Subcutaneous terbutaline

   Ans. a

5. Hypoglycemia in newborn is seen in:
   a. IUGR
   b. Mother with hypothyroidism
   c. Rh in compatibility
   d. Macrosomia
   e. Hyperthyroidism

   Ans. a, b, d

6. Birth weight of a baby can be increased by:
   a. Cessation of smoking
   b. Aspirin
   c. Ca and vitamin D supplementation
   d. Bed rest

   Ans. a

7. Which organ is spared in asymmetrical IUGR:
   a. Liver
   b. Muscle
   c. Subcutaneous fat
   d. Brain

   Ans. d

8. Difference between prematurity and IUGR is that premature baby has:
   a. Sole creases all over feet
   b. Breast nodule 2 mm
   c. Ear cartilage well formed - a good elastic recoil
   d. Skin glistening thin
   e. Poor muscle tone

   Ans. b, d, e

9. Intrauterine fetal distress is indicated by:
   a. Acceleration of 15/min
   b. Deceleration of 30/min
   c. Variable deceleration 5-25/min
   d. Fetal HR < 80 min
   e. Fetal HR > 160-180/min

   Ans. b, d, e

10. A lady of 150 cm height with Hb 11 gm%, BP of 160/110 mm Hg and 12 kg gain during her pregnancy delivered an IUGR baby, the causes in this case are:
    a. Maternal infection
    b. Short structure
    c. HTN
    d. Increased weight gain
    e. Decreased Hb%

    Ans. c

34 Hypertensive Disorders in Pregnancy

Science is organized knowledge, wisdom is organized life.

GENERAL CONSIDERATION

Hypertensive disorders are among the most common medical disorders during pregnancy. In developing countries 7-10% of all pregnancies are complicated by some form of hypertensive disease. High blood pressure is a sign, not a disease in itself, which reflect an increase in cardiac output or more commonly increase in total peripheral resistance. It can be caused by number of disorders that may have different effects on the pregnancy outcome. So the correct identification of the underlying hypertensive disorder is necessary for appropriate management.

Definition and Classification of Hypertensive Disorders in Pregnancy

Hypertension during pregnancy is defined as a sustained systolic blood pressure of 140 mm Hg or more and or a diastolic blood pressure of 90 mm Hg or more. This is best confirmed when evidence is present on two occasions at least 6 hours apart but within 7 days. *Proteinuria is defined as excretion of ≥ 0.3 gm protein in a 24 hours sample, which correlates with ≥ 30 mg/ dl or ≥ 1 + on dipstick in a random sample after excluding urinary tract infection.*

Classification

Various classifications of hypertensive disorders in pregnancy have been proposed. A recent classification recommended by National Institute of Health (NIH) working group on high blood pressure in pregnancy in 2000 has been summarized on Table 34.1.

Approximately two-third of a women with hypertension in pregnancy have preeclampsia or gestational hypertension, while one-third have chronic hypertension. The categories in above classification are easily distinguished by careful history, physical examination and laboratory findings.

Preeclampsia

Preeclampsia is a multisystem disorder of unknown etiology which is unique to pregnancy with onset after 20 weeks of gestation. It is defined by hypertension and proteinuria. For women who do not have chronic hypertension, an elevation above 140 mm Hg systolic or 90 mm Hg diastolic meets the criteria. The previous definition of increase in blood pressure above base line (a 30 mm Hg increase in systolic or a 15 mm Hg increase in diastolic) has been discarded in favor of the absolute definition of 140 mm Hg systolic and 90 mm Hg diastolic. *Edema of the face and hands which used to be a component of the diagnosis of preeclampsia has been dropped as criteria because of its poor predictive value.* Many pregnant women with normal blood pressure have hand and fascial edema.

Incidence and Risk Factors for Preeclampsia

Preeclampsia complicates 2-8% of pregnancies and is a major cause of maternal morbidity, perinatal death and premature delivery. The risk factors for the preeclampsia are as follows:
a. Nulliparity
b. Obesity
c. Multiple gestation
d. Family history of preeclampsia or eclampsia
e. Pre-existing hypertension or renal disease
f. Previous preeclampsia or eclampsia
g. Diabetes mellitus
h. Antiphospholipid antibody syndrome
i. Molar pregnancy
j. Nonimmune hydrops.

Etiopathogenesis

The exact etiology of preeclampsia remains unknown, many theories have been proposed most of which have

Table 34.1: Classification of hypertensive disorders of pregnancy

Gestational Hypertension	• Systolic BP ≥ 140 or diastolic BP ≥ mm Hg for first time during pregnancy • No proteinuria • BP returns to normal before 12 weeks postpartum • Final diagnosis made only postpartum • May have other signs or symptoms of preeclampsia, for e.g. epigastric discomfort or thrombocytopenia
Pre-eclampsia	*Minimum criteria:* • BP > 140/90 mm Hg after 20 weeks gestation • Proteinuria > 300 mg/24 hours or > 1 + dipstick *Increased certainty of preeclampsia:* • BP > 160/110 mm Hg • Proteinuria 2.0 g/24 hours or > 2 + dipstick • Serum creatinine > 1.2 mg/dl unless known to bee previously elevated • Platelets < 100,000/ μl • Microangiopathic hemolysis – increased LDH • Elevated serum transaminase levels – ALT or AST • Persistent headache or other cerebral or visual disturbance • Persistent epigastric pain
Eclampsia	• Seizures that cannot be attributed to other causes in a woman with preeclampsia
Superimposed preeclampsia on chronic hypertension	• New onset proteinuria > 300 mg/24 hours in hypertensive women but no proteinuria before 20 weeks gestation • A sudden increase in proteinuria or blood pressure or platelet count < 100,000/ μL in women with hypertension and proteinuria before 20 weeks gestation • BP ≥ 140/90 mm Hg before pregnancy or diagnosed before 20 weeks gestation not attributable to gestational trophoblastic disease or
Chronic hypertension	• Hypertension first diagnosed before 20 weeks gestation and persistent after 12 weeks postpartum

ALT – alanine aminotransferase; AST – aspartate aminotransferase; BP – blood pressure; LDH – lactate dehydrogenase.
National High Blood Pressure Education Program Working Group Report on High Pressure in Pregnancy (2000)

been discarded. Hypertension, proteinuria and other signs and symptoms of the illness are merely the outward manifestation of a systemic illness characterized by vasoconstriction and hypovolemia. All organs including the fetoplacental unit show evidence of poor perfusion. Following theories have been proposed:

a. *Immunologic response:* Inadequate maternal antibody response to the fetal allograft results in vascular damage from the circulating immune complexes. This theory is supported by an increased prevalence of the disease in pregnancies with limited prior exposure to antigen like young nullipara and in situations where there are increased fetal antigens – like twins, molar pregnancy, hydropic pregnancies and diabetic with large placentas.

b. *Circulating toxins:* Vasoconstriction substances have been extracted from blood, amniotic fluid and the placenta in women with preeclampsia.

c. *Endogenous vasoconstriction:* There is increased sensitivity to vasopressin, epinephrine and norepinephrine. Loss of normal third trimester resistance to angiotensin II has also been noted.

d. *Endothelial damage:* Primary endothelial damage results in a decrease in prostacyclin production, which is potent vasodilator and a relative increase in thromboxane A2 which is relative vasoconstrictor. But the cause of endothelial damage and prostaglandin change is unclear.

e. *Primary disseminated intravascular coagulation:* Microvascular thrombin formation and depositions have been noted, producing vessel damage especially in the kidney and the placenta.

f. *Oxidation stress:* There is growing evidence that preeclampsia is increased in women with elevated level of oxidized low density lipoproteins and triglycerides and abnormal increase of serum lipid peroxidase in preeclamptic women. These substances act by inhibiting prostaglandin synthetase and cause cellular damage.

Pathophysiology

Preeclampsia as a two stage disorder:
According to Redman et al (2009), preeclampsia is a two stage disorder. Stage 1 is caused by faulty endovascular trophoblastic remodelling which cause stage 2 clinical syndrome (Flow chart 34.1).

Flow chart 34.1: Two stage theory of preeclampsia

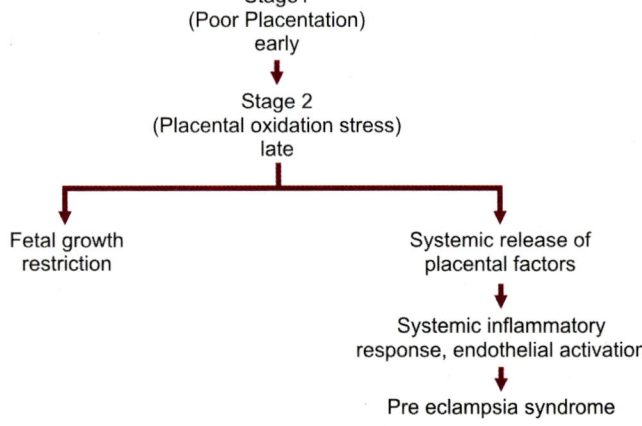

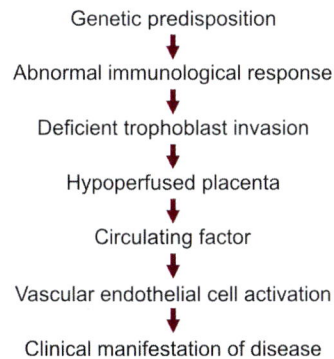

Flow chart 34.2: Proposed etiology of preeclampsia

Table 34.2: Specific changes associated with preeclampsia
Cardiovascular:
• Generalized vasospasm
• Increased peripheral resistance
• Reduced initial venous/pulmonary wedge pressure
Hematological:
• Platelet activation and depletion
• Coagulopathy
• Decreased plasma volume
• Increased blood viscosity
Renal:
• Proteinuria
• Decreased GFR
• Oliguria
Hepatic:
• Periportal necrosis
• Subcapsular hematoma
Central nervous system:
• Cerebral edema
• Cerebral hemorrhage

By strict definition preeclampsia and eclampsia fits in the definition of a syndrome, (i.e. a group of symptoms or pathological signs, which consistently occur together especially with an unknown cause). In preeclampsia the multiorgan involvement is consequence of vasospasm, endothelial dysfunction and ischemia (Flow chart 34.2), (Table 34.2).

Cardiovascular Changes

Preeclampsia is characterized by the absence of normal intravascular volume expansion, a reduction in normal circulating blood volume and loss of normal refractorines to endogenous vasopressors including angiotensin II. Reduction in normal circulating blood volume is due to constricted vasculature and extravasation, so preload may be normal or decreased. But the afterload is elevated because of raised vascular resistance. These patients are very sensitive to both plasma volume increase as well volume loss.

Hematologic Changes

In patients with preeclampsia there is increased hematocrit due to hemoconcentration and thrombocytopenia due to extravasation. There is low platelet count and decreased fibrinogen. There can be alteration in coagulation profile and hemolytic anemia may be present.

Morphological Changes

a. *Kidney:* The classic renal lesion of preeclampsia is **glomerular endotheliosis** which is characterized by swelling and enlargement of glomerular capillary endothelial cells leading to narrowing of capillary lumen. There is increased amount of cytoplasm containing lipid filled vacuoles. Immunoglobulin, complement, fibrin and fibrin degradation products have been observed in the glomerulus.

b. *Liver:* The pathological changes in the liver are periportal hemorrhage, ischemic lesions and fibrin deposition. Liver damage varies from mild hepatocellular necrosis to severe liver injury with marked increase in liver enzymes, subcapsular rupture and very rarely even liver rupture.

c. *Lungs:* Alteration in colloid oncotic pressure, capillary endothelial integrity and intravascular hydrostatic pressure in preeclampsia predispose to noncardiogenic pulmonary edema. In women with preeclampsia superimposed on chronic hypertension, pre-existing hypertensive cardiac disease may exacerbate the situation, superimposing cardiogenic pulmonary edema on noncardiogenic preeclampsia related pulmonary edema. If there is excessive administration of intravenous fluid and postpartum mobilization of accumulated extravascular fluid, it increases the risk of pulmonary edema. In eclampsia aspiration of gastric contents can cause pneumonia, pneumonitis, or adult respiratory distress syndrome.

d. *Placenta and uterus:* In preeclampsia there is increased incidence of infarcts, hematomas, congested chorionic villi, proliferative endarteritis and degeneration in the hypertensive group. On microscopy there are increased syncytial knots, cytotrophoblastic cellular proliferation, fibrinoid necrosis, endothelial proliferation and calcified and hyalinized vilous spots.

e. *Eyes:* Retinal vasospasm, retinal edema, serious retinal detachment and cortical blindness may occur in preeclampsia. Blindness is uncommon and usually transient, resolving within hours to days of delivery.

Prediction of Preeclampsia

Though many tests have been proposed for the prediction and early detection of preeclampsia, but at present there is no single screening test that can be considered reliable and cost effective for predicting preeclampsia. Following tests have been proposed:

a. ***Roll over test or supine pressor test:*** According to this test at 18-22 weeks gestation in normotensive women, if there is rise of diastolic blood pressure by 20 mm Hg or more within 5 minutes after changing from left lateral to supine position, that women is likely to develop hypertension later in pregnancy.
b. ***Isometric exercise:*** An increase of 15 mm Hg in systolic pressure during the handgrip test predicts the development of gestational hypertension with high sensitivity (55-70%) and specificity (85%).
c. ***Doppler study of uterine artery:*** If there is diastolic notching in the arcuate vessels of the uterus at 16-20 weeks of gestation, it predicts the development of preeclampsia.
d. ***Low level of PAPP-A:*** Low levels of PAPP-A in the first trimester have been found to be associated with a two fold risk of developing preeclampsia later in pregnancy.

Prevention of Preeclampsia

a. ***Aspirin and antiplatelet agent:*** Beneficial results with combined low molecular weight heparin with low dose aspirin in women with history of severe early onset preeclampsia and IUGR have been reported. Low dose aspirins as antiplatelet agent is found to reduce the risk of preeclampsia by 19%.
b. ***Diet and exercise:*** There is no reliable evidence that any change in diet or life style has any impact on the occurrence of preeclampsia.
c. Several studies on the therapeutic role of vitamins C and E (major antioxidants) in the prevention and treatment of preeclampsia are now in progress.

MANAGEMENT

The basic objective of management of any pregnancy complicated by PIH is:
a. Termination of pregnancy with least possible trauma to the mother and fetus.
b. Birth of an infant who subsequently thrives and who will not require intensive and prolonged neonatal care.
c. Complete restoration of health of mother.
The objective can be achieved by formulating a management plan that takes into consideration of following:
i. Severity of disease process.
ii. Fetal gestational age.
iii. Maternal and fetal status at time of initial evaluation.
iv. Presence of labor.
v. Cervical bishop score.

Severity of disease process: For assessing severity of disease process we have to define and classify the patients according to criteria summarized in Table 34.3.

Management of Mild PIH

Mild PIH near term: In general women with mild PIH developing at 37 weeks of gestation or longer have a pregnancy outcome similar to that found in normotensive pregnancy. Expectant management can be done in hospital or home until onset of labor or completion of 40 weeks gestation. Maternal and fetal evaluation should be performed twice weekly. However, following types of patients require induction of labor even in mild PIH:
a. Women having a favorable cervix at or near term and noncompliant patients.
b. Delivery is recommended in those with a gestational age of 34 weeks or more in the – (i) Presence of progressive labor, (ii) Rupture of membrane, (iii) Abnormal fetal testing, (iv) Fetal growth restriction.

Expectant Management in Mild PIH

All patients should have evaluation of maternal and fetal condition. Following should be observed:
1. Salt restriction, diuretics, anti-hypertensive drugs and sedatives are not used.
2. The patient should have relative rest, daily dipstick measurement of protein, daily blood pressure monitoring, 1-2 times per week fetal testing, laboratory evaluation of hematocrit and platelet, and liver function

Table 34.3: Classification of preeclampsia

Mild preeclampsia	Severe preeclampsia
• Blood pressure ≥ 140/90 mm Hg but < 160/110 6mm Hg on two occasion at least 6 hours apart while patient is on bed rest	• Blood pressure ≥ 160 mm Hg systolic or ≥ 110 mm Hg diastolic on two occasions at least 6 hours apart, while the patient is an bed rest
• Protein urea ≥ 300 mg/ 24 hour but < 5 g/ 24 hour	• Proteinuria of 5 gm or higher in 24 hours urine specimen or 3 + or greater on two random urine samples collected at least 4 hours apart oliguria < 500 ml in 24 hours, cerebral or visual disturbances. Pulmonary volume or cyanosis. Epigastric or right upper quadrant pain.
• Asymptomatic	• Impaired liver function
	• Thrombocytopenia
	• Fetal growth restriction

test 1-2 times a week. The patient should be educated about *preeclampsia warning signs as headache, visual disturbances, epigastric pain, and nausea and vomiting.* Mother should be instructed about daily kick count and labor signs or vaginal bleeding.
3. Fetal testing should consist of at least weekly nonstress test (NST) and measurement of amniotic fluid volume.
4. Ultrasound is performed every 10-14 days for fetal growth. Fetal testing is considered non reassuring if:
   a. NST is non reactive with abnormal fetal biophysical profile.
   b. NST shows late deceleration, moderate to severe variable deceleration or prolonged deceleration.
   c. Oligohydramnios.
   d. Estimated fetal weight is less than 10th percentile for gestational age.

Prompt hospitalization is needed if there is disease progression, acute hypertension, development of significant proteinuria (2 gm/ 24 hours) or abnormal fetal testing. Management plans for delivery is described in Flow chart 34.3.

Management in Severe Preeclampsia

Severe PIH is defined as – (i) Systolic blood pressure > 160 mm Hg or diastolic BP > 110 mg Hg on 2 occasions, 6 weeks apart, (ii) Proteinuria > 5 gm/ dl, (iii) Oliguria (urine output < 400 ml/ dl), (iv) Neurological symptoms as headache, scotomas, visual blurring, altered consciousness, (v) Pulmonary edema or cyanosis, (vi) Epigastric pain, (vii) Deranged liver function test, subcapsular liver hematoma, (viii) Thrombocytopenia (< 1 lack/μl), (viii) HELLP syndrome.

The definitive treatment of severe preeclampsia is delivery. For the fetus remote from term in certain cases prolongation of pregnancy might be more appropriate. The plan of management in severe PIH is summarized in Flow chart 34.4.

Pregnancy < 24 Weeks

In these situations various studies have clearly demonstrated that termination of delivery is the management of choice. Because maternal morbidity is severe and perinatal survival is less than 10% even for fetus remote from term. *Perinatal probability of fetal survival may be better in a well operated neonatal intensive care unit than when the fetus in utero.* These patients should be induced for delivery to reduce maternal risk and avoid prolonged hospitalization and intensive therapy that have little chance of success.

Pregnancy > 34 Weeks

Induction and delivery, steroid can be given for lung maturity and then deliver after 48 hours.

Pregnancy Between 24 and 34 Weeks

Expectant management is a modern concept for gestation between 24 and 34 weeks of pregnancy based on the fact that perinatal outcome is directly related to gestational age of fetus. Prolongation of pregnancy of even 7-14 days reduces the neonatal complications. But decision to continue the pregnancy with use of antihypertensive drug for achieving fetal maturity should be weighed against maternal compromise.

Flow chart 34.3: Management plans for delivery in mild pregnancy induced hypertension

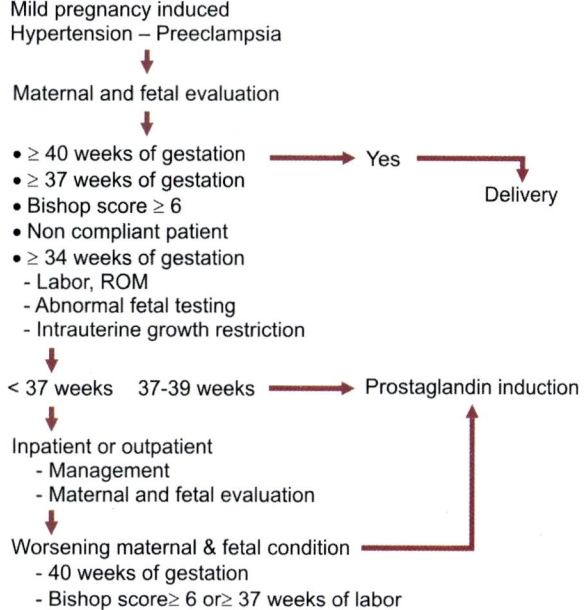

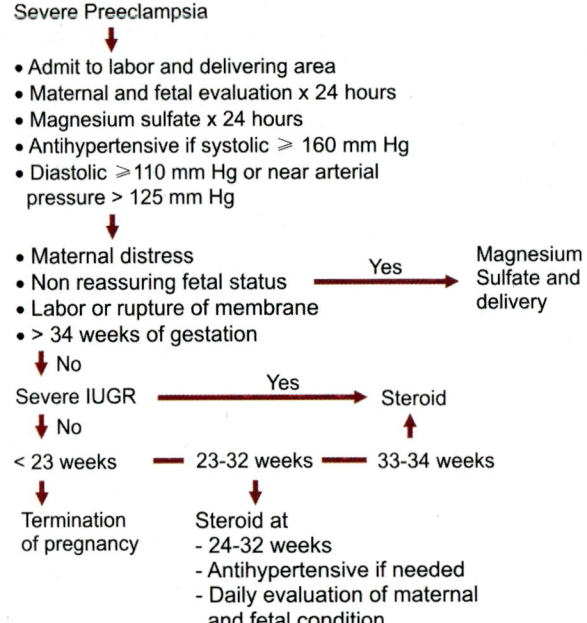

Flow chart 34.4: Management in severe PIH

Monitoring Protocol in Expectant Treatment

If patient is on expectant management close fetal and maternal monitoring is must. Signs of IUGR by clinical examination, fetal movement count and ultrasound should be observed repeatedly. **Suspected fetal compromise is indication for delivery.** In maternal monitoring, involvement of other organ system must be sought by following investigations:

a. **Platelet count:** Platelets are consumed due to endothelial activation. So a falling platelet count $<100 \times 10^9$/lit may indicate need to consider termination of delivery.
b. **Hematocrit and hemoglobin.**
c. **Uric acid** is measure of fine renal tubular function. So used to assess the disease severity. Spuriously high levels of uric acid are associated with acute fatty liver of pregnancy.
d. Serum urea and serum creatinine.
e. **Liver function test:** Liver transaminase, which can be raised in liver involvement like subcapsular hematoma, liver rupture and hepatic infarction. Liver, renal and hematologic evaluation is done at 24-48 hours interval. It should be remembered that normal range for transaminase is approximately 20% lower than the non-pregnant range.

Expectant Management of Severe Preeclampsia

Expectant management in severe PIH is appropriately only in a select group of patient and should be practiced only in a tertiary care center with facility of adequate maternal and neonatal intensive care facilities. A multidisciplinary approach with involvement of senior obstetrician, anesthetic, hematologist, physician and Neonatologist is needed. The main aspects of conservative management are as follows:

a. Bed rest
b. Daily weight measurement
c. Initial intravenous Magnesium sulfate for 24 hours as prophylaxis against development of convulsion.
d. Antihypertensive treatment:
   i. Nifedipine: 10-20 mg orally every 30 minutes to max 50 mg. then 10-20 mg every 4-6 hours (max 120 mg/day). It is calcium channel blocker.
   ii. Labetalol: It is beta blocker 20-40 mg bolus (max. dose 220 mg) then 200 mg orally every 8 hours (max. 600 mg every 6 hours).
   iii. Hydralazine: It is vasodilator 5-10 mg bolus every 20-30 minute (max. dose 20 mg).
   The aim is to maintain diastolic BP of 90-100 mm Hg and systolic BP 140-150 mm Hg. To achieve normal blood pressure is avoided because of risk of decreased uteroplacental perfusion. Adequate therapeutic response is expected in 12 hours.
e. **Steroid** is given for accelerating lung maturity and attempt to delay delivery at least for achieving steroid benefit.
f. **Daily fetal maternal testing is done:** Daily NST, fetal movement count is done. Mother is questioned about headache, visual disturbance, epigastric pain and fetal movement. Liver, renal, hematologic evaluation is at 24 or 48 hours interval. Amniotic fluid volume is

assessed every week and ultrasound for fetal growth at every 14 days.

Indications of Termination of Delivery in Severe PIH

If under observation patient exhibit one or more of the following conditions, indication of termination of delivery is considered:
a. Blood pressure persistently 160/100 or greater despite treatment.
b. Urine output < 400 ml in 24 hours.
c. Platelet count < 50,000/μl.
d. Progressive increase in serum creatinine.
e. LDH > 1000 IU/L.
f. Repetitive late deceleration with poor variability.
g. Severe IUGR with oligohydramnios.
h. Decreased fetal movement.
i. Reversed umbilical diastolic blood flow.

In women with preeclampsia without contraindication to labor, vaginal delivery is preferred. Cervical ripening agents and oxytocin are used as needed.

Intrapartum Management of Preeclampsia

The first priority is to assess and stabilize the maternal condition and then to evaluate fetal well being. The following things are to be followed in management of labor in PIH.

a. **In severe PIH:** Intravenous magnesium sulfate 6 gm loading dose over 20 minutes (6 gm in 150 ml, 5% dextrose in water) is given followed by maintenance dose of 2 gm/hour during labor and for 12-24 hours postpartum.
b. Strict fluid balance chart should be maintained in women with PIH. Total intake is restricted to 85-100 ml/hour to avoid pulmonary edema. If pulmonary edema is suspected, chest X-ray is performed and diuretic can be given. *Oliguria without a rising serum urea or creatinine is a manifestation of severe preeclampsia and not of incipient renal failure.* So administration of intravenous fluid in response to oliguria must be performed with caution. If CVP is high (>8 mm Hg) with persistent oliguria, a dopamine infusion at rate of 1 μ/kg/minute can be considered. Pulmonary artery catheterization is considered in difficult cases. Hemodilaysis or hemofiltration may be necessary if creatinine or potassium rises.
c. Epidural analgesia is preferred methods of pain relief for labor. General anesthetic is best avoided because it causes hypertension and laryngeal edema. In low platelet count, HELLP syndrome pudendal block and epidural are not advisable as they might result in hematoma formation.
d. Antacids are usually recommended in labor as they are at increased risk of operative delivery.
e. Close monitoring of maternal pulse, blood pressure and respiration should be done. Continuous CTG is recommended for fetal monitoring. Sign for magnesium toxicity is noted, and if present, it can be counteracted with 10 ml 10% calcium gluconate I/v.
f. **In 2nd stage of labor:** In moderate to severe PIH there should be low threshold for instrumental delivery, while in mild PIH, usually a normal second stage is conducted. Experienced medical aid should be ensured and there should be two experienced persons caring for women in labor room.
g. **Postpartum management:** Mother is observed for 12-24 hours in recovery room under magnesium sulfate coverage. Most patient show evidence of resolution of disease process within 24 hours after delivery. It is of importance to recognize that women with PIH are much less tolerant of blood loss than normotensive pregnant women. So an appreciable fall in blood pressure soon after delivery most often means excessive blood loss and not sudden dissolution of vasospasm. If oliguria develops following delivery, hematocrit should be promptly evaluated to detect excessive blood loss and should be treated appropriately by careful blood transfusion.
h. **Postnatal management:** At the postnatal follow-up both blood pressure and renal function test should be checked for cardiovascular and renal abnormalities. It is now clear that woman who had preeclampsia, have double risk of subsequent ischemic heart disease. So at postnatal visit the future pregnancies and need for screening for hypertension in later life should be discussed.

Complications of Preeclampsia

These are uncommon but potentially life-threatening. They can be:

Maternal Complications

a. **Eclampsia**
b. **Cerebrovascular accidents** usually intracerebral hemorrhage, this may be fatal or the women may be left with residual neurological deficit.
c. **Abruptio placentae** is an important and common complication of PIH.
d. **HELLP syndrome:** Hemolytic anemia, elevated liver enzymes, low platelet count.
e. Acute left ventricular failure.
f. Acute renal failure.
g. Liver hematoma with possible rupture.
h. Postpartum hemorrhage and wound or intra-abdominal hematoma.
i. DIC and multiorgan failure including liver, kidneys, and lungs (Adult respiratory distress syndrome).
j. Side effects of drug therapy.

Fetal Complications

a. Intrauterine death
b. Intrauterine growth restriction
c. Iatrogenic prematurity with associated complication
d. There can be antepartum and intrapartum asphyxia, which is due to anoxia associated with poor placental perfusion, maternal hypoxia in eclampsia and excessive therapy with sedation and anti convulsant.

HELLP SYNDROME

HELLP is an acronym for a syndrome of *hemolysis*, elevated liver function and or low platelets. It is thought to be a subcategory of severe preeclampsia. It occurs in 2-12% of severe preeclamptic patients.

Diagnosis

Patient has complaints of nausea and vomiting (50%), malaise of a few days' duration (90%), epigastric or right upper quadrant pain (65%). There can be vague abdominal pain, flank or shoulder pain, hematuria, gastrointestinal bleeding or gum bleeding. In 70% of cases onset is antepartum and in 30% postpartum usually within 48 hours of delivery. Hypertension and proteinuria is variable.

Investigation

Diagnosis is confirmed by following laboratory investigation:

a. Fragmented red blood cells on peripheral smear.
b. Increased bilirubin ≥ 1.2 mg/dl.
c. Increased lactic dehydrogenase level greater than 600 IU/lit.
d. Elevated liver enzyme SGOT > 70 IU/lit.
e. Low platelet less than $100 \times 10^3/\mu l$.

Management

Management is similar to severe preeclampsia. High dose parenteral corticosteroid have been found useful. *Dexamethasone I/v in 4 dose of 10 mg, 10 mg, 5 mg, 5 mg at 12 hours interval or in dose of 10 mg I/v at 12 hour interval, until improvement is recommended.* Antihypertensive and prophylactic anticonvulsant treatment is given. If platelet count is less than 40,000/μl, 6-10 unit of platelet transfusion is recommended. Termination of pregnancy is planned according to the gestation, favorability of cervix and severity of disease. The rate of recurrence of HELLP syndrome in subsequent pregnancies is from 2 to 19%.

ECLAMPSIA

Eclampsia is defined as the development of convulsions and or unexplained coma during pregnancy or postpartum in patients with signs and symptoms of preeclampsia. Incidence in developed countries is 1 in 2000, while in developing countries incidence is 1 in 100 to 1in 1700 cases.

Diagnosis

Symptoms and Signs

In impending eclampsia there is usually headache, visual disturbance, restlessness, nausea, vomiting and epigastric or right upper quadrant pain prior to eclampsia. If convulsion develops typical eclamptic seizure is described in 4 phases:

a. **Initial or prodromal phase:** There may be aura and convulsive movement which begins around mouth.
b. **Tonic phase:** The entire body become rigid, face contorted, arm flexed, fist clenched, respiration ceases for 15-20 seconds.
c. **Clonic phase:** There are jerky movement, start from facial muscle to involve entire body. There is frothing and may be cyanosed. This phase last for approximately 1 minute.
d. **Recovery:** The movement slowly subside. Respiration is resumed and patient passes into coma of variable duration.

Eclamptic seizures are more common in nullipara from low socioeconomic status and peak incidence is in the teenage group and again there is increased prevalence in women older than 35 years.

Management

a. *General measures:* The first priority in eclamptic women is to avoid maternal injury and attention to airways. The patient should be turned in left lateral position. An airway is inserted between teeth to avoid tongue bite and maintain airway. Oxygen should be given by mask at 8-10 l/minute to correct maternal and fetal hypoxia. Oxygen saturation should be monitored with pulse oxymeter. An I/v access is secured and treatment is tailored to control convulsion and blood pressure.
b. *Control of convulsion:*
   i. Drug of choice is magnesium sulfate. A total loading dose of 4 gm as I/v infusion 20 ml of 20% solution) over 15-20 minutes and 10 gm deep intramuscular, 5 gm in each buttock (10 ml of 50% solution) is given. This is followed by 5 gm I/m every 4 hours. Alternatively I/v infusion of 1-2 gm/ hour can be started after the loading intravenous dose in place of intramuscular injection. A low dose regimen has been tried in India considering lower body mass index of women. A loading dose of 4 gm I/v and 3 gm in each buttock (total 10 gm) followed by a maintenance dose of 2.5 gm 4 hourly. The suggested therapeutic plasma level of magnesium sulfate for treatment of eclampsia convulsion is 1.8-3.0 m mol/liter. *The first sign of toxicity is loss of patellar reflex, which corresponds to a plasma level of 3.5-5 m mol/ lit.* So repeat dose should be given only if the patellar reflex is present, respiratory rate is greater than 12

per minute and urine output is greater than 100 ml in previous 4 hours. If a patient develops sign of toxicity the infusion should be immediately discontinued, oxygen is administered and serum magnesium level is obtained and 10 ml of calcium gluconate solution should be infused slowly over a period of 3 minutes.
  ii. Diazepam is highly effective anticonvulsant but it can cause neonatal depression and maternal respiratory depression.
  iii. **Lytic cocktail:** The combination of chlorpromazine, promethazine and pethidine has been used in past but now no longer used because of risk of producing respiratory depression in mother and neonate.
  iv. **Phenytoin:** It is given I/v in initial loading dose of 15-18 mg/kg body weight followed by 100 mg I/v every 8 hours to prevent recurrence.
c. *Control of blood pressure:* Persistent and severely elevated blood pressure (≥ 160/110) mm Hg should be treated with antihypertensive to prevent cardiovascular accidents, pulmonary edema and renal failure. Hydralazine, labetalol, and nifedipine are drug of choice.
d. *Delivery:* The definitive treatment of eclampsia is delivery, irrespective of gestational age. But patient should be first stabilized with supportive treatment and patient should be transferred to well equipped tertiary care center. There is a fetal heart bradycardia and deceleration during fit, which usually resolve spontaneously after control of seizure. But if the fetal bradycardia and late deceleration present beyond 10-15 minutes, despite all resuscitation effort, the patient should be evaluated for hypertonus and abruptio. Vaginal delivery is safe option but cesarean section is choice of treatment if:
  i. If fetus is older than 34 weeks, mature and alive and patient is not in labor.
  ii. If contemplated induction delivery is going to be long.
  iii. Other obstetric reasons.

Gestational Hypertension

Hypertension occurring after 20 weeks of gestation but not accompanied by proteinuria is termed as gestational hypertension. Pregnancy outcome for patient with mild gestational hypertension is generally favorable.

Chronic Hypertension in Pregnancy

Chronic hypertension complicates as many as 50% of pregnancies. It is characterized by a history of high blood pressure before pregnancy, elevation of blood pressure during first half of pregnancy or high blood pressure that lasts for 12 weeks after delivery. Primary (essential) hypertension accounts for 90-95% of cases. In rest chronic hypertension is secondary to one or more underlying disorders as renal disease, collagen vascular disease, endocrine disorders or Coarctation of aorta. Causes of chronic hypertension are summarized in Table 34.4.

Table 34.4: Causes of chronic hypertension

Essential Hypertension
  Renal Disease
    Glomerular nephritis
    Polycystic disease
    Diabetic nephropathy
    Renal artery stenosis
Collagen Vascular Disease
    Systemic lupus erythematosus (SLE)
    Scleroderma
Coarctation of the Aorta
Endocrine Cause
    Pheochromocytoma
    Conn's syndrome
Risk Factors for Developing Superimposed Preeclampsia
Renal disease, Maternal age > 40 years, Diabetes, Connective tissue disease, e.g. SLE and antiphospholipid syndrome, Coarctation of the aorta, Blood pressure > 160/100 mm Hg in early pregnancy

Management

Ideally all women with chronic hypertension should be evaluated prior to pregnancy to determine the underlying pathology and optimize blood pressure control with suitable antihypertensive drugs. If ACE inhibitors are used it should be changed. Chronic hypertension in pregnancy can be low risk or high risk. *Low risk* has mild essential hypertension without any organ involvement and no previous perinatal loss. *High risk* are women with secondary hypertension with target organ damage, previous perinatal loss and women over age of 40 years.

Role of Anti-hypertensive

In women with low risk chronic hypertension, the benefits and risk of antihypertensive therapy is uncertain. However, the pregnancy should be monitored carefully to detect any rise in blood pressure or feature of preeclampsia or fetal growth restriction. Appropriate investigations like serum creatinine, electrolyte levels, liver function test, 24 hours urinary protein/creatinine clearance and renal scan should be done. Antihypertensive agents are recommended for high risk hypertensive women along with frequent evaluation of maternal and fetal well being (Flow chart 34.5). This reduces the risk of cerebrovascular accident, congestive heart failure, renal failure and helps in prolongation of pregnancy and improving perinatal outcome. *The aim of antihypertensive therapy is to keep systolic blood pressure between 140 and 110 mm Hg and diastolic blood pressure between 90 and 100 mm Hg in women without target organ damage. In presence of target*

Flow chart 34.5: Use of antihypertensive drugs in pregnancy with chronic hypertension

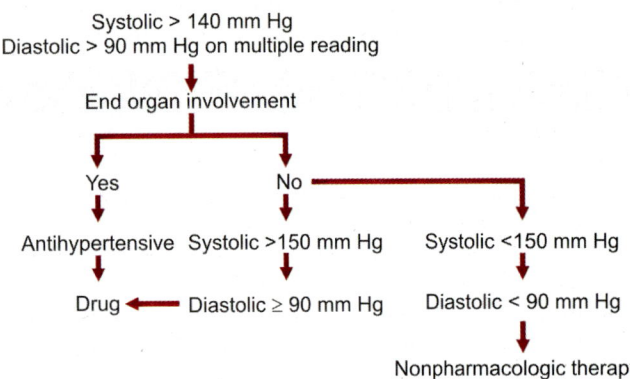

organ damage, blood pressure is kept below 140/90 mm Hg. A profound drop of maternal blood pressure in a short time should be avoided to prevent decreased placenta fetal perfusion.

Management for severe chronic hypertension is summarized in Flow chart 35.5. The choice of antihypertensive drug is *Alpha methyldopa* in dose of 500 mg to 2 gm in 2-4 divided doses. Sedation and postural hypotension are the most common side effects. *Labetalol* is a α_1 adrenergic blocker and a nonselective β adrenergic blocker. The usual starting dose is 100 mg BID and dose can be increased weekly to a maximum of 2400 mg daily.

Nifedipine is a calcium channel blocker; usually starting dose is 30 mg daily. If necessary, dose may be increased to 60-90 mg daily. Use of angiotensin converting enzyme inhibitor like enalapril captopril during pregnancy is associated with fetal malformation and fetal and neonatal deaths. These agents are contraindicated in pregnancy. Diuretic should also be avoided during pregnancy.

Prognosis

Usually the pregnancy outcome is good in patient with low risk category. IUGR, superimposed preeclampsia; placental abruptio and preterm delivery are the most common complication. But in high risk women the prognosis for pregnancy outcome is not favorable. Close monitoring for development of IUGR and superimposed preeclampsia is indicated.

MULTIPLE CHOICE QUESTIONS

1. Risk factors for preeclampsia:
   a. Chronic hypertension
   b. Obesity
   c. Placental ischemia
   d. Multigravida
   e. Antiphospholipid syndrome
   Ans. a, c, e

2. Which of the following are seen in preeclampsia:
   a. Hypertension
   b. Proteinuria
   c. Convulsions
   d. Pedal edema
   Ans. a, b

3. In PIH, impending sign of eclampsia is:
   a. Visual symptoms
   b. Weight gain of 2 lb per week
   c. Severe proteinuria of 10 gm
   d. Pedal edema
   Ans. a

4. All are prognostic indicators of PIH *except*:
   a. Low platelet count
   b. Serum Na
   c. Elevated liver enzymes
   d. Serum uric acid
   Ans. b

5. Which is not a feature of HELLP syndrome:
   a. Thrombocytopenia
   b. Eosinophilia
   c. Raised liver enzyme
   d. Hemolytic anemia
   Ans. b

6. Which is drug of choice for severe preeclampsia:
   a. Labetalol
   b. Metoprolol
   c. Alpha methyldopa
   d. Nifedipine
   Ans. a

7. A 27-year primigravida presents with PIH with blood pressure of 150/100 mm Hg at 32 weeks gestation with no other complications. Subsequently her BP is controlled on treatment. If there are no complications, pregnancy should be terminated at:
   a. 40 completed weeks
   b. 37 completed weeks
   c. 35 completed weeks
   d. 34 completed weeks
   Ans. b

8. In PIH, sudden vision loss is due to:
   a. Retinal detachment
   b. CRAO
   c. Vitreous hemorrhage
   d. CRVO
   Ans. a

9. Treatment of choice in eclampsia is:
   a. Diazepam
   b. Phenergam
   c. $MgSO_4$
   d. Phenobarbitone
   Ans. c

10. Magnesium sulfate is given to a pregnant lady with PIH, which of the following drug is contraindicated in this condition:
    a. Nifedipine
    b. Hydralazine
    c. Methyldopa
    d. Labetalol
    Ans. a

35. Third Trimester Bleeding

A person who is master of patience is master of everything.

GENERAL CONSIDERATION

Third trimester hemorrhage is one of the most ominous complications of pregnancy and requires evaluation in 5-10% of pregnancies. Third trimester obstetric hemorrhage is one of the three leading cause of maternal death and perinatal morbidity and mortality. There are certain non obstetric causes of bleeding and they must be differentiated from obstetric causes of bleeding which are more hazardous. Causes of third trimester bleeding are summarized in Table 35.1.

Table 35.1: Causes of third trimester bleeding

Obstetric cause	Nonobstetric cause
1. Bloody show	1. Cervical cancer or dysplasia
2. Placenta previa	2. Cervicitis
3. Abruptio placenta	3. Cervical polyp
4. Vasa previa	4. Cervical erosion
5. Disseminated intravascular coagulopathy	5. Vaginal laceration
6. Uterine rupture	6. Vaginitis
7. Marginal sinus bleeding	

In this chapter three major causes of hemorrhage are considered:
a. **Premature separation of placenta:** Abruptio placenta, circumvallate placenta and marginal sinus rupture are considered variants of premature separation of placenta.
b. **Placenta previa**
c. **Uterine rupture**

General Management of Antepartum Hemorrhage

When the patient is first seen with APH, the cause of bleeding is usually not obvious in most of cases. Following principles in any third trimester hemorrhage must be followed:
a. Women with third trimester hemorrhage must be evaluated in well equipped hospitals.
b. No vaginal or rectal examination should be performed until placenta previa has been ruled out.
c. Early recognition of hypovolemia is essential. Immediate resuscitation is first priority on arrival at hospital – Airway should be patent. Patient should be placed in trendelenberg position with left tilt, which will maximize venous return by preventing the gravid uterus from compressing the inferior vena cava. Two large bore intravenous catheters should be placed and fluid replacement with crystalloid or colloid volume expander is initiated. Blood should be arranged, when clinically indicated.
d. Vasoactive drugs should be used only when specific pharmacologic effect is desired and when volume expanders are not promptly available. Dopamine which is a mixed α and β adrenergic stimulant is given at rate of 2-5 $\mu g/kg/$minute and can be increased gradually to 20-50 $\mu g/kg/$minute.
e. Once the patient is stabilized, the cause of bleeding must be quickly identified by clinical examination and ultrasound examination. Laboratory investigation include blood type and cross match for complete blood count with platelet and baseline coagulation status by prothrombin time, partial thromboplastin time, dimmer or fibrin split products.
f. The further line of management depends upon the cause of obstetric hemorrhage, gestational age and condition of fetus and severity of hemorrhage.

PLACENTA PREVIA

Definition: When placenta is implanted in the lower uterine segment within the zone of effacement and dilatation of the cer1vix so that it covers or adjoins the internal os, is termed placenta previa.

Incidence: Incidence of placenta previa is 4-5/1000 pregnancies (0.5%). Only 20% of these are complete placenta praevia. However, incidence of placental tissues covering the internal cervical os at 18 weeks is 5-15%. Placenta previa seen in such early gestation has a 90% chance of resolution by term.

Classification of Placenta Previa

Placenta previa is classified according to its relation with internal os (Figs 35.1A to D).
  i. *Total or complete placenta previa* — The placenta completely covers the internal cervical os.
  ii. *Partial placenta previa* — The internal os is partially covered by placenta.
  iii. *Marginal placenta previa* — The placenta is implanted at the margin of the internal cervical os within 2 cm.
  iv. *Low lying placenta* — The placenta is on the lower uterine segment but does not reach as far as the os.

Each of the later 3 types is subdivided into Type A and Type B depending on whether the placenta mainly lies on the **anterior** or the **posterior** wall respectively. Posterior placenta is more common and is also more dangerous because it discourages engagement of head more often and during labor more liable to get compressed which impairs placental perfusion.

Etiology and Risk Factors

Though various risk factors have been identified with placenta previa, there is no definitive cause. It is presumed that as a result of some local aberration in uterine blood supply the distinction between chorion frondosum and chorion larvae does not occur in normal situation. The blastocyst which usually implants in the thicker and more receptive endometrium of the upper uterine segment, gets implanted in the endometrium of the isthmus or over a previous lower segment uterine scar. In such situation invasion by the trophoblast secures the embryo and when the uterus grows to form a lower segment later in pregnancy, the placenta remains in lower uterine segment.

Bleeding in the placenta previa may be due to any of the following causes—(a) Due to mechanical separation of the placenta from its implantation site during labor or formation of lower uterine segment. (b) Placentitis. (c) Rupture of poorly supported venous lakes in the decidua basalis that have become engorged with venous blood.

The risk factors of placenta previa are:
a. *Advancing maternal age* women older than 40 years have nearly nine fold greater risk than women at age of 20 years.
b. *Multiparity*
c. *Smoking* cigarette smoking increases risk of placenta previa probably due to defective decidual vascularization and hypoxemia which leads to compensatory hypertrophy of placenta.
d. *Maternal cocaine and opiate use* has been demonstrated with placenta previa.
e. *Multifetal gestation* — The rate of placenta previa is 40% higher among twin birth in comparison to singleton pregnancies because placenta is bigger size and has a greater chance of encroaching into the lower uterine segment.
f. *History of abortion* has increased risk for low lying placenta following uterine curettage.
g. *Previous uterine scar* — It is the strongest associated risk factor for placenta previa. The risk increases proportionately with the number of previous cesarean section to 10% in patient with 4 or more cesareans.
h. *Prior history of placenta previa* — The recurrence rate of placenta previa is 2.4%, which is an 8 fold increase compared to normal incidence.

Diagnosis

Symptoms and Signs

The most characteristic event in the placenta previa is *painless, causeless and recurrent hemorrhage; usually occur near the end of second trimester or after*. The initial bleeding is usually not profuse and ceases spontaneously only to recur. In approximately 10% of cases there is some initial pain, because of coexisting placental separation and localized uterine contraction. In 25% of cases spontaneous labor can be expected.

On **examination** the uterus is usually soft, relaxed and non tender. A high presenting part cannot be pressured into the pelvic inlet. The fetus will present in oblique or transverse lie in approximately 15% of cases. Fetal heart rate abnormalities are unlikely unless there are complications such as hypovolemic shock, placental separation or cord accidents.

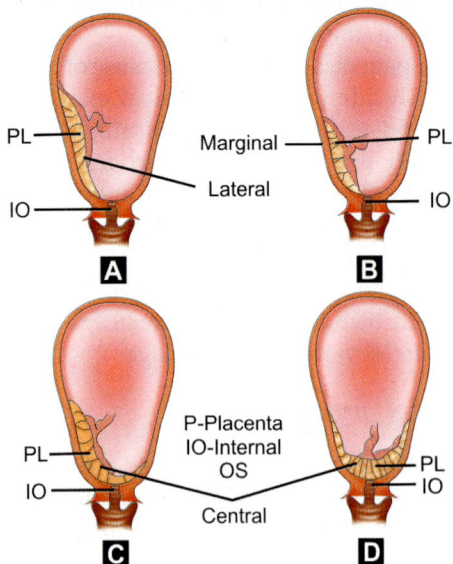

Figs 35.1A to D: Classification of degree of placenta previa: (A) Low lying placenta previa; (B) Marginal placenta previa; (C) Partial placenta previa; (D) Total or complete placenta previa

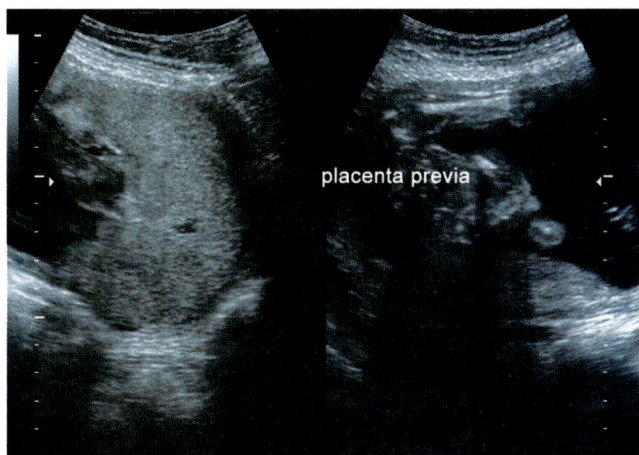

Fig. 35.2: Ultrasound image shows placenta covering the internal os (Central placenta previa)

Localization of Placenta

a. **Ultrasound:** The simplest, precise and safest method of placental localization is provided by transabdominal sonography (Fig. 35.2). False positive result can occur if bladder is over distended or there is pressure of myometrial contraction. Ultrasound seen in apparently positive cases should be repeated after emptying the bladder. An uncommon source of error is in cases when abundant placenta implanted in the fundus has been identified but one fail to appreciate that the placenta was large and extended downwards to internal os of the cervix. Transvaginal and transperenial scan has substantially improved diagnostic accuracy of placenta previa.
b. **Placental migration:** During middle of second trimester the placenta is observed by ultrasound to cover the internal cervical os in approximately 30% of cases. With development of the lower uterine segment almost all of these low implantation placenta will be carried to higher station. This phenomenon is called **placental migration.** An early diagnosis of placenta previa requires the confirmation at later date before any definitive diagnosis is made.
c. **MRI:** Though it is superior to ultrasound particularly if the placenta is posterior, but it is not recommended for routine clinical practice.

Differential diagnosis: The other causes of placental bleeding are partial premature separation of the normally implanted placenta or circumvallate placenta.

Treatment

As stated above maternal evaluation and stabilization are first priority. The obstetric treatment depends on the (a) amount of uterine bleeding (b) duration of pregnancy (c) viability of fetus (d) degree of placenta previa (e) the presentation, position and status of the fetus (f) the gravidity and parity of the patient (g) the status of the cervix (h) onset of labor.

The patient has to be admitted in the hospital for confirming the diagnosis and further management. Blood should be readily available in case of emergency.

a. **Expectant treatment:** The initial hemorrhage in placenta previa may occur before fetal pulmonary maturity is established. In such cases expectant management can be done to prolong pregnancy till the fetus is reasonably mature. Usually in placenta previa the first hemorrhage is not so profuse to be dangerous either for mother or fetus and soon stops practically in every case. The separated area of placenta becomes infarcted and the maternal vessels supplying the exposed portion of the placental site thromboses. Usually, the fetus develops some compensatory mechanism to meet its oxygen requirement in due time. So the small repeated hemorrhages are less dangerous than a single large one.

Expectant hospital management till delivery includes: (a) Rest, (b) Monitoring of mother and fetus, (c) Correcting anemia with blood transfusion, (d) Ultrasound localization of the placenta. Once active bleeding stops a per speculum examination is done to rule out local causes, (e) Tocolytic can be tried in selected cases to suppress uterine activity which can encourage bleeding.

After 34 week of gestational age the benefit of further maturation must be weighed against the risk of major hemorrhage. In selecting the optimum time for delivery, test of fetal lung maturation and ultrasound fetal biometry are important. If the patient is between 24-34 weeks gestational age, a single course of Betamethasone (2 doses of 12 mg I/M at 24 hours) or Dexamethasone (4 doses of 6 mg I/M every 12 hours) should be given to promote lung maturity. Because of high cost of hospitalization, patient with a presumptive diagnosis of placenta previa can be sent home on strict bed rest after their condition has become stable under ideal controlled circumstances. It is important in outpatient management that women and her family must fully appreciate the problem of placenta previa and be prepared to transport her to hospital immediately.

b. **Delivery:** Delivery should be conducted by a senior obstetrician along with experienced anesthetic in an institution where adequate blood banking facility and intensive care facility are available. The decision for route of delivery depends on the type of placenta previa, gestational age, maternal and fetal condition.

c. **Cesarean section:** Cesarean section is the method of choice with placenta previa. Cesarean section has proved to be the most important factor in lowering maternal and perinatal mortality rates. Hypovolemic shock should be corrected by I/V fluids and blood before start of operation. So that not only mother is better protected but at risk the fetus also recover more quickly in utero, than if born while the mothers is still in shock.

The **choice of anesthetic** depends on current and anticipated blood loss. Regional or epidural anesthetic is safe in small amount of hemorrhage and stable patient but in excessive bleeding, general anesthetic is suitable method.

The **choice of operation technique** is important because of low insertion of placenta and development of lower uterine segment. The anterior placenta should be spared from damage as far possible because the baby may lose a significant amount of blood before the cord is clamped. If there is marginal placenta it may be possible to find an edge to the placenta and push it aside in order to extract the baby rather than to deliver through it. With posterior implantation of placenta a low transverse incision is best. Some time in complete placenta previa a vertical incision is recommended. Cord should be clamped as soon as possible because of risk of fetal hemorrhage. In small percentage of cases, hemostasis in the placental bed is unsatisfactory because of the poor contractility of the lower uterine segment. **Mattress suturing of placental bed or packing may be required in addition to the usual oxytocin, prostaglandin and methylergometrine.** When placenta previa is complicated by degree of placenta accreta beside above methods, bilateral uterine artery ligation or even hysterectomy is required to control hemorrhage. Puerperal infection and anemia are the most likely postoperative complication.

d. **Vaginal delivery:** Vaginal delivery is to be considered only in very limited number of women with marginal implantation and cephalic presentation. If vaginal delivery is planned the membrane should be artificially ruptured prior to any oxytocin as it can cause further bleeding. Pressure of presenting part against the placenta edge usually reduces bleeding with progress of labor. Because of possibility of fetal hypoxemia, due to either placental separation or cord accident, continuous fetal monitoring must be used. If there are fetal heart rate abnormalities a rapid cesarean section should be performed until vaginal delivery is imminent. In 2nd stage of labor the vaginal delivery should be accomplished in easiest and fastest ways. Vacuum extraction is preferred to forceps as there is less risk of trauma to lower uterine segment. Patient should be carefully watched for postpartum hemorrhage and cervical laceration.

Double Set-up Examination

It refers to a pelvic examination for suspected placenta previa, performed when the diagnosis is not clear. The examination is also done in the operating room with the patient prepared and draped for immediate cesarean section, with anesthetist and obstetrician scrubbed and ready to do cesarean section, if required. Double setup examinations are not commonly done today because diagnosis of placenta previa is usually clear by ultrasound examination.

In today practice indications of double set-up examination are:
a. Facilities are not available for ultrasound assessment and delivery needs to be considered.
b. Despite ultrasound assessment, diagnosis is not clear.
c. When suspicion of a low accessory lobe of placenta where main body of the placenta is normally situated.
d. The placenta previa is of minor grade and decision regarding vaginal delivery is to be used.

Method

a. The team is assembled so if placenta previa is confirmed, a cesarean section can be done. It can be done under epidural anesthesia.
b. Blood must be cross matched in advance.
c. Woman is placed in lithotomy position. The urinary bladder is evacuated. Initially a vaginal examination is performed to palpate in each fornix. The placenta can be felt as sponginess between the fetal head and fornix. The whole 360° of cervix should be palpated against the fetal head. If no placenta is felt all over cervix, an index finger should be passed through the cervix and a gentle examination is performed to feel for the edge of placenta. If placenta is felt cesarean section is done. If fetal head is felt with no apparent placenta and bleeding, the membranes are ruptured and Syntocinon can be started. But if cervix is not favorable for delivery, cesarean section is safe option.

Complications of Placenta Previa

Maternal

a. Maternal hemorrhagic shock and even death may follow severe antepartum bleeding. Death can occur as a consequence of intrapartum and postpartum hemorrhage, operative trauma, infection or embolism.
b. There can be premature separation of a portion of placenta.
c. **Placenta previa accreta** is a serious condition, when sparse endometrium and myometrium of the lower uterine segment are penetrated by the trophoblast in a manner similar to higher in the uterus. Three degrees of adherence have been described—**accreta, increta and percreta,** which indicates that placenta adheres to or invades into or through the uterine wall respectively because of abnormal development of the decidua basalis.

Incidence and Risk Factors of Placenta Accreta

It occurs in 1 in 2500 deliveries and has increased 10 folds in the past decade. Uterine scar, submucosal leiomyoma, prior cesarean section, chronic endometritis and intrauterine synechia are predisposing factors for placenta accreta.

Uterine rupture, uterine inversion during placental removal and hysterectomy for incompletely removed placenta with maternal bleeding are complications associated with placenta accreta.

Diagnosis and Management of Placenta Accreta

In cases with a high index of suspicion, antenatal imaging should be performed for diagnosis of this condition. Ultrasound with color Doppler is the best imaging modality.

Maternal Serum Alpha Fetoprotein

Second trimester elevation of MSAFP with ultrasound evidence of placenta previa are associated with increased risk of placenta accreta, percreta and increta. As MSAFP is governed by both fetal production and placental transfer, abnormally deep invasion of the placenta results in elevation of MSAFP even in second trimester.

In diagnosed cases, there should be elective cesarean section. Manual removal of placenta is not recommended at time of cesarean. Prior to surgery an informed consent of anticipated complication, blood transfusion and alternative surgery like internal iliac artery ligation or hysterectomy should be obtained.

Fetal Complications in Placenta Previa

a. **Prematurity** (gestational age < 36 weeks) accounts for 60% of perinatal death due to placenta previa.
b. **Fetal hypoxia**.
c. **Birth injury**.
d. **Fetal hemorrhage** due to tearing of the placenta. Fetal blood loss is directly proportional to the time that elapses between lacerating the cotyledon and clamping the cord.

Prognosis

Maternal—With the increased use of cesarean section preceded by well organized expectant treatment, use of blood transfusion and expertly administered anesthetic, overall maternal mortality rate is less than 1 in 1000. There is eight fold increase of recurrence of placenta previa than in general population.

Fetal—The perinatal mortality rate associated with placenta previa has declined to approximately 4-8% in well equipped center and in ideal obstetric and neonatal care.

Velamentous Insertion of Cord and Vasa Previa

In velamentous insertion of cord, the umbilical vessels spread within the membrane at a distance from the placental margin, where they reach surrounded only by amnion. In some cases of velamentous insertion placental vessels overlie the cervix and are supported only by membranes. This is defined as vasa previa. This is uncommon (1 in 5000), but potentially dangerous, complication because vessels are liable to compression which lead to fetal anoxia and laceration which can cause fetal exsanguinations.

Risk Factors

1. Bilobate or succenturiate placenta
2. Second trimester placenta previa
3. IVF and multiple pregnancies.

Complications

1. There is higher incidence of congenital malformation like spina bifida, renal tract anomalies.
2. Increased risk of antepartum hemorrhage, miscarriage, prematurity, low birth weight.

Diagnosis, Symptoms and Signs

Usually it presents as vaginal bleeding after spontaneous or artificial rupture of membrane or sudden fetal heart irregularity after AROM. Sometimes examiner palpate a tubular fetal vessel in the membranes overlying the presenting part.

Investigations

1. On ultrasound echogenic parallel or circular lines can be seen overlying the cervix. Color Doppler examination is recommended, if vasa previa is suspected.
2. When there is suspected vasa previa, confirmation of fetal blood in the vagina can be done with various biochemical tests:
   a. Kleihauer test
   b. Apt test (NAOH)
   c. Modified Apt test
   d. Landerslot (0.1 NKOH).
   Every test relies on the increased resistance of fetal hemoglobin compared with maternal to denaturing alkaline reagents.
3. Hemoglobin electrophoresis is confirmatory but it takes long time.

Management

If antenatally diagnosed elective cesarean section should be done at 37 weeks of gestation. If diagnosis is made during labor, expedite delivery preferably by cesarean and aggressive neonatal resuscitation is mandatory. Unfortunately in many cases fetal death is virtually instantaneous with bleeding.

ABRUPTIO PLACENTA (ACCIDENTAL HEMORRHAGE, ABLATIO PLACENTA, PREMATURE SEPARATION OF PLACENTA)

Definition: Abruptio placenta is defined as premature separation of normally implanted placenta before delivery of the fetus.

Incidence: The incidence of abruptio placenta is around 0.6-1% of all birth. Abruptio can occur at any time in late pregnancy but occurs more commonly around 34 weeks. Depending on the extent and intensity of placental separation, it is a significant cause of perinatal mortality (15-20%) and maternal mortality (2-5%).

Types of Presentation

Placental abruptio is initiated by hemorrhage into the decidua basalis. This hemorrhage can eventually lead to the formation of a hematoma, which can contribute to further expansion of the abruptio.

Revealed bleeding or external hemorrhage when some of the bleeding of placental abruption insinuates itself between the membrane and uterus and then escapes through the cervix, it causes revealed bleeding or external hemorrhage. This presentation is found in 80% of cases of abruptio placenta.

Concealed hemorrhage when blood does not escape externally but is retained between the detached placenta and the uterus, it cause concealed hemorrhage. This presentation is in 20% of cases (Figs 35.3A and B).

Mixed variety: More commonly mixed type of presentation is seen.

Placental abruptio may be partial or total. In revealed form the blood drains through the cervix, so placental detachment is more likely to be incomplete and complications are fewer and less severe. In concealed form attachment of placenta may be complete and the complications are often severe. Ten percent of abruptio are associated with clinically significant coagulopathy.

Etiology and Risk Factors

The exact cause is not known but there are several risk factors:

a. **Multiparity:** Incidence of abruptio is four times higher in multipara as compared to primigravida and increase markedly after the fifth pregnancy.
b. Higher incidence in **lower socioeconomic status.**
c. **Hypertensive disorders in pregnancy:** These are most common associated factors in causing abruptio. The relative risk of abruptio is increased 3.8 fold for severe pre-eclampsia and 2.8 fold for chronic hypertension with superimposed pre-eclampsia.

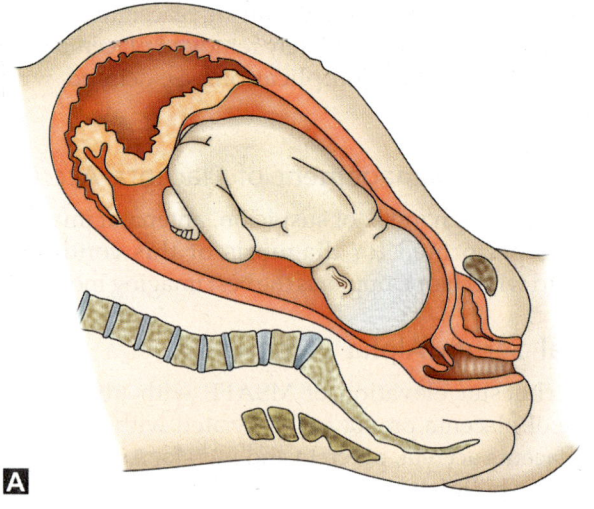

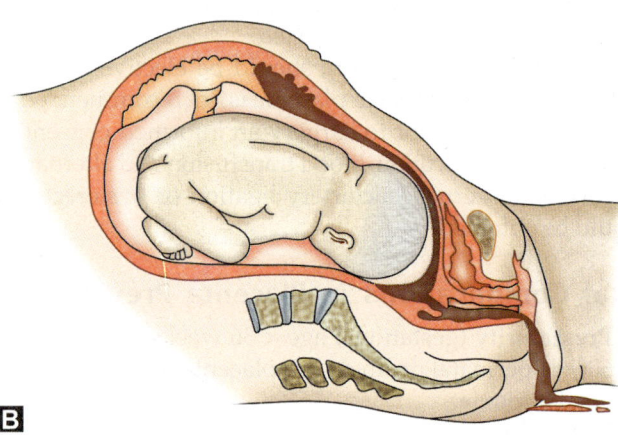

Figs 35.3A and B: (A) Placental abruption with concealed hemorrhage; (B) Placental abruption with revealed hemorrhage

d. **Preterm premature rupture of membrane** causes 3 fold increased chance of abruptio.
e. **Smoking:** It is an independent risk factor associated with 90% increase in risk of placental abruptio. Risk is proportionately increased with number of cigarettes.
f. **Multiple pregnancy:** The incidence of abruptio in twin pregnancy is twice than that of singleton pregnancies.
g. **Polyhydramnios:** Sudden rapid decompression after ROM in polyhydramnios leads to abruption.
h. **Thrombophilia:** The combination of thrombophilic factors like hyperhomocysteinemia with APC resistance, deficiency of protein C, protein S and genetic mutation of factor V Leiden increases the risk of abruptio.
i. **Folic acid deficiency:** It is believed to be risk factors for placental abruptio. Hyperhomocysteinemia is marker of folate deffiency, which is found to be associated with increased risk of pre-eclampsia and abruptio placenta.
j. **Trauma:** The trauma caused by road traffic accident, fall and domestic violence and obstetric procedure like external cephalic version increase the risk of abruptio to 1-5% in minor injuries and 40-50% in major injuries.

k. **Fibroids and uterine malformation:** Risk of abruptio is more especially with submucous fibroids and those with larger volume than 200 cc. The risk of abruptio is 8 times with uterine malformation.
l. **Increasing maternal age** is an independent risk factor for abruptio.
m. **Cocaine abuse** is major risk factor for placental abruption.
n. **Short cord** can bring out placental separation during labor by mechanical pull.
o. **History of prior abruptio:** Abruptio is 10-15 time more common in subsequent pregnancies.

Pathophysiology

Mechanisms of initiation of abruptio: Following mechanism is thought to be important in the pathophysiology of premature placental separation:
a. *Local vascular injury:* It results in vascular rupture into the decidua basalis, bleeding and hematoma formation. The hematoma shears off adjacent denuded vessels, which produce further bleeding and hematoma formation.
b. Abruptio can cause rise in uterine venous pressure, which is transmitted to intervillous space, resulting in engorgement of venous bed and separation of all or a portion of placenta.
c. Mechanical factor like sudden decompression causing separation of placenta in after delivery of first twin, rupture of membrane in polyhydramnios.
d. Initiation of coagulation cascade: Trauma may cause release of tissue thromboplastin, which initiates clot formation in the relative hemodynamic stasis occurring in placental pool.

Anatomical Changes

Anatomically placental abruption may occur by hemorrhage into the decidua basalis, which splits leaving a thin layer adjacent to the myometrium. This decidual hematoma leads to separation, compression and further bleeding. Alternatively a spiral artery may rupture, causing reteroplacental hematoma. In both ways bleeding occur, clot is formed and placental surface can no longer provide metabolic exchange between mother and fetus. The blood may rupture through the membranes or placenta and gain access to amniotic fluid. The tissue disruption by bleeding may allow maternofetal hemorrhage, fetomaternal hemorrhage, maternal bleeding into amniotic fluid or amniotic fluid embolus depending on the areas disrupted and their relative pressure difference.

Couvelaire Uterus

Occasionally extensive intra myometrial bleeding occurs in uteroplacental apoplexy, resulting in Couvelaire uterus. It characteristically shows ecchymosis on its serous surface

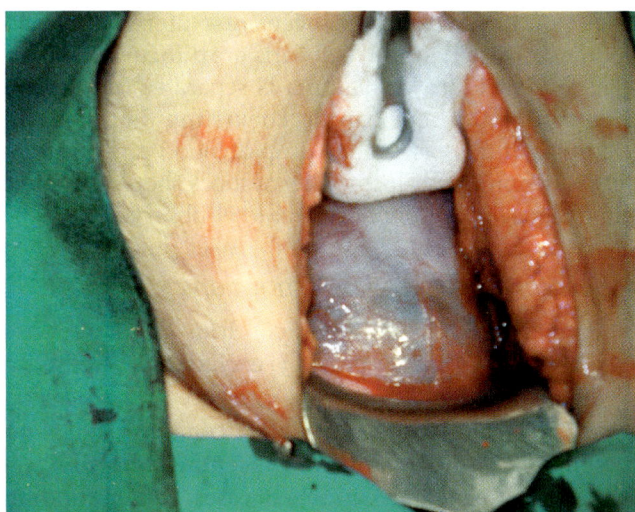

Fig. 35.4: Couvelaire uterus showing blue discoloration of uterus muscle and serosa

(Fig. 35.4). Bleeding may occur between layers of broad ligament and the muscle bundles of the uterine wall are heavily infiltrated with extravasated blood and edema fluid which cause uterine atony.

Coagulation Disorder

In more severe cases of separation there may be clinically significant amount of DIC associated with depletion of fibrinogen, platelet and other clotting factors. The patient can develop hemorrhagic diathesis which is presented as widespread petechiae, active bleeding, hypovolemic shock and failure of normal clotting mechanism. In addition fibrin deposits in small capillaries can result in potentially fatal complication like acute cor pulmonale, renal cortical and tubular necrosis and anterior pituitary infarction– Sheehan's syndrome. Pathological changes of pre-eclampsia may be found in liver, kidney and other organs. Fetal hypoxia and fetal death can occur depending on the amount and duration of placental separation.

Diagnosis

The clinical features depend on degree and speed of separation of placenta and amount of blood concealed in uterus cavity. **The classic symptoms are vaginal bleeding and abdominal pain.** Approximately 80% of patient will present with vaginal bleeding and 2/3rd will have uterine tenderness and abdominal or back pain. In 30% of cases separation is small and produces few or no symptoms. If process is extensive, evidence of fetal distress, uterine tetany, DIC or hypovolemic shock may be seen.

On Examination

If there is tense, tender uterus with or without uterine contraction, one should think of diagnosis of abruptio. The size of uterus may be disproportionately larger than expected for period of gestation. In severe case uterus is of hard wooden consistency and fetal parts are difficult to palpate. If more than 1/3rd of placenta is separated, the fetus is already dead. There can be coexisting signs of pre-eclampsia. If there is sudden drop of blood pressure from 190 to 110 mm Hg, the possibility of shock should be kept in mind. Signs of coagulopathy should be observed.

Laboratory Tests and Investigations

a. *Imaging:* Ultrasonography confirms the situation of placenta so placenta previa is excluded. It also aids in diagnosis of fetal maturity, presence of fetal cardiac activity, fetal presentation. **Ultrasound has poor sensitivity in diagnosing placental abruption and findings are negative in 50% of cases.** Possible findings are hyperechoic foci posterior to the placenta suggestive of a collection of fresh blood or a hypoechoic area suggestive of formed clot. Lack of USG findings does not rule out abruption and use of ultrasound should not be substituted for clinical judgment.
b. *Laboratory studies:*
   i. Maternal hematocrit may show anemia
   ii. Maternal peripheral smear will show a reduced platelet count
   iii. Clot observation test: It is simple bedside invaluable procedure. A venous blood sample is drawn every hour, placed in a clean test tube and observed for clot formation and lysis. *Failure of clot formation within 5-10 minutes or dissolution of a formed clot when the tube is gently shaken is proof of clotting deficiency.*
   iv. Clotting factor estimation: Prothrombin time, partial thromboplastin time, platelet count, fibrinogen and fibrin split products should be available in hospital as an emergency basis.
   v. Kleihauer Betke test is done in Rh negative mother for determination of quantity of Anti D vaccine.

Differential Diagnosis

a. Rupture uterus
b. A retroperitoneal hematoma
c. Hematoma of rectus abdominis
d. Acute polyhydramnios
e. Nonobstetrical acute abdominal condition like appendicitis
f. Placenta previa

Management

Management of abruptio placenta will depend on gestational age and status of mother and fetus. These patients should be managed in a well equipped hospital with resources capable of dealing with all the complication of abruptio placenta like coagulopathy.

A. *General measure:* As described earlier, a quick assessment of the general condition of the patient needs to be performed on admission. Initial measures are administration of I/V fluid, oxygen. Blood sample is taken for blood grouping and cross matching and for test for hematocrit, platelet count, peripheral smear, coagulation profile, liver and renal function test. Ultrasound should be performed for placental location, fetal gestational age and presentation. The patient is catheterized and urine output is monitored, urine is examined for protein, presence of cast or blood. Electronic fetal monitoring is preferred for continuous assessment of fetal well being. If patient is in shock vigorous blood and volume replacement with packed RBC and crystalloid should be done with the aim to maintain the hematocrit at or above 30% and the urinary output ≥ 0.5 ml/kg/hr.

B. *Expectant treatment:* Expectant management in suspected placental abruptio is the exception, not the rule. This can only be considered in mild cases of abruptio, when mother is stable, fetus is immature and fetal heart tracing is reassuring. The patient should be admitted in hospital for 24-48 hours and include the following:
   i. Regular assessment of maternal condition
   ii. Frequent assessment of maternal hematologic parameter and coagulation profile
   iii. Antepartum fetal surveillance with NST and biophysical profile
   iv. Administration of steroid
   v. Anti D if needed
   vi. Tocolysis in selected case: Tocolysis can be used in selected cases to prevent preterm labor and prolong pregnancy till steroid has been administered. Magnesium sulphate has been found to be safest. Once the patient is stable, the decision to manage the patient as an out patient basis should be tailored to the clinical situation. If out patient surveillance is selected the fetus should be closely followed with nonstress testing.

C. *Timing and mode of delivery:* The timing and method of delivery depend on the gestational age of the fetus and the severity of abruptio.
   a. *Vaginal delivery:* If pregnancy is at term, abruptio is mild and continuous fetal heart rate tracing is reassuring vaginal delivery may be attempted. If fetus is dead, effort should be made to achieve vaginal delivery with careful attention to coagulation status. Labor should be induced with artificial rupture of membrane and oxytocin. Amniotomy is considered advantageous because it may decrease extravasation of blood into the myometrium and entry of thromboplastic substances into the circulation. If the uterus is spastic, uterine contraction can not be clearly identified, the progress of labor must be judged by

observing cervical dilatation. Pudendal block anesthetic is recommended. A careful watch on progress of labor is must, as longer the interval between abruptio and delivery; the greater are chances of hypofibrinogenemia and shock. Active management of 3rd stage of labor is mandatory.

b. *Cesarean section:* Indication of cesarean section are as follows:
   i. Significant abruptio with alive and reasonably mature baby
   ii. Unstable maternal condition not responding to resuscitation measures
   iii. Uncontrolled hemorrhage
   iv. Biochemical evidence of DIC
   v. Fetal distress
   vi. Failure of labor to progress

Complications and Management of Abruptio

Disseminated Intravascular Coagulation

Placental abruptio can lead to initiation of the coagulation cascade by release of tissue thromboplastin into the maternal circulation. Consumption of coagulation factors and platelet is followed by coagulopathy hemorrhage. A vicious cycle is started as further bleeding worsens the depletion of coagulation factor, so continuous monitoring for evidence of clotting deficiency should be done every 4 hours until delivery. *Quantification of fibrin split products is the most sensitive lab test, but once raised, FSP are not helpful in guiding therapy.* Fibrinogen level and platelet count are more indicative of the ongoing process and are more useful in terms of management. Treatment will depend not only on the demonstration of hematologic deficiencies, but also on the amount of active bleeding and the anticipated route of delivery.

a. *Transfusion of blood and blood products:* Hemodynamic stabilization is the main stay of treatment. DIC should be treated by blood (to replace lost hemoglobin) and plasma expanders. Plasma expanders should consist not of synthetic maternal like Dextran because by Dextran the fibrinogen may be precipitated as fibrin or inactivated by forming a fibrinogen Dextran compound. It is also more difficult to cross match the patient blood for subsequent transfusion after infusing Dextran. *Component therapy is mainstay of treatment of DIC guided by hematologic investigation.*

Fresh whole blood: Fresh whole blood is generally reserved for massive hemorrhage (5-6 L blood loss in a 24 hours period). Each unit has a volume of 500 cc and contains red blood cells, white blood cells, coagulation factors and other plasma proteins. One unit of blood raises the hematocrit by 3%.

Packed red blood cells (PRBC): Packed red blood cells are satisfactory for immediate replacement of blood loss but they do not contain clotting factors. Each unit has a volume of 250 cc. The chances of transfusion reaction are decreased because amount of white blood cells and plasma protein is less.

Fresh frozen plasma: Fresh frozen plasma is a preparation of non-concentrated clotting factors without platelets. Each unit has a volume of 250 ml and raises any clotting factors by 2-3%. Fibrinogen concentration is raised by 10 mg% per unit.

Cryoprecipitate: Cryoprecipitate is prepared as fresh frozen plasma and contain all the necessary labile coagulation factors. Each unit has a volume of 40 cc. It is useful in avoiding fluid overload, while treating hypofibrogenemia.

Platelets: Each unit of platelet has a volume of 40-50 cc and can be expected to raise the platelet count by 10,000. Usually 6-8 unit of platelet concentrate is required.

Heparins: There is no role of heparin in treatment of DIC related to abruption.

b. *In preparation of surgery:* If cesarean section is indicated, preparation for surgery must be completed quickly. Two to four unit of PRBC should be reserved. Blood component should be ordered as per directed by investigation and clinical condition. In cases of uncontrollable hemorrhage, despite maximal attempt to correct coagulapathy, alternative management should be thought of like intrauterine balloon tympanode, whole pelvis embolization, uterine packing. Rarely hysterectomy is necessary to control bleeding even in the presence of some degree of coagulopathy.

Ischemic necrosis of distal organs

Ischemic necrosis of distal organs usually involves the kidney, liver, adrenal glands or pituitary glands. Ischemic necrosis of the kidney may take the form of acute tubular necrosis (ATN) or bilateral cortical necrosis. Both are characterized by oliguria or anuria.

The possibility of renal cortical or tubular necrosis must be considered if oliguria persist after an adequate blood volume has been restored. An attempt should be done to improve renal circulation and promote diuresis by increasing fluid volume with careful maintenance of input output chart. If there is continued impairment of renal function, peritoneal dialysis or hemodialysis is required. Bilateral cortical necrosis results in death from uremia within 1-2 weeks unless dialysis is initiated, whereas acute tubular necrosis usually resolves spontaneously.

Prognosis

Perinatal Outcome

Fetal implications include hypoxia, anemia, growth retardation, increased incidence of anamolies (especially of CNS) and death. Death of fetus occurs in 4 of 1000 abruptio and account for 15% of all perinatal death. In surviving infants after severe abruption, long term neurological sequele like cerebral palsy may be 4 times greater.

Maternal Outcome

Maternal mortality rates ranges from 0.5-5%. *Causes of death usually are excessive hemorrhage, cardiac or renal failure.* A high degree of suspicion, early diagnosis and definitive therapy should reduce the maternal mortality.

RUPTURE OF THE UTERUS

Rupture of the uterus is one of the most dreaded complications of child birth and is a major cause of maternal death.

Definition

Disruption in the continuity of the uterine wall any time beyond 28 weeks of pregnancy is called rupture of the uterus.

Incidence

In developed countries, uterus rupture is practically a complication related to previous cesarean section scar. It is 0.8% incidence in prior low transverse uterine scar and 4-8% for women with a prior classic scar. In developing world, uterus rupture is still common in unscarred uterus due to obstructed labor and multiparity.

Pathology and Classification

Uterus rupture may be complete or incomplete depending on whether or not the serous layer of uterus is involved in rupture. In **complete rupture** the serous layer is ruptured and fetus and occasionally placenta is extruded into the peritoneal cavity. In *incomplete rupture* usually there is rupture of lower segment scar or extension of a cervical tear into the lower uterine segment with formation of broad ligament hematoma.

Rupture may be:
a. Spontaneous
b. Traumatic

Spontaneous rupture: It is more common, it usually occurs in last few weeks of pregnancy. Mostly it is due to weakening of the uterine wall by previous operations like myomectomy, cesarean scar or old perforation following MTP.

Traumatic rupture: It is due to result of road traffic accidents, improper administration of oxytocic agents and obstetric maneuver like internal version, breech extraction, difficult forceps delivery or manual removal of the placenta.

Rupture during labor: Neglected obstructed labor may be responsible for uterus rupture. Causes of obstructed labor include contracted pelvis, fetal macrosomia, and brow or face presentation, hydrocephalus or tumors involving the birth canal. The vast majority of rupture during labor occurs in patient with previous uterine scar like cesarean or myomectomy scar or surgery done on the cervix or uterine anomalies.

Risk Factors for Uterus Rupture

a. **History:** History of uterine surgery like hysterotomy, Cesarean, myomectomy, metroplasty, cornual resection.
b. **Trauma:** Road traffic accidents, rotational forceps, extension of cervical tear.
c. **Uterine over distension:** Hydramnios, multiple gestation, fetal macrosomia.
d. **Uterine anomalies.**
e. **Adherent placenta** like placenta percreta.
f. **Choriocarcinoma:** Silent rupture is seen in classic cesarean and hysterotomy scar, placenta percreta, invasive mole, choriocarcinoma and cornual pregnancy.

Diagnosis

a. *Signs of impending uterine rupture:* There are no reliable sign of impending uterine rupture that occurs before labor. **Sudden appearance of gross hematuria and sudden abnormal fetal heart rate pattern on CTG are suggestive of impending uterine rupture.**
b. *Signs of rupture in unscarred uterus:* The patient classically presents with severe pain followed by cessation of uterine contractions. There is some vaginal external bleeding and signs of hypovolemic shock and fainting. A characteristic sign is loss of the presenting part from its former position within the pelvis. If fetus is expelled in abdominal cavity the fetal parts are palpable through the abdominal wall. The fetus usually dies and fetal heart sound are not found. In complete rupture, the empty and retracted uterus forms a firm swelling to the side of the fetus. In complete rupture, bulge of retroperitoneal hematoma in broad ligament can often be felt to one side of the uterus and ovary extend into the pelvis up to vagina.
c. *Scar dehiscence in labor:* It is more common. There may be no sign other than a rise in pulse rate. So in vaginal birth after cesarean section this sign is highly significant. Like wise fetal heart rate pattern associated with uterine rupture are recurrent variable or late deceleration and bradycardia. There may be local pain and tenderness with a small amount of vaginal bleeding.
d. *Uterine rupture detected in 3rd stage of labor:* Occasionally rupture occurs at the end of 2nd stage of labor so that vaginal delivery of the fetus occurs. *But after that there is characteristic sign of shortening of the cord. It is pathognomic of uterine rupture caused by extrusion of placenta into the abdominal cavity.* Beside this if a newly delivered patient exhibits persistent bleeding or shock the uterus must be carefully reexamined for signs of rupture. Uterus may be difficult to palpate because of soft irregular tissue surface. If bleeding is continued in spite of a well retracted uterus,

especially after operative delivery, cervical laceration should be looked for. Sometimes cervix is intact but bleeding occurs from a rupture of vaginal vault.

Differential Diagnosis

Other causes of acute abdominal catastrophe should be thought. **Abruptio placenta** is difficult to differentiate as it presents with pain, shock, absence of uterine contraction and disappearance of fetal heart sound. However, in abruptio the uterus is regular in outline and there is no other swelling caused by broad ligament hematoma or fetal parts. In patients presenting with postpartum collapse, possibility of **uterine inversion** should be excluded.

Treatment

Immediate laparotomy is indicated when the diagnosis of uterus rupture is made. With preceding or accompanying resuscitative measures and blood transfusion, quick surgery is strongly recommended. Surgery is directed by clinical scenario and can range from *simple repairing of defect* to removal of the uterus.

Hysterectomy is the best cure in cases of extensive rupture if it is potentially infected. Hysterectomy can be total or subtotal depending on site of rupture and patient's condition. The most difficult cases are when there is broad ligament hematoma, and uterine artery hemorrhage. Before proceeding to hysterectomy one should be fully satisfied that main source of hemorrhage is not a vaginal vault laceration. In these cases, care must be taken to avoid ureteral damage by blind suturing at the base of broad ligament. If there is a doubt about ureteral ligature in suture, it is best to perform cystotomy and observe the bilateral appearance of intravenously injected dye – indigocarmine. A retrograde ureteral catheter can be passed upward if still there is doubt.

Repair of Scar

In young patient, if child bearing is important and both short and long term risks are acceptable to patient, repair of rupture can be done (Figs 35.5A and B). Occult rupture of previous scar at repeat section can be treated by freshening the wound edges and secondary repair. After repair risk of uterine rupture in subsequent pregnancy is high and in next pregnancy elective cesarean section should be done just before term. No trial of labor should be done in next pregnancy.

Repair and Sterilization

Repair of rupture and sterilization is best treatment for young patient who are not desirous of further child bearing. The advantages are avoidance of potential complication of hysterectomy. In repair, uterus should be repaired with interrupted sutures in layers, starting with one traction

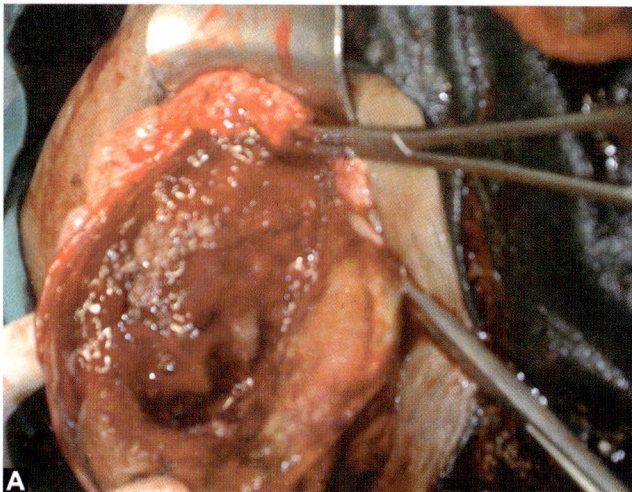
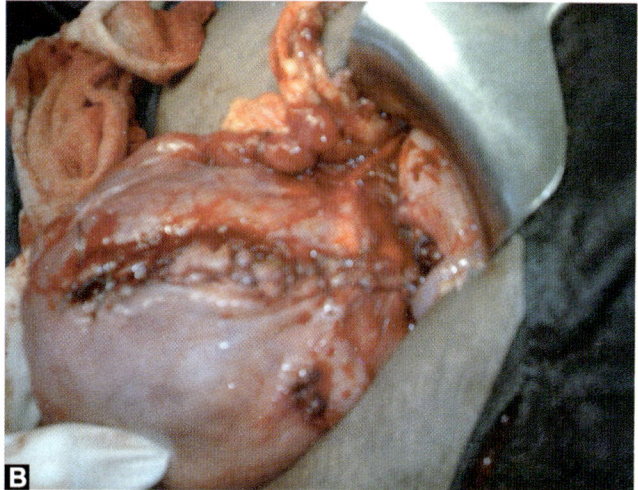

Figs 35.5A and B: (A) Rupture of uterus in upper uterine segment; (B) Repair of rupture uterus done in two layers

suture at the upper end of the rent and repairing from below upwards.

Complications of uterine rupture: They are hemorrhage, shock, postoperative infection, amniotic fluid embolism, DIC, pitutary failure and death.

Prognosis

The maternal mortality rate is 4-5%. The perinatal mortality rate is 46%.

Prevention

Good intrapartum care, timely intervention by cesarean section in obstructed labor and trial of vaginal birth after cesarean section in only selected cases and specialized instruction can prevent uterine rupture. Good transportation facility is also important to avoid uterus rupture in malpresentation and high risk cases. Once diagnosed, surgery with availability of blood transfusion and antibiotic reduce the maternal mortality caused by uterine rupture.

MULTIPLE CHOICE QUESTIONS

1. Placenta previa is associated with all except:
   a. Larger placenta
   b. Previous cesarean section scar
   c. Primigravida
   d. Previous placenta previa
   Ans. c

2. Classical presentation of placenta previa:
   a. Anterior
   b. Central
   c. Lateral
   d. Posterior
   Ans. d

3. A primigravida at 37 weeks reported to labor room with central placenta previa with heavy bleeding per vagina. The FHS was normal at time of examination. The best management option for her is:
   a. Expectant management
   b. Cesarean section
   c. Induction and vaginal delivery
   d. Induction and forceps delivery
   Ans. b

4. A second gravida P_1X_0 presented at 32 weeks of pregnancy with grade III placenta previa and contraction. Patient vital are normal. The treatment of choice is:
   a. Bed rest and sedation
   b. Bed rest and dexamethasone
   c. Rest, nifedipine and dexamethasone
   d. Bed rest and nifedipine
   Ans. c

5. Most death involving placenta previa results from:
   a. Infection
   b. Toxemia
   c. Hemorrhage
   d. Thrombophlebitis
   Ans. c

6. Fetal Hb is different from HbA in that it is:
   a. More sensitive to alkali denaturation
   b. More resistant to alkali denaturation
   c. More sensitive to acid denaturation
   d. All of the above
   Ans. b

7. The first consideration in the treatment of placental abruption:
   a. Immediate delivery
   b. Administration of fibrinogen
   c. Amniocentesis to establish diagnosis
   d. Prompt restoration of an effective circulation with I/V fluid
   Ans. d

8. One of the following is not true about vasa previa
   a. Blood of maternal origin
   b. May be a cause of antepartum hemorrhage
   c. Blood of fetal origin
   d. Singer's test positive
   Ans. a

9. Abruptio placenta occurs in all except:
   a. Smokers
   b. Alcoholics
   c. PET
   d. Folic acid deficiency
   Ans. b

10. All are true about abruption placenta except:
    a. Absent fetal heart
    b. Uterine tenderness
    c. Profuse bleeding
    d. Hypotension
    Ans. c

11. In placenta previa, conservative treatment is not done in case of:
    a. Active labor
    b. Anencephaly
    c. Dead baby
    d. Premature baby
    Ans. a, b, c

12. Couvelaire uterus is seen in:
    a. Placenta previa
    b. Accidental hemorrhage
    c. PIH
    d. PPH
    Ans. b

36
Multiple Pregnancy

What we learn with pleasure, we never forget.

INTRODUCTION

When more than one fetus simultaneously develops in the uterus, it is called multiple pregnancy. Simultaneous development of two fetuses (twins) is the commonest. Development of three fetuses (Triplets), four fetuses (quadruplets), five fetuses (quintuplets) or six fetuses (sextuplets) may also occur.

TWIN

Incidence of Twin Pregnancy

Traditionally the expected incidence of twin was calculated using Hellen's rule. Using this rule twin were expected 1 in 80 pregnancies, triplet 1 in 80^2 and so on. Twin occurs in 1 of 100 pregnancies among white women, 1 in 80 in black women and 1 in 155 in Asian pregnant women. Monozygotic twins (MZ) occur in 1 in 250 births and are independent of race, heredity, age and parity. Incidence of Dizygotic twin (DZ) is affected by each of these factors and also by fertility drugs. A woman who is a DZ twin is twice as likely to give birth to DZ twins. Assisted reproductive drugs and technology has increased the rate of multiple gestation. The rate is 16-40% with Gonadotrophin induction of ovulation, 25-30% with superovulation and 7-13% with Clomiphene therapy. In women undergoing IVF option multiple embryos are placed into the uterus, there are more chances of multiple gestation.

Genesis of Twins

A. *Identical twins (Monozygotic twins, Uniovular twin):* Identical or MZ twins arise from division of one fertilized ovum into two separate embryos. The timing of this division has important implications.
   i. *Diamniotic dichorionic monozygotic twins:* Division within 72 hours after conception results in a diamniotic dichorionic MZ twin pregnancy. As neither the inner cell mass nor the outer layer of blastocyst (destined to become chorion) has formed, each embryo will have a separate amnion and chorion. This occurs in about 30% of MZ twins and has the lowest mortality rate 9%.
   ii. *Diamniotic monochorionic twins:* If division of ovum occurs 4-8 days after fertilization, it results in diamniotic monochorionic twin. As the amnion is not yet differentiated there are separate amniotic sac but there is a shared chorion. This is the most frequent type of MZ twining (68%). Mortality can be as high as 25% due to complication of vascular anastomosis within the placentas.
   iii. *Mono amniotic monochorionic twins:* Division of ovum occurs 8-13 days after fertilization. These MZ twin occur least often 2% but have the highest mortality rate up to 50%.
   iv. *Conjoined twins:* Division occurs at 2 weeks after fertilization, after the amniotic sac and embryonic disc are formed but division of the embryonic disc is incomplete, resulting in conjoined twin. It is in order of 1 in 60,000 births. Conjoined twins are commonly referred to as *Siamese twins*. After Chang and Eng Bunker of Siam (Thailand). Joining of twins may begin at either pole and may produce characteristic forms like thoracopagus, cephalopagus, ischiopagus, omphalopagus. Of these parapagus is most common.
B. *Fraternal twins:* Fraternal or DZ twins arise from the fertilization of two separate ova. **Superfecundation** refers to fertilization of different ova in the same menstrual cycle at two separate episodes of intercourse.
C. *Superfetation:* Occurs when two ova are fertilized during separate menstrual cycle i.e. the second ovulation occurred after the first pregnancy was established. This is rare.

Methods of Establishing Zygosity

There are important differences in risk and outcome between dichorionic and monochorionic pregnancies, therefore determination of chorionicity of critical to good management.

Ultrasound Examination

i. Best diagnosed by ultrasound at 6-9 weeks of gestation. In dichorionic twins there is a thick septum between the chorionic sacs. It is best identified at the base of the membrane where a triangular projection is seen. This is known as *Lambda or twin peak signs. The sign indicates dichorionic placenta*. In monochorionic twins this sign is absent and the intertwine membrane join the uterine wall in T shape.
ii. If fetal gender can be identified on ultrasound, twins of opposite sex are almost always DZ.
iii. If the separating membrane between the twins measure > 2 m in thickness, the pregnancy is probably dichorionic. If two separate placentas are scanned, the pregnancy is DZ.

Placental Examination

Twins of the opposite sex (barring genetic abnormalities) are always dizygotic. Placental examination reveals zygosity in cases of like sex twins. Determination is based on the chorion/amnion states.

i. *Dizygotic twins*: There are two placenta either completely separated or more commonly found at the margin appearing to be one. There is no anastomosis between fetal vessels. Each fetus is surrounded by separate amnion and chorion. Intervening membrane consist of 4 layers – amnion chorion, chorion and amnion (Fig. 36.1).
ii. *Monozygotic twins*: The placenta is single, there is varying degree of free anastomosis between the two fetal vessels – each fetus is surrounded by a separate amniotic sac with the common chorionic layer, so the intervening membrane consist of two layers of amnion only.

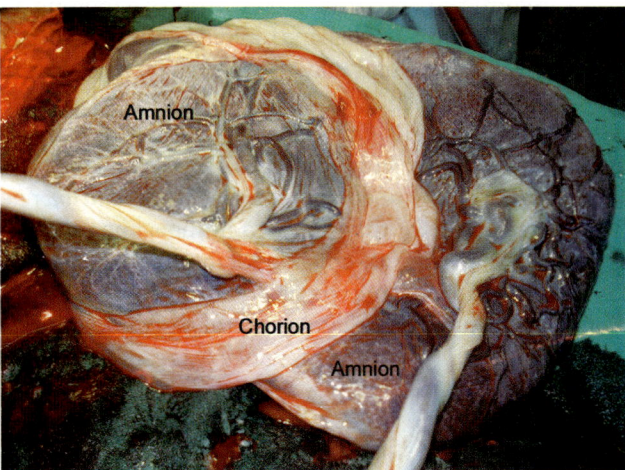

Fig. 36.1: Term placenta in dizygotic twin—Membrane portion consists of chorion

Diagnosis of Twin Pregnancy

Symptoms

Severity of common problems of pregnancy is more troublesome in multiple pregnancy. There are earlier and more severe complaints of nausea, vomiting, backache, varicosity, constipation, hemorrhoids, abdominal distension and breathing discomfort. Fetal activity is more in frequency and persistent in twin pregnancy.

Signs

The following signs should alert the physician to the possibility of definite presence of multiple pregnancies:
a. Uterus larger than expected (>4 cm) for dates
b. Excessive maternal weight gain that is not explained by edema or obesity
c. Polyhydramnios
d. Outline or ballottement of more than fetus
e. Multiplicity of small parts
f. Simultaneously recording of different fetal heart rate, each asynchronous with the mother pulse and with each other and varying by at least 8 bpm.

Investigations

Ultrasound examination: Ultrasound is done to assess following in multiple pregnancy.
a. An early ultrasound examination is important to confirm expected date of confinement and assess chorionicity (Fig. 36.2A).
b. If fetal size discrepancy exists, biometry of larger fetus is done for dating consideration. Serial ultrasounds are useful.
c. Fetal growth monitoring every 3-4 weeks interval.
d. Twin transfusion
e. Assessing amniotic fluid volume
f. Placental localization
g. Presentation and lie of the fetuses (Fig. 36.2B).
h. Chorionicity of the placenta at 6-9 weeks can be assessed by presence or absence of lambda sign.

Maternal hematocrit values: The hematocrit and hemoglobin values and red cell count usually are considerably reduced in direct relationship to the increased blood volume. Maternal hypochromic normocytic anemia is common because fetal demands for iron increase beyond the mother's ability to assimilate iron in the second trimester.
Maternal glucose screening: It should be done in multiple pregnancies.

Prenatal Testing

The usual indication for prenatal diagnosis and counseling in a singleton pregnancy also apply to twin and high order gestation. Maternal age of 33 can be used as an indicator.

sampled. As the placentas are often fused together, CVS has special challenges. *Selective termination* of an aneuploid fetus can be performed via ultrasound guided intra-cardiac injection of potassium chloride. The pregnancy then can be continued carrying the normal twin only.

Differential Diagnosis

Multiple pregnancies must be distinguished from following conditions:

a. *Single ton pregnancy:* With fetal macrosomia or mistaken dates.
b. *Polyhydramnios:* Either single or multiple pregnancy may be associated with excessive accumulation of fluid.
c. *Hydatidiform mole:* Can be easily diagnosed by ultrasound.
d. *Abdominal tumors complicating pregnancy:* Fibroid, ovarian tumor can be differentiated by ultrasound examination.
e. *Complicated twin pregnancy:* Vanishing twin, death of one twin, fetal papyra aceous is diagnosed by serial ultrasound scans.

Management

Prevention

Meticulous use of ovulation inducing drugs, less number of embryo transfer in ART procedure results in prevention of multiple pregnancy.

Complications of Multiple Pregnancies

Maternal Complications

a. *Anemia:* Due to iron defficiency is common because of increased fetal requirements. Rarely megaloblastic anemia from folic acid defficiency occurs. Additionally physiologic dilution from plasma volume expansion contributes.
b. *Preterm delivery:* In multiple pregnancy approximately 50% deliveries are preterm. Prematurity is the most common cause of neonatal morbidity and mortality in multiple gestation. Overall twins account for about 10% of all premature infants. The mean length of gestation in twins is 35 weeks, in triplets 33 weeks and quadruplets 31 weeks.
c. *Spontaneous abortion:* Spontaneous abortions are twice as often as singleton pregnancies. With increasing use of ultrasound, early abortion or resorption of one twin – *the vanishing twin syndrome* – has been observed to occur in 21-63% of spontaneous twin gestation.
d. *Hyperemesis* can occur.
e. *Pregnancy induced hypertension:* The incidence of gestational hypertension and pre-eclampsia is increased 2-3 fold. There is tendency to develop PIH earlier in pregnancy and more severe as compared with singleton

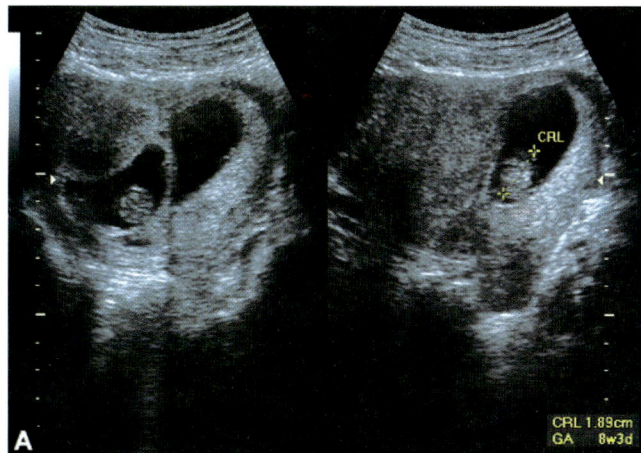
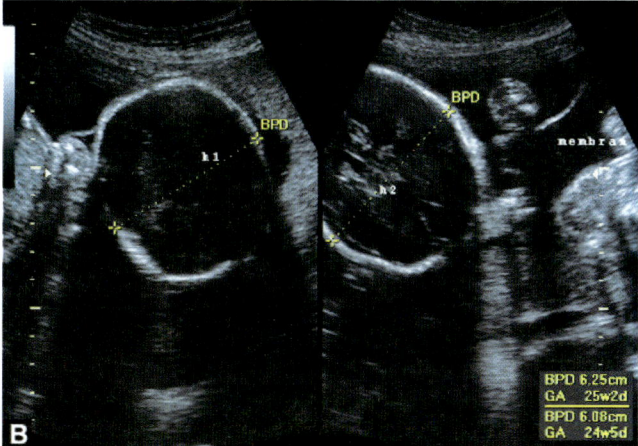

Figs 36.2A and B: (A) Twin gestation sac in early pregnancy; (B) Twin pregnancy in vertex-vertex presentation

A detailed second trimester ultrasound is very useful in risk assessment. More time must be allowed for scan. As monochorionic twins have a significantly increased risk of fetal anomalies, it is preferred that screening is done at specialized center. The use of other screening methods varies by institution. The combination of maternal age and *Nuchal Translucency* (NT) has been reported to detect 88% of fetuses with Down's syndrome. Second trimester *serum α feto protein* screening is accomplished by using mathematical models and yield approximately 51% detection rate. But maternal serum marker is not so effective in multiple pregnancy because the relative contribution from each twin to each serum marker can not be isolated. The optimal method of screening twin is **ultrasound**. The measurement of nuchal translucency at 12 weeks gestation allows each fetus to have an individualized assessment of risk. The combination of Nuchal thickness and first trimester estimation of PAPP-A and βhCG has resulted in a 75% detection rate at a false positive rate of 9% of pregnancies. Both *amniocentesis and chorionic villus sampling* (CVS) can be performed in women with multiple gestation in experienced centers. In dichorionic pregnancies it is essential that both fetuses are

pregnancies. It occurs with equal frequency in MZ and DZ twin pregnancies. There is increasing frequency with higher order gestation. The incidence of atypical form like HELLP and abruptio placenta also increases.

f. *Abruptio placenta:* Abruptio placenta may also occur beside PIH, due to sudden decompression of the uterus immediately after birth of first twin.

g. *Polyhydramnios:* Polyhydramnios in one or both sacs to a greater or lesser degree is found in 5-8% of twin pregnancies over all. It is more common in MZ sets, usually from the twin to twin transfusion syndrome.

h. *Placenta previa:* The placenta occupies a much larger area of the uterine cavity than in singleton pregnancies and therefore is more likely to cover the internal os of the cervix.

Fetal Complications

a. Vanishing twins (described).
b. **Congenital malformation:** Twice as frequent, increased risk is confined to MZ sets.
c. **Intrauterine growth restriction (IUGR):** It occurs in up to two-third of twins. Usually twin growth is similar to singleton gestation up to 28–30 weeks, after that point a fall off in the growth rate is expected. Growth restriction may occur in one or both fetus. Asymmetric or discordant growth is identified in 10-25% of twin pregnancies and carries a higher perinatal mortality. **Cause of IUGR** in multiple pregnancy can be: (a) Placental insufficiency, (b) Velamentous cord insertion, (c) Twin to twin transfusion, (d) Intrinsic fetal condition effecting any singleton pregnancy. IUGR is more common in MZ twins.
d. **Growth discordance:** It is defined as greater than 20% difference in the Estimated Fetal Weight (EFW) of the twins (based on the EFW of the larger twin). If the EFW is < the 10th percentile for gestational age, IUGR is diagnosed. These twins are followed with antepartum surveillance.
e. **Perinatal mortality:** Perinatal mortality is 5 times higher than singletons. The risk is higher for MZ twins and twins displaying discordant growth. The largest single cause of perinatal death is prematurity. Other causes of perinatal mortality are *congenital malformation, twin to twin transfusion syndrome, uteroplacental insufficiency, birth trauma or hypoxia*.

Other Complications Unique to Twin

a. **Twin to twin transfusion syndrome:** It occurs when one placenta is fed by an artery from the first twin and drained by a vein that leads to the second twin. This syndrome develops in 15% of MZ twins and varies in severity. In its full blown picture the donor twin is hypoperfused, anemic, under grown and hypotensive. Oligohydramnios develops and can be so severe that donor twin appears stuck (immobilized fetus). While the recipient fetus is polycyathemic, have hypertensive cardiac hypertrophy, edema and polyhydramnios. *The polyhydramnios oligohydramnios syndrome may result in IUGR, fetal contracture and pulmonary hypoplasia in one twin, with heart failure and PROM in other*. Perinatal mortality is high. If the fetus dies, significant problem may occur in the remaining twin like multicystic encephalopathy and renal cortical necrosis. The recipient placenta has more plethoric appearance and larger, whereas donor placenta appears pale and smaller.

b. **Acardiac twin:** It is also known as *Twin Reversed Arterial Perfusion (TRAP) sequence*. It is complication unique to MZ twins. Its incidence is 1 in 35,000 births. TRAP sequence is characterized by the presence of an acardius, a twin that does not have a normally formed heart and lacking multiple other structures as well. This is lethal anomaly.

Antenatal Care in Twin Pregnancies

Prenatal care in multiple pregnancy is based on following principles:

a. Early diagnosis is associated with an improved perinatal outcome.
b. Frequent antenatal visit at least every two weeks from 20-36 weeks.
c. Diet of additional calories (+ 300 Kcal/day) and protein (to 80 gm/day), 60-100 mg/day of iron supplementation, folic acid 1mg/day, weight gain 35-45 ponds.
d. Extra bed rest.
e. Educate the patient about the signs and symptoms of preterm labor. In each visits these symptoms should be questioned.
f. Prevent, recognize and aggressively treat preterm labor.
g. Fetal growth is followed by serial ultrasound examination to detect discordant growths, IUGR or twin to twin transfusion syndrome. It is reasonable to plan 4-6 weekly ultrasound scan in dichorionic twins but due to increased risk in monochorionic pregnancies fortnightly ultrasound is appropriate.
h. Watch for and treat pregnancy induced hypertension and pre-eclampsia as in singleton pregnancy.
i. Watch for and manage any complication like polyhydramnios, twin to twin transfusion syndrome and intrauterine death.
j. Institute antepartum testing if IUGR, growth discordance, oligohydramnios or polyhydramnios, preeclampsia, fetal anamolies or monoamniotic monochorionic twins are present.
k. Patients should be psychologically prepared for care of two babies.

Management of Specific Situations

Preterm Labor

Patient is managed on the same line as in singleton pregnancies with rest, hospitalization, frequent ultrasound cervical examinations and prophylactic cirlcage. The additional consideration in multiple pregnancy is that there is increased maternal plasma volume (as much as 50-60% of the non pregnant state vs 45% in singleton pregnancy) and cardiac output. So β mimetic therapy in women with twins entails a higher risk of pulmonary edema and other cardiac problem. *Magnesium sulphate may be the best initial tocolytic drug.* Strict monitoring of patient fluid volume is mandatory. The use of Nifedipine and Indomethacin can be tried. A single course of steroid therapy is recommended to accelerate fetal lung maturity in patients with documented preterm labor between 24-34 weeks of gestation.

Death of One Fetus in utero

If death of one fetus occurs in the first trimester, the dead fetus may be completely absorbed or may persist as a fetus papyraceaus (small, flattened died out fetus). If the patient did not have an ultrasound during this time, the twin gestation may not be identified. If death occurs in the second or third trimester (incidence 0.5-6.8%) the surviving fetus may face significant morbidity and mortality. Monozygotic twins with monoamniotic/ monochorionic or diamniotic/ monochorionic placentation are at highest risk of complications. In surviving monozygotic twins there are structural defects of the central nervous system, skin and kidney – cerebral palsy, microcephaly, multicystic encephalo malacia, renal cortical necrosis and aplasia cutis. Current explanation holds that such defects results from significant prolonged hypotension as the living twin looses blood to the dead twin through placental vascular anastomosis. Maternal morbidity from DIC is rare and usually does not occur until 4 or more weeks after fetal death. Early delivery does not prevent or decrease the risk of such complications, which are likely to have occurred at the time of demise. Delivery should be done for the usual obstetrical indications. Vaginal delivery is appropriate unless there is an obstetric indication for cesarean section (Fig. 36.3).

Twin to Twin Transfusion Syndrome (TTTS)

More than 90% of pregnancies complicated by TTTS end in miscarriage or severe preterm delivery due either to polyhydramnios or to intrauterine death of one or both fetus. With treatment, one or both babies survive in about 70% of pregnancies. Common method of treatment is amniocentesis every 1-2 weeks with the drainage of large amount of amniotic fluid. This treatment can prolong the pregnancy and improve survival. More recently some countries have used fetoscopically guided laser coagulation to disrupt the placental blood vessels that connect the circulation of the two fetuses.

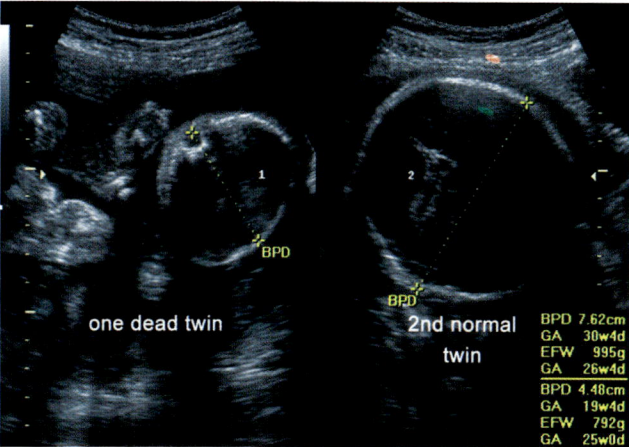

Figs 36.3: Ultrasound image showing death of one fetus and one alive fetus *in utero*

Management of Labor in Multiple Pregnancies

There can be increased risk of many complications of labor in multiple pregnancy which includes preterm labor, uterine contractile dysfunction, abnormal presentation, cord prolapse, abruptio placenta and postpartum hemorrhage. So certain special arrangements should be made in conduct of labor:
a. Presence of senior obstetrician.
b. Facility of continuous electric fetal monitoring of both twins. Specialized twin monitors should be used to ensure that both twin's heart rates are sampled.
c. Intravenous fluid access.
d. Surveillance of patient and fetus by a trained obstetrician and nurse.
e. Presence of anesthetist for any intervention manipulation or cesarean section.
f. Presence of two people skilled in neonatal resuscitation.

Management According to Presentation of Fetus

The two fetuses can present as in following combination of fetal positions (Figs 36.4A to D):

Vertex – Vertex	42%
Vertex – Breech	27%
Breech – Breech	5%
Vertex – Transverse	18%
Others	8%

Vertex-Vertex Twins

Vaginal delivery is recommended for most of the cases. After delivery of the first twin the cord is left clamped and no

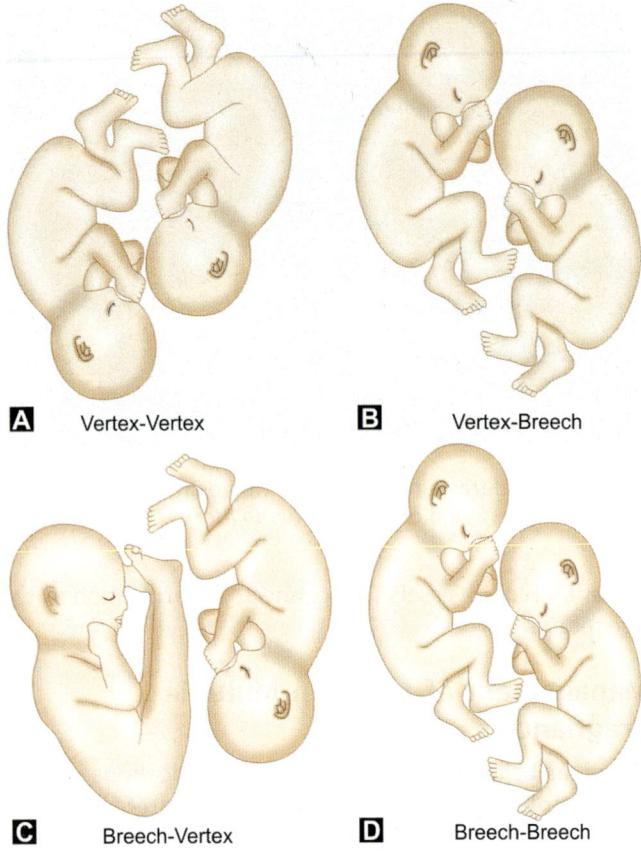

Figs 36.4A to D: Different presentations of fetuses in twin pregnancy

blood is taken as placental anastomosis may compromise the blood supply to the second twin. The presenting part of second twin, its size and relationship to pelvic is ascertained. Until the second twin's head is well engaged, its amniotic sac should be left intact. Under normal condition, the uterus is allowed to resume labor for delivery of the second twin. Oxytocin may be needed to restart uterine contractions. Generally, the second twin delivers within 15-30 minutes of the first twin. But this interval may be prolonged as long as the fetal heart tracing remains reassuring. If there is bleeding indicative of abruption or non reassuring heart rate pattern, delivery as with twin A, may be expedited by vacuum extraction or low forceps, if indicated.

Indication of cesarean in vertex–vertex twins should be reserved only for obstetric indications. In 5-6% patients cesarean section is needed for twin B because of cord prolapse, fetal distress, abruptio placenta or malpresentation which occur spontaneously some times.

Management of Labor in Vertex Breech

a. ***Cesarean section:*** Cesarean section is a safe option for vertex breech extraction especially if the obstetrician is not adequately trained in maneuver of breech extraction or external cephalic version.

b. ***Breech extraction of second twin:*** It is successful in 83-96% of attempts. The prerequiste for breech extraction are same as for singleton breech delivery – that is adequate pelvis, estimated fetal weight of 2000 – 3800 gm, flexed head. Experienced obstetrician, immediate availability of general anesthetic is mandatory for managing soft tissue dystocia or delivery of nuchal arms and after coming head. It is not preferred to attempt if estimated fetal weight of twin B is significantly greater than that of twin A.

c. ***External cephalic version of the second (breech) twin:*** ECV under ultrasound guidance is another option which is successful in 46-73% of attempts. Delivery then proceeds like singleton vertex delivery. The disadvantages are fetal distress secondary to the version and failure. In such case either breech extraction under general anesthetic or immediate cesarean section is performed.

Non-Vertex Twin A

When either twin A or both twins are non vertex, primary cesarean section should be performed.

Management of 3rd Stage in Multiple Pregnancy

Postpartum hemorrhage is anticipated in multiple pregnancy because of larger placental size, which may occupy lower segment and concomitant uterine inertia following its recent over distension. Active management of 3rd stage is recommended. Injection methylergometrine or prostaglandin is given after delivery of 2nd twin. 10-20 unit oxytocin infusion should be continued for 3-4 hours. After delivery of 2nd twin, if separation of placenta is delayed or bleeding is brisk, manual extraction of placenta is recommended. The placenta, cord and membrane should be sent to the pathology to assist in determining whether the fetuses are monozygotic or dizygotic.

Twin Locking

It is rare (1 in 817 twins). It occurs usually in **first breech second vertex** presentation as the vertex of second twin enters the brim in advance of after coming head of the first and two head become locked either chin to chin, occiput to chin, or occiput to occiput. Sometimes it occurs in **two vertex presentation**, when one head lies in advance after other, so the vertex of second twin enters the pelvis with neck of the first. If twin locking is not spontaneously disengaged, delivery must be done by cesarean section. While cesarean preparations are underway, the partially delivered first twin is elevated, and cord is protected.

Other complications of multiple pregnancies like PIH, Preterm labor, and PPROM is managed as in singleton pregnancy.

Chapter -36 ♦ Multiple Pregnancy

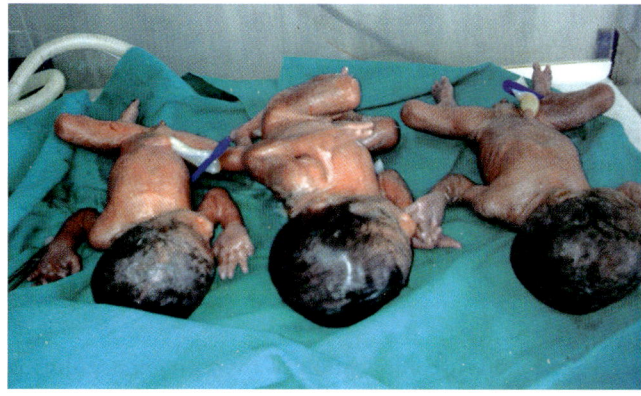

Fig. 36.5A: Preterm triplet born after cesarean section

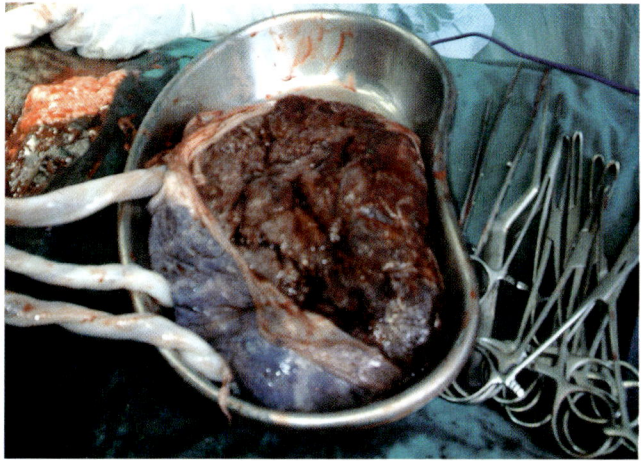

Fig. 36.5B: Placenta of triplet pregnancy

TRIPLETS AND HIGHER ORDER MULTIPLES

Over the past two decades the number of triplets and higher order multiples has increased due to greater use of assisted reproductive technologies. The problems of twin pregnancy are markedly intensified when there are additional fetuses. With increase in number of fetus, there is higher incidence of preterm labor (Figs 36.5A and B).

Antepartum Management

Antepartum management for a triplet pregnancy is generally similar to that for twins. Iron and folate supplementation are as for twin pregnancies. *The incidence of hypertension, particularly severe PIH is increased seven folds more that found in twin pregnancies.* Serial sonography in third trimester and antenatal visiting is done as in twin pregnancy. For any obstetrical complication patients should be promptly hospitalized.

Intrapartum Management

Delivery of high order pregnancy can be significantly more complicated than delivery of twins. Monitoring the fetal heart rate of triplet or higher order pregnancy is challenging. With vaginal delivery the first infant is usually born with little manipulation, but the delivery of the subsequent infant may require obstetrical maneuver like total breech extraction. There is increased risk of cord prolapse, placental hemorrhage, abruptio placenta and fetal hypoxia. For considering all reasons, cesarean section can be preferred method of delivery. Vaginal delivery is reserved only when following criteria are fulfilled:
a. Pelvic is adequate in size and shape
b. Cephalic presentation of first triplet
c. Unscarred uterus
d. Gestation > 32 weeks
e. No fetal compromise
f. Special circumstance, when survival of fetus is not expected because of marked prematurity of fetus.

Selective Reduction in Multiple Pregnancies

Multifetal pregnancy reduction was developed in an effort to improve the poor prognosis of higher order pregnancies complicated by quadruplets or greater. Pregnancy reduction is usually performed transabdominally *between 10-13 weeks gestation*. This time period is selected because the majority of early pregnancy losses have already occurred and the remaining fetuses are large enough for sonographic evaluation and amount of devitalized fetal tissue remaining after the procedure is relatively small. It is done with injection of *potassium chloride* into heart or thorax of each selected fetus under ultrasound guidance. Precaution is taken of not entering the sac of other fetus. Usually pregnancies are reduced to twins in order to increase the chance of delivery of at least one viable fetus. The risk of loss of the entire pregnancy after multifetal reduction is 8-12%.

Selective Termination

It implies termination of one or more anomalous fetus. It is not simple reduction of number of fetus in higher order multiple pregnancy. Indication of selection termination is only when anomaly of fetus is severe and estimated risk of continuing the pregnancy is greater than the risk of procedure.

MULTIPLE CHOICE QUESTIONS

1. According to Hellen's law, chances of twin in pregnancy are:
   a. 1 in 60
   b. 1 in 70
   c. 1 in 80
   d. 1 in 90
   Ans. c
2. Twin peak sign is seen in:
   a. Monochorionic diamniotic
   b. Dichorionic monoamniotic
   c. Conjoined twins
   d. Diamniotic dichorionic
   Ans. d

3. To say twin discordant, the difference in the two twins should be:
   a. 15% with larger twin as index
   b. 15% with smaller twin as index
   c. 25% with larger twin as index
   d. 25% with smaller twin as index
   Ans. c
4. Doppler USG in twins is used for:
   a. Twin to twin transfusion
   b. Conjoined twins
   c. Diagnosis of twins
   d. All of the above
   Ans. d
5. Most common cause of perinatal mortality in twin is:
   a. Dystonia
   b. Hemorrhage
   c. Anemia
   d. Prematurity
   Ans. d
6. Easiest method of determining zygosity is:
   a. Blood grouping
   b. Sex of fetus
   c. Placental examination
   d. Amniotic fluid examination
   Ans. c
7. Which types of twins have the highest mortality:
   a. Mono amniotic mono chronic
   b. Diamniotic dichorionic
   c. Binovular twins
   d. Siamese twins
   Ans. d
8. Multiple births are commonest among:
   a. Indian
   b. Mongols
   c. Caucasians
   d. Negroes
   Ans. d
9. The commonest complication of twin pregnancy during delivery includes:
   a. Interlocking
   b. Abruptio placenta
   c. Postpartum hemorrhage
   d. Obstructed labor
   Ans. c
10. Multiple pregnancies occurs most commonly with:
    a. Clomiphene
    b. Clomiphene with dexamethasone
    c. Dexamethasone
    d. Pulsatile GnRH therapy
    Ans. a

37. Disorders of Amniotic Fluid

It is easier to go downhill than up, but the view is from the top.

PHYSIOLOGY OF AMNIOTIC FLUID

Amniotic fluid provides a protective milieu for the growing fetus (Fig. 37.1). The amniotic fluid volume rises linearly from early gestation up to 32 weeks, after that it remains constant in the range of 700 to 800 ml until term. After 40 weeks gestation the volume declines at rate of 8% per week. By 42 weeks this volume decreases to approximately 400 ml. Composition and physiology of amniotic fluid is described in detail in Chapter 4.

Measurement of Amniotic Fluid by Ultrasound

Following three techniques are commonly used to measure amniotic fluid volume:
a. Amniotic fluid index (AFI)
b. Single deepest pocket
c. Two diameter pocket

Amniotic Fluid Index

The amniotic fluid index is measured by dividing the maternal abdomen into four quadrants. The umbilicus divides the uterus into upper and lower halves and the linea nigra divides the uterus into right and left halves. With the transducer perpendicular to the floor the deepest amniotic fluid pocket in each quadrant is identified. The AFI is total of the numbers obtained from each quadrant.

Single deepest pocket: It is measured by identifying the amniotic fluid pocket with the maximum vertical depth.

Two diameter pocket: It is measured by identifying the amniotic fluid pocket with the largest product of pocket depth multiplied with by pocket width.

Both oligohydramnios and polyhydramnios are associated with increased maternal and perinatal morbidity and mortality.

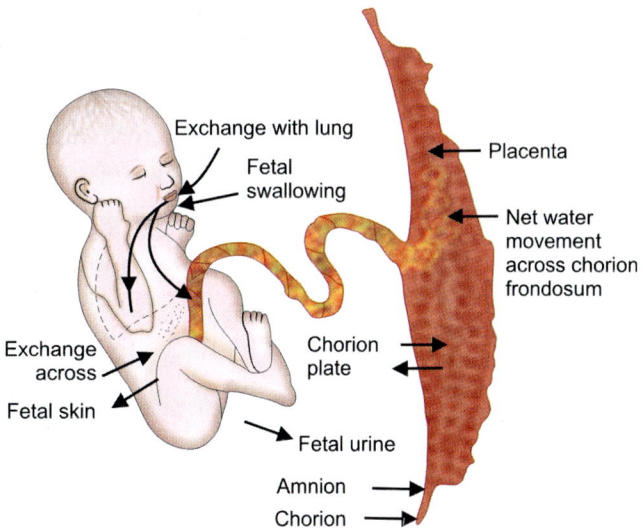

Fig. 37.1: Solute and water exchange in amniotic fluid

POLYHYDRAMNIOS

Definition

Amniotic fluid index ≥ 24 cm, AFI > 95% for a specific gestational age, single deepest pocket > 8 cm and two diameter pocket > 50 cm^2 are defined as polyhydramnios. Somewhat arbitarily more than 2 liters of amniotic fluid is considered as polyhydramnios.

Degree of Polyhydramnios: Depending on AFI
a. Mild   24.0 – 30.0 cm
b. Moderate   30.1 – 34.9 cm
c. Severe   ≥ 35.0 cm

Incidence: Polyhydramnios complicates approximately 1-3.5% of pregnancies.

Causes of Polyhydramnios

1. Idiopathic (66%)
2. Maternal diabetes (Pregestational and gestational (15%)
3. Fetal causes
    a. Congenital malformation (13%)
    b. Rh incompatibility (1%)
    c. Nonimmune Hydrops
    d. Multiple gestations (5%)
4. Placental
    a. Chorioangioma
    b. Arteriovenous fistula

Approximately 2/3rd of all cases of polyhydramnios are idiopathic. The congenital anomalies associated with polyhydramnios are central nervous system (CNS) and the gastrointestinal symptoms. The major GIT anomalies are esophageal and duodenal atresia and major CNS anomalies are anencephaly and primary neuromuscular disease. It is also noted with diaphragmatic hernia, cardiac valvular lesions and arhythmia.

Evaluation

Symptoms

Maternal symptoms accompanying polyhydramnios arise from the mechanical distension like dyspnea, edema.

Signs

Uterus is larger than gestational age. The abdomen is tense. Fetal parts and fetal heart sounds are difficult to define.

Investigations

Ultrasound: Diagnosis is confirmed by ultrasound evaluation of amniotic fluid. If polyhydramnios is seen, detailed sonogram for fetal anomalies, multiple pregnancy or evidence of Hydrops is performed.

Laboratory test: (i) ABO and Rh typing is must to asses probability of Rh isoimmunization, (ii) Postprandial blood sugar or glucose tolerance, (iii) Serological studies for maternal infection like CMV virus, rubella, syphilis and hemoglobinopathies should be performed.

Complications of Polyhydramnios

In general the more severe the degree of hydramnios, the higher is the perinatal mortality rate. *Even in idiopathic cases where fetus looks apparently normal, prognosis is still guarded because fetal malformation and chromosomal abnormalities are common.* There is increased risk of preterm labor and preterm premature rupture of fetal membrane due to overdistention of uterus or increased uterine volume. Other complications are associated with *erythroblastosis* in immune Hydrops, difficulties encountered in infants of *diabetic* mother, prolapse of umbilical cord on time of rupture of membrane. There is increased risk of *abruptio* placenta after ROM because uterus rapidly decreases in size. Abruptio placenta is the most frequent maternal complication in labor. Uterine dysfunction and *postpartum hemorrhage* result from uterine atony consequent to over distention. Malpresentation and operative interventions are more common.

Management

The treatment of polyhydramnios depends on the:
a. **Underlying etiology:** Like control of maternal diabetes, management of Hydrops. High resolution ultrasound should be performed to assess the degree of polyhydramnios, identify multiple pregnancies, and target assessment of fetal anomalies. Fetal assessment should include examination of fetal thorax, CNS, and gastrointestinal and renal system. Karyotyping can be offered if there is suspected structural anomaly. If viral infection is suspected, appropriate fetal and maternal samples should be obtained. When there is fetal anomaly, fetus is monitored or termination is offered in severe congenital anomalies. Mild degrees of polyhydramnios resolve spontaneously.
b. **Therapeutic amniocentesis:** It is reducing the amount of amniotic fluid through amniocentesis and is performed for relief of maternal symptoms like abdominal discomfort, dyspnea, or when preterm labor is not responding to drugs. Treatment is only recommended when there is severe polyhydramnios (AFI> 40 cm, SAP> 12 cm).

   Procedure: An 18-gauge spinal needle is inserted under ultrasound guidance into the uterus under full aseptic preparation and local anesthetic. When aspiration of amniotic fluid is confirmed, the stellate is withdrawn and needle is connected to I/v tubing. Fluid should be removed no faster than 1000 ml/ over 20 minutes. Procedure is stopped, when AFI is within normal range. Usually maternal relief is prompt. The procedure can be repeated if necessary under strict aseptic condition (Figs 37.2A and B).

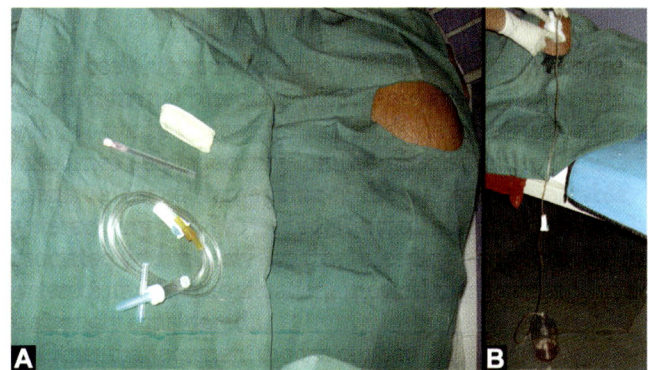

Figs 37.2A and B: Procedure of amniocentesis: (A) Equipment for amniocentesis; (B) Performing the amniocentesis

c. **Indomethacin:** Indomethacin is a prostaglandin synthetic inhibitor that decreases fetal urine output and may enhance resorption of lung liquid. The dose is 25 mg 4 times per day. It may be administered when the gestational age is less then 32 weeks, as treatment after this may result in premature closure of the ductus arteriosus. Indomethacin should not be used in trapped twin syndrome because of its adverse effects on the trapped twin. The AFI is monitored 2-3 times per week and treatment is stopped when the AFI returns to normal range. There are reports of renal failure, necrotizing enterocolitis and intracranial hemorrhage in infant treated with indomethacin *in utero*.

Management in Labor

There can be prolonged labor due to uterine inertia. Controlled artificial rupture of membrane should be done with slow release of liquor to avoid risk of sudden maternal hypotension, abruptio and cord prolapse. Active management of third stage of labor is strongly recommended because of risk of atonic PPH. After delivery neonate should be thoroughly examined for congenital anomalies. A Ryle's tube should be passed in neonate to exclude possibility of esophageal atresia.

OLIGOHYDRAMNIOS

Definition: Oligohydramnios can be defined in 4 ways AFI less than 5 cm, AFI less than 5% for a specific gestational age, single deepest pocket < 2 cm and 2 diameter pocket < 5 cm^2.

Incidence: It complicates approximately 3.9% of pregnancies.

Causes

Conditions associated with oligohydramnios is summarized in Table 37.1.

Oligohydramnios is almost always evident when there is either obstruction of the fetal urinary tract or renal agenesis. **Renal anomalies** accounts for 57% of cases with severe oligohydramnios presenting in the mid second trimester of pregnancy. In 15-20% of cases *other congenital anomalies* are associated with oligohydramnios like cardiac-Fallot's tetralogy, septal defect, chromosomal abnormalities like Triploidy, Trisomy 18, Turner's syndrome, cystic Hygroma, Diaphragmatic Hernia (Table 37.2).

Exposure to **angiotensin converting enzyme inhibitors** has been associated with oligohydramnios. A **chronic leak** from a defect in the membrane may reduce the volume of fluid appreciably. Preterm premature rupture of membrane occurs in approximately 3-17% of all pregnancy.

Prognosis: Fetal outcome is poor with early onset oligohydramnios and only half survive. Following fetal complication can occur:
a. *Pulmonary hypoplasia:* Pulmonary hypoplasia is associated with early onset oligohydramnios and occurs in ~ 15% of fetus with oligohydramnios in first-two trimesters.
b. *Fetal deformities:* It is associated with adhesion between amnion and fetal parts and may cause serious deformities including amputation and club foot.

Oligohydramnios in Late Pregnancy

An amniotic fluid index of less than 5 cm after 34 weeks is associated with an increased risk of adverse perinatal outcome. There is increased risk for variable heart rate deceleration, cesarean delivery for fetal distress and 5 minutes Apgar score of less than 7.

Management of Oligohydramnios

Management depends on the associated pregnancy complications and on the gestational age. The exclusion of congenital anomalies in combination with aneuploidy or isolated is mandatory. Clinical examination of mother may reveal the presence of chronic hypertension or preeclampsia.

Table 37.1: Conditions associated with oligohydramnios			
Fetal	Placental	Maternal	Drugs
• Chromosomal abnormalities • Congenital anomalies • Growth restriction • Fetal demise • Post-term pregnancy • Ruptured membrane	• Abruptio • Twin to twin transfer	• Uteroplacental insufficiency • Hypertension • Preeclampsia • Diabetes	• Prostaglandin • Synthetase inhibitor • Angiotensin converting enzymes • Idiopathic

Table 37.2: Congenital anomalies associated with oligohydramnios
Amniotic band syndrome
Cardiac: Fallot tetralogy, septal defects
Central nervous system: Holoprosencephaly, meningocele, encephalocele, microcephaly
Chromosomal abnormalities: Triploidy, Trisomy 18, Turner's syndrome
Cloacal dysgenesis
Cystic hygroma
Diaphragmatic hernia
Genitourinary: Renal agenesis, renal dysplasia, urethral obstruction, bladder exstrophy, Meckel-Gruber syndrome, ureteropelvic junction obstruction, prune-belly syndrome
Hypothyroidism
Skeletal: Sirenomelia, sacral agenesis, absent radius, facial clefting
TRAP (twin reverse arterial perfusion) sequence
Twin-twin transfusion
Vacterl (vertebral, anal, cardiac, tracheoesophageal, renal, limb) association
Adapted from McCurdy and Seeds (1993) and Peipert and Donnenfeld (1991)

Serial USG examinations are required to assess growth pattern of fetus to exclude congenital anomalies. When remote from term, the management is to prolong pregnancy with close fetal monitoring. Near term pregnancy termination is planned if fetus is at risk of adverse perinatal outcome shown by abnormal Doppler studies, or IUGR.

Maternal hydration has been found to increase amniotic fluid volume in some studies.

Aminoinfusion: In this technique normal saline is instilled into the amniotic cavity by the transabdominal route in antepartum period and transcervically in intrapartum period. It has been found to reduce the complication like risk of pulmonary hypoplasia, meconium aspiration syndrome and abnormal fetal heart rate pattern. However, AICOG (2006) concludes that routine prophylactic amnioinfusion for labor complicated by meconium stained amniotic fluid is not warranted. Amnioinfusion can be considered with oligohydramnios regardless of amniotic fluid meconium status.

MULTIPLY CHOICE QUESTIONS

1. Amniotic fluid is mainly produced by:
    a. Placenta
    b. Fetus
    c. Chorion
    d. Amnion
    Ans. b
2. The pH of amniotic fluid is:
    a. 6.8-6.9
    b. 7.1-7.3
    c. 7.4-7.6
    d. 6.7-6.8
    Ans. b
3. A case of 35 weeks pregnancy with polyhydramnios and marked respiratory distress is managed by:
    a. IV Furosemide
    b. Saline infusion
    c. Amniocentesis
    d. ARM
    Ans. c
4. Cause of polyhydramnios are:
    a. Anencephaly
    b. Esophageal atresia
    c. Renal agenesis
    d. Twins
    Ans. a, b, d
5. Oligohydramnios is associated with:
    a. Anencephaly
    b. Esophageal atresia
    c. Renal agenesis
    d. All
    Ans. c
6. Amniotic fluid is in balance by:
    a. Excretion by fetal kidneys
    b. Maternal hemostasis
    c. Fetal intestinal absorption
    d. Fetal sweating
    Ans. a, b, c, d
7. Indication of aminoinfusion is:
    a. Oligohydramnios
    b. Suspected renal anomalies
    c. To facilitate labor
    d. In case of fetal distress
    Ans. a, b, d
8. Bleeding of fetal origin in:
    a. Placenta previa
    b. Vasa previa
    c. Placenta accreta
    d. Abruption placenta
    Ans. b
9. Clinical signs of hydramnios can be demonstrated when fluid collection is more than:
    a. 1 liter
    b. 2 liter
    c. 3 liter
    d. 4 liter
    Ans. b
10. Placenta with umbilical cord attached to its margin is called:
    a. Battledore placenta
    b. Circumvallate placenta
    c. Succenturiate placenta
    d. Velamentous insertion
    Ans. a

38. Special Cases in Obstetrics

Prayers should be our key to the day, lock to the night.

ELDERLY PRIMIGRAVIDA

FIGO recommends that all women going through their first pregnancy over the age of 35 years should be considered high risk for pregnancy and defined as elderly primigravida. Incidence of elderly primigravida is rising due to changing socioeconomic scenario.

Complications of Pregnancy in Elderly Primigravida

a. Chances of spontaneous conception are reduced.
b. Incidence of abortion is higher because of cause of infertility like polycystic ovary syndrome, chromosomal abnormalities. The likelihood of Down syndrome is 1 in 400 at age of 35 years and 1 in 60 at age of 42 as compared to incidence less than 1 in 1000 in general population. So, prenatal diagnosis should be offered to these patients.
c. Hyperemesis is more common.
d. Increased incidence of preeclampsia and essential hypertension.
e. Incidence of gestational diabetes and type 2 diabetes mellitus is higher.
f. Placenta previa and placental abruptio are more common.
g. More chance of gynecological problem like presence of uterine fibroid.

Complications in Labor

a. More chance of preterm labor.
b. Prolonged labor and occiput posterior position are more common.
c. Maternal distress appears more readily in elder women.
d. More chances of operative delivery due to uterine inertia, less resilient maternal soft tissue. Incidence of cesarean section is increased 4 fold.

Management

a. Preconceptional counseling is desirable. Prenatal screen test, combined test should be offered at 16 weeks of gestation for chromosomal abnormality. Target ultrasound scan should be done in the late first trimester (11 to 12 weeks) and at about 18 weeks gestation to look for congenital malformation in the fetus. In high risk cases, chorionic villous sampling or amniocentesis should be offered.
b. Regular monitoring for blood pressure and blood sugar should be done.
c. Pelvis should be assessed at term and if not adequate cesarean section should be offered. The relative indications for cesarean section have to be extended. The elderly primigravida should not be allowed to go postdate. Induction if tried should be followed by cesarean section within 24 hours if it fails.
d. Psychological stress to be looked after in elderly primigravida by sympathetic but firm and confident handling.

GRAND MULTIPARA

Grand multipara includes those women who had 4 or more previous viable babies.

Complications of Pregnancy

The incidence of pregnancy complication is increased in women belonging to low socioeconomic status and delivery in low resource setting.

a. Abortion rate is increased.
b. Anemia is quite common.
c. Hiatus hernia is common. Hyperemesis is relatively uncommon in multipara, but if present should be taken seriously. Liver and thyroid function should be checked.
d. Hypertensive vascular disease is more due to patient's higher age group, but preeclampsia and eclampsia are

no more common in grand multipara. However, if eclampsia occurs, the mortality is 1.4 times higher than primigravida.
e. Incidence of twin pregnancy is 3 times more common in grand multiparity.
f. Placenta previa and abruptio placenta both are more common in grand multipara and effect of antepartum hemorrhage is more profound due to usual presence of iron deficient anemia.
g. Malpresentations are more common caused by pendulous abdomen and lordosis of lumbar spine.
h. Chromosomal abnormalities in fetus are more common due to age factor.
i. If Rh negative there are more chances to develop erythroblastosis fetalis.

Complications in Labor

a. Malpresentation are more common.
b. There can be cephalopelvic disproportion in grand multipara because of gradually increasing size of babies, increased inclination of the pelvic brim, subluxation forwards of the sacrum upon the sacroiliac joints and occasionally due to osteomalacia.
c. Uterus rupture is one of the gravest danger of high multiparity. Causes are increased strength of uterine contraction, reduced strength of myometrium to resist rupture and large size of baby. So, oxytocin should be administered very judiciously in these cases.
d. Postpartum hemorrhage is real risk because of rapid labor, hampering of full retraction of uterine muscles, by increased quantities of elastic tissue in uterine myometrium and more chances of abruptio placenta and adherent placenta.
e. More incidences of instrumental delivery and cesarean section due to higher incidence of fetal macrosomia and alteration in pelvic shape.

Management

a. In antenatal care good nutrition, prophylactic and therapeutic iron and folic acid therapy to prevent and treat iron and folic acid deficiency anemia is must.
b. Regular monitoring of blood pressure and blood sugar level is done.
c. Antenatal ultrasound scan should be offered to detect any abnormalities and asses fetal weight.
d. The grand multipara should be advised to deliver in hospital. Good evaluation of pelvis and fetal position should be done at onset of labor.
e. Oxytocin should either be not administered or in very low dosage as risk of uterus rupture is very high.
f. In complicated labor, early onset to cesarean section should be considered.
g. Active management of 3rd stage of labor is must.
h. After delivery the patient should be encouraged to adopt permanent method of sterilization or suitable contraception methods.

OBESITY

Obesity is defined as 20% increase in body weight. The body mass index (BMI) or Quetlet's index is calculated as weight in kg divided by height in meters in square. Women with BMI over 27 Kg/m^2 are overweight, whereas those with a BMI greater than 29 Kg/m^2 corresponding to 120% of ideal body weight is considered obese. Morbid obesity has been defined as 150% of ideal weight.

Complications in Pregnancy

a. There is strong association of obesity with hypertension and diabetes with its associated fetal and maternal complication. The incidence of hypertension is 2.2 to 21.4 times greater and preeclampsia 1.22 to 9.7 times more than normal weight women.
b. There is increased risk of venous thromboembolic disease, urinary tract infection and respiratory complication.
c. Obesity is an independent risk factor for neural tube defects, fetal mortality and preterm delivery.
d. Skin disorders, edema of lower extremity, dyspnea on exertion or secondary to bronchitis are more troublesome in obese pregnant women.
e. More chances of fetal macrosomia and postdatism with increased risk of operative intervention and long-term risk of childhood obesity and associated morbidity.
f. Malpresentation are more common, harder to diagnose and are corrected by external cephalic version.

Complications in Labor

a. Need for induction is more common due to hypertension, preeclampsia, diabetes and postmaturity.
b. Incoordinate uterine action and uterine inertia are more common.
c. Higher incidence of fetal macrosomia, so shoulder dystocia and birth asphyxia is higher.
d. Incidence of operative intervention, primary cesarean section is doubled in case of obesity.
e. Postoperative complications are more common like wound infection, chest complication, venous stasis and embolism.
f. Postpartum hemorrhage is also more common and veins are less accessible for transfusion.
g. There are more chances of inappropriate lactation.
h. The babies have higher perinatal mortality because of maternal hypertension, diabetes and difficult delivery.

Management

a. **Diet:** Obese women should receive a properly supervised diet of 20 to 25 Kcal/kg body weight. More than a modest reduction in calories is not recommended as this may lead to IUGR. Appropriate exercise required for increasing energy consumption is important with a balanced high protein, low fat and carbohydrate diet. Appetite reducing drugs and tranquilizers are not recommended.

b. The mother should be carefully monitored for development of high blood pressure and preeclampsia. Blood pressure should be measured with an appropriate size of cuff. If the standard cuff is used to measure blood pressure, it can give artificially high reading.
c. Obesity is a risk factor for carbohydrate intolerance so screening for gestational diabetes needs to be performed at 24 weeks and again at 32 to 34 weeks if earlier screening tests are negative. Association of obesity, hypertension and diabetes may be manifestation of X syndrome.
d. Repeated ultrasound monitoring of fetal well-being and growth is essential to detect fetal macrosomia, IUGR, malpresentation and condition of liquor.
e. For fetal macrosomia, PIH, diabetes or postdatism induction of labor is needed more frequently. Cephalopelvic disproportion should be ruled out before induction.
f. In labor, close fetal and maternal surveillance is needed. Need of forceps delivery and cesarean section is almost doubled.
g. In cesarean section, regional anesthesia is preferred to general anesthetic. It is better to leave a subcutaneous drain for first 2 days to facilitate drainage of any collected fluid. It promotes wound healing. Prophylactic antibiotics are recommended as thickness of abdominal wall hinders wound healing and liable to get infected. Postoperative chest complication should be treated appropriately. In selected cases, prophylactic administration of low molecular weight heparin is considered after delivery until the patient is fully ambulatory.
h. Active management of 3rd stage of labor is recommended.
i. Neonate should be carefully observed for any complication.
j. To treat morbid obesity certain surgical procedure like gastroplasty and adjustable gastric banding before pregnancy has been tried with reported lesser complications in subsequent pregnancies.

An obese pregnant woman need especial sympathy and helps not only to detect and treat complication but also to rehabilitate self-respect and moral confidence.

39 Diabetes Mellitus and Pregnancy

One's first step to wisdom is to question everything, and one's last is to come to term with everything.

GENERAL CONSIDERATIONS

Diabetes mellitus is a chronic metabolic disorder due to either insulin deficiency which may be relative or absolute or due to peripheral tissue resistance to the action of insulin, which results in hyperglycemia. Two types of diabetes is recognized.

Type I Insulin Dependent Diabetes Mellitus

It is characterized by young age (Juvenile) and absolute insulinopenia. There is genetic predisposition and auto-antibodies are present against insulin producing cells.

Type II Noninsulin Dependent Diabetes Mellitus

It is characterized by late age onset, overweight women and peripheral tissue insulin resistance, i.e. hyperinsulinemia. There is also genetic predisposition in this type.

Incidence

Incidence of diabetes mellitus varies from 1-14%, depending on ethnicity, selection criteria and diagnostic test. Asian population has incidence of around 5-8%. Before invention of insulin and in cases of uncontrolled diabetes, infertility was rule and if patient conceived, there was very high maternal morbidity and mortality rate. Perinatal mortality was as high as 60%. With introduction of insulin and better understanding of the pathophysiology of the disease and advanced maternal and fetal monitoring, the maternal and perinatal complications have been markedly reduced, even though the fetus and neonate are still at high risk than the general population. So management of diabetes mellitus in pregnancy requires a team approach including the obstetrician, diabetologist, the dietist, and neonatologist.

PATHOPHYSIOLOGY: GLUCOSE METABOLISM IN NORMAL AND DIABETIC PREGNANCY

Insulin is an anabolic hormone with essential roles in carbohydrate, fat and protein metabolism. It promotes the uptake of glucose, storage of glucose as glycogen, lipogenesis and uptake and utilization of amino acids. Where there is lack of insulin, it results in hyperglycemia and lipolysis. Elevation of free fatty acids leads to an increase in formation of ketone bodies, acetoacetate and α hydroxybutyrate. When blood glucose level exceeds the renal threshold for absorption of filtered glucose, glycosuria occurs and causes osmotic diuresis with dehydration and electrolyte losses.

Maternal Glucose Homeostasis in Normal Pregnancy

Many metabolic changes occur in carbohydrate, protein and lipid metabolism in the normal pregnant individual, which helps in increasing nutrient supply to the fetus and also increase maternal body stores to meet demands of pregnancy and lactation. In the first trimester increasing maternal estrogen and progesterone level are associated with decrease in fasting glucose levels which reach a nadir (lowest value) by the 12th week. The decrease is average 15 mg/dl, so the fasting value of 70-80 mg/dl is common by 10th week of pregnancy. In advancing gestation, the basal as well postprandial insulin level increases progressively, this reaches almost twice the level of non pregnant level by the third trimester. There is also parallel insulin resistance, which is at its peak around 34-36 weeks. Insulin resistance is caused by high level of maternal and placental hormones particularly human chorionic Somatomammotropin, estrogen, progesterone, prolactin and cortisol. The net effect of all changes is lowering of maternal fasting blood glucose level, but a sustained and significant increase in postprandial glucose levels which is preferentially diverted to the fetus. The hepatic glucose production is increased by 15-30%, which maintains the fetal nutrition in fasting stage.

During pregnancy, there is an increase in glomerular filtration rate as results of increased renal blood flow. This increase result in increase in the amount of glucose delivered to the kidneys. Associated with this is a reduction in the renal threshold for glucose. In the nonpregnant woman, the total urine glucose excretion rarely exceeds 0.55 mmol/24 hours but during pregnancy about a third of women excrete more than 5.5 mmol/24 hours. Since most commonly available commercial glucose oxidase/peroxidase strips have a sensitivity of approximately 5.5 mmol/lit. So they will detect glycosuria in between 5-50% of the pregnant population. The routine use of urinalysis for monitoring of glycemic control during pregnancy is therefore unreliable.

Fetal Glucose Homeostasis in Normal Pregnancy

Glucose is crossed through the placenta by facilitated transport, so the fetal glucose level are about 10 mg/dl lower to maternal blood glucose level. Maternal insulin does not cross the placenta and the fetus produces its own insulin from the first trimester. But the fetal insulin response in normal pregnancy is sluggish and fetal insulin plays lesser role in glucose homeostasis and more perhaps in promoting growth.

Maternal and Fetal Glucose Homeostasis in Diabetic Mother

In women with gestational diabetes the insulin secretion and basal production of glucose is the same as in non diabetic women, but insulin is less effective in suppressing hepatic gluconeogenesis and there is a marked increase in the peripheral resistance to insulin. Both result in increased plasma level of glucose, which positively correlates with the fetal weight and other fetal and neonatal complications.

In diabetic mother, the fetal blood glucose does not increase to the same extent as the mother because the system of facilitated diffusion is cut off at maternal plasma glucose level above 200 mg/dl. But the fetal insulin response becomes sharper in response to glucose and amino acid. Paderson has proposed the theory of '*Hyperglycemic hyperinsulinism*'. According to this maternal hyperglycemia leads to fetal hyperglycemia which in term stimulates fetal pancreatic β cells to hypertrophy resulting in fetal hyperinsulinemia.

Elevated blood glucose level are toxic to developing fetus in first trimester causing increase in rate of miscarriage and major congenital malformation. They are preventable by preconceptional glucose control. *The fetal hyperinsulinemia causes increased fat deposition and macrosomia, organomegaly especially of liver and heart, increased erythropoietin production and decreased surfactant production.*

The fetal macrosomia causes an increased risk of birth trauma and intrapartum asphyxia, respiratory distress syndrome and polycythemia in newborn. Neonatal hypoglycemia results from the direct effect of high insulin level in the fetus. In gestational diabetes if maternal glucose level can be maintained in a normoglycemic state, the adverse effect of fetal hyperinsulinemia can be reduced and fetal and neonatal outcome is improved.

Diagnostic Criteria for Diabetes Mellitus Prior to Pregnancy

There are three ways of diagnosing pre-existing diabetes mellitus:
a. Classic symptom of diabetes which are polyuria, polydipsia and unexplained weight loss, with random plasma glucose concentration equal to or greater than 200 mg/dl.
b. Fasting plasma glucose level equal to or greater than 126 mg/dl. Fasting is defined as no caloric intake for at least 8 hours.
c. Two hours post load glucose level equal to or greater than 200 mg/dl during an oral glucose tolerance test (OGTT) using >50 gm anhydrous glucose dissolved in water.

In the absence of unequivocal hyperglycemia, these criteria should be confirmed by repeat testing on different day.

Gestational Diabetes Mellitus

Gestational diabetes is defined as carbohydrate intolerance of variable severity with onset or first recognition during pregnancy. This definition applies irrespective of whether or not insulin is used for treatment or the condition persists after pregnancy. It also does not exclude the possibility that unrecognized glucose intolerance may have predated the pregnancy. There can be following type of gestational diabetes:
a. **Class A1:** Diet controlled fasting glucose level less than 95 mg/dl, 2 hours postprandial glucose less than 120 mg/dl.
b. **Class A2:** Diet and insulin or Glyburide- elevated fasting and or postprandial glucose level.

Screening and Diagnosis for Gestational Diabetes

a. *Risk assessment:* Risk assessment for gestational diabetes mellitus is performed at the first prenatal visit in all women who do not already have diagnosed diabetes. The risk factors are as follows:
   a. Obesity (nonpregnant body mass index ≥ 30)
   b. Prior history of GDM
   c. Heavy glycosuria (>2++)
   d. Unexplained stillbirth, prior infant with congenital malformation

e. Family history of diabetes in first degree relation
   f. Previous macrosomic infant (>4000 gm)
   g. History of recurrent pre-eclampsia
   h. History of recurrent moniliasis
   i. Maternal age over 30

Low risk women are:
   i. Maternal age less than 25 years
   ii. Normal body weight
   iii. No family history of diabetes in first degree relation
   iv. No history of abnormal glucose metabolism
   v. No history of poor obstetric outcome
   vi. Not a member of an ethnic/racial group with high prevalence of diabetes

b. *Screening methods and guidelines:*
   a. Women with risk factors should be screened for diabetes mellitus as early as possible. However, all women of ordinary or high risk should be screened for glucose intolerance in between 24-28 weeks.
   b. *50 gm glucose load with plasma glucose estimation is done after 1 hour, between 24-28 weeks, irrespective of the day or time of last meal. This should be done in all pregnant women, who have not been tested before.* Value ≥ 140 mg/dl indicates the need for a full diagnostic glucose tolerance test (GTT). This has a sensitivity of 90% with a cut off of 130 mg/dl, sensitivity is nearly 100% but 25% of patient require a GTT.
   c. A plasma glucose measurement ≥ 200 mg/dl outside the context of formal glucose challenge test or a truly fasting plasma glucose ≥ 126 mg/dl suggest the diabetic state and warrants further investigation.

Diagnostic Criteria

1. 100 gm oral glucose load is administered in the morning after overnight fast for at least 8 hours but not more than 14 hours and following at least 3 days of unrestricted diet and usual physical activity. Venus plasma glucose level is measured – fasting 1, 2 and 3 hours. *Value of fasting 105 mg/dl at 1 hr, 190 mg/dl at 2 hr, 165 mg/dl at 3 hr and 145 mg/dl or more must be met for a positive diagnosis.*
2. GTT is repeated at 32–34 weeks in patients with the abnormal value.

Management

Prepregnancy Counseling

Prevention of hyperglycemia through rigorous control of blood glucose level is the mainstay of treatment in the pregnant women with pregestational diabetes. **In these patients, careful preconceptional glycemic control and achievement of normal glycilated hemoglobin A1c level, diet and regular exercise reduces the risk of congenital anomalies and other complications during pregnancy.** Till now the recommendation is that Type II diabetes on oral hypoglycemic agent should be changed to insulin prior to pregnancy. Folic acid supplementation should be advised in the dosage recommended for high risk women in dose of 4 mg/day.

Diabetic retinopathy and nephropathy can deteriorate during pregnancy. So a base line fundus examination should be done prior to pregnancy and thereafter in each trimester. Proliferative retinopathy should be treated prior to pregnancy by laser photocoagulation. A base line kidney function test must be done in all pregestational diabetes, including 24 hours urine for albumin. In prepregnancy state, any infection like urinary tract infection and dental caries should be screened and treated. But antihypertensive medication if are being taken should be reviewed and ACE inhibitor should be replaced by safer drugs like methyldopa, lobetal or nifedipine. Lipid lowering drugs like satin are contraindicated in first trimester. In patients with Type I diabetes mellitus thyroid function should be evaluated because of increased risk of thyroid disease.

Antepartum Management

Option for Termination of Pregnancy

Diabetes mellitus per se is not an indication for therapeutic abortion except in following situations:
i. Severe diabetic nephropathy which causes a high perinatal mortality.
ii. Women with high risk of congenital malformation with elevated HbA1c level may opt for termination of pregnancy.

Program of Care

Antenatal visit should be at every two weeks until 36 weeks gestation, than weekly.

Dietary Recommendation

Plan should be 3 meals with bed time snack. Diet—2000 – 2200 Kcal/day, Normal weight—30 Kcal/kg ideal pregnancy body weight, Lean —35 Kcal/kg ideal pregnancy body weight, Obese—25 Kcal/kg ideal pregnancy body weight.

Composition of diet: *It should have high fiber carbohydrate diet 40-50%, protein 20% and fat 30-40% (10% saturated).*

Weight gain should be 9 kg in average size women and 7.25 kg for obese women.

Regular Exercise

Regular exercise should be encouraged. 20-30 minutes brisk walking, 3-4 times/week.

Surveillance of Maternal Diabetes

i. Self monitoring of capillary blood glucose to check fasting and 1 hour or 2 hours postprandial glucose level, to assess efficacy of diet and exercise control.

ii. If fasting plasma glucose value is > 95 mg/dl and 1 hour value is >140 mg/dl, and or 2 hours value is > 120 mg/dl, insulin therapy is required.

Insulin Therapy

It can be tailored in two ways:
1. ***Multiple injection (usually 3) of regular short acting insulin before the three major meals and bed time injection of intermediate acting insulin (NPH).*** This regimen is easier to manipulate and give more consistent mean blood sugar level. The pre meal insulin dose can be increased usually 2 units at a time, depending on the corresponding post meal value of blood sugar and NPH insulin is increased if fasting glucose is high.
2. ***Combination of regular and NPH insulin*** Two-third of total insulin dose given in the morning before breakfast and one-third in the evening before dinner. The morning dose is constituted by two-third NPH and one-third regular insulin and in evening dose one half NPH and one half regular insulin is combined.
3. ***Subcutaneous insulin infusion or insulin pump therapy*** can be used as an alternative in women who are not well controlled on alone regimen.

Regular insulin should be administered about 30 minutes before meal. Regular insulin has a peak effect at 2-3 hours and duration of action is 8-10 hours. Intermediate acting insulin (NPH) has its peak effect in 4-10 hours and its effective duration is 12-18 hours. Recombinant human insulin is preferred in pregnancy.

Cautions in Insulin Therapy

a. There can be fasting hypoglycemia, if there is inadequate insulin dose at bed time. So insulin dose to be increased in such situation.
b. ***Somogyi effect:*** When there is hypoglycemia at night it may stimulate endogenous glucose release which causes a rebound hyperglycemia in the morning, which is called Somogyi effect. It is seen more with use of regular insulin. To confirm the Somogyi effect, a night blood glucose level around 3 AM should be taken. If it is confirmed the night dose of insulin may be reduced a little or the bed time NPH may be given little later to postpone the peak.
c. ***Education of patient:*** Patient is to be educated in technique of taking insulin injection properly. They should also be made aware of the symptoms of hypoglycemia and advised to carry some glucose biscuits in the morning.
d. ***Oral hypoglycemic agent:*** Older oral hypoglycemic agent **Sulphonylurea** cross the placenta and can be potentially teratogenic. Newer agent like **Glyburide** do not cross placenta. Though not routinely recommended, limited trial has found Glyburide effective and safe in pregnancy. Glyburide is given in starting dose of 2.5 mg orally with morning meal. Dose can be increased if necessary by 2.5 mg per week increment until 10 mg per day, then switched to twice daily dose until maximum of 20 mg per day is reached. If 20 mg per day does not achieve glucose control patient should be switched to insulin.

Metformin has been used as a treatment of polycystic ovarian disease and has been reported to reduce the incidence of gestational diabetes in women who used the drug throughout the pregnancy. Still it is usually recommended that Metformin should be discontinued once the pregnancy is diagnosed. Yet the recent studies shows that Metformin use is not associated with increased perinatal complication.

Obstetric Management

The patient with pre-existing diabetes should have antenatal visit at 15 days interval throughout pregnancy and weekly in the third trimester. At first visit beside routine investigation, baseline kidney function, urine culture, Glycosylated hemoglobin and fundus examination should be done. *A first trimester ultrasound should be offered around 12 weeks for nuchal translucency and for accurate dating.* Early USG dating is important because most diabetic patient require induction of labor. *Ultrasound scan for fetal anomalies and morphology should be performed at 18-20 weeks.* Fetal echocardiography can be referred if there is doubt on four chamber view of the heart. A triple screen test at 16-18 weeks is usually offered to all as a screening test for Down syndrome and neural tube defect. *Ultrasound are done at 28-30 weeks and repeated at 34-36 weeks. If there is fetal macrosomia or polyhydramnios, insulin therapy dose should be readjusted.*

Fetal Surveillance

Close surveillance for fetal well-being is started at 32 weeks gestation using twice weekly non stress test or modified fetal biophysical profile (BPP) measuring the fetal heart rate and amniotic fluid volume. Women with diet controlled gestational diabetes usually begin testing at 36-40 weeks until delivered. Maternal fetal movement counting using a count to 10 is recommended for all pregnant women, including those with diabetes to reduce the still birth rate. Doppler velocimetry of the umbilical artery is useful in monitoring pregnancies in women with vasculopathy or if there is intrauterine growth retardation. In diabetes, entire clinical picture and result of serial fetal surveillance should be taken into consideration, while making an assessment of fetal well-being.

Time and Mode of Delivery

Patient with gestational diabetes controlled on diet can be followed till term, at which time induction is done if patient is not already in labor. Patients of gestational diabetes mellitus on insulin pregnancy are preferably terminated at

38-39 weeks because of higher risk of perinatal morbidity and mortality. If there is associated hypertension or compromised fetal testing, pregnancy may need to be terminated earlier. In such situations, antenatal corticosteroids should be administered. Though it can affect glycemic control adversely. So strict monitoring of blood sugar level is recommended. If there is fetal macrosomia detected by clinical estimation and ultrasound index, cesarean section should be considered to avoid risk of shoulder dystocia.

Intrapartum Management

a. Indications of cesarean section in diabetic pregnancy are fetal macrosomia, obstetric indications and advanced diabetes. Elective cesarean is best planned as first case in the morning. The night dose of regular and NPH insulin are given, omitting the morning dose. Trial of labor has no place in diabetic patients.
b. Monitoring of labor:
   i. Good analgesia should be ensured as pain stimulates adrenergic pathways and disturbs blood sugar control.
   ii. If induction of labor is decided, the method used depends on favorability of cervix. If Bishop Score is poor, local prostaglandin are administered and the patient is allowed to take her regular meals and insulin till patient goes into labor. If cervix is favorable, oxytocin induction should be started in the morning, omitting the morning insulin and meal and I/V infusion is started.
   iii. Once labor is started, mean blood glucose level should be maintained around 80-100 mg/dl. Constant insulin infusion by calibrated pump is best. I/V infusion with 5% dextrose is given at rate of 100-125 ml fluid per hour. An insulin infusion with 50 units of insulin added to 50 ml of normal saline (1 unit/ml) is started with another I/V line. With this concentration one unit of insulin/ hour is equal to infusion rate of 1 ml/hour. Blood glucose level is checked in every 1-2 hours by glucometer and insulin infusion is regulated according to it. If blood glucose level is > 250 mg/dl the 5% dextrose solution is changed to normal saline.
   iv. Fetal heart rate is closely monitored, preferably with electronic fetal monitoring.
   v. Expert obstetrician should be at hand at time of delivery to manage any complications, particularly shoulder dystocia. There is higher risk of instrumental delivery and emergency cesarean section.

Postpartum Care

In postpartum period there is a sharp fall in the patient's insulin requirement. So insulin dose is readjusted based on self monitoring of blood glucose level. The general rule is to give two-third of the pre pregnancy dose or one half of the present dose. If patient had cesarean section, sliding scale may be implemented until oral intake can be established. Infection must be promptly detected and treated. **All gestational diabetic should be advised to undergo glucose tolerance test at 6 weeks.** They should be counseled regarding diet, exercise and weight reduction, which can reduce their chance of developing type two diabetes, which is 50-60% within 10-15 years. Breastfeeding should be encouraged in all diabetic women as it improves glycemic control and insulin is continued for these women. Oral hypoglycemic agent can be used in non breastfeeding women.

Contraception

Diabetic women without vascular complication can use all contraception as nondiabetics. In women with an increased risk for embolism, hormonal contraception containing estrogen is not recommended, but progesterone only method including levonorgesterol intrauterine system can be used. Permanent sterilization should be offered with diabetics who have completed childbearing.

Complications of Diabetes in Pregnancy

Maternal and fetal complications of diabetes in pregnancy are summarized in Table 39.1.
Congenital anomalies in infant of women with diabetes are summarized in Box 39.1.

Box 39.1: Congenital malformation in infant of women with overt diabetes

i.	Caudal regression
ii.	Situs inversus
iii.	Spina bifida, hydrocephalic or other CNS defects
iv.	Anencephaly
v.	Cardiac anomalies
vi.	Anal/rectal atresia
vii.	Renal anomalies—Renal agenesis, Cystic kidney, Duplex ureter

Chapter -39 ♦ Diabetes Mellitus and Pregnancy

Table 39.1: Maternal and fetal complications of diabetes mellitus

Maternal	Fetal
• Retinopathy (Progressive) • Neuropathy (Temporarily worsening) • Coronary artery disease • Hyperglycemia, hypoglycemia, kotoacidosis • Preeclampsia • Infection • Thromboembolic disease • Recurrent vulvo vaginal infection • Increased incidence of operative delivery • Obstructed labor	• Congenital abnormalities—Cardiac and neural tube defect • Macrosomia leading to birth asphyxia, and traumatic birth injury like brachial plexus • Respiratory distress syndrome • Hypoglycemia • Hypomagnesemia • Polycythemia • Hyperbilirubinemia

MULTIPLE CHOICE QUESTIONS

1. Pregnant diabetic female on oral hypoglycemic is shifted to insulin. All of the following are true *except*:
   a. Insulin does not cross placenta
   b. During pregnancy insulin requirement increases and can not be provided with sulfonylurea
   c. Tolbutamide crossed placenta
   d. Tolbutamide causes PIH
   Ans. d

2. Late hyperglycemia in pregnancy is associated with:
   a. Macrosomia
   b. IUGR
   c. Postmaturity
   d. Congenital malformation
   Ans. a

3. AG2P1+0 diabetic mother presents at 32 weeks of pregnancy. There is history of full term fetal demise in last pregnancy. Her vitals are stable, sugar is controlled and fetus is stable. Which among the following will be most appropriate management:
   a. To induce at 38 weeks
   b. To induce at 40 weeks
   c. Cesarean section at 38 weeks
   d. To wait for spontaneous delivery
   Ans. a

4. A lady with 8 weeks pregnancy is presented with random blood sugar level of 177 mg/dl. The treatment is:
   a. Phenformin
   b. Sulfonylurea
   c. Insulin
   d. Glipizide
   Ans. c

5. Infants of diabetic mother are likely to have the following cardiac anomaly:
   a. Coarctation of aorta
   b. Fallot's tetralogy
   c. Ventricular septal defect
   d. Transposition of great arteries
   Ans. c, d

6. Which is the best method to access fetal damage in a diabetic mother in 1st trimester is:
   a. Blood sugar estimation
   b. Urine ketone assay
   c. Amniocentesis for sugar level
   d. Glycosylated Hb
   Ans. d

7. The complication seen in fetus of a diabetic mother:
   a. β cell hyperplasia
   b. Hyperglycemia
   c. Small fetus
   d. β cell hyperplasia
   Ans. a

8. All are features of infant born to diabetic mother *except*:
   a. Obesity
   b. Hearing disability
   c. Ketotic hypoglycemia
   d. Future diabetes mellitus
   Ans. b

9. Fetal abnormality in pregnancy with diabetes is:
   a. Sacral agenesis
   b. Hydrocephalus
   c. RDS
   d. Phocomelia
   Ans. a

10. Which is the most common complication during vaginal delivery is a diabetic women:
    a. Uterine inertia
    b. Shoulder dystocia
    c. PPH
    d. Excessive moulding of head
    Ans. b

40 Hematological Disorders in Pregnancy

It is easier to find persons who will volunteer to die than to find who are willing to endure pain with patience.

ANEMIA

Anemia is one of the major public health problems in the developing world. In South East Asia, 40-90% of pregnant women are considered anemic. One of the primary aims of antenatal care is to prevent and treat anemia during pregnancy and lactation period.

Definition

Anemia is a pathological condition in which the oxygen carrying capacity of red blood cells is insufficient to meet the body's needs. *The center for disease control defines anemia as a hemoglobin concentration of less than 11 gm/dl (hematocrit < 33%) in the first or third trimester or a hemoglobin concentration of less than 10.5 gm/dl (hematocrit < 32%) in the second trimester.* The degree of anemia is graded according to the hemoglobin level (Hb) level as:

Moderate : 7.0–10.9 gm/dl
Severe : 4 - 6.9 gm/dl
Very severe : <4 gm/dl

Physiological Hemodynamic Changes in Pregnancy and Erythropoiesis

The normal physiological changes of pregnancy are:
a. Increased blood volume
b. Increased cardiac output
c. Increased heart rate
d. Decreased blood pressure

In general maternal blood volume increases up to 50% above nonpregnant levels. Blood volume begins to increase in the first trimester and continues until approximately 32 weeks of gestation. After that it remains constant until delivery. Maternal plasma volume increases by 50% while maternal red blood cell mass increases by 20%. This discrepancy causes dilutional or physiologic anemia of pregnancy. The hormonal mechanisms responsible for this increase are: Steroid hormones of pregnancy, increased plasma renin activity and hyperaldosteronism.

Cardiac Output

Cardiac output begins to increase in the first trimester and peaks at 30-50% above nonpregnant level by 20 weeks gestation. After that it remains constant until term. At 38 - 40 weeks gestation cardiac output decreases. Early in pregnancy an increased stroke volume is responsible for the changes in cardiac output, while in later period of gestation an increased heart rate is responsible.

Blood Pressure

In a normal pregnancy there is a slight decrease in systolic blood pressure and a moderate increase in diastolic pressure. The nadir occurs in mid trimester and then there can be a slow increase to the patient's nonpregnant blood pressure. Physiological changes in pregnancy are summarized in Table 40.1.

Erythropoiesis

In adult erythropoiesis is confined to bone marrow. Red blood cells are formed through stages of pronormoblast-normoblast-reticulocytes—to mature non-nucleated

Table 40.1: Physiological and hematological changes in pregnancy
a. Plasma volume increase by 50%.
b. Red cell mass increase by 25% causing hemodilution.
c. Mean cell volume increase secondary to erythropoiesis.
d. MCHC is stable.
e. Serum iron and ferritin concentration decrease secondary to increased utilization.
f. Total iron binding capacity increases.
g. Iron requirement increase from 2.5 mg/day in first trimester to 6.6 mg/day in the third trimester.
h. There is moderate increase in iron absorption.
i. Folate requirement increases in pregnancy.
j. There is no major effect on B_{12} stores, although levels decrease because of preferential active transport to the fetus.

erythrocytes. The average *lifespan* of red cells is about 120 days, after which RBC degenerates and hemoglobin is broken down into hemosiderin and bile pigments. For proper erythropoiesis following are needed:

a. **Minerals:** Iron is essential and main element in the synthesis of hemoglobin. Traces of copper and cobalt are also required.
b. **Vitamins:** Vitamin B_{12}, folic acid and vitamin C are needed for erythropoiesis. Folic acid and vitamin B_{12} are essential in the synthesis of nucleoproteins, particularly of erythropoietin cells. *Vitamin B_{12} acts at an early stage in the synthesis of RNA and folic acid acts at a later stage in the synthesis of DNA.* Thus deficiency of vitamin B_{12} results in defective synthesis of both RNA and DNA. While the deficiency of the folic acid results in defective synthesis of DNA only. Vitamin C is essential for conversion of folic acid to folinic acid.
c. **Protein:** The protein gives amino acids for the synthesis of globin molecule.
d. **Erythropoietin:** It is a glycoprotein with a molecular weight of 55,000 KD produced by kidney (90%) and liver (10%). It acts on the erythroblast to stimulate the marrow production and release of RBC.

Normal red cell survival is about 100-120 days in circulation, which causes the normal reticulocyte count of 1-1.5%. As RBC age, they develop a senescent antigen, which is recognized by the reticuloendothelial system in the spleen. The red cell disintegrates and hemoglobin is broken down into hemosiderin and bile pigments. The iron core re-enters the storage pool in the form of ferritin or hemosiderin, which is now again available for new hemoglobin synthesis. Daily RBC production requires about 30-35 mg of iron per day, most of which is derived from the recycling of storage pool iron. Only about 1 to 2 mg of daily loss of iron from the body requires replenishment.

ANEMIA IN PREGNANCY

The following types of anemia are associated with pregnancy:
a. Iron deficiency
b. Megaloblastic
c. Aplastic variety
d. Hemoglobinopathies
e. Hemolytic
f. Secondary to repeated bleeding, chronic infection, Hodgkin's disease.

Iron Deficiency Anemia

Iron deficiency anemia is the most common type. Depending upon the socioeconomic status it may be found in 50-90% of all pregnancies. Commonly iron deficiency and blood loss in pregnancy are closely related because blood loss causes concomitant loss of hemoglobin, iron and exhaustion of iron stores.

Physiology of Iron Metabolism in Pregnancy

The demand for iron in pregnancy is about 900 mg out of which about 500-600 mg goes to the uterus and its contents. About 150-200 mg is lost in the average blood loss at delivery and same amount is expanded in lactation. There is an increased maternal hemoglobin mass which consumes about 500 mg, but this iron is returned to the stores after delivery. On the other hand, there is an average gain of about 225 mg as a result of amenorrhea during pregnancy. *So in pregnancy there is a likely iron deficiency of about 600-700 mg.* Thus in pregnancy a women's iron requirement is approximately 4-6 mg/day in the 2nd trimester and 6-8 mg/day in the 3rd trimester. Out of which 1 mg/day of iron is available in normal diet and additional requirement should be met by supplementation of at least 40-60 mg/day of elemental iron (10% of which is absorbed).

Cause of Iron Deficiency Anemia

a. **Dietary deficiency:** Diet lacking in iron like green vegetables, fruits like apple, banana and cereals can cause iron deficiency. Beside this, diet rich in carbohydrates have high phosphate and phytic acid which results in insoluble iron phosphates and phytates in the gut, which reduce iron absorption.
b. **Deficient iron absorption:** Iron absorption is increased by the presence of hydrochloric acid in the stomach. On the contrary achlorhydria and copius intake of antacids reduce iron absorption. Intestinal disorders like chronic diarrhea interfere with iron absorption.
c. **Iron loss:** Worm infestation, menorrhagia, chronic malaria, repeated pregnancies at short duration can further aggravate severity of iron deficiency anemia.
d. **Chronic infection:** Chronic infection can cause iron deficiency anemia resistant to dietary and iron therapy. Urinary tract infection and latent pyelonephritis is particularly common.

Diagnosis of Iron Deficiency Anemia

The clinical feature depends on the degree of severity of anemia. The patients may be asymptomatic and detected during antenatal examination and investigation. There may be vague or nonspecific symptoms like pallor, easy fatiguability, headache, palpitation, breathlessness. There can be anorexia and indigestion. In advanced stage, there can be generalized edema. On examination there is pallor, edema. Hemic murmur or cardiomegaly can be present in advanced cases. Angular stomatitis, glossitis, koilonychias (spoon shaped nails) may be present in long standing severe anemia.

Laboratory Findings

Hematological examination: Denotes severity and type of anemia. The following examination can be done.

a. *Hemoglobin:* Anemia is classified according to level of hemoglobin in mild, moderate and severe category.
b. *RBC count:* It is considered normal when more than 3.2 million/cc. It may be decreased in iron deficiency anemia.
c. *Packed cell volume:* It is normal at 37-47%. It is considered low when falls below 32%.
d. *Mean corpuscular volume (MCV):* It is 78 to 92 cubic microns. In iron deficiency anemia the value is low while in megaloblastic anemia value is high.
e. *Mean corpuscular hemoglobin concentration (MCHC):* It is 26-30%. It is decreased in iron deficiency anemia. MCHC is one of the most sensitive index of iron deficiency anemia.
f. *Peripheral smear:* In well made peripheral blood smear stained with Leishman stain, the morphology of the red cells gives an idea about type of anemia. Microcytic hypochromic cells are found in iron deficiency anemia, while macrocytic cells are found in folate and vitamin B_{12} deficiency. Variation in size of RBC (Anisocytosis) and shape (Poikilocytosis) is found in iron deficiency and hemolytic anemia. In smears malaria parasite or Leishmania can be seen. Platelet count is also appreciated in smear.

Ferrokinetic Studies

Normal value of the ferrokinetic parameter are as follows:

Serum iron	: 60-120 µg/dl
Total iron binding capacity	: 325-400 µg/dl
Transfusion situation	: 20-50%
Serum ferritin level	: >15 µg/dl

In iron deficiency anemia the serum iron is usually below 30 µg/100 ml, total iron binding capacity above 400 µg/100 ml and serum ferritin level is below 15 µg/dl.

Investigations for Etiology of Anemia

a. Stool examination to detect worm infestation.
b. Urine is examined for protein, sugar and pus cells and mid stream specimen of urine for culture and sensitivity.
c. Chest X-ray in suspected case of tuberculosis.
d. Estimation of serum protein in hypoproteinemia
e. Osmotic fragility in hereditary spherocytosis or hemoglobinopathic disorders.
f. Bone marrow study is not done as a routine but indicated only:
    i. Cases not responding to therapy directed by hematological studies.
    ii. To diagnose hypoplastic anemia.
    iii. To diagnose kala-azar by detecting LD bodies

In iron deficiency anemia the bone marrow is normoblastic in character and there is absence of hemosiderin granules when stained with Prussion blue.

Differential Diagnosis

Anemia due to chronic disease or an inflammatory process (e.g. Rheumatoid arthritis) may be hypochromic microcytic. *Anemia due to thalassemia trait can be differentiated from iron deficiency anemia by normal serum iron levels and the presence of stainable iron in the marrow and elevated level of hemoglobin A2.* Other less common causes of microcytic hypochromic anemia are sideroblastic anemia and anemia due to lead poisoning.

Complications of Anemia

a. **Maternal:** Women with chronic mild anemia are well compensated and do not endanger pregnancy. Women with moderate to severe anemia are pone to following complications:
    i. Preterm labor
    ii. Pregnancy induced hypertension
    iii. Predisposition to infection
    iv. Obstetric shock and inability to withstand hemorrhage
    v. Abruptio placenta
    vi. In severe anemia there can be congestive cardiac failure
    vii. Puerperal sepsis and inappropriate lactation.
b. **Fetal effect:** The fetus is at increased risk of preterm birth, intrauterine growth restriction, stillbirth, neonatal anemia. If anemia is moderate to severe, there is three fold increase of perinatal mortality rate.

Prophylaxis

Indian diet usually contains only 1.5 gm iron per day of which only 10% is available for absorption, so there is definite role of prophylactic iron supplementation in pregnant women in developing countries. Women should be advised to consume diet rich in iron as peas, green leafy vegetable, sprouts, jaggery (gur), and certain diet fruits like apricots, eggs, fish and meat for nonvegetarian persons. Vitamin C helps in reducing ferric to ferrous iron, so fresh vegetables should be advised. The policy of routine iron prophylaxis in pregnancy varies in different countries. The National Nutritional Anemia Control Program of India recommends 100 mg of elemental iron and 500 µg of folic acid for prophylactic supplementation for 100 days starting in the second trimester to postpartum period. WHO recommendation is based on the prevalence of anemia, 60 mg elemental iron with 400 µg of folic acid per day is recommended for 6 months where prevalence of anemia is < 40% and this dose to be supplemented for another 3 months postpartum in area where prevalence is > 40%.

Treatment of Iron Deficiency Anemia

The objective of treatment is correction of the deficit in hemoglobin mass and eventually restitution of iron stores.

Oral iron therapy: Ferrous sulphate 300 mg (containing 60 mg of elemental iron of which 10% is absorbed) should be given 3 times a day. Therapy should be continued for approximately 3 months after hemoglobin values returns to normal in order to replenish iron stores. Hemoglobin level should increase by at least 0.3 gm/dl/week if the patient is responding to therapy. Iron is best absorbed in the ferrous form or reduced form in an empty stomach. Administering ascorbic acid at the time of iron supplementation creates a mildly acidic environment that aids the iron absorption. If ferrous sulfate is not tolerated, ferrous fumarate or gluconate should be prescribed. Recently carbonyl iron and iron III hydroxide carbohydrate complex containing ferric iron complex with polymaltose has been shown to be effective with lesser gastrointestinal side effects. But there is no additional hematologic benefit with these preparation compared to cheaper salts.

Parenteral Iron

Indication: Parenteral iron administration is indicated in women who do not tolerate oral iron, in case of inflammatory bowel disease or poor response to oral therapy or patient is not compliant. Parenteral iron should ideally be given after documenting iron deficiency. Aggressive iron therapy is positively contraindicated where there is iron overload like thalassemias.

Parenteral iron preperation: There are two commonly used compounds—**Iron dextran** which can be given both intramuscularly and intravenously and **iron sorbitol citric acid complex,** which is used only for intramuscular therapy. Iron dextran is available in 2 ml vial, providing 100 mg of elemental iron. After a 0.5 ml test dose iron dextran can be administered intramuscularly or intravenously at a rate not to exceed 100 mg/day of elemental iron. Intramuscular injection must always be given into the muscle mass of the upper outer quadrant of the buttock with a 2" 20 gauge needle using the Z technique (Pulling the skin and superficial musculature to one side before inserting the needle to prevent leakage of the solution and subsequent tattooing of the skin). There is only slightly faster hemoglobin rise due to slow and occasionally incomplete mobilization of iron from the muscle.

Risks of parenteral iron administration are anaphylactic reaction, muscle necrosis and phlebitis.

Iron sucrose is newer preparation for intravenous iron administration. A new preparation of iron sucrose (Ferose) is now licensed for total dose iron replacement in the second and third trimesters. It is given as a single infusion in normal saline and takes 4-6 hours to complete.

Erythropoietin

Recombinant human erythropoietin is mainly used for the anemia associated with erythropoietin deficiency in chronic renal failure but can also be used to increase auto logous production of blood in normal individuals. It has been used in cases of severe postpartum anemia with success and has been life-saving in cases when blood transfusion is declined. It has also been used during pregnancy in a small number of renal patients.

Severe Anemia in Late Pregnancy and Labor

In Indian subcontinent, 7% of women have severe anemia which is associated with 5 fold increase in maternal mortality. Severe anemia in late pregnancy and labor is dangerous one due to risk of congestive cardiac failure. Blood transfusion can be life-saving for severely anemic women presenting in last 4 weeks of pregnancy. But these patients have pronounced myocardial ischemia and cardiomegaly. To avoid any added strain on heart, packed cells should be slowly transfused with simultaneous diuretic administration. The patient is kept in propped up position and oxygen inhalation is given as per the requirement. If patient with severe anemia presents in labor, intravenous access is placed during labor and cross-matched blood should be in hand if there is any hemorrhage. Blood should be transfused after delivery. Active management of third stage, avoidance of unnecessary episiotomy, early repair of tears and cutting short the 2nd stage of labor by prophylactic forceps or Ventouse should be done to reduce maternal exhaustion and blood loss. Intravenous ergometrine should be avoided. Prophylactic antibiotic and thrombo-prophylaxis should be considered in appropriate cases.

Megaloblastic Anemia

In megaloblastic anemia there is derangement in red cell maturation with the production in the bone marrow of abnormal precursors known as megaloblast due to impaired DNA synthesis. Megaloblastic anemia is a deficiency disease caused by lack of either vitamin B_{12} or folate or both. Vitamin B_{12} requirement in nonpregnant condition is 2 µg and during pregnancy is 3 µg. Vitamin B_{12} deficiency is rare in pregnancy. So megaloblastic anemia is almost always due to folic acid deficiency. *Vitamin B_{12} deficient megaloblastic anemia is seen in women with gastrectomy or bowel resection or with previous anemia.*

Incidence

Incidence of megaloblastic anemia is 0.2 to 5%.

Etiopathogenesis

In nonpregnant women the minimum daily requirement of folate necessary for hematopoiesis and to maintain store is

50 mg. In pregnancy this requirement is increased. In order to meet pregnancy requirement and to decrease neural tube defect associated with folic acid deficiency, a dietary supplement of at least 400 µg per day of folic acid is recommended.

In situation when there is increased demand like multifetal gestation or hemolytic condition like sickle cell anemia, malaria, hereditary spherocytosis, require additional folate supplementation in order to meet the demands imposed by increased hematopoiesis. Impaired absorption or metabolism of folic acid can occur by use of oral contraceptive, phenytoin, barbiturates, or alcohol consumption. Jejunal bypass surgery or malabsorption syndrome also can impair folic acid absorption.

Diagnosis

a. ***Symptoms and signs:*** The symptoms are nonspecific, e.g. lassitude, anorexia, nausea and vomiting, diarrhea and depression. Pallor often is not marked. A sore mouth or tongue may be present. Sometimes purpura is a clinical manifestation. *Megaloblastic anemia should be suspected and diagnosed if iron deficiency anemia does not respond to iron therapy.* In severe case spleen and liver may be enlarged. Megaloblastic anemia of pregnancy may continue in postnatal period and may be diagnosed only in puerperium when it becomes evident after any hemorrhage or delivery.

b. ***Laboratory findings:***
   i. **Hematologic finding:** Folic acid deficiency result in a hematologic picture similar to that of true pernicious anemia (due to vitamin B_{12} deficiency) which is extremely rare in reproductive age group. In severe cases, hemoglobin level may be as low as 4-6 mg/dl and red cell count may be less than 2 million/ml. The *red cells* are macrocytic, *MCV* is usually > 100 fl, and appear as **macrovalocytes** on *peripheral blood smear.* The **peripheral white blood cells** are hypersegmented. There are more than 5% neutrophil with 5 or more lobes. However, this finding can be seen in 25% of normal pregnant patients.
   ii. **Ferrokinetic findings:** Serum folate level less than 3 ng/ml are suggestive of folic acid depletion. Erythrocyte folate activity of less than 20 ng/ml (50 nmol/lt) usually indicates folic acid deficiency. But in 30% of patients values overlap, serum iron and B_{12} level are normal.
   iii. **Bone marrow study:** It demonstrate megaloblastic erythropoiesis but usually it is not necessary for diagnosis.

Treatment

Clinically full blown and megaloblastic anemia can be more dangerous for a patient than iron deficiency anemia so treatment should be energetic. In case of established anemia 1-5 mg/day orally folic acid is given. *Folic acid in this dose should be given when treating any acute anemia presenting in later months of pregnancy and with parenteral iron, while awaiting the result of investigation and in all cases of multifetal pregnancy.* Once megaloblastic hemopoiesis is established, the treatment of folic acid deficiency becomes more difficult, as there is impaired absorption of folic acid due to megaloblastic changes in the gastrointestinal tract. Oral treatment with 1-5 mg of folic acid per day should raise the hematocrit approximately 1% each day, beginning on 5-6 days of therapy. The reticulocyte count should be increased after 3-4 days of therapy and is earliest morphologic signs of response. Iron supplementation should be administered as indicated by hematologic findings. If oral treatment is ineffective parenteral treatment should be tried. Women on anticonvulsant drugs should review folate supplementation before and during conception.

Blood transfusion: Antepartum hemorrhage in the uncorrected state of megaloblastic anemia is an indication for blood transfusion. But before blood transfusion peripheral blood smear should be prepared for correct diagnosis.

Prognosis

In adequately treated case, megaloblastic anemia due to folate deficiency has a good prognosis. Usually anemia is mild, unless associated with multifetal pregnancy, systemic infection, or hemolytic disease. Low birth weight and fetal neural tube defects are known to be associated with maternal folic acid deficiency. The association with placental abruptio, spontaneous abortion and pre-eclampsia is not universally accepted. This anemia even without treatment usually resolves after delivery, when folate demands come to normal in non pregnant state.

Vitamin B_{12} Deficiency

Addisonian pernicious anemia caused by vitamin B_{12} deficiency does not usually occur with pregnancy. It may be associated with chronic tropical sprue. The absorption of vitamin B_{12} is normally unaltered in pregnancy. The recommended dose of vitamin B_{12} is 2 µg/day in non pregnant state and 3 µg/day during pregnancy. This dietary requirement will be met by almost any diet that contains animal product. Strict vegetarian may require supplementation in pregnancy.

Aplastic Anemia

It is rare in pregnancy. Anemia may be secondary to exposure to known bone marrow toxic agents like chloramphenicol, phenylbutazone and insecticide. *Idiopathic aplastic anemia in pregnancy may have a spontaneous remission following* delivery or pregnancy termination but may recur in subsequent pregnancies. The condition is likely to be immunological mediated.

Clinical Findings

There is rapidly developing anemia causing pallor, fatigue, tachycardia, painful ulceration of throat and fever.

Laboratory Investigations

There is pancytopenia and empty bone marrow on biopsy.

Treatment

Patient must avoid any bone marrow toxic agents. Blood product replacement with packed red blood cells and platelet should be utilized as per requirement. Infection must be treated aggressively with appropriate antibiotics. Bone marrow transplantation is performed if remission does not occur following delivery or termination of pregnancy.

Hemoglobinopathies

Hemoglobin itself is a conjugated protein with a molecular weight of about 68,000 dalton which contains a globin fraction bound to 4 heme molecules. In hemoglobinopathies there are disorders within polypeptide chains that effect globin fraction. There are 4 possible chains—normal alpha, beta, gamma and delta. There are large numbers of variants of the hemoglobin molecule. Thalassemia is particularly common in certain population as North West part of India, Pakistan and Mediterranean region and sickle cell anemia is common in eastern India and Africa.

In adult, 90% of hemoglobin is HbA which is constituted by $\alpha_2\beta_2$ chain and 3% is HbA2 constituted by $\alpha_2\delta_2$ chain. Fetal hemoglobin has a globin protein of 2 alpha and 2 gamma chains ($\alpha_2\gamma_2$). At time of birth 80% of hemoglobin is fetal. In first year of life the fetal hemoglobin is gradually replaced by normal adult hemoglobin (HbA). There are two types of HbA synthesis abnormality:
a. Quantitative: Thalassemia syndrome
b. Qualitative: Sickle cell disease

Thalassemia: It is genetically defined disorder of reduced synthesis of one or more of the structurally normal globin chain in hemoglobin. Thalassemia are inherited as an autosomal recessive trait.

Pathophysiology: In beta-thalassemia, hemoglobin β chain syntheses is defective but α chains are produced normally. In alpha thalassemia the reverse is true. If 4 defective alpha globin genes are present it causes Hb Bart Hydrops which is incompatible with survival. This unbalanced synthesis results in a relative excess of normally produced chains. The normal globin chain then forms teramers which precipitate within red blood cells precursors in the bone marrow. It causes ineffective erythropoiesis, red cell sequestration and destruction and hypochromic anemia.

In **thalassemia, major (homozygous form)** both α chains are missing. There is severe anemia and secondary organ damage. In **thalassemia minor (heterozygous form)** only one locus of the globin chain is missing, which results in microcytosis without significant anemia. A third intermediate state is where both β chains are missing but an inherited defect is at the alpha locus which results in parallel reduction in the α chains. These patients may be moderately anemic but do not need blood transfusion.

Management of Thalassemia in Pregnancy

Thalassemia in Intermediate and Minor

Women with thalassemia trait present in pregnancy with a characteristic low MCV and MCHC with near normal or low hemoglobin. In women belonging to ethnic population in which thalassemia is predisposed, a high index of suspicion is required even with mild anemia. Diagnosis is confirmed by raised concentration of HbA2 with or without raised HbF. If the patient is having thalassemia, the partner should also be tested. If both partners have trait, prenatal diagnosis should be offered. There are 25% chances that the fetus will be affected with thalassemia major. These cases can be offered termination of pregnancy.

In thalassemia minor, there is very little danger of hemochromatosis with usual iron and folate supplementation. *But these patients should never receive parenteral preparation.* Iron supplementation may not be necessary if ferritin levels are adequate.

Thalassemia Major

In the past-pregnancy in women with β thalassemia major was rarity due to short lifespan, reduced fertility multiple organ defects iron deposition. Usually, women with thalassemia major are having hypogonadotropic hypogonadism with primary or secondary amenorrhea, resulting from iron deposition in hypothalamus and pituitary. In last decade with improved management, pregnancy is now possible.

Preconceptional counseling is vital to assess systemic evaluation. Pregnancy in these women is associated with marked anemia, increased transfusion requirement and high cesarean section rate. Cardiac failure can be precipitated. There is high rate of pregnancy loss, prematurity and IUGR. To maintain hemoglobin level of 10 gm/dl, thalassemic women require repeated blood transfusion, which have to be carefully monitored to prevent cardiac overload. Desferrioxamine is discontinued because of harmful effect on the fetus and risk of iron deficiency in neonate. **Folic acid supplements should be continued but iron supplements and vitamin C should not be given.** Fetal growth should be carefully monitored. Labor management is like that of a patient with severe anemia. Desferrioxamine should be restarted within the first weeks of puerperium and breastfeeding is continued. Contraceptive counseling is important. In splenectomized women oral contraceptive should be avoided as they have a high-risk of thrombosis.

Sickle Cell Disease

Sickle cell hemoglobin (HbS) *results from a genetic subscription of valine for glutamic acid at codon 6 of the globin chains.* Decreased oxygen tension causes hemoglobin S to form insoluble polymers in curvilinear strands. These polymers deform the normal biconcave structure of the erythrocytes. The process is reversible but eventually lead to cell membrane damage and permanent sickling. Homozygous patients for HbS genes have sickle cell anemia (SS disease) and heterozygous have sickle cell trait. Women who are heterozygous for both S and C genes have hemoglobin SC disease. In hemoglobin S/beta thalassemia disease, the patient is heterozygous for both hemoglobin S and B thalassemia.

Diagnosis

Symptoms and Signs

a. **Chronic anemia:** Any cause of refractory anemia especially in women with a good social class from high prevalence ethnic group should be investigated.
b. **Sickling of red blood cells:** Intravascular sickling leads to vaso-occlusion and infarction, resulting in ischemic pain, necrosis and organ damage.
c. **Sickle cells crisis:**
   i. Pain crisis involve bone and joints, which is precipitated by dehydration, acidosis or infection.
   ii. Aplastic crisis is characterized by rapidly developing anemia. Hemoglobin may be as low as 2-3 gm%.
   iii. Acute splenic sequestration crisis is associated with severe anemia and hypovolemic shock which is caused by sudden massive trapping of red blood cells within the splenic sinusoids.
   iv. Other manifestation can be increased susceptibility to bacterial infection, myocardial damage and cardiomegaly, hematuria, headache, convulsion, etc.

Laboratory Findings

Screening for abnormal hemoglobin is imperative in the population at risk. There are two tests:
a. **Sodium metabisulfate test:** One drop of fresh 2% reagent is mixed on a slide with 1 drop of blood. Sickling of most red cells occur in few minute both in cases of sickle cell trait and disease.
b. **Sickle dextest:** In this, 20 µL of blood is mixed with 2 ml of sodium dithionite reagent. Clouding of the solution indicates the presence of hemoglobin S. If test is positive, the homozygous and heterozygous status must be differentiated by hemoglobin electrophoresis.

Complication in Pregnancy

There is increased maternal mortality and morbidity from hemolysis, folic acid deficiency, frequent crisis, congestive heart failure, infection and PIH. There is increased incidence of early fetal loss, stillbirth, preterm delivery and IUGR.

Management

Prenatal Counseling

Women with sickle cell disease must be appropriately counseled on the advisability of pregnancy. The complications should be told, the partner's hemoglobin electrophoresis should be done and prenatal diagnosis should be offered. Patient receiving hydroxyurea to mitigate the severity of disease should be counseled regarding the risk to the fetus such as craniofacial, neural abnormalities and IUGR.

Antenatal Management

It is a joint venture by hematologist and obstetrician. At the booking visit, a careful examination should be undertaken with special reference to the complications of sickle cell disease like proliferative retinopathy, blood group, antibody screen, base line liver, kidney function. *Folate requirement* is increased because of RBC destruction and 5 mg/day of folic acid is needed throughout the pregnancy. *Iron supplementation* is given when serum ferritin level is low. If serum ferritin level is elevated or there is history of iron overload, an echocardiograph and cardiac assessment should be performed to exclude cardiomyopathy. Careful surveillance of asymptomatic bacteriuria and cure is important for preventing pyelonephritis. *Pneumococcal and influenza vaccine* can be considered. Penicillin prophylaxis throughout pregnancy should be instituted. *Blood transfusion should be considered if hematocrit level falls to less than 25% to prevent crisis.* But decision should be guided by patient's history and clinical examination. *Exchange transfusion* in which two units are removed by every 3-4 unit transfused, is helpful in cases of stroke, renal papillary necrosis or painful crisis. By exchange transfusion percentage of sickle hemoglobin is reduced but transfusion carries the risk of allergic reaction, delayed hemolytic reaction, isoimmunization and transmission of infection. Thus, need of blood transfusion should be carefully weighted.

Fetal surveillance should be instituted to detect IUGR and fetal well-being. In management of crisis, the common predisposing factors like infection, dehydration and hypoxia should be evaluated and treated. Symptomatic treatment of pain is done with intravenous fluid, oxygen supplementation and adequate analgesic. Bacterial pneumonia and pyelonephritis must be treated vigorously with intravenous antibiotics.

Labor Management
Optimal hydration, oxygenation and asepsis should be maintained. Cesarean section is done only for obstetric indication. Epidural anesthetic can be given but care is needed to avoid hypotension and hypoxemia.

Puerperal Care and Contraception
In the puerperium, antibiotic cover and thromboprophylaxis should be considered. Oral contraceptive pills can cause the thrombosis and crisis. Progesterone only method are best as they reduce the incidence of sickling crisis. Intrauterine device is not contraindicated. For women with completed family, permanent sterilization is best.

Hemorrhagic Disorders

Thrombocytopenia
Thrombocytopenia is defined as a platelet count of 150×10^9/liter ($150,000/\mu l$) which occurs in up to 15% of pregnancies (Table 40.2).

Causes of Thrombocytopenia
Low platelet count in pregnancy may be associated with large variety of disorders like acquired hemolytic anemia, severe PIH, severe obstetrical hemorrhage, consumptive coagulopathy, septicemia, antiphospholipid antibodies syndrome, viral infection. But here we focus on other causes of thrombocytopenia.
a. **Gestational thrombocytopenia:** It constitute 74% of cases of thrombocytopenia in pregnancy. Gestational thrombocytopenia affects 5% of pregnancy. It is characterized by mild asymptomatic thrombocytopenia with platelet levels usually greater than $70000/\mu l$ (70×10^9/lit). It usually occurs in later gestational age and resolves spontaneously after delivery. Its etiology is unclear and routine obstetric management is enough.
b. **Immune thrombocytopenia perpura (ITP):** It is secondary to circulating immunoglobulin (IgG) anti platelet antibody that crosses the placenta and may affect fetal platelet.

Clinical Features
The clinical picture varies from asymptomatic to minor bruises or patechiae, bleeding from mucosal sites or rarely fatal intracranial bleeding. It is caused by small unsealed endothelial lesions. By contrast patients with inherited bleeding disorders do not have patechial or excessive bleeding from small cuts because platelet adhesion and aggregation tends to be sufficient. The diagnosis is made when there is demonstration of isolated thrombocytopenia and other causes like drug or HIV have been excluded.

Table 40.2: Causes of thrombocytopenia in pregnancy

a. Pregnancy associated thrombocytopenia (PAT)—74%
b. Hypertensive disorders of pregnancy—21%
c. Immune disorder—4%
d. Other—Disseminated intravascular coagulation, thrombotic thrombocytopenic purpura (TTP), HELLP syndrome, acute fatty liver—2%

Treatment
The treatment is initiated when the platelet count falls to less than $30000\text{-}50000/\mu l$.

Glucocorticoids
Prednisolone is used as a first line therapy in a dose of 1mg/kg/day. Response occurs in 3-7 days and reaches maximum within 2-3 weeks. Once the desired platelet count is achieved, it is slowly tapered and maintained at the lowest dose required to sustain a platelet count greater than 50×10^9/l ($50,000 \mu l$).

Intravenous Immunoglobulin
It is effective in cases from refractory to steroids and in more urgent situation like platelet below 10×10^9/lit. IVIG is given is dose of 0.4 gm/kg/day for 5 days or 1 gm/kg/day for 2 days.

Splenectomy
Splenectomy is rarely required in pregnancy, when medical therapy fails. If indicated it is best performed in the second trimester.

Transfusion of Platelet and Whole Blood
It may be necessary to restore losses from acute hemorrhage or to normalize low perioperative platelet count ($< 50,000/\mu l$).

Complications
Maternal IgG antiplatelet antibodies cross the placenta, so the fetus is at risk for severe thrombocytopenia. But only 10% of infants born to women with ITP have platelet count less than 50×10^9/lit at birth. Maternal treatment with corticosteroid and immunoglobulin does not affect the fetal platelet count. In labor fetal blood sampling, invasive fetal monitoring, ventouse application should be avoided because of risk of cephalohematoma. Cesarean section is not considered beneficial. Cord blood platelet count is usually not routinely recommended. Nadir of the neonatal platelet count occurs on day 4-7 so platelet count and pediatric assessment is needed. But in event of bleeding or platelet count is below 20×10^9/lit the infant can be treated with IVIg and platelet transfusion can be given if there is active hemorrhage.

MULTIPLE CHOICE QUESTIONS

1. According to WHO, anemia in pregnancy is diagnosed when hemoglobin is less than:
   a. 11.0 gm%
   b. 10.0 gm%
   c. 12.0 gm%
   d. 9.0 gm%
   Ans. a

2. Which of the following tests is most sensitive for the detection of iron depletion in pregnancy:
   a. Serum iron
   b. Serum ferritin
   c. Serum transferrin
   d. Serum iron binding capacity
   Ans. b

3. In pregnancy which types of anemia is not common in India:
   a. Vitamin B_{12} anemia
   b. Folic acid deficiency anemia
   c. Iron + folic acid anemia
   d. Iron deficiency anemia
   Ans. a

4. Fetal requirement of iron is:
   a. 200 mg
   b. 300 mg
   c. 400 mg
   d. 500 mg
   Ans. b

5. How much iron a patient can tolerate at a time given intravenously:
   a. 1000 mg
   b. 2000 mg
   c. 2500 mg
   d. 3000 mg
   Ans. c

6. With oral iron therapy, rise in Hb% can be seen after:
   a. 1 week
   b. 3 weeks
   c. 4 weeks
   d. 6 weeks
   Ans. b

7. What is the value of color index in microcytic hypochromic anemia associated with pregnancy?
   a. 1
   b. <1
   c. >1
   d. 3
   Ans. b

8. With iron treatment, Hb increases by:
   a. 2 gm/week
   b. 1 gm/week
   c. 2 gm/month
   d. 1 gm/month
   Ans. b

9. Which is the safest contraceptive method for a woman with sickle cell anemia:
   a. IUCD
   b. Low dose progesterone pill
   c. Condom or diaphragm
   d. Low dose estrogen progesterone
   Ans. c

10. The following complications are likely to increase in a case of severe anemia during the pregnancy, *except*:
    a. Pre-eclampsia
    b. Heart failure
    c. Preterm labor
    d. Subinvolution
    Ans. d

41 Cardiac Disease in Pregnancy

Extreme remedies are most appropriate for extreme disease.

INTRODUCTION

Cardiovascular disease is a fourth leading nonobstetric cause of maternal death and maternal morbidity both in antepartum and postpartum period.

Incidence and Types of Cardiac Disease in Pregnancy

Cardiac disease in pregnancy can be congenital or acquired. The acquired group includes rheumatic heart disease, cardiomyopathy and ischemic heart disease. **Rheumatic heart disease is most common in developing countries, whereas cardiomyopathies and congenital heart disease are more common in developed countries.** Out of rheumatic valvular heart disease mitral stenosis is predominant and account for nearly 75% of cases. Predominantly aortic lesions are found in less than 5% of cases. Cardiomyopathies are being increasingly recognized. The three main types are—dilated, restrictive and hypertrophic variety.

Physiological Changes in Pregnancy and Effect of Cardiac Disease on Pregnancy

The physiological hemodynamic changes in the pregnancy have been described in previous chapter (Basic science). These hemodynamic changes have a profound effect on underlying heart disease in pregnancy. The most important consideration is that during pregnancy cardiac output is increased by as much as 30-50%, out of which half of the total increase occurs by 8 weeks and is maximized by mid-pregnancy. It results from increased stroke volume associated with decreased vascular resistance and corresponding diminished blood pressure. Later in pregnancy, there is added increased pulse rate and more increase in stroke volume, which is caused by increased diastolic filling from augmented blood volume. As significant hemodynamic alterations are apparent early in pregnancy, women with severe cardiac dysfunction may experience worsening of heart failure before mid-pregnancy. In other women heart failure develops in the third trimester, when the normal hypovolemia of pregnancy is maximum. In majority heart failure develops around labor, because during uterine contraction 300-500 ml of blood is shifted from the uterus to maternal systemic circulation. Because of this autotransfusion, systemic venous pressure and right ventricular pressure increases. Maternal pain and anxiety result in increased adrenaline, which decreases maternal blood pressure and heart rate. Following delivery, venal caval compression is decreased and blood volume is increased. These changes cause 10-25% increase in circulating cardiac output. During peripartum period, the chance of heart failure is maximum.

Diagnostic Evaluation of Heart Disease in Pregnancy

Many of the physiological changes of normal pregnancy tend to make the diagnosis of heart disease more difficult like fatigue, shortness of breath, orthopnea and peripheral edema can be found in normal pregnancy. However, following symptoms and clinical findings are suggestive of heart disease during pregnancy:

Symptoms:
a. Progressive dyspnea or orthopnea
b. Nocturnal cough
c. Hemoptysis
d. Syncope
e. Chest pain.

Signs:
a. Cyanosis
b. Clubbing of fingers
c. Persistent neck vein engorgement
d. Systolic murmur grade 3/6 or greater
e. Diastolic murmur
f. Cardiomegaly
g. Persistent arrhythmia
h. Persistent split second sound.

Pregnant women who have none of these findings rarely have serious heart disease.

Diagnostic Studies

Most diagnostic cardiovascular studies are noninvasive and can be conducted safely in pregnant women. Conventional testing includes:
a. Electrocardiography
b. Echocardiography
c. Chest radiography.

Electrocardiography

There are several pregnancy induced changes that need to be considered while interpreting ECG. As the diaphragm is elevated in advancing pregnancy, there is an average 15° left axis deviation in the ECG. There can be T wave inversion and dysrhythmias in heart disease in ECG finding.

Echocardiography

Echocardiography allows accurate and noninvasive diagnosis of most heart disease during pregnancy. In normal pregnancy, there is mild tricuspid regurgitation and significantly increased left atrial size. By echocardiography structural abnormalities like ASD, VSD, valve anatomy, valve area, valve function, left ventricular ejection fraction and pulmonary artery systole can be detected.

Chest X-ray

Anteroposterior and lateral chest radiography may be very useful when heart disease is suspected clinically. When used with a lead apron shield, fetal radiation exposure is minimized. Cardiomegaly, increased pulmonary vascular markings and enlarged pulmonary veins can be detected by chest X-ray.

Exercise Stress Testing

Stress testing usually is indicated for preconceptional workup for estimation of myocardial reserve to determine that if a woman can safely carry a pregnancy to term.

Cardiac Catheterization

Pulmonary artery catheterization without fluoroscopy at the bedside is a relatively safe procedure and allows for hemodynamic monitoring in labor and delivery in patients with significant heart disease.

Clinical Classification

New York Heart Association classification of heart disease has been summarized in Table 41.1. It is based upon the cardiac response to physical activity.

Table 41.1: New York Heart Association Classification of Heart Disease

Grade 1	Uncompromised = No limitation of physical activity.
Grade 2	Slight limitation of physical activity. The patients are comfortable at rest but ordinary physical activity causes discomfort.
Grade 3	Marked limitation of physical activity. The patients are comfortable at rest but less than ordinary activity causes discomfort by excessive fatigue, palpitation, dyspnea or anginal pain.
Grade 4	Severely compromised. Inability to perform any physical activity without discomfort. There are symptoms of cardiac insufficiency or angina may develop even at rest.

This classification is important to assess the functional capacity of the heart rather than structural damage. But its value is limited by its subjective nature and individual variation. So, it is important to have a precise anatomic diagnosis by physical signs and echocardiography.

Management of Cardiac Disease in Pregnancy

Prepregnancy Counseling

It has a major preventive role in ensuring an optimal pregnancy outcome. It is best done in joint consultation with cardiologist. Following points should be considered in prepregnancy counseling:
a. Desirability of future conception in the presence of the cardiac disease.
b. The current fitness and status of the patient and anticipated complication in pregnancy.
c. Any potential sources of infection should be looked for and treated fully like infection in genital tract, dental roots, urinary tract infection.
d. Women receiving drugs like ACE inhibitors should be switched to drugs which are safe in pregnancy. The need for direction should be reassessed in women with prosthetic heart valve, who are on anticoagulant drugs. Switch over from oral anticoagulant to heparin at about 6 weeks gestation should be considered.

Antenatal Management

The patient cardiac functional class should be decided during the first four months of pregnancy as management will depend on the class:

A. General management:
a. Advice on diet, rest and fresh air should be given.
b. Iron, folic acid and vitamins should be prescribed to all cases with adequate intake of calcium through milk and supplementation.
c. Ample rest should be ensured and exertion should be permitted only to a degree that falls just short of producing dyspnea.

d. Infection is very important in precipitating cardiac failure. As far as possible, steps should be taken to avoid infection and any febrile illness should be treated aggressively. Prophylactic antibiotics may be necessary. Any dental procedure should be done under antibiotic cover. Pneumococcal and influenza vaccine can be recommended.
e. Cigarette smoking is prohibited.
f. Special attention should be directed towards prevention and early recognition of heart failure. ***The first warning sign of congestive heart failure is persistent basilar rales, accompanied by nocturnal cough. A sudden decrease in ability to carry out usual duties, increasing dyspnea on exertion, and attacks of smothering with cough are symptoms of serious heart failure. Clinical findings are hemoptysis, progressive edema and tachycardia.***

It is better that patient is reassessed by the cardiologist for her cardiac status between 28th and 32nd weeks. The principles of treatment are the same as in the nonpregnant individuals. The women should be admitted and the diagnosis should be confirmed by clinical examinations for signs of heart failure and echocardiography. Drug given can include diuretics, vasodilators and digoxin. Oxygen and morphine may also be required. Dysrhythymias also require urgent correction and drug therapy adenosine for supra-ventricular tachycardia and selective beta adrenergic blocker may be required. In all cases, assessment of fetal well-being is done with ultrasound and fetal electro-cardiography. In cases of intractable cardiac failure the risk to the mother of continuing the pregnancy and risk to the fetus of premature delivery must be carefully weighed.
g. Anemia should be diagnosed early and vigorously treated as it has the potential to aggravate infection and heart failure.
h. In class I and II patient, who have no other complications should preferably be admitted to hospital in last 15 days of pregnancy, if they live at a considerable distance.

Management of Labor and Delivery

In general, delivery should be accomplished vaginally unless there are obstetric indications for cesarean delivery. **Induction of labor is not indicated in cardiac patient because of the inherent risk of infection, fluid overload failure and possibility of cesarean section.** However, if induction is needed for other obstetric indication, oxytocin infusion in concentrated drip is method of choice. Amniotomy is deferred for fear of ascending infection. Prostaglandin E2 is a potent vasodilator and causes a marked rise in cardiac output. So, prostaglandin should be used with extensive caution and in minimum dose if required.

Management of First Stage of Labor

a. The pregnant cardiac women should be in lateral supine position to avoid the hemodynamic impairment caused by supine position. Sedation should be liberal.
b. Epidural analgesic can be given but care has to be taken in patients on anticoagulants. Parenteral analgesic provides satisfactory pain relief. For vaginal delivery epidural analgesic along with intravenous sedation is sufficient.
c. Cardiac patient in labor should be continuously monitored with pulse oxymeter. In a women with severe heart disease pulmonary artery catheterization may be indicated for continuous hemodynamic monitoring.
d. Fluid overload should be avoided. Almost all cardiac patients in labor should be kept on dry side and I/V fluid should be restricted to no more than 75ml/hr. According to American Heart Association antibiotic prophylaxis is recommended. **In Ampicillin 2 gm IV/IM and Gentamicin 1.5 mg/kg within 30 minute before delivery followed by Ampicillin 1 gm I/v/I/m or orally 6 hours later. In patient allergic to Ampicillin, Vancomycin 1 gm I/v over 1-2 hours with Gentamicin can be given.**
e. During labor if there is increase in pulse rate much above 100/minute or the respiratory rate above 24, it may suggest impending ventricular failure. With any evidence of heart failure intensive medical management must be instituted immediately.

Management of Second Stage of Labor

The patient should not be encouraged to bear down forcibly. Usually, labor in cardiac women is easy. Prophylactic forceps are usually not required. An episiotomy may be given to facilitate easy delivery. Vacuum extractor is a good alternative to forceps applications. Rate of instrumental delivery is usually high (≈25%) in class IV patient.

Third Stage of Labor

It should never be hurried. Routine use of ***methyl ergometrine is barred,*** as it will increase cardiac load by causing additional blood to be squeezed back into circulation and shut down the uterine arteriovenous shunt. Oxytocin infusion in compensated patient and simultaneous Furasemide 40 mg I/v is preferred. After completion of delivery the patient should be propped up, which increases venous pooling in the lower extremity and decrease venous return to the heart and there is more gradual adaptation to the postpartum hemodynamics.

Indication of Cesarean Section

There is 2-3 times higher mortality rate in cardiac patients in cesarean section as compared to vaginal delivery. It is only indicated for obstetric reasons like cephalopelvic disproportion, malpresentation. In class IV and sicker patients, elective cesarean section can be considered as it allows better control over the ventilation and fluid management and prevents the additional stress caused by labor. For cesarean section, epidural anesthetic is preferred by most clinicians. Spinal anesthetic is contraindicated in some lesions. Major danger of regional anesthetic is maternal hypotension. Finally general anesthetic with thiopental, succinylcholine, nitrous oxide and oxygen is a satisfactory choice.

Puerperium

As there is risk of decompensated cardiac failure after delivery, it is important that meticulous care should be continued into the puerperium. In cardiac patient, postpartum hemorrhage, anemia, infection and thromboembolism can be serious and precipitate heart failure. If tubal sterilization is to be done after delivery, it is best to delay the procedure till the woman is afebrile and not anemic. Postnatal contraception advice should be given to these women. Injection depot medroxy progesterone acetate 150 mg is a good choice. Low dose oral contraceptive pills can also be considered in the stable patients, 6 months after delivery.

SPECIFIC HEART DISEASE DURING PREGNANCY AND MANAGEMENT

Mitral Stenosis

a. *Pathophysiology:* Rheumatic fever is the leading cause of mitral stenosis. It impedes the flow of blood from the left atrium to the left ventricle during diastole. These patients usually have a fixed cardiac output. Normal area of mitral valve is 4-5 cm^2. When valve area is <2.5 cm^2, women experiences symptoms with exertion. When valve area is <1.5 cm^2, a woman experiences symptoms at rest. During pregnancy, increased blood volume increases venous return, which causes pulmonary congestion instead of increased cardiac output. Tachycardia of pregnancy shortens diastole and decreases left ventricular filling and cardiac output.

b. *Management:* In antepartum period, management is focused on maintaining cardiac output and decreasing pulmonary congestion. This is achieved with diuretic and beta blocker therapy. Good pain control during labor is important to reduce maternal heart rate. Antibiotic prophylaxis to prevent endocarditis is must and 2nd stage of labor should be cut short by operative delivery. In postpartum period, diuresis is recommended.

Aortic Stenosis

a. *Pathophysiology:* Usually, there is a combination of congenital lesions and rheumatic fever. Normal aortic valve area is 3-4 cm^2. Aortic stenosis becomes significant, when the valve area is < 1 cm^2. As stenosis progresses, the left ventricle initially hypertrophies in response to increased pressure gradient. Finally, there is dilatation of left ventricle. Presenting symptoms are angina, syncope and congestive heart failure.

b. *Management in pregnancy and labor:* As women with aortic stenosis have a fixed cardiac output so their preload should be maintained throughout. Any hypotension can cause sudden death. During labor, they may require central hemodynamic monitoring. Regional anesthetic should be used with extreme caution as there is a risk of hypotension. Stage of labor should be shortened. Antibiotic prophylaxis is given. Postpartum blood loss can significantly reduce preload and resuscitation with fluid or blood may be needed.

Mitral Regurgitation

Usually it is result of rheumatic disease, but other cause may be genetic defect in collagen synthesis (Marfan's syndrome) or following endocarditis of a previously abnormal valve. They usually better tolerate the physiologic changes of pregnancy as compared to mitral stenosis. But, there is risk of atrial fibrillation and endocarditis. In management, symptomatic prolapse should be treated with β blockers. Myocardial depressants should be avoided and arrhythmias should be treated.

Congenital Ventricle Septal Defect or Atrial Septal Defect

Women with ASD and left to right shunt usually do well in pregnancy. Peripheral vasodilatation of pregnancy decreases the left to right shunts. Women with ASD are not at risk for bacterial endocarditis and do not need antibiotic prophylaxis. Women with VSD and left to right shunt also do well in pregnancy. These patients are less prone to arrhythmia but are at significant risk of endocarditis, so they need antibiotics prophylaxis during labor and delivery.

Eisenmenger's Syndrome

Pathophysiology: It is a congenital communication between the pulmonary and systemic circulation causing increased pulmonary vascular resistance (PVR) either to systemic level or greater than systemic level. Once the PVR is greater than systemic vascular resistance, a right to left shunt develops along with significant pulmonary hypertension. The most common cause of Eisenmenger's syndrome is large VSD. These women have a mortality rate of 50%, fetal mortality rate of 50% and preterm delivery is 85%.

Management: They should be counseled regarding risk of pregnancy. Management during pregnancy revolves around maintaining pulmonary blood flow. Antenatal care is on ample rest, oxygen therapy and possibly pulmonary dilators. Delivery should be planned with central hemodynamic monitoring. Second stage should be assisted. Cesarean is advised only for obstetric indication.

Coarctation of Aorta

The maternal risks are aortic dissection, bacterial endocarditis and cerebral hemorrhage due to ruptured intracranial aneurysm. **Maternal mortality is high (3-8%). Fetal loss is 25%. Surgical correction should be done prior to pregnancy.** Termination of pregnancy should be seriously considered. Elective cesarean section is preferred to minimize dissection associated with labor.

Primary Pulmonary Hypertension

Women with severe pulmonary hypertension have an obstruction to right ventricular outflow. The major physiological concern is to maintain pulmonary blood flow. Women with this condition should be strongly advised against pregnancy. **The mortality rate is 50%.** Antenatal care is centered around limitation of physical activity, oxygen therapy and possibly pulmonary vasodilators.

Peripartum Cardiomyopathy

It occurs in 1 in 1500 to 1 in 15000 pregnancies. It is a dilated cardiomyopathy of an unknown cause. Patient usually presents with symptoms of congestive heart failure late in pregnancy or in early postpartum period in the absence of prior heart disease. Echocardiography is indicative of left ventricular dysfunction.

Treatment

Treatment is rest, fluid and salt restrictions, diuretic, vasodilators, digitalis and β blockers. In addition prophylactic anticoagulation during pregnancy and full anticoagulation for 1-2 week after delivery is recommended.

Prognosis

Cardiac function normalizes within 6 months of delivery in approximately half of patients. But in women whose left ventricular size and function remain abnormal 6 month after delivery have a 5 year mortality of 50-85%. These women should be counseled against subsequent pregnancies. Women who have normal left ventricular size and function within 6 months of delivery have greatly reduced 5 year mortality but they also have a 25% recurrence rate during a subsequent pregnancy.

MECHANICAL HEART VALVES

The problem for pregnant women with metal heart valve replacement is that they require life long anticoagulant and this must be continued in pregnancy because of increased risk of thrombosis. Warfarin is associated with warfarin embryopathy and increased risk of miscarriage, stillbirth and fetal intracerebral hemorrhage.

There are three broad strategies for use of anticoagulants in pregnancy:

i. The safest option for mother to continue warfarin throughout pregnancy.
ii. Other management strategies are to replace warfarin with high dose unfractionated or low molecular weight heparin either from 6-12 weeks of pregnancy to avoid warfarin embryopathy and to continue warfarin throughout pregnancy.
iii. Third option is to give heparin throughout pregnancy whichever option is chosen, warfarin should be discontinued and substituted with heparin 10 days prior to delivery to allow clearance of warfarin from fetal circulation. At the time of delivery, heparin therapy is interrupted and warfarin is started 2-3 days postpartum. If there is sudden bleeding or urgent delivery, warfarin can be reversed with fresh frozen plasmas, vitamin K. Heparin can be reversed with protamine sulphate. In addition, low dose aspirin 75-100 mg daily should be orally administered.

Valve replacement during pregnancy: Usually valve replacement is postponed until after delivery but in some situation valve replacement may be life saving. Studies confirm that surgery on the heart or great vessels is associated with major maternal and fetal morbidity and mortality.

Mitral valvotomy during pregnancy: Tight mitral stenosis requiring intervention during pregnancy was previously treated by closed mitral valvotomy. In the past decade, percutaneous transcatheter balloon dilatation of the mitral valve has largely replaced valvotomy during pregnancy, preferably done at 14-18 weeks of gestation.

MULTIPLE CHOICE QUESTIONS

1. Signs of heart disease in pregnancy are:
   a. Diastolic murmur
   b. Systolic murmur
   c. Tachycardia
   d. Dyspnea on exertion
   e. Nervousness or syncope on exertion
   Ans. a, d, e
2. Most common heart disease associated with pregnancy is:
   a. Mitral stenosis
   b. Mitral regurgitation
   c. Patent ductus arteriosis
   d. Tetralogy of Fallot
   Ans. a
3. A pregnant woman with heart disease, all of the following are to be done *except*:
   a. I/v methergine after delivery
   b. Prophylactic antibiotic
   c. I/v Furasemide postpartum
   d. Cut short 2nd stage of labor
   Ans. a

4. In which of the following heart disease is maternal mortality during pregnancy found to be highest:
   a. Coarctation of aorta
   b. Eisenmenger syndrome
   c. AS
   d. MS

   Ans. b

5. Cardiac failure is most likely in pregnancy at:
   a. 32 weeks
   b. 1st stage of labor
   c. 3rd stage of labor
   d. 4th stage of labor

   Ans. d

6. Tubectomy in heart patient, who has recently delivered is best done after:
   a. 48 hours
   b. 1 week
   c. 2 week
   d. Immediately

   Ans. b

7. To suppress lactation in the mother with rheumatic heart disease, treatment of choice is:
   a. D-Norgesterol
   b. Pyridoxine
   c. Bromocriptine
   d. DMPA

   Ans. c

8. During pregnancy, corrective cardiac surgery is commonly indicated in:
   a. Mitral stenosis
   b. Active stenosis
   c. Atrial septal defect
   d. Ventricular septal defect

   Ans. a

9. Surgery for mitral stenosis during pregnancy is ideally done at:
   a. 14 weeks
   b. 20 weeks
   c. 28 weeks
   d. 32 weeks

   Ans. a

10. A para 4, poorly compensated cardiac patient has delivered 2 days back. You will advice her to:
    a. Undergo sterilization after 1 week
    b. Undergo sterilization after 6 week
    c. Suggest her husband to undergo vasectomy
    d. Take oral contraceptive pills after 6 months

    Ans. c

42 Thyroid Dysfunction with Pregnancy

The price of greatness is responsibility.

GENERAL CONSIDERATION

The thyroid gland is altered by the metabolic and hormonal changes of pregnancy. Likewise the reproductive outcome may be affected by disease of this organ, since all forms of thyroid disease are 3-4 times more common in women than in men. Disorders of this gland are not uncommon during pregnancy.

Thyroid Physiology During Normal Pregnancy

Both total thyroxine (T_4) and triiodothyronine (T_3) levels increase because the level of their carrier, thyroxine binding globulin (TBG) becomes elevated. Estrogen cause increased TBG synthesis and decreased TBG clearance. The concentration of free thyroxine (FT_4) and free triiodothyronine (FT_3) fluctuate and are within normal range. The thyrotropin stimulating hormone (TSH) level decreases and even can be low in some patients—13% in the first trimester, 4.5% in the second trimester and 1.2% in the third trimester. *The TSH level is lowest and FT_4 level is highest when the human chorionic gonadotrophins level is at its peak.* Serum thyroglobulin level increases more towards the end of the pregnancy. During pregnancy iodide clearance by the kidney increases. For this reason plus the iodide loss to the fetus, the prevalence of goiter is increased in area of iodine deficiency. In iodine deficient areas, pregnancy may increase risk of iodine deficiency. The fetal hypothalamic pituitary thyroid axis becomes functional towards the end of the first trimester. Until then the fetus is dependent on local monodeiodination of transferred maternal T_4 to T_3. *The small but effective transfer of T_4 from mother to fetus seems to be important for fetal growth, particularly for early brain development.* TSH does not cross the placenta. Thyrotropin releasing hormone (TRH) crosses the placenta but it does not have a known effect on fetal thyroid function. Iodine also crosses the placenta and the fetal thyroid starts concentrating it by 10-12 weeks. Excess iodine causes fetal goiter and hypothyroidism. At birth thyroid hormone profile reaches normal value after a few hours. Normal thyroid hormone level in the newborn is crucial for subsequent brain maturation and intellectual development.

Laboratory reference values in pregnancy are summarized in Table 42.1.

Table 42.1: Reference values in pregnancy	
Test	Pregnancy changes
Thyroid stimulating hormone	None
Thyroid binding globulin	Increases
Total thyroxine (T_4)	Increases
Total triiodothyronine (T_3)	Increases
T_3 total resin uptake (T_3RU)	Decreases
Free T_4	None
Free T_3	None

Indications of Thyroid Function Test During Pregnancy

Indications of thyroid function test during pregnancy are as follows:
a. Women on thyroid hormones
b. Family history of autoimmune thyroiditis
c. Presence of goiter
d. Past history of radiation to thyroid
e. Type 1 diabetes.

HYPERTHYROIDISM IN PREGNANCY

Incidence and Causes

Hyperthyroidism affects 1:2000 pregnancies. *Grave's disease* accounts for 90% of cases. Other causes of hyperthyroidism in pregnancy are—toxic adenoma, subacute thyroiditis, iatrogenic ingestion of thyroxine, transient hyperthyroidism secondary to hyperemesis gravidarum and gestational trophoblastic disease.

Complications of Hyperthyroidism in Pregnancy

a. *Maternal:* Maternal complications are spontaneous abortion, pregnancy induced hypertension, preterm delivery, anemia, higher susceptibility to infection, placental abruptio. In untreated and severe cases, there can be cardiac arrhythmias, congestive heart failure and thyroid storm.
b. *Fetal:* There can be fetal and neonatal hyperthyroidism, intrauterine growth restriction (IUGR), stillbirth, prematurity and morbidity related to antithyroid medications. Most maternal and neonatal complications are seen in cases of uncontrolled or untreated hyperthyroidism.

Graves' Disease

Etiopathogenesis

Graves' disease is caused by maternal thyroid stimulating antibody (TsAb) belonging to immunoglobulin (IgG) class which binds with high affinity to TSH receptors. TsAb can cross the placenta, bind to fetal TSH receptors and cause fetal or neonatal hyperthyroidism. However, the placenta acts as a partial barrier, so usually only those with high titers are likely to be affected.

Diagnosis

Clinical presentation: The diagnosis may not be easy, particular in mild cases because normal pregnant women may experience symptoms resembling thyrotoxicosis as heat intolerance, warm and moist skin, tachycardia and systolic flow murmur on cardiac auscultation. The following signs should raise a suspicion—goiter, tachycardia on awakening from sleep or resting pulse >100 bpm, eye involvement, weight loss or failure to gain weight despite a good appetite. The thyroid enlargement usually is diffuse with a firm consistency. Hand tremors, proximal muscle weakness, hyperkinesis and hyperdynamic cardiovascular system may be present.

Laboratory Investigation

It will confirm elevated FT_4, T_3 and FT_3 levels and a suppressed or undetectable TSH level. Thyroid stimulating antibody titers (TsAb) will be elevated in significant number of cases.

Treatment

Treatment during pregnancy almost always consists of *antithyroid medications*. The aim of treatment should be to maintain mild hyperthyroidism in the mother to avoid thyroid dysfunction in the fetus. **The principal group of drug used is thionamides which include prophylthiouracil, methimazole and carbimazole**. They block the synthesis of T_4 and T_3 and also cause immunosuppression. *Prophylthiouracil* is drug of choice. Therapy is initiated at a dose of 200–450 mg/day and then reduced to minimum effective dose; once euthyroidism is achieved (maintenance dose is usually 50-300 mg/day).

Methimazole: It is an alternative treatment. It is not the first line drug due to reports of scalp defects (aplasia cutis) and esophageal or choanal atresia in newborns exposed to methimazole.* Dose is 10-45 mg, but starting at lower dose of 10-15 mg reduces the incidence of side effects like skin rash.

Monitoring of Women on Antithyroid Drug

Thyroid function test should be done during pregnancy using TSH and FT_4 every 2-8 weeks depending on the control. *Women who are euthyroid on small dose (PTU ≤ 100 mg/day, methimazole ≤ 10 mg/day) for 4 weeks can stop taking the medication by 32-34 weeks gestation under supervision.* This minimizes the risk of fetal or neonatal hypothyroidism. Therapy can be resumed if symptoms recur. Women with large goiter, long standing hyperthyroidism or significant eye involvement should remain on treatment throughout the pregnancy. Other side effects of antithyroid drugs are—pruritis, skin rash, urticaria, cholestatic side effect and polyarthritis. Leukopenia may be a medication effect but is also seen in untreated Graves' disease, so a WBC count should be obtained before start of treatment. *Agranulocytosis is the serious complication but uncommon.* So a sore throat should be thoroughly investigated. Beta-blockers propranalol 20-40 mg every 6-8 hours can be used for symptomatic relief in severe cases but only for short period and before 34-36 weeks gestation.

Fetal Monitoring

The Graves' disease in pregnancy poses a dual risk to the fetus. PTU can cross the placenta and iatrogenic fetal hypothyroidism can be produced. Beside this there can be fetal thyrotoxicosis due to transplacental transfer of thyroid stimulating antibodies. Thus, it is recommended that fetal thyroid size should be monitored by periodic ultrasound examination from 20 weeks onward. There is role of cord blood sampling if:
a. Ultrasound shows fetal goiter
b. Growth restriction
c. Hydrops
d. High maternal antibodies level. Women who have had Graves' disease treated by surgery may be euthyroid but still have active antibodies. So, TSH receptor antibodies should be measured in these women and women with active Graves' disease. If antibody levels are low,

---

* In recent studies, the relationship found between aplasia cutis and methimazole is not proved.

involvement of fetus is unlikely. If antibody levels are high, fetal and neonatal thyroid function should be checked by cord sampling and in peripheral samples respectively.

e. *Uncertain fetal thyroid status. Fetal hyperthyroidism is treated by increasing maternal antithyroid medication and hypothyroidism is treated by reducing dose of antithyroid drugs.*

Breastfeeding is allowed if the total daily dose of PTU is < 150 mg or methimazole < 10 mg. The medication should be given immediately after each feeding and the infant should be monitored periodically.

Role of Surgical Treatment

Surgery is performed only in exceptional situations as— (a) Allergic reaction to all drugs (b) Lack of response to large dosage, drug resistance and noncompliance. *Radioactive iodine therapy for gland ablation is contraindicated in pregnancy.*

Effect of Pregnancy on Graves' Disease

Patient tends to have aggravation of symptoms during the first half, followed by amelioration of symptoms during the second half of pregnancy. There is again recurrence of symptoms in postpartum period. This is thought to be due to relative immunosuppression of pregnancy.

Neonatal Assessment

Close monitoring is required in babies born to hyperthyroid mother. There can be transient thyrotoxicosis 7-10 days after birth, once the antithyroid drugs have cleared from the fetal plasma due to the presence of circulating maternal autoantibodies. In this situation newborn may have symptom like vomiting, diarrhea, dehydration, weight loss, irritability and poor feeding. Usually the condition is self limiting but symptomatic and supportive treatment is required. *In untreated newborn, mortality can be 15%.*

Thyroid Storm

It is a hypermetabolic state, fever and change in mental status. This is life threatening complication which can occur during labor or cesarean section or infection in antenatal or postnatal period or in patients with gestational trophoblastic disease. It is treated with symptomatic and supportive treatment of fever, tachycardia, and severe dehydration. Mainstays of therapy are—(a) Thionamide (b) PTU (c) β blocking agent (d) Steroid (e) Iodine (f) Ipodate (to block thyroid hormone release). Any associated hypertension, infection or anemia is treated.

HYPOTHYROIDISM IN PREGNANCY

Serious hypothyroidism is rare in pregnancy because of associated anovulation and infertility. *Overt hypo-thyroidism has been reported 1 in 1000 to 1 in 1600 deliveries, but subclinical hypothyroidism (elevated TSH, normal T4) is found in 0.19-2.5% of pregnancies.*

Cause of Maternal Hypothyroidism

Most common cause is autoimmune thyroid disease. Goitrous form is more common than atrophic form. Other causes are previous treatment of Graves' disease by radioactive iodine or subtotal thyroidectomy or excessive doses of PTU for Graves' disease.

Effect of Hypothyroidism of Pregnancy

a. *Effect on mother:* There is significantly increased risk of spontaneous abortion, pregnancy induced hypertension, placental abruptio, preterm labor, postpartum hemorrhage and cardiac dysfunction.
b. *Effect on fetus:* Preterm delivery, low birth weight and perinatal death.

Clinical Diagnosis

Symptoms and Signs

Symptoms may include fatigue, sleepiness, lethargy and mental slowing, sadness, and cold intolerance, weight gain despite poor appetite, arthralgia, and muscle pain. **Signs** can be dry and pale skin, hoarse voice, bradycardia, hyporeflexia, carpal tunnel syndrome and a diffuse or nodular goiter.

Laboratory Investigation

The best laboratory test is TSH level. It allows very early diagnosis and accurate treatment monitoring. Other tests include Free T4 and antibody titers. Anemia is present in 30-40% of cases.

Management

a. *Prepregnancy management:* Hypothyroid women should have prepregnancy counseling. The thyroxine dose is adjusted to achieve TSH level below 2.5 µ/lit. Women with autoimmune thyroid disease and other autoimmune disease like type 1 diabetes should be screened for TSH.
b. *Antenatal management:* Fetal thyroid starts functioning by 12-14 weeks, the fetal serum T4 level gradually increasing up to 18 weeks. As fetus is entirely dependent on the mother for its thyroid supply in 1st trimester and later for iodine. Supplemental thyroxine should be given from early pregnancy. Treatment is 1.6 µg/kg of levothyroxine with variation on an individual basis. Usually women being already treated for hypothyroidism require an increase (20-50%) in thyroxine during pregnancy. In postpartum period, the dose

should be immediately decreased to prepregnancy level. All women should undergo a thyroid function test 4-6 weeks after delivery.

c. **Neonatal assessment:** There seems to have no significant effect on neonatal thyroid function. Undiagnosed or untreated maternal hypothyroidism is associated with lower intelligence quotient and poor cognitive function in offspring. However, neonatal hypothyroidism unrelated to maternal disease occurs in about 1 in 3500 newborn and routine screening is performed in many developed countries.

Hypothyroidism in Iodine Deficient Area

In iodine deficiency, the maternal thyroid gland has a greater affinity for iodide than placenta thus fetus is prone to cretinism. **It is the leading preventable cause of mental retardation worldwide.** Iodine administration prior to conception and up to second trimester improves neonatal outcome by protecting the fetal brain. Iodination of water, salt or flour can easily supplement this deficiency. But high level of iodine intake can cause fetal hyperthyroidism.

Postpartum Thyroiditis

It occurs 1-8 months in postpartum period. It may affect 5% of parturient.

Etiopathogenesis

Autoimmune thyroid disease is suppressed to some degree by the immunologic changes in pregnancy. In postpartum period, there is destructive thyroiditis associated with thyroid microsomal autoantibodies. *Women at risk are with a personal or family history of autoimmune disease, or history of previous postpartum episode of thyroiditis and insulin requiring diabetes mellitus.*

Clinical Presentation

Usually, there is initial hyperthyroidism (1-4 month), followed by hypothyroidism (5-8 months). Hyperthyroidism is similarly diagnosed by a low TSH and presence of antibodies. On investigation, diagnosis is confirmed by elevated TSH and antithyroid peroxidase (TPO) antibodies (Hypothyroid state).

Treatment

Spontaneous resolution usually occurs in most of the patients. Treatment in immediate postpartum period is only symptomatic that is β blockers for the hyperthyroid phase and low dose levothyroxine or triiodothyronine for the hypothyroid phase.

Prognosis

The risk of recurrence in subsequent pregnancies is up to 70%. Long-term risk of developing hypothyroidism is 2-5% per year, so monitoring of thyroid function must be continued after every pregnancy and after that yearly.

Solitary Thyroid Nodule During Pregnancy

Ultrasound examination reveals the cystic and solid nature of nodule. Solid nodules are more likely to be malignant and fine needle aspiration or tissue biopsy should be done. Surgery of nodule during second trimester has a low complication rate. ***Radioactive iodine should never be given during pregnancy.***

43 Jaundice, Hepatitis and Gastrointestinal Disorders in Pregnancy

*He who becomes the master of all,
becomes the rightful pioneer of the great.*

JAUNDICE AND HEPATITIS IN PREGNANCY

Jaundice can be caused by many diseases, but viral hepatitis is the most common cause of jaundice in pregnancy. In India, jaundice is seen in 1 in 1000 pregnancy.

Physiological Changes in Liver During Pregnancy

The liver is not palpable in normal pregnancy. There is moderate increase in alkaline phosphatase, cholesterol and serum globulin in last trimester, so there is mild cholestasis in normal pregnancy but serum bilirubin and transaminase level are within normal limit. *10-15% of normal women may have bilirubin level over 1.0 mg% due to delayed excretion of bilirubin which cause pruritis in pregnancy.*

Causes of Jaundice in Pregnancy

They may be related or a coincidental cause of jaundice in pregnancy. Table 43.1 describes causes of jaundice in pregnancy.

Table 43.1: Causes of jaundice in pregnancy

I. Intercurrent jaundice in pregnancy:
   a. Viral hepatitis A to E
   b. Cholelithiasis
   c. Hepatotoxic drugs
II. Jaundice specific to pregnancy:
   a. Acute fatty liver of pregnancy
   b. Intrahepatic cholestasis of pregnancy
   c. Severe PIH and eclampsia
   d. Severe hyperemesis
III. Pregnancy superimposed on pre-existing liver disease:
   a. Familial hemolytic jaundice
   b. Crigler-Najjar syndrome

Liver Disease Unrelated to Pregnancy

Viral Hepatitis

Viral hepatitis is the most common cause of jaundice in pregnancy in the tropics. Hepatitis is more common in ill-nourished mothers, living in unhygienic environment. In tropic, it can occur as an epidemic form. At present 6 distinct types of highly contagious hepatitis virus have been identified.

a. **Hepatitis A:** It may occur sporadically or in epidemics. The primary mode of transmission is oral fecal route. A generalized viremia occurs with the infection that is predominantly hepatic. Disease is usually self-limited and fulminant hepatitis is rare. Both blood and stool are infectious during the 2-6 weeks incubation period. Perinatal transmission does not occur.

b. **Hepatitis B:** It is global health problem. Hepatitis B is transmitted by inoculation of infected blood and blood products or sexual intercourse. The virus is contained in most body secretions. Infection occurs by parenteral and sexual contact. *The risk of transmission to fetus ranges from 10% in first trimester to as high as 90% in third trimester and it is specially high (90%) from those mother who are seropositive to hepatitis B surface antigen (HbSAg) and e antigen (HbeAg).*[*]
Approximately 10% of the infected patients will go to the chronic state. They are at high risk of developing chronic active hepatitis, cirrhosis and hepatocellular carcinoma. *Neonatal transmission mainly occurs at or*

---

[*] The likelihood of prenatal transmission of HBV correlates with the presence of Hbe antigen. 90% of Hbe antigen positive mothers but only 10-15% of anti-Hbe positive mother will transmit HBV infection to the offspring.

around the time of birth through mixing of maternal blood and genital secretion. Approximately 25% of the carrier neonate will die from cirrhosis or hepatic carcinoma between late childhood to early adulthood. HBV is not teratogenic.

Maternal infection: The acute infection is manifested by flu like illness as malaise, anorexia, nausea and vomiting. There may be arthralgia and skin rash. In majority, it remains asymptomatic. Jaundice is rare and fever is uncommon. Spontaneous resolution occurs in 90% and about 1% will die of fulminating hepatitis.

Diagnosis of hepatitis B: Diagnosis is confirmed by serological detection of HbSAg, HbeAg (denote high infectivity) and antibodies to hepatitis B core antigen (HbCAg). Chronic carriers are diagnosed by presence of HbSAg and Anti-HBC antibody 6 months after initial dose.

Screening of hepatitis B: All pregnant women should be screened for hepatitis B viruses infection at first antenatal visit and it should be repeated in third trimester for high risk group like I/v drug abusers.

c. **Hepatitis C:** It is recognized as the major cause of Non-A, Non-B hepatitis. Transmission is mainly blood borne and to a lesser extent by fecal oral route. It can cause chronic active hepatitis and hepatocellular failure. *Perinatal transmission is 10-40%.* Detection can be done by recombinant immunoblot assay (RIBA—3).

d. **Hepatitis D:** It is an RNA virus. This agent can cause infection only when HbSAg positivity exists. Hepatitis D is isolated in up to 50% of cases of fulminant hepatitis B infection. Hepatitis D antigen (HDAg) and hepatitis D antibody (HDAb) are serologic markers for the disease.

e. **Hepatitis E:** It is transmitted via oral fecal route. It can be endemic in developing countries. The disease is self-limited, does not result in a chronic carrier state. In pregnancy if acutely infected can have a 15% risk of fulminant liver failure with a 5% mortality rate.

f. **Hepatitis G:** It is more likely to be found in people infected with hepatitis B or C or with a history of injection drug use. There is no chronic carrier state. There can be vertical transmission.

Clinical Features

The clinical picture of hepatitis is highly variable. Most patients have asymptomatic infection but few may present with fulminant disease. Interestingly viruses are not actually hepatotoxic. *It is the immune response to virus that causes hepatocellular necrosis.* It has usually following phase:

a. *Prodromal phase:* In this phase there are constitutional symptoms like nausea, vomiting, low grade fever, fatigue, loss of appetite and upper abdominal pain. The pain is due to stretching of the peritoneum over enlarged liver. Myalgia and arthralgia sometime precede the onset of jaundice by 1-2 weeks. Patient may notice dark colored or yellow urine.

b. *Icteric phase:* In this phase temperature subsides and clinical jaundice appears. Liver may be palpable and tender. The spleen is palpable in about 20% of cases.

c. *Recovery phase:* The jaundice recedes, the urine and stool regain their color and the liver enlargement regresses. It may take 6-12 weeks for complete recovery. Most fatalities are due to fulminant hepatic necrosis, which in later pregnancy must be differentiated from acute fatty liver. Hepatic encephalopathy is the usual presentation of patients with fulminant hepatitis with mortality of 80%. About 50% of patient with fulminant hepatitis have infection with hepatitis B viruses.

Laboratory Investigations

a. *Liver function test:* The plasma bilirubin levels affect the severity of jaundice. There is a fall in serum albumin with an increase in gamma globulin. The alkaline phosphatase activity is either normal or mildly raised. Prolonged prothrombin time is a reliable indication of severe liver damage. Bilirubinuria is an early finding and continues till convalescent period. Serum bilirubin level usually peak at 5-20 mg/dl. Serum aminotransferase level varies. Peak level of 400-40000/liter is usually reached by the time jaundice develops. Serum alkaline phosphatase remains normal or initially elevated.

b. *Serologic markers:* Anti-HA IgM, HbSAg, HC PCR, anti-HbC IgM, HDPCR, Anti-HE IgM and Anti-HG IgM are serological markers for defining type of hepatitis. They can be done as guided by clinical situations.

c. *Ultrasound examination:* Ultrasound examination of liver and biliary tract is helpful in the diagnosis of other causes of jaundice in pregnancy such as fatty liver, obstructive jaundice or chronic liver disease.

Management

Treatment of acute viral hepatitis is supportive. Rest should be instituted during the acute phase of illness. If nausea, vomiting or anorexia is prominent, intravenous hydration and general supportive measures are instituted. Drug metabolized by liver should be avoided. Ursodeoxycholic acid or cholestyramine may be used if there is marked pruritis. Antepartum fetal assessment should be instituted in the third trimester because of the increased risk for premature delivery and stillbirth. **There is no place for termination of pregnancy.** In labor vitamin K 5 mg intramuscularly is given to raise the prothrombin time. Prophylactic ergometrine is to be given.

For prevention of complications: Hypokalemia, hypoglycemia and hypocalcemia are corrected by regular blood check up. Lactulose (15-30 ml three times daily) reduces colonic amonia absorption and acts as an osmotic laxative.

Prevention and Prophylaxis

Immunoglobulin prophylaxis should be given to pregnant women within 2 weeks of exposure to hepatitis A. Two hepatitis A vaccines using inactivated viruses are available and can be used during pregnancy but its use in developing country is very limited. Hepatitis B Ig can be given to patients who are parenterally or sexually exposed to blood or secretions from hepatitis B infected individuals. Hepatitis B vaccine also should be administered to HBSAg negative patients. Hepatitis B Ig 0.5 ml intramuscularly and hepatitis B vaccine with a repeat dose at 1 and 6 months should be administered to neonates born of HbSAg positive mothers, to decrease the risk of vertical transmission. Passive and active immunization of the newborn is 85-95% effective in preventing perinatal transmission of hepatitis B virus. Breastfeeding is not contraindicated with hepatitis B as long as the infant has been immunized.

LIVER PROBLEMS UNIQUE TO PREGNANCY

Intrahepatic Cholestasis of Pregnancy

Intrahepatic cholestasis of pregnancy occurs usually in the third trimester of pregnancy but can begin earlier. The most characteristic symptom is pruritis, which is more severe at night. Laboratory test shows mild hyperbilirubinemia, elevated level of bile acids. Alkaline phosphatase level is moderately increased and serum aminotransferase are normal or only minimally elevated. The intrahepatic cholestasis of pregnancy generally progresses until time of delivery. After delivery pruritis disappears usually within 24-48 hours. ICP may recur in subsequent pregnancies in 60-70% of cases. Cholestasis may return with use of oral contraceptive pill.

Effect of ICP on Pregnancy

The long-term prognosis for mother is good, though these women have higher incidence of gallstones. The fetus can be affected adversely. There is a high risk of premature labor and delivery, fetal distress during labor (19-60%) and Meconium aspiration (35-45%). The mechanisms of adverse fetal effect are not known but these events are attributed to elevated bile acids in circulation which increases uterine contraction and fetal colonic muscle contraction.

Treatment

Treatment is primarily symptomatic for pruritis. Ursodeoxycholic acid (UDCA) is a hydrophilic bile acid that improves cholestasis by stimulating biliary excretion of toxic acids. UDCA is safe in pregnancy and given in dose of 15-20 mg/kg/day.

Fetal surveillance is necessary in all women with ICP, especially in case of twin pregnancy with biweekly nonstress test and biophysical profile. *Pregnancy is usually terminated electively at 38 weeks and earlier for women who have jaundice, after fetal lung maturity has been documented.*

Acute Fatty Liver of Pregnancy (AFLP)

It is a rare complication in pregnancy (incidence is 1 in 5000 to 1 in 13000), which occurs in the third trimester.

Etiopathogenesis

Current evidence suggests that recessively inherited mitochondrial abnormalities of fatty acid oxidation such as deficiency of long chain 3-hydroxyacyl-coenzyme (LCHAD) predisposes women to fatty liver in pregnancy.

Clinical Presentation

It usually manifests late in pregnancy, more common in nulliparous and multifetal gestation. Typically, there is onset over several days to weeks of malaise, anorexia, nausea and vomiting, epigastric pain and progressive jaundice. Vomiting may be presenting symptom. There may be signs suggestive of pre-eclampsia.

Diagnosis

Laboratory values shows markedly elevated **AST** and **ALT** levels (up to 7 times normal) and may show markedly elevated bilirubin level and prolonged prothrombin time. There is hypoglycemia in 30% of cases, low platelet count and fibrinogen level. There is elevated serum creatinine level and elevated liver enzyme level.

Complications

Acute renal failure, DIC, encephalopathy and sepsis.

Management

Supportive care and prompt delivery is the principal of management. Intravenous glucose, blood products, broad spectrum antibiotic coverage and pulmonary support are critical. The total bilirubin level may continue to rise for up to 10 days after delivery and this should not be taken as an indication for liver transplant, which is not needed in acute fatty liver of pregnancy. During recovery, there can be evidence for transient diabetes insipidus, pancreatitis and ascites.

Prognosis

Termination of pregnancy and extensive supportive therapy has reduced the mortality rate to approximately 5-10%.

HELLP SYNDROME

HELLP syndrome in some respects mimics acute fatty liver of pregnancy. This liver derangement is a variant of severe pre-eclampsia or eclampsia. This disorder occurs in the last trimester of pregnancy.

CHOLELITHIASIS IN PREGNANCY

Cholelithiasis is noted in 6% of pregnant women. Pregnancy induced changes in the bile composition is decreased bile salt pool in the second trimester, increased cholesterol level and slow emptying of the gallbladder. All these factors increase the risk of cholelithiasis. Laparoscopic cholecystectomy for biliary colic can be safely performed in the first and early second trimester of pregnancy.

OTHER DISORDERS OF GASTROINTESTINAL TRACT IN PREGNANCY

Reflux Esophagitis

Heartburn is common symptoms in late pregnancy. This retrosternal burning sensation is caused by esophagitis of the lower gastroesophageal reflux related to relaxation of the lower esophageal sphincter. Raising the head of the bed and ingestion of oral antacid usually relieve the symptoms. In unresponsive patient, H_2 receptor antagonist is prescribed. Both cemitidine and ranitidine are safe.

Peptic Ulcer

During pregnancy, there is remission of symptoms in women with proven peptic ulcer disease. Because during pregnancy gastric secretion is reduced, motility is decreased and there is considerably increased mucus secretion. Antacids are first line therapy and H_2 receptor blockers are prescribed for those who do not respond. Proton pump inhibitors such as Omperazole are not recommended during pregnancy. Sucralfate provides a protective coating at the ulcer base and is considered safe. Supportive advice can be given regarding rest, avoidance of stress, bland frequent diet and cessation of smoking. Eradication of *Helicobacter pylori* if indicated can be treated with Azithromycin and bismuth compound. Endoscopy, if indicated, can be performed.

Inflammatory Bowel Disease

These disorders are two forms of intestinal inflammation as **ulcerative colitis and Crohn's disease**. Pregnancy does not increase the likelihood of an attack of inflammatory bowel disease but active disease at conception increases the probability of poor pregnancy outcome. So women with inflammatory bowel disease should be encouraged to conceive during period of disease remission. Management is not effected by pregnancy. Oral or rectal salazopyrin, mesalazine and steroid can be safely used throughout pregnancy and breastfeeding.

ACUTE ABDOMINAL PAIN RESULTING FROM NONOBSTETRIC CAUSES

Introduction

Evaluation and treatment of the pregnant women with acute abdominal pain represents a challenging clinical dilemma that demands great care and judgment. The etiology of acute abdominal pain in pregnancy can be separated into obstetric related and nonobstetric causes (Table 43.2). Here we will deal with nonobstetric causes of acute abdomen pain. Management is also more difficult because intervention may adversely affect the pregnancy outcome and concern about harming the fetus may delay treatment.

Table 43.2: Causes of acute abdomen pain during pregnancy	
Pregnancy related	Nonobstetrical causes
• Abortion • Ectopic pregnancy • Cystitis, Pyelonephritis • Torsion of ovarian cyst • Degenerating myoma • Abruptio placenta • Pre-eclampsia • Chorioamnionitis • Preterm labor • Uterine rupture	• Appendicitis • Cholecystitis • Intestinal obstruction • Pancreatitis • Renal/ureteric colic • Acid peptic disease

Pathophysiology Changes During Pregnancy

These changes may modify symptoms and clinical responses from that of nonpregnant status. At 12 weeks gestation the uterine fundus rises from the pelvis and becomes an abdominal organ. The intestines and omentum are displaced superiorly and laterally. Appendix is more likely to be closer to gallbladder, than to McBurney's point by late pregnancy. Leukocyte count is elevated up to 12000-16000/ml. Levels which overlap with intra-abdominal inflammatory condition such as appendicitis.

Fetal Consideration

In optimal care of pregnant surgical patient the potential hazards to the fetus should be minimized. So risk associated with maternal disease, diagnostic radiologic procedures, drugs, anesthetic and surgery to fetus should be considered. Ultrasound and MRI are considered safe to fetus. Limited diagnostic CT or X-ray procedure can be undertaken with lead shielding of fetus.

Diagnostic Consideration

a. *Pain:* Pain is the most prominent symptoms encountered with acute abdominal pain. Generalized abdominal pain, guarding and rebound tenderness suggest peritonitis. Cramping with lower central abdominal pain suggest a uterine disorder. Lower abdominal pain on either side suggests torsion, rupture or hemorrhage of ovarian cyst or tumor. Mild abdominal pain early in gestation suggests an intestinal origin. Upper abdominal pain is often related to the liver, spleen, gallbladder, stomach, duodenum or pancreas.

b. *Other symptoms:* Abdominal pain with nausea and vomiting after first trimester usually suggests a gastrointestinal disorder. **Nausea, vomiting with inability to pass flatus or stool points to an intestinal obstruction.** Associated syncope with signs of peritoneal irritation indicates an acute abdominal emergency with rupture of viscera or hemorrhage. A high grade temperature suggests infection. Vaginal bleeding usually points to an intrauterine problem.

c. *History taking and examination:* The patient with an acute abdomen should undergo careful assessment of reproductive organs and her vital signs. General condition, bowel sounds, abdominal rigidity, tenderness and presence or absence of mass should be carefully noted. Examination should be gentle and slow using the flat part of hand and starting from an asymptomatic area.

Principle of Surgical Management

a. Delay in diagnosis and performance of surgery is the factor primarily responsible for increased maternal morbidity and mortality and perinatal loss. When there are unmistakable signs of peritonitis, intestinal strangulation and intra-abdominal hemorrhage, immediate surgical exploration is indicated.
b. In subacute condition, caution should be used in deciding to proceed with surgery.
c. Essential of good preoperative care are adequate hydration, availability of blood transfusion and appropriate preoperative medication that will not decrease oxygenation for mother and fetus.
d. At operation, the least extensive procedure necessary should be performed with as little manipulation of the uterus as possible.
e. In postoperative care, over sedation, and fluid and electrolyte imbalance are to be avoided. Fetal monitoring should be done in last 4 months of pregnancy.
f. In recent times, laparoscopic surgery can be performed during pregnancy. The benefits of this approach are decreased hospitalization time, decreased use of narcotics and faster return to normal diet.
g. **Anesthetic risk:**
   - Delayed gastric emptying time and increased residual gastric volume, which increases risk of aspiration of gastric contents during intubation.
   - There can be difficult intubation due to hyperemia.
   - Risk of supine maternal and fetal hypotension.
   - Decreased functional residual capacity may lower oxygen reserve enough to significantly lower pO_2 in short period of apnea. So, 100% oxygen is given prior to attempt at intubation.

Management of Specific Condition

Appendicitis: Incidence of acute appendicitis is 0.1-1.4/1000 pregnancy (1 in 1500 deliveries). Appendicitis more often occur in the middle trimester and perforation of the appendix is more towards later pregnancy. The clinical presentation is same as in nonpregnant patient. There is vague pain on right side of the abdomen, nausea and vomiting. There is leukocytosis. MRI imaging and appendiceal computed tomography is more sensitive and accurate than ultrasound to confirm suspected appendicitis.

Treatment: **Treatment of nonperforated acute appendicitis complicating pregnancy is appendicectomy.** Antibiotics are generally administered prior to and after surgery. Under appropriate conditions, laparoscopic appendectomy is as safe as open appendectomy.

Prognosis: With appropriate following of principles of management, maternal mortality is quite low and perinatal loss in 13-25%.

Acute intestinal obstruction: It is estimated to occur in approximately one-third of every 10,000 pregnancies. But it is the third most common nonobstetric reason for laparotomy during pregnancy (following appendicitis and biliary tract disease). The most common causes of mechanical obstruction are adhesion (60%) and volvulus (25%) followed by intussusception, hernia and neoplasm.

Clinical findings: The classical triad of abdominal pain, vomiting and obstipation is observed in pregnant and non-pregnant women with intestinal obstruction. Diagnosis is confirmed by radiological studies, which should be done when intestinal obstruction is suspected.

Treatment: It is same as in nonpregnant state. The basic of treatment are bowel decompression, intravenous hydration, correction of electrolyte imbalance, Ryle's tube aspiration of gastric contents and timely surgery when indicated. *Surgery is indicated if perforation or gangrenous bowel is suspected or when the patient symptoms do not resolve with medical management.* A vertical midline incision is preferred. The entire bowel should be examined carefully because there may be more than one area of obstruction or limited bowel viability.

Prognosis: Intestinal obstruction in pregnancy is associated with a maternal mortality rate of 6%. Causes of mortality are secondary to infection and irreversible shock. Early diagnosis and treatment is essential for improving the outcome. Perinatal mortality is approximately 20% and result from maternal hypotension and resultant fetal hypoxia and acidosis.

Cholecystitis and Cholelithiasis

Asymptomatic cholelithiasis occurs in 3-4% of pregnant women and is cause of over 90% of cases of cholecystitis in pregnancy. Steady right upper abdominal pain with nausea and anorexia are presenting symptoms. Ultrasound confirms the diagnosis.

Treatment: Medical treatment is preferred in pregnancy. Initial treatment is no oral intake, I/v hydration, rest, pain relief and antibiotic, if febrile. Most women respond to this treatment. However, surgery if needed for failed medical treatment is the best performed in the second trimester.

Ovarian Cyst and Adnexal Torsion

Ovarian cyst may cause acute abdominal pain because of torsion or rupture. Adnexal torsion may occur with normal adnexa, but usually occurs with adnexal cystic lesions, neoplastic lesions, or hyperstimulated ovaries. The majority of torsion occurs in the first half of the pregnancy.

Diagnosis: Patient usually presents with unilateral pelvic pain with vomiting. Ultrasound may demonstrate a pelvic mass and absent flow on Doppler evaluation.

Treatment: Adnexal torsion is a surgical emergency because of the potential danger of permanent destruction of the organ involved, peritonitis and even death. The traditional treatment is surgical removal of adnexa. Untwisting and preservation of ovary has also been found successful.

Pancreatitis

Acute pancreatitis complicates 1 in 1000 -10000 pregnancies. Gallbladder disease is the most common cause. Medication, infection and hyperlipidemia are less frequent causes. Signs and symptoms are like in nonpregnant state.

Treatment: Patients with pancreatic abscess, ruptured pseudocyst or hemorrhagic pancreatitis may require surgical treatment.

Surgical Condition with Left Upper Quadrant Pain

a. *Splenic rupture:* The hypovolemia and relative anemia associated with pregnancy contributes to hypersplenism and increased risk for spontaneous rupture.
b. *Splenic artery aneurysm rupture:* This is rare catastrophic event but 25% of these cases occur in pregnant women. Diseased vessels are further compromised by the moderate displacement of the spleen by the gravid uterus and pregnancy induced hypersplenism.

Immediate laparotomy is warranted. Despite prompt treatment, mortality is high.

Hemorrhoids in Pregnancy

Approximately one-third of pregnant patients suffer from hemorrhoid. It is due to secondary to increased tendency of constipation, increased rectal venous pressure and increased intra-abdominal pressure. Mild hemorrhoids respond well to increased dietary fiber intake and hemorrhoidal suppository. Severe hemorrhoids can be treated with banding. When there is complication of thrombosis or severe pain, hemorrhoidectomy is indicated.

Uterine Leiomyoma

Acute pain from myoma during pregnancy is usually caused by degeneration secondary to inadequacy of blood supply to the myoma. Pain and tenderness are generally localized and can be severe. Low grade fever and leukocytosis can occur. Ultrasound helps in making the diagnosis. *Management is nonsurgical with use of analgesic, rest, I/v hydration and observation for preterm labor.*

44 Renal Disorders in Pregnancy

When I have listened to my mistake, I have grown.

GENERAL CONSIDERATION

Anatomical Changes in Renal System During Pregnancy

During normal pregnancy, the kidney enlarge approximately 1 cm in length with the right kidney enlarging slightly more than left kidney. By the second month of pregnancy the renal pelvis and ureter also begin to increase in size, more so on the right side. The ureter increases in diameter by 2 cm and right and left renal pelvis dilates on average 15 mm and 5 mm respectively. The dilatation in urinary tract is caused by mechanical obstruction by growing uterus and smooth muscle relaxation from increasing progesterone levels. It increases the incidence of asymptomatic bacteriuria and pyelonephritis. Moreover these changes should be considered in urologic studies.

Physiological Changes in Renal Hemodynamics in Pregnancy

By the second trimester, renal plasma flow increases approximately 75% above baseline and than increases by the end of the third trimester. The glomerular filtration rate is increased almost 50% by end of first trimester and this rate is maintained throughout pregnancy. In women with moderate to severe renal insufficiency, this normal rise in GFR fails to occur. Because of increased GFR there is increased filtration. So the average plasma creatinine and urea level falls by 20-30% as compared to the nonpregnant values. So level in the normal nonpregnant range for, e.g. creatinine level of more than 0.8 mg/dl is usually taken as abnormal in pregnancy.

The serum angiotensin system is stimulated which leads to sodium and water retention resulting in edema in nearly 80% of antenatal woman, though there is no changes in serum sodium concentration. Protein secretion is increased in pregnancy due to increased filtration, so urinary protein up to 300 mg/24 hrs is considered normal in pregnancy.

URINARY TRACT INFECTIONS

Asymptomatic bacteriuria, acute cystitis and acute pyelonephritis are common disorders in pregnancy. The anatomical and physiological changes of pregnancy—which are ureteric dilatation, increased bladder volume and decreased bladder tone, with decreased ureteral tone, glycosuria and increase in urinary amino acids—all contributes to increased chances of urinary tract infection in pregnancy.

Asymptomatic Bacteriuria

This is defined as the presence of actively multiplying bacteria in the urinary tract (count of 10^5/ml bacteria of same species) in the midstream sample of urine on two occasions. The prevalence of asymptomatic bacteriuria in pregnant women is 2.5-11% (VS 3-8% in nonpregnant women). Risk factors for developing asymptomatic bacteriuria are low socioeconomic status, parity, age, sexual practice, and medical conditions such as diabetes and sickle cell trait.

Effect on Pregnancy

If asymptomatic bacteriuria is left untreated in pregnancy, up to 40% of patients will develop symptoms of urinary tract infection (UTI) and 25-30% of women will develop acute pyelonephritis. While if asymptomatic bacteriuria adequately treated, the rate of UTI is only 10%. Asymptomatic bacteriuria has been associated with preterm delivery, fetal loss and pre-eclampsia.

Diagnosis

It is based on isolation of microorganism with a colony count >10^5 organism per ml of urine in a clean catch specimen. The *Escherichia coli* is the most common organism (approximately 80% of cases) found for asymptomatic bacteriuria. The other organisms are *Klebsiella*.

Enterobacteria group, *Gr B Streptococcus* and *Proteus* are responsible for remainder of cases. Urine culture is the gold standard but the draw back are time lag and high cost. Advantages are identification of causative organism and determination of antibiotic sensitivities. Less expensive methods are—Dipstick test for nitrite and leukocyte esterase. But it has relatively poor predictive value. In routine urine microscopy presence of protein, white and red blood cells and bacteria are suggestive of UTI but have a sensitivity of 25-67%.

Table 44.1: Antibiotic regimen for treatment of asymptomatic bacteriuria

Antibiotic	Drug category in pregnancy	Dosage
Cephalexin	B	250 mg 2-4 times daily
Erythromycin	B	250-500 mg 4 times daily
Nitrofurantoin	B	50-100 mg 4 times daily
Amoxicillin Clavulanic acid	B	250 mg 4 times daily

Treatment

The initial antibiotic selection should be empirical. As most common causative organism is *E. coli*, sulfonamides, nitrofurantoin or cephalosporins are good choice and safe for mother and fetus. A 5-14 days course of one of these drugs will effectively eradicate asymptomatic bacteriuria in majority of cases. A urine culture should be repeated 1-2 weeks after therapy is started and monthly for rest of pregnancy. The recurrence rate for all regimens is about 30%. The drug regimen is listed in Table 44.1. Sulfa drugs are best avoided in pregnancy because of increased likelihood of neonatal hyperbilirubinemia. Tetracycline is contraindicated because of risk of dental staining in exposed child. Trimethoprim is a folic acid antagonist so trimethoprim sulfamethoxazole is generally avoided in period of organogenesis.

Acute Cystitis

It is uncommon in pregnancy (1%). The causative organisms are same as that of asymptomatic bacteriuria. The symptoms are increased urinary frequency, dysuria, and urgency and suprapubic discomfort. Urine is often cloudy and malodorous. Diagnosis is confirmed with urine culture and sensitivity. The *treatment* is same as that of asymptomatic bacteriuria (Table 44.1).

Acute Pyelonephritis

It occurs in 1-2% of all pregnant women, and is associated with risk to the mother and fetus. It develops most commonly in the second trimester and in young nulliparous women.

Symptoms

Onset is usually abrupt with fever with chills, flank pain, nausea, headache, increased urinary frequency and dysuria.

Diagnosis

Urine examination shows significant bacteriuria with pyuria and white blood cell cast in the urinary sediments. Diagnosis is confirmed by urine culture. Associated hematuria may indicate urinary calculi.

Effect on Pregnancy and Complication

Complication can be serious and are primarily caused by bacterial endotoxin damage. Endotoxic shock, anemia, leukocytosis, thrombocytopenia, renal insufficiency, adult respiratory distress syndrome can occur if not treated. There can be preterm labor and IUGR and fetal death may be seen in severe cases.

Treatment

Hospitalization is indicated if there are signs of sepsis, vomiting and unable to maintain hydration. Intravenous hydration is given to ensure adequate urinary output. Antibiotics are started as soon as clinical diagnosis is made. Acetaminophen can be used as antipyretic if required. Vital signs including respiratory rate and fluid intake output chart are closely monitored. A first generation cephalosporin as *Cefazolin 1 gm I/V every 8 hours* is effective. *Ceftriaxone 1 gm I/V every 24 hours* is effective for most enterobacteriacia, if there is suspected antibiotic resistance. After that treatment is guided according to culture sensitivity report. When patient is afebrile for 48 hours, parenteral therapy may be changed to an effective oral antibiotic for 14 days. If there is no clinical response in 48-72 hours, a resistant organism can be treated by adding an *aminoglycosides as Gentamicin 3-5 mg/kg per 24 hours in every 8 hours* can be given. Failure to respond may be caused by urolithiasis or a structural urinary tract abnormality. In these cases ultrasound imaging of kidney and urinary tract should be done. Ultrasound also can diagnose perinephric abscess, which is usually due to obstruction complicated by infection. The perinephric abscess must be drained surgically in addition to parenteral antibiotic.

Follow-up and Prognosis

After one episode of pyelonephritis, there are 28% chances of recurrence of bacteriuria and 10% chances of recurrence of pyelonephritis, so antibiotic suppressive therapy with Nitrofurantoin 100 mg orally at bed time or Cephalexin 250 mg daily is continued through pregnancy and puerperium. Periodic culture of urine assists in detection of recurrence.

Relapse

It is defined as the recurrent infection from the same species and type specific strain of organism present before treatment. This presents *treatment failure.*

Reinfection

It is recurrent infection due to a different strain of bacteria following successful treatment of the initial infection occurring >3 weeks after the completion of therapy.

Urinary Calculi

The incidence of urinary calculi is not altered by pregnancy. The incidence is 0.03 to 0.35% of pregnancies. The diagnosis can be made by urine microscopy, by straining urine presence of stones and by ultrasound. If a patient is diagnosed with urolithiasis, serum phosphorus and calcium level estimation can be considered for hyperparathyroidism.

ACUTE RENAL FAILURE

Acute renal failure is defined as urine output less than 400 ml in 24 hours. It occurs infrequently in pregnancy but carries a high mortality rate. So it must be prevented, where possible and treated aggressively.

Causes

Prerenal

a. **Renal hypoperfusion** due to maternal hypotension like obstetrical hemorrhage, septicemia.
b. **Circulating nephrotoxins** (Aminoglycosides)
c. **Mismatched blood transfusion**.
d. **Pre-eclampsia, eclampsia.**
e. **DIC**
f. **Hypoxemia** in chronic lung disease and heart failure.

Renal Type

Intrinsic renal disease like acute glomerulonephritis, pyelonephritis

Post-renal Type

Urinary obstruction from ureteric stone, or retroperitoneal tumor.

Prevention

a. Prompt and vigorous replacement of blood in instances of massive hemorrhage.
b. Termination of pregnancies complicated by severe pre-eclampsia and eclampsia.
c. Close observation for early signs of septic shock in women with pyelonephritis, septic abortion, chorioamnionitis
d. Avoidance of potent diuretic to treat oliguria, before starting appropriate effort to ensure cardiac output for renal perfusion.
e. Avoidance of vasoconstrictors to treat hypotension.

Clinical Course

It is in three phases:
a. **Oliguric phase:** In which urine output drops to < 30 ml/hours with increase in blood urea, nitrogen and potassium.
b. **Diuretic phase:** Large volume of dilute urine are passed with loss of electrolytes due to absence of function of renal tubule.
c. **Recovery phase:** As tubular function returns to normal, the volume and composition of urine normalize.

Clinical Manifestation and Complication

Clinical manifestation and complications are anorexia, nausea, and vomiting, lethargy, cardiac arrhythmia secondary to electrolyte disturbance, anemia, renal or extra-renal infection, thrombocytopenia, metabolic acidosis. Electrolyte imbalance reveals Hyperkalemia, hyponatremia, hypermagnesemia, hyperphosphatemia, and hypocalcemia.

Treatment

Prevention should be aim in obstetric practice. Specific treatment is as follows:
a. **Emergency treatment:** Emergency treatment of underlying cause of acute renal failure.
b. **Surgical measures:** Determination of any obstetric uropathy or sepsis due to infection which should be treated properly.
c. **Routine measures:** It include achieving fluid and electrolyte balance. Strict input output chart must be maintained. Hyperkalemia is controlled by giving glucose and insulin. The diet should be high in calories and carbohydrate but low in protein and electrolytes. Infection is treated with antibiotic without renal toxicity.
d. **Dialysis:** Dialysis is indicated if serum K level > 7 meq/lit, serum sodium level > 130 meq/lit. Serum bicarbonate is more than 120 mg/dl or daily increment of 30 mg/dl. *In obstetrics dialysis is indicated earlier in process, commonly advised if blood urea nitrogen level is 60 mg/dl.*

CHRONIC RENAL DISEASE

When counseling the women with chronic renal disease regarding fertility and risk of a complicated pregnancy, it is important to determine the degree of functional impairment and presence or absence of hypertension.

Types of Chronic Renal Diseases

The four major clinical glomerulopathic syndromes are—acute rapidly progressive glomerulonephritis, nephrotic syndrome, asymptomatic abnormalities of the urinary sediment and chronic glomerulopathies. The majority of these diseases are encountered in young women of reproductive age and thus they may complicate pregnancy.

Effect of Pregnancy on Chronic Renal Disease

In general the long-term effects of pregnancy on renal disease are unclear. In patient with mild renal disease (serum creatinine < 1.4 mg/dl) pregnancy should not cause a worsening of renal function but these patients are at greater risk for pyelonephritis. Patients with moderate to severe renal insufficiency (serum creatinine >1.4 mg/dl and >2.5 mg/dl respectively) can experience deterioration of renal function that may not improve after delivery. Comorbid condition as hypertension and diabetes can also increase the risk of irreversible renal function with pregnancy. Worsening proteinuria is common and this makes the diagnosis of superimposed pre-eclampsia difficult.

Effect of Chronic Renal Disease in Pregnancy Outcome

These patients are at greater risk for miscarriage, IUGR, pre-eclampsia and preterm delivery. Perinatal mortality is significantly increased in patients with moderate to severe renal dysfunctions. Though prognosis has improved with advancements in antepartum surveillance, steroids and neonatal care.

Management

Women with chronic renal disease should have frequent prenatal visit to determine blood pressure. Serial creatinine measurement and protein excretion is monitored. Women should be screened and treated for bacteriuria to decrease the risk of acute pyelonephritis. In pregnancy protein restricted diet is not recommended. Hypertension, IUGR is managed accordingly. Anemia associated with chronic renal insufficiency respond to recombinant erythropoietin S/C but hypertension is well documented side effect.

Prognosis

Prognosis for a successful pregnancy outcome in general is related not to the underlying kidney disorder, but to the degree of functional impairment. Women with normal renal function and blood pressure before pregnancy usually have a normal outcome. But if renal impairment worsens, there is more likelihood of pregnancy complications like worsening of hypertension, or superimposed pre-eclampsia.

Dialysis During Pregnancy

For those women requiring dialysis, increased dialysis time may improve pregnancy outcome. The improvement with type of dialysis—Hemodialysis vs Peritoneal does not appear significantly different.

PREGNANCY AFTER RENAL TRANSPLANTATION

Many women who experienced oligomenorrhea with chronic renal disease regain fertility as renal function improves after renal transplantation. It is recommended that following criteria should be present before attempting the pregnancy:

a. The women should be in good general health, without severe hypertension for at least 2 years after transplant. Because graft rejection is more common during the period.
b. There should be stable renal function without severe renal insufficiency.
c. Drug therapy is reduced to maintenance levels, i.e. Prednisolone dosage 15 mg/day or less, Azathioprine 2mg/kg per day or less, cyclosporine 5 mg/kg/day or less.

Management

Bacteriuria must be treated and if recurrent, suppressive treatment is given for remainder of pregnancy. Serial hepatic enzyme level and blood counts are monitored for toxic effect of Azathioprine and cyclosporine. Renal function is monitored with serum creatinine, if serum creatinine is abnormal, 24 hrs. creatinine clearance is performed. Throughout pregnancy women is carefully monitored for development of PIH and management is accordingly as in nontransplanted patients. Graft infection or rejection should prompt admission for aggressive management. Fetal surveillance is indicated because of significantly increased risk of IUGR and preterm delivery. Cesarean delivery is reserved only for obstetrical indication, unless the transplanted kidney is expected to obstruct labor.

ADULT POLYCYSTIC KIDNEY DISEASE

It is an autosomal dominant disorder with an incidence of 1 in 400 to 1000, usually present in the 4th or 5th decade of life. The disease is associated with hypertension and pregnancy could worsen the hypertension. In general pregnancy does not appear to worsen the course of this disease.

45 Nervous System Disorders in Pregnancy

*The world is like a mirror, if you smile, it smiles,
if you frown, it frowns back.*

EPILEPSY AND SEIZURE DISORDER

A seizure is defined as a paroxysmal disorder of the central nervous system, characterized by an abnormal neuronal discharge with or without loss of consciousness. *Epilepsy* is defined as a condition characterized by a tendency for two or more recurrent seizures unprovoked by any known proximate insult. This excludes seizures due to active systemic metabolic derangement or to an acute central nervous system insult.

Cause of Seizure in Pregnancy

a. Eclampsia.
b. Epilepsy.
c. Encephalitis/meningitis.
d. Space-occupying leisons like tuberculoma, toxoplasmosis.
e. Cerebrovascular accidents.
f. Thrombotic thrombocytopenic purpura.
g. Drug withdrawal.
h. Metabolic disturbances.

Incidence: Epilepsy complicates approximately 1 in 200 pregnancies. Convulsive disorders are the second most prevalent and certainly the most serious common neurological condition encountered in pregnant women.

Types of Epileptic Seizures

a. **Generalized convulsive:** Tonic, clonic or grandmal.
b. **Complex partial:** Loss of awareness or staring with mild motor movements.
c. **Focal motor or sensory:** Jacksonian with no loss of awareness.
d. **Absence or petit mal:** Brief eye blinking with no after confusion.
e. Myoclonic jerk.
f. Aura of fear or abnormal odos.

Diagnosis

A detailed history from the patient and observer should be taken to differentiate true seizures from other form of loss of consciousness as syncopal episodes, hysteric attacks or hyperventilation. Seizures may result from drug withdrawal, medication, or exposure to toxic substances, so appropriate physical examination and screening for toxic substances are important in patients suffering an apparent first seizure during pregnancy.

Investigation

In general the pregnant women should receive the same evaluation as any one else. Identifiable cause of convulsive disorder need to be ruled out. Both cranial computed tomography and magnetic resonance imaging are believed safe in pregnancy and should be utilized if needed. EEG is useful to confirm the type of epilepsy and therefore guiding the appropriate drug therapy.

Effect of Seizure Disorders on Pregnancy and Vice Versa

Between 25 and 50% of women with idiopathic epilepsy have an increase in seizure frequency during pregnancy, usually during the first trimester. Rests have no change in seizure pattern. Patients with frequent seizures before pregnancy are likely to experience worsening of seizure control during pregnancy. Likewise good seizure control before pregnancy usually correlates with a lower risk of exacerbation during pregnancy. The cause of increased seizure frequency is unclear. Possible causes are poor seizure control before conception, no prepregnancy counseling, poor compliance and lower serum levels of anticonvulsant during pregnancy. Increased seizure activity during one pregnancy does not predict a similar response in future pregnancies. However, there is only mildly increased risks of obstetric complications like pre-eclampsia, preterm labor and stillbirth reported in some studies. Vaginal bleeding is more common in epileptic probably secondary to anticonvulsant therapy including vitamin K deficiency.

Gestational epilepsy: It is idiopathic epilepsy diagnosed for the first time during pregnancy, 25% of these newly diagnosed epileptic are known as *gestational epileptics*. Gestational epilepsy in one pregnancy is not predictive of recurrence in future pregnancies.

Management

Management is guided by specific aims before, during and after pregnancy.

Preconceptional Counseling

The offspring of epileptic women are at increased risk to have certain congenital malformation caused by epilepsy itself, the anticonvulsant drugs or combination of both. On average 7% of the offspring of epileptic women have major congenital abnormalities compared with 3% of the general population. So the treatment of epileptic women should ideally begin preconceptionally:

a. Patient's seizures should be assessed to ascertain whether or not she truly needs an anticonvulsant drug.
b. If antiepileptic drugs to be withdrawn, they should be withdrawn at least 6 months prior to pregnancy to see if there is relapse.
c. When possible, monotherapy should be used and lowest plasma antiepileptic drug level that prevents seizures should be determined. The use of divided dose or slow release preparation result in lower peak levels and may reduce the risk of malformation.
d. Folic acid in dose of 4 mg per day should be given with antiepileptic drug in preconceptional period.

Antenatal Care

Care should be carried out by an obstetrician with special interest in epilepsy or high risk pregnancy jointly with a neurologist. The major aim of pregnancy is to keep the women seizure free.

a. **General care:** Patient may need treatment for nausea and vomiting, she should avoid seizure provoking stimuli.
b. **A mid pregnancy targeted ultrasound examination** may identify fetal anomalies. Antepartum fetal surveillance is indicated if there is poor fetal growth, inadequate seizure control or comorbid maternal conditions. A fetal cardiac scan may be warranted at 22 weeks gestation.

Anticonvulsant Therapy

Treatment of epilepsy should consist of the medications that have been the most beneficial for the patient and at the lowest possible dose to maintain seizure control. *During pregnancy anticonvulsant drug level change as a result of decreased protein binding, increased plasma volume, and alteration in the absorption and excretion of drugs.* Lamotrigine, phenytoin, phenobarbitone and carbamazepine have an increased plasma clearance that is related to high hepatic metabolism in pregnancy. These factors can lead to low antiseizure plasma levels. Beside this noncompliance, morning sickness and hyperemesis in pregnancy can also cause low drug levels, therefore ideally blood level measurement of antiseizure medication should be done to monitor and maintain therapeutic range. *Levels should be checked at least each trimester and prior to delivery. Because of decreased protein binding, serum free drug levels rather than routine serum levels will be more accurate.*

Choice of Drugs

Anticonvulsant drugs in general should not be considered safe during pregnancy. But uncontrolled seizures are dangerous for both the women and fetus, supporting their judicious use when needed. So choice and dose of medicine should be tailored. Frequently prescribed anticonvulsants are summarized in Table 45.1. Drug level monitoring may not need to be carried out as a routine but many clinicians

Table 45.1: Frequently prescribed anticonvulsant

Medication	Nonpregnant dose	Therapeutic level	Toxicity
Carbamazepine (Tagretol)	600-1200 mg/day in 3-4 d.d.	4-10	Ataxia, drowsiness nystagmus, agitation
Phenytoin (Dilantin)	300-500 mg/day in single or d.d. dose	10-20	Ataxia, slurred speech, vertigo, nystagmus
Phenobarbitol (Phenobarbitol)	90-180 mg/day in 2-3 d.d.	15-40	Ataxia, drowsiness
Primidone (Primidone) Primidone is metabolized to phenobarbitone so combined use of phenobarbitol and primidone should be avoided.	750-1500 mg/day in 3 d.d.	5-15	Ataxia, vertigo, nystagmus
Valproic acid	550-2000 mg/day in 3-4 d.d.	50-100	

may like to have a starting level of antiepileptic drug. Antiepileptic drug level should be performed in following situations:
a. Suspected noncompliance
b. Increasing seizure frequency.
c. Concerns over toxic side effects.
d. Patient is on other drugs.

Risks of Antiepileptic Drugs

Risks of various antiepileptic drugs are summarized in Table 45.1.

Neonatal Complications with the Anticonvulsant Drugs

a. *Fetal hydantoin (Phenytoin) syndrome:* It consist of various combination of craniofascial and limb abnormalities. As this pattern is also associated with other anticonvulsant and combination of major anomalies—like microcephaly, growth retardation, midface hypoplasia and digital hypoplasia - also known as **anticonvulsant embryopathy.**
b. *Phenobarbitol:* It has been associated with some birth defects; *its major risk is neonatal addiction and withdrawal symptoms.*
c. *Carbamazepine:* Though, its use is considered safe but recent data suggest that Carbamazepine may be associated with an increased incidence of craniofascial defects, developmental delay and NTDs.
d. *Valproic acid:* It is a teratogenic drug. When exposure is between 17 and 30 days after conception, the risk of NTD is 1-2%. So women exposed during the critical period should be closely screened.
e. Newer anticonvulsant drugs like Felbamate, Gabapentin, and Lamotrigine categorized as 'C' type in pregnancy. Still their routine use is not recommended without more supporting evidence.
f. *Trimethadione:* Trimethadione is associated with a greater risk of anomalies as compared with other anticonvulsant and cause *Trimethadione syndrome* in fetus. So, its use is contraindicated in pregnancy.

Role of Epoxide Hydrolase Enzyme in Development of Congenital Malformation

Epoxide hydrolase is an enzyme within a metabolic pathway. Genetic heterogeneity within this enzyme can affect its overall efficacy. Homozygosity in the fetus for the genes producing lowered efficacy of this enzyme is associated with highest development rate for feature of congenital phenytoin syndrome. Beside this it remains unclear whether the increased risk is due solely to the medications. It is possible that idiopathic epilepsy itself is associated with a risk of fetal anomalies. Treatment with two or more antiseizure medication approximately doubles the risk of malformation so monotherapy is preferred.

Vitamin K Administration to Mother and Neonate

If the patient is taking an antiseizure medication, metabolized by the P450 liver enzyme system, she should be given vitamin K 10 mg/day from 36 weeks until delivery to prevent hemorrhage in her baby. Beside this intramuscular vitamin K should be given to infant and neonate should be closely observed for signs of clotting abnormality. Carbamazepine and Valproic acid are not associated with this effect.

Intrapartum Care

Induction of labor and cesarean section are indicated for the usual obstetric indication. Vaginal delivery should be the aim. In labor there is higher risk of seizure due to sleep disturbance, reduced intake and absorption of antiepileptic drug and hyperventilation. So anticonvulsant drug should be given during labor. *Epileptic seizures during labor are best controlled with intravenous benzodiazepines* (Clonazepam or diazepam). Seizure during labor is not indication for cesarean section but status epilepticus or recurrent seizures in labor may warrant abdominal delivery.

Postnatal Care

Antiepileptic drugs pass into the breast milk in varying degrees depending on protein binding characteristics. The benefit of breast milk usually outweighs the small risk from the medication to the infant. If a breastfed infant is too sedated and not feeding well, presumably due to medication in the milk, breastfeeding can be suspended and supplemented with formula. Mother with frequent seizure should be counseled on seizure and infant safety. A single 1 mg intramuscular vitamin K neonatal supplement is advised in order to prevent hemorrhagic disease of newborn. Following special advice is given for epileptic mothers:
a. Extra help if sleep is disturbed.
b. Ensuring somebody's presence while bathing the baby.
c. Surround mother with pillow while holding baby.

Regarding contraception: Anticonvulsant drugs induce hepatic P450 microsomal enzyme system, which increase estrogen metabolism so COC containing 50 µg (not 30 µg) should be prescribed. *Barrier method, IUCD, progestin pill, injection and COC with 50 µg of ethinyl estradiol are good choices for contraception.*

Risk of Epilepsy in Child

In general a child has 3% risk of epilepsy. The risk may be higher if the parental seizure etiology is unknown, the mother is affected parent or the child has febrile seizure.

HEADACHE

Headache is the most common neurologic complaint during pregnancy. More than 90% of headaches are either tension or migraine headache.

Tension Headache

They are characterized by tightness and pain in the back of the neck and head that can persist for hours. There are no associated neurological disturbances. Diagnosis is made on clinical feature in absence of any underlying neurological abnormalities. This may also be a symptom of depression.

Management

Rest, massage, anti-inflammatory medication or mild tranquilizer are effective. Counseling about stress management is beneficial.

Migraine Headache

Chronic migraine headache decreases during pregnancy in 50-80% of affected patients presumably because of high estrogen level in pregnancy. Almost 15% of migraine headache appear for the first time during pregnancy and they are more likely to be classical.

Clinical Presentation

Migraine is term which describes periodic, hemicranial, throbbing headache that is often accompanied by nausea and vomiting. There are 4 types of migraine headache:

a. *Common migraine* is often familial, usually characterized by a unilateral headache, nausea and vomiting and scalp tenderness.
b. *Classical migraine:* It has similar symptoms but is preceded by aura.
c. *Basilar migraine:* It includes vertigo, dysarthria and diplopia.
d. *Complicated migraine:* Includes more severe transient neurological symptoms and may mimic an ischemic event.

As migraine is frequently a diagnosis of exclusion, the initial attack should prompt a full neurological workup to rule out other pathology.

Management

a. *Abortive:* Most migraine headache respond to single analgesic as aspirin, acetaminophen. Antiemetic are frequently needed. For severe headache codeine or meperidine is given along with promethazine. Ergotamine preparations are potent vasoconstrictors and should be avoided in pregnancy. Sumatriptan – a seratonin receptor agonist relieves migraine headache but safety in pregnancy is not proven.
b. *Prophylactic:* Prophylactic medication should be instituted, if abortive therapy is only partially effective and disabling migraine are occurring more than once per week. Amytriptilene 10-150 mg/day, Propranolol 20-80 mg three times daily can be given.

46 Asthma in Pregnancy

When fear ceases to scare you, it cannot stay.

PULMONARY DISORDERS IN PREGNANCY

Physiological Changes in Pulmonary System in Pregnancy

Physiological changes in pulmonary system have been described in chapter previously.

Dyspnea of Pregnancy

Most pregnant women (up to 70%) complain of dyspnea. Progesterone levels are increased in pregnancy and progesterone stimulate the respiratory center, which may cause breathlessness. Despite this being a common complaint, it is important to evaluate the patient for pathologic causes of dyspnea.

ASTHMA IN PREGNANCY

Asthma is a disorder in which paroxysmal dyspnea occurs due to the spasmodic contraction of hyper-reactive air passages, mucus hypersecretion and mucosal edema.

Incidence

The general prevalence of asthma appears to be increasing. Incidence is about 1-4% of all pregnant women.

Effect of Pregnancy in Asthma

Recent information suggests that during pregnancy up to 70% of patients with asthma shows improvement, approximately 20% shows no change and up to 10% experience worsening of symptoms. In adolescents asthmatic, who become pregnant have a higher percentage of exacerbations. Noncompliance of treatment and respiratory tract infections are factors associated with asthma flares.

Effect of Asthma on Pregnancy

There is conflicting evidence. In well controlled and actively managed asthmatics perinatal mortality is not affected. But there may be increased risk of preterm labor, PROM, pre-eclampsia, IUGR and neonatal hypoxia. Maternal complications can be hyperemesis, pneumonia, pre-eclampsia, vaginal bleeding, more complicated labor and more cesarean deliveries. Women with severe asthma are at the higher risk. However, mothers also are at little or no increased risk when the disease is effectively treated and controlled.

Classification of Asthma

Classification of asthma is according to severity:
a. Mild intermittent.
b. Mild persistent.
c. Moderately persistent.
d. Severe persistent.

Diagnosis

Diagnosis is based mainly on clinical grounds.

Symptoms

Symptoms are cough, dyspnea, chest tightness and wheezing.

Investigation

Pulmonary function studies should be part of initial investigation. *Sequential measurement of the forced expiratory volume in one second (FEV1) from maximum expiration is the single best measure to reflect severity of disease.* An FEV1 less than 1 liter or less than 20% of predicted value correlates well with severe disease as manifested by hypoxia, poor response to therapy and a high relapse rate. *The peak expiratory flow rate (PEFR) correlates well with FEV1 and it can be measured reliably with inexpensive portable peak flow meters.*

Management

Most patients with asthma can be managed effectively during pregnancy, and complications are generally confined to the patients with uncontrolled asthma. In most cases the disease is well controlled with **inhaled β_2 agonist** like salbutamol, terbutaline, fenoterol, which relieves and **corticosteroid** like Betamethasone, which prevents.*

Mild Intermittent Asthma

These patients do not need daily medication. When symptoms occur 2-4 puffs of a short acting inhaled β_2 agonist like salbutamol, terbutaline, fenoterol can be used as needed.

Mild Persistent Asthma

a. The preferred therapy for this group of patients is a low dose inhaled corticosteroids. Beclomethasone or Budesonide inhalations are administered every 3-4 hours. Inhaled corticosteroids suppress and may even prevent airway inflammation.
b. Cromolyn sodium: It is anti-inflammatory drug but its efficacy is less predictable than inhaled corticosteroids.

Moderate Persistent Asthma

The preferred treatment is a combination of *low dose or medium dose inhaled corticosteroids and a long acting β_2 agonist.*

Severe Persistent Asthma

The preferred treatment is a **high dose inhaled corticosteroids and a long acting inhaled β_2 agonist as well as a systemic corticosteroids such as 2 mg/kg/day of Prednisolone or equivalent steroid not to exceed 60 mg/day** with an attempt to reduce the minimal effective dose. An alternative but not preferred treatment includes a high dose inhaled corticosteroids and sustained release theophylline.

Treatment of Acute Asthmatic Attacks

Treatment of acute asthma during pregnancy is similar to that for the nonpregnant asthmatic. An exception is significantly lowered threshold for hospitalization of the pregnant women. Status asthmaticus is a severe asthma exacerbation in which oxygenation is difficult despite therapy. Therapy is:

A. Humidified oxygen 30-40%.
B. Nebulised beta agonist.
C. Subcutaneous catecholamine–epinephrine or terbutaline.
D. Intravenous steroid are used if the patient doesn't respond to subcutaneous catecholamine.

During treatment, fetal monitoring should be used if patients are more than 24 weeks pregnancy. Assessment of maternal oxygenation is also done to guide effectiveness of therapy. If the patient does not respond with these measures and it is difficult to maintain adequate oxygenation, intubation becomes necessary.

Management During Labor and Delivery

Regularly scheduled asthma medications are continued throughout labor and delivery. Low dose corticosteroids are administered to any women receiving systemic steroid therapy within the preceding 4 weeks. The usual drug therapy is 100 mg of hydrocortisone given intravenously every 8 hours. PEFR should be determined on admission. If asthma symptoms develop then serial measurement are made after treatment.

For labor analgesia, a nonhistamine releasing narcotic such as fentanyl may be preferred to meperidine or morphine. Epidural analgesia for labor is ideal. For surgical delivery, conduction analgesia is preferred because tracheal intubation can trigger severe bronchospasm. Syntocinon is better than ergometrine because of bronchoconstrictor effect of ergometrine. **PGF2 should not be used as it precipitates bronchospasm.** PGE1 and PGE2 compound can be used locally for induction of labor.

Aspirin and nonsteroidal anti-inflammatory drugs like Indomethacin may trigger severe bronchospasm as well as ocular, nasal, dermal and gastrointestinal inflammation in 3-8% of asthmatic patients and are best avoided. Inhaled β_2 agonist cromolyn sodium, steroids are safe while breastfeeding.

TUBERCULOSIS

Tuberculosis is a chronic bacterial infection caused by *Mycobacterial tuberculosis* or *M. bovis,* which is transmitted by respiratory droplet and spread from person to person via air. South East Asia region has the highest number of cases among all WHO regions. India alone accounts for 20% of the global burden of the disease. As most cases occur in the younger age group, a large number of women with pregnancy would invariably be affected.

---

*The teratogenic risk and possible harmful fetal effects of maternal steroid treatment remains an area of controversy. However, the committee on safety of medicines has concluded that, there is no evidence that systemic corticosteroid increase the incidence of congenital abnormalities as cleft lip and palate. But prolonged or repeated doses increase the risk of IUGR.

Chapter - 46 ♦ Asthma in Pregnancy

Table 46.1: Dosages of anti-tuberculosis drugs

Drug	Daily dose	Major side effects
Isoniazid + Pyridoxin	5 mg/kg up to 300 mg +50 mg daily	Hepatitis, peripheral neuropathy, hepatic enzyme elevation, hypersensitivity
Rifampicin	10 mg/kg up to 600 mg	Nausea, vomiting, hepatitis, orange color of urine
Ethambutol	15 mg/kg up to 2.5 gm	Skin rash, optic neuritis, decreased visual activity
Pyrazinamide	15-30 mg/kg up to 2 gm	Hepatic toxicity, skin rash, arthralgia

Effect of Pregnancy on Tuberculosis

There is no evidence to show that pregnancy makes women more likely to develop tuberculosis or have a poorer prognosis if tuberculosis is diagnosed during pregnancy, provided if they are treated promptly.

Effect of Tuberculosis on Pregnancy

It is difficult to decide that how much effect the disease per se has on pregnancy, or from the malnutrition, anemia and poor living conditions that predispose to developing the disease. Data shows that women, who are diagnosed and start treatment before pregnancy or in early part of pregnancy, have a better pregnancy outcome as compared to those who are diagnosed late in pregnancy and in postpartum period. Neonates born to women with tuberculosis were found to have higher risk of prematurity, low birth weight and perinatal death.

Diagnosis

Symptoms and Signs

Typical symptoms includes cough, weight loss, fatigue, night sweats and anorexia. However, some patients may have very few symptoms.

Laboratory Findings

a. **Tuberculin skin test**: It is done with purified protein derivate (PPD) and important screening test for tuberculosis. An induration of ≥ 10 mm is usually considered positive but in HIV infected persons ≥ 5 mm is taken as positive. A strongly positive mantoux (Mx) response is suggestive of active disease. India and in areas where the disease is endemic, the tuberculin positivity is high because of either due to latent infection or due to BCG vaccine.
b. **Chest X-ray** is useful for diagnosis of pulmonary tuberculosis, which may show infiltration or cavities.
c. **Bacteriological examination**: Definitive diagnosis is made after positive identification of the bacilli by Ziehl-Neelson staining and a positive culture. A specimen can be obtained from sputum or secretion observed by bronchoscope or gastric lavage. According to guidelines of Revised National Tuberculosis Control Program of India, 3 sputum smears should be tested for acid-fast bacilli.

Treatment

The indications of treatment are the same in pregnancy as those in the nonpregnant women. Treatment should not be delayed due to fetal or maternal concerns, whatever may be the period of gestation. Most of the drugs used as first line treatment for tuberculosis like **Isoniazid, Rifampicin, and Ethambutol have been found to be safe with incidence of congenital malformation well within the range of control population.** Pyrazinamide has also been used in pregnancy but its safety profile has not been proven beyond doubt. Hepatotoxicity is the common adverse effect in patient on Antitubercular treatment reported in 10% of patients. So liver function tests should be done every month. Revised National Tuberculosis Control Program in India has advocated Directly Observed Treatment Short Course (DOTS) treating tuberculosis. *Because of risk for fetal and maternal ototoxicity, streptomycin, kanamycin, and capreomycin should not be used.* The dosage of anti-tuberculosis drugs are shown in Table 46.1.

Most treatment plans have 3 drug regimen Isoniazid, ethambutol and rifampicin for 8 weeks and isoniazid and rifampicin for 9 months. Pyridoxine 50 mg. should be given to prevent INH induced neuritis due to vitamin B_6 deficiency.

Obstetric Management

It includes adequate rest and nutrition, family support, correction of anemia if present and regular follow-up visit. Other management is no different from other pregnant women, once tuberculosis is well managed, with anti-tuberculosis drugs.

Breastfeeding

In only *active* lesions the breastfeeding is contraindicated. Baby should be isolated from the mother following delivery and baby should be given prophylactic Isoniazid 10-20 mg/kg/day for 3 months when the mother is suffering from active disease. But a women already on anti-tuberculosis drug, breastfeeding is not contraindicated. BCG should be given to the baby as early as possible.

Contraception

Spacing can be achieved by any methods acceptable to the couple. *Oral contraceptive* should be avoided when Rifampicin is used. Puerperal sterilization should be considered if family is complete.

Chemoprophylaxis for Pregnant Women

Isoniazid prophylaxis is highly effective and not shown to be teratogenic in standard dosage. Chemoprophylaxis is recommended in women with positive Mantoux test in the following situations:

a. Documented recent conversion of tuberculin test within preceding two years.
b. In close contact of persons with active tuberculosis.
c. Immunocompromised, e.g. HIV positive.

Liver function test must be performed monthly and pyridoxine should be supplemented to avoid the risk of peripheral neuropathy.

47 Local Abnormalities

Mind like muscle is developed by use.

LOCAL GYNECOLOGICAL ABNORMALITIES ASSOCIATED WITH PREGNANCY

A variety of coincidental gynecologist conditions may present during pregnancy which may need to be dealt during pregnancy. Some of the common conditions are discussed here.

Congenital Uterine Anomalies

In grosser form of Müllerian development pregnancy is rare. In general population the prevalence of uterine anomalies is 0.5%. In women with recurrent pregnancy loss and poor pregnancy outcome the incidence is 3 fold (3-6.9%).

Obstetric Problem in Congenital Uterine Anomaly

a. Preterm delivery
b. Miscarriage
c. Recurrent malpresentation
d. Rarely torsion in gravid horn of uterus didelphys.

Diagnosis

The diagnosis is usually made between pregnancies:
a. Hysterosalpingogram is usually made for indication like recurrent pregnancy loss.
b. Ultrasound has a reported accuracy of 90-92% in diagnosing Mullerian anomalies. Transvaginal ultrasound gives better special resolution.
c. MRI is costly but by far is the best imaging modality for uterine malformation with accuracy of 100%.

Treatment

Surgical correction of uterine anomalies like septate uterus provides excellent result in terms of reproductive outcome. Cervical incompetence is a common accompaniment of malformed uterus (30%). Cervical circlage is recommended in all pregnant patients with anomalous uterus.

Retroversion Uterus

The uterus lies in retroverted position in 15-25% of women. In most of cases spontaneous correction occurs between 12-16 weeks of pregnancy. In unusual events the uterus remains retroverted and can get incarcerated in the hollow of sacrum or there can be sacculation of anterior uterine wall due to asymmetric expansion. Incarceration is predisposed by presence of fibroids, Müllerian anomalies and pelvic adhesion. Incidence of incarceration in gravid uterus in second trimester occurs in 1 in 3000 pregnancies. The **symptoms of incarceration** are mainly due to effect on urinary bladder. There is increased urinary frequency, dysuria and finally retention of urine. In extreme cases there can be overflow incontinence. Rectal pressure and tenesmus can also be present. Spontaneous abortion, preterm labor and uterine dystocia can ensue.

Diagnosis

On clinical examination, retroverted uterus occupies pelvic cavity, cervix is pulled high up and anterior vaginal wall is stretched. Urinary meatus is drawn up and urinary bladder is palpable suprapubically.

Treatment

Urinary retention is relieved by indwelling catheterization. Patient is asked to lie in prone position which helps in spontaneous correction. Manual reposition is indicated if it fails to correct impaction.

Pendulous Abdomen

Acute anteversion of the pregnant uterus can occur with pendulous abdomen. The pendulous abdomen is due to weak abdominal muscles with wide divarication of rectus muscles between which uterus herniates. It is associated with marked lordosis of spine. Malpresentation and unstable lie are more common. The condition makes the women more uncomfortable. Properly designed corset can help in reducing discomfort.

Fibroid in Pregnancy

Incidence of fibroids in pregnancy is 0.1-3.9%.

Effect of Fibroids on Pregnancy

They are as follows:
a. The risk of spontaneous abortion and recurrent pregnancy loss is increased particularly with submucous fibroids. Preconceptional myomectomy is justified in these cases if there is no other identifiable cause.
b. Increased risk of antepartum hemorrhage
   a. Placenta previa
   b. Abruptio placenta particularly with fundal fibroid.
c. Increased risk of malpresentation and malposition.
d. Preterm delivery
e. Risk of IUGR by causing mechanical obstruction of labor.
f. Increased risk of dysfunctional labor.
g. Increased risk of cesarean delivery and difficult cesarean section.
h. Increased risk of postpartum hemorrhage.
i. Delayed involution in puerperium.
j. Increased chances of secondary postpartum hemorrhage.

Effect of Pregnancy on Fibroids

a. There can be increase in size of fibroid due to increased vascularity, edema, hypertrophy and hyperplasia of fibromuscular tissue. But also there can be arrested growth of fibroid and fibroid may atrophy in puerperium.
b. Fibroid becomes softened, tends to become more discoid and flattened shape.
c. The degenerative changes especially **Red degeneration**, which predominantly occurs in large fibroid during second half of pregnancy or puerperium.
   Incidence: 5-15% of women with fibroid require hospitalization for pain related to fibroid.
   Etiology: The fibroid suffers from relative ischemia because blood supply is preferably diverted to the rest of the pregnant uterus resulting in necrosis within fibroid. Larger fibroids are more prone to degenerate.
   Symptoms: There is onset of abdominal pain of all grades of severity. Usually there is acute onset of pain with temperature raised and frequently associated vomiting.
   Signs: There is localization of tenderness at the site of the fibroid, so diagnosis is enormously assisted by prior knowledge of existence of fibroid.
   Treatment: Rest, analgesic and good hydration is a main stay of treatment. The symptoms usually clear off within 10 days. When laparotomy is done for mistaken diagnosis, abdomen is to be closed without doing anything. Pedunculated subserous fibroids however may be removed.
d. Torsion of the pedunculated subserous fibroid.
e. Infection and polypoidal changes are more in puerperium.

Management

Diagnosis

In pregnancy the diagnosis of fibroid is difficult unless tumor is large and discrete. In *early pregnancy*, apparent asymmetry of uterus should raise the possibility of fibroids. Sonography confirms the diagnosis with certainty.

Differential Diagnosis

a. Retroverted gravid uterus has to be distinguished from a posterior fibroid.
b. Multiple pregnancy.
c. Ovarian tumor which has to be confirmed by ultrasound because in ovarian tumors treatment is surgical while conservative treatment is indicated for fibroid.
d. Nongravid half of variety of double uterus.

Treatment

The basic principle in management of pregnancy complicated by fibroid is wait and observe and not to do anything. Usual antenatal care is followed. All cases are assessed at 38 weeks to formulate the method of delivery. Fibroid situated above the presenting part usually results in uneventful vaginal delivery. In fibroid situated below the presenting part vaginal delivery is possible but if there is any difficulty cesarean section should be done. One should be alert for postpartum hemorrhage, retained placenta. Patient is followed closely for puerperium fever.

Role of Myomectomy in Pregnancy

Myomectomy should not be performed during pregnancy because of risk of uncontrollable hemorrhage either in antenatal period or during cesarean section. The only exception is pedunculated leiomyoma with a narrow stalk.

Adnexal Mass in Pregnancy

The incidental finding of an adnexal mass in pregnancy has become more common with the routine use of ultrasonography. 1-4% of pregnant women are diagnosed with adnexal mass. Common cause of Adnexal mass in pregnancy is summarized in Table 47.1. The line of management is as follows:
a. More than 90% of unilateral, noncomplex masses less than 5 cm in diameter, noted in first trimester are functional or corpus luteal cyst and resolve spontaneously by 16 weeks.
b. The pathologic ovarian neoplasm tends not to resolve. The most common pathologic ovarian neoplasm during pregnancy are:
   i. Benign cystic teratoma (21%).
   ii. Serous cystadenoma (21%)
   iii. Cystic corpus luteum (18%).
   iv. Mucinous cystadenoma—Of all the persistent adnexal mass 1-10% will be malignant (Table 47.1).

> **Table 47.1: Common cause of adnexal mass in pregnancy**
> - Functional cyst
> - Mature teratoma (dermoid)
> - Cystic tumor (serous and mucinous)
> - Paraovarian cyst
> - Endometriosis
> - Leiomyoma
> - Malignancy

Differential Diagnosis

Ovarian mass must be differentiated from—(a) Lesion of colon, (b) Pedunculated leiomyoma, (c) Pelvic kidney, (d) Congenital abnormalities of the uterus. *Ultrasound usually facilitates delineation of the size and consistency of adnexal mass.*

Management

Conservative

If the adnexal mass is unilateral, mobile, cystic, operation can be deferred and close follow-up of its size and complication if any is done.

Indication of Surgery

Surgical treatment is indicated when there is risk of—rupture (2%), torsion (0-7%) or malignancy. The risk of malignancy should be further assessed by ultrasound characteristics of masses. The decision of clinician is to be weighed for each individual patient against risk of abdominal surgery during the pregnancy. The risks of surgery in pregnancy are abortion, preterm labor and PPROM.

The ideal time of surgery is 14-18 weeks via laparotomy or laparoscopy because the risk of postoperative abortion is much reduced. Only in cases where symptoms and signs are highly suggestive of torsion or highly aggressive malignancy indicate need for immediate intervention. After this time the access to mass is difficult because of the size of the uterus. If the cyst is discovered within the last 5 weeks of pregnancy the best course is to wait until term and performing cesarean section and removal of mass at the same time. It reduces the difficulty in access, incidence of repeat surgery and preterm labor.

To summarize **any adnexal lesion that is *present after 14 weeks of gestation, growing in size on serial ultrasound evaluation, contains solid and complex components or internal papillae, is fixed, surrounded by abdominal ascites, or is symptomatic warrants surgical exploration and pathologic diagnosis.***

Solid ovarian tumor discovered during pregnancy should be treated generally with surgery because of low but significant incidence (1-10%) of cancer.

Carcinoma of Ovary

It occurs in less than 0.1% all gestation. Between 1 and 10% of all ovarian tumors complicating pregnancies are malignant. Most neoplasm in reproductive age are:

a. Germ cell tumor (dysgerminoma, endodermal sinus tumors, malignant teratoma, embryonal carcinoma and choriocarcinoma).
b. Cystadenocarcinoma

Treatment

Treatment of carcinoma of ovary is like for nonpregnant status. A generous surgical incision is given to explore the abdomen and to reduce uterine manipulation. Surgical staging is done and adequate tissue is obtained for histologic diagnosis. Conservative surgery is appropriate for encapsulated tumors if there is no evidence of uterine or contralateral ovary involvement.

In More Advanced Stage

The extent of surgery including tumor debulking will depend upon gestational age and patient wish with regard to the pregnancy. Neoadjuvant chemotherapy may offer an interim treatment for selected patients diagnosed at mid gestation to allow for fetal maturity prior to extensive surgical cytoreduction.

If tumor is benign, residual ovarian tissues are conserved if possible. The contralateral ovary must always be carefully evaluated to rule out disease. If surgical extirpation of corpus luteum is required in first trimester *progestin support is recommended.*

Torsion of Adnexa

Torsion of adnexa can involve the ovary, tubes and ancillary structure either separately or together. The most *common time* is 6-14 weeks of gestation and puerperium.

Symptoms and Signs

a. Acute abdominal pain and tenderness which is sudden in onset due to occlusion of the vascular supply to the twisted organ.
b. There can be shock and peritonitis.

Diagnosis

Diagnosis is confirmed by ultrasound, which shows an adnexal mass and altered blood flow on Doppler studies.

Treatment

Prompt operation is necessary to prevent tissue necrosis, preterm labor and potential perinatal death. Previously untwisting of adnexal mass was not advocated because of concern for potentially fatal thromboembolic complication. But nowadays recent studies demonstrate that derotation can safely be done followed by appropriate removal of mass, e.g. cystectomy.

These adnexa are capable of recovering and becoming functional. Salpingo-oophorectomy can be reserved for the management of active bleeding or suspicious neoplasm.

Premalignant and Malignant Lesions of Cervix

Carcinoma cervix is the most common genital tract malignancy encountered in pregnancy with an estimated incidence of 1 in 200 to 1 in 10000.

Clinical Presentation

Majority of patients in stage one are diagnosed on routine examination. The practice of routine Pap test during pregnancy reveals suspicious tumors in 0.5% of women. When symptomatic patient presents with bleeding which may be profuse and to a lesser extent with discharge and a diagnosis of threatened abortion may be made, so a perspeculum examination of cervix is must if bleeding persists for more than 5-7 days.

Diagnosis

In pregnancy women should undergo routine cervical cytology screening at their first prenatal visit. The reliability of the PAP smear is the same as in nonpregnant women. The incidence of abnormal smear in the pregnancy is 5-8%. Any abnormality repeated in the Pap smear must be followed by colposcopy. In colposcopy the physiological changes of pregnancy render the transformation zone easily accessible for satisfactory colposcopy by 20 weeks gestation. But one should keep in mind that change in cervical epithelium may mimic those of dysplasia. Colposcopic directed ectocervical biopsy can be performed safely with minimal increase in risk of significant bleeding. Endocervical curettage is not recommended during pregnancy because the columnar cells are sampled easily from the surface smear and increase the risk of abortion. Repeat biopsies are only performed for progressive lesions.

Management

Premalignant Lesions

In women with preinvasive lesions confirmed in histology a close follow-up throughout the pregnancy must be maintained with cytology and colposcopy every 6-8 weeks. Further treatment is deferred till postpartum period. Even high grade lesions discovered during pregnancy have a high rate or regression in the postpartum period. *Conisation* is only indicated if early invasive disease is suspected. The risk of cone biopsy is—abortion, hemorrhage, infection, incompetent cervix. Cone biopsy is shallower in pregnancy.

Re-evaluation must be done 6-8 weeks postpartum. Delivery in patients with cervical dysplasia and carcinoma *in situ* may be via the vaginal route.

Carcinoma Cervix During Pregnancy

Invasive cervical cancer complicate 0.05% of pregnancies. Pregnancy does not appear to affect the prognosis for women with cervical cancer and the fetus is not affected by maternal disease but may suffer morbidity from its treatment.

Treatment in stage Ia, Ib1, IIa1: In pregnancy, early radical hysterectomy with therapeutic pelvic lymphadenectomy can be performed with fetus *in situ* unless the patient is unwilling to terminate the pregnancy. In first trimester external beam radiation can be started with fetus *in situ* followed by intracavitary brachytherapy following abortion. Usually spontaneous abortion occurs. In second trimester interruption of pregnancy by hysterotomy prior to radiation therapy is preferred. Surgery is performed as the treatment of choice in young women because it prevents radiation induced vaginal stricture and radiation associated morbidity. Besides ovarian function can be preserved.

In women at a gestational age closer to fetal viability, the patient may continue the pregnancy with careful decision of maternal risk. Cesarean radical hysterectomy is performed as soon as the fetus can be salvaged. Antenatal steroid to the mother would help fetal lung maturation. Patient with invasive cervical cancer should be delivered by classical cesarean section to avoid potential cervical hemorrhage and dissemination of tumor cells during vaginal delivery.

Late stage Ib2 IIb, IIIb: Treatment in pregnancy with late stage should be planned with a multidisciplinary approach. *Radiotherapy with or without chemotherapy* is treatment of choice. In early pregnancy radiotherapy can be started with fetus *in situ*. In late pregnancy fetus should be delivered by cesarean section. Whole pelvic external radiation may be started immediately postpartum followed by intracavitary irradiation.

If the mother does not wish to terminate pregnancy and the fetus is immature, the option of neoadjuvant chemotherapy may be discussed with the mother to postpone definitive treatment explaining the risk of teratogenesis and IUGR.

Other Lesions of Cervix

Scarring of Cervix

It is caused by a previous conization as in Manchester operation, or deep cauterization of cervix. These patients should be delivered in hospital as rate of cesarean section is very high due to cervical dystocia. There are more chances of preterm labor and recurrent abortion.

Cervical Polyp

Cervical polyp can cause intermittent bleeding during pregnancy and their removal is advisable. If there is persistent bleeding following polyp removal, hemostatic drug and gentle local pressure usually can control it.

Vaginal Discharge in Pregnancy

Physiological Vaginal Discharge of Pregnancy

During pregnancy there is hyperemia as a result of hormonal stimulation so there is increase in vaginal transudate. Microscopic examination of wet specimen of this discharge reveals large number of well cornified squamous cells and very few pus cells. For this no treatment is indicated except for personal hygiene.

Other Causes of Vaginal Discharge

Vulvovaginal Candidiasis

It is relatively more common in pregnancy because of acidic pH of vagina in pregnancy. It is caused by yeast like organism *Candida albicans*. Complaints are pruritis vulva, thick curdy white vaginal discharge and dysuria. On examination vulva may be swollen and excoriated. Per speculum examination shows thick curdy discharge and vaginitis.

Treatment: Local antifungal preparation containing polyene (Nystatin) or Imidazoles (Clotrimazole, Miconazole, Econazole, Terconazole) are effective in uncomplicated candidiasis. The same antifungal cream can be used for local application in case of vulvar candidiasis twice a day for 7-14 days. Oral Fluconazole is not recommended in pregnancy (category C drug).

Trichomonas Vaginitis

It is not uncommon in pregnancy which presents as foul smelling frothy discharge with vaginal irritation or itching. Diagnosis is confirmed by per speculum examination and microscopy of wet smear, which shows motile Trichomonads.

Treatment: Metronidazole 200 mg three times a day for 7 days to both partners. Metronidazole should be preferably avoided in the first trimester.

Bacterial Vaginosis

It is a condition in which the normal vaginal flora (lactobacilli) is replaced by anaerobes like *Gardnella vaginalis*, *Mycoplasma hominis* and anaerobes. Women with bacterial vaginosis may complain of whitish or grayish vaginal discharge with an unpleasant fish like odor. Amsel criteria are standard criteria used for clinical diagnosis. 3 out of 4 criteria should met for diagnosis—(a) Milky homogenous discharge, (b) Vaginal pH > 4.5, (c) Release of fishy odor on adding alkali (10% iron), (d) Presence of clue cells in the vaginal fluid under light microscopy.

Treatment: Symptomatic women can be treated by metronidazole tablet 250 mg three times daily or Clindamycin tablet 300 mg twice daily for 7 days. Topical therapy is not recommended during pregnancy.

Cervical erosion: Due to hyperestrogenism there is hyperemia and ectopy of the squamocolumnar junction at the external cervical os. This forms excessive secretion of mucoid discharge. No active treatment is needed. Spontaneous regression occurs usually 6-8 weeks postpartum.

Genital Prolapse in Pregnancy

Incidence of prolapse with pregnancy is about 1 in 250 pregnancies.

Effect of Pregnancy on Prolapse

There is aggravation of the morbid anatomical change in prolapse as marked by hypertrophy and edema of the cervix. There is aggravation of grade of prolapse. These changes are marked during early pregnancy due to weight of the uterus and increased vascularity. Vaginal discharge is increased and there is chance of incarceration, if uterus fails to rise above the pelvis by 16th week of pregnancy.

Effect of Prolapse on Pregnancy

a. There is increased chance of abortion, discomfort, PROM, intrauterine infection.
b. In labor, increased chance of PROM, cervical dystocia, operation interference.
c. Puerperium—Subinvolution, uterine sepsis.

Treatment

a. During pregnancy:
   - If the cervix is outside the introitus, cervix is reposited inside the vagina, packing done with gauge soaked with glycerin and acriflavin. Treatment is continued till 18-20 weeks of pregnancy till prolapsed mass is reduced in size and replaced inside the vagina.
b. If there is irreducible prolapse and incarceration of uterus, termination of pregnancy may have to be done.

Labor: Prophylactic antibiotic is given. Manual stretching of cervix or pushing up the cystocele or rectocele part the presenting part during uterus contraction facilitates progressive descent of head. If head is deeply engaged but cervix remains undilated but thin, cesarean section is done. In low resource setting Duhressen's incision at 2 and 10'o clock followed by Ventouse extraction can be done. If head is high and cervix remains edematous, thick or undilated—cesarean section should be done.

Puerperium: Reposition of prolapse with glycerin and acriflavin packing is done and prophylactic antibiotic is given. If there is subinvolution a ring pessary can be given. Surgical repair of prolapse is offered after 3-6 months.

Other Malignancies During Pregnancy

Breast Cancer

About 15% of breast cancer occurs in women under the age of 40 years and 1% of these occur in pregnant women.

Clinical Presentation

A painless lump is the most common presentation. Bloody nipple discharge may be presenting symptoms and require work up. Any mass found by the patient or by the obstetrician should be fully evaluated without the under delay.

Investigation

a. When localized lesion is present breast *ultrasonography* is the preferred first imaging modality during pregnancy. It is safe and helpful in distinguishing between cystic and solid mass.
b. Mammography: The sensitivity of mammography is diminished by the breast changes in pregnancy but in inconclusive clinical examination, low dose mammography with appropriate shedding of fetus is advisable.
c. MRI can be done, but experience of MRI in pregnancy is limited.
d. Cystic lesion should be aspirated and fluid is examined cytologically.
e. FNAC, core biopsy can be done.
f. Excisional biopsy is the most appropriate for clinically suspicious or cytologically abnormal lesions.

Management

It is difficult because it requires careful consideration of both mother and fetus. The general approach is like in non-pregnant patients and should not be delayed because of pregnancy:
a. *Modified radical mastectomy* is preferred local management in pregnancy, so that adjuvant radiation may not be required.
b. *Breast conserving surgery* with adjuvant radiation is limited to patients in third trimester.
c. *Chemotherapy:* Indication of adjuvant chemotherapy to pregnant women are same as for nonpregnant patients: Cyclophosphamide, Doxorubicin, and 5 fluorouracil have been given successfully during the second and third trimester, with no increase in congenital malformation. Neoadjuvant chemotherapy may be a treatment option in select patients with locally, advanced or metastatic gestational breast cancer.
Breastfeeding: Breastfeeding should be avoided during chemotherapy, hormone therapy or radiation. Otherwise there is no contraindication to breastfeeding after completion of therapy for breast cancer.

Prognosis

a. The result of treatment are same stage for stage as they are in nonpregnant patient but pregnancy associated breast cancer tend to be more advanced at diagnosis, because of large tumor size, more frequently involved lymph nodes, which result in an overall worse prognosis for this group of patients as a whole.
b. Subsequent pregnancy does not increase the risk of recurrence or death from breast cancer after a suitable period of recuperation and observation.
c. For women who are breast cancer antigen (Br CA-1) or (Br CA-2) mutation carriers, there is no evidence that pregnancy decrease the breast cancer risk.

MULTIPLE CHOICE QUESTIONS

1. Treatment of red degeneration of fibroid in pregnancy:
   a. Analgesic
   b. Laparotomy
   c. Termination of pregnancy
   d. Removal at cesarean section
   Ans. a
2. Most Common tumor in pregnancy is:
   a. Granulosa cell tumor
   b. Mucinous cystadenoma
   c. Mature dermoid
   d. Fibroid
   Ans. c
3. Acute retention in gravid retroverted uterus occur in:
   a. 12-14 weeks
   b. 20-24 weeks
   c. 16-20 weeks
   d. 24-28 weeks
   Ans. a
4. A pregnant woman with fibroid uterus develops acute pain in abdomen with low grade fever and mild leukocytosis at 28 weeks. The most likely diagnosis is:
   a. Preterm labor
   b. Torsion of fibroid
   c. Red degeneration of fibroid
   d. Infection in fibroid
   Ans. c
5. Which one of the following is the best drug of choice for treatment of bacterial vaginosis during pregnancy?
   a. Clindamycin
   b. Metronidazole
   c. Erythromycin
   d. Rovamycin
   Ans. b
6. A patient comes with gravida 4, living one with 22 weeks of pregnancy with carcinoma *in situ*. The treatment of choice is:
   a. Conisation of cervix
   b. MTP and hysterectomy
   c. MTP and radiotherapy
   d. Allow the baby to be born and then hysterectomy is done
   Ans. d

7. Procedure of choice in a woman with 12 weeks pregnancy and abnormal Pap smear is:
   a. Cone biopsy
   b. MTP with cone biopsy
   c. Hysterectomy
   d. Colposcopy
   Ans. d
8. Fibroids in pregnancy should be removed:
   a. In pregnancy
   b. During cesarean section
   c. In the early puerperium
   d. Should not be removed
   Ans. d
9. Which female genital malignancy is most common in pregnancy?
   a. Ovarian cancer
   b. Vaginal vulvar cancer
   c. Endometrial cancer
   d. Cervical cancer
   Ans. d
10. A patient with 10 weeks of pregnancy has an ovarian cyst of size 5 inches. The treatment of choice:
    a. Removal of cyst at 14 weeks
    b. Terminate pregnancy and cyst removed
    c. Cesarean section at term and removal of cyst
    d. Removal at puerperium
    Ans. a
11. All are true about retroversion of uterus in the pregnancy *except*:
    a. Surgery is the only treatment of choice
    b. Leads to retention of urine
    c. May lead to abortion
    d. Spontaneously corrects during pregnancy
    Ans. a

48 Infection During Pregnancy

Today I don't want to live for, I want to live.

GENERAL CONSIDERATION

Maternal infection during pregnancy can have adverse effect both on the health of the mother and fetus. Pregnancy per se does not predispose women to increased risk of infection. Infection during pregnancy is important for two reasons—some infection can cause significant maternal morbidity or even mortality (Pneumococcal Pneunomia). Other infections may be of little or no clinical significance to the mother but can harm the fetus through fetoplacental infection e.g. toxoplasmosis. The following viral, protozoal, and bacterial infection which can have perinatal complications, are discussed in this chapter:
a. TORCH infection
b. HIV virus
c. Varicella zoster
d. Malaria
e. Parvovirus

TORCH INFECTION—GENERAL CONSIDERATION

Toxoplasmosis

It is a zoonotic disease caused by *Toxoplasma gondii*, an intracellular parasite. It is transmitted by ingestion of undercooked meat or consumption of unpasteurized goat milk or exposure to infected cat's feces. Incidence of primary infection during pregnancy is less than 0.1%. The prevalence of seropositivity during reproductive years is 10-40%.

Clinical Presentation

a. **Mother:** Most acute infection in mother and newborn are asymptomatic and can be detected only by prenatal or newborn serology. Maternal symptoms may be fatigue, muscle pain and sometimes lymphadenopathy. In Immunocompetent normal adult initial infection confers immunity and pre pregnancy infection eliminates any risk of vertical transmission.

b. **Fetal significance:** If fetal infection occurs early in gestation that is most likely to cause fetal sequelae. If infection occurs late in pregnancy, the more likely the infection will pass to fetus causing congenital infection in neonate. There is a wide range of fetal effects from toxoplasmosis which include subclinical disease, growth retardation and severe effects on multiple systems including the central nervous system.

Management

a. Prior maternal exposure to *T. gondii* provides protection against fetal infection. Simple protection steps like avoiding poorly prepared meal, proper hand washing before handling food and avoiding cat litter.
b. There is no consensus on the most appropriate screening or treatment strategy. If antitoxoplasma IgG antibody is confirmed before pregnancy, the incidence of congenital toxoplasmosis in fetus/neonate is nil. **Acute infection may be documented by seroconversion of IgG and IgM antibodies or by a greater than 4 fold rise in paired samples.** In addition a PCR assay with high specificity and sensitivity has been developed. **A high PCR quantitative parasite load before 20 weeks has greatest risk for a poor fetal outcome.**
c. **Treatment:** Treatment of pregnant women with Spiramycin reduces but does not eliminate the risk of congenital infection. When fetal infection is diagnosed by prenatal testing, Pyrimathamine, Sulfonamide and folinic acid are added to Spiramycin to eradicate parasites in the placenta and fetus.

Rubella (German Measles)

This is single stranded RNA virus, which cause infection of minor importance in absence of pregnancy and confers life long immunity. During pregnancy it has been directly responsible for abortion and severe congenital malformation.

Clinical Presentation

It is transmitted by air droplet (respiratory route). It causes a mild febrile illness in adults with a generalized maculopapular rash, with or without arthralgia and lymphadenopathy. 20-50% of infection can be asymptomatic. Fetal infection is more likely if maternal illness occurs early in pregnancy and fetal infection in first trimester is more likely to lead to serious sequele. There can be—(i) Spontaneous abortion, (ii) Congenital rubella syndrome, which constitutes symmetric IUGR, congenital heart disease, hepatosplenomegaly and thrombocytopenic purpura, (iii) CNS manifestation like deafness, eye lesion, e.g. congenital cataract, retinopathy, microphthalmia, microcephaly, panencephalitis, brain calcification and psychomotor disorder.

Diagnosis

a. **Mother:** Positive IgG and IgM titers are present in mother. IgM titer makes its appearance at the onset of rash and disappears in 4-8 weeks. The IgG titer begins with the onset of rash and remains elevated for life. In recent infection there is four fold increase in paired samples of IgG titers taken 2 weeks apart.
b. **Neonate:** Umbilical cord blood at birth reveals a positive IgG titer. A positive IgG titer at 5 months of age is diagnostic as maternal passive antibodies should disappear by that age.
c. **Fetal diagnosis:** In confirmed cases of maternal rubella in first half of pregnancy, confirmation of fetal infection can be done by PCR or viral culture of chorionic villi, amniotic fluid or fetal blood.

Management

To eradicate rubella and prevent congenital rubella syndrome a comprehensive approach is recommended for minimizing the adult population. The MMR vaccine should be offered to all women of childbearing age, who do not have evidence of immunity. Pregnancy after the vaccine should be avoided for one month as it contains live attenuated virus.

Cytomegalovirus—General Consideration

It is a DNA virus that belongs to herpes virus family. The infection is systemic with a tendency to lifelong latency. It is the most common cause of perinatal infection in the developed world. **CMV is present in body fluids and person to person transmission usually occurs through sexual or close and intimate contact. There can be fetal intrauterine infection, intrapartum infection or postpartum infection from breastfeeding. Day care centers are a common source of infection.**

Diagnosis

Mother

Clinical symptoms: Usually there are asymptomatic infection. Symptomatic infection may mimic infectious mononucleosis like syndrome with fever, pharyngitis, lymphadenopathy and polyarthritis. Following primary infection, the virus becomes latent. Maternal immunity to CMV does not prevent recurrence which may be due to reactivation or exogenous reinfection. It can cause congenital infection in fetus.

Fetal

Primary CMV infection is transmitted to fetus in 40% of cases and can cause severe morbidity in the fetus. Fetal infection is more likely with maternal infection during the first half of pregnancy. In recurrent maternal infection or reactivation, the risk of congenital fetal infection is less than 1%. *Symptomatic congenital CMV infection is a syndrome that includes low birth weight, microcephaly, intracranial calcification, chorioretinitis, mental and motor retardation, sensorineural deficit, hepatosplenomegaly, jaundice, hemolytic anemia and thrombocytopenia purpura.* Only 5-6% of infected neonates are symptomatic with mortality rate of 10-15%. **Asymptomatic infected fetus:** 7% of asymptomatic fetus can develop sensorineural hearing loss or developmental delay during first two year of life.

Investigation

Routine screening for maternal antibody is not recommended because most women have antibodies and presence of antibodies does not provide immunity against future infection. Even in cases of suspected acute maternal infection, antibody titer is of limited value. **Direct sampling of fetal umbilical cord blood through cordocentesis, detection of IgM in cord blood after delivery and detection of IgM in infant's blood after the age of 5 months support the diagnosis.**

Management

1. Prevention: Counseling should be done to observe meticulous hygiene in high risk setting like neonatal nursing, day care center.
2. Women with recent primary infection should be offered prenatal diagnosis with ultrasonography and amniocentesis.
3. There is no treatment for maternal primary CMV infection nor there is any fetal prophylaxis or treatment. There is neither an available CMV vaccine nor an effective mode of passive prophylaxis.
4. Intravenous ganciclovir administered for 6 weeks to the neonate with central nervous system disease prevents hearing deterioration at 6 months and possibility even at one year and beyond.

Herpes Simplex Virus—General Consideration

Genital herpes simplex virus infection is one of the most common viral sexually transmitted diseases HSV I and HSV II are two of 8 viruses in the human herpes virus family. They are DNA virus with considerable hemology. Antibodies to one virus provide some cross protection against the other viruses. Both HSV I and HSV II can cause clinical maternal and neonatal disease. Whereas most orolabial lesion are secondary to HSV I, genital lesions may be caused by either virus.

Transmission of HSV I and HSV II is primarily from genital contact or orogenital contact and there can be vertical transmission from mother to neonate. The incubation period is ~ 2-12 days. The virus replicates at the point of entry and then enters the nervous system. It is transported along axons to the sensorineuron cell body and virion remains there for whole of the life of the host. Periodic reactivation is common and may lead to clinically apparent disease or asymptomatic refection.

Neonatal Infection

The fetus is infected only by contact with virus shed from the cervix or lower genital tract during birth. Newborn infection has three forms:
a. Disseminated with involvement of major viscera.
b. Localized involvement confined to the central nervous system, eyes, skin or mucosa.
c. Asymptomatic: *There is 50% risk of neonatal infection with primary maternal infection but only 0-5% with recurrent infection.*
   Localized infection has good outcome but in disseminated infection there is 50% mortality rate.

Diagnosis

The diagnosis is often made clinically. **Isolation of virus by cell culture is the most sensitive test widely available.** Type specific serology can be done as antibodies begin to develop within 2-3 weeks of infection. Other genital ulcer disease as chancroid, syphilis may present with manifestation similar to HSV. Evaluation for other STD should be done.

Management

a. **Antenatal:** Systemic antiviral such as acyclovir and valaciclovir may be used to attenuate signs and symptoms of NSV. Prophylactic acylovir therapy in later part of pregnancy from 36 weeks gestation until delivery can reduce the rate of clinical HSV recurrences at delivery and rate of asymptomatic shedding at delivery. For intense discomfort analgesic and topical anesthetic can be added.
b. **Intrapartum: According to ACOG guide line, cesarean delivery is indicated in women with active genital lesions or in those with a typical prodrome of an impending out break.** So cesarean delivery is performed only if primary or recurrent lesions are visualized near the time of labor or when the membranes are ruptured.
c. **Postpartum** breastfeeding is allowed with advice to avoid any contact between lesions, hands and baby.

OTHER VIRAL INFECTIONS IN PREGNANCY

Varicella Zoster

Acute varicella infection (or chickenpox) and herpes zoster (or shingles) are both caused by the varicella zoster virus. The initial infection with varicella usually involves skin alone causing typical maculopapular and vesicular rash. Secondary streptococcal or staphylococcal skin infection is the most common complication. Varicella pneumonitis can develop in 5-10% of cases and cause serious morbidity or even mortality. Subsequent reactivation of the dormant virus can lead to zoster usually affecting a single unilateral dermatome. *In pregnancy* acute maternal varicella infection can be a serious illness for both the mother and fetus. Adult generally have greater morbidity from varicella infection than do children or adolescent.

Fetal Effect

There is risk to the fetus only if maternal infection occurs during 13-20 weeks or at the time of delivery. Infection in the second trimester can cause **congenital varicella syndrome** which results from transplacental infection of the fetus. The features of this syndrome are chorioretinitis, cerebral cortical atrophy, hydronephrosis and bony leg defects. Peripartum exposure can lead to neonatal varicella infection. Zoster outbreak during pregnancy can cause maternal discomfort but do not pose risk to the fetus.

Prevention

a. **Passive immunization:** In a pregnant women who has a negative or uncertain history of varicella, has significant exposure, serology test can be performed. For susceptible or e xposed women without serology test result VZIg (Varicella zoster immunoglobulin) should be administered to prevent or moderate maternal infection. Infant born to mother who develop varicella between 5 days before and 2 days after delivery should receive 125 IU VZIG to ameliorate a potentially serious infection (varicella zoster immunoglobulin).

Varicella Vaccination

A live attenuated varicella vaccine is available which if given within 72 hours after varicella exposure can prevent or significantly modify disease. *Vaccine is contraindicated in pregnancy.*

Parvovirus B19 Infection

Parvovirus B19 is a single stranded DNA virus. In the normal host B19 infection can manifest as:
a. Asymptomatic or subclinical infection.
b. Erythema infectiosum (EI) or fifth disease.
c. As an arthropathy.
d. In patients with thalassemia or sickle cell disease B19 infection can cause transient aplastic crisis.
e. In fetus B19 infection is associated with anemia, non-immune hydrops and fetal death.

Diagnosis

It is done by serology. An individual is susceptible in the absence of documented IgM and IgG. The presence of only IgG denotes an immune individual. The presence of only IgM denotes a very recent infection, whereas the presence of both IgM and IgG is typical of patient with recent exposure.

Management

In an event that a pregnant patient has complaints potentially consistent with B19 infection, serology should be performed. Serial ultrasound scans should be done. In the event of hydropic changes and Doppler velocimetry showing fetal anemia—intrauterine transfusion may be necessary. *There is no B19 vaccination.*

HUMAN IMMUNE DEFICIENCY VIRUS

It is described in chapter of Gynecological Infection. The points to remember in management of pregnant women with HIV are as follows:
a. All pregnant women should be routinely screened for HIV infection. Targeted testing of only women with risk factors, misses too many cases.
b. The likelihood of vertical transmission to fetus is directly related to maternal viral load. Before starting therapy the risk of these drugs during pregnancy as well as benefit for infected women and reducing the risk for HIV–1 transmission to her infants should be explained. Regimens of antiretroviral drugs are guided by viral load and CD4 count.
c. Cesarean section reduces the rate of transmission in women with higher viral loads.
d. Vaginal delivery if opted than membranes should be left intact for as long as possible. Use of invasive procedure like fetal electrodes should be avoided. Antiretroviral (ARV) drugs to be continued throughout labor. Cord should be clamped as early as possible and baby should be bathed immediately after birth.
e. After delivery the women as well neonate should have proper assessment. Infant should be given prophylactic antiretroviral drug.
f. WHO recommends that breastfeeding is not recommended in developed countries. But in developing countries where infectious disease and malnutrition are primary causes of infant death, exclusive breastfeeding for 6 months with abrupt weaning is supported. Mixed feeding is not advised, as it increases the risk of transmission.

OTHER INFECTIONS

Syphilis

Syphilis is a sexually transmitted disease caused by *Treponema pallidum*. Overall frequency of vertical transmission (that is congenital syphilis) is high in primary and secondary (50%) syphilis.

Fetal Effect

Depending upon the intensity and time of occurrence of infection there can be following sequelae:
a. Abortion
b. Preterm birth
c. Intrauterine death
d. Delivery of highly infected baby with early neonatal death
e. Survival with congenital syphilis.

Diagnosis

In obstetric history there is serial improvement in obstetric performance. A classic history shows **late abortion—still-birth—congenital syphilitic baby—healthy baby**.

Laboratory Investigation

VDRL should be routinely done in all pregnant women. A positive VDRL test should be confirmed by fluorescent treponemal antibody absorption test (FTA – Abs) which is specific. Spouse should also be tested. *Fetal infection* can be diagnosed by polymerase chain reaction of *Treponema pallidum* in amniotic fluid, fetal serum or cerebrospinal fluid.

Management

Treatment is the same for pregnant and nonpregnant women. According to CDC 2002 patients with early syphilis should receive a single intramuscular dose of 2.4 million unit of Benzathine Penicillin. For pregnant women with late latent syphilis of more than 1 year duration or with cardiovascular syphilis, Benzathine penicillin G 2.4 million unit intramuscularly should be given weekly for 3 weeks. Pregnant women with neurosyphylis should receive aqueous crystalline penicillin G 18-24 million unit/day by I/v dosage of 3-4 million unit every 4 hours for 10-14 days. An alternative outpatient program is of giving intramuscular procaine penicillin 2.4 million/day with 500 mg oral probenecid 4 times daily for 10-14 days.

Fetus should be monitored by ultrasound to look for hydrops, ascites, skin edema and hepatomegaly. With sonographic abnormalities, neonatologist and maternal fetal medicine specialist should be consulted.

In patient allergic to penicillin, skin testing and referral for penicillin desensitization is preferred. Treatment of newborn with congenital syphilis is 100,000 – 150,000 unit/kg/day of aqueous crystalline penicillin G daily at 50,000 unit/kg/dose every hour, or 50,000 unit/kg of procaine penicillin intramuscularly once daily for 10 days.

Prevention

The mainstays of prevention of congenital syphilis are early detection, appropriate treatment and follow-up. All pregnant women should have serological testing at their first prenatal visit and women in high risk areas again in the third trimester of pregnancy. All serological positive test cases should be treated. Finally all patients with syphilis should be counseled about the risk of HIV infection and be encouraged to be tested for HIV antibody.

Group β Streptococcal

General Consideration

Between 10-30% of pregnant women are colonized with group β *Streptococcus*. Colonization may result in symptomatic infection in some women, commonly manifested as chorioamnionitis, postpartum endometritis or urinary tract infection. Intrapartum and postpartum bacteremia can occur. Neonates may be colonized and develop symptomatic infection via transmission from mother. These neonatal infections including localized infection—meningitis or septicemia carry high risk of sequelae and are potentially fatal.

Diagnosis and Management

The most accurate mode of diagnosis is by means of culture from cervix, vaginal fornix and rectum.

Prevention Strategies

There are two prevention strategies advocated by CDC and ACOG:
a. *Risk based approach:* In this intrapartum prophylaxis is given to women with preterm labor, preterm premature rupture of membrane and rupture of membrane more than 18 hours, intrapartum fever and previous sibling with Gr B streptococcal disease.
b. *Culture based approach:* All women are screened for Gr β streptococcal colonization at 35-37 weeks and intrapartum antibiotics given in carriers. Recommended regimens are as follows:

a. In penicillin 5 million units I/V followed by 2.5 million unit I/v every 4 hour. Alternative is 2 gm I/V followed by 1 gm every 4 hours.
b. In cases that have risk for allergy – Cefazolin 2 gm I/V followed by 1 gm I/V every 8 hour. Clindamycin 500 mg I/V every 8 hour or erythromycin 500 mg I/V every 6 hour.
c. In resistant cases vancomycin 1 gm every 12 hours.
All antibiotics should be discontinued following delivery in the absence of clinical diagnosis of maternal infection.

Other Genital Infections

Bacterial vaginosis has been associated with preterm birth and treatment of bacterial vaginosis in high risk women may reduce the incidence of preterm birth. Other genital infections as *Trichomonas*, gonorrhea and *Chlamydia* have been inconsistently associated with preterm premature rupture of membrane and or preterm delivery.

Malaria—General Consideration

Malaria is a protozoal disease caused by 4 species of *Plasmodium — Vivax, Ovale, Malariae* and *falciparum*. Organisms are transmitted by the bite of female anopheles mosquito. Nearly 300-500 million persons world wide are infected at any given time and disease causes 1-3 million deaths annually.

Effect of Pregnancy on Malaria and Vice Versa

Malarial episode increases by 3 fold during the last two trimesters of pregnancy and two months postpartum. Pregnancy enhances the severity of falciparum malaria, especially in nonimmune nulliparous women. The incidence of abortion and preterm labor is increased with malaria. The malaria parasites have an affinity for decidual vessels and may involve the placenta extensively without affecting the fetus. Placental and fetal infection may cause stillbirth. Neonatal infection is uncommon with congenital malaria developing in up to 7% of neonates born to non-immune mother.

Clinical Presentation

It is characterized by high grade fever with chills and rigors, myalgia which may occur at interval. Malaria may be associated with anemia and jaundice and falciparum infections may cause kidney failure, coma and death.

Diagnosis

It is based on clinical symptoms and identification of intracellular malaria organism on a blood smear.

Treatment

a. **Prevention:** From mosquito bite using mosquito nets and repellants.
b. **Prophylaxis:** Chloroquine 300 mg base orally once a week continued till 4 weeks when a pregnant woman is traveling to endemic areas.
c. **Treatment:** Commonly used antimalarial drugs are not contraindicated during pregnancy. Chloroquine is treatment of choice for all forms of malaria except chloroquine resistant *P. falciparum* and newly emerging strains of resistant *P. vivax*. Chloroquine is given in dose of 10 mg/kg at 24 hours and 5 mg/kg at 48 hours. For women with chloroquine resistant infection mefloquine is given orally. For severe resistant malaria quinine or quinidine is given intravenously.

Leprosy in Pregnancy

Latent infection by *M. leprae* may become overt for the first time during pregnancy or within few months following delivery. With established leprosy there is chance of exacerbation of the lesion during pregnancy. Pregnancy may be regarded as a test of cure. Failure of signs of the disease to reappear during or after pregnancy indicates that leprosy is definitely arrested. Congenital infection of baby is unlikely. However, in active disease the baby should be separated from the infected mother immediately after delivery.

Treatment

Dapsone and Clofazimine appear safe in pregnancy. Rifampicin may also be used. IUGR is a common problem.

Gonorrhea in Pregnancy

Gonorrhea results from *N. gonorrhoeae*. The prevalence varies during pregnancy but may be as high as 7%. Risk factors are adolescence, poverty, drug abuse, prostitution, and other STD. Gonorrhea infection increases the risk of *preterm labor, PROM, intrapartum, and postpartum infection*. The baby may be affected during labor while passing through the infected birth canal resulting in *ophthalmia neonatarum*.
Treatment: Ceftriaxone 125 mg I/m as a single dose or Cefixime 400 mg orally in a single dose. Possible concomitant *Chlamydia* infection should be treated. Infected neonate is treated with single dose of ceftriaxone 50 mg/kg I/m.

MULTIPLE CHOICE QUESTIONS

1. Which of the following perinatal infection has the highest risk of fetal infection in the first trimester?
   a. Hepatitis B virus
   b. Syphilis
   c. Toxoplasmosis
   d. Rubella
   Ans. d

2. A pregnant woman is diagnosed to be HbSAg +ve. Which of the following is the best way to prevent infection to the child?
   a. Hepatitis vaccine to the child
   b. Full course of hepatitis B vaccine and immunoglobulin to the child
   c. Hepatitis B immunoglobulin to the mother
   d. Hepatitis B immunization to mother
   Ans. b

3. With which of the following types of viral hepatitis infection in pregnancy the maternal mortality is highest?
   a. Hepatitis A
   b. Hepatitis B
   c. Hepatitis C
   d. Hepatitis E
   Ans. d

4. Highest transmission of hepatitis B from mother to fetus occurs if the mother is infected during:
   a. 1st trimester
   b. 2nd trimester
   c. 3rd trimester
   d. At the time of implantation
   Ans. c

5. A G_2P_1 with 10 weeks pregnancy has come to you. She had one live child with ocular toxoplasmosis. The risk of present baby to get infected is:
   a. 50%
   b. 25%
   c. 100%
   d. Nil
   Ans. d

6. A pregnant lady acquires chicken pox 3 days prior to delivery. She delivers by normal vaginal route, which of the following statement is true:
   a. Both mother and baby are safe
   b. Give antiviral treatment to mother before delivery
   c. Give antiviral treatment to baby
   d. Baby will develop neonatal varicella syndrome
   Ans. d

7. Which of the following abnormality is commonly seen in fetus with congenital CMV infection?
   a. Colitis
   b. Myocarditis
   c. Blood dyscrasias
   d. Pulmonary cyst
   Ans. c

8. Congenital infection affection fetus with minimal teratogenic risk is:
   a. HIV
   b. Rubella
   c. Varicella
   d. CMV
   Ans. a

9. Which drug is given to prevent HIV transmission from mother to child?
   a. Nevirapine
   b. Lamivudine
   c. Stavidine
   d. Abacavir
   Ans. a
10. Syphilis is transmitted in which gestational age:
    a. 4th week
    b. 8th week
    c. 16th week
    d. 28th week
    Ans. c
11. Cesarean section is preferred in:
    a. Toxoplasmosis
    b. Herpes
    c. CMV
    d. Varicella zoster virus
    Ans. b

49 Normal Labor

Should you shield the canyons from windstorm, you would never see the beauty of their carving.

GENERAL CONSIDERATION

Labor is the process by which a fetus of viable age is expelled from the uterus. It varies greatly in duration, severity and risk involved to mother and fetus. **WHO defines Normal Labor as one in which fetus presents by the vertex, begins spontaneously at term and terminates naturally without artificial aid and without complications.**

Abnormal labor is somewhat difficult to define but for practical purpose, it may include all cases in which some part other than the vertex presents and all vertex cases in which maternal or fetal complications arise. The role of obstetric caregivers should be based on evidence based practice, modified/obstetric skill and women's personal preferences. One should avoid unnecessary intervention in course of normal labor, but at the same time identify and intervene in difficult situations.

Calculation of Date of Labor

The date at which labor may be expected can not be predicted with certainty. A calculation of date of labor is usually based on the date of last menstrual period. Calculation is made by adding 7 days to the date of last menstrual period and counting forward a calendar months or counting back 3 months. When the date of last menstrual period is not known or women conceive in lactational amenorrhea, ultrasound dating especially if done in early pregnancy plays important role in calculation of date of labor. Clinical estimation of symphysis fundal height and date of quickening also helps.

Cause of Onset of Labor

The physiological process that regulates parturition and onset of labor is still not definite. Onset of labor represents the culmination of series of biochemical changes in uterus that results from endocrine and paracrine signals coming from both the mothers and fetus. Some of the factors which play an important role in initiation of labor are:

a. Uterine sensitivity to chemicohormonal influence and stretch.
b. Fetal anterior pituitary adrenal system.
c. Placenta estrogen and progestogen formation.
d. Maternal estrogen, progestogen, oxytocin and prostaglandin production.

Presently we can explain onset of labor after and ongoing clinical and preclinical research work in the way that increasing fetal anterior pituitary adrenal activity brings about increasing production of estrogen and of surfactant. Surfactant causes lung maturation while estrogen combined with oxytocin is responsible for release of prostaglandin from decidual and myometrial cells. The release is delayed until level of progesterone falls to a level, which is now no longer effective in its inhibitory action. Causes of onset of labor has been summarized in Flow chart 49.1.

FEMALE PELVIS

Obstetrical anatomy of female pelvis has been discussed in chapter of anatomy.

FETAL DIMENSION AND DISPOSITION

The journey of fetus from maternal passage to outer world is considered most dangerous and difficult one of the human life. Dimensions, disposition and specific characteristics of fetus in relation to maternal passage is critical to route of delivery. So let's review the facts and diagnosis of fetal positions in laboring women.

Fetal Lie

It denotes the relation of long axis of fetus to that of uterine ovoid. It may be longitudinal or transverse or occasionally oblique at 45° angle which is considered unstable and always becomes longitudinal or transverse in course of labor. Longitudinal lie are present in over 99% of labor at term. When long axis of fetal and uterine ovoid correspond, lie is said to be longitudinal. It may be both head (97%) or breech

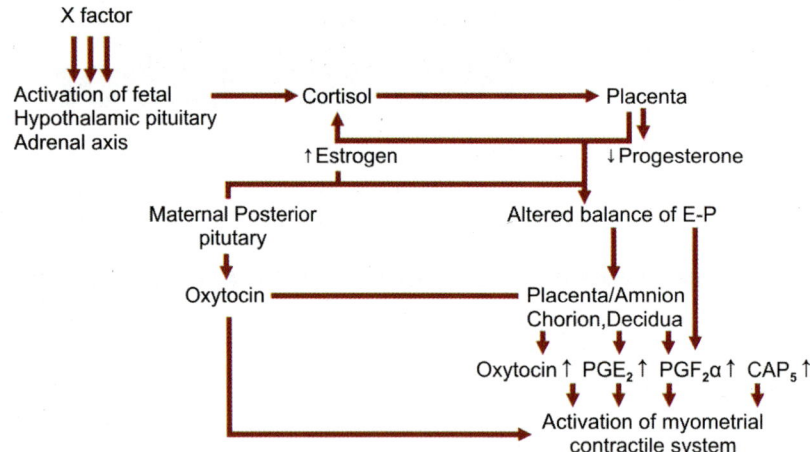

Flow chart 49.1: Sequele in onset of labor

below (2.5%), transverse or oblique lie is said when long axis of fetus and uterine ovoid do not correspond (0.5%).

Fetal Presentation

Part of fetus which lies below and presents at pelvic brim is called fetal presentation which may be (a) cephalic, (b) breech, (c) shoulder.

Presenting Part of Fetus

It is more precisely the particular part of fetal presentation, which first enters the pelvic brim and like wise first to be felt by examining finger during pelvic examinations. In majority of cephalic presentation it is vertex presentation.

Disposition of Fetus—Fetal Attitude or Posture

During last weeks of pregnancy the head, trunk and limb of fetus are packed up into smallest possible space in a regular and fairly constant arrangement of generalized flexion—this is termed as **fetal attitude**. Fetus become folded or bent upon itself in such a manner that back becomes convex, chin is almost in contact with chest, thighs are flexed over abdomen, legs are bent at knees and the arches of feet rest upon the anterior surfaces of the legs, arms are closed over thorax and umbilical cord lies in the space between them and lower extremities (Fig. 49.1).

This characteristic fetal posture results from mode of growth of fetus and its accommodation to uterine cavity. If fetal head become extended from vertex to face presentation, it results in progressive change in fetal attitude from a convex (flexed) to a concave (extended) contour of the vertebral column.

Fetal Skull

From obstetrical point of view the characteristic of fetal skull and size of fetal head is important because firstly head is presenting part in more than 90% of labor and secondly an essential feature of labor is the adaptation between the fetal head and maternal bony pelvis. Ossification of the fetal skull at term pregnancy is incomplete, especially of the vault bones. So bones of base of fetal skull are firm and incompressible, while the tabular bones of vault remain thin and pliable. These pliable vault bones are separated at their edges by interval of unossified membranes, which form the sutures and fontanelle.

Sutures

a. **Sagittal suture:** It cross the vault of skull in middle line, in an anteroposterior direction between two parietal bones (Fig. 49.2—a).
b. **Frontal suture:** Sagittal suture continues in front beyond the anterior fontanelle, in the same plane between two halves of frontal bones (Fig. 49.2—f).
c. **Coronal suture:** It separates the frontal from parietal bones meeting the sagittal and frontal suture at the anterior fontanelle (Fig. 49.2—d).

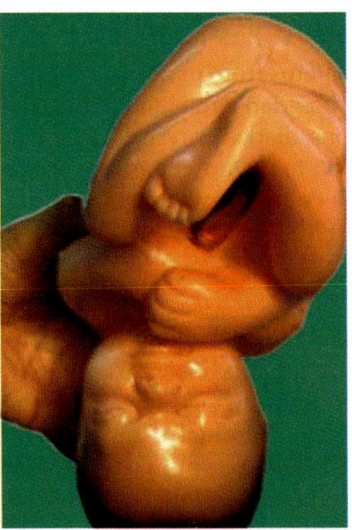

Fig. 49.1: Fetal attitude of generalized flexion

Chapter -49 ♦ Normal Labor

d. **Lambdoidal suture:** It separates the parietal bone from the tabular portion of the occipital bone (Fig. 49.2—b).

Fontanelles

Where several sutures meet, an irregular space forms, which is enclosed by a membrane and designated as fontanelle. Six fontanelle exist on the fetal skull at term, but only two—anterior and posterior fontanelle are of practical importance.

Anterior Fontanelle (Bregma)

It is an unequal sided kite shaped piece of unossified membrane, lying in mesial plane between two halves of frontal and two parietal bones. Its angle are continuous with frontal, sagittal and right and left halves of the coronal suture. It measures 3 cm in anteroposterior and 2 cm in transverse diameter. As it lies a little below the general level of the skull, it can felt on the surface as a shallow depression (Fig. 49.2—e).

Posterior Fontanelle

It is a small triangular depressed area at the intersection of the sagittal and lambdoid suture. It is to be noted that it is not an unossified piece of membrane at all but depression, except in a premature fetus (Fig. 49.2—c). Temporal or cesarean fontanelle have no diagnostic significance.

Obstetrical Significance of Anterior and Posterior Fontanelle

These two fontanelle are of great clinical obstetrical significance because they can be recognized during labor via its special characteristics and from them valuable information can be obtained regarding position and attitude of the fetal head. Table 49.1 illustrates the differentiating feature of anterior and posterior fontanelle.

Diameters and Circumference of Fetal Head

General shape of the fetal head is that of an ovoid with a long anteroposterior diameter. In a normal attitude of complete flexion, long diameter of fetal head ovoid forms a very acute angle with that of body ovoid. If head lies mid way between flexion and extension, the two long diameter cross each other at right angles. And if head is fully extended, the angle formed is obtuse and the face becomes the lowest part (Figs 49.3A to D). This relationship of head with body is basis of different diameter of engagement in cephalic presentations.

Girdle of contact is that part of circumference of head which first comes in contact with pelvic brim. Diameter of girdle of contact is called **diameter of engagement**.

Vertex is area of vault of skull which is bounded in front by anterior fontanelle and coronal suture behind by posterior fontanelle and lambdoid suture and laterally by lines passing through parietal eminences.

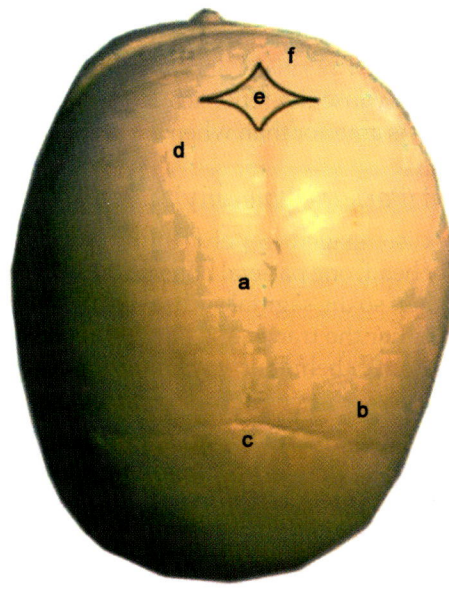

Fig. 49.2: Fetal vault—suture fontanelle

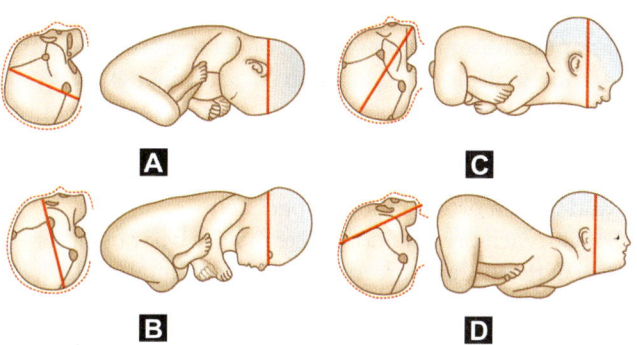

Figs 49.3A to D: Different diameters of engagement with varying attitudes of fetal head: (A) Completely flexed vertex: engagement of suboccipitobregmatic diameter; (B) Extended vertex: engagement of occipitofrontal-diameter; (C) Brow presentation: engagement of mentovertical diameter; (D) Completely extended face: engagement of submentobregmatic diameter

	Table 49.1: Differentiating characteristics of anterior and posterior fontanelle	
	Anterior fontanelle	*Posterior fontanelle*
1. Shape	Lozenge	Triangular
2. Consistency	Soft membranous	Hard floor
3. Presence of suture	Four sutures running from its angle	Three connecting sutures

It is most common and favored cephalic presentation occurs in fully flexed head presenting suboccipitobregmatic diameter for engagement which is shortest diameter of fetal skull. Different diameters of engagement with different cephalic presentation are illustrated in Table 49.2.

TRANSVERSE DIAMETER OF FETAL SKULL

- **Biparietal diameter**—9.4 cm, between two parietal eminence.
- **Bitemporal diameter**—8.1 cm, between anteroinferior ends of coronal suture.
- **Bimastoid**—7.5 cm, between tip of mastoid process.

Facts of Obstetrical Significance

1. Greatest circumference of head, corresponds to plane of occipitofrontal diameter, average 34.5 cm, is too large to fit through pelvis without flexion.
2. Smallest circumference correspond to plane of suboccipitobregmatic diameter is 32 cm.
3. As vault is compressible, all diameters can be reduced in length to an appreciable extent during passage of head through pelvis.
4. **Moulding:** As the bones of the cranium are normally connected only by a thin layer of fibrous tissue that allows considerable shifting or sliding of each bone to accommodate size and shape of maternal pelvis. This intrapartum process is termed moulding. It can result in reduction of all diameters.

Fetal Position and Denominator

Fetal denominator *is* a bony point on fetal presenting part in reslation to designated location of maternal pelvis.

Position refers to the relationship of denominator to right or left side of maternal birth canal. Fetal occiput, chin (mentum) and sacrum are the determining point in vertex, face and breech presentation respectively.

So with each presentation, there may be two positions—right or left. So there are right or left occipital, right left mentum and right and left sacral presentation.

Varieties of Presentation and Positions

For still more accurate orientation, the relationship of a given position of the presenting part to the anterior, transverse or posterior part of maternal pelvis is considered. As the presenting part in right or left positions may be directed Anteriorly (A), Transversely (T) or Posteriorly (P), there are six variables of each of three presentations. Thus in occiput presentation the presentation, position and variety may be abbreviated in clockwise fashion.

- 1st position—LOA
- 2nd position—ROA
- 3rd position—ROP
- 4th position—LOP

In majority of cases the vertex enters the pelvis with sagittal suture lying in transverse pelvic diameter. The fetus enters into pelvis in left occiput transverse (LOA) positions in 40% of labor and in right occiput transverse (ROT) position in 20%. In occiput anterior position (LOA or ROA), the head either enters the pelvis with occiput rotated 45%, anteriorly from the transverse position or subsequently does so. In 20% of labor the fetus enters the pelvis in an occiput posterior (OP) positions (Figs 49.4A and B).

While the mechanism of labor in transverse and anterior position are usually similar, posterior position are more often associated with narrow forepelvis.

Vertex engage in right oblique diameter much oftener than left because left oblique diameter is encroached upon by pelvic colon and rectum.

Approximately 2/3rd of all vertex presentation are in left occiput position (Ist position) and one third in right (IInd position), it is because the fetus lies more easily in uterus, when the back is anterior than when back is posterior.

Asynclitism (Parietal Obliquity)

When vertex is engaged in pelvic brim, owing to lateral inclination of head, one parietal bone usually lies at a lower level than other, so the sagittal suture does not correspond precisely to either the transverse or oblique diameter, but lies either in front or behind it. It is known as asynclitism or parietal obliquity.

Table 49.2: Different diameters of engagement in different cephalic presentation

Diameter of engagement	Diameter	Presentation	Attitude
1. Suboccipitobregmatic (nape of neck to center of bregma)	9.4 cm	Vertex flexed	Fully
2. Suboccipitofrontal (nape of neck to anterior end of bregma)	10 cm	Deflexed vertex	Incomplete flexion of head
3. Occipitofrontal (occipital protuberance to root of nose)	11.3 cm	Extended vertex	Extended
4. Mentovertical (point of chin to one inch in front of posterior fontanelle in the sagittal suture)	13.8 cm	Brow	Incomplete extension
5. Submentovertical (Angle between neck and chin to center of sagittal suture)	11.3 cm	Incomplete extended face	Partially extended face
6. Submentobregmatic (angle between neck and chin to center of bregma)	9.4 cm	Complete extended face	Fully extended face

CHAPTER -49 ♦ Normal Labor

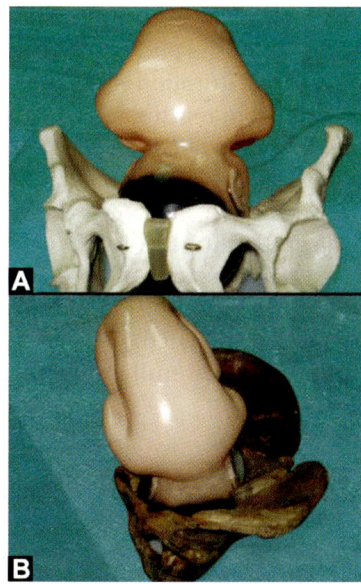

Figs 49.4A and B: Variants of positions of fetus: (A) Occiput anterior; (B) Occiput posterior

a. **Anterior asynclitism:** If sagittal suture approaches the sacral promontory, anterior parietal bone is below the posterior and presents itself to the examining finger. It is called anterior asynclitism, or anterior parietal obliquity or Naegele's obliquity. It is found chiefly in multipara (Fig. 49.5A).

b. **Posterior asynclitism:** If sagittal suture lies close to symphysis, posterior parietal bone will be below the anterior and present to examining finger. It is called posterior asynclitism, posterior parietal obliquity or Litzman's obliquity. It is found chiefly in primigravida because in primigravida the relatively tense abdominal wall tends to keep the uterus back and so prevent body of fetus from coming forward into line of axis of the brim (Fig. 49.5B).

Moderate degrees of asynclitism are rule in normal labor. But severe and persistent asynclitism is abnormal and only occurs with varieties of contracted pelvis.

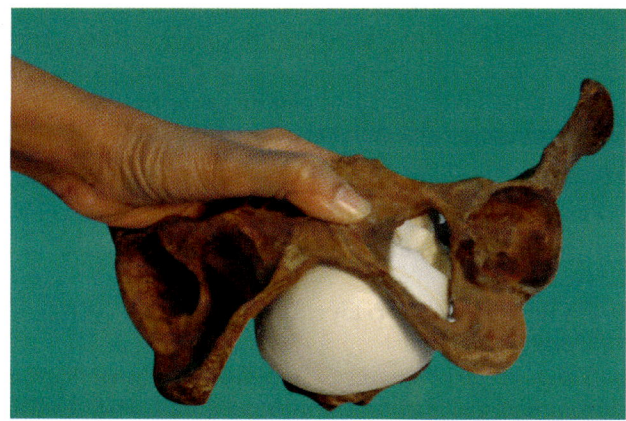

Fig. 49.5A: Anterior asynclitism

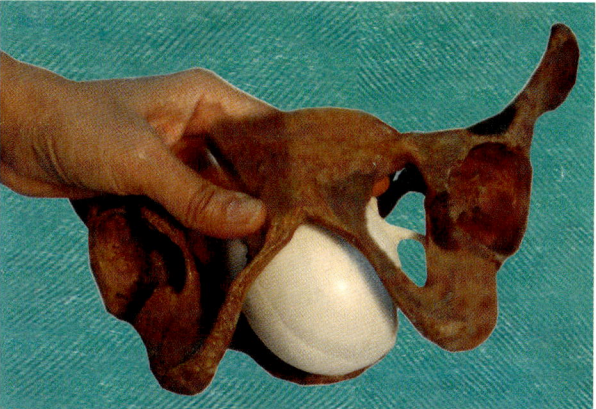

Fig. 49.5B: Posterior asynclitism

PHASES OF LABOR (PARTURITION)

Physiological process of parturition is divided into following phases, which correspond to major physiological transition of myometrium and cervix during pregnancy.

a. **Phase zero:** It is characterized by uterus smooth muscles quiescence with maintainenence of structural integrity. It is continued till near the end of the pregnancy.

b. **Phase one:** *Physiological preparation of labor*—Near end of pregnancy myometrium is awakened or activated. This represents the sequence of change of uterus during last 6-8 weeks of pregnancy. These changes are as follows:

   i. *Lightening:* The settling of the fetal head into the brim of the pelvis is known as lightening, which usually occurs two or more weeks before labor in first pregnancy. In multigravida lightening often does not occur until early labor. The descent of fetus is often accompanied by a decrease in discomfort associated with pressure on abdominal organs like heart burn, breathlessness and increase in pelvic discomfort and frequency of urination.

   ii. *Increased uterine contraction:* During last 4-8 weeks of pregnancy generally painless uterine contraction occurs with slowly increasing frequency and intensity. It is because of alteration in expression of key protein that control myometrial contractility which are termed CAPs (Contraction Associated Proteins) and there is striking increase in myometrial oxytocin receptors which results in increased uterine contraction and responsiveness to uterotonics. When these contractions occur early in third trimester, they must be distinguished from true preterm labor. In late third trimester they are common cause of *false labor*, which is distinguished by lack of cervical changes in response to contraction.

   iii. *Cervical changes:* During the course of several days to several weeks before the onset of true labor, the cervix begins to soften, efface and dilate. These cervical changes are due to increase in collagen break down and rearrangement of collagen fibers bundles. There is striking increase in amount of hyaluronic acid and water in the cervix with decrease in dermaton sulfate needed for collagen fiber cross linking. Simultaneous increase of uterine contractility and dilatation of cervix causes formation of lower uterine segment in phase one.

c. **Onset of labor:** The signs on which start of labor is diagnosed should be clearly understood as it is important to diagnose true labor from false labor. These signs are as follows:

  i. *Painful uterine contraction:* True labor pain contractions are more regular, gradually increasing in severity, more prolonged and palpable on uterus palpation. False labor pains causes mild discomfort but not accompanied by retraction responsible for dilatation of cervix.

  ii. *Show - slight uterine hemorrhage:* It is per vaginal discharge of blood stained mucus which comes from abundantly secreted cervical mucus during labor and hemorrhage caused by separation of membrane from lower uterine segment at beginning of cervical dilatation.

  iii. *Dilatation of internal os:* At term, the ripe cervix is soft, effaced, slightly patulous and closely applied to head. Dilatation of internal os is accompanied by stretching of lowest part of the lower uterine segment so the cervix will be found shortened. Start of dilatation of internal os of the cervix is a sign of onset of labor especially in primigravida. In multigravida a slightly dilated cervix may be found even before onset of labor.

  iv. *Formation of bag of water:* On dilatation of cervix, the lower side of fetal membrane—chorion and amnion which has been already separated few weeks before actual onset of labor by stretching of lower uterine segment, now bulge into the cervical canal. This bulge of membrane which contains little liquor amni is called the presence of bag of water, which becomes tense and convex during uterine contraction and disappears with passing off the pain.

d. Active labor.

STAGES OF LABOR

Conventionally events of labor are divided into three stages:

a. **First stage:** It start from onset of true labor and ends with full dilatation of the cervix. Its average duration is 12 hours in primigravida and 6 hours in multigravida.

b. **Second stage:** It starts from the full dilatation of the cervix and ends with expulsion of the fetus from the birth canal. It can be divided in two phase.

  i. *Propulsive phase:* This starts from full dilatation to descent of the presenting part up to the pelvic floor.

  ii. *Expulsion phase:* It is distinguished by maternal bearing down efforts and ends with delivery of the baby. Its average duration is 2 hours in primigravida and 30 minutes in multipara.

c. **Third stage:** It begins after expulsion of the fetus and ends with expulsion of the placenta and membranes. It's average duration is about 15 minutes in both primigravida and multipara.

d. **Fourth stage:** It is the stage of observation for at least one hour after expulsion of the placenta. During this period general condition of the patient and the behavior of the uterus are to be carefully watched.

First Stage of Labor

Friedman developed the concept of three functional division of labor to describe the physiological objective of each division:

a. *Preparatory division:* In this phase there is little dilatation of the cervix but connective tissue component of cervix change considerably. Duration of the latent phase is more variable. *Oxytocin infusion or AROM can reduce duration of this stage. Sedation and conduction analgesia are capable of arresting this division of labor.*

b. *Dilatational division:* In this phase cervical dilatation proceed at its most rapid rate and this is unaffected by sedation or conduction analgesia.

c. *Pelvic division:* It starts with deceleration phase of cervical dilatation. The classical mechanism of labor that include the cardinal fetal movement of the cephalic presentation that is – *engagement, flexion, descent, internal rotation, extension and external rotation* takes place principally during the pelvic division.

Friedman Curve

Friedman plotted the active division of labor in form of graph. These phases of normal labor take the shape of sigmoid curve. The latent phase corresponds to preparatory division and active phase correspond to dilatational division. Friedman popularized the use of an objective measure of labor progress over 30 years ago. Friedman curves plot *cervical dilatation against* time passed with varying expectation for nulliparous and multiparous patient used in conjunction with *fetal descent*. This curve provides clinical feedback about the normalcy of the progress in labor (Fig. 49.6).

Cervical dilatation: Friedman subdivided the active phase into further three phases:
a. Acceleration phase.
b. Phase of maximum slope.
c. Deceleration phase.

The average length of active phase is within the limits of normal being 2 and 6 hours in multipara and nullipara respectively.

CHAPTER -49 ♦ Normal Labor

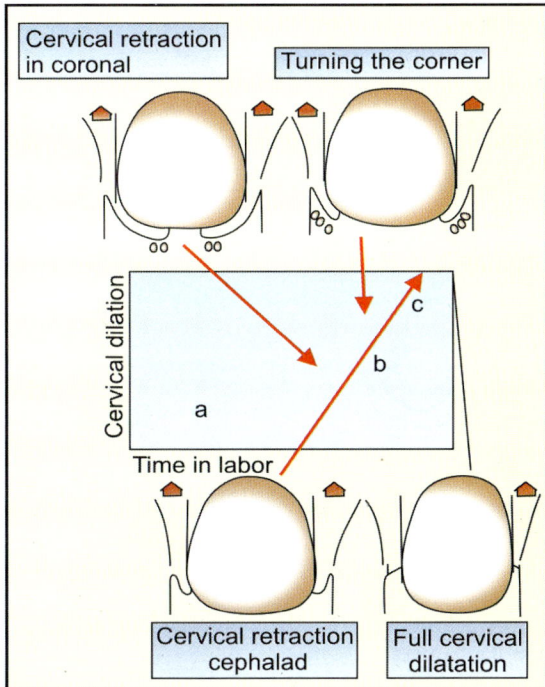

Fig. 49.6: Graphic display progress of labor with gradual dilatation of cervix in first stage of labor (a—Preparatory division, b—Dilatational division, c—Pelvic division)

Descent of presenting part: During latent and early active phase of cervical dilatation, fetal descent may be small. Once the phase of rapid cervical dilatation starts, steady fetal descent usually begins. The main part of the descent takes place when the cervix is near full dilatation and in the second stage of labor. Once descent begins it should be progressive.

Abnormal active phase: Friedman subdivided active phase problem into:
a. **Protraction disorder:** It is defined as a slow rate of cervical dilatation or descent which for nullipara is less than 1.2 cm dilatation per hour or less than 1 cm descent per hour. For multipara protraction was defined as less than 1.5 cm dilatation per hour or less than 2 cm descent per hour.
b. **Arrest of dilatation:** It is defined as 2 hours with no cervical changes in dilatation and arrest of descent as one hour without fetal descent. Factors contributing to both protraction and arrest disorders were *excessive sedation, analgesic, fetal malposition, and undetected cephalopelvic disproportion.*

Second Stage of Labor

This stage begins when cervical dilatation is complete and ends with fetal delivery. In this stage uterus, cervix and vagina is merged into a single broad channel and vagina is gradually dilated from above downwards by the passage through it of the head. The following events occur in second stage:

a. **Uterine contraction:** Uterine contractions become severe, last 60-90 seconds and occur every 2-3 minutes.
b. **Bearing down pains:** These occur due to voluntary expulsive effort by the patient. It is due to nerve reflex initiated by the stretching of the vaginal wall by the presenting part. The main expulsive effort is from the abdominal muscles and the diaphragm. They contract simultaneously during uterine contraction to push the baby down against the perineum. The patient holds her breath, grunts, braces her feet to push down by contracting her abdominal muscles. The bearing down nature of the pain herald the onset of the second stage.
a. **Descent of fetus:** Because of descent of fetus there is stretching of perineal body, anus become turgid and heavy, scalp appears at vulva. When head is about to emerge there is gaping of anus, exposing 1-2" of anterior rectal wall, fourchette is thinned and there may be a certain degree of laceration of post vaginal wall.
b. **Crowning of head:** The head is said to be crowned when its maximum diameters stretches the vulvar outlet and does not recede in between uterine contraction.
c. **Delivery of baby:** After crowning, the actual expulsion of fetal head is accompanied by a very prolonged and severe contraction or series of powerful uterus contractions accompanied by violent straining. After delivery of head there is short pause, immediately to be followed by return of pain in 1-2 minutes, which expel first the shoulder, then trunk and lower extremities. As the body of fetus is delivered, there is a gush of blood stained liquor amni follows, which represents the portion of fluid which has been retained in uterus along with trunk and limbs.

Duration of Second Stage of Labor

Duration of second stage is 1-2 hours in primigravida and 15 minutes to 1 hour in multigravida. But it may last much longer, when pains are relatively feeble or with malposition. Current review suggests that arbitrary time limit on second stage should be abandoned, providing there are no fetal or maternal problems and progress is occurring.

Third Stage of Labor

The third stage starts at the birth of the baby and ends with complete expulsion of placenta and fetal membranes. When fetus is delivered, there is sudden and striking reduction in size of uterus and the placental bed is reduced to one third of its size in pregnancy. The placenta itself remains unchanged. So the shearing effect starts separating the placenta and cause retroplacental bleeding from the torn blood vessels in the intervillous spaces. It separates the placenta further through the cleavage plane of deep spongy layer of the decidua basalis.

The signs of separation of placenta are as follows:
a. Uterus becomes smaller, harder, and more globular in shape and more freely mobile.

b. The level of fundus which is hard and retracted rises and the lower segment felt above pubis, is soft and bulging from presence in it of placenta.
c. A certain amount of gush of blood is seen.
d. True lengthening of cord is noted.

Duration of Third Stage

The average duration of third stage is 5-15 minutes. These sequences of changes become more rapid and associated with less bleeding when an oxytocin is administered in labor in second stage or at beginning of the third stage of labor. The delivery of the placenta is accompanied by an insensible loss of blood, which normally should not be more than 300 ml. The uterus retracts strongly after birth of the baby and because of the lattice type of arrangement of the uterus musculature; the blood vessels supplying the placental bed get occluded, which prevent further blood loss.

Fourth Stage of Labor

The fourth stage (Golden hour) is essentially a stage of observation following the completion of the third stage of labor. The signs to be observed are:
a. To ensure that uterus is not relaxed.
b. Vaginal bleeding.
c. Maternal vital signs.
d. To start breastfeeding.

Total Duration of Labor

Normal duration of labor varies a great deal from one patient to the other. Labor exceeding 16-24 hours in a primigravida is considered prolonged, whereas in multigravida 8-12 hours is considered upper limit for normal progress of labor.

MECHANISM OF LABOR

The positional change in the presenting part required to navigate the pelvic canal constitute the mechanism of labor. These series of movement of fetus alter its relationship to the pelvic canal. Customarily these movements are described as movement of head, but virtually head is the only index of movement, trunk also initiates and participates in some movements.

Cardinal Movement of Labor

a. Engagement.
b. Descent.
c. Flexion.
d. Internal rotation.
e. Extension.
f. External rotation.
g. Expulsion.

It should be understood that these movements are sequential as well overlap and concomitant uterus contraction modify fetal attitude (Figs 49.7A to H).

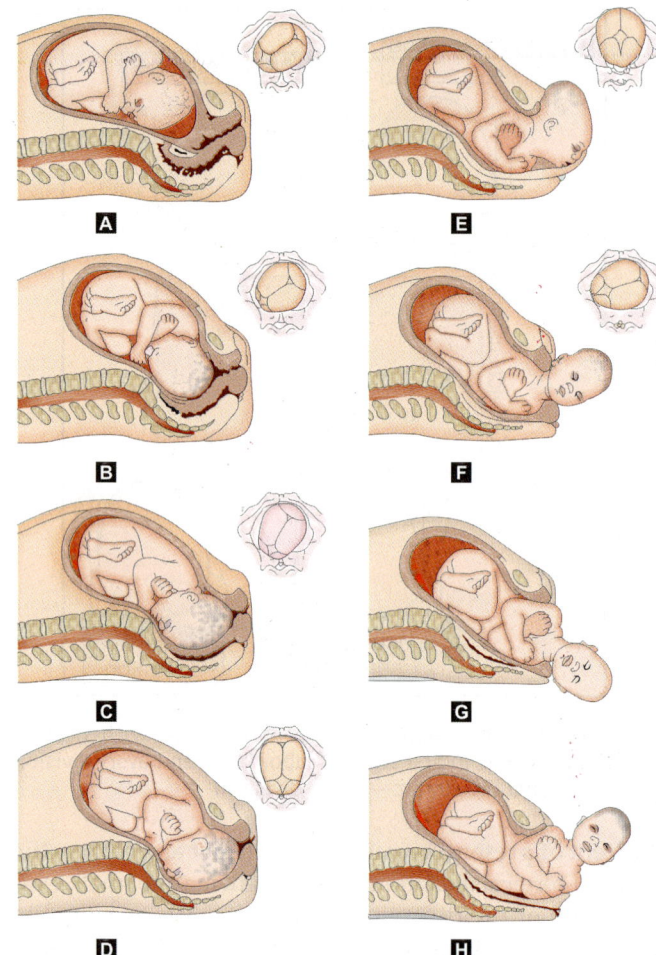

Figs 49.7A to H: Cardinal movement of labor: (A) Engagement; (B and C) Descent flexion; (D) Internal rotation; (E and F) Head delivered by extension; (G and H) Delivery of anterior and posterior shoulder

Engagement

The fetal head is said to have engaged when the maximum transverse (biparietal – 9.5 cm) and anteroposterior (which varies with the degree of flexion or extension of the head) diameter have crossed the plane of the pelvic brim. In a primigravida the engagement of the fetal head occurs mostly before onset of labor, while in multipara the head engages in the first stage. With engagement *anterior or posterior asynclitism* occurs which is a lateral deflection of head to a more anterior or posterior position in the pelvis. Successive shifting from posterior to anterior asynclitism helps in descent.

Descent

Throughout first and second stage of labor there is more or less continuous movement of descent. Descent of fetus is first requisite for birth of newborn. Descent is brought about by following forces:
a. Pressure of the amniotic fluid.
b. Direct pressure of the fundus upon the breech with contraction.

c. Bearing down effort of abdominal muscles.
d. Extension and straightening of fetal body.

Flexion

Flexion is primarily an attitude of fetus but usually at onset of labor head enters in pelvic brim in an attitude of deficient flexion. With start of labor flexion is increased, because of following facts:

a. *Head lever action:* With descent of head, when at start of labor the head begins to meet resistance during its passage through the birth canal, flexion is increased. It occurs because fetal head represents a two armed lever with fulcrum at occipitoatlantoid joint and whose anterior arm is longer than the posterior, so when fetal head meets resistance, long arm of lever ascends and short arm descends, which brings occiput lower than forehead and increasing flexion.
b. *Strong uterine contraction* encourages flexion.
c. *Shape of head:* The slope of the occipital regions of the head is much steeper than that of the forehead. So occiput can descend more easily with less friction. Any ovoid when pushed through a tube tends to adapt its long diameter to the long axis of the tube. When head is completely flexed, its longest diameter verticomental diameter is lying in the long axis of the birth canal.
d. *Point of flexion:* Point at which movement of increased flexion occurs, varies. Normally, it occurs at level of pelvic floor but where there is disproportion between head and pelvis, flexion can occur at level of contracted pelvis.

Internal Rotation

The head normally engages in the transverse diameter of the pelvis. Internal rotation refers to the anterior rotation of the head. This brings the occiput into one of the oblique diameter followed by complete rotation to bring the occiput directly behind the symphysis pubis. This movement carries the large diameter of head into the anteroposterior diameter, which is the largest diameter of the pelvic outlet. The internal rotation is determined by following anatomical and dynamic factors:

a. *Sloping characteristic of pelvic floor* caused by downward and forward direction of levator ani muscle. These directions are imparted to any movable part impinging upon the pelvic floor, driven by a force from above. When the head is flexed, the occiput reaches the pelvic floor first.
b. *Shape of the pelvic floor:* The pelvic floor is deficient anteriorly due to wide pubic arch. The part of the head which moves forward is moving in the direction of least resistance.
c. *Unequal flexibility of the different parts of the fetus:* In case of oblique anterior position the occiput rotates by one eighth of circle (45°) whereas in occiput lateral position there is rotation by 2/8th of circle (90°). The more posterior the position of the occiput, when it reaches the

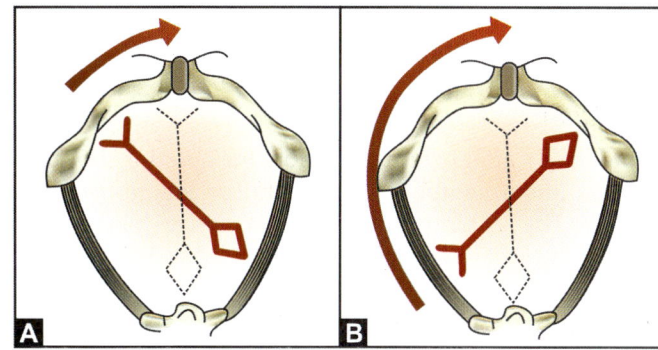

Figs 49.8A and B: Anterior rotation from ROA and ROP position: (A) 1/4th of circle; (B) 3/8th of circle

pelvic floor, the longer is the arc of rotation. In oblique posterior position the rotation amounts to 3/8th of a circle (135°). The fetal head must be well flexed and there must be good uterine contraction for internal rotation to occur (Figs 49.8A and B).

Extension

In the second stage of labor two forces act on the head:
a. Uterine force acts downwards
b. Force of resistant pelvic floor and symphysis act upward and forward. The downward and upward force counterbalances each other, the resultant force pushes the head forwards. It cannot go forward as the nape of the neck is fixed against the symphysis pubis; the head therefore follows the curves of the birth canal by the process of extension. As a result the chin leaves the chest and the vertex stretches the vaginal outlet, which is called *crowning of head*. With progressive distension of perineum and vaginal opening, an increasing large portion of occiput gradually appears and head is born in following sequences with movement of extension – *Occiput – Bregma – Forehead – Nose – Mouth – finally Chin passes successively over anterior margin of perineum.*

Restitution

When head emerges in AP diameter of outlet, the shoulder engage in oblique diameter of brim, so there is slight twist of the neck. When head is delivered, there is a slight movement, so neck is back into normal relation to the bisacromial diameter. *This passive movement of head is called restitution.* If occiput was originally directed towards left, head rotate towards left ischial tuberosity, if occiput was originally directed towards right, occiput rotate to the right.

External Rotation

This movement primarily occurs at the shoulders to bring them into A-P diameter of the pelvis and can also be called the internal rotation of the shoulders. This is reflected externally as a passive movement of the head which rotates further in the same direction as during restitution and is called external rotation.

Expulsion

Immediately after external rotation, the anterior shoulder appears under symphysis pubis and perineum becomes distended by posterior shoulder. After delivery of shoulder rest of body is delivered quickly.

MANAGEMENT OF LABOR

Antenatal supervision and intranatal care forms a continuum of planned responsibility. The ideal management of labor and delivery requires two potentially opposing view points to be kept in mind. First is that labor or birthing should be recognized as a normal physiological process that most women experience without implication. Other point is that intrapartum complications often arise quickly and unexpectedly and they have to be anticipated and intervened.

Objective of Intranatal Care

a. General care of mother.
b. Prevention of infection.
c. Diagnosis and monitoring of maternal and fetal condition and progress of labor.
d. Control of pain.
e. Management of abnormal progress of labor—use of uterine stimulant.
f. Technique of delivering of fetus and placenta.
g. After care of mother and baby.

Birth Environment

Birth environment in pre labor and labor ward should be clean, tidy, spacious and airy. Usually a fetal heart monitoring device, stethoscope or Doppler and gloves with antiseptic is needed for admission checkup of women. Verbal support, relaxed, calm and quiet surroundings helps in release of pain killing endorphins.

Admission Procedure

Whenever a women is evaluated for labor, the following factors should be assessed and recorded:

a. Time of onset of frequency of uterine contraction, status of membrane, any history of bleeding and any fetal movements.
b. History of allergies, use of medication, time and content of last oral intake.
c. Prenatal records with special attention to prenatal laboratory results that impact intrapartum and immediate postpartum management, e.g. HIV and hepatitis B virus, blood hematocrit, and Rh type.
d. Maternal vital signs, urinary protein and glucose.
e. Fetal heart rate, presentation and clinically estimated fetal weight.
f. Status of membrane, cervical dilatation and effacement (unless contraindicated like placenta previa) and station of presenting part.

Examination of Patient in Labor

1. *General examination:* Maternal pulse rate, temperature, and blood pressure should be recorded at least every 2 hours and more frequently when there is any deviation from normal.
2. *Abdominal examination:* It is to be emphasized that nearly all information required at this stage can be obtained by examination of abdomen. Abdominal examination is entirely without risk, noninvasive, painless so that it may be freely employed. During examination the mother should be supine, with knees slightly bent and abdomen uncovered. Hand should be warm and used with gentleness. Examination should be suspended during the uterine contraction. Steps of abdominal examinations are as follows:
   a. The size of contour of the uterus and height of fundus to assess baby size and lie of fetus.
   b. At the same time strength and frequency of uterine contraction should be assessed and recorded.
   c. **Leopold maneuver:** Abdominal examination can be conducted systematically employing the four maneuvers devised by Leopold and Sporlin in 1899 (Figs 49.9A to E).
      i. *First maneuver (Fundal palpation):* This maneuver permits identification of which fetal pole – breech or head occupies the uterine fundus. For this fundus of uterus is palpated with two hands laid flat upon it, obstetrician stands facing the patient. *Breech is felt as large firm, irregular body continuous with trunk of fetus and not so hard.* While the *head* is harder *than breech,* better defined in outline, more mobile and *ballotable,* head is separated from trunk by groove corresponding to neck (Fig. 49.9A).
      ii. *Second maneuver:* It is lateral palpation after determination of fetal lie. Palms are placed on either side of maternal abdomen with gentle and deep pressure. On one side back is felt as hard resistant structure and fetal limbs as irregular mobile parts in other side (Figs 49.9 B and C).
      iii. *Third maneuver (First pelvic grip):* The lower position of the maternal abdomen is grasped using thumb and finger of one hand. If presenting part is not engaged, a movable mass will be felt, usually the head. Head and breech is differentiated as in first maneuver. If presenting part is deeply engaged, it indicates that lower fetal pole is in the pelvis (Fig. 49.9D).

Chapter 49 ♦ Normal Labor

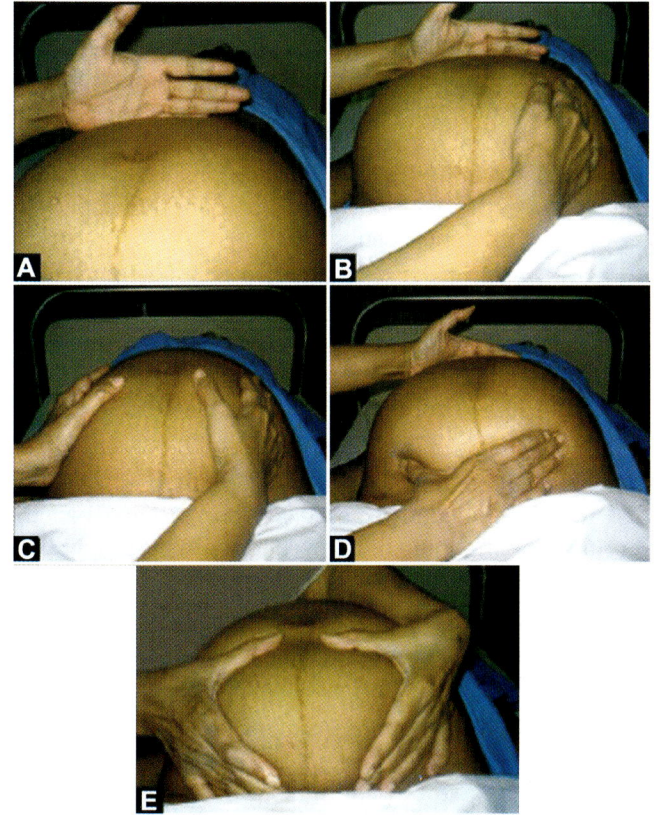

Figs 49.9A to E: Leopold maneuvers: (A) Fundal palpation; (B and C) Lateral palpation; (D) First pelvic grip; (E) Second pelvic grip

iv. *Fourth maneuver (Second pelvic grip):* The examiner faces the mother feet and with the tip of first three fingers of each hand exerts deep pressure in the direction of the axis of the pelvic inlet. When head has descended into the pelvis, the anterior shoulder may be differentiated by this maneuver (Fig. 49.9E).

3. *Auscultation of fetal heart sound:* Fetal heart sound should be auscultated at the time of admission and throughout the labor during the first and second stage of labor. Presence, rate, rhythms and intensity of fetal heart denote whether the fetal condition is good or disturbed. Location over which fetal heart sound is audible additionally helps in establishing the lie, presentation and position of fetus. Auscultation can be done by a stethoscope, pinards or ultrasound fetal Doppler. Table 49.3 and Figure 49.10 depicts the location of best fetal heart sound in different position of vertex.

4. *Vaginal examination:* Most often, unless there has been bleeding in excess of bloody show, a vaginal examination under aseptic condition is performed. The number of vaginal examination during labor correlates with infectious morbidity, especially in cases of early membrane rupture. Therefore these examinations should only be done, when the information gained is useful.

Table 49.3: Place of best heard FHS in respect to fetal position

Position of vertex	Place of fetal heart sound
1st Position (LOA)	Between umbilicus and left anterior superior iliac spine
2nd Position (ROA)	Often in middle line half way between pubes and umbilicus
3rd Position (ROP)	Slightly higher level, further from middle line toward the flank or near umbilicus
4th Position (LOP)	Most difficult to hear. Well towards left flank

Information to be gained during admission vaginal examination of women in normal labor:
a. *Amniotic fluid:* If there is suspicion of membrane rupture, a sterile speculum is carefully inserted and fluid is sought in the posterior vaginal fornix. Any fluid is observed for vernix or meconium.
b. *Cervix:* Softness, degree of effacement, extent of dilatation, and location of the cervix with respect to the presenting part and vagina are ascertained. One can feel the presence of membrane with or without amniotic fluid below the presenting part by careful palpation.
c. *Presenting part:* The nature of presenting part and its position should be positively determined and documented.
d. *Station:* The degree of descent of the presenting part into the birth canal is identified. If the fetal head is high (above the level of ischial spine), the effect of firm fundal pressure on descent of fetal head is tested (Munrokerr method).
e. *Pelvic architecture:* The diagonal conjugate, ischial spine, pelvic side walls and sacrum are evaluated for adequacy.

By above abdominal and pelvic examination fetal lie, presentation, attitude and position of the fetus is determined:

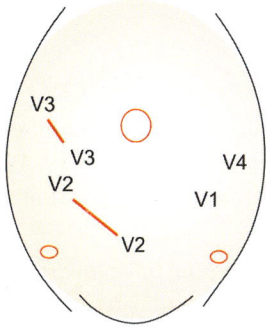

Fig. 49.10: Site of fetal heart sound, best heard in four different positions: (V1) 1st position (LOA); (V2) 2nd position (ROA); (V3) 3rd position (ROP); (V4) 4th position (LOP)

Fetal lie: The lie indicate relationship of long axis of the fetus to that of the mother and it can be longitudinal, transverse or oblique.

Fetal presentation: The presenting part is that portion of the body of the fetus that is either foremost or in closest proximity to the birth canal. In longitudinal lie, the presenting part is either the fetal head or the fetal buttock or legs, which cause cephalic and breech presentation respectively.

In cephalic presentation: When head is flexed sharply, the vertex is the presentation when posterior fontanelle is presenting part. When fetal neck is sharply extended, occiput and back come in contact and *face is presenting part*. The fetal head may assume a position between these extremes, either *Sinciput or Brow presentation* which are usually transient and convert with vertex or face presentation as labor progresses.

Fetal attitude or positions: In late months, the fetus assumes an attitude of generalized flexion.

Fetal position: Position refers to the relation of an arbitrarily chosen portion of the fetal presenting part to the right or left side of the maternal birth canal so with each presentation there may be two positions—right or left. The fetal occiput, chin (mentum) and sacrum are the determining points in cephalic, face and breech presentations respectively. At or near term the incidence of the various presentations are as follows—**Cephalic 96%, Breech 3.5%, Face 0.3%, Shoulder 0.4%**. The fetus enters the pelvis in left occipito transverse position (LOT) in 40% of labor, compared with 20% in right occiput transverse position (ROT). In about 20% of labor the fetus enters in pelvis in occipito posterior (OP) with right occiput posterior (ROP) being slightly more common than the left (LOP). Approximate 10% of LOP presentation persist until delivery.

Management of First Stage of Labor

It is mandatory for optimal pregnancy outcome that a well defined protocol should be established which provides careful surveillance of the maternal and fetal well-being.

General Management of Mother

Maternal vital signs: Maternal temperature, pulse and blood pressure is evaluated at least every 4 hours. If there is premature rupture of membrane, hourly temperature is checked.

Oral intake: A women can have low residue or high calorie snacks as toast, dalia, biscuits, fruit juice, etc. in 1st stage of labor. Encouraging women to fast in normal labor is not evidence based and is not recommended. Fasting in labor can lead to poor progress, unpleasant hunger sensation, ketonuria. In more active phase, most women do not wish to eat. At this stage, food can be withheld as gastric emptying time is remarkably prolonged, once labor is established. So ingested food and medicine remain in the stomach and not absorbed. At this stage sips of clear fluid can be given. Women who are at high risk of emergency cesarean section, regular antacid or hydrogen ion inhibitor should be given, which reduces the risk of aspiration pneumonitis especially associated with general anesthesia.

Intravenous fluids: It is customary to establish an I/V infusion lines early in labor. It is advantageous in oxytocin augmentation or active management of third stage of labor. With longer labor administration of crystalloid solution at rate of 60-120 ml/hour is helpful to prevent dehydration and acidosis.

Maternal position during labor: The normal laboring women need not be confined to bed early in labor. When in bed, the laboring women should be allowed to assume a comfortable position and should minimize lying supine.

Care of bladder and bowel: The mother is encouraged to pass urine every 2 hours. Enema can be given to prevent soiling of perineum during second stage of labor.

Relief of pain during labor: Analgesic should be initiated on the basis of maternal discomfort. The type of analgesic, amount and frequency of administration should be based on the need to reduce pain and discomfort on one hand and the likelihood of delivering a depressed infant on the other. Beside this aim of anesthetic and analgesic in vaginal delivery is to block nociceptive pathways while preserving motor functions so that laboring women is comfortable and also can actively participate in end stage expulsion efforts. Following options can be considered:

a. *Nonpharmacological:* In highly motivated patients non pharmacological methods such as relaxation, gentle massage, breathing exercise can reduce or discourage use of pain medication. Labor support personnel are among the most effective nonpharmacological method of pain relief in labor. Other methods are hydrotherapy, water bath, maternal movement, positioning, acupunctures, and electric nerve stimulation with varying degree of efficacy.

b. *Pharmacological method:* Indications, doses, risk and limitation is summarized in Table 49.4.

Monitoring Progress of Labor

The progress of labor is documented by:

1. **Uterine contraction:** Are monitored by palpation every 30 minutes to assess their frequency, duration and intensity. For at risk patient uterine contraction is measured along with fetal heart rate by using external cardiotocodynamometer.
2. **Per vaginal examination:** The progress of labor is measured in terms of descent of the presenting part and dilatation of the cervix. During latent phase, vaginal

Table 49.4: Comparative summary of various pharmacological analgesic and anesthetic in vaginal delivery

	Local injection (Field block)	Peripheral nerve block	Regional block epidural/spinal (Pudendal, Paracervical block)	Systemic IV, IM	General anesthesia
1. Indication	1. Before episiotomy 2. For repair of episiotomy or perineal tear	1. 1st stage of labor 2. Supplement during 2nd stage 3. Low forceps application	Maternal request for pain control in 1st stage of labor	Maternal request	In urgent situation like shoulder dystocia, head arrest
2. Agent and application	1 to 2% Lidocaine 1 to 3% Chloroprocaine max. dose = 4.5 mg/kg/dose	Paracervical - 4.5 ml local anesthetic, into lateral vaginal fornices at a depth of 2-3 mm around 2, 10/ 4, 8 o' Clock Pudendal – 7-10 ml of local anesthetic injected laterally through transvaginal approach injected laterally and posteriorly to ischial spine	Epidural catheter is introduced into lumbar epidural space through epidural needle, usual dose is 3ml of 1.5% lignocaine with rep. bolus dose if required Spinal or combined spinoepidural is usually for cesarean delivery	Fentanyl I/M Meperidine Butorphanol	1. Preoperative antacid 2. Preoxygenation with 100% oxygen for 3 to 5 minutes 3. Follow by IV agent with endotracheal intubation
3. Advantages	1. Good pain relief for procedure 2. No systemic complication after correct administration	Highly effective	Effective anesthetic yet allow patient to participate in labor and delivery	Pain relief to certain extent	Rapid onset of uterine relaxation which is desirable in emergencies
4. Limitation	May not be complete pain relief	May not provide the necessary anesthetic	Difficult in availability of person and monitoring	With inhalation agent amnesia can occur	Loss of consciousness, inhalation agent cross the placenta and can cause respiratory depression in neonates
5. Complication	Inadvertent injection into bloodstream	1. Inadvertent intravascular injection of anesthetic 2. Hematoma formation 3. Infection 4. Fetal bradycardia is common side effect	1. Infection 2. Neurological – spinal headache, back pain, Drug-related systemic toxicity, Hypotension, More incidence of operative delivery	Mother may have respiratory depression and increased risk of aspiration	1. Related to intubation - aspiration hypoxia 2. Drug-related complication of maternal depression 3. Fetal respiratory depression 4. Source of inhalation agent cause uterine relaxation and then predispose to PPH

examination should be done sparingly. While in active phase; the cervix should be assessed approximately at every 2 hours. In vaginal examination following things are recorded:
a. Position, effacement, dilatation of cervix.
b. **Presenting part:** Position, station in relation to ischial spines, presence of caput or moulding. *Moulding* of fetal head is assessed at sagittal and lambdoidal suture and graded as follows:
+ suture opposed
++ suture overlap but reducible
+++ suture overlapped but irreducible
3. **Station of head** is described as the position of the lowermost part of head in relation to ischial spines in

the centimeter —1 indicating 1 cm above the spine +1 indicating 1 cm below the spines. O indicating at the level of spine.

4. Presence of cord or limbs (any compound presentation).
5. Color of liquor.

Documentation of Progress of Labor by Partogram

Partogram is graphic display record of cervical dilatation and descent of head against duration of labor in hours. It also gives information about fetal and maternal condition recorded on a single sheet of paper.

The component of partogram:
a. Patient's identification
b. Time – Zero time for spontaneous labor is the time of admission in labor ward, and for induced labor is the time for induction.
c. Fetal heart rate – ½ hourly recorded.
d. Status of membrane and color of liquor: It is marked I for intact membrane, 'C' for clear and 'M' for Meconium stained liquor.
e. Uterine contraction: The squares in vertical column are shaded according to duration and intensity.
f. Drug and fluid given.
g. BP recorded at every 2 hours and pulse every 30 minutes.
h. Temperature
i. Oxytocin concentration if given.
j. **Cervicograph** is most important part of partogram, where cervical dilatation and descent of head is displayed at 1-2 hourly intervals against time in hours. On cervicograph standard *alert line* devised by Philpott and Castle is shown, which starts at 3 cm of cervical dilatation and ends at 10 cm dilatation at rate of 1 cm/ hours. The action line is drawn 3-4 hours to the right and parallel to the alert line. In a normal labor the cervicograph should be either in the alert line or to the left of it. When it falls in zone 2, it is abnormal and demands critical evaluation of labor (Fig. 49.11). When it falls in zone 3 case should be reassessed by a senior persons and decision is to be made either for cesarean section or augmentation of labor by oxytocin or AROM.

Advantage of Partograph

Partogram helps in detection of abnormal labor even by junior person or paramedicals without any increase in cost. Beside this it is helpful to see all details of necessary information at a glance in a busy labor room. It also facilitates handover procedure. Use of partogram has been shown to reduce maternal morbidity, prolonged labor, cesarean section rate and perinatal morbidity and mortality.

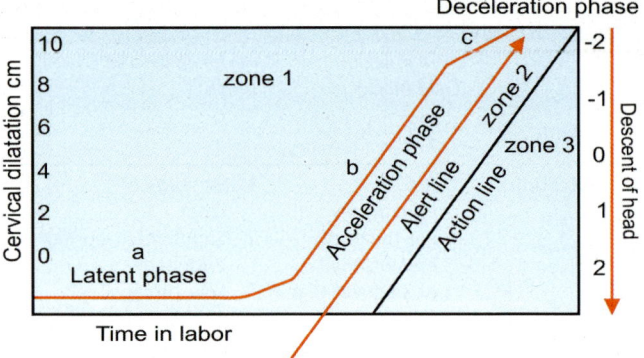

Fig. 49.11: Partograph—graphic display of labor

Fetal Monitoring in Labor

Fetal heart rate is auscultated with a suitable stethoscope or any of a variety of Doppler ultrasonic devices or by electronic fetal heart rate monitoring machines. It is recommended by **ACOG and AAP (1997) that during the first stage of labor in the absence of any abnormalities, the fetal heart rate should be checked immediately after contraction at least every 30 minutes and then every 15 minutes during the 2nd stage.** If continuous electronic monitoring is used, the tracing is evaluated at least every 30 minutes during first stage and at least every 15 minutes during 2nd stage of labor. In high risk pregnancies fetal heart rate auscultation should be done at 15 minutes interval in first stage of labor and at every 5 minutes during 2nd stage.

Electronic Cardiotocography (CTG)

The following features are to be critically observed in any CTG tracing:
a. Baseline FHR.
b. Baseline variability of FHR.
c. Any acceleration.
d. Any deceleration.

Categorization of the components of CTG and Management of abnormal fetal heart rate patterns is discussed in chapter of Fetal Surveillance.

Artificial Rupture of Membrane (Amniotomy)

AROM increases the risk of chorioamnionitis and need for antibiotic, so amniotomy should not be performed routinely. It can be used when enhancement of uterine contractility in the active phase of labor is indicated and when information of amount of liquor Amni or presence or absence of Meconium is to be confirmed. One should be careful to palpate for umbilical cord before and after AROM. Fetal heart should be recorded before, during and immediately after procedure. AROM have been largely not recommended for induction when used alone.

Management of Second Stage of Labor and Conduct of Delivery

With full dilatation of the cervix which signifies the onset of the second stage of labor, the women typically begin to bear down and with descent of the presenting part; she develops the urge to defecate. Uterine contraction and the accompanying expulsive forces may last for 30 seconds and recur at time after a myometrial resting phase of no more than a minute. The duration of second stage as stated earlier is 50 minutes in nulliparous and 20 minutes in multiparous. Duration can be highly variable depending on the size of infant, presence of cephalopelvic disproportion, or impairment of expulsion effort based on analgesic.

Following things to be observed in second stage of labor:
a. **Risk assessment must be continued:** Fetal heart rate must be heard for 60 second after a contraction every 5 minutes in the early second stage and after each contraction, when the patient is pushing actively.
b. **Position:** Patient should be allowed to adopt whatever position they feel comfortable to push. Upright postures increase pelvic outlet diameters and increase the efficiency of maternal expulsive effort thus reducing the length of second stage.
c. **Bladder and bowel:** Sips of oral fluid should be encouraged. If the bladder is full, and patient is unable to void, catheterization must be considered.
d. **Preparation for delivery:** The most widely used position for delivery of baby is dorsal lithotomy position. For better exposure leg holder or stirrups are often used.
e. **Ritgen's maneuver:** When head is crowned and head distends the vulva and perineum the vaginal introitus is opened to a diameter of 5 cm or more during uterine contraction, a towel draped glove hand is used to exert forward pressure on the chin of the fetus through the perineum just in front of the coccyx. At the same time the other hand exerts pressure superiorly against the occiput. This allows controlled delivery of the head. This is called Ritgen's maneuver (Figs 49.12F and G). Advantage of it is that this allows controlled delivery of the head and also favors extension so that head is delivered with its smallest diameter passing through the introitus and over the perineum. The head is delivered slowly with the base of the occiput rotating around the lower margin of symphysis pubic as a fulcrum, while the bregma (anterior fontanelle), brow, and face pass successively over the perineum.
f. **Episiotomy:** Episiotomy is mediolateral incision of perineum. It should be considered in case of a complicated vaginal delivery like breech, shoulder dystocia, instrumental delivery, or when the perineal tear is imminent due to rigidity or scarring (Figs 49.12C and D).
g. **Delivery of shoulders:** Mostly the shoulder appear at the vulva just after external rotation and are born spontaneously. Occasionally if delay occurs, immediate extraction of shoulder may be advisable. For this situation, the sides of the head are grasped with the two hands and gentle downward traction is applied, until the anterior shoulder appears under the pubic arch. After that by an upward movement the posterior shoulder is delivered.
h. **Delivery of body:** Rest of body is usually easily and rapidly delivered, but in case of moderate delay, its birth may be hastened by moderate traction on the head and moderate pressure on the uterus fundus. Hooking the fingers in axilla should be avoided because this may injure the nerves of upper extremity, which can produces transient or even permanent paralysis. Beside this traction on the body should be exerted only in the direction of the long axis of the infant. If oblique traction is applied, it can cause bending of neck and excessive stretching of brachial plexus.
i. **Clearing of nasopharynx:** After delivering the thorax, face is quickly wiped and nose and mouth suctioned with a bulb syringe to minimize aspiration of amniotic fluid, particulate matter and blood (Fig. 49.12H).
j. **Nuchal cord:** After delivery of anterior shoulder, a finger should be passed to the fetal neck to determine the presence of nuchal cord which is found in 25% of deliveries and usually do no harm. If a coil of cord is felt, it should be drawn down between the fingers. If cord loop is loose, it is slipped over the infant head. If cord is too tightly applied to the neck and can not be slipped over infant's head, cord should be cut between two clamps and infant is promptly delivered.
k. **Cord clamping:** Cord is cut between two clamps placed 4-5 cm from the fetal abdomen. Later after initial care of newborn, an umbilical cord clamp is applied 2-3 cm from the fetal abdomen (Fig. 49.12I).
l. The new born is not elevated above the introitus at vaginal delivery.

All the steps of conduct of delivery is shown in Figures 49.12A to J.

Management of Third Stage of Labor

After delivery of newborn the height of uterus fundus and its consistency are ascertained. Sign of placental separation are noted. In physiological management, after separation of placenta, the mother is asked to bear down and intraabdominal pressure is adequate to expel the placenta or pressure is exerted with the hand on the fundus to propel the detached placenta into the vagina. **Traction on the umbilical cord must not be used to pull the placenta out of uterus before placental separation**. As it may cause inversion of uterus which is one of the grave complication associated with delivery. The gentle traction with counter pressure between the symphysis and fundus to prevent

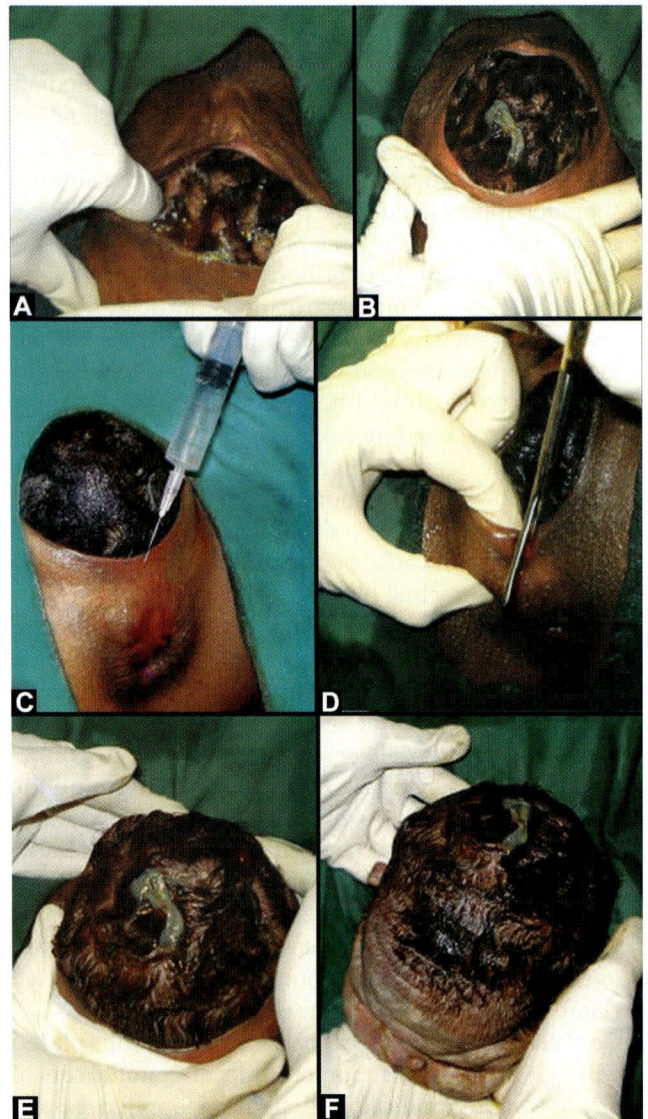
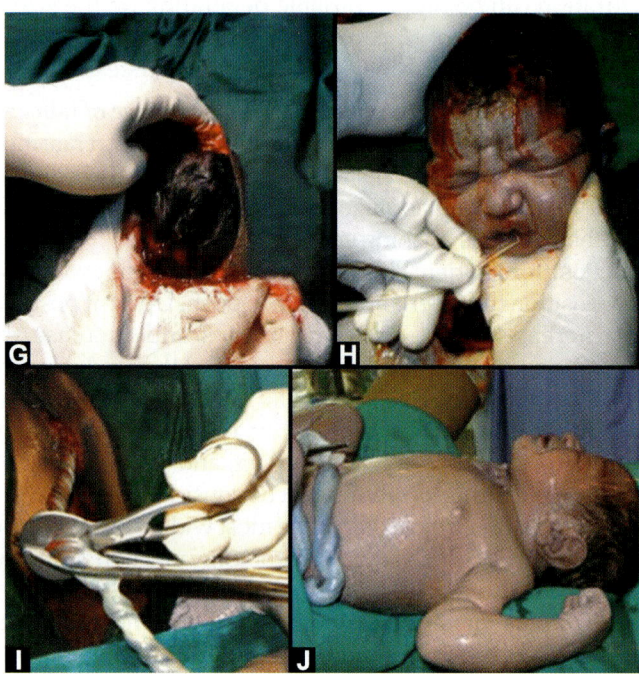

Figs 49.12A to J: (A) Ironing of perineum; (B) support of perineum; (C) Infiltration of local anesthetic; (D) Episiotomy; (E) Controlled delivery of baby head; (F) Ritgen's maneuver; (G) Aspiration of baby secretion; (H and I) Clamping and cutting of cord; (J) Receiving the baby in head low

descent of uterus facilitates delivery of the placenta. Active management of third stage of labor is described at the end of chapter. It should be practiced in all cases to reduce chances of postpartum hemorrhage (Figs 49.13A and B).

Management of Fourth Stage of Labor

After delivery of the placenta, placental membrane and umbilical cord should be examined for completeness. Patient should be watched for any excessive bleeding and uterine contraction. Uterine contraction can be enhanced with uterine massage or infusion of oxytocin infusion. Cervix and vagina should be inspected for active bleeding, laceration and surgical repair should be performed as needed. Mother's vital signs are monitored immediately after delivery and every 15 minutes for the first hour. In normal newborn breastfeeding should be initiated in this period.

Active Management of Labor

O'Driscoll and colleague in Dublin (1984) pioneered the concept that a disciplined standardized labor management protocol enhanced the satisfaction of the primigravida mother by ensuring that labor did not last more than 12 hours and it lowered the cesarean section rate by 5-7%. This active labor management protocol is as follows:
a. Patient is admitted in active labor defined as when cervical dilatation is of 3-4 cm or more in presence of uterine contraction or when ruptured membrane is confirmed.

Chapter -49 ♦ Normal Labor

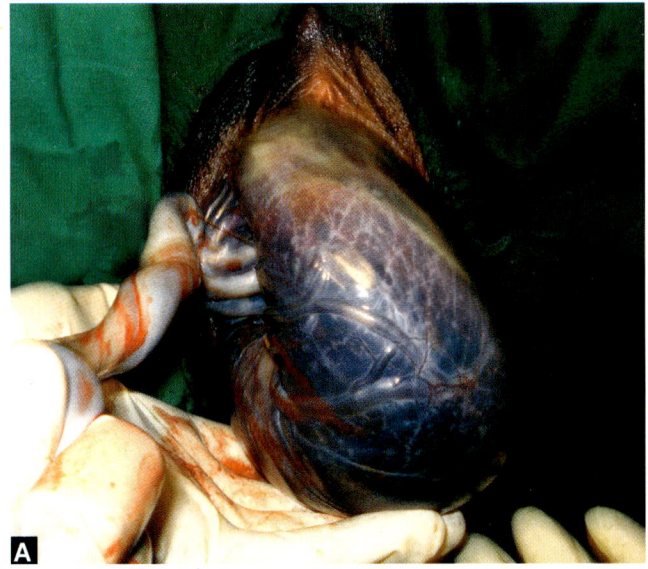
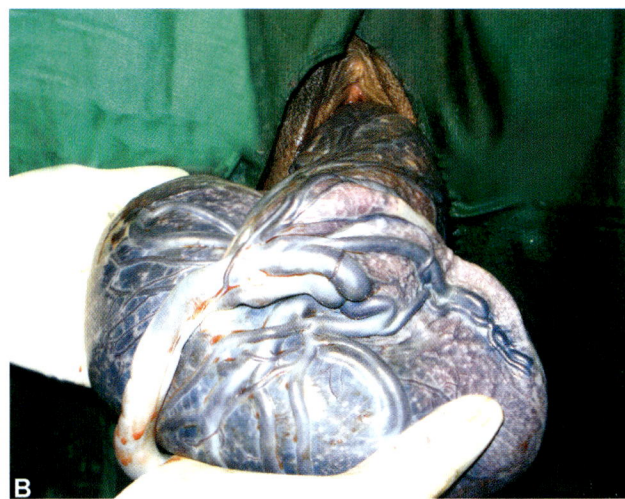

Figs 49.13A and B: Delivery of placenta—3rd stage of labor

b. Pelvic examinations are performed at approximately every two hours and cervical dilatation is charted in WHO partogram. Labor is grafted and assessed including use of alert and action line.
c. Amniotomy is performed if cervix does not dilate within about two hours of admission and after that progress of labor is evaluated at next two hours.
d. If there is hypotonic uterus and there is slow or no progress in cervical dilatation after 3-4 hours, oxytocin augmentation is done with 10 units of oxytocin in one liter of ringer lactate.
e. Dilatation rate of 1-2 cm/hour is accepted as evidence of progress after satisfactory uterine contraction has been established with oxytocin.
f. Expected duration of total of <12 hours for first stage of labor and 2 hours of 2nd stage of labor is considered.
g. If after amniotomy and oxytocin infusion, there is no progress of labor up to 8 hours or more, cesarean section is considered for dystocia.

Outcome of Active Management of Labor

Initial studies suggested that active management of labor could lower the rate of cesarean section due to dystocia. But recent review have shown that although there is a significant decrease in duration of labor and reduction in incidence of prolonged labor, there is no significant difference in cesarean section rate.

Traditional and active management of labor is summarized in Box 49.1 and Flow chart 49.2.

Active Management of Third Stage of Labor (AMTSL)

The active management of third stage of labor differed from physiologic or expectant management. In the expectant

Box 49.1: Traditional management of labor

1st Stage
- Diagnosis of onset of labor
- Maternal evaluation of pulse, BP, temperature and hydration
- Fetal evaluation by intermittent auscultation or EFM/ admission cardiotocography
- Evaluation of liquor
  — Allowed to ambulate
  — Oral food allowed
  — Partographic progress of labor
  — Per vaginal examination to assess labor, cervical dilatation, and station of presenting part, presentation

2nd Stage
- Oral fluid allowed
- FHS every 5 minutes and after every contraction
- No routine episiotomy
- Allow to adopting any posture

3rd Stage
- Oxytocin 10 unit in infusion or ergometrine 0.2 mg/IM or syntometrine IM or IV
- Placenta delivered after sign of separation of placenta by cord traction

Flow chart 49.2: Active management of labor

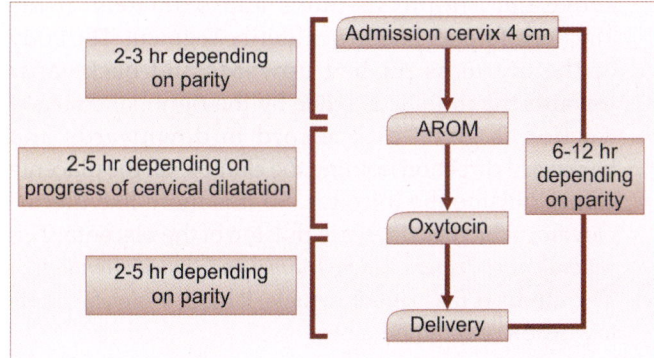

management placenta is allowed to deliver spontaneously by gradually or maternal effort. In active management, there are three components which intend to augment uterine contraction and prevent postpartum hemorrhage:
a. Administration of uterotonic agent within one minute of birth.
b. Controlled cord traction.
c. Uterus massage after delivery of the placenta where appropriate.

Uterotonic drug administration within one minute of birth has the greatest impact on the prevention of PPH. Following drugs can be used.

i. **Oxytocin infusion:** 10 unit of oxytocin in 500 ml of ringer lactate is started. Oxytocin in the uniject TM device is a prefilled, easy to use, nonreusable syringe. It is advancement in the method of delivering oxytocin. This method ensures that correct dose is given with little preparation and there is no medical waste.

ii. **Ergometrine (Methyl ergometrine, methyl ergonovine):** It is given in 0.2 mg I/M injection. It acts within 6-7 minute and effect last 2-4 hours. It is contraindicated in women with history of hypertension, heart disease, retained placenta or PIH. Side effects are nausea, vomiting and headache.

iii. **Syntometrine (Oxytocin plus ergometrine):** It is effective but side effects like nausea, vomiting, headache and high blood pressure are more. Beside this ergometrine is contraindicated in certain maternal situation like pregnancy induced hypertension and requires proper storage condition.

iv. **Misoprostol:** It is prostaglandin E1, analog. It is inexpensive, readily available and cheap. It also does not require special storage or transfer condition. Beside this it can be given orally or rectally. But still oxytocin is preferred to oral misoprostol for active management of 3rd stage of labor. Dosage is 200-600 µg tablets orally or rectally.

v. **Controlled cord traction (Modified Brandt-Andrew's Method):** In this after delivery of placenta, the fundus of the uterus is palpated to confirm that it is firmly contracted. Only then controlled cord traction is applied. The palmer surface of the fingers of the left hand is placed above the symphysis pubis approximately at the junction of upper and lower uterine segment. The body of the uterus is pushed upwards and backwards towards the umbilicus while by the right hand steady traction is given on the cord in downwards and backward direction holding the clamps, till the placenta comes outside the introitus. So it is more like uterine elevator which facilitates expulsion of the placenta. *This should only be conducted by trained and skilled attendant.*

vi. **The uterus is massaged:** to make it hard, which facilitate expulsion of retained clots.

MULTIPLE CHOICE QUESTIONS

1. Sensitivity of uterine musculature is:
   a. Enhanced by progesterone
   b. Enhanced by estrogen
   c. Inhibited by estrogen
   d. Enhanced by estrogen and inhibited by progesterone
   Ans. d

2. Cardinal movement of labor are:
   a. Engagement – Descent – Flexion – Internal rotation – Extension – Restitution – External rotation – Expulsion.
   b. Engagement – Flexion – Descent – Internal rotation – External rotation – Extension – Expulsion
   c. Engagement – Flexion – Descent – External Rotation – Expulsion
   d. Engagement – Extension – Internal rotation – External rotation – Expulsion
   Ans. a

3. Duration of active phase of labor is affected by:
   a. Early use of conduction anesthetic and sedation
   b. Unripe cervix
   c. Hypertonic uterine contraction
   d. Pre-eclampsia
   Ans. a,b

4. Living ligature of uterus is:
   a. Endometrium
   b. Middle layer of myometrium
   c. Inner layer of myometrium
   d. Perimetrium
   Ans. b

5. Assessment of progress of labor is best done by:
   a. Station of head
   b. Rupture of membrane
   c. Contraction of uterus
   d. Partogram
   Ans. d

6. Most common cause of non engagement at term in primigravida is:
   a. Cephalopelvic disproportion
   b. Hydramnios
   c. Brow presentation
   d. Breech
   Ans. a

7. During active phase of labor cervical dilatation per hour in primigravida is:
   a. 1.2 cm
   b. 1.5 cm
   c. 1.7 cm
   d. 2 cm
   Ans. a

8. Immediately following delivery the height of the uterus corresponds to … weeks:
   a. 32
   b. 20
   c. 25
   d. 12
   Ans. b

9. The earliest sign of placental separation is:
    a. Change in shape and consistency of uterus
    b. Sudden gush of blood
    c. Prolongation of umbilical cord
    d. Cessation of cord pulsation
    e. Increased height of fundus
    Ans. a
10. First stage of labor is up to:
    a. Rupture of membranes
    b. 3/5th dilatation of cervix
    c. Full dilatation of cervix
    d. Crowing of head
    Ans. c
11. Engagement of fetal head is with reference to:
    a. Biparietal diameter
    b. Bitemporal diameter
    c. Occipitofrontal diameter
    d. Suboccipitofrontal diameter
    Ans. a
12. Which is most common diameter of engagement:
    a. Suboccipitofrontal
    b. Mentovertical
    c. Occipitofrontal
    d. Submentovertical
    Ans. a
13. Normal partogram include the following, *except*:
    a. Cervical dilatation in X axis
    b. Descent of head in Y axis
    c. Sigmoid shaped curve
    d. Alert line followed 4 hours later by active line
    Ans. a
14. Signs of placenta separation in stage 3 of parturition is:
    a. Gushing of blood
    b. Lengthening of cord
    c. Fitting of placenta in vagina
    d. Increased BP
    Ans. a,b
15. True labor differs from false labor by all, *except*:
    a. Absence of bag of water
    b. Painful uterine contraction
    c. Progressive effacement and dilatation of cervix.
    d. Pain often felt in front of the abdomen or radiating towards the thigh
    Ans. a

50 Malpresentation and Malposition

Nothing is life is to be feared, it is only to be understood.

MALPRESENTATION

Malpresentations are defined as any presentation of the body other than vertex such as breech, face or brow presentation, transverse lie or shoulder presentation.

MALPOSITION

Malposition is a term for presentation whereby the vertex is in abnormal position. So the diameter of fetal skull in relation to the pelvic opening is greater than normal, e.g. the occiput posterior position or an asynclitism where the fetal head is tilted laterally so that the parietal bone presents first.

The women presenting in labor with malpresentation and malposition has to undergo difficult and prolonged labor, there are more chances of operative intervention and increased maternal and neonatal morbidity.

Types of Malpresentation

More than 95% of fetus at term present with the vertex. The malpresentation can be of following types:
a. **Breech:** Most common incidence 3-5%
b. **Brow**
c. **Face**
d. **Shoulder**
e. **Arm**
f. **Cord.**

Causes of Malpresentation

1. *Maternal:*
   a. Multiparity
   b. Pelvic tumors
   c. Congenital uterine anomalies
   d. Contracted pelvis.
2. *Fetal:*
   a. Prematurity
   b. Multiple pregnancy
   c. Intrauterine death
   d. Macrosomia
   e. Fetal abnormality including hydrocephalus, anencephaly, cystic hygroma.
3. *Placental:*
   a. Placenta previa
   b. Polyhydramnios
   c. Amniotic bands.

BREECH PRESENTATION

Breech presentation is when the lie of the baby is longitudinal and pelvic or podalic extremity of fetus presents at the brim and cephalic extremity at the fundus. The term probably derives from the word 'Britches' which describes a cloth covering the loin and thigh.

Types of Breech Presentation

The varying relation between the lower extremities and buttocks of breech presentation form the following types of breech presentation:
a. **Frank breech:** It is most common type of breech presentation. In this both hips are flexed and both knees are extended.
b. **Complete breech:** If one or both knees are flexed, it is termed as complete breech.
c. **Incomplete breech:** If either hip is extended, leading to foot or knee presentation—it is called incomplete breech.

In breech presentations sacrum is denominator and following four positions are described (Figs 50.1A to D).

1st position...............left sacroanterior...............LSA
2nd position...............right sacroanterior...............RSA
3rd position...............right sacroposterior...............RSP
4th position...............left sacroposterior...............LSP

Diagnosis of Breech Presentation

a. **Palpation and ballottement:** Performance of leopard's maneuver and ballottement of the uterus can confirm breech presentation. The softer, more ill defined breech

Chapter - 50 ♦ Malpresentation and Malposition

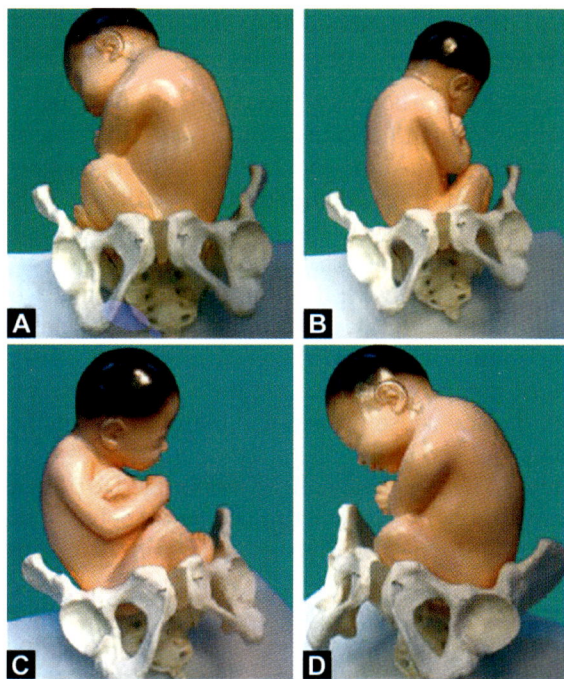

Figs 50.1A to D: Position of breech presentation
(A: LSA, B: RSA, C: RSP, D: LSP)

may be felt in the lower uterine segment above the pelvic inlet.

b. **Pelvic examination:** In labor during vaginal examination, the soft irregular breech will be felt. If no presenting part is defined, further studies like ultrasound are needed.

c. **Radiographic studies:** X-ray will differentiate breech presentation from cephalic. But because of risk of radiation exposure ultrasonography is now used instead of radiography.

d. **Ultrasound:** Ultrasonography scan will document fetal presentation. Beside this attitude of fetus, multiple pregnancy, fetal weight, location of the placenta and amniotic fluid volume is assessed. Which guide the mode of delivery in breech presentation. It will also reveal skeletal and soft tissue malformation of the fetus.

Management

Antepartum Management

Following confirmation of breech presentation, the mother must be closely followed to evaluate for spontaneous version to cephalic presentation. If breech presentation persists beyond 36 weeks, external cephalic version should be considered.

External Cephalic Version (ECV)

It is a technique in which one or two people attempt to maneuver the fetus into a cephalic presentation by applying pressure to the maternal abdomen. The technique is performed under ultrasound guidance to assist the operation and to help monitor the fetus. Tocolytic agent and regional anesthetic helps in the procedure by relaxing the uterus and to ensure patient comfort respectively.

Contraindications to ECV are: (a) **Absolute**—placenta previa or abruptio, (b) **Relative**—patient in labor, oligohydramnios, IUGR, and nonreassuring fetal heart rate pattern. Prior cesarean section is not a contraindication to version. *Rh negative mother should receive anti-D immunoglobulin to prevent immunization.* **Risks of ECV** are fetal distress, placenta abruptio and amniotic fluid embolism. So preparation of an emergency cesarean has to be kept ready. Success rate varies from 35 to 85%.

Management During Labor

1. **Examination:** Patients with singleton breech presentation are admitted in hospital early with onset of labor because of increased risk of cord complication. Upon admission a repeat ultrasound is performed to confirm breech and type of breech presentation and to rule out any fetal congenital anomaly. Careful assessment of pelvis is made.

2. **Role of cesarean section:** ACOG (2000) shows that planned cesarean delivery decreases perinatal and neonatal morbidity and mortality verses planned vaginal breech delivery. So cesarean delivery has now become choice of mode of delivery by most obstetrician and patients.

3. **Trial of labor/vaginal delivery in breech presentation:**
   a. Vaginal delivery is an option when a patient presents with advanced labor with breech presentation and when second twin presents as breech presentation. Delivery is accomplished by assisted breech delivery or breech extraction.
   b. If trial of labor is decided by doctor or patients, following guidelines should be followed:
      i. The estimated fetal weight is 2000–3500 gm at onset of labor.
      ii. The estimated gestational age of the fetus is 37-42 weeks.
      iii. The fetus is in frank or complete breech presentation.
      iv. CT pelvimetry or bedside ultrasound confirms that the fetal head is not hyperextended and arms are flexed upon the fetal chest.
      v. Pelvis should be adequate, that is, interspinous diameter at the midpelvis is more than 10 cm and anterior-posterior diameter at the pelvic inlet is more than 11 cm and transverse diameter at the pelvic inlet is more than 12 cm.
      vi. An experienced obstetrician, neonatologist and anesthesiologist should be present in conduct of vaginal breech delivery.

Types of Vaginal Breech Delivery

Spontaneously Vaginal Delivery

It is termed when there is delivery of an infant in breech presentation without assistance and no obstetric maneuvers are applied to the body. The fetus negotiate the maternal pelvis in following steps and operator simply supports the body of fetus as it delivers:

a. *Descent and engagement:* Engagement occurs when bitrochanteric diameter (measuring 4 inches or 10 cm) of the fetus has passed the plane of pelvic inlet.
b. *Internal rotation:* When buttocks reach the levator ani muscles of the maternal pelvis, internal rotation occurs. So the anterior hip rotates beneath the pubic symphysis resulting in sacrum transverse position. Now the bitrochanteric diameter of the fetal pelvis is now in an Anteroposterior diameter within the maternal pelvis. The breech then presents at the pelvic outlet and upon emerging rotates from a sacrum transverse to sacrum anterior.
c. *Delivery of breech:* Crowing occurs when the bitrochanteric diameter passes under the pubic symphysis. Breech is then delivered by movement of *the descent with lateral flexion of the spine around the pubis.* The anterior hip is first disengaged; the posterior distends the perineum and follows it.
d. *Delivery of shoulder and trunk:* As descent occurs; the bisacromial diameter rotates to an oblique or anteroposterior diameter until the anterior shoulder rests beneath the pubic symphysis. Delivery of the anterior shoulder occurs as it steps beneath the pubic symphysis. Upward flexion of the body allows for easy delivery of the posterior shoulder over the perineum.
e. *Delivery of head:* As the shoulder descends, the head engages in the pelvic inlet in a transverse or oblique position. Rotation of the head to occiput anterior position occurs as it enters the midpelvis. The occiput then steps beneath the pubic symphysis and the remainder of the head is delivered by flexion as the chin, mouth, nose and forehead steps over the maternal perineum.

Difficulty in Spontaneous Breech Delivery

In breech delivery, increasingly larger diameter (bitrochanteric, bisacromial, biparietal) of the body enters the pelvis, whereas in cephalic presentation, the largest diameter (biparietal diameter) enters the pelvis first. Particularly in preterm labor, the head is considerably larger than the body and provides a better dilating wedge, as it passes through the cervix and into the pelvis. *The smaller bitrochanteric and bisacromial diameter may descend into the pelvis through a partially dilated cervix, but the larger biparietal diameter may be trapped.* These difficult situations in vaginal breech delivery are dealt with following obstetric maneuver.

Partial Breech Extraction (Assisted Breech Extraction)

It is used when the body is allowed to deliver spontaneously up to the level of the umbilicus. But assisted in delivering of leg, shoulders, arm and head. In this situation, the operator presumes that spontaneous delivery will not occur or expeditious delivery is indicated for fetal or maternal reasons. The steps are as follows:

a. **Step 1 (Episiotomy):** It is important adjuvant to every breech delivery. It saves a perineal laceration and more importantly it relieves the head in breech delivery of that quick compression and sudden release during birth, which may cause intracranial injury and hemorrhage (Figs 50.2A to E).
b. **Step 2:** The mother should be encouraged to push as the cord is drawn well down into maternal pelvis. If cord is short, it must be divided between two artery forceps and time is noted.
c. **Step 3:** As the fetus continues to descend, the legs are sequentially delivered by splinting the medial aspect of each femur. While the operator finger is positioned

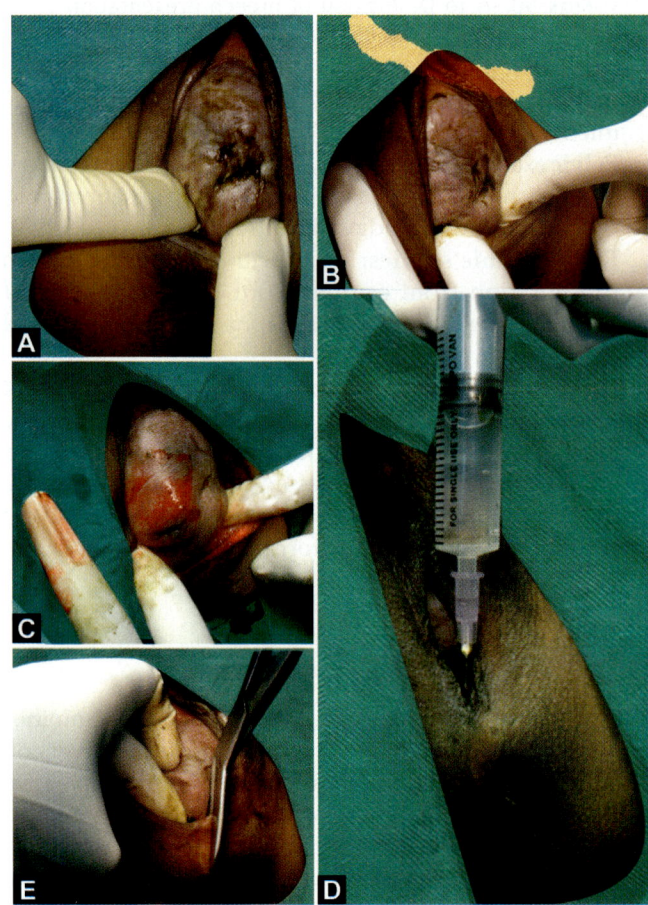

Figs 50.2A to E: Breech delivery: (A and B) Rumping of breech and distension of perineum; (C) Ironing out of vagina; (D and E) performance of episiotomy during conduct of breech delivery

parallel to each femur, once by exerting pressure laterally so each leg is sweeped away from the midline. After delivery of leg, the fetal trunk is wrapped in warm towel to support to the body. The fingers should rest on the anterior-superior iliac crest and the thumb on the sacrum, which minimizes the chances of fetal abdominal soft injury. When both scapulas are visible, the body is rotated counter-clockwise. The operator locates the right humerus and laterally sweeps the arm across the chest and out the perineum. In a similar fashion, the body is rotated clockwise to deliver the left arm (Figs 50.3 and 50.4).

d. **Step 4:** After delivering of both arm, the corresponding shoulder appears leaving the fetus hanging by neck. Head can spontaneously deliver or following maneuver can be used for delivery of after-coming-head.

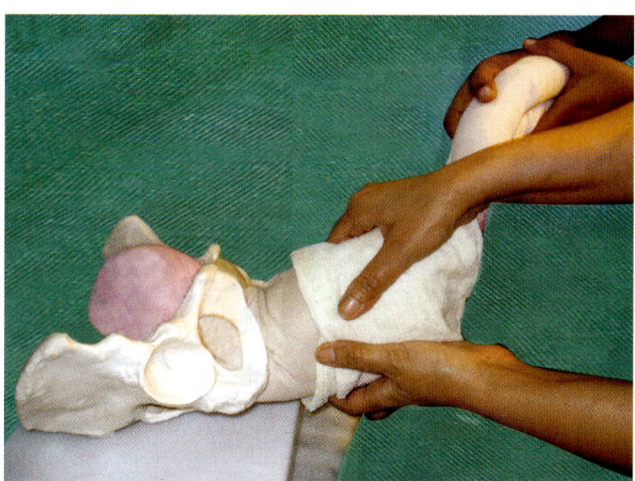

Fig. 50.3: Delivery of breech with movement of descent and lateral flexion

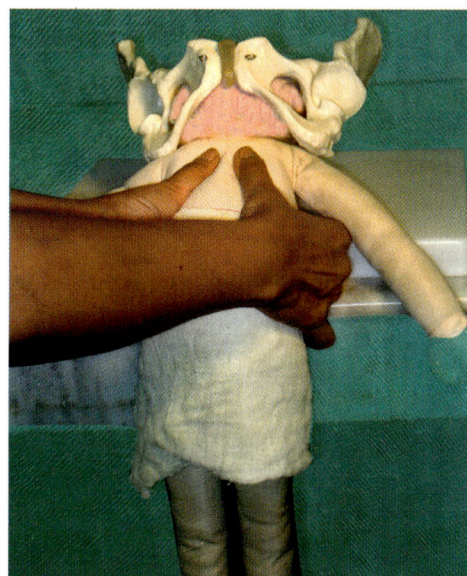

Fig. 50.4: Delivery in breech presentation— head entering brim in fully flexed position

Special Maneuvers for Delivery of Head

a. ***Burns-Marshall method:*** It is the most commonly used method to assist delivery of head. The baby is allowed to hang by its own weight from the vulva, the women is in lithotomy position. It encourages flexion of head. At this time, some suprapubic pressure is given to help its descent. When nape of child neck becomes visible, the obstetrician stands with back to the patients left leg, take the child's leg in the right hand, placing the middle finger between the two ankles. The obstetrician applies traction and at the same time lifts the fetal trunk through 3/4th of circle up over the mother abdomen (Figs 50.5A to E). The left hand of the obstetrician protects the perineum which prevents too quick delivery of head. The maneuver maintains flexion of head and occiput is thrust firmly against the back of symphysis pubis. As soon as the mouth and nose of baby are free, the baby can now breathe and the airways should be cleared by removing the debris from nose and mouth. The head is now delivered slowly and carefully. If this maneuver is done before head is safely low enough, then there is real danger of injury to the fetal spine.

b. ***Mauriceau-Smellie-Viet maneuver:*** If Burns-Marshall method fails, this maneuver can be used. In this procedure the index and middle finger of one hand are applied over the maxillae to flex the head, while the fetal body rest on the palm of hand and forearm. The forearm is straddled by the fetal legs. Two fingers of other hand then are hooked over the fetal neck and grasping the shoulder, downward traction is applied, until the suboccipital region appears under the symphysis. Simultaneously gentle pressure is applied suprapubically by assistant to keep the head flexed (Fig. 50.6). The body is then elevated towards the maternal abdomen and mouth, nose, brow and eventually occiput emerges successively over the perineum.

c. ***Modified Prague's maneuver:*** If after delivery of the body the spine remains in the posterior position and rotation is unsuccessful, extraction of head in persistent occipitoposterior position may be accomplished by *Modified Prague's maneuver;* one hand of the operator supports the shoulder from below, while the other hand gently elevates the body upward toward the maternal abdomen. This action flexes the head within the birth canal and results in delivering of the occiput over the perineum.

d. ***Application of forceps in after-coming-head:*** Pipers forceps or standard forceps can be used if:
   i. Cervix is completely dilated.
   ii. Head is engaged in the pelvis.
   iii. Ideally head is in direct occiput anterior position. An assistant supports and slightly elevates the fetal trunk while the operator places each forceps blade alongside the fetal parietal bones (Fig. 50.7). When

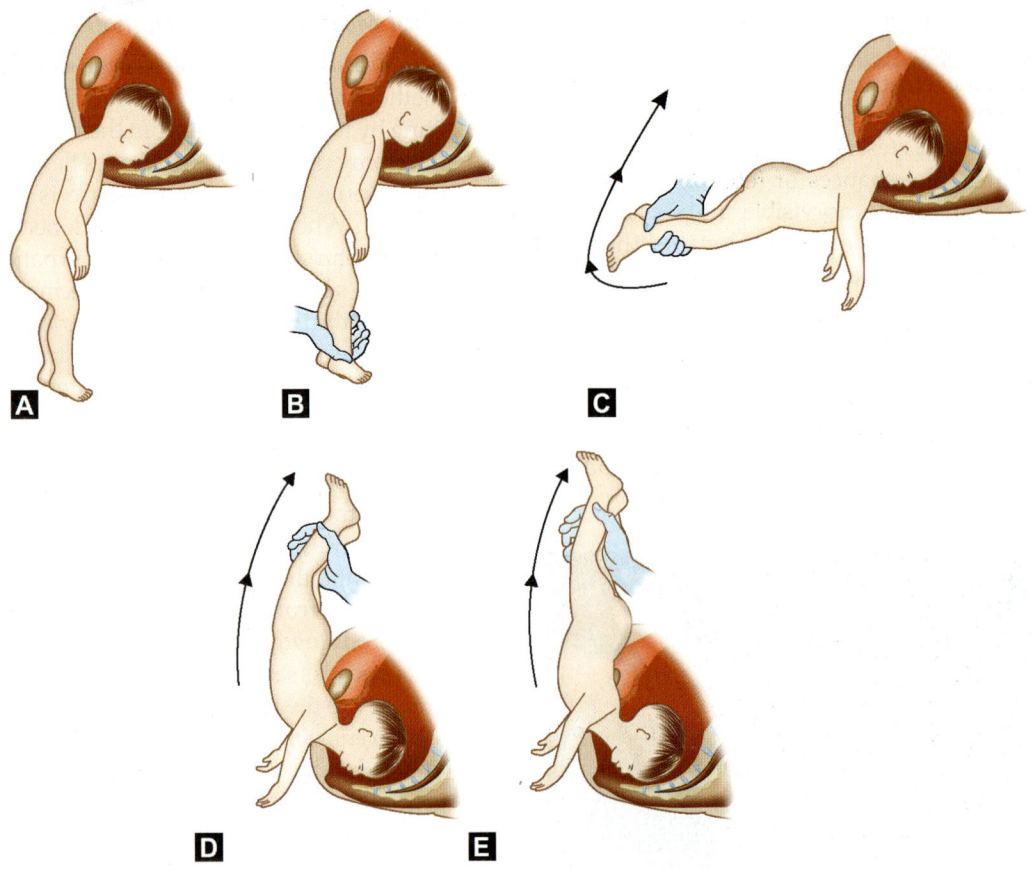

Figs 50.5A to E: Burns-Marshall maneuver for the delivery of after-coming-head

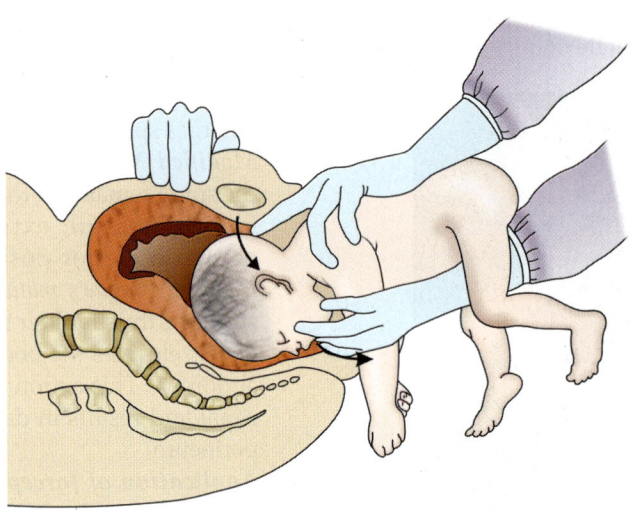

Fig. 50.6: Mauriceau-Smellie-Veit maneuver for delivery of the head

Chapter - 50 ♦ Malpresentation and Malposition

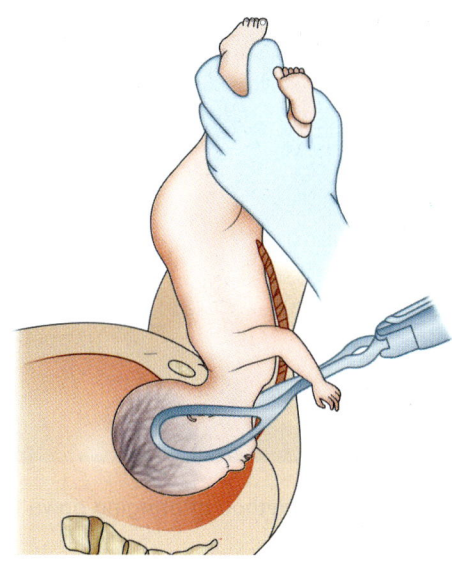

Fig. 50.7: Delivery of after-coming-head by forceps application

proper placement is confirmed, the forceps are locked and gentle traction is applied to flex and deliver the head over the perineum.

e. *Duhrssen's incision:* Occasionally, especially in preterm fetus the incompletely dilated cervix does not allow delivery of the after-coming-head. ***In this situation as an emergent situation to preserve fetal life, incisions are made in the posterior cervix at 6 o'clock position to loosen the entrapped head.*** Occasionally, additional incisions are made at 3 and 10 o'clock position. This incision relieves the fetal head but maternal consequence may be severe with resultant hemorrhage. After delivery of entrapped head, incisions are repaired like cervical tears.

f. *Zavanelli's maneuver:* If all attempts fail at delivery of after-coming-head in breech, the fetus is replaced higher into the vagina and uterus followed by cesarean delivery.

Total Breech Extraction

In total breech extraction, the entire body is manually delivered. This procedure is used only occasionally when there is fetal distress and rapid delivery is indicated, or in delivering of second twin. ***In today's obstetrics, total breech extraction is virtually replaced by cesarean section***. It is done with patient fully relaxed under anesthesia, in lithotomy position and by confirming with full surgical precaution.

Incomplete or Foot Ling Presentation

The both feet are grasped; gentle downward pressure is made, until buttocks are delivered. A generous episiotomy is made. The operator gently grasps the fetal pelvis with both thumb placed directly in either side of sacrum. The spine is rotated if necessary, until rests under pubic symphysis. Gentle firm downward pressure is applied to the body until both scapulas are visible. The shoulder arm and head are delivered as in partial breech extraction. In frank breech extraction groin traction is made to deliver the legs.

Difficulties Encountered During Breech Delivery

Delay in Descent of Breech

a. The breech may be arrested at the pelvic floor due to insufficient uterine contraction or unforeseen disproportion. Augmentation with oxytocin can be done to facilitate contraction. If fetopelvic disproportion is anticipated cesarean delivery is preferred.
b. If breech is arrested at outlet, groin traction is applied.

Bringing Down Leg

When there is difficult delivery of leg, following procedure can be applied:

a. *Pinard's maneuver:* In this the first and second fingers are placed over the thigh and pressed against the trunk. This flexes the knee which brings the foot lower and easier to grasp.
b. *Classical maneuver:* The anterior buttock must be pushed up to the level of the top of the symphysis pubis before the popliteal fossa can be properly reached, the leg flexed and the foot slowly extracted. *These methods are only permissible in situations where facility of cesarean section is not available.*

Extended Arms

If after delivery of baby up to umbilicus, the arms are hooked across the chest, in which case they can be taken out very easily. But if extended, arms should be brought down immediately.

a. *Classical method:* Preferably an anesthetic is rapidly induced, and body of the fetus is pulled to the side opposite to what was its posterior and slightly upwards. The operator hand is passed up the child's body to reach the shoulder and fingers are reached along the arm to the elbow. Flexion of elbow is produced and arm is brought down in front of the face of the baby. The similar procedure is carried out on the other side. *It is important that no traction is applied until the elbow has reached and properly flexed, otherwise humerus is likely to be fractured* (Fig. 50.8).
b. *Lovset's maneuver:* The principle of this maneuver is that the posterior shoulder is below the promontory of

the sacrum when the anterior shoulder is above the symphysis pubis. So when the inferior angle of the anterior scapula is seen, the baby is gently pulled downwards and at the same time rotated so that the back looks upwards. Rotation is continued till posterior shoulder turns and being in the pelvis already is seen under symphysis pubis. When rotation of posterior shoulder is complete, the trunk is suddenly lowered. Thus, one shoulder which was posterior lying below the brim, emerges anteriorly still below the brim, and so delivered beneath the symphysis pubis. After delivery of one shoulder the child is turned in the opposite direction which brings the former anterior shoulder under pubic symphysis (Figs 50.9A to D). *It is easy to learn, does not require internal manipulation, and works when arm is extended or nuchally displaced.*

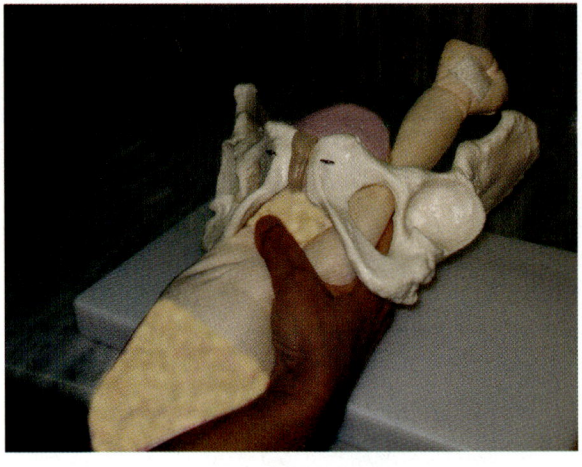

Fig. 50.8: Classical method of bringing down the arm

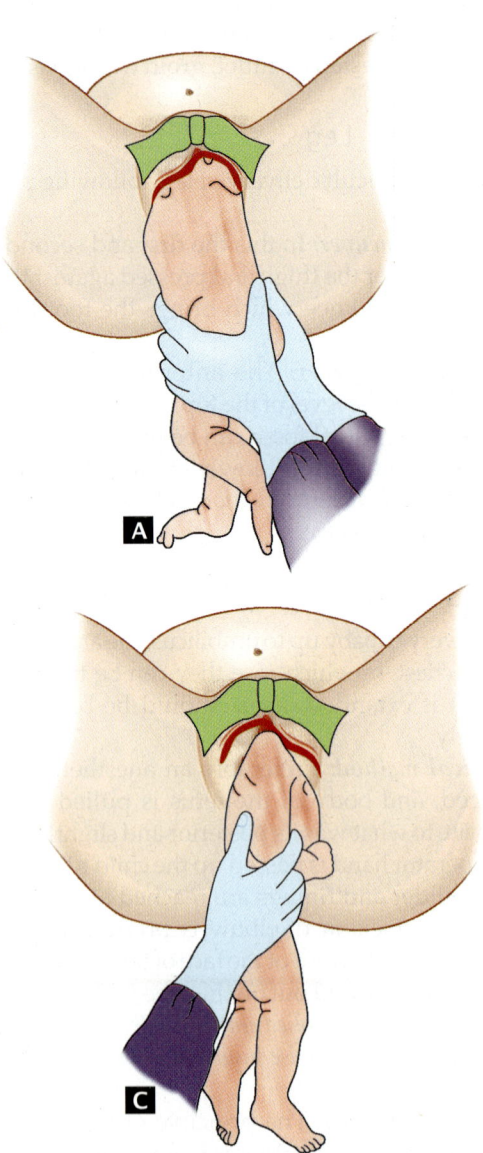
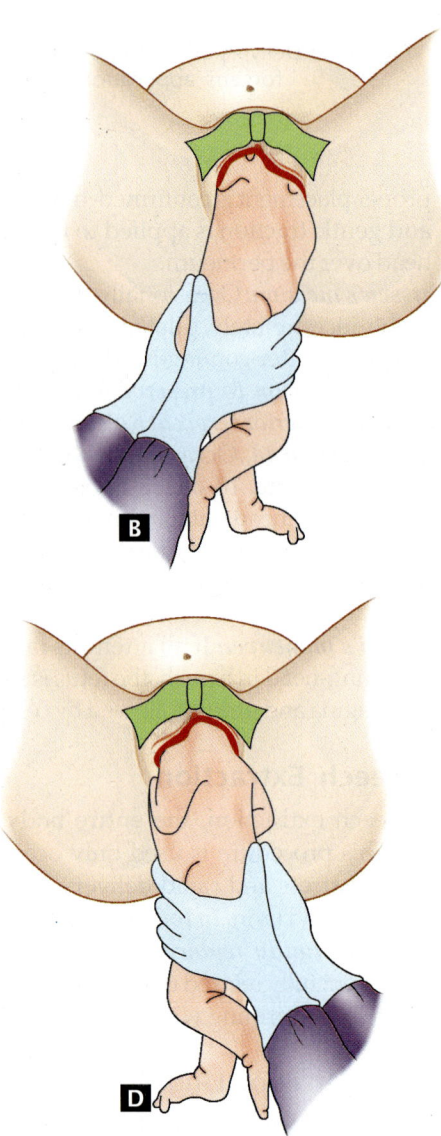

Figs 50.9A to D: Loveset's maneuver for delivery of extended arm

Difficulty in Delivery of After-Coming-Head

It can result from:
a. Large size of fetal head
b. Extension or backward rotation
c. Pelvic contraction
d. Imperfectly dilated cervix
e. Resistant perineum.

When head is arrested above the brim or high in the pelvic cavity. The choice of treatment can be:
i. Jaw and shoulder traction.
ii. Allowing the fetus to hang unsupported for a short time. Both methods are accentuated by fundal pressure.
iii. Application of obstetric forceps: If backward rotation has occurred an attempt should be made to rotate the head and trunk so as to bring occiput forwards or sometimes head is delivered in occiput posterior position.
iv. Perforation can be considered when the fetus is dead.
v. In hydrocephalic head the body is pulled down, and a transverse incision is made over the highest available cervical spine of the fetus. A straight catheter can then be introduced into the spinal canal and thrust through the foramen magnum to drain the excess cerebrospinal fluid. When the baby can be salvaged cesarean section is the choice.

Preterm Breech

In preterm breech babies, there is much more increased risk of intrapartum asphyxia, cord prolapse and entrapment of after-coming-head. There are contradictory reports of benefit of cesarean section in babies weighing 500–2500 gm over vaginal delivery. Though cesarean section is preferred approach in preterm breech but in developing countries, where NICU facilities and after care of preterm babies is not optimal, the decision should be guarded and tailored according to parents' desires and facility.

Cesarean Section Delivery in Breech Presentation

The delivery of fetus in cesarean delivery has the same fundamental principles as vaginal delivery. Upon entering the abdominal cavity the fetus is palpated; a transverse uterine incision usually suffices. In opening the uterus, great care is taken to avoid fetal laceration. An Allis' clamp can be used to elevate the myometrium away from the fetus. A simple snap is used to rupture the membrane. The fetal buttocks are positioned at the incision. Fundal pressure is given by assistant, the fetal scapula is reached and the shoulders are delivered by rotation. After-coming-head is delivered by direct fundal pressure to maintain cranial flexion. In preterm breech, the low vertical incision can be considered. If there is difficulty in delivery of head, Mauriceau-Smellie-Viet maneuver can be used.

Complications in Breech Delivery

Maternal

a. Increased frequency of operative delivery including cesarean section.
b. Increased risk of infection.
c. Increased risk of genital tract laceration.
d. Uterine atony and postpartum hemorrhage.

Fetal

The fetal risk in term of perinatal morbidity and mortality is higher in breech delivery. **The overall perinatal mortality in breech is 9-25% as compared with 1-2% for nonbreech delivery.** The complicated factors beside breech presentation are prematurity and congenital malformation. The corrected perinatal mortality ranges from 5-35/1000 birth. The factors influencing the fetal risk are:
i. Weight and gestational age of fetus
ii. Skill of obstetrician
iii. Position of legs
iv. Type of pelvis

The fetal mortality is least in frank breech and maximum in footling presentation because of cord complication. Gynecoid and anthropoid pelvis is favorable for after-coming-head. Fetal dangers in vaginal breech delivery are as follows:

i. **Intracranial hemorrhage:** Compression followed by decompression during delivery of the unmolded after-coming-head results in tear of tentorium cerebelli and hemorrhage in the subarachnoid space. The risk is more in preterm breech.
ii. **Fetal hypoxia:** It is due to—(i) Cord compression, a delay of more than 10 minute in delivery of head of baby produces fetal hypoxia of varying degree, (ii) Retraction of placental site, (iii) Premature start of respiration while head is still inside, (iv) Delayed delivery of head, (v) Cord prolapse.
iii. **Fetal injuries:** (i) Hematoma of thigh or sternomastoid region, (ii) Fracture of femur, humerus, clavicle, odontoid process, (iii) Visceral injury which includes rupture of liver, kidney, adrenal gland, lungs, and hemorrhage in the testicles, (iv) Nerve injury—spinal cord injury or stretching of the brachial plexus leading to Erb's or Klumpke's palsy. Possibility of long-term handicap and neurological morbidity should always be kept in mind.

Fetal hazards can be prevented by:
a. Use of external cephalic version whenever possible.
b. Use of elective cesarean section after exclusion of congenital anomalies.
c. Availability of skilled obstetrician with organized team of anesthetist, neonatologist and assistant nurses.

Prognosis

The incidence of cesarean section for breech delivery has been steadily increasing for approximately 30% in 1970 to 80% in 1999. The term breech trial collaborate group recently conducted a randomized controlled trial and found that a policy of planned cesarean section will result in seven cesarean birth to avoid one infant death or serious morbidity, **so ACOG recommends planned cesarean delivery for persistent breech presentation at term.**

FACE PRESENTATION

In face presentation the head is hyperextended so that occiput is in contact with fetal back and chin (mentum) is presenting and becomes denominator (Fig. 50.10). A face presentation can develop from an occipitoposterior position during 2nd stage of labor.

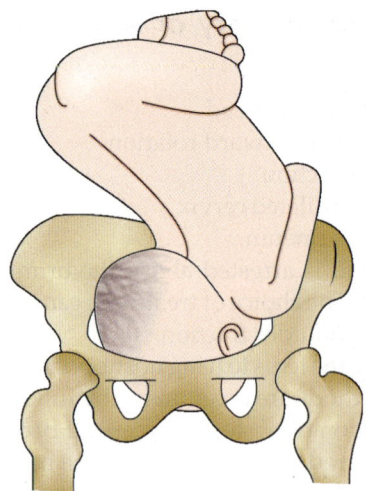

Fig. 50.10: Face presentation in second position, note that spine in extended

Incidence

Face presentation constitute 0.1 to 0.2% vaginal birth. Out of which 50% are diagnosed during 2nd stage of labor. Two-third of face presentation are found in nulliparous women.

Labor in Face Presentation

In face presentation chin is denominator. There can be four positions relative to maternal symphysis pubis:

    1st position – Right mentoposterior – RMP
    2nd position – Left mentoposterior – LMP
    3rd position – Left mentoanterior – LMA
    4th position – Right mentoanterior – RMA

Left mentoanterior 3rd position is the commonest one which usually results from complete extension occurring in occipitoposterior position. In a mentoanterior position the face engages and descends with increasing extension. When the chin reaches the pelvic floor, there is internal rotation through one eighth of circle. This is favorable for a vaginal delivery as the head fits in the sacral hollow and the submental region comes to lie under the pubic arch. **The head is born by movement of flexion,** the submentovertical diameter distending the vulva. The rest of the delivery follows the normal mechanism of labor. In a mentoposterior position, the chin has to undergo the long rotation anteriorly through 3/8th of circle for a safe vaginal delivery. If chin rotates **posteriorly into the sacral hollow, vaginal delivery can not be expected.** The head is unable to enter the pelvis and the labor becomes obstructed.

Diagnosis

a. **Abdominal palpation:** It is not easy to recognize a face presentation by abdominal palpation alone. If there is marked protuberance, e.g. the occiput on the same side as the fetal back, it strongly suggests the diagnosis.
b. **Vaginal examination:** Most face presentation are diagnosed in labor on vaginal examination. It should be suspected in unusually large bag of water and high presenting part. In advanced labor, one can feel alveolar margins and mouth, nose and supraorbital ridge on examination. It can be confused with *breech presentation* if there is lot of facial edema. It is important to confirm the mouth and chin very carefully so as to exclude a brow presentation.
c. **Ultrasound examination:** It should be done in suspected face presentation to exclude fetal anomaly.

Management

a. **Mentoanterior position:** In this case, spontaneous delivery occurs in over 50% of cases. Labor is usually longer because facial bones cannot mold as in vertex presentation. Oxytocin augmentation is not contraindicated if fetopelvic disproportion has been excluded. Delivery of fully rotated mentoanterior face presenting at the outlet can be assisted with forceps if required. Continuous fetal heart monitoring is recommended because there is higher incidence of fetal heart rate abnormalities and low 5 minute APGAR score.
b. **Mentoposterior position:** The only chance of vaginal delivery in a case of mentoposterior presentation is if it rotates spontaneously to mentoanterior, which may not occur till the 2nd stage of labor. Following procedures can be done:
   i. *Wait and watch policy:* In 30% of cases there will be spontaneous rotation to mentoanterior position and can have a spontaneous or easy forceps delivery.
   ii. *Cesarean section:* If there is persistent mentoposterior position, cesarean section should be performed without delay. Manual rotation or rotation with Kielland's forceps is not advocated.

CHAPTER - 50 ♦ Malpresentation and Malposition

BROW PRESENTATION

Brow presentation is rarest, and quoted as 1 in 1500. **Brow presentation is diagnosed when the position of fetal head is between the orbital ridge and anterior fontanelle present at the pelvic inlet.** Thus fetal head occupies position of midway between full flexion (occiput) and extension (mento or face).

It is an unstable presentation and will usually convert to a face or vertex presentation prior to birth. This is the most unfavorable of all cephalic presentation because its presenting diameter is the largest possible that is **mentovertical—13.5 cm.**

Diagnosis

a. *Abdominal examination* is less certain. Only head is not engaged and felt large.
b. *Ultrasound* is useful to exclude fetal malformation and fetal macrosomia.
c. *Vaginal examination,* brow presentation may be missed on vaginal examination until the cervix is well dilated. **The brow presentation is then recognized by the anterior fontanelle at one end of the presenting part and the supraorbital ridges and root of the nose at the other end.** These landmarks must be identified before clinical diagnosis (Fig. 50.11). It is to be noted that neither mouth, nose, chin is within reach. *Any multipara who demonstrates a delay in labor with high head* should raise the suspicion of brow presentation. A full bladder should be excluded by catheterization which also facilitates delivery.

Management

a. In transient brow presentation, the outcome for vaginal delivery depends on the ultimate presentation. *More than 50% of brow presentation converts by flexion to vertex or extension to face presentation.* Expectant management can be pursued if the labor is well in progress and fetal heart is reassuring.
b. If labor is prolonged, cesarean section should be done. *As a brow presentation is undeliverable, instrumental delivery or manual conversion to vertex or face or symphysiotomy are dangerous and should not be attempted.*

TRANSVERSE LIE/OBLIQUE AND SHOULDER PRESENTATION

Transverse lie of the fetus is defined when the long axis of the fetus is approximately perpendicular to that of mother. When long axis forms an acute angle with that of mother, oblique lie results. Oblique lie is called an unstable lie, as with onset of labor either a longitudinal or transverse lie commonly results (Fig. 50.12).

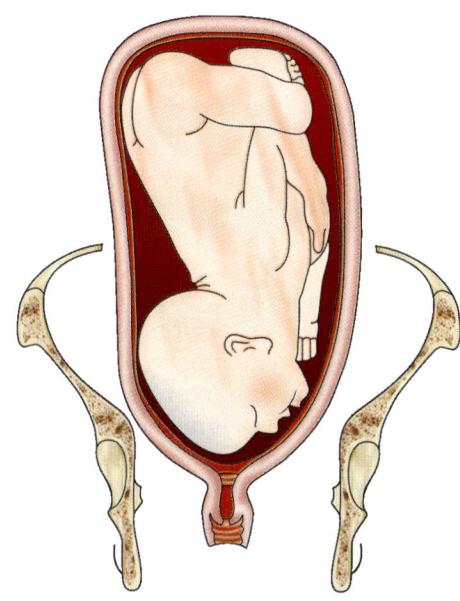

Fig. 50.11: Brow presentation. Head is not engaged. The mentovertical diameter of the head is trying to engage in transverse diameter at the brim

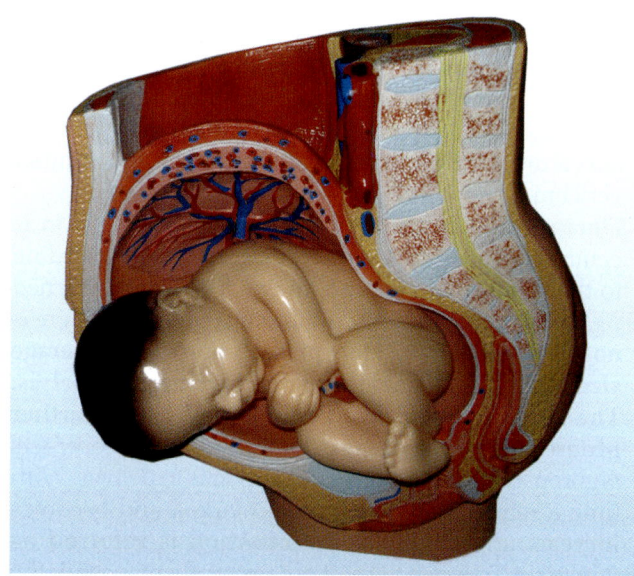

Fig. 50.12: Attitude and position in transverse lie

Incidence and Etiology

Transverse lie of the fetus occurs in approximately 1 in 300 pregnancies. All conditions which prevent the ready descent of the fetal head into the pelvic brim may cause shoulder presentation like:

a. Abdominal wall relaxation from high parity
b. Preterm fetus
c. Pelvic contraction
d. Hydramnios
e. Placenta previa
f. Multiple pregnancy

g. Extreme uterine obliquity
h. Bicornuate uterus.

Diagnosis

a. **Abdominal examination:** The abdomen is enlarged transversely, the fundal height is lower and the pelvic grip is empty. The ballottable head is found in one iliac fossa and breech in the other. In dorsoanterior position, the back is identified easily while in dorsoposterior position the irregular nodulation, representing the small parts are felt through abdominal wall.
b. **Vaginal examination:** The most important finding is negative as the clinician feels neither the fetal head nor fetal breech. The presenting part is often high; there is elongated bag of water, and tendency to early rupture of membrane. After rupture of membrane gridiron feel of the ribs, scapula and clavicle are distinguished. If woman comes late in labor, the shoulder will become tightly wedged in the pelvic canal and head and arm frequently prolapses into the vagina and through the vulva.

Attitude, Position and Mechanism of Labor

The position is determined by the direction of back, which is the denominator. The position may be:
a. **Dorsoanterior: (60% most common)**, because the fetus accommodates itself better in that position to the forward curvature of the maternal lower dorsal and lumbar vertebra.
b. **Dorsoposterior:** In this chance of fetal extension is common with increased risk of arm prolapse. According to the position of the head, the fetal position is turned right or left, the left being commoner than right. **There is no mechanism in shoulder presentation and an average size baby fails to pass through an average size pelvis. The shoulder is wedged in the pelvis, and further progress of fetus ceases.** The uterus then contracts vigorously in the unsuccessful attempts to deliver. With time a retraction ring becomes marked and becomes increasingly higher. This situation is referred as '*Neglected Transverse Lie.*' If not promptly managed, the uterus eventually rupture, which causes mother and fetus at grave risk. Rarely early in labor, before rupture of membrane, there may be *spontaneous rectification or spontaneous version* in which transverse lie is transformed into head or breech presentation respectively. Exceptionally in very premature and dead fetus, there can be *spontaneous evolution or spontaneous expulsion* when baby is delivered doubled up.

Management

External Cephalic Version

External cephalic version can be tried antenatally at term or even in early labor if contracted pelvis, placenta previa and uterus anomaly is ruled out. If ECV is successful, close supervision is needed till the time the head is settled in the lower uterine segment. AAFP 2000/2001, note that ECV can be tried in a second twin who presents as transverse lie at full dilatation. It is easier as the uterus is initially relaxed.

Cesarean Section

In general, the onset of active labor in *women with a transverse lie is an indication for cesarean section.* It is the safest course even if the baby is dead. An immediate cesarean section is indicated if there is cord prolapse, unsuccessful external cephalic version and neglected transverse lie.

Internal Podalic Version

It is often considered hazardous for the baby and a cesarean section is the preferred option. Version is only recommended in second twin with transverse lie only if there is sufficient liquor amni and uterus is well relaxed between the pains.

Complications

a. The perinatal morbidity in transverse lie is considerably increased due to birth asphyxia and severe acidosis as compared to vertex and even breech. Risk of premature rupture of membrane and spontaneous cord prolapse is very high.
b. Maternal morbidity is high because of increased operative intervention, risk of obstructed labor, infection and uterine rupture.

UNSTABLE LIE

It is a condition where the presentation of the fetus is constantly changed even beyond 36th weeks of pregnancy, when it should have been stabilized.

Causes

Grand multiparity with pendulous belly is the commonest cause. Polyhydramnios, contracted pelvis, placenta previa and pelvic tumors are condition which prevents presenting part to be fixed in the lower pole of the uterus and causing unstable lie.

Management

a. **External cephalic version:** ECV can attempt near term. If version is successful, the patient can be managed expectantly for spontaneous wait of labor or stabilizing induction with amniotomy. If version fails, elective cesarean should be done at 38 weeks.
b. **Hospital admission:** There is risk of spontaneous and rapid labor with uncorrected malpresentation. So it is preferable to admit the patient in hospital near term, so that women is safe and can wait for spontaneous labor. If there is active labor with transverse lie or cord prolapse, *immediate cesarean section should be done.*

COMPOUND PRESENTATION

In compound presentation, there is presentation or prolapse of either hand or foot along with the presenting part and both presents in the pelvis simultaneously (Fig. 50.13).

Incidence and Cause

Incidence is about 1 in 1000. Causes are again all the conditions which prevent complete occlusion of the pelvic inlet by the fetal head including preterm birth.

Diagnosis

On per vaginal examination in active labor one can feel the limb by the side of presenting part, especially after rupture of membrane. Cord prolapse is to be excluded because of its frequent association (10-15%).

Management

a. **Expectant treatment:** In most cases the prolapsed part should be left alone. If arm is prolapsed along side the head, one should observe to ascertain that arm retracts out of the way with descent of presenting part. If arm fails to retract, the prolapsed arm should be pushed gently upward and head is simultaneously pushed downwards by fundal pressure.
b. **Cesarean section:** Mature singleton fetus associated with contracted pelvis or cord prolapse with the fetus alive should be delivered by cesarean section.

CORD PROLAPSE

Umbilical cord prolapse is defined as descent of the umbilical cord into the lower uterine segment, beside or below the presenting part. If the membranes are intact, this is known as *cord prolapse*. If cord is adjacent to presenting part, it is called *occult*. In this, umbilical cord cannot be palpated during pelvic examination. In *Frank prolapse*, the cord is below presenting part and can be easily palpated through the membranes. **Overt cord prolapse** is associated with rupture of membrane and displacement of the umbilical cord into the vagina, often through the introitus.

Incidence: Incidence of cord prolapse is 0.2-0.6%. The incidence is decreasing because of increased use of elective cesarean section in malpresentation.

Causes and Risk Factors

a. Any obstetric condition that predisposes to poor application of the fetal presenting part to the cervix can result in prolapse of the umbilical cord. Cord prolapse is associated with prematurity (<34 week gestation), abnormal presentation (breech, brow, face, transverse), multiparity, cephalopelvic disproportion, placenta previa.

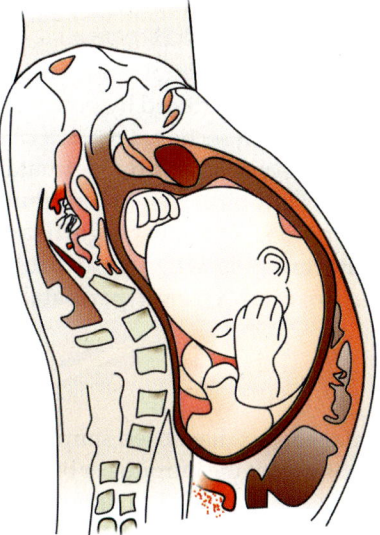

Fig. 50.13: Compound presentation

b. Hydramnios, multiple gestation or premature rupture of the membrane occurring before engagement of the presenting part are other risk factors.
c. Obstetric intervention like artificial rupture of the membrane is direct cause in 50% of cases. Scalp electrode application, attempted external cephalic version and expectant management of preterm premature rupture of membrane are associated with increased chance of cord prolapse.
d. When fetus is dead, low pressure in blood vessels of the cord reduces its turgidity and become limp and prolapses more readily.
e. An abnormal long cord predisposes to cord prolapse.

Fetal and Maternal Risk

1. **Maternal risk:** Cord prolapse does not increase the maternal risk except when prompt easy vaginal delivery is not possible. In these cases, the maternal risk would be directly proportional to the extent of operative assistance. Maternal risks include laceration of cervix, vagina or perineum because of hastily performed delivery. There is increased rate of cesarean with its associated morbidity.
2. **Fetal risk:** The fetus is in great danger of death from anoxia because prolapsed cord is likely to be compressed between the presenting part and the pelvic brim or cervix and blood flow within it, therefore, becomes restricted or obstructed. However, fetal death can occur even in absence of pressure on cord, probably due to spasm of the vessels. The fetal risk is more when:
   a. Cord prolapse in 1st stage (70% as compared to 30% in 2nd stage).
   b. Vertex presentation.

c. Descent in front of head.
d. Primigravida.

Though the risk of perinatal mortality and morbidity has been considerably reduced by policy of emergency delivery and cesarean section, *umbilical cord prolapse* is in *important independent risk* for perinatal mortality. Prematurity and low birth weight contributes to overall perinatal mortality. **The most significant factor for perinatal mortality is when cord prolapse** *occurs* **outside the hospital. Overall perinatal mortality is about 50%.**

Diagnosis

Overt cord prolapse: It is diagnosed simply by visualizing the cord prolapsing from the introitus or by palpating loops of cord in vaginal canal. AROM or spontaneous prelabor rupture of membrane can be complicated by sudden cord prolapse, especially if done in high presenting part or malpresentation.

Occult cord prolapse: It is suspected when there is sudden fetal heart rate changes like variable deceleration, bradycardia or both associated with intermittent compression of the umbilical cord detected during monitoring.

Management

Prevention

Patient at high risk for cord prolapse should be considered for ultrasonographic examination at the onset of labor to determine fetal lie and cord position. **In high risk cases, AROM should be avoided and continuous fetal monitoring should be done.** At the time of rupture of membrane a careful pelvic examination should be done to rule out cord prolapse. If amniotomy has to be done, carefully needling and slow release of amniotic fluid should be performed until the presenting part sites against the cervix.

Management

Cord prolapse and cord presentation are managed in the same way. The principle of management are:
a. To release pressure on the cord.
b. To find out if fetus is alive or dead.
c. If alive to deliver expeditiously.
d. If fetus dead and pelvis and presentation are favorable, spontaneous delivery is awaited.

Release Pressure on Cord

For this following method can be used:
a. The gloved hand is inserted into the vagina and presenting part is lifted off the cord, leaving the cord where it is. At the same time cord pulsation, cervical dilatation, station and presenting part is confirmed.
b. Alternative method is the woman is positioned in knee chest position to reduce the pressure caused by the presenting part (Fig. 50.14).
c. Maternal bladder is filled with 400-700 ml normal saline by 16F foley's catheter. This not only relieves the cord compression but also inhibit uterine activity.

By above method one can see that after relief of pressure there is return of fetal heart activity.

Subsequent decision making will depend on:
(a) Status of fetus, (b) Degree of cervical dilatation, (c) Station of presenting part.

If fetus is alive: The principle is to deliver the fetus as expeditiously as possible:
i. **In 2nd stage:** If cervix is fully dilated, head is engaged; forceps delivery in vertex presentation and breech extraction in breech presentation by experienced obstetrician should be done. Pediatrician should be present for immediate resuscitation of the newborn if necessary.
ii. **In cervix, less than 3/4th dilated** or there are some other adverse factors like cephalopelvic disproportion, *immediate cesarean section* must be resorted. Pressure over the cord must be released while preparations are being made for cesarean section. This is done by elevating the presenting part by hand in vagina until uterus is incised or bladder filling and keeping the patient in moderate trendelenburg position. At the same time continuous fetal heart rate monitoring is continued.

OCCIPITOPOSTERIOR POSITION

General Consideration

Occipitoposterior position of the vertex was once looked upon as the betanoir of obstetric practice. It is one of the most common malposition. **At the time of onset of labor, the two posterior positions taken together are found in about 25% of all vertex presentation. In the 2nd stage of labor, the majority of posterior position converts into anterior position by the forward rotation of the occiput.**

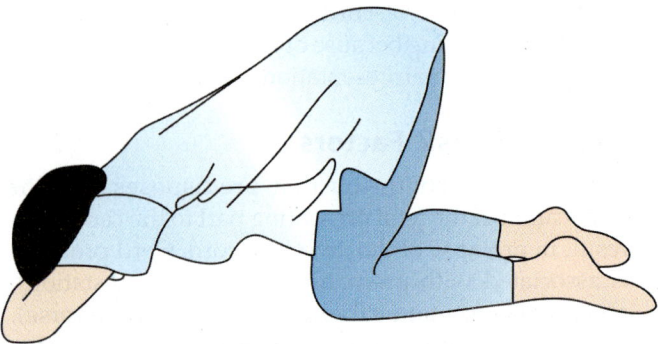

Fig. 50.14: Knee chest position to reduce pressure of the cord by presenting part

Such a rectification of position occurs in about 80-90% of cases. If head does not rotate, persistent occipitoposterior position may result in dystocia. It occurs in 4-5% of occipitoposterior position.

Cause of Occipitoposterior Position

The following factors may be responsible for occipitoposterior position:

Anthropoid, Android Pelvis or Minor Degree of Pelvic Contraction

In these types of pelvis a narrowed transverse diameter of the outlet may directly interfere with a long rotation of the head.

Deficient Flexion of Head

It is the most important cause of failure to rotate in occipitoposterior position.

Causes of deflexion are:
a. **High pelvic inclination**.
b. **Anterior position of placenta:** Extension of head is more liable to occur in posterior than in anterior position because the attitude of generalized flexion of fetus is disturbed by some degree of extension of the spine, which results from the opposition of the two convexities of the fetal back and maternal lumbar vertebra.
c. **Weak uterine contraction:** Flexion of head and movement of rotation is facilitated by strong uterine contraction as it increases the resistance which the head meets on pelvic floor. That's why uterine inertia is commonly associated with persistent occipito posteriorpositions.
d. **PROM/oligohydramnios:** In premature rupture of membrane or oligohydramnios, the trunk is so closely embraced by the retracting uterus that its freedom of movement is interfered with and internal rotation of head is impeded.

Diagnosis

The diagnosis of occipitoposterior position depends on the suspicion of the problem.

Symptoms

There can be deep back discomfort during labor and early spontaneous rupture of membrane.

Signs of Palpation

(i) Limbs are felt with unusual ease and back is difficult to locate, (ii) On pelvic grip, the head is not engaged and sinciput–cephalic prominence is not felt so prominent as in occipitoanterior positions.

Vaginal Examination

(i) There can be elongated bag of membrane, (ii) Anterior fontanelle is easily reached and at a lower level than posterior level, (iii) In late labor the diagnosis is difficult because of caput formation. *In such case ear should be located as unfolded pinna points towards the occiput* (Fig. 50.15), (iv) There can be shortened cervix or edematous cervix with deflexed head of the occipitoposterior position.

Mechanism of Labor in Occipitoposterior Position

Normal course of labor in occipitoposterior position: The head engage through the right oblique diameter in ROP and left oblique diameter in LOP. The engaging transverse diameter of the head is biparietal—9.5 cm and that of anteroposterior diameter is **suboccipitofrontal (10 cm) or occipitofrontal (11.5 cm)**. Because of deflexion engagement is delayed. In 90% cases of favorable circumstances following course occurs:

a. *Flexion:* Good uterine contraction aids descent and food flexion.
b. *Internal rotation of the head:* Occiput rotates 3/8th of the circle (135°) anteriorly to lie behind the symphysis pubis (Figs 50.16A and B).
c. Further course of labor is usually identical with that of primary anterior position. In difficult flexion and weak uterine contraction, there is delayed anterior rotation.

Abnormal Course of Labor

Due to weak uterine action, faulty shape of the pelvis, or deflexion of head, the above normal mechanism of labor fails to occur and can result in following situations:
a. Where head engage in the pelvis in oblique occiput posterior position and remains unrotated.

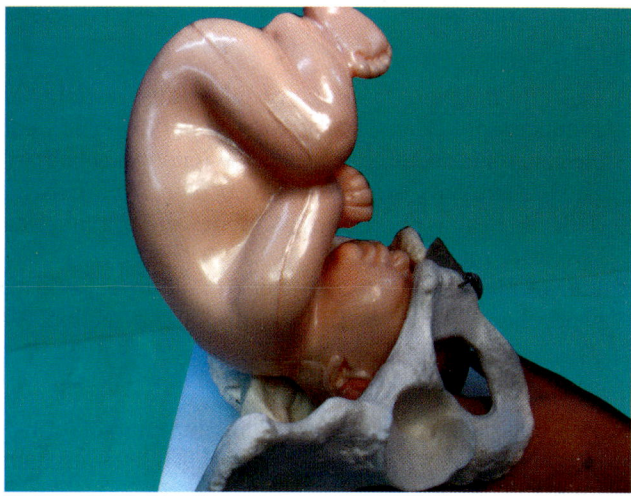

Fig. 50.15: Persistent occipitoposterior position—Ear can be landmark to confirm position

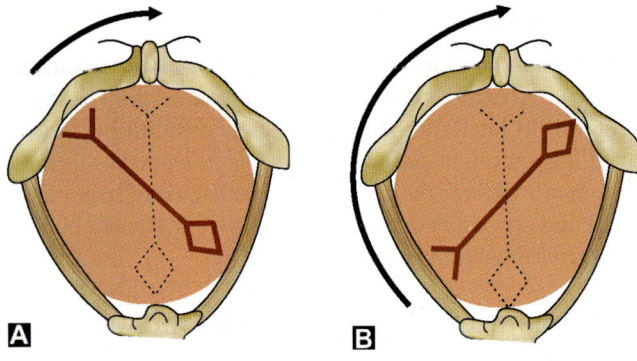

Figs 50.16A and B: Long internal rotation in occipitoposterior position (B) as compared to occipitoanterior position (A) (A: 1/4th circle B: 3/8th circle)

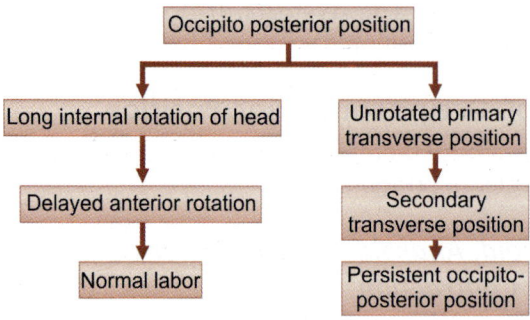

Flow chart 50.1: Various courses of labor in occipitoposterior position

Causes-
1. Deficient flexion of head
2. Weak uterine action
3. PROM
4. Anthropoid/Android pelvis

b. When forward rotation of the occiput from an oblique posterior position is arrested in secondary transverse position. **Deep transverse arrest** is more common in android pelvis.
c. When a short backward rotation of the occiput from oblique posterior position into the hollow of sacrum, which results in **persistent occipitoposterior position (Fig. 50.15)**. In favorable circumstances in posterior occipitoposterior position spontaneous delivery may occur in **'face to pubes'** position. In this, root of the nose hinges under the symphysis pubis. Flexion of head occurs which releases successively the brow, vertex and occiput out of the stretched perineum and then **face is born by extension. Face to pubes delivery is more common in anthropoid pelvis (Fig. 50.17).** Course of labor in occipitoposterior position is summarized in Flow chart 50.1.
d. If face to pubes delivery does not occur, there can be arrest which is called occiput sacral arrest (Fig. 50.17).

Maternal and Fetal Risk

In 1st Stage

a. There is delayed 1st stage of labor due to delay in engagement because persistence of deflexion of head increases diameter of engagement (occipitofrontal 11.5 cm).
b. There is tendency of early rupture of membrane because deflexed head is ovoid and cannot fit well into spherical lower uterine segment.
c. Weak uterine contraction because of ill fitting deflexed head, there is less of stimuli for uterine contraction.

In 2nd Stage

a. The 2nd stage is delayed due to long internal rotation or malrotation with at times arrest of head. If left untreated, there can be obstructed labor.
b. There is increased rate of instrumental delivery rate (43.7%) and cesarean section (41.7%) compared to

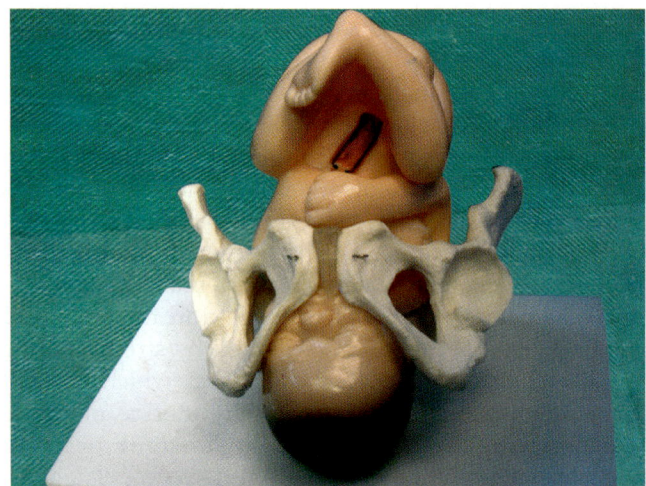

Fig. 50.17: Face to pubes delivery in persistent occipitoposterior position

occipitoanterior position (24.4% and 13.7% respectively). Because of increased need of operative intervention maternal morbidity is higher.

Third Stage

Because of prolonged labor and operative intervention, there is increased incidence of postoperative hemorrhage.

Neonatal Risk

Because of delayed course of labor, early rupture of membrane and increased operative intervention, neonate is adversely affected and there is increased incidence of low APGAR scores, umbilical cord acidemia, meconium staining, birth trauma and longer neonatal stay in the hospital.

Management of Labor

Principle of Management in the Occipitoposterior Position

a. Early diagnosis.
b. Strict vigilance with watchful expectancy hoping for descent and anterior rotation of the occiput.
c. Judicious and timely interference.

Management of 1st Stage

a. Psychological preparation of women for labor of indeterminate length. Light food should be given to avoid dehydration and ketoacidosis. Mobilization and upright posture is preferred because it increases pelvic outlet diameter.
b. Partographic documentation of progress of labor and fetal heart rate pattern for early detection of abnormal course of labor and need for interference.
c. If there is weak uterine contraction, persistence of deflexion and nonrotation of occiput—oxytocin infusion can be started for augmentation of labor.
d. Cesarean section should be considered if—(i) There is arrest of labor and failure of rotation, (ii) Incoordinate uterine action, (iii) Fetal distress.

Management of 2nd Stage of Labor

a. In majority anterior rotation of the occiput is completed and delivery is either spontaneous or can be accomplished by low forceps or ventouse.
b. In unrotated and malrotated head, if fetal and maternal status is satisfactory, one should have a watchful expectancy approach for anterior rotation of head and descent of head. In occiput sacral position, there can be *Face to Pubes delivery*. In such cases, delivery should be properly conducted and **liberal episiotomy should be done to prevent complete perineal tear. Because in face to pubes delivery the diameter of engagement is occipitofrontal measuring 11.5 cm, which is larger than suboccipitobregmatic diameter of 9.5 cm found in occipitoanterior position.** In general many patients need obstetric assistance, so incidence of instrumentally assisted vaginal delivery or cesarean section is increased.

Management of 3rd Stage

Active management of 3rd stage is indicated. Following vaginal operative delivery meticulous inspection of cervix and lower genital tract should be made to detect any injury.

Management of Persistent Occipitoposterior Position

If there is failure to progress after full cervical dilatation instead of good uterine contraction for too long period (2 hours for nullipara, 50 minutes for multipara), interference is indicated. Following protocol should be followed:

1. Good assessment of fetal heart rate, size of baby, engagement, station of head, position of sagittal suture and occiput, degree of molding and caput formation, assessment of pelvis.

   After thorough assessment, decision for following intervention is taken:

   a. **Ventouse (vacuum extractor):** Its use is helpful when pelvis is adequate and nonrotation is either due to weak uterine contraction or lack of tone of pelvic floor muscles. The ventouse cup is applied to the fetal head near the occiput end of vertex. It promotes flexion and head rotate smoothly as it descends (Fig. 50.18).
   b. **Manual rotation followed by forceps application:** The objectives are first to rotate the head manually until the occiput is placed behind the symphysis pubis and secondly in that position forceps blades are applied. For this maneuver, there must be no cephalopelvic disproportion and liquor should be adequate to facilitate manual rotation.
   c. **Forceps rotation and extraction by use of Kielland forceps in expert hands:** The procedure can be dangerous in inexpert hands.
   d. **Face to pubes delivery:** By forceps application. If head is engaged and occiput descends below the ischial spine. Liberal episiotomy should be given to avoid perineal tear (Fig. 50.19).
   e. **Cesarean section:** If occiput is above level of ischial spine, cesarean section should be considered. If there is mild pelvic contraction and unsuitable for above maneuvers or there is fetal or maternal distress, cesarean section is much safer even in 2nd stage.
   f. **If the baby is dead, craniotomy** can be considered. It is rarely required.

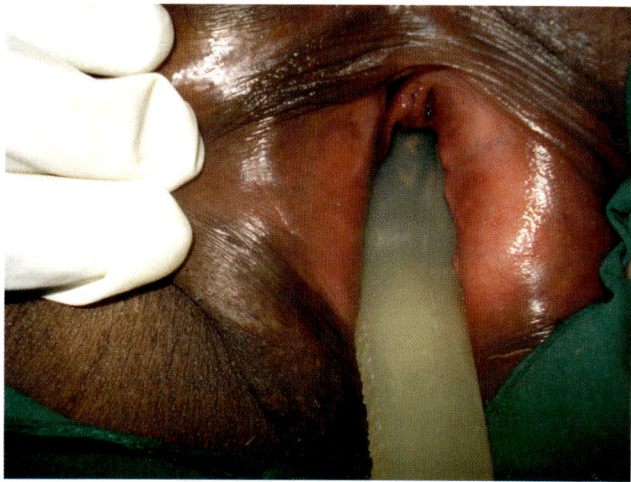

Fig. 50.18: Ventouse cup application in occipitoposterior position

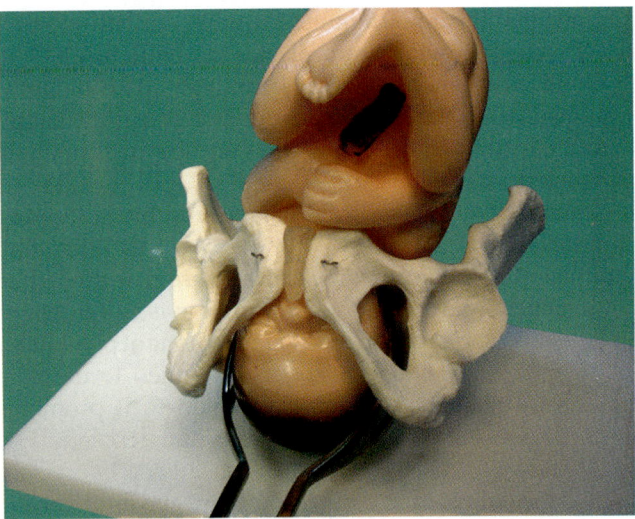

Fig. 50.19: Forceps application in unrotated head with face to pubes delivery

Management in Deep Transverse Arrest

If the head is deep into pelvic cavity, sagittal suture is placed in transverse bispinous diameter. Anterior fontanelle is easily felt and there is no progress in descent of head after a long time (arbitary limit of 1-2 hours) following full dilatation of the cervix. The diagnosis of deep transverse arrest is made. There can be associated faulty architecture of pelvis. Management is on the same line as persistent occipitoposterior position. Following protocol is recommended:

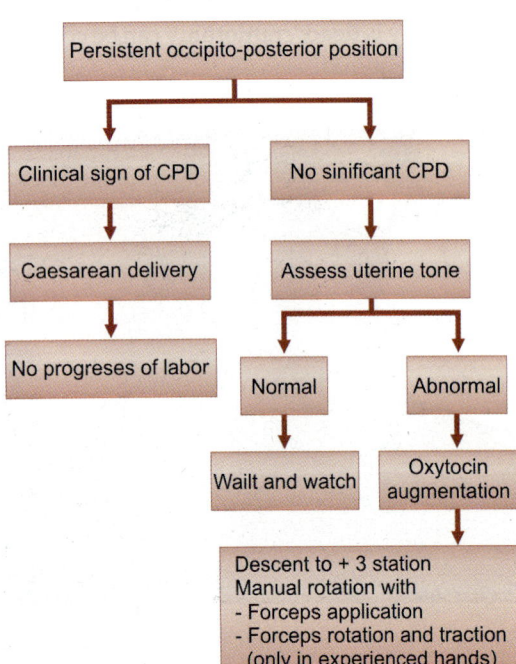

Flow chart 50.2: Management of persistent occipitoposterior position

1. If vaginal delivery is anticipated safe:
   a. Ventouse application.
   b. Manual rotation and forceps application.
   c. Forceps rotation and delivery of head with Kielland's forceps in expert hands.
   d. Craniotomy in dead baby.
2. **If vaginal delivery is not safe:** Like cephalopelvic disproportion, severe fetal and maternal distress, cesarean section should be done.

Management protocol for occipitoposterior position is summarized in Flow chart 50.2.

MULTIPLE CHOICE QUESTIONS

1. The commonest cause of breech presentation is:
   a. Prematurity
   b. Hydrocephalus
   c. Placenta previa
   d. Polyhydramnios
   Ans. a
2. All of the following are associated with breech presentation at normal full term pregnancy except:
   a. Placenta accreta
   b. Fetal malformation
   c. Uterine anomaly
   d. Cornual implantation of placenta
   Ans. a
3. Cause of fetal death in breech delivery:
   a. Intracranial hemorrhage
   b. Aspiration
   c. Atlantoaxial dislocation
   d. Asphyxia
   Ans. a, c, d
4. Best method to deliver arms in breech:
   a. Lovset's method
   b. Smellie veit
   c. Pinard
   d. Any of the above
   Ans. a
5. The after-coming-head of breech, chin to pubes is delivered by:
   a. Mauriceau-Smellie-Veit
   b. Burns-Marshall maneuver
   c. Lovset's method
   d. Manual rotation and extraction by piper's forceps
   Ans. d
6. Breech presentation with hydrocephalus can be managed by:
   a. Cesarean section
   b. Transabdominal decompression
   c. Pervaginal decompression
   d. Craniotomy of after-coming-head
   Ans. a, b, c, d
7. True about frank breech:
   a. Thigh extended, leg extended
   b. Thigh flexed, knee extended
   c. Both are flexed
   d. Common in primigravida
   Ans. b, d

Chapter - 50 ♦ Malpresentation and Malposition

8. Incidence of cord prolapse is least in:
   a. Frank breech
   b. Footling presentation
   c. Transverse lie
   d. Brow presentation
   Ans. a
9. In an after-coming-head, the following bone is perforated during decapitation:
   a. Occiput
   b. Parietal
   c. Palate
   d. Frontal
   Ans. a
10. Which one of the following terminologies is NOT correctly matched:
    a. Breech delivery—Burns-Marshall Technique
    b. Neglected shoulder presentation—Bandl's ring or retraction ring
    c. Retained placenta—True knot of cord
    d. Reverse rotation to occipitosacral position—face to pubes delivery
    Ans. c
11. Face to pubes delivery is possible with which cephalic presentation?
    a. Mentoanterior
    b. Mentoposterior
    c. Occipitosacral
    d. Brow presentation
    Ans. c
12. In a case of direct occipitoposterior delivery (face to pubis delivery) the most commonly encountered problem is:
    a. Intracranial injury
    b. Cephalhematoma
    c. Periurethral tears
    d. Complete perineal tears
    Ans. d
13. The commonest cause of occipitoposterior position of fetal head during labor is:
    a. Maternal obesity
    b. Deflexion of fetal head
    c. Multiparity
    d. Android pelvis
    Ans. d
14. Cause of face presentation are:
    a. Anencephaly
    b. Prematurity
    c. Hydramnios
    d. Contracted pelvis
    Ans. a, b, d
15. Diameter of engagement in face presentation:
    a. Mentovertical
    b. Submentovertical
    c. Suboccipitobregmatic
    d. Submentobregmatic
    Ans. b, d
16. In brow presentation, presenting diameter are:
    a. Submentovertical
    b. Occipitofrontal
    c. Mentovertical
    d. Suboccipitobregmatic
    Ans. c
17. Most common congenital anomaly associated with face presentation:
    a. Anencephaly
    b. Microcephaly
    c. Hydrocephalus
    d. Macrosomia
    Ans. a
18. In deep transverse arrest, the delivery of baby is conducted by:
    a. Cesarean section
    b. Vacuum extraction
    c. Kielland's forceps
    d. Manual rotation and forceps delivery
    e. All
    Ans. e
19. In a primigravida with 38 weeks pregnancy in early labor with transverse presentation, treatment of choice is:
    a. Allow for cervical dilatation
    b. Internal podalic version
    c. LSCS
    d. Forceps
    Ans. c
20. On per vaginal examination, anterior fontanelle and supraorbital ridge is felt in the second stage of labor. The presentation is:
    a. Brow presentation
    b. Deflexed head
    c. Flexed head
    d. Face presentation
    Ans. a

51 Dystocia and Cephalopelvic Disproportion

When faced with a challenge, look for a way, not a way out.

DYSTOCIA

Dystocia literally means difficult labor and is characterized by abnormally slow progress of labor. It is the consequence of abnormalities in three categories, as simplified by ACOG (1995) :

a. Abnormalities of the power (uterine contractility) and maternal expulsive efforts.
b. Abnormalities of the passage—maternal bony pelvis and soft part.
c. Abnormalities of passenger—fetus or a combination of these factors.

Any deviation of normal pattern of labor can be designated as dystocia. Overall the incidence of labor disorder is approximately 25% in primigravida and 10% in multigravida. It is one of most common indication for cesarean section.

Abnormal Pattern of Labor

Freidman described four abnormal patterns of labor:
I. Prolonged latent phase.
II. Protracted disorder.
III. Arrest disorder.
IV. Precipitate labor disorders.

Prolonged Latent Phase

The duration of latent phase that is from onset of uterine contraction to beginning of active phase of cervical dilatation is 6.4 hours in nullipara and 4.8 hours in multipara. The latent phase is said to be prolonged if it lasts more than 20 hours in nulliparous or 14 hours in multipara.

Causes of Prolonged Latent Phase

a. Excessive sedation.
b. Use of conduction anesthetic before active phase of labor.
c. Labor starting with unfavorable cervix.
d. Ineffective uterine contraction.
e. Weak irregular uncoordinated uterine dysfunction.

Treatment of Prolonged Labor

It may be therapeutic rest or active management of labor.

a. **Rest with sedation and hydration:** Usually after 6-12 hours of rest, 85% of patients spontaneously enter the active phase of labor. In 10% of patients there is false labor and can be sent home for *await the onset of labor,* if there is no other indication of delivery.
b. **Augmentation with oxytocin:** In remaining 5% of patients uterine contraction remain ineffective in producing dilatation and augmentation with oxytocin may be effective in progression to active phase of labor. Usually prognosis for vaginal delivery after treatment is excellent and usually patients are not at any greater risk of developing subsequent labor disorders.

Protracted Disorders

Protracted active phase dilation is characterized by an abnormally slow rate of dilatation in the active phase, that is less than 1.2 cm/ hour in nullipara or less than 1.5 cm/hour in multiparous. *Protracted descent of* the fetus is characterized by a rate of descent less than 1 cm/hour in nullipara or less than 2 cm/hour in multipara. The *2nd stage of labor is protracted* when the stage exceeds 2 hours in nullipara or 1 hour in multipara or 2 and 3 hours respectively in the presence of conduction anesthetic.

Causes of Protracted Disorders

Causes are multifactorial. *Fetopelvic disproportion* is cause in approximately one-third of patients. Other factors are: *minor malposition as occipitoposterior, epidural anesthetic, excessive sedation and pelvic tumors obstructing the birth canal.*

Diagnosis

Diagnosis is made by time chart. The use of partogram alerts the obstetrician to possibility of prolongation of labor.

Treatment

Treatment depends on the:
a. Presence or absence of fetopelvic disproportion.
b. Adequacy of uterine contraction.
c. Fetal status.

If there is confirmed fetopelvic disproportion or signs of fetal distress, *cesarean section* is indicated. In case of poor uterine activity *oxytocin infusion* can be tried with close supervision. Oxytocin augmentation along with support and close observation carry a good prognosis for vaginal delivery which is achieved in approximately two-third of the patients. In protracted disorders vaginal examination should be kept to minimum, if done all sterile precaution to be strictly observed. Prophylactic antibiotic should be given if the membranes are ruptured and delivery is likely to be delayed.

Arrest Disorders

There are two patterns of arrest disorders:
a. Secondary arrest of dilatation with no progressive cervical dilatation in the active phase of labor for two hours or more.
b. Arrest of descent with descent failing to progress for 1 hour or more.

Causes

Causes are the same as protracted disorder that is fetopelvic disproportion, fetal malposition, sedation and use of inappropriate anesthetic.

Treatment

When arrest disorder is diagnosed, a thorough evaluation of pelvis and estimation of fetal weight is done. If fetopelvic disproportion is estimated prompt cesarean section is warranted. If fetopelvic disproportion is not present and uterine activity is less than optimal, oxytocin augmentation can be done. Arrest disorders in the presence of good uterine contraction carry a poor prognosis for vaginal delivery and if allowed to continue are associated with increased perinatal morbidity. But if postarrest rate of cervical dilatation and descent is equal or greater than prearrest rate, prognosis for vaginal delivery is excellent.

Precipitate Labor

It is defined as delivery in less than 3 hours from onset of contraction. *Precipitate dilatation* can be defined as cervical dilatation occurring at a rate of 5 cm or more per hour in a Primipara or 10 cm or more per hour in multipara.

Causes

It is caused by:
a. Extremely strong uterine contraction and low resistance of birth canal.
b. Iatrogenic by use of oxytocic drugs.

Treatment

a. If oxytocin administration is being used, it should be stopped and patient to be placed in lateral position.
b. If there is a fetal heart rate abnormality, despite withdrawal of oxytocin, beta mimetic as 125-250 μg of Terbutaline or Ritodrine can be given.

Complications

a. Maternal complications are rare. Sometimes when birth canal is rigid and uterus hypertonus occurs, there can be uterine rupture. Lacerations of birth canal are common and incidence of postpartum hemorrhage is increased.
b. Perinatal mortality and morbidity is increased because of:
   i. Decreased uteroplacental flow.
   ii. Possibility of intracranial hemorrhage.
   iii. Risk associated with unattended delivery as resuscitation equipment may not be available.

CONTRACTED PELVIS AND CEPHALOPELVIC DISPROPORTION

Contracted Pelvis

Definition

Anatomically contracted pelvis is defined as one where essential diameters of one or more planes are shortened by 0.5 cm. *Obstetric definition* is more important according to which there is such alteration in size and shape of the pelvis of sufficient degree so as to alter the normal mechanism of labor in an average size baby.

Cephalopelvic Disproportion

Definition

Presence of disparity between the diameters of fetal head and the dimensions of maternal pelvis is called *cephalopelvic disproportion*. It is considered *absolute* if the disparity between fetal head and pelvis exist when optimal fetal head diameter are present. *Relative* CPD is considered when an abnormal position of the fetal head results in the presentation of a head diameter too large to pass through pelvis.

Variation of Female Pelvis

Using X-ray studies Caldwell and Moloy classified the four major types of adult pelvis:

a. **Gynecoid**: It is considered the most typically 'female' pelvis and is most favorable for uncomplicated vaginal delivery, found in approximately 50% of all women. The pelvic inlet has an *oval* configuration, transverse diameter slightly larger than Anteroposterior diameter. Pelvic side walls are straight, the ischial spines are not prominent, the subpubic arch is wide, and sacrum is concave.

b. **Android or male:** In this inlet is wedge shaped with convergent side walls, the ischial spines are prominent, the subpubic arch is narrowed and sacrum is inclined anteriorly in its lower third. The android pelvis is associated *with persistent occiput posterior position and deep transverse arrest.*

c. **Anthropoid pelvis:** Inlet is oval with anteroposterior diameter slightly greater than transverse diameter. Pelvic side walls are divergent, sacrum is inclined posteriorly. This is most commonly associated with persistent occipitoposterior position.

d. **Platypelloid:** It is present in fewer than 3% of all women. The pelvis is characterized by transverse diameter that is wide with respect to the anteroposterior diameter. *Deep transverse arrest* pattern of labor are commonly associated with this pelvic type.

Comparison of the four types of pelvis is summarized in Table 51.1.

Causes of Contracted Pelvis

Beside variant of type of pelvis in women other feature can cause contracted pelvis in one or more diameter. These causes can be:

1. **Nutritional and environmental defects:** Minor variations are common. In major defects rachitic and osteomalacic pelvis can result. **Rachitic** flat pelvic is caused by rickets

Table 51.1: Features of various types of pelvis (Caldwell and Moloy—1933)

	Gynecoid	Android	Anthropoid	Platypelloid
Shape of brim	Well rounded	Triangle with base towards sacrum	Oval	Flat
Relation of hind pelvis and fore pelvis	Area of hind pelvis is only somewhat less than that of fore pelvis limiting use of posterior space by fetal head	Postsagittal segment or hind pelvis is shorter	Hind pelvis and fore pelvis are almost equal	Short anteroposterior and transverse diameter
Sidewall	No convergence or parallel	Convergent downwards		Divergent downwards
Ischial spines	Not prominent	Often prominent	No distinguished feature	Not prominent
Subpubic angle	Not ≥ 85°	Narrow		> than 90°
Subpubic arch	Normal	Narrow		Wide
Sacral angle	Exceeds 90°	> than 90°		> than 90°
Labor complication	Normal	• Persistent occipito Posteior position of head • Less tendency to injury to bladder neck	• Direct occipito-posterior or anterior • Face to pubes delivery	• At brim difficulty in engagement • Outlet dystocia • Asynclitism is usually present sometimes resulting in secondary face presentation • Tendency to bladder neck injury
Approximate incidence	50%	19%	27%	4%
Body build	Feminine	Thick and heavy built somewhat masculine	Tall, long headed, wide shouldered	Average height

- Intermediate form are more common that pure parent type
- Slight degree of contraction in any of nongynecoid group have more difficulty in labor than in more perfectly adapted female type.

which is a disease of early childhood when the bones remains soft and unossified. At this time if the child lies or sits in the bed, change occurs in the soft pelvis due to weight bearing. **Osteomalacic** pelvis is caused by softening of pubic bones due to calcium and vitamin D defficiency and lack of exposure to sunrays. In this shape inlet becomes triradiate and there is generalized contracted pelvis.

2. **Diseases and injuries:** Which affects the bones of the pelvis are fracture, tumor, and tubercular arthritis. *Spine*- kyphosis, scoliosis, spondylosthesis. Coccygeal deformity or *lower limb* like poliomyelitis, hip joint disease. The deformity can cause asymmetrical or obliquely contracted pelvis. Other asymmetrical pelvis of importance are:
   a. *Naegele's pelvis*: It is produced due to assisted development of one ala of the sacrum. It may be conjugated or acquired due to osteitis of sacroiliac joint.
   b. *Robert's pelvis (Transversely contracted pelvis):* In this ala of both sides are absent and the sacrum is fused with innominate bones.
   In both types cesarean section is required.

Diagnosis of Contracted Pelvis

Clinical History and Physical Examination

History of fracture, rickets, osteomalacia, tuberculosis of spine or pelvic joint, poliomyelitis is to be enquired. Height and weight of women is also important. A small woman of less than 5 feet is likely to have a small pelvis.

Clinical Pelvimetry

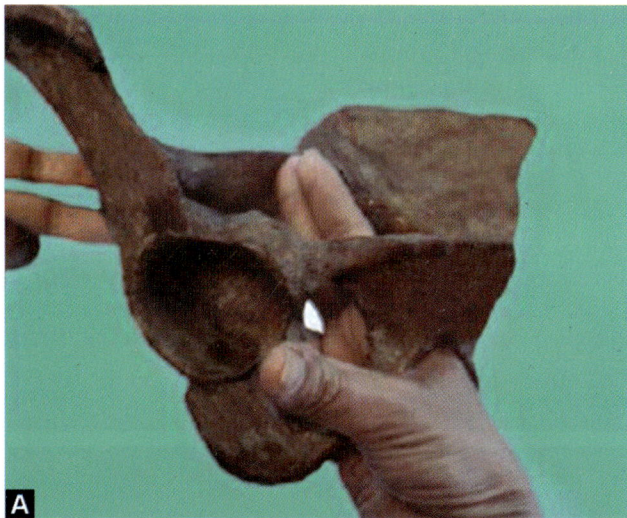

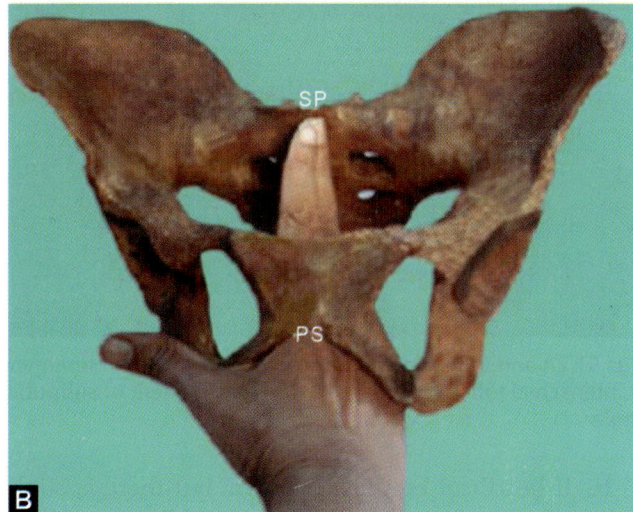

Figs 51.1A and B: Measurement of diagonal conjugate

It is most commonly done to estimate pelvic dimensions.
  i. **To assess the pelvic inlet:** The diagonal conjugate is obtained by measuring the distance from the lower edge of the symphysis pubis to the sacral promontory (Figs 51.1A and B). The obstetric conjugate is the distance from the most prominent portion of the symphysis pubis to the sacral promontory, which measures 1.5-2.0 cm less than the diagonal conjugate. *The obstetric conjugate should measure grater than 10 cm.*
 ii. The mid pelvis is evaluated clinically based on convergence of side wall, prominence of ischial spines and concavity of sacrum.
iii. The pelvic outlet is measured by measuring intertuberous diameters and palpating the subpubic arch. The intertuberous diameter greater than 8 cm and a wide subpubic arch characterize an adequate pelvis outlet (Figs 51.2A and B).
 iv. **Hill's Muller test**: For this during pelvic examination when the uterus contraction is at its peak, an attempt is made to push presenting part into the pelvis by pressing on the uterine fundus with the free hand. The hand in the vagina is used to determine whether or not there is downward mobility of the presenting part. If the presenting part moves easily into the pelvis the possibility of disproportion is low. If presenting part does not move or move very little, the possibility of CPD is high.
  v. **Abdominal method:** The patient is placed in dorsal position with thighs slightly flexed and separated. The head is grasped by left hand. Index and middle fingers of the right hand are placed above the symphysis pubis keeping the inner surface of the finger in the line with the anterior surface of the symphysis pubis to note the degree of overlapping if any, when head is pushed downwards and backwards:
    a. If head can be pushed down in the pelvis without overlapping of the parietal bone on the symphysis pubis—no disproportion.

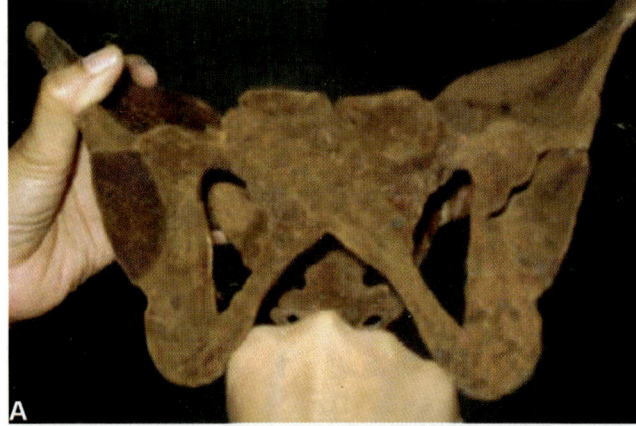

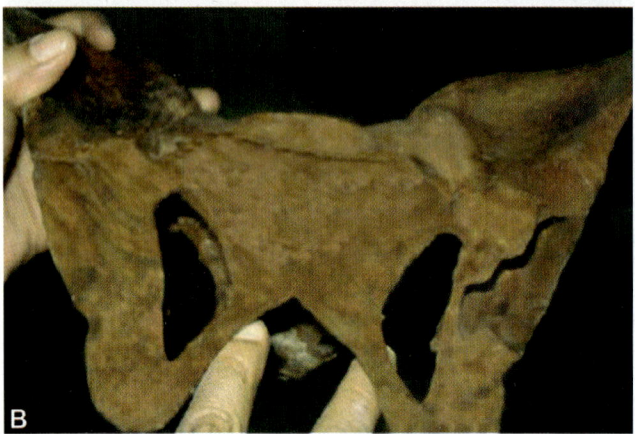

Figs 51.2A and B: Measurement of pelvic outlet: (A) Measurement of interischial tuberous diameter; (B) Measurement of subpubic angle

b. If head can be pushed down, but there is slight overlapping of parietal bone (0.5 cm or ¼") – moderate disproportion.
c. If head can not be pushed down and parietal bone overhangs the symphysis pubis – severe disproportion.

Abdominal method is a screening procedure and difficult to elicit when there is deflexed head, **thick abdominal wall, irritable uterus and high floating head.**

X-ray Pelvimetry

Now, its use has been very limited because evidence suggests that technique is not accurate with added risk of fetal exposure to radiation and may even increase cesarean section rate. Its role has been limited in evaluation of pelvis for the feasibility of *vaginal breech delivery* and in *assessment of gross body distortion*. If abnormal architecture is noted based on history and physical examination, imaging studies may be warranted. In this category traumatic pelvic fracture are most common abnormalities. Others are rachitic pelvis, chondrodystrophic dwarf pelvis, kyphotic and scoliotic pelvis, exostosis and bony neoplasm.

Computed Tomographic (CT) Scanning

Advantages of CT over conventional X-ray pelvimetry are less radiation exposure, greater accuracy and easier performance. But it is not useful for routine clinical purpose because of high cost and uncertain decision.

Magnetic Resonance Imaging (MRI)

The advantages of MRI pelvimetry includes lack of imaging radiation, accurate measurement, complete fetal imaging and potential for evaluating soft tissue dystocia. But still its use is markedly limited in clinical obstetrics because of exposure time involved for adequate imaging studies and equipment availability.

Course of Labor in Contracted Pelvis

a. Pelvic contraction may present as a *floating vertex* presentation with no descent during labor, as malpresentation or cord prolapse.
b. In *prolonged* labor complicated by contracted pelvis there can be considerable moulding of fetal head, caput succedaneum formation and prolonged rupture of membrane.
c. If allowed to continue in labor there can be thinning of lower uterine segment, development of Bandl's retraction ring. If still not attended there can be uterus rupture.
d. With severely prolonged 2nd stage, vesicovaginal or rectovaginal fistula may form due to pressure necrosis of the surrounding tissue of the birth canal by fetal head. Signs of cephalopelvic disproportion are summarized in Box 51.1.

Management of Labor in CPD

Due to contracted pelvis there is choice of following methods:

Box 51.1: Signs of cephalopelvic disproportion

Abdominal examination
- Large fetal size
- Fetal head overriding the pubic symphysis

Pelvic examination
- Cervix shrinking after amniotomy
- Edema of cervix
- Head not well applied against the cervix
- Head not engaged
- Caput formation
- Molding
- Deflexion
- Asynclitism

Others
- Maternal pushing before complete dilatation
- Early deceleration
    a. Negative Hills Muller test
    b. Reverse Hills Muller test

Elective Cesarean Section

i. This is the method of choice in all cases where degree of pelvic contraction is gross. Any pelvis with a true conjugate of less than 9 cm is severely contracted and a normal size baby cannot be expected to deliver and cesarean delivery should be done.
ii. In special cases like elderly primigravida even in borderline disproportion cesarean section should be done.
iii. All malpresentation associated with contracted pelvis should be taken for cesarean section.
iv. Any significant degree of outlet contraction should be treated by cesarean section.

Premature Induction of Labor

It is more a theoretical possibility because it is difficult to be certain of degree of disproportion and effective uterine action. The only cases where induction can be considered are when there is only borderline disproportion and a history of previous delivery is available.

Trial of Labor

Trial of labor is done with close monitoring and with full facilities for the safe performance of cesarean section. It is carried only up to limit when safety of mother as well fetus is not compromised. In conduct of trial of labor following are recommended approach:

a. The onset of labor should preferably spontaneous and not induced.
b. After rupture of membrane, per vaginal examination is performed to assess descent of presenting part and to exclude cord or compound presentation.
c. Intravenous hydration is maintained, prophylactic antibiotic should be given. Progress of labor should preferably be documented partographically.
d. Usually a trial of labor should not extend beyond 6-8 hours.
e. If head gradually descends and there is prolonged 2nd stage forceps or vacuum assistance can be required.
f. If there is delay in 1st stage of labor, sign of fetal or maternal distress and or one anticipate difficult instrumental delivery, cesarean section is resorted.

Contraindications to Trial of Labor

a. Elderly primigravida.
b. Malpresentation.
c. Outlet contraction.
d. Preeclampsia or hypertensive disease.
e. Cardiac or pulmonary disease.
f. True conjugate less than 9 cm.
g. Failed previous trial of labor.

Incoordinate Uterine Action

Hypertonic status of uterine contraction can result from:

a. Spastic lower segment
b. Constriction ring
c. Cervical dystocia
d. Generalized tonic contraction of uterus
e. Bandl's ring.

Spastic Lower Segment

In this fundal dominance of uterine contraction is lacking and there is reverse polarity. There is inadequate relaxation between contractions. Basal uterine pressure is raised above the critical level of 20 mm Hg.

Diagnosis: Patient complaints of severe pain referring to back. On **abdominal examination** uterus is tender and tense. Palpation of fetal part is difficult and fetal distress appears early. On **pelvic examination**, cervix is thick, edematous, hangs like a curtain. Membranes are absent. There can be caput succedaneum and meconium stained liquor.

Management: Dehydration is corrected by rapid infusion of Ringer's lactate. Cesarean section is done in majority of cases.

Constriction Ring

In this there is localized spastic contraction of a ring of circular muscle fibers of the uterus. Ring is usually situated at the junction of upper and lower segment around a constricted part of fetus usually around neck in cephalic presentation. It may appear in all stages of labor. Its presence can be associated with injudicious administration of oxytocin, PROM and premature attempt at instrumental delivery.

Diagnosis: It is difficult, ring is not felt per abdominally like retraction ring. It is revealed during cesarean section in first stage, during forceps application in 2nd stage and during manual removal in third stage. There is fetal distress due to hypertonic status.

Treatment: If found during cesarean section, sometimes the ring needs cutting to deliver the baby. In 2nd stage cesarean section is better option. Sometimes forceps delivery is possible with deepening of the plane of general anesthetic (Fig. 51.3).

Cervical Dystocia

Cervical dystocia, i.e. failure of cervical dilatation can be primary due to inefficient uterine contraction or malposition or secondary to excess scarring or rigidity of cervix from effect of previous operation or disease.

Cesarean section is usually preferred treatment.

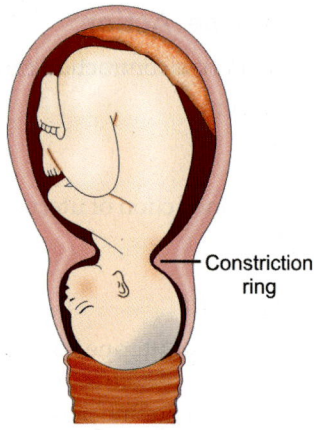

Fig. 51.3: Localized constriction ring at junction of upper and lower uterus segment

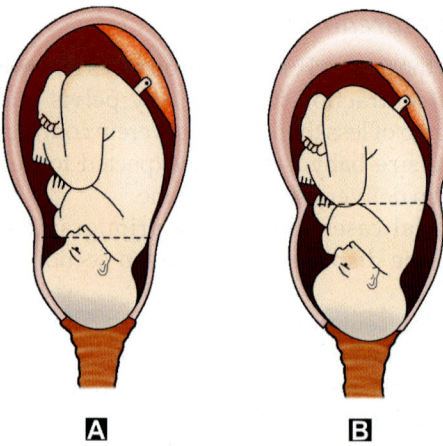

Figs 51.4A and B: Rising retraction ring as labor advances

Generalized Tonic Contraction (Uterine Tetany)

In this condition there is no physiological differentiation of the active upper segment and passive lower segment of the uterus. Causes are injudicious administration of oxytocin.

Diagnosis: Patient is in prolonged labor, uterus is small in size, tense and tender. Fetal parts and fetal heart sounds are not well-defined. On pelvic examination there is jammed head with caput and dry and edematous vagina.

Treatment: Correction of dehydration and ketoacidosis by intravenous fluid, antibiotic, analgesic. Oxytocics are stopped, tocolytic can be given. Cesarean delivery is usually preferred treatment.

Bandl's (Pathological Retraction) Ring

It is seen predominantly in obstructed labor. There is graduall increase in intensity, duration and frequency of uterine contraction and relaxation phase is less and less. The lower segment elongates and become progressively thinner to accommodate the fetus driven from the upper segment. Bandl's ring appears as circular groove encircling the uterus in between upper and lower uterine segment. It is palpable per abdominally.

In primigravida usually further retraction ceases in response to obstruction and there is nonprogress of labor with sign of maternal distress. In multigravida, there is continued retraction, progressive rise of Bandl's ring moving nearer and nearer to umbilicus and ultimately the lower segment rupture.

i. **Prevention:** It is preventable with watch on progress of labor and use of partogram.
ii. **Treatment:** Correction of dehydration with intravenous fluid, analgesic, antibiotic followed by cesarean delivery (Figs 51.4A and B).

MULTIPLE CHOICE QUESTIONS

1. All of the following are contraindications for trial of labor, *except*:
    a. Breech presentation
    b. Outlet contraction
    c. Primigravida
    d. Postcesarean pregnancy
    Ans. c
2. Critical obstetric conjugate for trial of labor is:
    a. 8.5 cm
    b. 9.0 cm
    c. 9.5 cm
    d. 10.0 cm
    Ans. d
3. Trial of labor is indicated in:
    a. Face presentation
    b. Breech presentation
    c. Mild CPD
    d. Severe CPD
    Ans. c
4. Trial of labor is contraindicated in:
    a. Elderly primigravida
    b. Minor disproportion
    c. Major disproportion
    d. Severe PET
    Ans. a, c, d
5. Bandl's ring is also called as:
    a. Constriction ring
    b. Schroeder's ring
    c. Retraction ring
    d. Cervical dystocia
    Ans. c
6. Labor is termed as precipitate if it occurs under:
    a. 1 hour
    b. 2 hours

Chapter - 51 ♦ Dystocia and Cephalopelvic Disproportion

    c. ½ hour
    d. 4 hours
    Ans. b
7. Cervical dystocia is usually present in:
    a. Level of external os
    b. Level of internal os
    c. Level of os
    d. Level of cervical canal
    Ans. a
8. Hypertonic dysfunctional labor is characterized by which of the following:
    a. Fetal distress occurs early
    b. Reaction to oxytocin is favorable
    c. Sedation is of little value
    d. Occurs in the active phase
    Ans. a, d
9. Construction ring in uterus is seen in:
    a. Obstructed labor
    b. Normal labor
    c. Both
    d. None
    Ans. d
10. All are true of constriction ring, *except*:
    a. Also called Schroeder's ring
    b. Can be caused by injudicious oxytocin use
    c. Ring can be palpated perabdomen
    d. Inhalation of amyl nitrate relaxes the ring
    Ans. c
11. All of following are feature of obstructed labor, *except*:
    a. Hot dry vagina
    b. Bandl's ring
    c. Unruptured membrane present
    d. Tonic contracted uterus
    Ans. c
12. One of the following features can be used to define contracted pelvis:
    a. Transverse diameter of inlet is 10 cm
    b. AP diameter of inlet is 12 cm
    c. Platypelloid pelvis
    d. Gynecoid pelvis
    Ans. a
13. Triradiate pelvis is seen in:
    a. Rickets
    b. Chondrodystrophy
    c. Osteoporosis
    d. Hyperparathyroidism
    Ans. a
14. Which type of pelvis is associated with increased incidence of face to pubes delivery?
    a. Gynecoid
    b. Anthropoid
    c. Android
    d. Platypelloid
    Ans. b
15. AP diameter is maximum in which type of pelvis:
    a. Platypelloid
    b. Android
    c. Anthropoid
    d. Gynecoid
    Ans. c
16. Dystocia dystrophia syndrome is found in:
    a. Android pelvis
    b. Platypelloid pelvis
    c. Anthropoid
    d. Gynecoid
    Ans. a
17. The following is true of Naegele's pelvis:
    a. Absence of one Ala
    b. Both Ala absent
    c. Kyphotic spine
    d. Triradiate pelvis
    Ans. a
18. The most common type of pelvis associated with direct occipito-posterior position is:
    a. Gynecoid
    b. Platypelloid
    c. Anthropoid
    d. Android
    Ans. c
19. True about anthropoid pelvis sacrosciatic notch is:
    a. Wide and shallow
    b. Wide and deep
    c. Narrow and shallow
    d. Narrow and deep
    Ans. a
20. The following is true of Robert's pelvis:
    a. Triradiate pelvis
    b. Single ala absent
    c. Both ala absent
    d. Wide pelvic brim
    Ans. c

52. Postpartum Hemorrhage

Adversity introduces a man to himself.

GENERAL CONSIDERATION

Traditionally postpartum hemorrhage has been defined as the loss of 500 ml or more of blood after vaginal delivery or 1000 ml or more after cesarean delivery. Usually the term is applied to pregnancies beyond 20 weeks of gestation.

Incidence

The incidence of primary postpartum hemorrhage is 5-8%. It is the most common cause of obstetric hemorrhage, leading cause of maternal mortality in developing countries and third leading cause of maternal mortality in developed world and most common cause of blood transfusion.

Physiology of Third Stage of Labor

1. *Systemic physiology:* The women with normal pregnancy induced hypervolemia usually increases her blood volume by 30-60% that amounts to 1-2 liter in average sized women. A woman can tolerate a physiological blood loss at time of delivery (usually 500 ml at vaginal delivery and 1000 ml at cesarean delivery) without any detrimental effect. These changes are compromised in complicated pregnancies as pre-eclampsia. Beside this the blood coagulation system is activated which reduces the risk of extensive blood loss during delivery. There is slight reduction of hemoglobin after delivery in first 3 days due to redistribution of extracellular fluid, after which it increases gradually and returns to normal by 6 weeks.
2. *Uterine changes in 3rd stage:*
   a. **Method of separation of placenta:** The reason for placenta separation is the mechanical effect of shearing because the bulk of the placenta cannot accommodate itself to the placental site, which is reduced to 10 cm or less after delivery of fetus. In normal cases there is not much resistance in the decidua at the plane of cleavage. As the placenta is separated, the blood from the implantation site may escape into the vagina immediately that is *Duncan's method.* In this whole of placenta is sheared off the uterine wall and presents with inferior margin. In *Schultz method of separation* the central portion of placenta is separated, so bleeding is concealed behind the placenta and placenta bulges into view presenting the center of fetal surface.
   b. **Physiological prevention of PPH:** Approximately 600 ml/minute of blood flows through the intervillous space. With separation of the placenta many uterine arteries and veins that carry blood to and from the placenta are severed abruptly. At the placental implantation site contraction and retraction of the myometrium to compress the vessels and obliterate their lumens are required to control hemorrhage. If the myometrium at and adjacent to the denuded implantation site contracts and retracts vigorously, excessive hemorrhage from the placental implantation site is unlikely even when the coagulation mechanism is severely impaired. Adherent piece of placenta or large blood clot will prevent effective myometrial contraction and retraction and thereby impair hemostasis at the implantation site.

Classification of Postpartum Hemorrhage

Conventional Temporal Classification

Based on timing of onset of hemorrhage in relation to time of delivery.

a. **Primary hemorrhage:** Hemorrhage within the first 24 hours of vaginal delivery is termed either early or primary postpartum hemorrhage.
b. **Secondary postpartum hemorrhage:** Bleeding occurring after 24 hours of delivery to within 12 weeks of delivery is termed late or secondary postpartum hemorrhage. It is common and affects 1-3% of all deliveries.

Classification Based on Quantification of Blood Loss

a. The International statistical classification of disease describes PPH as blood loss of 500 ml or more for vaginal delivery and 750 ml or more in association with cesarean delivery.
b. Change in hematocrit: ACOG defines of either a 10% change in hematocrit between the antenatal and postpartum period or a need for erythrocyte transfusion.
c. Rapidity of blood loss: Severe hemorrhage is classified as blood loss > 150 ml/minute, or sudden blood loss > 1500-2000 ml.
d. Benedetti's classification: It reflect the volume deficit (Table 52.1).

Table 52.1: Benedetti's classification of hemorrhage

Hemorrhage class	Acute blood loss	% loss
1	900 ml	15
2	1200– 500 ml	20-25
3	1800-2100 ml	30-35
4	2400 ml	40

ETIOLOGY OF POSTPARTUM HEMORRHAGE

Primary postpartum hemorrhage is traditionally considered as a disorder of one or more of the four processes:
a. Uterine atony: **Tonus**
b. Retained clots or placental debris: **Tissue**
c. Genital trauma: **Trauma**
d. Disorders of coagulation: **Thrombin**

Uterine Atony

Uterine atony alone accounts for 50% of cases of postpartum hemorrhage. Predisposing causes are: (a) Uterine over distention, (b) Operative delivery or intrauterine manipulation of uterus, (c) Rapid or prolonged labor, (d) Grand multiparity, (e) General anesthetic especially halogenated anesthetic, (f) Uterine fibroids, (g) Uterine infection, (h) Oxytocin to induce labor (i) History of previous hemorrhage in the 3rd stage.

Genital Trauma

Excessive bleeding from an episiotomy, laceration or both causes approximately 20% of postpartum hemorrhage. There can be vulvar, vaginal, cervical or uterine laceration. They usually result from precipitous or uncontrolled delivery or operative delivery of large infant but can occur after any delivery. Laceration of blood vessels underneath the vaginal and vulvar epithelium results in hematomas. The bleeding is concealed and can be particularly dangerous, because it may go unrecognized and presents only as hemorrhagic shock. **Persistent fresh bright red color bleeding with well contracted firm uterus suggests genital tract laceration.**

Retained Placental Tissue or Blood Clot

Retained placental tissues and membrane are the causes in 5-10% of postpartum hemorrhage. It can occur in placenta accreta, in manual removal of the placenta, mismanagement of 3rd stage of labor and unrecognized succenturiate lobe.

Coagulation Defects

Coagulopathy in pregnancy may be acquired in several obstetric disorders as in abruptio placenta, excess thromboplastin from a retained dead fetus, amniotic fluid embolism, severe pre-eclampsia and sepsis. These coagulatopathies may present as hypofibrinogenemia, thrombocytopenia, and disseminated intravascular coagulation. Transfusion of more than 8 unit of blood in itself may induce a dilutional coagulopathy. There can be primary problem like von Willebrand's disease, women on anticoagulant therapy.

MANAGEMENT OF POSTPARTUM HEMORRHAGE

Prophylaxis for Postpartum Hemorrhage

a. High risk cases should be identified and they should be delivered in institutions which have facility and skill to manage obstetric hemorrhage.
b. Good antenatal care and anemia prevention is an important measure to ensure the patients against possible ill effect of hemorrhage.
c. All obstetric patients should have blood hemoglobin and group types and screened on admission. In high risk cases on admission blood typed and crossmatching should be done.
d. A large bore intravenous catheter should be usually taped.
e. Delivery room personal should be alerted to the risk of hemorrhage.

Proper management of 2nd stage of labor: It is important in prevention of postpartum hemorrhage. It is important to deliver the baby's trunk slowly in to allow a little time for uterine retraction to follow the egress of the baby's body.

Active management of 3rd stage of labor: It is defined in the recent IFM/FIGO joint statement as the: (a) Administration of uterotonic agent, (b) Controlled cord traction, (c) Uterine massage. **Active management of 3rd stage of labor should be offered to all women because the risk factor usually cannot predict PPH.** This reduces the incidence of postpartum hemorrhage and quantity of blood loss.

Management in Postpartum Hemorrhage

Treatment of placental site hemorrhage before delivery of placenta:

The placenta typically separates from the uterus and is delivered within 5-15 minutes of delivery of the infant. **Spontaneous placental separation is impending if uterus is round and firm, uterus seems to rise in the abdomen, a sudden gush of blood comes from the vagina and there is true lengthening of umbilical cord**. There is no need to speed separation of placenta. If there are signs of placental separation, *Brandt-Andrews* method of controlled *cord traction can be done*. It is gentle steady downward traction on the cord which is combined with upward pressure on the lower uterine segment and placenta is delivered. Adherent membrane can be removed by gentle traction with ring forceps. The placenta is inspected for completeness immediately after delivery.

Manual Removal of the Placenta

a. *Timing:* In the presence of hemorrhage, manual removal of placenta should be considered without delay. In the absence of bleeding, manual removal of placenta is advocated 30 minutes after delivery of the placenta.

b. *Technique:*
   a. Adequate anesthetic or full fledged anesthetic is needed.
   b. Aseptic surgical technique is followed
   c. Bladder is evacuated by catheterization.
   d. The uterus is stabilized by grasping fundus with a hand placed on the abdomen; the other hand is introduced in the vagina and passed into the uterus along the umbilical cord. As soon as the placenta is reached, its margin is located and ulnar border of hand is insinuated between it and uterine wall. Then with back of hand in contact with the uterus, the placenta is peeled off its uterine attachment by a motion, similar to that used in separating the leaves of book. After its complete separation the placenta is grasped with the entire hand, which is than gradually withdrawn (Figs 52.1A to F).
   e. The fetal and maternal side of the placenta is inspected to ensure its completeness. If there is evidence of incomplete removal, the uterus must be re-explored and any small adherent piece of placenta is removed.
   f. The methergine or prostaglandin can be given at end of separation of placenta. After delivery of placenta uterus is massaged until a firm myometrial tone is achieved.
   g. Prophylactic antibiotic should be given.

Management of PPH After Delivery of Placenta

After delivery of placenta, the fundus should be palpated to make certain that uterus is well contracted. Routine use of oxytocin 10-20 U/liter in isotonic saline by slow intravenous injection reduces the blood loss at delivery and decreases the chance of postpartum hemorrhage. Ergot alkaloids

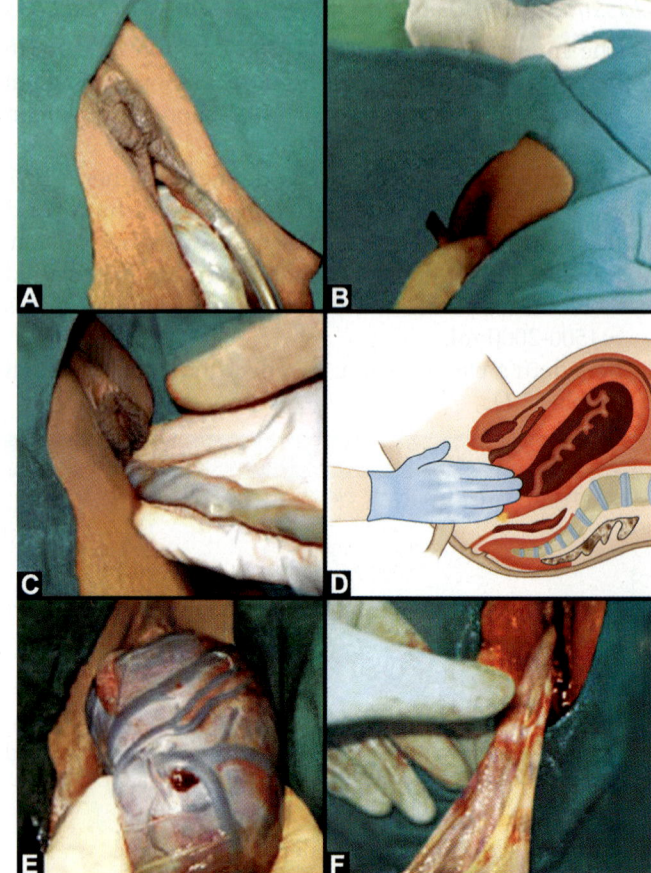

Figs 52.1A to F: Steps of manual removal of placenta: (A) Preliminary catheterization; (B) Grasping the fundus of uterus through abdominal wall; (C) Other hand introduced into vagina to uterus along the umbilical cord; (D) Placenta is peeled off its uterine attachment; (E) Placenta is gradually withdrawn; (F) Membranes are removed carefully

(Methyl ergotamine maleate 0.2 mg IM) can also be routinely used except in women with hypertension or cardiac disease.
Prostaglandin: The 15 methyl derivative of prostaglandin F2 α may be used for treatment of uterus atony. The recommended dose is 250 µg (0.25 mg) given intramuscular and can be repeated if necessary at 15-90 minutes interval up to maximum of 8 doses. Side effects of prostaglandin are airways and vascular contraction, diarrhea, hypertension, vomiting, fever, flushing and tachycardia.
Misoprostol: A prostaglandin E1 analog misoprostol in dose of 400 – 800 µg is rapidly absorbed orally or rectally and can effectively prevent and treat uterine atony. The side effects are shivering and fever. It is not associated with bronchospasm and safe for asthmatic patients. Its use is not routinely recommended but *is useful as it does not require refrigeration, storage is easy especially in tropical countries and it does not require I/v line.*
Genital tract laceration: If the bleeding prevents despite a firm, well contracted uterus, the cause of the hemorrhage is most likely from laceration. To ascertain the role of laceration

as a cause of bleeding, **careful inspection of the vagina, cervix and uterus is essential.** Good lighting, good assistant and anesthetic help in thorough exploration of genital tract. Examination of the uterine cavity, the cervix, and the entire vagina is essential after obstetric maneuver like breech extraction, internal cephalic version, or vaginal delivery after cesarean section. Beside this PPH can be caused by both atony and trauma, so inspection of cervix and vagina should be performed in every case of postpartum hemorrhage (Fig. 52.2).

Repair of Laceration

Episiotomy or perineal tear is quickly repaired after confirmation of uterine contraction. A pack is placed in the vagina above tear, which keeps the field dry, attaching the free end of the pack to the adjacent drapes, so operator is reminded to remove it after completion of repair. **It is important that tear should be repaired above the highest extent of the laceration because bleeding vessels tends to retract.** The highest suture is also used to provide gentle traction so that laceration can be visualized properly. Hemostatic ligatures are placed appropriately. *Deep cervical tear* should always be inspected in case of profuse hemorrhage. The extent of injury is inspected only after adequate exposure by use of one or two right angle vaginal retractor by assistant, while the operator grasps the cervix with a pair of ring forceps. In the repair, the first suture is applied just above the angle. Suturing is done towards the operator. Repair is done by absorbable suture by continuous interlocking or interrupted suture (Figs 52.3A to C).*

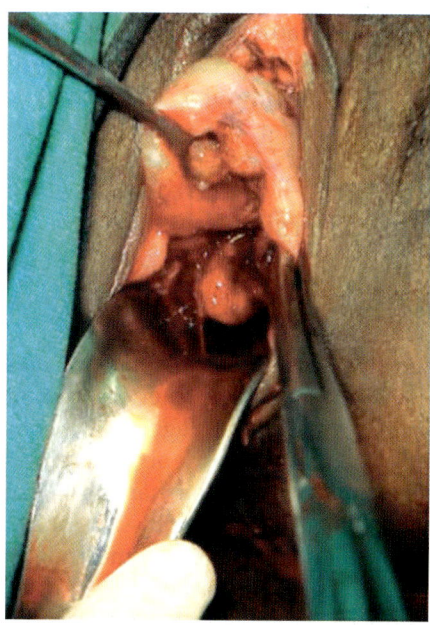

Fig. 52.2: Inspection of cervix, vagina and vault under good illumination to confirm cause of PPH

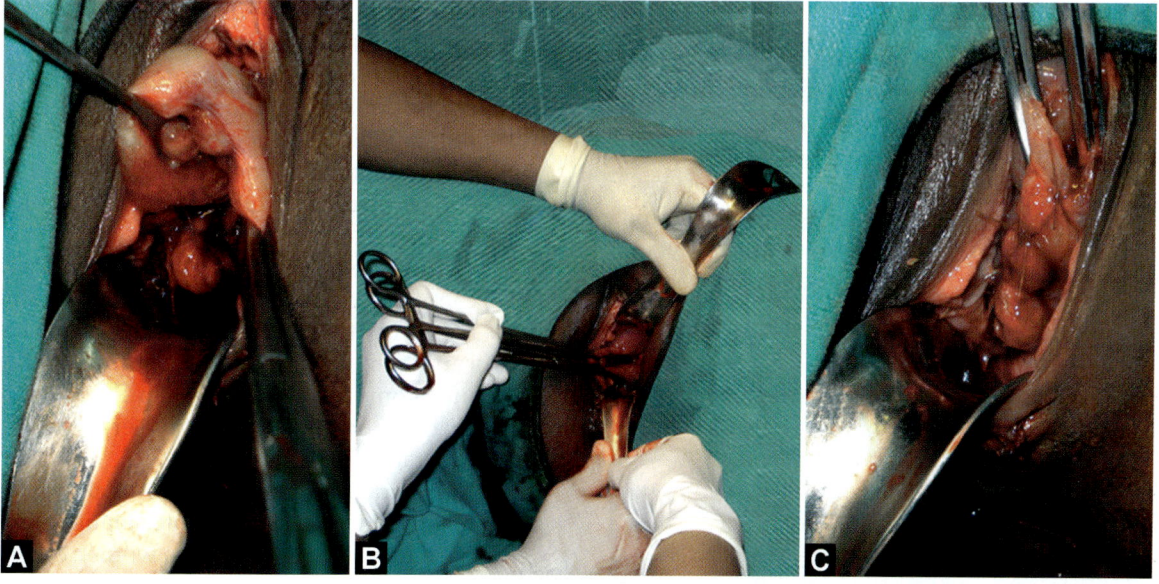

Figs 52.3A to C: Repair of cervical tear: (A) Visualization of cervical tear; (B) Holding of cervical lip with sponge forceps; (C) Stitching of cervical tear

---

* If the apex of tear is difficult to visualize, suturing can be started at its proximal end using the suture for traction to expose the most distal position of the cervix until the apex is in view.

Large or expanding hematoma of vaginal wall requires operative management. Smaller vulvar **hematoma** can be left as such, but if it is enlarging or painful, hematoma is incised at the point of maximum distention. Blood is evacuated and bleeding points are ligated. The cavity may be obliterated with mattress suture or cavity is packed for 12-14 hours. With hematomas of the genital tract, blood loss is nearly always considerable more than the clinical estimate. Hypovolemia and severe anemia should be prevented by adequate blood replacement (Figs 52.4A and B).

Evaluation of Persistent Bleeding

If vaginal bleeding persists despite above measures, aggressive treatment should be initiated. The following steps should be undertaken without delay:

1. *Bimanual compression of uterus and massage:* The clenched fist is placed in the anterior fornix and the body of the uterus is compressed against it by a hand placed behind the uterus through the abdominal wall. Massage of the uterus is done with both hands while maintaining compression. Prolonged compression for 20-30 minutes may be required but in atonic hemorrhage it is always successful in controlling bleeding.
2. *Foley's catheter* is inserted before bimanual compression for: (a) To watch urine output, (b) Vigorous fluid and blood replacement cause diuresis, (c) Distended bladder will interfere with compression and massage, (d) Distended bladder may itself cause uterine atony.
3. **Obtain help of full team senior obstetrician, nurse and anesthetic**.
4. **Manual exploration of the uterus:** Manual exploration of uterus after delivery of the placenta should be considered in following circumstances:
   a. Vaginal delivery after previous cesarean section to rule out possibility of scar dehiscence.
   b. When obstetric maneuver has been performed like internal podalic version or breech extraction.
   c. If malpresentation has occurred during labor or delivery.
   d. After delivery of a premature infant.
   e. If there has been abnormal contour of uterus before or after delivery.

   In exploration hand with double glove is introduced into shape of cone through the cervix while other hand stabilizes the fundus of uterus. All exploration should be gentle because the postpartum uterus is soft and easily perforated. Placental piece or membrane if found is removed. Uterine rupture detected by manual exploration, require immediate laparotomy.

   f. **Curettage:** Curettage of a large soft, postpartum uterus can be dangerous because the risk of perforation is high and the procedure commonly results in increased rather than decreased bleeding. So curettage should be delayed, unless bleeding can not be controlled by compression and massage alone. A large blunt curette – Banzo curette, probably is the safest instrument for curettage of postpartum uterus. Later on it can result in formation of adhesion and Asherman's syndrome (amenorrhea and secondary infertility). It is better to perform ultrasound evaluation to distinguish those patients who will benefit from curettage from those who should be managed without it.
   g. **Uterine tamponade:** Although uterine packing was advocated for treating PPH, it fell out of use because of possibility of concealed hemorrhage and uterine over distention. In recent years several modification of uterine tamponade has been found effective. Balloon tamponade using either a Foley's catheter or Sengstaken-Blakemore tube has been used with efficacy. Both have open tops, which permit the continuous drainage from the uterus. Condom catheter can also be prepared in low resource setting where catheter is connected to IV fluid at one end and condom at other. The hydrostatic pressure acts as tamponade.
   h. **Other measures:** Insert second intravenous camulae for administration of blood or fluid, obtain blood for typing and crossmatching, begin fluid replacement with crystalloid and blood, use uterotonic agent by oxytocin IV infusion in 10-20 U/lit in crystalloid, methyl ergonovine, and/or prostaglandin injection.
   i. **Radiographic embolization of pelvic vessels:** In institution with trained interventional radiologist, the technique can be used in women of low parity as an alternative to hysterectomy. Under local anesthetic, a catheter is placed in the aorta and fluoroscopy is used to identify the bleeding vessels. Pieces of absorbable gelatin sponge (gelfoam) are injected into the damaged vessels or into the internal iliac vessels. **Complications of this procedure are— local hematoma formation, infection, ischemic**

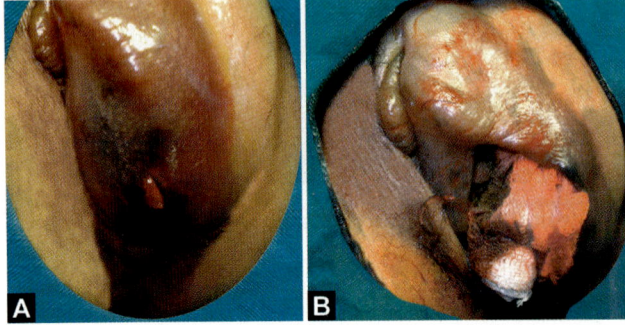

Figs 52.4A and B: (A) Vulvar hematoma; (B) Hematoma drained and packed

phenomena including uterine necrosis and contrast related adverse effects.

j. **Operative management:** When mechanical and medical measures fails to control postpartum hemorrhage, surgical intervention is required. This should be undertaken sooner than later before the patient is too sick to undergo any surgical procedure. These measures can be: (a) Presume occlusion of the aorta, (b) Stepwise uterine devascularization, (c) Undersuturing the placental bed, (d) Compressive suture, (e) Internal iliac ligation, (f) Hysterectomy.
   – **Presume occlusion of the aorta:** Immediate temporary control of bleeding can be obtained at laparotomy by pressure occlusion of the aorta, which will provide valuable time to treat hypotension and arrangement for other procedure.
   – **Selective uterine devascularization:** The principle behind it is that the vascularity to the uterus may be reduced in a stepwise maneuver tying the feeding vessels one by one till the bleeding is stopped. The five steps are as follows:
      i. Unilateral uterine vessel ligation
      ii. Bilateral uterine vessel ligation
      iii. Low uterine vessels ligation
      iv. Unilateral ovarian vessel ligation
      v. Bilateral ovarian vessels ligation.

Technique: The uterus is lifted upward and away from the side to be ligated. Absorbable suture on a large needle is placed avoiding the ascending uterine artery and vein on the one side of the uterus, passing through the myometrium 2-4 cm medial to the vessels and through the avascular area of broad ligament. The suture includes the myometrium to fix the suture and to avoid tearing the vessels. The procedure is repeated on opposite side. Bilateral uteroovarian ligation is performed with absorbable suture near the point of anastomosis between the ovarian arteries and the ascending uterine artery at uteroovarian ligament.

Ligation of anterior branch of internal iliac artery: This procedure requires expert surgical skill and clear knowledge of retroperitoneal anatomy. It is recommended in hemodynamically stable patient, so that there is time to proceed to another procedure if it fails.

Technique: The peritoneum lateral to the infundibulopelvic ligament is incised parallel with ligament. The ureter is retracted medially. The common iliac artery bifurcates into the external and internal iliac arteries at the level of pelvic brim with ureter crossing the bifurcation. The internal iliac artery is dissected until the posterior branch is identified. Distal to this point anterior division of internal iliac artery is ligated with ligature of 1-0 vicryl suture using a right angled clamp (Fig. 52.5). Pulsation of the external iliac artery must be checked to confirm that blood supply to this vessel has not been compromised.

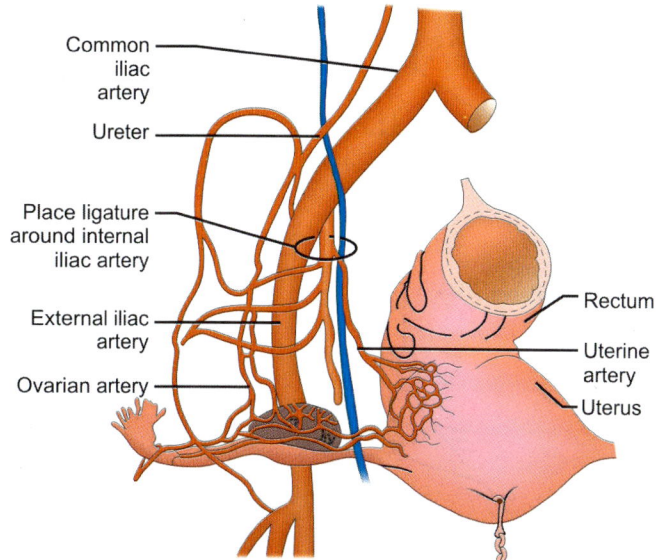

Fig. 52.5: Site of ligation of anterior division of internal iliac artery

Under Suturing the Placental Bed

Bleeding from the lower uterine segment, particularly in case of placenta previa may occur from large sinus and may not be controlled by uterine contraction. These are needed to be under sutured with sutures in the placental bed. If lower segment is thin, full thickness sutures into the myometrium can be taken; with care that cervical canal is not obliterated.

Compression Suture

a. **B lynch suture technique** involves a pair of vertical brace suture around the uterus to oppose the anterior and posterior wall of the uterus. *It can be tried if uterus compression effectively controls bleeding.* In this vertical brace suture using no. 2 catgut is applied (Figs 52.6A and B).
b. **Hayman and Cho suture** are modified compression suture, in which hysterotomy is not required.

Hysterectomy

If all effort fails, hysterectomy is needed. The decision for hysterectomy should not be delayed to the point that DIC sets it. In obstetric emergencies a subtotal hysterectomy is usually performed, which is quick and adequate to control hemorrhage. Total hysterectomy may be required in case of placenta previa and laceration extending into the lower uterine segment.

BLOOD TRANSFUSION AND FLUID REPLACEMENT

Blood and fluid replacement are required for successful management of postpartum hemorrhage. **Crystalloid**

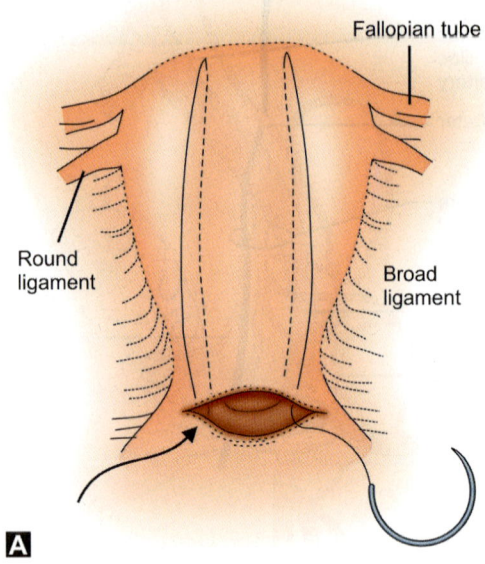

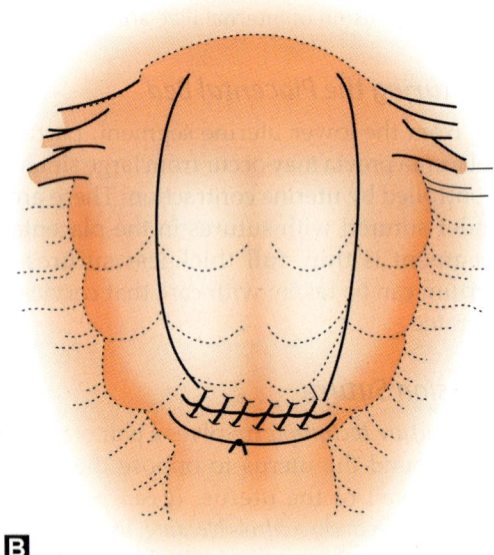

Figs 52.6A and B: (A) B-Lynch brace suture; (B) Compressed uterus after B-lynch suture—Anterior view

solution is preferred for fluid replacement either normal saline (N/S) or ringer lactate solution. Dextran containing solution has no role in the management of PPH. Loss of 1 liter blood requires replacement with 4-5 liter of crystalloid because most of the infused fluid is not retained in the intravascular space but shifts to interstitial space. Massive transfusion may be necessary in patients with severe hemorrhage. Component therapy is advocated with transfusion of packed cells, platelets, fresh frozen plasma and cryoprecipitate as indicated. *If there are abnormal coagulation findings with ongoing bleeding or oozing from puncture sites, fresh frozen plasma is given.* Cryoprecipitate may be useful with FFP, if there are markedly depressed fibrinogen levels. Blood products should be given without delay when required, because postponing transfusion may only contribute to development of DIC.

SECONDARY POSTPARTUM HEMORRHAGE

When bleeding occurs after an interval of 24 hours or more following delivery, it is called secondary postpartum hemorrhage.

Clinical Presentation

Uterine hemorrhage may occur within first-two weeks after the delivery. Occasionaly this bleeding may be severe and life-threatening.

Etiology: It is almost always due to subinvolution of the placenta bed or retained placental fragments. Involution of the placental site is normally delayed when compared with rest of the endometrium. In subinvoluted uterus for unknown reasons the adjacent endometrium and the decidua basalis is not regenerated to cover the placental implantation site. The thrombosis and hyalinization which occurs in normal involution, fails to occur in subinvoluted uterus, so bleeding may occur with only minimal trauma or other stimuli. Causes of subinvolution can be: (a) Idiopathic, (b) Faulty placental implantation, (c) Implantation in poorly vascularized lower uterine segment, (d) Persistent infection at placental site.

Management

a. In situation of active bleeding uterine compression and bimanual massage controls bleeding.
b. Ultrasound examination is done to look for retained placental product. If USG shows intracavitary tissue curettage is warranted.
c. Broad spectrum antibiotic should be started. The material removed is to be sent for histological examination.
d. Oxytocin 10-20 Iu/lit intravenous solution, 15 methyl PcF2 α every 2 hours or ergot alkaloids-Methyl-ergonovine maleate 0.2 mg orally every 6 hours should be administered for at least 48 hours.
e. Presence of bleeding from the sloughing wound of cervicovaginal canal should be controlled by hemostatic sutures.
f. Secondary hemorrhage following cesarean section may at times require laparotomy. The bleeding from uterine wound can be controlled by hemostatic suture, may rarely require ligation of the internal iliac artery or may end in hysterectomy.

RETAINED PLACENTA

The retained placenta is said to be retained when it is not expelled out even 30 minutes after birth of the baby.

Etiology: There are three phases *involved in normal expulsion* of the placenta: (a) Separation through the spongy layer of

the decidua, (b) Descent into the lower segment and vagina, (c) Finally its expulsion to outside. Interference in any of these physiologic process results in retention:
a. Placenta completely separated but retained due to lack of voluntary expulsion force.
b. Simple adherent placenta due to atonic uterus.
c. Morbid adherent placenta.
d. Placenta incarcerated due to constriction ring (hour glass contraction), premature attempt to deliver the placenta before separation.

Diagnosis

It is made by selecting and setting time limit of 30-40 minutes following delivery of the baby.
Complications of retained placenta:
a. Hemorrhage
b. Shock
c. Puerperal sepsis
d. Recurrence in next pregnancy.

Management

During the period of arbitrary time limit of half an hour the patient is to be watched carefully for incidence of any bleeding. Oxytocin in crystalloid solution is to be continually administered. When the placenta is not expelled, manual removal of placenta is done under anesthetic (as described).

PLACENTA ACCRETA (ADHERENT PLACENTA)

There is physiological line of cleavage between the placental villi and myometrium through the decidual spongy layer. When placenta is directly adhered to the myometrium without an intervening decidual layer, it is termed placenta accreta.

Classification

By Degree of Adherence

a. Placenta accreta Vera: Villi adhere to the superficial myometrium.
b. Placenta increta: Villi invade the myometrium.
c. Placenta percreta: Villi penetrate the full thickness of the myometrium.

By Amount of Placental Involvement

a. Focal adherence: A single cotyledon is involved.
b. Partial adherence: One or more cotyledons are involved.
c. Total adherence: The entire placenta is involved.

Incidence

It varies from 1 in 2000 to 1 in 7000 delivery. Placenta accreta vera accounts for approximately 80% of abnormally adherent placenta, placenta increta accounts for 15% and placenta percreta for 5%. The incidence has risen slightly due to increased cesarean rate.

Etiopathogenesis

Histological examination shows absence of decidua and Nitabuch's layer at site of placental implantation. Excessive permeability of the trophoblast and defecting and missing decidua basalis can cause placenta accreta. The clinical situations associated with placenta accreta are previous cesarean section, placenta previa, grand multiparity, previous uterine curettage and previously treated Asherman's syndrome.

Diagnosis

a. **Ultrasound** examination shows lack of hypoechoic area normally seen beneath the placental implantation site which can give clue to diagnosis of adherent placenta prior to delivery.
b. **MRI** has also aided in diagnosis.
c. **Presentation:** Delayed spontaneous separation of the placenta or profuse hemorrhage when delivery of the placenta is attempted. Focal or partial involvement may be manifested as difficulty in establishing a cleavage plane during manual removal of the placenta. Persistent effort to manually remove a totally adherent placenta are futile and they result in even more blood loss, so preparation for hysterectomy should begin as soon as the diagnosis is suspected.

Management

1. Fluid and blood replacement should begin as soon as excessive blood loss is diagnosed.
2. In 72% of cases Prompt hysterectomy has to be done.
3. Alternative measures are as follows:
    i. Uterine or internal iliac artery ligation.
    ii. Angiographic embolization.
    iii. Sometimes successful conservative approach that placenta is left to remain *in situ* in the hope that it will gradually disappear by lysis can be an option. It should be considered only when focal defects are present, blood loss is not excessive and patient wishes to preserve fertility.*
4. In placenta percreta sometimes additional resection of adjacent organs as partial cystectomy may be necessary.

---

* When fertility is desired a variety of uterus conserving technique can be considered. These techniques include delayed manual removal of placenta, packing of lower uterine segment, curettage, oversewing of the placental implantation site, uterine artery embolization and use of methotrexate.

Transfusion of blood and other Components in Obstetrical Hemorrhage

a. *Red blood cell transfusion:* The fresh whole blood replaces both blood volume and fibrinogen.
b. *Fresh frozen plasma:* It has volume of 250 ml and 30 minutes thawing is needed before use. It contains colloid and 600-700 mg fibrinogen, but no platelets. It restores circulating volume and fibrinogen.
c. *Packed RBC:* It has 250 ml volume and addition solution. It contains only RBC with no fibrinogen and platelets. It is ideal in severely anemic, cardiac patient when fluid overload is not required.
d. *Cryoprecipitate:* It is frozen 15 ml, contains 200 mg fibrinogen with other clotting factors but no platelets. About 3000-4000 mg total is needed to restore maternal fibrinogen to >150 mg/dl.
e. *Platelet concentrate:* Platelet concentrate has volume of 50 ml, stored at room temperature, one unit releases platelet count of 50,000 µl. Usually 6-10 unit are transfused when needed.

UTERINE INVERSION

Definition: Uterine inversion is prolapse of the fundus of uterus to or through the cervix so that the uterus is in effect turned inside out.
Incidence: It is a rare event, complicating approximately 1 in 2500 deliveries.
Etiology: There is no agreement on the etiology of this condition. Though following factors are associated with its occurrence:
1. Mismanagement of 3rd stage of labor either by inappropriate traction during controlled cord traction or too rapid removal of placenta during manual removal.
2. Maternal age more than 25 years.
3. A sudden rise in intra-abdominal pressure in the presence of relaxed uterus.
4. A fundally placed placenta with short umbilical cord.
5. Uterine inversion is more common in women with collagen disorders.

Degree of Uterine Inversion

First degree: The fundus inverts in body of uterus but does not herniate through internal os.
Second degree: The fundus passes through the cervix and lies within the vagina.
Third degree: In this entire uterus is turned inside out and hangs outside of vulva taking vagina with it. It is least common (Fig. 52.7).

Diagnosis

Uterine inversion should be suspected when there is sudden postpartum hemorrhage in association with absent palpable fundus

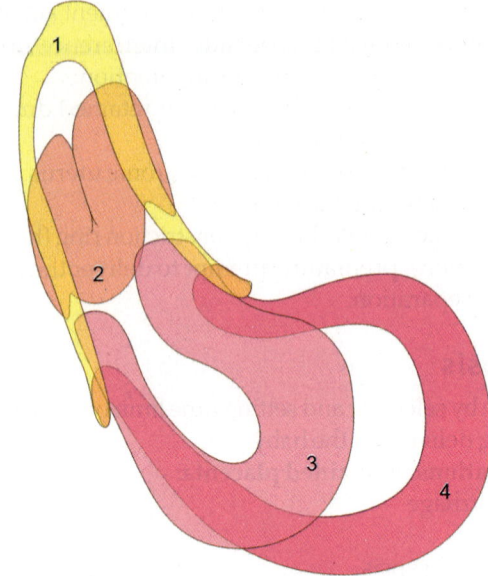

Fig. 52.7: Degree of uterine inversion

of uterus abdominally and unstable hemodynamic condition of mother. It may occur before or after placental detachment.

The diagnosis is made clinically with bimanual examination in which fundus of uterus is palpated in lower uterine segment or vagina. Bed side sonography can be used to confirm the diagnosis, if clinical examination is unclear.

Risk of Inversion

The *immediate* risks are due to postpartum hemorrhage and shock due to hypovolemia. The *late* risks are puerperal sepsis. Anuria and Sheehan's syndrome can be caused due to severe shock.

Management

a. *Manual repositioning of uterus:* Once diagnosed, uterine inversion require rapid intervention to restore maternal hemodynamic stability and to control hemorrhage. Maternal fluid resuscitation through large bore intravenous cannula is recommended with quick replacement of uterus to its proper position.
This is best done in operation theater with the assistance of anesthesiologist. The uterus and cervix should initially be relaxed with tocolytic agent ($MGSO_4$, β mimetic, Nitroglycerine). Once relaxed, gentle manual pressure is applied to uterine fundus in order to return to its proper abdominal location (Figs 52.8A to C).
Antibiotic should be started at earliest. After replacement, uterotonic therapy like oxytocin drip, prostaglandin should be started to assist with uterine contraction and prevent recurrence of inversion for 24 hours. In postoperative care hematocrit level should be assessed for need of blood replacement and iron therapy.

Chapter -52 ♦ Postpartum Hemorrhage

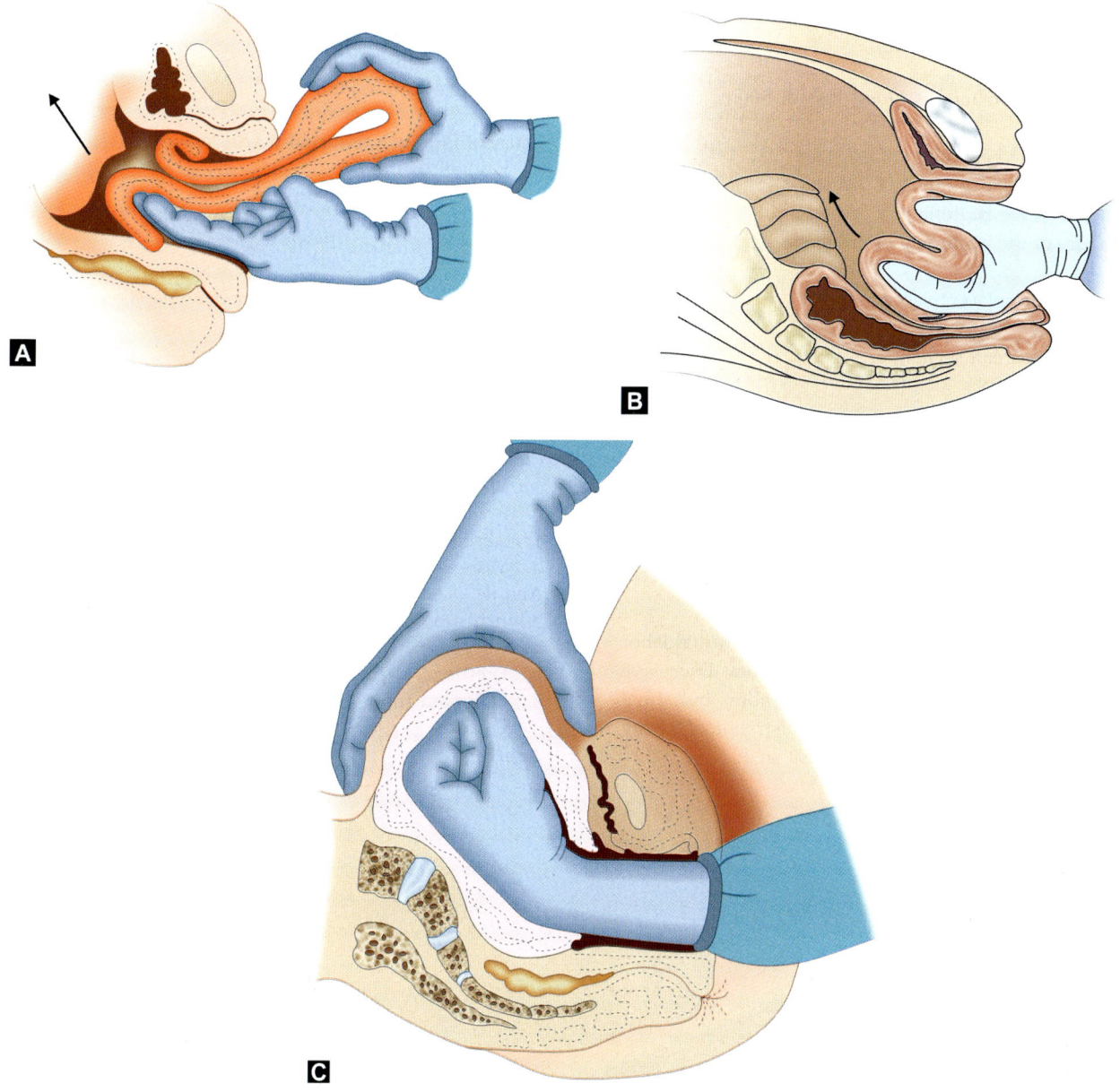

Figs 52.8A to C: Replacement of inverted uterus

b. *Hydrostatic pressure:* If manual repositioning is unsuccessful, hydrostatic pressure can be applied. In this a silicon cup is placed into vagina and warmed saline is infused in order to create increased intravaginal pressure which results in correction of inversion.

c. *Surgical repositioning of uterus:* It is nowadays rarely required. It can be lifesaving. It is done by giving a vertical incision through the lower uterine segment (Haultain's method) the uterus is repositied by either pulling from above or very rarely pushing from below. The incision is repaired like any uterine incision. Blood replacement antibiotic and careful monitoring is mandatory.

MULTIPLE CHOICE QUESTIONS

1. The following components during pregnancy increases the risk of PPH *except*:
   a. Hypertension
   b. Macrosomia
   c. Twin pregnancy
   d. Hydramnios
   Ans. a

2. All of the following drugs are used for the management of PPH *except*:
   a. Misoprostol
   b. Oxytocin

c. Prostaglandin
d. RU 486

Ans. d

3. Postpartum hemorrhage is blood loss of 500 cc or more within:
   a. 6 hours of the beginning of 3rd stage
   b. 12 hours of the beginning of 3rd stage
   c. 12 hours of the beginning of 3rd stage
   d. 24 hours of the beginning of 3rd stage

   Ans. d

4. All predispose to placenta accreta *except*:
   a. Multiparity
   b. Previous cesarean section
   c. Placenta previa
   d. Previous D & C

   Ans. a

5. During PPH internal iliac ligation is done at:
   a. Origin of internal iliac artery
   b. Anterior division of internal iliac artery
   c. Posterior division of internal iliac artery
   d. Common iliac artery

   Ans. b

6. A 30-year-old P6 delivers vaginally following normal labor with spontaneous delivery of intact placenta. Excessive bleeding continues despite manual exploration, bimanual massage, intravenous oxytocin and administration of 0.2 mg methergine I/v which should be the next step:
   a. Packing the uterus
   b. Immediate hysterectomy
   c. Bilateral internal iliac ligation
   d. I/m injection of $PGE_2\alpha$

   Ans. d

7. Cause of PPH in a retracted uterus is:
   a. Vaginal tear
   b. Cervical laceration
   c. Retained placenta
   d. Atony of uterus

   Ans. a,b

8. Attempts to express the placenta before separation may lead to
   a. Trapping of placenta
   b. Incomplete separation of placenta
   c. Inversion of uterus
   d. All of the above

   Ans. d

9. Which is not true of placenta accreta:
   a. May penetrate serosa
   b. Invades myometrium
   c. Absence of Nitabuch's layer
   d. More common in primigravida

   Ans. d

10. B-lynch suture is applied on:
    a. Cervix
    b. Uterus
    c. Fallopian tube
    d. Ovaries

    Ans. b

53 Operative Obstetrics

*Truth is not something that can be glanced from book,
it can be learned and known by practice.*

INTRODUCTION

Operative obstetric is unique and peculiar as this combines the fine judging and decision-making of obstetric situations and surgical skills usually required in difficult situations either for mother or fetus or both.

This chapter covers minor operative procedure like Episiotomy, Perineal tears, Instrumental delivery–Forceps, Ventouse, Induction of labor, shoulder dystocia and finally cesarean section which is one of the most common operation done in woman worldwide.

EPISIOTOMY

Definition

Episiotomy is a surgically planned incision on the perineum and posterior vaginal wall during second stage of labor with a view to facilitate the passage of fetal head and prevent uncontrolled tear of the perineal tissue.

Indication

According to current studies, routine use of episiotomy is not recommended. The procedure should be applied selectively for appropriate indication as:
a. It is obvious that failure to perform episiotomy will result in perineal trauma.
b. In shoulder dystocia.
c. Breech deliveries.
d. Occipitoposterior position.
e. Instrumental delivery.
f. Fetal distress in 2nd stage of labor.
g. Previous perineal surgery like pelvic floor repair, perineal reconstruction surgery.

Timing of Episiotomy

The episiotomy should be performed when presenting part is bulging in the perineum and is about to crown or at least 3-4 cm of diameter of head is visible during contraction. In case of instrumental application, the episiotomy should be given after the application and locking of blade of forceps or after application of vacuum cup. If applied too early it results in significant blood loss. If applied too late perineal laceration will not be prevented.

Types of Episiotomy

Several varieties of episiotomy are given.
a. **Midline (Median):** In this the incision is started from the center of fourchette and extended posteriorly along the midline for about 2.5 cm. In this repair is simple, bleeding is less and anatomical approximation is good. The disadvantage is that any extension by tearing will involve the anal sphincter or canal.
b. **Lateral episiotomy:** The incision starts from about 1 cm away from the center of fourchette and extended laterally. It has many drawbacks. There can be excessive bleeding, Bartholin's gland or duct may be injured, and accurate alignment of divided structure is difficult.
c. **Mediolateral (Posterolateral):** The incision is made downward and outwards from the midpoint of the fourchette either in the right or left. It is directed diagonally in a straight line which seems about 2.5 cm away from the anus (midpoint between anus and ischial tuberosity). It is slightly more difficult in repair than midline episiotomy. The advantage is that it avoids damage to the anal sphincter.
d. **J shaped episiotomy:** The incision begins in the center of the fourchette and is directed posteriorly along the midline for about 1.5 cm and then directed downwards and outwards along 5 or 7 o' clock position to avoid the anal sphincter. In this the tissue approximation is not perfect and repaired wound tends to be puckered. Usually in practice mediolateral or median episiotomy is done commonly.

Advantage and disadvantage of midline and mediolateral episiotomy is compared in Table 53.1.

Table 53.1: Comparative characteristics of midline and mediolateral episiotomy		
Characteristic	Midline	Mediolateral
1. Surgical repair	Easy	More difficult
2. Healing	Good	Less
3. PO pain	Less	More
4. Anatomical approximation	Good	Occasionally faulty
5. Blood loss	Less	More
6. Dyspareunia	Rare	Occasional
7. Extension	Common	Uncommon

Analgesia for Episiotomy

Episiotomy should always be given and repaired under analgesic. Lignocaine 1% is infiltrated in line of proposed cut unless the patient has been already under epidural anesthesia. One should always remember that local anesthetic takes sometime to be effective. Women may choose to combine Entonox and local or regional anesthesia.

Repair of Episiotomy

Timing: Usually episiotomy is repaired after delivery of the placenta but it can be repaired even before delivery of placenta to save time and blood loss.

Technique

a. The surgical principal of hemostasis and anatomical repair without excessive suturing are essential prerequisites for success.
b. The suture material can be 1-0 or 2-0 chronic catgut or 3-0 polyglycolic acid (delayed absorbable synthetic).
c. Episiotomy is sutured in following layers (Figs 53.1A to C).
   i. **Vaginal mucosa:** The apex of incision is identified and suture is started above the apex with chromic catgut or Vicryl Rapide as a continuous suture till the hymenal edges are approximated. Here suture is tied and cut. One should not use blanket or locking stitches.
   ii. **Muscle layer:** Perineal muscles are approximated with 3-4 interrupted sutures in one or two layers.
   iii. **Skin:** Skin is closed by mattress sutures or Subcuticular stitches.

After Care of Episiotomy

One should check and remove if any tampoon has been inserted before start of repair of episiotomy and after cleaning the wound local antiseptic cream is applied. Postoperative antibiotic, analgesic are given for 5-7 days which helps in pain relief and prevention of infection. If there is persistent and severe pain, vaginal hematoma should be ruled out. A stool softener can be given to allay discomfort during defecation.

Complications of Episiotomy

a. **Extension of incision** to involve anal sphincter or anal canal. It is more common in median episiotomy or during delivery of undiagnosed occipitoposterior position.
b. **Infection:** Patient may complain of pain, swelling and discharge from stitch line. Treatment is by cutting one or two stitch to facilitate drainage of pus, local dressing with antibiotic after cleaning wound with mild antiseptic solution and antibiotic, anti-inflammatory drug.

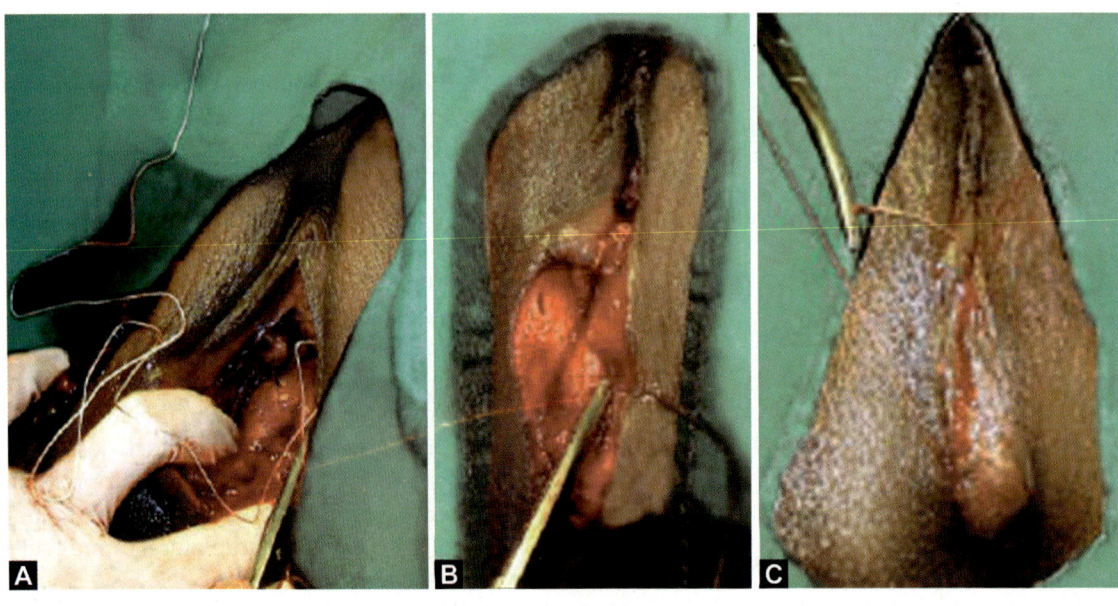

Figs 53.1A to C: A. Identification of apex of vaginal mucosa and suturing 1cm above the apex; (B) Interrupted suturing of muscle; C. Subcuticular skin suture

c. **Vulvar hematoma.**
d. **Wound dehiscence:** It may be due to infection, hematoma formation or faulty repair. Treatment is daily cleaning and dressing with antibiotic until the local infection subsides and healthy granulation tissue forms in the margin. After that secondary sutures are given under local anesthetic, which is again followed by postoperative cleaning and dressing.
e. **Injury to anal sphincter.**
f. **Rarely necrotizing fascitis** in women who are diabetic or immunocompromised.

Remote Complication
a. **Dyspareunia:** It is due to a narrow vaginal introitus which may result from faulty technique of repair or painful perineum scar.
b. Chance of perineal laceration in next labor.
c. Rarely scar endometriosis, implantation dermoid.

PERINEAL LACERATION

Lacerations of perineum are caused by overstretching or too rapid stretching of the tissues especially if they are poorly extensile and rigid. Perineal injuries are more common in primigravida, malpresentation, occipito-posterior, android pelvis and in instrumental delivery.

Classification of Perineal Laceration

- 1st degree: Involving just skin
- 2nd degree: Involving skin and muscle
- 3rd degree: Involving skin, muscle and extending into anal sphincter.
  – 3a: Perineal tear of anal sphincter involving less than 50% thickness.
  – 3b: Complete tear of anal sphincter
  – 3c: Internal sphincter torn
- 4th degree: Involving skin, muscle and extending into the anal sphincter and rectal mucosa.

Prevention of perineal tear: Episiotomy by creating a simple clear cut incision in perineum prevents ragged perineal tear. A careful ironing out of perineum and pelvic floor before operative delivery is also protective.

Suture of perineal laceration
a. First and second degree perineal tears are repaired like episiotomy wound.
b. In third degree perineal tears the suturing should be preferably done in general anesthetic in OT setup with good light in following layers:
   i. Anal mucosa is repaired either running or interrupted suture 3-0 or 4-0 vicryl or catgut. The superior extent of anterior anal laceration is identified and suture is placed through submucosa of the anorectum, approximately 0.5 cm apart down to anal verge.
   ii. Second layer of stitch is placed through the rectal muscle using 3-0 vicryl suture. It incorporates the torn end of anal sphincter.
   iii. Finally the cut ends of anal sphincter are isolated, approximated and sutured together with 3-4 interrupted stitches.
   The remainder of repair is done as an episiotomy. Stool softener should be prescribed for a week.

INDUCTION OF LABOR

Induction of labor is the process of initiating labor by artificial means.
Augmentation: Augmentation of labor is the artificial stimulation of labor that has begun spontaneously.

Principle of Induction of Labor

a. Labor induction should be performed only after appropriate assessment of the mother and fetus.
b. Additionally the risk, benefits and alternatives to induction in each case must be evaluated and explained to the patient.
c. In the absence of medical indication for induction, fetal maturity must be confirmed by exact pregnancy dating, first trimester ultrasound measurement and or amniotic fluid analysis.
d. Evaluation of the cervical status in terms of effacement and softening is important in predicting success of induction and must before any elective induction.

Indication of Induction of Labor

Induction is indicated in situations when the benefits to either the mother or the fetus outweigh those of continuing the pregnancy. Indications are summarized in Table 53.2.

Table 53.2: Indication of induction of labor	
Obstetric indication	*Medical indication*
1. Postdated pregnancy or postmaturity	1. Chronic nephritis
2. Pre-eclampsia and eclampsia	2. Hypertension
3. Previous unexplained intrauterine fetal death	3. Diabetes
4. Intrauterine growth restriction	
5. Prelabor rupture of membrane	
6. Rh isoimmunization	
7. Malformed fetus	
8. Severe hydramnios	
9. Abruptio placenta	
10. Intrauterine death of fetus	

Contraindications of Induction of Labor

Contraindications to labor induction are similar to those that preclude spontaneous labor or delivery. *Maternal contraindications* are related to:
a. Cephalopelvic disproportion.
b. Active genital herpes infection, placenta previa.
c. Uterus upper segment scar.
d. Myomectomy entering the endometrium.
e. Hysterotomy or unification surgery.

Fetal contraindications are fetal malpresentation, appreciable fetal macrosomia.

Induction of labor should be done with caution in cases of grand multiparity, oligohydramnios, multiple gestation and prematurity.

Complication of Induction of Labor

Maternal Complication

In many cases induction of labor exposes the mothers to more distress and discomfort than judicious delay and subsequent vaginal or cesarean delivery. Complication can be as follows:
a. Failed induction with increased risk of cesarean delivery.
b. Tumulus labor with hypertonus of uterus which may cause abruptio placenta, rupture of uterus and cervical laceration.
c. Intrauterine infection.
d. Postpartum hemorrhage.

Fetal Complication

a. Induced delivery exposes the fetus to risk of prematurity if gestational age has not been accurately estimated.
b. Cord prolapse can occur following AROM.
c. Injudicious administration of oxytocic drug during induction can lead to fetal distress or delivery of baby with low APGAR score.
d. Precipitous delivery may result in physical injury.

Methods of Induction of Labor

Induction of labor has two important components:
a. Cervical ripening.
b. Stimulation of uterine contraction to achieve dilatation of cervix and delivery of the fetus.

Preinduction Cervical Assessment

The condition of the cervix or favorability is important to assess chances of success of labor induction. Quantifiable method predictive of outcome of labor induction is introduced by Bishop (1964), modified by Calder (1974). It is summarized in Table 53.3. A score of more than 7 suggests high likelihood for successful induction while Bishop score of 4 or less identifies an unfavorable cervix. In this situation cervical ripening should be done (Table 53.3).

Table 53.3: Modified Bishop score (Calder score)

Cervical feature	Pelvic score			
	0	1	2	3
Dilatation of cervix	< 1 cm	1-2 cm	2-4 cm	> 4 cm
Length of cervix	4 cm	2-4 cm	1-2 cm	< 1 cm
Station of presenting part (relative to ischial spines)	-3 cm	-2 cm	-1/0 cm	+1/+2 cm
Consistency of position of cervix	Firm posterior	Average mid anterior	Soft	—

Test score: 0-5 unfavorable, 6-12 favorable

Methods of Cervical Ripening

Pharmacological Method

a. *Prostaglandin:* Two forms of prostaglandins are commonly used for cervical ripening prior to induction of labor: (a) Dinoprostone – PGE2 – PGE2 gel is available in 2.5 ml syringe for an intracervical application of 0.5 mg of Dinoprostone. **PGE2 should not be used in patients with a history of asthma, glaucoma or myocardial infarction.** Usually 12 hours is allowed for cervical ripening.
b. *Misoprostol (PGE1):* Misoprostol is available as 100 μg unscored, 200 μg scored tablet, and also 25 μg. tablet that can be administered orally, vaginally or rectally. Misoprostol is stable at room temperature and cheap as compared to Dinoprostone gel. The usual dosage is 25-50 μg 4-6 hourly. Prostaglandins should always be administered with close fetal heart rate and uterine activity monitoring. Side effects are fetal distress, uterine hypertonus, nausea, vomiting, fever and peripartum infection.
c. *Relaxin:* It is a polypeptide hormone that is produced in the human corpus luteum, decidua and chorion. Purified protein Relaxin 2 mg in tylose gel, given vaginally or intracervically is reported to induce labor in 80% of cases.

Mechanical Method

a. *Balloon catheter:* A Foley's catheter with 25-50 ml balloon is passed into the endocervix above the internal os using tissue forceps. The balloon is then inflated with sterile saline and the catheter is withdrawn gently to the level of internal cervical os. This method should induce cervical ripening over 8-12 hours.
b. *Hygroscopic Dilators:*
   i. Natural Laminaria tents are made from seaweed. When placed in the endocervix for 6-12 hours, the tent increases in diameter 3-4 fold by extracting water from cervical tissue, swells and expands the cervical canal.

ii. **Synthetic Lamicel** is a polyvinyl alcohol sponge impregnated with 450 mg of magnesium sulfate and Dilapan. It is made from a stable nontoxic hydrophil polymer and has been found to be highly effective in mechanical cervical dilatation.

Induction of Labor and Augmentation

a. **Oxytocin:** Dilute infusion of oxytocin is the most effective medical means of inducing labor. Dosages must be individualized. Usually 10 unit of oxytocin is given in 1 liter of Ringer's lactate solution or 5% Dextrose in water. Infusion is started at 1 mU/minute and increased every 30 minutes till good contractions are achieved. Oxytocin infusion is discontinued whenever there is evidence of hyperstimulation or fetal distress. But can be restarted with careful supervision when reassuring fetal heart rate and uterine activity patterns are restored.

b. **Amniotomy:** AROM can be used to induce labor but it implies a commitment to delivery. AROM may be an effective way to induce labor in selected cases with high Bishop scores. Release of amniotic fluid shortens the muscles bundle of the myometrium and increase strength and duration of uterine contraction. *It is recommended that AROM should only be done when patient has entered in active phase of labor.* The membrane should be ruptured with full sterile precaution with help of amniohook. To minimize the risk of cord prolapse, care should be taken to avoid dislodging the fetal head. Fundal or suprapubic pressure or both may reduce the risk of cord prolapse.

c. **Amniotomy with oxytocin augmentation:** Amniotomy with oxytocin augmentation for arrested active phase of labor shortens the induction to delivery interval without any increase in cesarean section rate.

OPERATIVE VAGINAL DELIVERY

Operative vaginal delivery refers to an obstetric procedure in which active measures are taken to accomplish delivery. Operative delivery can be divided into operative vaginal delivery and cesarean delivery. In last several years there has been a decrease in the operative vaginal delivery rate but rise in cesarean section rate. The success and safety of these procedures are based upon operator's skills, proper timing, and ensuring the proper prerequisite.

FORCEPS OPERATIONS

Design of Forceps

The obstetric forceps consist of two matched parts that articulate or lock. Each part is composed of – Blade, Shank, Lock, and Handle. Each blade is designed, so that it possess two curves – *the cephalic curve*, which conforms to the shape of fetal head and *pelvic curve*, which conforms to the curved axis of maternal pelvis. The blades are connected to the handle by shank. The blades are referred to the left and right according to the side of the mother's pelvis on which they lie after application. When blades are inserted in right order the right shank comes to a lie atop of the left so that the forceps articulate or lock as the handles are closed. Lock may be English types which are fixed or sliding type as seen in Kielland's forceps.

Types of Forceps

There have been various modifications of forceps depending upon need and situation. Though there are about 600 kinds of forceps described but usually following types of forceps are in use

a. *Wrigley's forceps:* These are light weighted short curved forceps, having generous cephalic curve. This is most commonly used outlet forceps in today's obstetric practice.

b. *Kielland's forceps:* It has sliding lock and peculiar shape, which can rotate and deliver a malrotated head in skilled and experienced hands.

c. *Piper's forceps:* It is recommended for delivery of after coming head in breech presentation. It has a reverse pelvic curve compared to other forceps.

d. *Simpson's forceps:* It is suited for application to the molded fetal head.

Diag: Varieties of obstetric forceps are shown in Figures 53.2A to C.

Classification of Forceps Delivery

The current classification proposed by ACOG is summarized in Box 53.1. The classification is based on two most important discriminators of risk for both mother and infant:

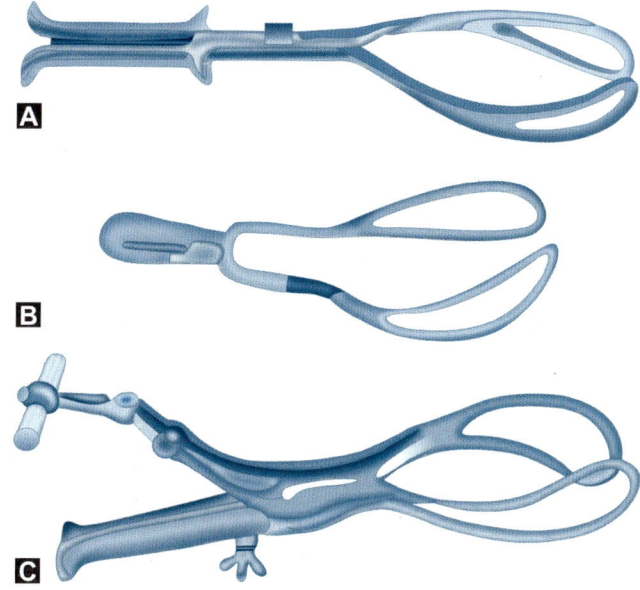

Figs 53.2A to C: (A) Kielland's forceps, (B) Wrigley's forceps, (C) Milne-Murray's axis traction forceps

> **Box 53.1:** Classification of forceps and vacuum delivery according to station and rotation

1. Outlet	•	Scalp is visible at introitus without separating the labia
	•	Fetal skull has reached pelvic floor
	•	Sagittal suture in anteroposterior diameter or right or left occiput anterior or posterior position
	•	Fetal head is at or on the perineum
	•	Rotation does not exceed 45°
2. Low	•	Leading point of fetal skull is station at + 2 cm, and not on pelvic floor
	•	Rotation is 45° or less (Left or right occiput anterior to occiput anterior or left or right occiput posterior to occiput posterior
	•	Rotation is greater than 45°
3. Mid pelvic	•	Station above + 2 cm but head is engaged
4. High	•	Not included in classification

a. Station of fetal head in relation to ischial spine.
b. Degree of rotation of head.

Forceps deliveries are categorized as outlet, low and mid forceps operations. Only rarely should an attempt be made at forceps delivery above station – 2 like unusual circumstances as sudden onset of severe fetal or maternal compromise or transverse arrest with full preparation ready for cesarean delivery in case of failed attempt. *Under no circumstances should forceps be applied to an unengaged head.*

Indications of Forceps Delivery

Maternal Indication

a. Maternal exhaustion and distress in 2nd stage of labor.
b. Prolonged 2nd stage which is considered more than 1 hour of active pushing in multiparous women and more than 2 hours in primiparous women.
c. Medical indication when active bearing down or Valsalva's maneuver is to be avoided – like severe cardiac disease, hypertensive crisis, uncorrected cerebrovascular malformation.
d. Pushing is not possible like paraplegia.

Fetal Indication

a. Fetal distress in 2nd stage of labor.
b. Cord prolapse in 2nd stage of labor in cephalic presentation.
c. To control after coming head in breech presentation.

Prerequisites for Forceps Applications

Following criteria should be satisfied before attempting a forceps delivery.
a. Fetal head must be engaged.
b. The presentation should be suitable -vertex or face with chin anterior.
c. Head should be flexed and preferably well rotated.
d. Cervix must be fully dilated, effaced.
e. Membranes should be ruptured.
f. There should be no suspected cephalopelvic disproportion.
g. There should not be complete uterine inertia. Uterine contraction is to be confirmed otherwise there is risk of failed forceps and postpartum hemorrhage.
h. The bladder must be empty.

Preparation for Forceps Delivery

a. The patient is placed in the dorsal lithotomy position with leg comfortably placed.
b. All sterile surgical precautions are made.
c. **Preliminary examination** is done to assess fetal position, station, and adequacy of pelvic diameters and to see that all prerequisites are fulfilled.
d. For **anesthesia** if pudendal block or local infiltration is to be used, it should be administered after the preliminary examination has been performed. If conduction anesthetic epidural is to be used, it must be administered prior to the positioning of patient.
e. **Application of forceps:** A major concept to bear in the mind is that the application of forceps should use finesse rather than forces. It is vital to ensure that forceps blades consist of complete and matched sets and they articulate easily before application. In occiput anterior position the steps of forceps applications are as follows:
   i. The left handle is held between the thumb and fingers of left hand and two or more fingers of the right hand are introduced inside vagina beside the fetal head. The left blade of forceps is guided to its correct positions on the left side of the fetal head. Left blade is held by assistant.
   ii. For application of right blade two or more fingers of left hand is introduced into vagina to serve as a guide for right blade. Right blade is held in right hand and introduced into vagina. The handles are depressed slightly before locking, in order to place the blades properly along the optimal diameter of the fetal head (Figs 53.3A to I). If the application is accurate, the blades are easily locked. If the force is needed to achieve locking the application may be faulty and positions must be rechecked. If simple manipulation of the blades does not permit easy articulation, the forceps should be removed and position verified by feeling ear, if necessary and the blades are applied correctly. After these 3 checks have been adequately performed, traction can be applied.
f. **Traction:** When it is certain that the blades are placed satisfactorily. The traction is made gently in horizontal direction until the perineum begins to bulge. As the vulva is distended by the occiput, episiotomy may be given.

Chapter - 53 ♦ Operative Obstetrics

is required, the cause can be cephalopelvic disproportion or asynclitism.

ii. Traction should be intermittent with uterine contraction.

iii. When head begins to distend the perineum, the amount of traction and direction must be altered. The faster the head advances, the resistance of pelvis and soft part is reduced so only minimal traction is applied. The head negotiates the final position of the pelvic curve by extension. At this time obstetrician should simulate this movement by elevating the handles of forceps more and more as the head crowns (Figs 53.4A and B).

g. After crowing of head, it is preferable to **remove the forceps** in the reverse order of their application by first disarticulating the forceps and raising the right handle until the blade is removed. The left blade is than removed

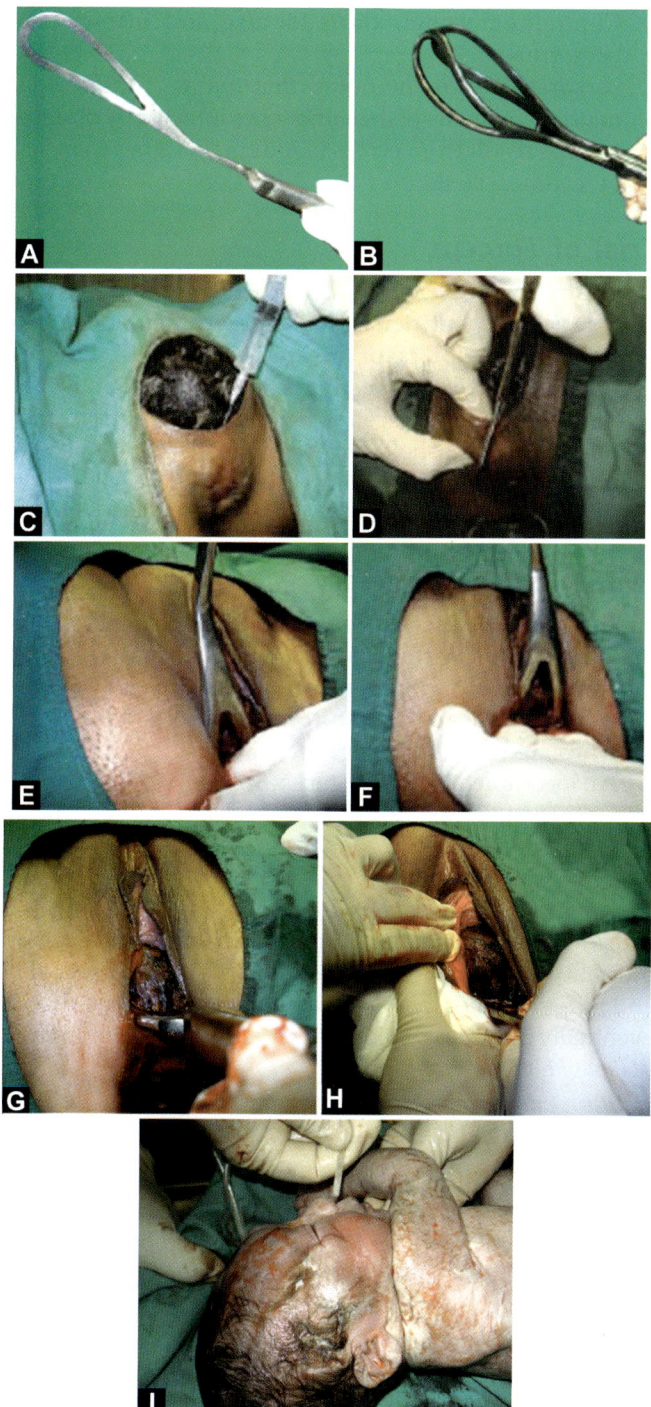

Figs 53.3A to I: Steps of forceps delivery: (A and B) Check the blades and lock of forceps before application; (C and D) Infiltration of local anesthetic and episiotomy; (E) Application of right blade; (F) Application of left blade; (G and H) Steady traction and perineal support; (I) Delivery of baby.

While giving traction following points should be kept in mind:

i. The force should not be more than that can be exerted by flexed forearms. Use of back muscles or bracing of feet should be discouraged, because if greater force

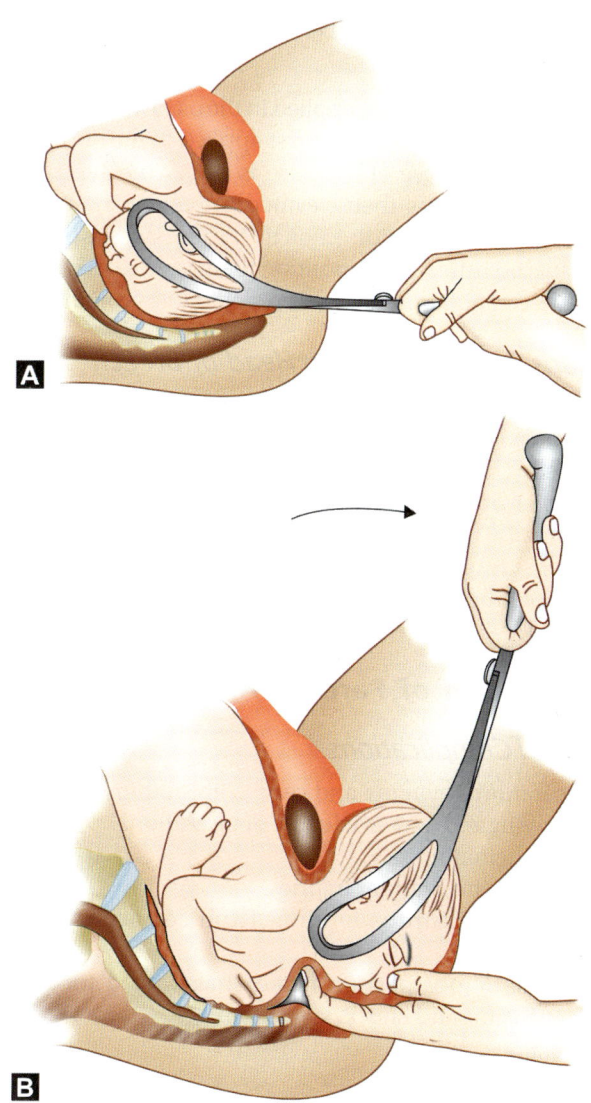

Figs 53.4A and B: Direction of traction in low forceps application: (A) Initially forward; (B) Later forward and upward

in similar fashion. Early removal of forceps reduces size of the mass that must pass through the introitus and so there is reduced chance of perineal laceration or extension of episiotomies. After removal of forceps, head can be delivered by use of Ritgen's maneuver during the next contraction. Some operator keeps the forceps till delivery of the head for control of movement of head.

Forceps Application in Face Presentation

Only in mentum anterior position forceps are occasionally used. The blades are applied to the sides of the head along the occipitomental diameter with pelvic curve directed to the neck. Downward traction is exerted till chin appears under the symphysis. Than by upward movement the face is slowly delivered, with nose, eyes, brows and occiput appear in succession over the anterior margin of the perineum. *Forceps is not applied in mentoposterior position.*

Forceps Application in Direct Occipitoposterior Position

In this position forceps are applied in the usual fashion. After locking the handle, traction is first applied in the horizontal direction till the base of the nose is under the symphysis pubis. The handle is then elevated to deliver the occiput followed by downward direction till the face sweeps over the vulva successfully. In this position there is increased risk of perineal laceration so a generous episiotomy is recommended.

Forceps in After Coming Head of Breech

In all breech vaginal delivery the forceps should be available in advance. The head should be brought as low down as possible by hanging the body of child downward till the occiput lies up against the back of the symphysis pubis. An assistant raise the leg of child and forceps blades are applied on either side of the baby's head from underneath its body. An episiotomy is given. Advantage is controlled delivery of fetal head.

Complication of Forceps Application

Maternal Complications

a. Laceration of vagina and cervix, episiotomy extension involving 3rd and 4th degree of laceration.
b. Pelvic hematomas.
c. Urethral and bladder injuries.
d. Uterine rupture extending from cervical or vault laceration.
e. Traumatic postpartum hemorrhage, need for blood transfusion and shock.
f. Infection.

Fetal Complications

a. Facial laceration, forceps marks.
b. Facial and brachial plexus palsies.
c. Cephalhematoma, skull facture and intracranial hemorrhage.
d. Seizures: It must be noted that many of the serious injuries and many of the minor ones inflicted by obstetric forceps result from errors in judgment rather than lack of technical skills.

Trial of Forceps

This term is used when it is not possible to determine with sufficient confidence that an instrumental delivery will be successful. Trial of forceps is done in OT with full preparation of cesarean section. If there is easy application of blade and baby descends with gentle traction, then delivery is accomplished vaginally with the forceps. If there is difficulty in any stage, then forceps blades are withdrawn and cesarean section is done.

Failed Forceps Delivery

Failed forceps is used to denote an unsuccessful attempt to deliver with the forceps. Failed forceps may be due to inability to apply to forceps or inability to deliver after application. Cause of failed forceps may be:
a. Unrotated occipitoposterior position.
b. An incompletely dilated cervix.
c. Constriction ring dystocia.
d. Disproportion.
e. Premature interference.

In past failed forceps has been associated with a considerable maternal and high perinatal morbidity and mortality. But now forceps operation is a procedure of skill and judgment, not the force. So term failed forceps should eventually disappear but only term *failed trial of forceps should be thought.*

VENTOUSE (VACUUM EXTRACTOR)

Ventouse is an instrumental device designed to assist delivery by creating a vacuum between it and fetal scalp. The pulling force is dragging the cranium while in forceps the pulling force is directly transmitted to the base of the skull.

Instrument Design

The vacuum extractor has got following components (Figs 53.5A and 53.6):
a. **Cups:** Initially metal cups of three sizes – 40 mm, 50 mm and 60 mm was used, which are smaller at rim than above the brim. Now soft cup, silicone cup are in use Cochrane review conclude that the soft vacuum extractor cup were associated with an increase in rate of failure but a significant reduction in scalp trauma.
b. **Hollow rubber tubing** by which air is evacuated.
c. Glass trap bottle with manometer.
d. **Chain attached to cup** which passes through the tubing and attaches to a cross bar and handle used for traction.
e. Suction hand pump or electric pump (Fig. 53.6).

Indication and Contraindication of Ventouse

Generally the indication for vacuum use are *similar to those of forceps application*, i.e.:
a. As an alternative to forceps application.
b. As an alternative to rotational forceps as in occipito-transverse or occipitoposterior position.
c. Delay in descent of head in case of second baby of twin.
d. Delay in 1st stage of labor due to uterine inertia.

Contraindications to vacuum delivery:
a. Face presentation.
b. Breech presentation.
c. Gestational age less than 34 weeks or estimated fetal weight less than 2000 gm.
d. Cephalopelvic disproportion.
e. Congenital anomalies of the fetal head, e.g. hydrocephalus.
f. Estimated fetal weight greater than 4000 gm and an unengaged fetal head.
g. Fetal coagulopathy.
h. Recent fetal scalp blood sampling.

Advantages of Ventouse Over Forceps Application

Certain advantages of Ventouse over forceps in specific situations are as follows:
a. Ventouse can be applied in un-rotated and malrotated occipitoposterior position of the head.
b. It can be applied even though cervix is a little less than fully dilated.
c. It does not occupy space like forceps application.
d. It can be used even where head is a little high.
e. It is comfortable to mother.
f. Chances of genital tract laceration are less as compared to forceps.
g. Lesser traction force is needed.

Disadvantages of Ventouse Over Forceps Application

a. Ventouse take longer time in delivery so in case of fetal distress, forceps operation can quickly deliver the fetus as compared to Ventouse.
b. Forceps can be applied in premature baby, mento-anterior face and after coming head of breech.
c. Ventouse can produce more fetal injuries like scalp laceration, cephalhematoma, intracranial hemorrhage.
d. More failure rates as compared to forceps.

Procedure of Vacuum Application

A. The **prerequisite for vacuum applications** are:
   i. Presenting part should be cephalic and preferably well flexed.
   ii. No evidence of cephalopelvic disproportion.
   iii. Head should be preferably well engaged. In modern obstetrics vacuum application in high station that is above ± 2 is no longer favored, except in case of second twin.

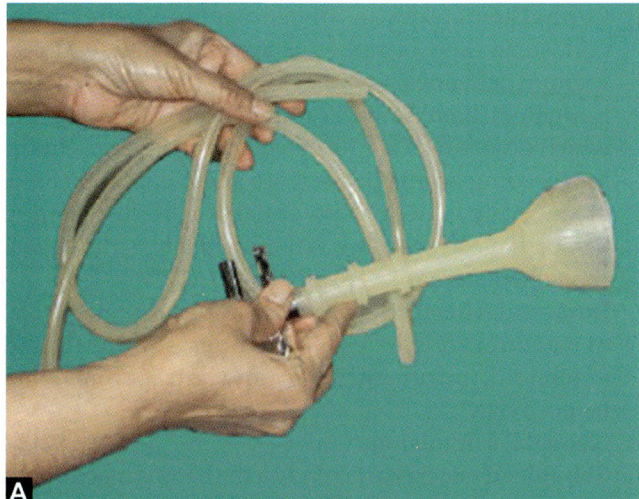
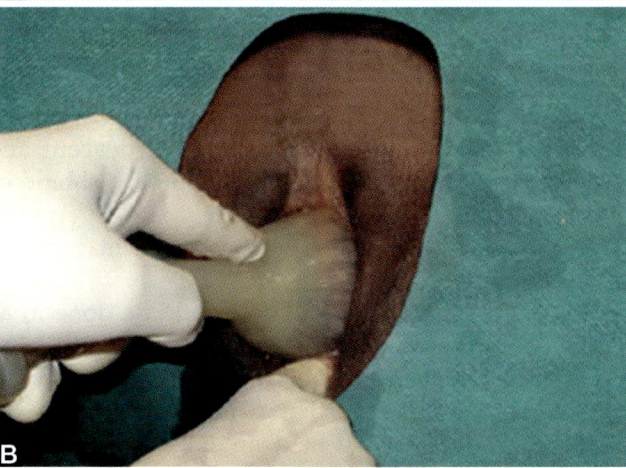

Figs 53.5A and B: (A) Ventouse with cup, hallow rubber tubing; (B) Application of ventouse

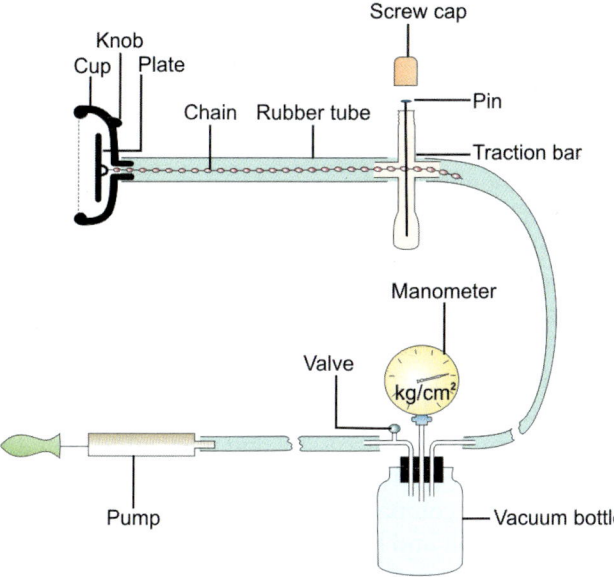

Fig 53.6: Vacuum extractor with malmstrom cup

iv. The cervix is almost fully dilated.
v. The obstetrician should be well versed to the instrument application.

B. **Application of ventouse:** The patient is prepared with full sterile surgical precaution and placed in dorsal lithotomy position. Before application the vacuum system is assembled to ensure that no leak is present.
   i. Pudendal block anesthesia usually is sufficient.
   ii. The cup is inserted into the vagina by directing pressure towards the posterior aspect of the vagina. So the cup is directly placed over the sagittal suture, at approximately 3 cm anterior to the posterior frontonelle. This application allows adequate maintenance of flexion of the fetal head during the procedure (Fig. 53.5B).
   iii. Prior to vacuum application one should be certain that no maternal tissue is included under the cup margin. Cup is placed at right site, and marker or vacuum part of the suction cup is pointed towards the occiput.
   iv. Traction: while the cup is held firmly against the fetal head, the suction is created at 0.2 kg/cm gradually increased to 0.2 kg/cm every 2 minutes, so as to induce a maximum negative pressure of 0.8 kg/cm. Traction is applied intermittently coinciding with uterine contraction and supplemented with maternal bearing down efforts. Duration of traction is along the pelvic axis. If more than 1 traction is necessary the vacuum pressure can be decreased to low level between the contractions.
   v. Delivery is usually affected with 4-6 pulls given over period of 15-20 minutes. While the head is delivering the cup should assure a 90° orientation to the horizontal as the head is extended. Once the head has completely delivered through the vagina, the suction is withdrawn and cup is removed. Delivery of baby is completed as in normal labor.

Complication of Ventouse

Maternal
i. Soft tissue genital tract injury can occur.
ii. Traumatic postpartum hemorrhage.
iii. Infection.

Fetal Complication
i. An artificial caput or chignon is routinely created during vacuum extraction. Use of vacuum has been associated with a variety of neonatal injuries from benign superficial scalp markings to serious and potentially life-threatening intracranial hemorrhage.
ii. The most common neonatal complication is retinal hemorrhage which may occur in as many as 50% of deliveries. Usually it is self-resolving.
iii. **Cephalhematoma** involves bleeding beneath the periosteum and complicates approximately 6% of all vacuum deliveries.
iv. **Subgaleal hematoma** is more serious complication which occurs in 50 of 10000 vacuum deliveries. In this the bleeding occurs in the loose subaponeurotic tissue of the scalp. There is potential for life-threatening hemorrhage as bleeding is not limited by sutures as in cephalhematoma.
v. **Intracranial hemorrhage** occurs in approximately 0.35% of vacuum deliveries. It includes subdural, sub-arachnoid, intraventricular and intraparenchymal hemorrhage.
vi. **Neonatal convulsion.**
vii. **Shoulder dystocia** particularly if the baby is macrosomic.

Precaution in Ventouse Application to Avoid Complication

a. Vacuum extraction should be considered as a trial and without early and clear evidence of descent and delivery, an alternative delivery approach should be considered.
b. Traction should be applied only when patient is actively pushing.
c. No torsion or twisting of cup should be done in an attempt to rotate the head.
d. Duration of time from application of cup to delivering should not exceed more than 20 minutes.
e. The procedure should be abandoned if the cup has dislodged from the fetal head twice.
f. Under no circumstances, the operator should switch from vacuum to forceps or vice versa. As greatest incidence of neonatal injury occurs in babies when both vacuum and forceps are used.
g. The clinician must be prepared to risk of shoulder dystocia which is increased with instrumental delivery more with vacuum as compared to forceps delivery.
h. Neonatal staff should be present at the time of instrumental delivery (forceps as well Ventouse).

Although both forceps and vacuum have proved to be useful in assisting with vaginal delivery, the vacuum in certain states is becoming the preferred instrument of choice. Both forceps and vacuum have the potential to cause maternal and fetal complications. In order to minimize both maternal and fetal risk, operator must be familiar with the indication, contraindication, application and use of particular instrument. It must be kept in mind that successful and uneventful operative vaginal deliveries have a much lower morbidity and mortality as compared to emergency cesarean section, but a difficult and heroic instrumental delivery can be extensively traumatic resulting in potentially grave maternal and fetal complications.

SHOULDER DYSTOCIA

Shoulder dystocia is an obstetrical complication which has potential for causing significant life long injury to newborn. It is obstetrician's nightmare because of its unpredictability, potential complications and legal implications.

Definition

Shoulder dystocia occurs when the fetal anterior shoulder impacts against the maternal pubic bone. Typically shoulder dystocia is defined as a delivery in which additional maneuvers are required to deliver the fetus after normal gentle downward traction has failed (Fig. 53.7). Less commonly, shoulder dystocia results from impaction of the posterior shoulder on the sacral promontory.

Incidence and Risk Factors

The incidence of shoulder dystocia is 0.6 – 1.4% of vaginal birth. There has been considerable evolution in obstetrical thinking about identification of – Preconceptual antepartum and intrapartum risk factors and preventability of shoulder dystocia in the past decade.

Preconceptual Risk Factors

a. **Previous shoulder dystocia:** The risk of a woman having a repeat shoulder dystocia, once having had one is 11 – 12%. Because of this increased risk some obstetricians have proposed "once a shoulder dystocia, always a cesarean". However, ACOG (2002) recommends that estimated fetal weight, gestational age, maternal glucose tolerance test, and severity of prior neonatal injury should be evaluated and risk and benefit of cesarean section discussed with any women with a history of shoulder dystocia.

b. **Maternal obesity:** Though relative risk of shoulder dystocia in women with a prepregnancy weight of greater than 82 kg is 2.3. Despite that, research concludes that any intervention undertaken based solely on the relationship between maternal weight and macrosomia would be without justification in majority of women.

Antepartum Risk Factor

a. **Fetal macrosomia:** ACOG (2002) recommended that performing cesarean delivery for all women suspected of carrying a macrosomic fetus is not appropriate, except possibly for estimated fetal weight over 5 kg in non-diabetic mother and over 4.5 kg in those with diabetic. ACOG bulletin also state that ultrasound has a sensitivity of only 21-44% and a positive predictive value of only 30-40% in predicting macrosomia.

b. **Diabetes:** Next to macrosomia, the factor most closely associated with shoulder dystocia is maternal diabetes in pregnancy. Babies of diabetic mother had a 3 – 4 fold increased risk of shoulder dystocia compared to babies of nondiabetic mothers in each weight category. Cause may be different body configuration of infant in diabetic mother.

c. **Maternal weight gain,** multiparity male sex of fetus and postdatism are only secondary risk factor.

Intrapartum Risk Factor

a. **Labor abnormalities:** Prolonged first and second stage of labor were not found to be useful clinical predictor of shoulder dystocia. This may be secondary to fetal macrosomia.

b. **Assisted delivery:** Shoulder dystocia is more likely to occur when labor is induced, accelerated with oxytocic and assisted delivery even in smaller babies.

c. **Experience of deliverer and episiotomy** has not been found to be significantly related with incidence of shoulder dystocia.

Prediction and Prevention of Shoulder Dystocia

Till now the answer to question "Can shoulder dystocia be reliably predicted is No".

Recently Dr Emuly Hamilton has described a tool based on sophisticated statistical and maternal analysis, which is claimed to identify 50 – 70% of patients destined to have shoulder dystocia with a false positive rate of only 2.7%.

To perform elective cesarean section for fetal macrosomia in high risk mother, to attempt to limit maternal weight gain, and careful management of 1st and 2nd stage of labor (prophylactic McRoberts' maneuver), can be appropriate preventive measure to reduce chances of shoulder dystocia.

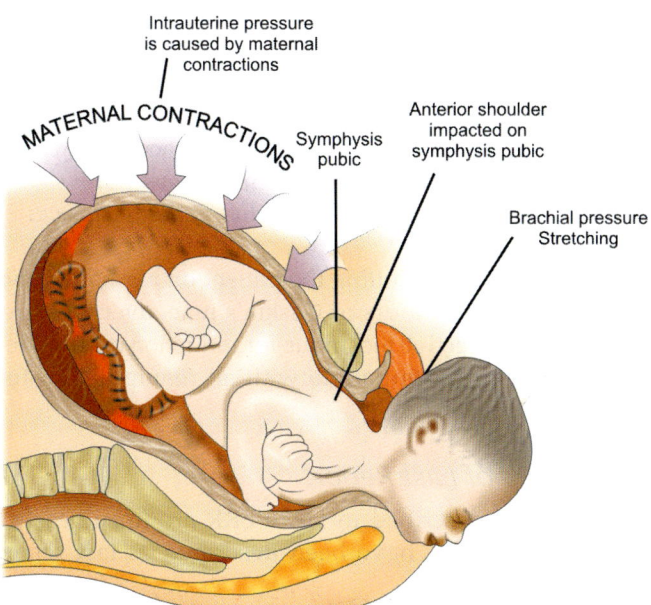

Fig. 53.7: Position in shoulder dystocia

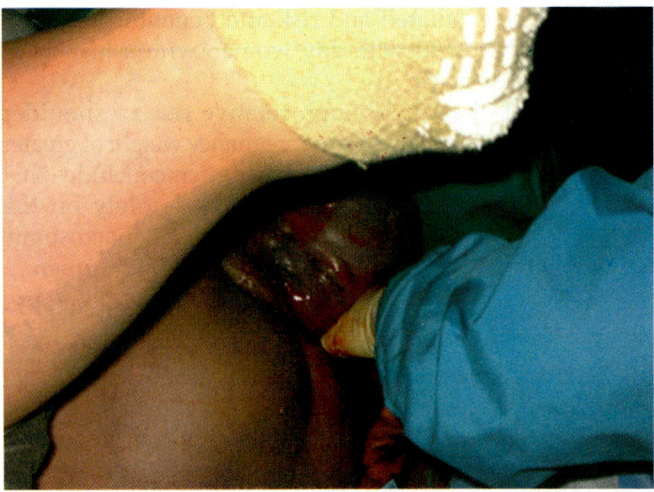

Fig. 53.8: Turtle sign in shoulder dystocia

Symptoms and Sign

Sign and symptoms preceding shoulder dystocia are summarized as follows:
a. Suspected large baby.
b. Slow progress from 7 to 10 cm, despite good contraction.
c. Slow progress in 2nd stage or precipitate labor.
d. Instrumental delivery.
e. Slow advancement and slow crowning and delivery of head.
f. Fetal head emerges and than retracts against the perineum referred to as "turtle sign" (Fig. 53.8).

Practice Recommendation/Maneuvers

Because shoulder dystocia cannot be predicted, the clinician must be well versed in the management principle of this occasionally devastating complication.

The HELPERR mnemonic is a clinical tool that offers structured framework for coping with shoulder dystocia (Box 53.2).

Box 53.2: HELPERR Drill in shoulder dystocia

H – Help-call emergency number for direct access to senior obstetrician, nurse, anesthetic and neonatologist
E – Evaluate for episiotomy
L – Leg hyperflexed (McRoberts maneuver)
P – Pressure suprapubic
E – Enter the vagina – internal maneuver (Woodscrew, Robin II, Reverse wood screw)
R – Remove the posterior arm
R – Roll on all four
These maneuvers are designed to do one of the three things:
1. Increase the functional size of the bony pelvis, through flattening of the lumbar lordosis and cephalad rotation of symphysis.
2. Decrease the bisacromial diameter of fetus through suprapubic pressure.
3. Change the relationship of the bisacromial diameter within the bony pelvis through internal rotation maneuver.

HELPERR have become a formalized and accepted approach to management of shoulder dystocia.

a. *Call for help:* To all concerned persons. The primary physician or obstetrician should direct the activities and one person should record the timing and event.
b. *Episiotomy:* Episiotomy by itself will not release the impaction because the primary problem is a bony impaction. It should be evaluated considering need of internal maneuver.
c. *McRoberts maneuver:* It involves removing the legs from the stirrup and sharply flexing the legs upon the maternal abdomen. By this symphysis pubis is rotated cephalad and sacrum is straightened.
d. *Suprapubic pressure:* Suprapubic pressure in conjunction with McRoberts maneuver is successful in 50–60% cases of shoulder dystocia. *Fundal pressure is contraindicated, as it may worsen the condition or cause uterus rupture.*
e. *Rubin I maneuver:* The clinician stands on the same side as the baby's back and direct pressure towards the midline, in order to help shift the impacted shoulder.
f. *Rubin II maneuver:* It consist of inserting the fingers of one hand vaginally behind the posterior aspect of the anterior shoulder of the fetus and rotating the shoulder towards the fetal chest. This results in adduction of shoulder girdle reducing its diameter.
g. *Woodscrew maneuver:* If Rubin II maneuver is unsuccessful, the Woodscrew maneuver can be attempted. The obstetrician places at least two fingers on the anterior aspect of the fetal posterior shoulder, applying gentle upward pressure around the circumference of the arc in the same direction as with Rubin II maneuver. If it also fails, reverse Wood Corkscrew maneuver may be tried. In this the physician fingers are placed on the back of the posterior shoulder of the fetus and fetus is rotated in the opposite direction. (Figs 53.9A to E).
h. **Delivery of posterior shoulder:** It consist of carefully sweeping the posterior arm of the fetus across the chest, followed by delivery of the arm. *The upper arm should never be grasped and pulled directly, as this may result in fracture humerus.*
i. **Roll the patient:** Rolling the patient on her hands and knees on the all fours or Gaskin's maneuver is a safe, rapid and effective technique for reduction of shoulder dystocia. It is compatible with all manipulation for shoulder dystocia.

Maneuvers of Last Report

If maneuvers described in HELPERR are unsuccessful, several techniques have been described as last resort maneuver.
1. *Deliberate clavicle fracture:* Clavicular fracture will heal rapidly and not as serious as brachial nerve injury, asphyxia or death.

Chapter -53 ♦ Operative Obstetrics

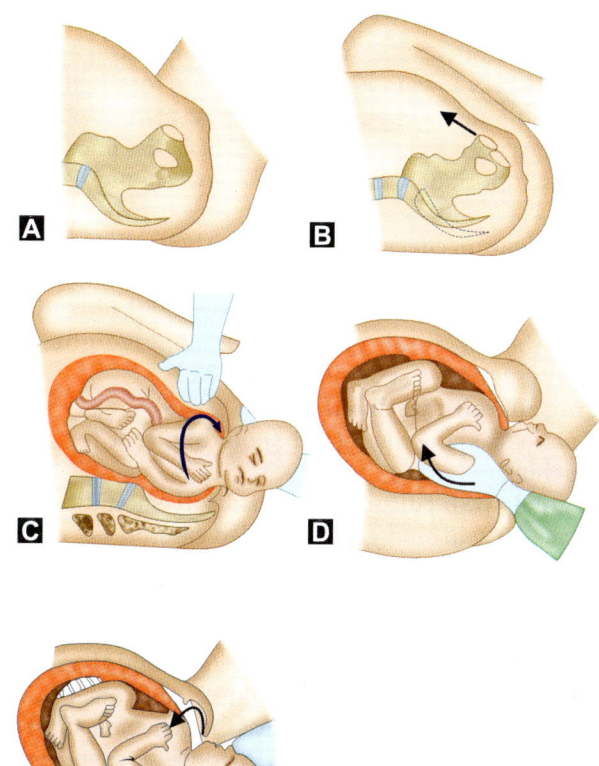

Figs 53.9A to E: Shoulder Dystocia: (A and B) McRoberts maneuver; (C) Suprapubic pressure; (D and E) Woodscrew and reverse Woodscrew method

2. *Zavenelli's maneuver:* It is the cephalic replacement into the pelvis in occiput anterior or occiput posterior position and then cesarean delivery. Terbutaline 250 μg S/C can be given to produce uterine relaxation. This procedure should never be attempted if a nuchal cord previously has been clamped and cut.
3. *Abdominal surgery with hysterotomy:* In general anesthesia cesarean incision is given, after which surgeon rotates the infant transabdominally through incision, like Woodscrew maneuver. Vaginal extraction is then accompanied by another physician.
4. *Cleidotomy:* Can be only in dead fetus.
5. *Symphysiotomy*.

After care: The couple should be offered the opportunity to discuss the events of shoulder dystocia and any long-term effect and prospects for future pregnancy.

Documentation and Litigation

Documentation of delivery is essential to reducing legal liability. An accurate and honest delivery note should be written by the attending physician Box 53.3.

Box 53.3: Documentation of Shoulder Dystocia

a. Position of fetal head at delivery.
b. Which shoulder was the anterior shoulder.
c. Time of delivery of the fetal head.
d. Staff present at time of delivery.
e. Maneuvers used to achieve delivery.
f. Newborn weight and Apgar score.
g. Any difficult motion of the extremities.
h. Disposition of newborn.
i. Any maternal injury.
j. Cord blood pH.

All of this information is important, e.g. sometime injury occur in posterior shoulder, which suggest that they did not occur during actual delivery but before delivery of fetal head. Normal Apgar score or cord pH greater than 7.0 would suggest that if newborn or child develops some sort of CNS injury, it is not the result of hypoxia during delivery.

Maternal and fetal complications of shoulder dystocia are summarized in Table 53.4.

CESAREAN SECTION

A cesarean section refers to the delivery of a fetus, placenta and membranes through an abdominal and uterine incision. This definition does not include removal of fetus from the abdominal cavity in the case of rupture of the uterus or in case of abdominal pregnancy.

Indications

Cesarean section is used in cases where vaginal delivery either is not feasible or would induce risk to the mother or baby. Some of the indications for cesarean sections are clear and straight forward, whereas others are relative. In some cases, fine obstetric judgment is necessary to determine whether cesarean section is indicated. The most common indication for cesarean section is presumed fetal distress (22%), failure to progress in labor (20%), repeat cesarean section (14%) and breech presentation (14%). In last decade maternal request is also coming as an emerging indication. Indication of cesarean section can be enumerated as follows:

Table 53.4: Complication of shoulder dystocia

Maternal:
1. Postpartum hemorrhage
2. Rectovaginal fistula
3. Symphyseal separation or diathesis with or without transient femoral neuropathy
4. 3rd or 4th degree perineal tear
5. Uterus rupture

Fetal:
1. Brachial plexus injury (4-15%, < 10% permanent)
2. Clavicular fracture
3. Fetal death
4. Fetal hypoxia with or without permanent neurological damage
5. Fracture humerus

a. **Maternal indication:** Maternal illness (severe pre-eclampsia), failed induction of labor, active genital herpes and strong maternal request.
b. **Fetal indication:** Fetal distress, malpresentation (breech presentation, transverse lie, some face presentation), some multifetal pregnancies, fetal macrosomia, maternal HIV infection to prevent vertical transmission of HIV in newborn and in some cases of intrauterine growth restriction.
c. **Maternal and fetal:** Arrest of labor and dystocia.
d. **Placental and umbilical cord:** Placenta previa, vasa previa, placental abruptio with fetal compromise, umbilical cord prolapse, umbilical cord presentation.
e. **Pelvic:** Anatomical abnormality which prevents vaginal delivery, pelvic mass obstructing the birth canal, e.g. adnexal mass, uterine myoma, history of complicated maternal birth injury like fourth degree laceration, rectovaginal fistula, history of pelvic reconstructive surgery, e.g. fistula repair.
f. **Uterine:** Previously scarred uterus, e.g. vertical uterine incision, prior myomectomy involving the uterine cavity.
Indication of cesarean section according to absolute/relative and maternal/fetal has been summarized in Tables 53.5 and 53.6.

Table 53.5: Absolute/relative indications of cesarean section

Absolute	Relative
• Severe cephalopelvic disproportion	• Fetal distress
• Major degree of placenta previa	• Antepartum hemorrhage
• History of repair for fistula	• Cervical dystocia
• Cancer cervix	• Pregnancy induced hypertension resistant to treatment
• Vaginal atresia	• Cord accident
• Transverse lie uncorrected by ECV	• Previous cesarean
• Previous history of classical cesarean scar	• Intrauterine growth retardation

Table 53.6: Fetal/maternal indications of cesarean section

Fetal	Maternal	Maternal-fetal
Nonreassuring FHR	Obstructive benign and malignant tumors	Cephalopelvic disproportion
Breech	Large vulvar condyloma	Failure to progress
Prematurity	Abdominal cervical cerclage	Placental abruption
IUGR	Vaginal stenosis/atresia	Placenta previa
Herpes simplex virus		
Congenital anomalies		
Maternal HIV infection		

Preoperative Preparation

Cesarean section is done in varied situation. It can be clean elective surgery to very high risk situation for mother and baby. Beside this women can easily pass from low risk to high risk category. So preoperative check list in cesarean section is important, the following points should be check listed:

a. **Investigation checklist:** The patient hemoglobin, blood Gr/Rh factor, blood sugar level, Hepatitis BAg, HIV I and II, (after voluntary counseling), and ultrasound records for fetal gestational age, weight and malpresentation are reviewed.
b. **Drug allergies are noted.**
c. If patient is anemic, blood should be sent for cross-matching.
d. **Vaginal swab culture and sensitivity** should be sent, particularly in emergency handled cases.
e. **The stomach should be preferably empty:** Non-particulate antacid (0.3 molar sodium citrate 30 ml) is given orally before surgery to neutralize existing gastric acid. Injection Metoclopromide hydrochloride and H_2 receptor antagonist like Ranitidine injection is given half to one hour before surgery. It safeguards the patients against the complication of acid aspiration (Mandelsen's syndrome).
f. **Informed consent is taken**, which should mention the indication of cesarean, any additional risk for mother and fetus, and names of the team of cesarean mentioning anesthetist and pediatrician.
g. Abdominal wall and vulva of patient are shaved from umbilicus to mons pubis laterally up to iliac crest and antiseptic is applied.
h. **Preoperative catheterization is must:** Catheter is kept in place till the end of operation.
i. Fetal heart sound should be checked once more at this stage.
j. Obstetric team for cesarean section includes – senior consultant, junior resident, anesthetist, neonatologist, and trained paramedical staff for assisting, running and neonatal management.

Anesthetic for Cesarean Section

The anesthetic choices are:
a. **Spinal:** Intrathecal administration of 0.8 to 1.0 ml of 5% xylocaine.
b. **Epidural:** Single shot or continuous with the help of an epidural catheter using 0.5% Marcaine or 5% Xylocaine.
c. **General anesthetic:** Induction with 250 mg Thiopentol followed by intravenous Scoline and endotracheal intubation. The tube is connected to Boyle's apparatus, which administers a combination of nitrous oxide and oxygen.
d. **Local anesthetic:** Only in bad emergency situation where anesthetic is not available, where layer wise infiltration with 0.5% xylocaine with Adrenaline is used.

Position for Cesarean Section

The patient is placed in supine position for surgery. It is better to have a 15% tilt to her side to prevent supine hypotension syndrome and maintain satisfactory placental perfusion.

Steps of Cesarean Section

A. **Abdominal incision:** Type of abdominal incision should be guided by operator's experience, site of previous operation scar and obstetric need of the patient. Following types of abdominal incision can be made.
   a. Vertical: It is infraumbilical and placed in midline or peramedian. It gives the fastest access to lower uterine segment, good exposure, less blood loss. So in emergency situation like cord prolapse, severe fetal distress, impending uterine rupture and severe maternal hemorrhage this can be choice of incision.
   b. Transverse: They are incision of choice because they are cosmetically superior, chance of incisional hernia is rare and postoperative recovery is fast. The various types of transverse incision are:
      i. Pfannensteil: It is curvilinear, 15 cm long given at pubic crease.
      ii. Joel Cohen: Straight, 2 finger breadth above Pfannensteil incision.

   Advantage and limitation of transverse incision in cesarean section is summarized in Table 53.7.

B. **Uterine incision:** After opening the abdominal cavity, the Doyen's or Morris retractor is introduced. The intestines are packed away using sponges draped in warm saline. Any dextrorotation of the uterus is noted and corrected so that uterine incision is centered. Now following type of incision can be given:
   a. Low transverse cesarean section: It is the most common incision used in practice. It is associated with less blood loss, gives adequate access to effect delivery and it provides the strongest postoperative repair. In this after peritoneal cavity is opened, the bladder fold of peritoneum is identified by visualizing loose peritoneum covering lower uterine segment, picked up with tissue forceps and incised transversely. The bladder is bluntly separated from the anterior aspect of the uterus inferiorly for a distance of 3-4 cm. A transverse incision is made through anterior uterine wall with scalpel. Using either scissors or fingers the transverse incision is extended in similar fashion and extended superiorly at the lateral edges in order to avoid the uterine vessels. *It is very important to make uterine incision large enough to allow delivery of fetal head and trunk of fetus without tearing into uterine vessels that course in lateral margin of uterus.*

Table 53.7: Advantage and limitations of transverse incision in cesarean section

Advantages	Limitations
1. Preferred cosmetically	1. A little longer time
2. Less painful	2. Limitation of view of upper abdomen
3. Allow early ambulation	3. Difficult if ovarian tumor and large myoma
4. Lower risk of subsequent herniation	4. A little less space in delivery of large baby/malpresentation

C. **Delivery of baby:** The membrane are ruptured, if intact. The blood mixed amniotic fluid is sucked out by continuous suction. The retractor is removed. The head is delivered by hooking the hand with the fingers which are carefully insinuated between the lower uterine flap and head until the palm is placed below the head. As the head is down to the incision line, the assistant applies pressure on the fundus. If head is located deep in the pelvis, the head can be safely pushed up by an assistant inserting a hand into the vagina to elevate the fetal head for ease of delivery. To minimize the aspiration by the fetus of the amniotic fluid and its content, the exposed nose and mouth are aspirated with mucus extractor, before thorax is delivered. The shoulders are than delivered using gentle traction plus fundal pressure. The rest of body is readily delivered.

D. **Delivery of placenta:** As soon as the shoulder is delivered, an intravenous infusion containing about 20 unit of oxytocin per liter is allowed at rate of 10 ml/minute, till uterus contracts satisfactorily. **Placenta should be allowed to deliver spontaneously.** It cause less blood loss and reduced incidence of postcesarean endometritis as compared to manual removal of placenta. Care must be taken to strip the membrane completely along with vernix caseosa. Dilatation of internal os is not required. Exploration of the uterine cavity is desirable.

E. **Suturing of uterus:** After delivery of baby and placenta, the uterus is exteriorized and full margin of lower uterine segment is followed. The uterine incision is generally closed in two layers using no 1 or 1.0 Vicryl or chromic catgut no. 1 on round body needle. It is undesirable to penetrate the decidual layer because of possibility of infection. Adequate hemostasis is achieved.

F. Bladder peritoneum can be reapproximated with suture or left in place.

G. **Adnexa are observed for any pathology,** uterine is reposited in the peritoneal cavity. Peritoneal toilet is done, and instrument and sponge count is done.

H. **Abdomen is closed in layers;** wound is dressed with sterile transparent dressing.

I. **Vaginal toilet is done,** uterine contractility is assured and any unusual bleeding is noted and treated. At the

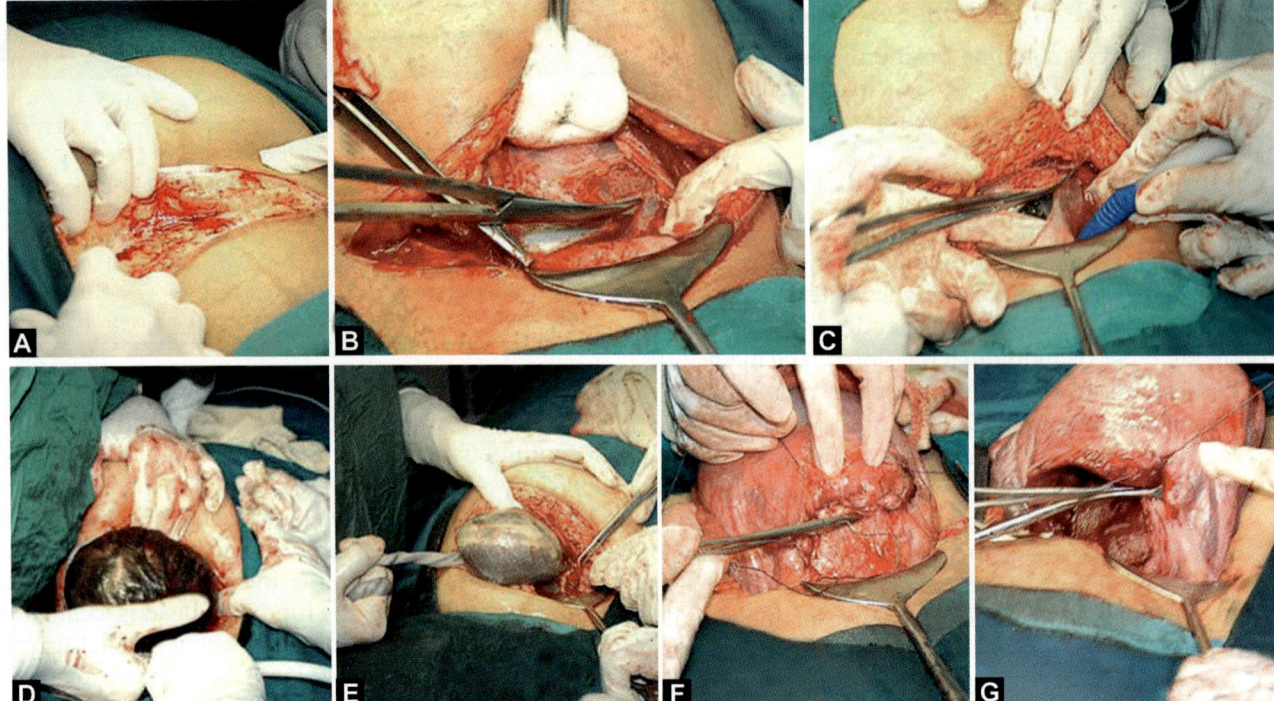

Figs 53.10A to G: (A) Abdominal incision by transverse Joel Cohen; (B) Dissection of bladder from anterior surface of uterus; (C) Uterus is incised transversely in lower uterine segment; (D) Delivery of baby; (E) Spontaneous delivery of placenta; (F and G) Suturing of uterus in two layers

same time presence of clear urine in catheter is looked for. If there is more than a faint degree of hematuria, indwelling catheterization is advocated.

Steps of cesarean section are shown in Figures 53.10A to G.

Other types of Uterine Incision

A. **Low vertical uterine incision:** It is sometime needed in preterm babies, where lower segment is poorly found, low vertical incision can be given, as it may be extended upwards if needed.
B. **High vertical incision:** Women with high vertical incision and classic cesarean section are at greater risk of uterine rupture with subsequent pregnancies and should be advised strongly for elective cesarean in next pregnancy.

The indications of high vertical or classic uterine incision in today's obstetrics are:

a. Placenta previa with highly vascular lower uterine segment.
b. In some cases of transverse lie with back down.
c. Preterm delivery.
d. In cancer cervix.
e. Lower segment can not be reached due to adhesions, presence of fibroids or marked contraction of the pelvis.
f. Threatened rupture or dehiscence of previous classical scar.
g. Rare case of conjoined twins.

Complication of Cesarean Section

Beside inherent anesthetic complication, the maternal complication of cesarean section can be as follows:

Preoperative

a. Postpartum hemorrhage.
b. Wound infection and endometritis. Administration of prophylactic antibiotics and ensuring hemostasis prior to closure of abdomen decreases the incidence of these complications.
c. Injury to uterus, ovaries, tubes, bowel, bladder or ureters.

Uterine incision can be extended, there may be hematoma formation. **Bladder** injury can occur, during opening of parietal peritoneum or during mobilization of urinary bladder. **Ureteric** injury occurs, where incision of lower uterine segment is extended laterally and without proper identification attempts are made to suture it. **Bowel** injury can occur during opening of parietal peritoneum or during adhesion dissection particularly in cases of prior abdominal surgery.

Postoperative Complication

a. Postpartum hemorrhage: Average blood loss during cesarean section is 1000 ml. There can be significant blood loss requiring blood transfusion.
b. Obstetric shock: Usually it is related to the blood loss but it may occur when cesarean operation is done following prolonged labor without correcting pre-existing dehydration and ketoacidosis.
c. Anesthetic: Aspiration atelectasis or aspiration pneumonitis.

d. Infection: Endomyometritis, urinary tract infection, and wound infection can occur. Risk factors are prolonged duration of labor and rupture of membrane before surgery, number of vaginal examination. Prophylactic antibiotic reduces the risk significantly.
e. Fistula.
f. Paralytic ileus or adhesive intestinal obstruction.
g. Wound complication like sanguineous or purulent discharge, hematoma, and dehiscence and burst abdomen.

Remote Complications

a. Incisional hernia.
b. Chronic pain in abdomen due to adhesions.
c. Rupture of scar in subsequent pregnancies: The incidence of uterine rupture is approximately 4-9% in classic uterus incision and 0.1-1.5% in low transverse scars. Rupture of classic scar usually is catastrophic and present as hemorrhagic shock. Rupture of low transverse scar is usually more subtle and almost always occurring during active labor. The most common presenting feature is sudden change in fetal heart rate pattern, vaginal bleeding and pain at prior incision site. If rupture is suspected, prompt surgery is warranted.

Perinatal Morbidity

It may appear that cesarean delivery is the safest for the baby but this may be not be the case. Following fetal problems can occur associated with cesarean delivery:
a. Transient tachypnea of newborn is more common with cesarean delivery.
b. Iatrogenic prematurity.
c. Development of respiratory distress syndrome is more common with elective cesarean section.
d. The risk of fetal hemorrhage and hypoxia is present when the placenta is encountered below the uterine incision.
e. Fetal laceration of baby at the time of making uterine incision (0.2-0.4%).
Because of potential fetal problem in cesarean section, each infant must be examined by a trained professional at the time of cesarean section.

Additional Surgery with Cesarean Section

a. *Adnexal surgery:* Adnexal surgery can be undertaken during cesarean section, after delivery of the newborn and repair of uterus.
b. *Myomectomy:* Generally myomectomy is *Not* preformed at time of cesarean section because of excessive blood loss and potential difficulty with hemostasis. But if location of the myoma interferes with closure of the uterus incision, myomectomy may be necessary.
c. *Elective cesarean hysterectomy with known uterus pathology:* With cesarean hysterectomy elective or emergent cases there is increased risk of morbidity compared with elective hysterectomy of a nonpregnant uterus. Generally elective cesarean hysterectomy is performed only in cases of malignancies (cervical, ovarian) when delay in therapy could worsen the prognosis. Other uterine pathologies such as myoma can be surgically treated after recovery from the cesarean section, when the pelvic organs and blood flow have returned to their prepregnant state.

Indication of cesarean hysterectomy are:
a. Uncontrollable bleeding due to atony 43%.
b. Uterine rupture when repair is impossible or carries unacceptable morbidity (13%).
c. Extension of low transverse incision (10%).
d. Some cases of placenta accreta, increta or percreta.
e. Leiomyomata preventing uterine closure and hemostasis
f. Malignancy.

Maternal Mortality

Overall maternal mortality rate for cesarean section is 3-30 per 100,000 depending on the population studies and the circumstances surrounding the cesarean section. The figure is comparable to mortality rate for vaginal delivery. The major cases of death are:
a. Hemorrhagic shock.
b. Anesthetic hazards.
c. Infection.
d. Thromboembolic disorders.

Perinatal Mortality

It ranges from 5 to 10% and cause is mostly related to complications which are indication of cesarean section. The major cause of perinatal mortality are:
a. Fetal asphyxia usually pre-existing.
b. Prematurity.
c. Infection.
d. Intracranial hemorrhage while attempting breech delivery through small incision.

VAGINAL BIRTH AFTER CESAREAN SECTION

Initially concern over rupture of uterine scar in future pregnancy led to the recommendation not to attempt normal labor after one cesarean section but to go for repeat cesarean section. This was summarized that once a cesarean section, always a cesarean section. In last 10 years, this thought has been reexamined. As overall switching of upper uterus segment scar to lower segment incision reduced the incidence of scar rupture in subsequent delivery from 22-32% to 6.4%. Beside this prophylactic antibiotic, good surgical technique has further reduced the risk of scar rupture. So now it is predicted that most of the women with one prior cesarean section should be considered for vaginal delivery in a well equipped place. Women attempting a vaginal birth after cesarean are said to be undergoing trial of labor.

Selection for a Candidate for Vaginal Birth After Cesarean

ACOG recommends following criteria for selection of vaginal birth after cesarean section:
a. One or two prior low transverse incision cesarean.
b. Clinically adequate pelvis.
c. No other uterine scar or previous rupture.
d. Physician availability and close fetal monitoring system.
e. Availability of anesthetist and personnel for immediate cesarean delivery.
f. There is no other contraindication to vaginal delivery, e.g. placenta previa or malpresentation.
g. Appropriate counseling regarding risk of attempting vaginal birth after cesarean.

In suitable candidate and high level setup success rate of vaginal delivery is 60-80% with 1% risk of uterine rupture.

Management of Vaginal Birth After Cesarean

1. Antenatal follow-up, good clinical examination and counseling of patient is done.
2. In history the specific factors associated with high risk of uterus rupture are identified. These risk factors are:
   a. Upper uterine segment incision.
   b. More number of cesarean.
   c. No history of vaginal delivery.
   d. Shorten interdelivery period
   e. Uterine anomalies.
   f. Fetal macrosomia.
3. It is always better to allow natural onset of labor than induction. Though oxytocin induction as well augmentation is not contraindicated in vaginal birth after cesarean but close following of fetal heart rate and uterine activity by cardiotocography is must.
4. Vigilant monitoring of maternal and fetal status with facility of immediate cesarean section if need arise.
5. Routine uterus exploration after delivery of baby is not recommended but should be done if there is:
   a. Excessive bleeding.
   b. Hematuria.
   c. Persistent or unusual pain.
   d. Sudden hypotension.

DILEMMA OF VAGINAL BIRTH AFTER CESAREAN

The women should be appropriately counseled. The argument in favor of vaginal birth after cesarean is that successful vaginal birth after cesarean section allows the mother to avoid maternal and fetal risk of cesarean section. Many women also value the experience of vaginal delivery. But the strongest argument against attempting vaginal birth after cesarean is the risk of uterine rupture and potential for morbidity and even fetal mortality that goes along with the uterus rupture. It is uncommon- less than 1% in properly selected case, but it is potentially disastrous. Many women

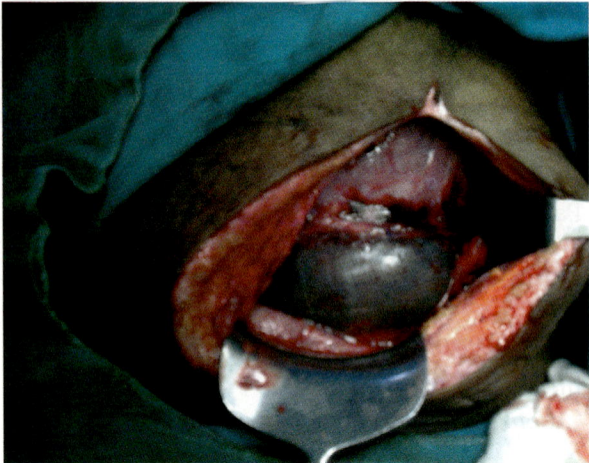

Figs 53.11: Scar dehiscence from previous lower segment scar showing bulge of amniotic membrane

and physician are also reluctant to subject themselves to a possible long labor and finally to go for cesarean section (Fig. 53.11).

MULTIPLE CHOICE QUESTIONS

1. Contraindication of Ventouse extraction is:
   a. Prematurity
   b. Brow presentation
   c. Fetal distress
   d. Floating head
   Ans. a
2. Which statement is true regarding Ventouse:
   a. Minor scalp abrasions and subgaleal hematoma to newborn are more frequent than forceps
   b. Can be applied when fetal head is above the level of ischial spine
   c. Maternal trauma is more frequent than forceps
   d. Cannot be used when fetal head is not rotated
   Ans. a
3. Last complication in outlet forceps is:
   a. Complete perineal tear
   b. Vulvar hematoma
   c. Extension of episiotomy
   d. Cervical tear
   Ans. d
4. In heart disease prophylactic forceps is applied at head status of:
   a. –1
   b. +1
   c. 0
   d. +2
   Ans. d
5. All of the following statement are true for episiotomy *except*:
   a. Allows widening of birth canal
   b. Can be either midline or mediolateral
   c. Involvement of anal sphincter is classified 3rd–4th degree perineal tear
   d. Midline episiotomy bleed less, are easier to repair and heal more quickly
   Ans. a

6. Contraindication to Ventouse delivery include all of the following *except*:
   a. Fetal coagulopathy
   b. Extreme prematurity
   c. Mentotransverse position
   d. Occipitotransverse position
   Ans. d
7. The following is always an indication of cesarean section *except*:
   a. Abruption placenta
   b. Untreated stage of Ib Ca cervix
   c. Active primary genital herpes
   d. Type IV placenta previa (major previa)
   Ans. a
8. An absolute indication for LSCS in cases of a heart disease is:
   a. Coarctation of aorta
   b. Eisenmenger syndrome
   c. Ebstein's anomaly
   d. Pulmonary stenosis
   Ans. a
9. Episiotomy is best done:
   a. Medially
   b. Laterally
   c. Mediolaterally
   d. J shaped
   Ans. c
10. Paracervical block is associated with the danger of:
    a. Inhibition of labor
    b. Fetal bradycardia
    c. Increased blood loss
    d. Atony of uterus
    Ans. b
11. The most important treatment of badly infected episiotomy is:
    a. Securing culture
    b. Antibiotic
    c. Hot sitz bath
    d. Drainage
    Ans. d
12. Absolute indication of LSCS is:
    a. Previous LSCS for transverse lie
    b. Plastic repair of VVF
    c. Myomectomy scar after 2 years
    d. Previous LSCS for APH
    Ans. b
13. Indication of classical cesarean section is:
    a. Obstructed labor
    b. Ca Cx
    c. Placenta previa
    d. Twin pregnancy
    Ans. b
14. The preferred management for neglected shoulder presentation in rural hospital in India is:
    a. Wait for spontaneous delivery
    b. Embryotomy
    c. Cesarean section
    d. None of the above
    Ans. c
15. A woman delivers a 9 lb infant with a midline episiotomy and suffers a third degree perineal tear. Inspection shows which of the following structure is intact:
    a. Anal sphincter
    b. Perineal body
    c. Perineal muscle
    d. Rectal mucosa
    Ans. d
16. A patient with third degree perineal tear presenting after 1 week repair should be done:
    a. Immediately
    b. 2 weeks
    c. After 6 weeks
    d. After 12 weeks
    Ans. d
17. Most suitable method of treating 4" size episiotomy hematoma is by:
    a. Evacuation
    b. Magsulf compression
    c. Cold compression
    d. Marsupialization
    Ans. a
18. Third degree perineal tear is involvement of:
    a. Vaginal mucosa
    b. Urethral mucosa
    c. Levator Ani muscle
    d. Anal sphincter
    Ans. d
19. In Bishop scores all are included *except*:
    a. Effacement of cervix
    b. Dilatation of cervix
    c. Station of head
    d. Interspinal diameter
    Ans. d
20. All of the following are used for induction of labor *except*:
    a. $PGF_2\alpha$ tablet
    b. PGE_2 tablet
    c. PGE_2 gel
    d. Misoprostol
    Ans. a
21. All of the following drugs are effective for cervical ripening during pregnancy *except*:
    a. Prostaglandin E_2
    b. Oxytocin
    c. Progesterone
    d. Misoprostol
    Ans. c
22. AROM is contraindicated in:
    a. Placenta previa
    b. Hydramnios
    c. Accidental hemorrhage
    d. Twins
    Ans. a
23. Indication of induction of labor is:
    a. Placenta previa
    b. PIH at term
    c. Heart disease
    d. Breech
    Ans. b

54 Puerperium

It may seem a strange principle to enunciate that the very prerequirement of a hospital is that it should do the sick no harm.

GENERAL CONSIDERATION

The puerperium or the postpartum period is the period of time immediately after delivery until 6 weeks postpartum. It is the period of adjustment after delivery when the anatomic and physiologic changes of pregnancy are reversed and body returns to the normal nonpregnant state. The postpartum period has been arbitrarily divided into three parts:

a. **Immediate puerperium:** In first 24 hours after parturition when acute postanesthetic or postdelivery complication may occur.
b. **Early puerperium:** This extends until the first week postpartum.
c. **Remote puerperium:** Which include the period of time required for involution of genital organs and return of menstruation usually by 6 weeks in nonlactating women and return of normal cardiovascular and psychological function, which may require months.

Anatomical and Physiological Changes in Puerperium

a. **Uterus:** The uterus weigh 1000 – 1200 gm immediately after delivery. As a result of involution it shrinks to 50-100 gm in four weeks. It is accomplished by reduction in the size of uterus muscle fibers, marked reduction in vascularity of uterus due to thrombosis in uterine vascular system. The superficial endometrial layer sloughs contributing to the lochia. Regeneration of the new endometrial glands and stroma from the basal layer begins in the first week and by the third postpartum week the entire endometrium is restored except at the placental site which takes about 6 weeks.
b. **Lochia:** It is physiological postpartum uterine discharge consisting of blood and necrotic decidua. Initially it is *Lochia rubra*. It is reddish in color, it change to brownish color and serous consistency the *lochia serosa*, which last for 1 week and then become *lochia alba*, which is whitish turbid fluid. The lochial discharge usually persists for about 4 weeks and may continue to 8 weeks after delivery.
c. **Cervix:** Cervix contract slowly and by end of first week a canal is formed. There is some degree of laceration of cervix so that a multiparous circular external os become slit like in parous women.
d. **Vagina:** Vagina diminishes in size and caliber and resumes its normal rugosities but prepregnant size and elasticity of tissue is never regained.
e. **Ovulation:** Ovulation suppression is related to persistently elevated prolactin levels in the lactating female. They remain elevated up to 6 weeks postpartum, where as in nonlactating female, they normalize by 3 weeks. Additionally estrogen levels remain low in a lactating mother while estrogen begins to rise and reach normal level 2-3 weeks after delivery in nonlactating women.
f. **Urinary tract:** Elevated glomerular filtration rate and renal plasma flow returns to normal by 6 weeks. Dilatation of renal calyces, pelvis and ureter resolves by 8 weeks postpartum.
g. **Abdominal wall:** Abdominal wall become flabby and remains soft and poorly toned for many weeks. Striae gravidarum become depigmented and lighter in color known as striae albicans. No treatment has been found to be effective in prevention and treatment of these striae.
h. **Cardiovascular system:** Change in heart rate, cardiac output and blood volume during pregnancy return to baseline by 6 weeks after delivery.
i. **Lactation and breastfeeding:** The preparation of lactogenesis starts in the third trimester when the lobuloalveolar complex is stimulated to increase the synthesis of enzyme necessary for production of milk components. Estrogen, progesterone, cortisol, insulin, prolactin and human placental lactogen all stimulate growth and development of mammary gland. After delivery estrogen and progesterone level decline rapidly and release the inhibitory influence over prolactin and lactation is started.

Care During Puerperium

Objective in management of puerperium are:
a. Restoration of health to prepregnancy status.
b. Promote lactation.
c. Prevent infection.
d. Care of infant and advice on immunization.

Immediate Care

In this period women is observed to ensure that women is stable, has a quick recovery and learns to take care of newborn.

a. **Pulse and blood pressure is monitored frequently** for first hour which is the most critical time for postpartum hemorrhage. Amount of bleeding, size and contractility of uterus is noted.
b. **Care of vulva and episiotomy:** Routine cleaning is done and analgesic with antibiotics is administered. In extended tears sitz bath is given to reduce swelling. Stool softeners can be given to promote a normal bowel movement. If patient is experiencing an excessive pain, it is important to examine her perineum to rule out hematoma or infection.

Conduct and Management of Normal Puerperium

Most patients will benefit from 2-4 days of hospitalization after delivery. Only 3% of women with a vaginal delivery and 9% of women having cesarean section have a childbirth related complications requiring prolonged postpartum hospitalization or readmission. Earlier discharge is acceptable in select mother and infant who have uncomplicated labors and delivery, discharge criteria should be met and follow-up care provided. The puerperal care includes the following:

a. **Early ambulation:** Early ambulation reduces incidence of bladder complication, constipation, puerperal venous thrombosis and pulmonary embolism. Exercise can be gradually resumed as soon as medically and physically safe.
b. **Bladder care:** In obstetric patients there is chance of over distention of bladder especially if there has been difficult labor, use of oxytocic drug and reduced sensation of urinary bladder because of epidural analgesia or reflex spasm due to pain in episiotomy or vaginal laceration. All puerperal patients must be encouraged to void within 4 hours of delivery. Women who cannot void it is best to leave an indwelling catheter for 24 hours. The incidence of true asymptomatic bacteriuria is approximately 5% in the early puerperium. In case of confirmed bacteriuria antibiotic treatment should be given, otherwise bacteriuria will persist in nearly 30% of patient. Three days of therapy is sufficient and prolonged antibiotic exposure to the lactating mother is avoided.
c. **Bowel function:** Constipation may occur in the early puerperium because of decreased tone of bowel during pregnancy, postpartum fluid loss by other routes and decreased food intake during labor, reflex spasm due to episiotomy or painful, hemorrhoids. High fiber diet, mild laxative are usually effective.
d. **Diet:** A regular diet and early feeding is encouraged as soon as the patient regains her appetite. Proteins food, fruits, vegetable, milk products and high fluid intake are recommended especially for lactating mother. Daily vitamin mineral iron supplement should be continued in early puerperium. Following cesarean section also early intake of solid food is desirable.
e. **Care of vulva and puerperium:** An episiotomy or repaired laceration should be inspected daily. Vulva is cleaned always from above downwards moving towards the anus. Ice pack, Sitz's bath can be given in episiotomy wound with use of pain killers and local anesthetic spray.
f. **Resumption of coitus:** Sexual activity can be resumed when all lochial discharge has cleared and woman is recovered and comfortable. It usually takes 6 weeks or longer time.
g. **Postpartum immunization:** The Rh-D negative woman who is not immunized and whose infant is D positive is given 300 μg of anti-D immunoglobulin shortly after delivery. Women who are not already immune to rubella should be offered vaccination before discharge. Unless contraindicated Diphtheria, tetanus, toxoid booster injection can be given.

Contraception and sterilization: During hospital stay the various contraceptive methods suitable for the patient depending on breastfeeding should be discussed. In exclusive breastfeeding women there is less than 2% risk of pregnancy. The contraceptive methods appropriate for lactating mothers are progestin only pill, depot medroxyprogesterone acetate (DMPA) injection, intrauterine contraceptive device or barrier methods such as diaphragms or condoms. Combined oral contraceptives are not recommended in breastfeeding women for first six months. Tubal sterilization is the procedure of choice for women desiring permanent sterilization. It can be performed easily at time of cesarean section and 24-48 hours after an uncomplicated vaginal delivery. Sterilization is not recommended in young women of low parity or when neonatal outcome is in doubt. Postponing tubal sterilization for 6-8 weeks may be desirable for many couple, because it allows time to ensure that infant is healthy and to fully understand the implication of permanent sterilization.

Discharge examination and instruction: Before discharge the women should receive instruction concerning the anticipated normal physiological changes of the puerperium including lochial pattern, weight loss and technique and common problems of breastfeeding and other problems like fever, excessive vaginal bleeding, leg pain, swelling and tenderness.

Follow-up Visits

At the postpartum visit, 4-6 weeks after discharge from hospital, the patient weight, blood pressure should be recorded. A suitable diet may be prescribed if the patient has not returned to her approximate prepregnancy weight. If patient was anemic previously, the complete blood count should be determined. Persistence of uterine bleeding demands investigation and definitive treatment. The breast should be examined for appropriate lactation and presence of any mass or nipple laceration. The episiotomy incision and repaired laceration should be examined. The patient may resume full activity or employment if her course to this point has been uneventful. Once again contraception should be discussed. The postnatal visit is an important opportunity to consider general disorders as backache, depression, infant feeding and immunization. The rapport established between the obstetrician and the patient during the prenatal and postpartum period provide a unique opportunity to establish preventive health programs in subsequent years.

ABNORMAL PUERPERIUM

Puerperal Fever

Puerperal fever is defined as a temperature of 38°C (100.4°F) or higher on any two of the first 10 days postpartum excluding the first 24 hours. Mildly elevated temperature is not uncommon in the first 24 hours but any fever associated with tachycardia warrants investigation.

Incidence

Puerperal infectious morbidity affects 2-8% of pregnant women and is more common in those of low socioeconomic status, who have undergone operative delivery with premature rupture of membrane, long labor and who have multiple pelvic examination.

Cause of Postpartum and Puerperal Fever

The common causes are:
a. Endometritis.
b. Thrombophlebitis.
c. Mastitis.
d. Urinary tract infection.
e. Wound infection.
f. Pulmonary infection.

Endometritis: The most common cause of postpartum fever is endometritis. It is a major problem in women delivered by cesarean section. The common *pathogen* responsible are Gr β *Streptococcus, Bacteroides, Enterococci, E. coli, Klebsiella* and *Proteus* (Table 54.1).

Symptoms are fever and chills, lower abdominal pain, and malodorous vaginal discharge.

Risk factors for infection are enumerated in (Table 54.2).

On *examination* the patient has *abdominal tenderness*, mucopurulent vaginal discharge and uterine tenderness on palpation (Table 54.3).

Table 54.1: Organism associated with puerperal genital infection

1. Aerobes
   a. Gram-positive:
      i. Hemolytic *Streptococcus*
      ii. *Staphylococcus epidermics*
   b. Gram-negative:
      i. *E. coli*
      ii. *Hemophilus influenzae*
      iii. *Klebsiella pneumoniae*
      iv. *Pseudomonas aeruginosa*
      v. *Proteus mirabilis*
2. Anaerobes
   a. *Peptococcus sp*
   b. *Peptostreptococcus sp*
   c. *Bacteroides*
   d. *Fusobacterium sp*
   e. *Fusobacterium*
3. Miscellaneous
   a. *Chlamydia trachomatis*
   b. *Mycoplasma hominis*
   c. *Ureaplasma urealyticum*

Table 54.2: Risk factor for puerperal infection

- Antenatal intrapartum infection
- Cesarean section
- Prolonged rupture of membranes
- Prolonged labor
- Multiple vaginal examination
- Internal fetal monitoring
- Instrumental delivery
- Manual removal of the placenta
- Retained product of conception
- Nonobstetric, e.g. obesity, diabetes, HIV

Table 54.3: Symptom and sign of puerperal pelvic infection

Symptoms:
- Malaise, headache, fever, rigor
- Abdominal discomfort, vomiting and diarrhea
- Offensive lochia
- Secondary postpartum hemorrhage

Sign of Puerperal Pelvis Infection:
- Pyrexia and tachycardia
- Uterus—Boggy, tender and larger
- Infected wound—cesarean/perineal
- Peritonism
- Paralytic ileus
- Indurated adnexa (perimetritis)
- Bogginess in pelvic (abscess)

Table 54.4: Investigation for puerperal genital infection	
Investigation	Abnormalities detected
• Full blood count	• Anemia, leukocytosis, thrombocytopenia
• Urea and electrolytes	• Fluid and electrolyte imbalance
• High vaginal swab and blood culture	• Infection screen
• Pelvic ultrasound	• Retained products, pelvic abscess
• Clotting screen (hemorrhage or shock)	• Disseminated intravascular coagulation
• Arterial blood gas (shock)	• Acidosis and hypoxia

Investigations

Table 54.4 summarizes possible investigations in puerperal genital infection which shouldbe guided by clinical situation.

Treatment: It is usually treated with intravenous Clindamycin and Gentamicin combination to provide coverage of most aerobic and anaerobic organism. Once symptoms have subsided and the patient is afebrile for 24-48 hours, I/V antibiotic therapy can be discontinued. It is not necessary to continue with oral antibiotics.

Complications: Potential complications from postpartum endometritis include :
a. Septic thrombophlebitis.
b. Pelvic peritonitis.
c. Sepsis and septic shock.
d. Pelvic abscess.
e. Future infertility.
f. Chronic pelvic pain.

Prevention:
a. Prophylactic antibiotic for all cesarean section. Antibiotic are administered after cord clamping. Cefezolin (1 gm) or Clindamycin can be given.
b. Gentle tissue handling.
c. Meticulous hemostasis.
d. Wound irrigation.
e. Intrapartum treatment of intra-amniotic infection.
f. Adherence to protocol for active management of labor.

Septic Pelvic Thrombophlebitis

Septic pelvic thrombophlebitis complicates 1 in 2000 to 3000 deliveries. It is more common following cesarean delivery and preceded by bacterial infection in the placental implantation site or the uterine incision. **It is a diagnosis of exclusion** and made when a patient on antibiotics for endometritis continue to exhibit spiked temperature and all other sources of fever have been ruled out. MRI may show obstructed pelvic veins but it is usually not necessary.

Management: The antimicrobial therapy for postpartum endometritis should be continued. Therapeutic heparin may be added and defervescence usually occurs within 72 hours of therapeutic heparin and most patients do not need anticoagulation on discharge.

Mastitis

Mastitis is a localized infection of the breast that usually occurs between the first and fifth weeks of postpartum, but can happen any time. Approximately 1-2% of breastfeeding women experience mastitis. The symptoms are sore reddened area on one breast which may become indurated or erythematous. The patient can experience high grade fever with chills and malaise.

Causative Organism

The most common organism is *Staphylococcus aureus*, other are *H. Influenzae, Klebsiella pneumoniae, E. coli, Enterococcus faecalis,* and *Enterobacter cloacae.*

Treatment

First line treatment is Dicloxacillin 500 mg 4 times a day. Women who are allergic to penicillin should be given Erythromycin. Analgesic, rest, good fluid intake and are given for symptomatic relief of fever and discomfort. It is also important to encourage patients to continue breast-feeding.

Breast Abscess

Breast abscess may occur in 0.4-0.5% of lactating mother.
Symptoms and signs: Patient is febrile in spite of antibiotics. On examination there is palpable mass and fluctuation, which may or may not be tender.
Treatment: Surgical incision and drainage under adequate anesthetic is essential.

Urinary Tract Infection

It occurs in 3-10% of patient and only 2% of patients are symptomatic. Most common organism is *E. coli* and Gr B streptococci followed by staphylococci and saprophyticus, *E. faecalis, Proteus* and *Klebsiella.*
Symptoms: Symptoms are dysuria, frequency, urgency, and low grade fever.
Management: Urine culture should be obtained. Treatment can be given empirically according to the common pathogens. If symptoms are severe, antibiotics with specific activity against the common organisms are the cornerstone of therapy. The most common drugs are nitrofurantoins, trimethoprim sulfamethoxazole, oral cephalosporin and Ampicillin. Sulfa-antibiotics can be used safely in women who are breastfeeding if the infants are term without

hyperbilirubinemia or suspected glucose 6 phosphate dehydrogenase deficiency. High fluid intake is encouraged.

Wound Infection

Perineal infection: Wound infections of episiotomy are infrequent (0.5-3%). The excellent local blood supply is suggested as an explanation for this. Risk factors are poor perineal hygiene, infected lochia and faecal contamination. Symptoms are perineal pain, discomfort, swelling and unhealthy discharge from wound. Common organisms are *Staphylococcus aureus*.
Treatment: A swab can be taken for culture and sensitivity. Broad spectrum antibiotics can be started empirically and changed if required according to culture and sensitivity report. Analgesic and hot fomentation, sitz bath is soothing. If there is pus, the stitches should be opened to allow drainage.
Cesarean wound infection: It occurs in 4-12% of cesarean patients. Use of prophylactic antibiotic has significantly reduced the incidence. Risk factors are obesity, diabetes, prolonged hospitalization, and prolonged rupture of membranes, chorioamnionitis, endomyometritis, prolonged labor, emergency cesarean section and anemia. **Causative organisms** are contamination from the vagina. *S. aureus* is most common followed by *Streptococcus*, *E. coli* and other gram-negative organism. **Symptoms** are abdominal wound induration, erythema, purulent discharge and fever.
Treatment: Broad spectrum antibiotic and drainage if there is a collection at the wound site.

Respiratory Tract Infection

Respiratory tract infection after cesarean section has been reported in 0.5-5% of women. Atelectasis occurs is the first 72 hours postoperatively. It persists with low grade fever and basilar rales. If left untreated, it may progress to pneumonitis.
Treatment: Deep breathing exercise, early ambulation reduces the progression. Broad spectrum antibiotic like erythromycin, cephalosporin and steam inhalation should be advised. In prevalent area tuberculosis should be ruled out by X-ray, sputum acid fast bacilli examination.

Puerperal Venous Thrombosis

The incidence of thrombosis in pregnancy is 1 in 1000 pregnancies of these nearly 50% present in puerperal period. Cesarean delivery, delayed ambulation, smoking, pre-eclampsia and thrombophilias are risk factors.

Postpartum Neuropsychiatric Complications

Peripheral nerve palsy: Nerve palsies involving pelvic nerves or parts of the lumbosacral plexus results from pressure by the presenting part or trauma by obstetric forceps. Typically the palsy occurs after prolonged labor in a nullipara and presents as unilateral foot drop. Most cases resolve spontaneously in days or weeks.

Seizures: Postpartum seizures immediately raise the possibility of eclampsia, but if the interval since delivery is more than 48 hours, other etiologies should be considered. In the absence of history of pregnancy induced hypertension or epilepsy, a thorough evaluation is done to determine the cause of seizures.
Postpartum blues: There is transient depressive illness found in approximately 30-70% of women. It appears as tearfulness, anxiety, irritation, restlessness, forgetfulness within first week of delivery. It is self-limiting, and usually resolves spontaneously by postpartum day 10. No treatment is necessary. Reassurance and increased rest is beneficial. According to Kaplan the sudden decrease in estrogen and progesterone immediately after delivery may also contribute to the disorder, but treatment with these hormones are not effective.
Postpartum depression: The incidence of true postpartum depression is 8-15%. The women with prior history of depressive disorder are more prone to PPD and there is 50-100% recurrence rate in subsequent pregnancies. Symptoms are like nonpregnant state as feeling of worthlessness, markedly diminished interest in all activities, pessimism, and fatigue. In addition the new mother may exhibit ambivalence towards her infant.
Treatment: It comprises of supportive care from health care professional and family. Serotonin reuptake inhibitor as Fluoxetine, Paroxetine, and Sertraline have been found to be effective in treatment of PPD. If symptoms do not lessen promptly with medication, consultation with a psychiatrist is advised.

Postpartum Psychosis

It is a severe mental disorder which occurs in 0.1-0.2% of all postpartum women. It primarily presents within 10-14 days after delivery. Women affected with psychosis loose touch with reality and can be potentially dangerous to themselves and the newborn. Symptoms are like acute psychosis. Women with underlying psychotic disorder and history of depression are highly susceptible.
Treatment: Antipsychotic drugs are mainstay of treatment. Treatment should be supervised by a psychiatrist and require hospitalization. Risk of future puerperal psychosis is 57% and nonpuerperal psychosis is 62%.

Postpartum Thyroiditis

It is autoimmune disorder characterized by a destructive lymphocytic thyroiditis mediated by thyroid microsomal autoantibodies. It is found in 5-10% of postpartum women and usually begins approximately 1-4 months postpartum. Patient presents with complaint of fatigue, palpitation and a goiter may be present.
Management: Prophylthiouracil is ineffective and treatment is only symptomatic relief with alpha blocker. Approximately two third of women return to a euthyroid state and

one-third experience hypothyroidism between 4-8 months postpartum.

Symptoms of hypothyroidism are depression, impaired memory and concentration. At this phase goiter is more common. In this phase thyroxine replacement is given for 12-18 months after which it can gradually be withdrawn. Approximately 10-30% of patients who experience thyroid dysfunction during the postpartum will have permanent hypothyroidism.

MULTIPLE CHOICE QUESTIONS

1. An ovarian cyst is identified in the immediate postpartum period. Time of surgery:
   a. 2 weeks
   b. 6 weeks
   c. 3 months
   d. Immediately
   Ans. d
2. Postpartum decidual secretions present are referred to as:
   a. Lochia
   b. Bleeding per vaginam
   c. Vasa previa
   d. Decidua capsularis
   Ans. a
3. Puerperal pyrexia is fever for 24 hours or more after childbirth if temperature is:
   a. 99°F
   b. 99.5°F
   c. 100°F
   d. 100.4°F
   Ans. d
4. Most common cause of postpartum endometritis is:
   a. *E. coli*
   b. *Gonococcus*
   c. *Streptococcus*
   d. *Proteins*
   Ans. c
5. Postabortal sepsis causing renal failure is likely to be due to:
   a. *Proteus*
   b. *E. coli*
   c. *Clostridium*
   d. *Pseudomonas*
   Ans. c
6. The most common site of puerperal infection is:
   a. Episiotomy wound
   b. Placental site
   c. Vaginal laceration
   d. Cervical laceration
   Ans. b
7. The most common cause predisposing to puerperal sepsis is:
   a. Iron deficiency
   b. Poor nutrition
   c. Maternal exhaustion
   d. Tissue trauma
   Ans. b
8. About colostrums true statements are:
   a. Started after 10 days of childbirth
   b. Rich in immunoglobulin
   c. Contains less fat
   d. Daily secretion is about 10 ml/day
   Ans. b, c, d
9. All are complications of formula fed baby over human milk fed baby *except*:
   a. Necrotizing enterocolitis
   b. Otitis media
   c. Hypocalcemia
   d. Vitamin K deficiency
   Ans. d
10. The cause of postpartum blues is:
    a. Decreased estrogen
    b. Decreased progesterone
    c. Increased prolactin
    d. Decreased estrogen and progesterone
    Ans. d
11. Common route of spread of puerperal sepsis:
    a. Lymphatic
    b. Direct invasion
    c. Skin lesion
    d. Hematogenous
    Ans. b
12. Without breastfeeding the first menstrual flow usually begins - weeks after delivery:
    a. 2-4 weeks
    b. 4-6 weeks
    c. 6-8 weeks
    d. 8-10 weeks
    Ans. C
13. Which of the following sets of conditions is attributed to normal physiology of puerperium:
    a. Tachycardia and weight gain
    b. Retention of urine, constipation and weight gain
    c. Constipation, tachycardia and retention of urine
    d. Retention of urine and constipation
    Ans. d

55 Essential of Normal Newborn Assessment and Care

Knowledge comes but wisdom lingers.

GENERAL CONSIDERATION

A healthy full term newborn is a baby born at 37 weeks or more gestation, should have an average birth weight usually exceeding 2.5 kg, cries immediately following birth, establishes independent rhythmic respiration and quickly adapts to changed environment. Term newborn is evaluated in the delivery room immediately following birth to assure that they do not require respiratory or circulatory support, have no birth related trauma or congenital anomalies requiring immediate intervention and transitioning as expected to extrauterine life.

Delivery Room Management

a. In every delivery room there should be at least one person whose primary responsibility is attending to the newborn.
b. Before and during delivery careful consideration must be given to prenatal and intrapartum history as it may alter care in the immediate postpartum period. Following points should be kept in mind and communicated to neonatologist that is:
    i. Health status of mother.
    ii. Suspected fetal malformation.
    iii. Labor complication.
    iv. Gestational age.
    v. Duration of labor and ruptured membrane.
    vi. Medication and anesthetic drug given.
    vii. Any difficulty with delivery.
c. Routine care of newborn in delivery room is given to all newborn. It includes (Figs 55.1A to E):
    i. The baby is received in dry sterilized sheet, with head slightly low and tilt, cord is cut with cord cutting scissor at distance of 5 cm.
    ii. Baby is placed in a warm environment, either in radiant heat warmer or mother chest skin to skin contact.
    iii. Airway is cleared by suctioning the mouth and nose with a bulb syringe or a suction catheter connected to mechanical suction. If newborn is completely normal, airway can be cleared simply by wiping the mouth and nose with towel.
    iv. Gastric lavage is done if required.
    v. Vitamin K is administered to prevent hemorrhagic disease of newborn in a single dose of 1 mg (Phytonadione).

One and five minutes APGAR score is evaluated to determine any need for intervention. APGAR score was developed by Virginia APGAR, to quantify the newborn's response to extrauterine environment and to resuscitation. The APGAR score is assigned at 1 and 5 minutes after birth. When the 5 minutes score is <7, additional score should be given every 5 minutes up to 20 minutes Table 55.1.

APGAR Score

Score 8-10—Normal,
    5-7—Mild asphyxia,
    4 or below—Severe asphyxia.

It is important to note that APGAR score is not what determines the need for resuscitation, nor should intervention for a depressed infant be delayed until the 1 minute assessment. However, the change between the scores at 1 and 5 minutes is a meaningful measure of the effectiveness of the resuscitation effort and 5 minutes score of 0-3 is associated with increased mortality in both preterm and full term infants.

Table 55.1: APGAR scoring			
Sign	0	1	2
Heart rate	Absent	Slow (<100 bpm)	≥100 bpm
Respiration	Absent	Slow, irregular	Good, crying
Muscle tone	Limp	Some flexion	Active mother
Reflex irritability	No response	Grimace	Cough, vigorous cry
Skin color	Blue or pale	Pink body Blue extremities	Completely pink

Chapter -55 ♦ Essential of Normal Newborn Assessment and Care

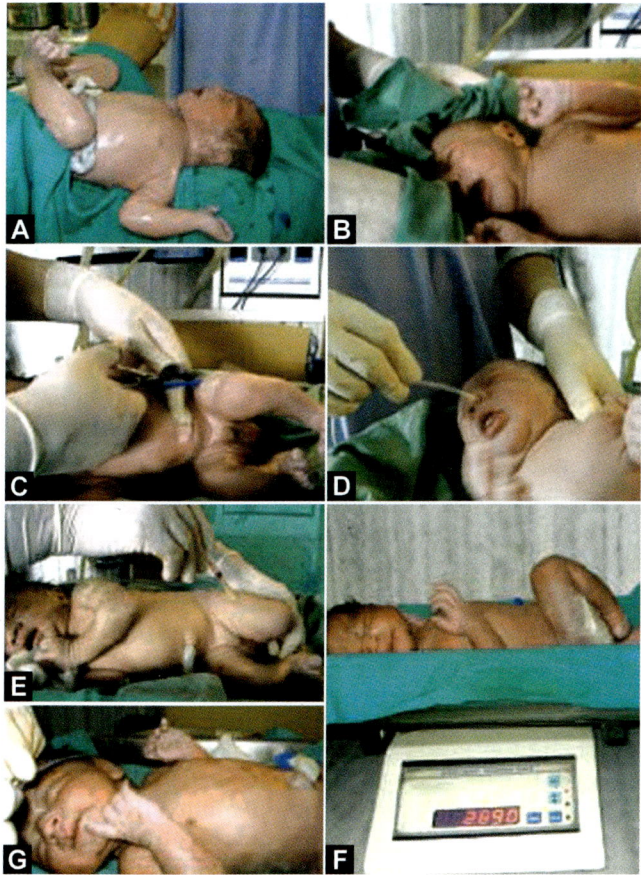

Figs 55.1A to G: Routine care of newborn at time of birth: (A) Baby received in dry sheet with head a little lower; (B) Drying of baby gently in radiant heat warmer; (C) Cord cutting with scissor at distance of 5 cm, after putting umbilical cord clamp; (D) Gastric lavage is done as and if required; (E) Vitamin K prophylaxis given; (F) Birth weight measurement; (G) Measurement of head circumference after 24 hours of birth

Measurement

i. **Weight:** Weight is measured in kg, in of undressed infant. Babies whose weight are either above 10th or below 10th percentile for gestational age are at risk of becoming hypoglycemic—In these cases blood glucose estimation should be done.
ii. **Head circumference:** It measure about 35 cm and biparietal diameter measures about 9.5 cm.
iii. **Length is 50-52 cm.** The length is a more reliable criteria of gestational age than weight.
iv. **Top to toe check of newborn:** Assess color, firm tone, response to handling, and established respiration with normal heart rate.
v. Head for moulding, caput, hematoma and birth trauma. The suture lines may be open or slightly overiding, but premature fusion requires intervention as it presents a constraints to brain growth. The anterior fontanelle should be soft, nontense or bulging in a quiet and calm newborn. It is typically 1-4 cm in size, and may be enlarged with hypothyroidism or increased intracranial pressure. The posterior fontanelle is typically less than 1 cm and may not palpable. **Caput succedaneum** (scalp edema) can be easily differentiated from **cephalhematoma** which is localized collection of blood under the dura mater.

Cephalhematoma is typically confined by suture line unlike caput succedaneum. Cephalhematoma should raise awareness for the possible development of hyperbilirubinemia because collected blood is hemolyzed and resorbed. Skull fracture should be looked for carefully.

vi. Eyes for stickiness, cataract, subconjunctival hemorrhage, albinism and the location.
vii. Ears for tags shape and position.
viii. Mouth for cleft lip, cleft palate, congenital teeth.
ix. Chest for shape, recession, nipple location, respiration pattern, clavicle fracture.
x. Abdomen for hernia, shape, umbilical clamp, 3 vessels in cord.
xi. Genitalia passing of urine and meconium, boys for hypospadias, hydrocele, descended testis. Girls for urethra, vagina.
xii. Back to check vertebra, skin, spina bifida, sacrococcygeal dimple, anus, passage of meconium.
xiii. Limbs for symmetry, fingers and toe count, palmer crease, webbing, overlapping digits, talipes.
xiv. Skin for laceration, birth marks, rashes, bruising, birth trauma.

Pediatrician should note any thing of significance and document in clinical notes.

Newborn Screening and Prophylaxis

The initial newborn may appear normal despite the presence of serious occult illness. Signs of complex congenital heart disease, renal pathology, gastrointestinal obstruction, significant jaundice, inborn error of metabolism and other illness may not be present until the second and third day of life at the earliest. Screening is done in the hope of early diagnosis before a patient becomes symptomatic. Screening in newborn is usually reserved for process that has worse prognosis if not detected early and for which we have effective therapy. Standard newborn screening test are the following:

a. Phenylketonuria by Guthrie test for phenylalanine level.
b. Congenital hypothyroidism by thyroid function test.
c. Congenital syphilis by either rapid plasma reagent as VDRL.
d. ABO incompatibility by infant blood type and direct Coombs' test.
e. Hearing loss (evaluated by auditory brain stem response or otoacoustic emission).

Sites			Gestational age	
	≤ 36 weeks	37-38 weeks	≥ 39 weeks	
1. Sole crease	Anterior transverse crease only	Occasional crease in anterior two-third	Sole covered with crease	
2. Breast nodule diameter	2 mm	4 mm	7 mm	
3. Scalp hair	Fine and fuzzy	Fine and fuzzy	Coarse and silky	
4. Ear nose	Pliable, no cartilage	Some cartilage	Stiff thick cartilage	
5. Testes and scrotum	Testes in lower canal, scrotum small, few rugae	Intermediate	Testes pendular, scrotum full, extensive rugae	

Table 55.2: Rapid estimation of gestational age of newborn infant

Routine Care of Newborn

1. **Estimation of gestational age of infant** is made very soon after delivery by examining certain characteristic of the newborn. A more definite estimation can be made in a few days with help of neurological examination. Though in preterm and growth restricted infants clinical gestational age estimation may be inaccurate. Table 55.2 shows rapid estimation of gestational age.
2. **Temperature:** During first few days of life the infant's temperature is unstable responding to slight stimuli with considerable fluctuation. So temperature of room should be monitored. Infant is encouraged to be on mother side.
3. **Care of cord:** There is loss of water from Wharton's jelly of cord. Within 24 hours cord loses its characteristic bluish color with moist appearance and becomes dry and black. In 3-45 days the stump sloughs, leaving a small granulating wound which after healing form umbilicus. Strict aseptic precaution should be observed in immediate care of cord by sprit or triple dye application. Umbilical infection can be caused by staphylococcal and should be treated with appropriate antibiotic.
4. **Skin care:** Excess vernix as well as blood and meconium is gently wiped off. Remaining vernix is absorbed readily by the skin and disappears entirely within 24 hours. Newborn should not be washed until temperature is stabilized.
5. **Feeding:** The benefit of breast feeding are enormous and as follows:
   a. Human milk is the ideal composition for easy digestion with low osmotic load.
   b. It protects against infection as it confers passive immunity to the baby as the milk contains protective antibodies and contains lysozone, leukocyte, complement which prevent viral infection, gastroenteritis.
   c. It contains vitamin D which prevents rickets.
   d. It is readily available, sterile and convenient.
   e. Psychological benefit by establishing mother child relationship.
   f. It acts as natural contraception if exclusive breast-feeding for first 6 months is practiced.

   Mother should be counseled in prenatal period about the benefit of breastfeeding and encouraged by their obstetric caregivers. The first feed should be started ½-1 hour following normal delivery. Feeding is encouraged at interval of 2-3 hours and demand feeding is encouraged. Proper positioning of infant and burping after each feed should be taught by obstetric caregivers.

   Contraindications of Breastfeeding
   i. HIV infection
   ii. Active tuberculosis infection
   iii. Use of certain medication like illicit drug cocaine, heroin, marijuana, chemotherapeutic agents and radioactive compound.

6. **Voiding and stooling:** Voiding should be closely monitored as change in baby's weight and frequency of urination can be used to assess the hydration status and adequacy of fluid intake in a breastfeeding baby. The time of first void of urine and stool should be documented. Failure to void in the first 24 hours of life should prompt an evaluation of renal function and hydration status. Meconium stooling is seen is 90% of newborn within first 24 hours and in rest within 36 hours. Failure to pass stool in the first 48 hours of life should prompt an evaluation for possible bowel obstruction. Obstruction can result from condition such as bowel atresia, stenosis, Hirschsprung's disease and meconium ileus.
7. **Weight:** In first 3-4 days of birth most infant loss weight. In normal infant birth weight is usually regained at the end of 10 day. There after the weight typically increases steadily at the rate of about 25 gm/day for first few months. Birth weight doubles by 5 months of age and triples by end of one year.
8. **Icterus neonatorum:** About one-third of all infants between 2nd and 5th day of life develops physiological jaundice of newborn. Serum bilirubin level at birth is 1.8-2.8 mg/dl, which rises to 5-10 mg/dl in next 3-4 days. Bilirubin level above this concentration can cause physiological jaundice. In preterm infant jaundice is more common, more severe and prolonged than in term infant because of less hepatic enzymatic maturity.

Enhanced erythrocyte destruction due to any cause also contributes to hyperbilirubinemia.

9. **Immunization:** CDC recommends routine immunizations of all newborn against hepatitis B prior to hospital discharge. If mother is hepatitis B positive, the neonate should also be passively immunized with hepatitis B immunoglobin. Immunization schedule is summarized in Table 55.3. This chart should be handed over to infant's guardian for follow-up of vaccination schedule.

NEONATAL RESUSCITATION

Birth asphyxia is responsible for approximately 1 million neonatal deaths each year worldwide. Ten percent of newborn require some assistance to begin breathing at birth. One percent requires extensive resuscitation and neonatal intensive care to survive.

Asphyxia

It is defined as significant and progressive hypoxemia, hypercapnia and metabolic acidemia that can affect the function of vital organs and can lead to permanent brain damage and death.

In Utero

In utero there is high pulmonary vascular resistance because small pulmonary arteries are compressed by the fluid filled alveolar space. Low estrogen production, low oxygen tension promotes the synthesis of vasoconstrictors such as endothelin -1 and inhibits the production of vasodilators such as Nitric oxide and prostacyclin. Because of high pulmonary vascular resistance, the fetal lung receives approximately 8% of combined ventricular output. Beside this most of the blood from the right side of the heart flows through the ductus arteriosus into the aorta, bypassing the lungs. In uterus fetus, normally has an arterial oxygen tension of 20-25 mm Hg. But fetus can grow and mature in this relative hypoxic environment secondary to several specific adaptations which are unique to the fetus that is fetal hemoglobin oxygen binding, fetal oxygen extraction, and local influence of respiratory acidosis.

After Birth

The primary stimuli for increasing pulmonary blood flow to the lungs are ventilation of the lungs and increase in oxygen tension.

Primary and Secondary Apnea

When significant oxygen deprivation occurs in a newborn, a sequence of events resulting in abnormalities of the heart rate and respiratory pattern occur. After an initial period of oxygen deprivation the infant develop a rapid breathing pattern associated with a decrease in the heart rate, followed by a period of *primary apnea*. If infant is stimulated and given oxygen at this point, normal respiration will resume and heart rate will increase. But if oxygen deprivation continues, the infant will develop irregular gasping with decreasing heart rate and blood pressure leading to *secondary apnea*. During secondary apnea positive pressure ventilation must be initiated to reverse the process.

Table 55.3: Immunization schedule from birth to 2 years

Time	Vaccine
At birth	BCG, oral polio, hepatitis B-1
6-8 weeks	Triple 1, oral polio 2, Hib vaccine, Hepatitis B vaccine 2
10-12 weeks	Triple 2, oral polio 3, Hib vaccine 2
14-16 weeks	Triple 3, oral polio 4, Hib vaccine 3
6 months	Hepatitis B vaccine 3
9 months	Measles vaccine, oral polio 5
15-24 months	MMR (15 Months), Triple and oral polio booster (18 months), Typhoid (24 months)

Triple—Diphtheria, Pertussis, Tetanus
Hib—Hemophilia B
MMR—Mumps, Measles and Rubella
IAP use of Hib vaccine is optional

Causes of Compromised Neonatal Infant

Many causes have been associated with a potentially compromised infant at birth. These can be divided into maternal, fetal and intrapartum. The causes are summarized in Table 55.4.

Equipment: Right and reliable equipment is paramount to a successful resuscitation. Table 55.5 summarizes list of essential equipment within the hospital setting. All essential equipment should be kept readily in radiant heat warmer. A clock is attached. Usually two sources of oxygen with two outlet should be available. Air supplies are available on some resuscitation units. Suction apparatus is intrinsic in resuscitation equipment.

Protocol of Neonatal Resuscitation

The component of neonatal resuscitation is TABCD of resuscitation:
a. **Temperature** control.
b. Clean the airway and establish the **airway**.
c. Establish **breathing** with adequate spontaneous or assisted ventilation.
d. **Circulation**—assist heart rate and circulation.
e. **Drugs**.

Table 55.4: Common causes for compromised newborn infant

a. Maternal:
- Chronic ill health
- Hypertension
- Diabetes mellitus
- Anatomical abnormalities
- Placenta previa

b. Fetal:
- Multiple pregnancies
- Prematurity
- Post-term
- Intrauterine growth restriction
- Congenital abnormalities
- Liquor abnormality (Oligo-or Polyhydramnios)
- Hydrops
- Isoimmunization
- Intrauterine infection

c. Intrapartum:
- Fetal distress
- Abnormal presentation
- Cord prolapse
- Antepartum hemorrhage
- Prolonged rupture of membrane
- Thick meconium
- Instrumental delivery

Table 55.5: Essential equipment for neonatal resuscitation

i. Light source
ii. Source of warmth (heater or warmed linen)
iii. Clock
iv. Flat surface (Radiant heat warmer)
v. Suction apparatus able to deliver suction up to 100 mm Hg
vi. Suction catheter
vii. Oxygen supply
viii. Ventilation system—(bag valve mask or mask and T piece)
ix. Endotracheal tube of various size—2.5-4.0 mm diameter
x. Inductory stylet
xi. Fixation kit for endotracheal tube
xii. Laryngoscope with straight blade and spare bulb
xiii. Oropharyngeal airway
xiv. Umbilical venous catheter
xv. Syringes and needles
xvi. Fluid and medication

Basic Steps of Neonatal Resuscitation

The following is summary of the guideline for neonatal resuscitation (ACOG 2002, 2003):

a. Infant is placed *in warm environment* in radiant warmer, amniotic fluid is dried. Room temperature must be moderate.

b. Airway is *cleared* by suctioning the mouth and nose if no meconium is present. If meconium is present endotracheal intubation is recommended so that airway can be suctioned before further resuscitation efforts are performed.

c. Evaluation for respiratory effort, heart rate and color within 20 seconds or less. In most instances the infant will take a breath within a few second of birth and cry within 30 seconds. If infant is breathing, heart rate greater than 100 beat/minute and skin of the central body and mucous membrane is pink than only supportive care is given.

d. If there is apnea, gasping respiration, bradycardia beyond 30 seconds after delivery—*Positive pressure ventilation* should be applied. The recommended assisted ventilation rate is 40-60 breaths per minute and 30 per minute if chest compressions are also being delivered. Adequate ventilation is indicated by bilateral rise of chest and auscultation of breath seconds with improvement in heart rate and color. Chest compression to ventilation rate is 3:1 that is 3 chest compression followed by a pause for one ventilation. Simultaneous chest compression and lung inflation may impede effective ventilation. Figures 55.2A to E summarizes the steps of neonatal resuscitation.

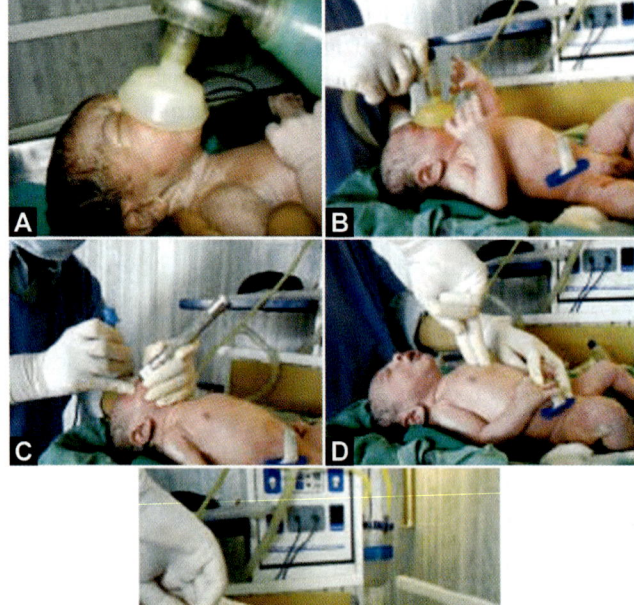

Figs 55.2A to E: Neonatal resuscitation: (A) Bag and mask ventilation with ambu bag; (B) Bag and mask ventilation with resuscitation machine; (C) Intubation with slightly extended neck, visualization of oropharynx with help of pediatric laryngoscope; (D and E) Method of giving cardiac massage

Chapter -55 ♦ Essential of Normal Newborn Assessment and Care

If newborn is failed to establish effective respiration following cause should be kept in mind:
a. Fetal immaturity.
b. Fetal hypoxemia from any cases.
c. Drugs administered to mother.
d. Upper airway obstruction.
e. Pneumothorax or other intrinsic factor as lung hypoplasia or extrinsic diaphragmatic hernia.
f. Aspiration of meconium stained amniotic fluid.
g. Central nervous system abnormalities.
h. Septicemia.

Chemical Resuscitation

Chemical resuscitation consist of:
a. Epinephrine
b. Volume expansion
c. Naloxone

Epinephrine: Recommended dose of epinephrine in neonate is 1:10,000 concentration given endotrachealy or intravenously at 0.1-0.3 mg/kg.

Volume expansion: Volume expansion with 10 ml/kg whole blood, normal Ringer lactate is given intravenously over 5 to 10 minute in cases where hypovolemia is suspected. Albumin is not recommended for neonatal resuscitation due to increased risk of infection and increased risk of mortality.

Sodium bicarbonate: Routine use of sodium bicarbonate during neonatal resuscitation is controversial. The hyperosmolarity and CO_2 generating properties of bicarbonates may be detrimental to myocardial and cerebral function. If sodium bicarbonate is used during prolonged arrest and unresponsive to other therapy, it should be given only after establishment of adequate ventilation and circulation in dose of 4.2% solution (0.5 mEq/ml) slowly over at least 2 minutes.

Naloxone: Naloxone hydrochloride is given for infants with marked respiratory depression and a maternal history of recent narcotic administration. Adequate ventilation should always be established prior to Naloxone administration. Naloxone is given in dose of 0.1 mg/kg preferably intravenously or intratracheally. Because the duration of action of narcotic may exceed that of Naloxone, continued monitoring of respiratory function is essential and repeat dose may be necessary to prevent recurrent apnea. **Prophylactic Naloxone administration in absence of respiratory distress does not confer any clinical benefit.** It is important to note that Naloxone is not to be given in mother with suspected chronic use of narcotic drug as it may precipitate withdrawl signs as seizures in such infants.

Endotracheal Intubation

Endotracheal intubation is indicated in following condition:

a. When meconium is present and the infant is not vigorous or tracheal suction is required.
b. When there is prolonged and ineffective bag and mask ventilation.
c. If chest compression is needed to improve cardiovascular status.
d. To administer epinephrine if required for persistent bradycardia.
e. **Known history of diaphragmatic hernia:** In these cases bag and mask ventilation should not be given and immediate intubation is done.

Technique of Endotracheal Intubation

1. A laryngoscope with a straight blade size 0 for preterm infant, size 1 for term infant is introduced at the side of the mouth and then directed posteriorly towards the esophagus.
2. The laryngoscope is moved gently into the space between the base of the tongue and epiglottis. Gentle elevation of the tip of laryngoscope will raise the epiglottis and expose the glottis and vocal cards.
3. The endotracheal tube of appropriate size 3-4 (usually) is taken. The size of endotracheal tube is descriptive of the internal diameter of the tube and is estimated by the neonate weight and gestational age. When intubating an infant the endotracheal tube should pass through the vocal cord into the trachea without resistance. The chart of endotracheal tube size estimation is in Table 55.6. One should always ensure that endotracheal tube is positioned on the trachea and not the esophagus which is done by:
   a. Observing symmetrical chest wall motion.
   b. Listening for equal breath sounds bilaterally.
   c. Mist in endotracheal tube.
   d. Absence of breath sounds or gurgling sound over stomach.
   e. Good response to intubation is important in skin color and heart rate. If there is no response in skin color and heart rate position of endotracheal tube should be checked. In trachea the tip of endotracheal tube should be mid trachea, half way between the vocal cords and the carina. Tip to lip location is roughly determined by adding 6 to infant's birth weight.
4. Any foreign material like blood, mucous, meconium encountered in tracheal tube should be suctioned immediately.
5. The resuscitation using an appropriate ventilation bag is attached to the tracheal tube, which should deliver

Table 55.6: Endotracheal tube size

Tube size	Weight	Gestational age (weeks)
2.5	<1000	<28
3.0	1000-2000	28-34
3.5	2000-3500	34-38
4.0	>3500	>38

oxygen rich air into tube at 1-2 seconds interval with force of ≃ 25-35 cm H$_2$O which is adequate to lift the chest wall gently, without causing pneumothorax or pneumomediastinum.

Ethical Issues in Neonatal Resuscitation

a. *Discontinuation of resuscitation:* Infants with cardiopulmonary arrest who do not respond promptly to resuscitation are at great risk for mortality and if survive can have severe morbidity. According to current recommendation discontinuation of resuscitation effort may be appropriate if resuscitation after cardiopulmonary arrest does not result in *spontaneous circulation within 15 minutes.*

b. In certain circumstances no intubation or discontinuation of resuscitation can be appropriate like extreme prematurity (< 23 weeks), very low birth weight (≤ 400 gm) and known underlying condition (anencephaly, Trisomy 13 or 18). After confirmation of disorder and counseling of the family, it may be appropriate to let nature take its course.

MULTIPLE CHOICE QUESTIONS

1. A premature baby of 34 weeks was delivered, had bullous lesions on the body, X-ray shows periostitis. What is the next step:
   a. VDRL for mother and baby
   b. Elisa for HIV
   c. PCR for TB
   d. HbS Ag for mother
   Ans. a

2. Vaginal bleeding in a female neonate is commonly due to:
   a. Sarcoma boytroides
   b. Trauma of delivery
   c. Hormonal withdrawal
   d. Viral infection
   Ans. c

3. Commonest cause of neonatal death in India is:
   a. Prematurity
   b. Congenital malformation
   c. Metabolic disease
   d. Birth injury
   Ans. a

4. Alkali resistant hemoglobin is:
   a. HbA
   b. HbA, C
   c. HbS
   d. HbF
   Ans. d

5. The umbilical cord stumps of a newborn most frequently sloughs off about the:
   a. 2nd day after delivery
   b. Fifth day after delivery
   c. 10th day after delivery
   d. 15th day after delivery
   Ans. c

6. Meconium is excreted by a newborn till - day:
   a. 2
   b. 3
   c. 6
   d. 4
   Ans. b

7. In a well baby clinic a neonate is brought with liver two fingers enlarged. The cause is:
   a. Normal phenomenon
   b. Hepatitis
   c. Choledochal cyst
   d. Biliary atresia
   Ans. a

8. Breastfeeding should be started in normal delivery:
   a. Soon after delivery
   b. After 2 hours
   c. After 6 hours
   d. After 4 hours
   Ans. a

9. Consider the following is a newborn (at heart rate of 110, slow and irregular respiratory effort, flaccid muscle tone, no reflex irritability, blue color) what is APGAR Score in this case:
   a. 1
   b. 3
   c. 5
   d. 7
   Ans. b

10. Considers the following statements regarding a Cephalhematoma - i. Present at birth, ii. It can occur after normal delivery, iii. The commonest site is over parietal bone, iv. The bleeding is subperiosteal. Which of the statement given above are correct:
    a. 1,4
    b. 1,2
    c. 1,2,3
    d. 2,3,4
    Ans. d

56 Special Topics in Obstetrics

The only way of discovering the limit of the possible is to venture a little way past them into the impossible.

INTRODUCTION

In last decade, there has been important advancement in routine obstetric management. Few of these topics are covered in this chapter. Obstetric analgesia and anesthesia has been developed in itself a specialized branch of anesthesia. Antepartum and intrapartum fetal surveillance is not only essential for high risk obstetrics but should be practiced in all cases as fetus is considered as second patient. Ultrasound in obstetrics is integral part of obstetrics right from conception, even before conception to emergency ultrasound in labor room or OT in critical situations.

Accidents, suicide attempts, trauma and other injuries are on the rise in the society due to change in socioeconomic cultural scenario. These risks are being faced increasingly by pregnant woman and has to be dealt by clinicians. This chapter briefly and clearly describes the approaches to be followed in management of such situations.

Obstetric Anesthesia and Analgesia

Concept of obstetric analgesia and anesthesia has evolved into own subspecialty in last two decades. In the past beside sympathetic support and few drugs, there was nothing to be offered to laboring women by medical profession. On quantification labor pain is greater than a fractured arm and cancer pain. Labor pain is severe, described as sharp, cramping, aching throbbing, stabbing, hot, shooting, and tight and every woman has right to demand for reduction in suffering of labor pain.

Cause of Pain During Labor

Cause and Location of Pain in 1st Stage of Labor

i. The pain in first stage of labor is primarily caused by distension and stretching of cervix during cervical dilatation. Stage first pain generally occurs during uterine contraction when fetal head pushes against the cervix and causes dilatation.

ii. There is also pain from pressure and stretching of the uterine muscles which activate the high threshold mechanoreceptors.

Location: The pain is visceral, strong and dull. Sites of pain are lower abdomen between the umbilicus and the symphysis pubis laterally over the iliac crest and posteriorly in the skin and soft tissue over the lower lumbar spines. This pain is *referred* pain. The sensory nerves of the uterus leave the cervix and join the sympathetic nerves as they pass through the hypogastric plexus to the sympathetic chain, synapsing with dorsal horn of the spinal cord at T_{10}, T_{11}, T_{12} and L_1. These are high threshold afferent nerves. In this region there are also low threshold cutaneous afferents of the skin from T_{10}, T_{11}, T_{12} and L_1, Because in the same area of cord there is convergence of both somatic and visceral fibers, the laboring women feels the pain in the area as originating from the cutaneous afferents of these spinal segments (Fig. 56.1).

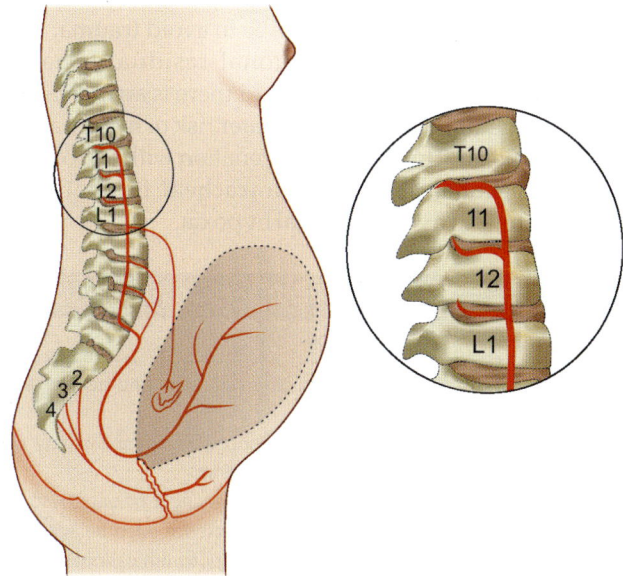

Fig. 56.1: Cause and location of pain in labor

Cause and Location of Labor Pain in 2nd Stage of Labor

It occurs as the fetus descends through the birth canal. **It is somatic pain which is caused by stretching and tearing of fascia, skin and subcutaneous tissue.** The somatic pain is transmitted through the pudendal nerve. The pudendal nerve is derived from the anterior primary division of sacral nerves S2, S3, and S4. In transitional stage of first and second stage when fetus descends in first stage of labor, usually the mother experience both visceral and somatic pain.

Requisites of Ideal Analgesia and Anesthesia in Labor

a. Analgesic should be easy to administer
b. Provides reversible, predictable and good analgesia
c. Safe for mother and baby
d. Allow the patient to ambulate
e. Should not interfere with uterine contraction
f. Should not affect the conscious level of laboring women
g. Should not have any long term effect on women

Physiological Changes of Pregnancy Significant in Relation to Obstetric Analgesia and Anesthesia

Hormonal factor as well mechanical effects of enlarging uterus cause major changes in maternal physiology throughout pregnancy which effect choice and dose of anesthetic agent (Table 56.1)

Respiratory Changes

a. Pregnancy cause congestion, oedema and increased vascularity of the mucosa of the respiratory tract so during endotracheal intubation in general anesthetic it is wiser to use a small sized tube to avoid trauma.
b. Because of lowered functional residual capacity hyperventilation is common and there is an increase in oxygen demand. So there is greater risk of maternal and fetal hypoxia. Thus, hyperoxygenation with full oxygen for 3 minutes prior to endotracheal intubation is mandatory to avoid maternal hypoxia.
c. Also in regional anesthetic it is advisable to give supplementary oxygen throughout the procedure to prevent hypoxia.

Cardiovascular Changes

a. Circulatory blood volume is increased by 40% during pregnancy, so induction and emergence from general anesthesia is more rapid during pregnancy.
b. Engorgement of the veins in the epidural space reduces the available space. So the dose of anesthetic drug in spinal or epidural anesthetic is reduced during pregnancy.
c. Supine hypotension syndrome is caused by aortocaval compression in pregnancy. In regional anesthetic there can be marked fall of maternal blood pressure due to loss of sympathetic tone. So it is preferred to position the patient at lateral tilt of 15°.

Gastrointestinal Changes

Because of delayed gastric emptying time and reduced sphincter tone there is more risk of regurgitation and aspiration of stomach contents, causing Mandelsen's syndrome. To prevent this complication following measures are taken:
a. Only light food is given in labor.
b. Preoperative non particulate antacid is given with H2 receptor antagonist.
c. Positive pressure ventilation before intubation is avoided.
d. Extubation is delayed until the patient has recovered sufficiently from the anesthetic effect.

Nonpharmacological Method of Pain Relief

Psychological Factors Influencing Labor Pains

Anxiety is powerful factor in reducing pain tolerance.

Attention can either enhance or diminish painful experience.

Motivation has a marked influence on the physiological factors, behavioral and affective aspect of pain. These factors can be best addressed by nonpharmacological method and knowledge imparted to laboring women. These methods

Table 56.1: Important maternal physiological changes in relation to anesthetic consideration		
Organ system	Physiologic changes	Anesthetic implication
Cardiovascular	Down regulation of alpha and beta receptors.	Decreased responsiveness to vasopressor and chronotopic agents.
Respiratory	Decreased functional residual capacity and increased oxygen consumption.	Vulnerable to hypoxia with induction of general anesthetic.
Gastrointestinal	Gravid uterus alters angle of gastroesophageal junction, leading to incompetence .also delays gastric emptying.	Full stomach consideration.
Neurologic	Increased sensitivity to inhalational agents and local anesthetic.	Anesthetic requirement decrease by 40%.

are useful in changing attitude of mother towards the labor pain experienced in child birth. Following non-pharmacological methods have been used:
a. **Psychoprophylaxis:** Breathing exercise, prepared child birth, hypnosis.
b. **Modification of labor room environment:** Presence of relative, soothing music.
c. **Physical modalities** like acupuncture, massaging, warm bath.
d. **Transcutaneous electric nerve stimulation (TENS).**

These methods as only method of pain relief best work only in highly motivated pregnant mother.

Pharmacological Method of Obstetric Analgesia and Anesthesia

Table 49.4 summarizes pharmacological analgesic and anesthetic used in obstetrics.
A. Inhalational agent.
B. Systemic injection of opioid or similar drugs.
C. Regional nerve blocks.

Inhalational Analgesia

Inhalational analgesia for labor can be defined as administration of sub anesthetic concentration of inhaled anesthetics to relieve pain during labor. In this premixed 50% nitrous oxide in oxygen (entonox) is self administered from a piped or cylinder supply by face mask or mouth piece with a diamond valve. Correct use is important. The mask should be used with deep but slow respiration at the onset of a contraction and before pain is experienced.

Advantages

a. It has a rapid onset of action.
b. Non cumulative because of the low blood gas solubility of nitrous oxide.
c. Self administration prevents excessive sedation.

Disadvantages

a. Unreliable at time.
b. Risk of maternal aspiration.

Opioids Injection

Demerol, Pentazocine and Tramadol are common drugs used for labor analgesia where epidural analgesia is unavailable or contraindicated. Opioids can provide adequate pain relief only in first and early second stage of labor. Usually frequent small doses are preferable to large doses given less frequently.

Tramadol is a synthetic opioid derivative with excellent analgesic properties but with minimal side effects of cardiovascular and respiratory depression. It's action is reached in 30 minutes and persists for 10-12 hours. So usually repeat dose is not needed. Morphine is no longer used in clinical obstetric practice.

Side Effects

a. Maternal hypotension, nausea, vomiting.
b. Greatest drawback is respiratory depression and obtounded reflex in newborn. *Pethidine or morphine induced respiratory depression in the newborn can be counteracted effectively with the administration of Naloxone/Nalorphine or Lethidrone.*

Local Analgesia

Local infiltration with local anesthetic* drug is of special value in following conditions:
a. Before episiotomy and delivery
b. After delivery into site of laceration to be repaired
c. Around the episiotomy wound.

Regional Anesthetic Technique

Paracervical Block

This is a safe method which can provide complete pain relief in first stage of labor in 80% of cases. In operation of dilatation and curettage local anesthetic 10 ml of 1% lidocaine or 0.25% Bupivacaine is injected submucosally into the fornix of vagina laterally to the cervix at 3° clock and 9° clock position.

Disadvantage: Somatic sensory nerves of perineum are not blocked, and there is high incidence of fetal bradycardia.

Pudendal Block

In this, local anesthetic agent is given below the ischial spine where there is approximate location of pudendal nerve. This block is given during second stage of labor. It alleviates the pain from distension of lower vagina, vulva and perineum. It is useful for vaginal delivery, repair of episiotomy and low forceps/vacuum delivery.

Lumbar Epidural Block

It is the most popular and relives pain in first and second stage.

Method: In this the epidural space is located peripherally to the dura mater. This space extends from the foramen magnum to sacral hiatus. The ligamentum flavum forms the posterior boundary. The contents of epidural space are

---

* Local anesthesia couse reversible blockade of neural conduction. Their molecular structure consists of an aromatic ring, a linking chain and a carbon chain bearing an amino group. *Esters* have a linking chain of the COO configuration. *Para-aminobenzoic* acid is a metabolic and an allergen. *Amide* are local anesthetics have a linking chain of NHCO configuration. Of the esters 2 choloroprocaine is used most frequently in obstetric anesthetic. Of the Amides bupivacane, ripivocaine and lidocaine are most widely used.

nerve roots, fat, lymphatic tissue and blood vessels. The epidural space is entered with 18/16 G thin catheter and local anesthetic is injected. Usually Bupivacaine 10-20 ml (0.125%) + Fentanyl 50-100 µg m is given. After the test dose subsequent analgesia can be provided by intermittent bolus dose of Bupivacaine 5-10 ml.

Complications of epidural analgesia:
  i. **Pain** at site of needle insertion.
  ii. **Hypotension** caused by sympathetic blockade is the second most common complication—Intravenous hydration may attenuate decrease in blood pressure. Sometimes medication usually ephedrine—a mixed alpha and beta agonist or Phenylephrine —a pure alpha agonist is given.
  iii. **Spinal headache:** If there is unintended dural puncture. It incidence is 1-2% of all epidural performed.
  iv. **Neurological injury:** The more common injured nerves are lumbosacral trunk, lateral femoral cutaneous nerve, femoral nerve, and common perineal tissue.

Spinal Block

It is highly effective but single shot technique with limited analgesia. In this dura mater and arachnoid mater is punctured and local anesthetic with or without opioid is administered in subarachnoid space.

Combined Spinal Epidural Block

In this epidural space is located with epidural needle, a long spinal needle is advanced through epidural space until cerebrospinal fluid is obtained. Local anesthetic or opioid is injected. After that spinal needle is removed and a catheter is threaded into epidural space.

Advantage: It has quick onset of action and limitless analgesic. It is also called as walking epidural.

Side Effects of Regional Anesthesia

Bladder dysfunction
It is often seen in patients who receive opioid in epidural anesthetic for pain relief. Some patients may require catheterization.

Effect of epidural anesthetic on course of labor: Recent studies have shown that it may result in longer first and second stage of labor, increased risk of instrumental and assisted delivery, increased need of oxytocin use but no increase in cesarean section rate. Satisfaction rate was more in patient using epidural anesthetic as compared to parenteral opioid.

Contraindications of Epidural Anesthetic

a. Patients refusal
b. Hypovolemia
c. Fever
d. Local infection/sepsis
e. Thrombocytopenia
f. Coagulation disorder
g. Certain neurological disorder
h. Severe cardiomyopathy and valvular heart disease.

Anesthetic Option for Cesarean Delivery

1. **General anesthesia:** It is most often used in—(a) Emergency delivery, (b) If there is any contraindication to regional anesthetic, (c) Patient refusal for regional anesthetic. General Anesthetia requires less than 2 minutes to prepare the patient for surgical incision, so **in severe degree of fetal or maternal distress, in hypovolemic shock and impending rupture of uterus general anesthetic is preferred.**

   Technique of general anesthesia:
   a. All patients should be pre oxygenated with 100% oxygen via a closefitting face mask for 3 minute prior to induction.
   b. A rapid sequence induction is done with thiopentone (3-5 mg/kg) or ketamine (1.5-2 mg/kg). Ketamine is used only in hypotension. Induction is followed by suxamethonium (1.5 mg/kg). Cricoid pressure is applied by the assistant. When air way is secure intubation is done. If intubation can not be performed, cricoid pressure should be continued and gentle mask ventilation is instituted to maintain oxygenation till the patient is breathing spontaneously.
   c. **Maintenance:** Anesthetic is maintained with a 50% mixture of nitrous oxide and oxygen with or without supplemental low concentration of halothane (0.5% or isofluorane 0.5%). But high concentration of volatile agents should be avoided because they may decrease uterine tone causing postpartum hemorrhage and also neonatal depression.
   d. **Further relaxation:** Further relaxation can be achieved with use of non depolarizing muscle relaxant of which the commonly used are— vecuronium, rocuonium and atracurium. These agents do not cross the placenta to any appreciable extent. Once the baby is delivered and cord is clamped, opioid as morphine 5-15 mg or Pentazocine can be given slowly intravenously and oxygen inspired concentration is reduced by 33-35%.
   e. **Reversal:** At the end of surgery, muscle relaxation is reversed with standard dose of neostigmine, atropine or glycopyrrolate. The endotracheal tube is removed only when laryngeal reflexes have returned and spontaneous respiration has resumed. Postoperative analgesic is given, and intravenous hydration is maintained.
2. **Spinal anesthesia:** It is a single shot technique that is rapid in onset. It requires approximately 5-10 minute before the patient is ready for incision.

3. **Epidural anesthesia:** It requires 10 minute to place. If already epidural catheter is in place, surgical anesthetic can be obtained within 2-4 minutes.

Risks of General Anesthesia

a. Difficulty in intubation in pregnancy because of mucosal hyperemia of nasal, oral pharynx, larynx and trachea.
b. There is reduced functional residual capacity (20% reduction) in pregnancy and increased (20-30%) oxygen consumption in pregnancy. So the pregnant women are vulnerable to rapid development of hypoxemia during periods of apnoea. Quick intubation should be accomplished.
c. *Aspiration*: Aspiration occurs when content of stomach gain access to the lungs especially when pH of the aspirated fluid is less than 2.5 and more common in right lower lobe. Aspiration pneumonitis can be fatal. Evidence for respiratory distress can occur immediately or as long as several hours after aspiration. Signs are decreased oxygenation, tachypnoea, bronchospasm, rhonchi, rales, atelectesis, cyanosis, tachycardia and hypotension.

Preventive measures to avoid aspiration:
i. Refrain from solid meals on onset of active labor.
ii. Use of non particulates antacid as sodium bicitrate.
iii. H2 blockers administration decreases gastric pH but requires > 40 minutes to become effective.
iv. Metaclopromide decreases gastric volume in 30 minutes and increases gastroesophageal sphincter tone immediately.
v. Sellick maneuver—Pressure on cricoid cartilage occludes the oesophagus and prevents passive regurgitation.
vi. Proper airway evaluation during induction of general anesthesia.
vii. Passage of nasogastric tube after intubation and during surgery in high risk cases. Additional antacids can be given through nasogastric tube. The stomach should be emptied and nasogastric tube usually can be pulled immediately before extubation.
viii. Extubation should be delayed till reflexes are returned with women lying on her side with her head lowered.
ix. Patient with difficult airways should be identified and treated with alternative techniques like regional anesthetic.

Treatment of aspiration pneumonitis: Respiratory rate and oxygen saturation are the most sensitive indicators of injury. Saline lavage, steroid and prophylactic antibiotic therapy has not been shown to be beneficial. If acute respiratory distress syndrome appears, mechanical ventilation with positive end expiratory pressure may be life saving.

Neonatal outcome in regional vs general anesthetic: The infant born to mother with GA have lower Apgar score at 1 minute with little difference at 5 minute. The induction delivery interval is directly proportional to depressed Apgar score.

TRAUMA IN PREGNANCY

Trauma either accidental or intentional, e.g. suicide, homicides or domestic violence) is a leading cause of death in women of reproductive age. It is estimated that physical trauma complicates approximately 1 in every 12 pregnancies. Trauma is leading cause of non obstetric maternal death.

Causes of Trauma

a. Physical abuse and domestic violence
b. Sexual assault
c. Automobile accident
d. Penetrating injuries—suicidal, homicidal assault
e. Accidental violence
f. Burns.

Risk of trauma is increasing for pregnant women because of more incidences of active employment and mobility with increased exposure to violent behaviors.

Complications Related to Trauma

Maternal

a. Abruptio placenta, DIC and shock
b. Hemorrhage, hypovolemia and shock
c. Uterus rupture
d. Respiratory distress
e. Spinal cord injury, brain death or mortality.

Fetal

a. Preterm labor, premature rupture of membrane and delivery.
b. Placental abruptio with fetomaternal hemorrhage and death.
c. Fetal skull injury especially when fetal head is engaged and there is pelvic fracture.
d. Fetal hypoxia secondary to maternal respiratory distress, shock DIC, thermal injury or maternal cardiopulmonary arrest.

The principles of management of trauma in pregnancy are as follows:

Management

a. Treatment priorities are directed towards the injured pregnant women as for non pregnant patients. Basic rules of resuscitation are followed including establishing ventilation and control of hemorrhage along with treatment for hypovolemia with crystalloids and blood products. An important aspect of management is deflection of large uterus away from the great vessels to diminish their effect on decreased cardiac output.

b. Following emergency resuscitation, evaluation is continued for fracture, internal injuries, bleeding sites as well as uterus injuries and fetal injuries.
c. **Indication of direct peritoneal lavage (DPL):** It is controversial but most trauma surgeon respect the 98% accuracy of DPL. The following are indications of direct peritoneal lavage in pregnancy.
   - Abdominal sign and symptom suggestive of intraperitoneal bleeding.
   - Altered sensorium.
   - Unexplained shock.
   - Major thoracic injuries.
   - Multiple major orthopedic injuries.
d. **If patient is relatively stable:**
   - CT scan can be preferred as it is less invasive, provides injury specific data and is superior to the evaluation of retroperitoneal injuries. But its sensitivity is less than DPL and in abdominopelvic CT employs a radiation dose (3.5 rad) near the threshold of fetal effect.
   - Ultrasound is increasingly being used in trauma setting and has no radiation exposures.
   - Radiologic imaging: If necessary for optimal treatment of bone injuries, X-ray can be performed with shielding of fetus whenever possible.
   - Exploratory laparotomy: Exploration is mandatory for abdominal gunshot found or when patient's clinical situation warrants exploration.
e. **Fetal monitoring:** In addition to standard workup, following facts about fetus and maternal condition should be observed in a pregnant traumatic patients:
   i. Estimated gestational age based on estimated date of conception, history, clinical examination and ultrasound.
   ii. Fetal status with ultrasound and external fetal monitoring.
   iii. Assessments of labor, uterine contraction, rupture of membrane. It is important that 20% of women who have more frequent contraction have an associated placental abruption. In these cases fetal tachycardia and deceleration are common. Fetal monitoring should be started as soon as the maternal condition is stabilized.
f. **Patient is to be observed** for 2-6 hour for clinical symptoms and signs of abruption placenta, or onset of labor. Monitoring should be continued as long as there are uterine contraction, non reassuring fetal heart rate pattern, vaginal bleeding, uterine tenderness, serious maternal injury or ruptured membranes.
g. Blood type and Kleihaur Betke testing should be obtained in pregnant trauma patient. In Rh negative women 300 µg of Rh immune globulin should be given. The KB test determines which Rh –ve unsensitized women have more than 30 ml transfusion. In those patients addition D immunoglobulin is administered. This appears to effectively prevent alloimmunization when administered within 72 hours post trauma.
h. Following measures are performed to maximize utero placental perfusion during evaluation and treatment of the pregnant trauma patients.
   i. Left uterine displacement
   ii. Administration of oxygen to the mother
   iii. I/V hydration
   iv. Military anti shock trousers to treat shock can be used especially in splinting fracture.

Indication of Cesarean Section in Trauma

1. Damage to uterine vessels, laceration or rupture of uterus. In these cases cesarean hysterectomy may be necessary.
2. Mechanical obstruction by gravid uterus, which prevents exposure for surgical repair.
3. Risk of potential injury to fetus in continuing the pregnancy.
4. Unstable thoracolumbar spinal injury with mature fetus.
5. Evidence of worsening DIC.
6. Persistent maternal shock/imminent maternal death, severe dislocated or unstable fracture.

Intrauterine death is not an indication for cesarean delivery.

Burn Victim in Pregnancy

Pregnancy does not appear to have an impact on maternal outcome. Fetal prognosis is related to the extent of the burn and development of maternal complication. If more than two third of the surface is involved in burn there is extremely high maternal mortality. Fetal survival is strongly influenced by the development of maternal complication like hypoxia, hypotension and sepsis.

Electrical Injury

The uterus and amniotic fluid offer low resistance to passage of electricity. The risk of fetal mortality is approximately 50%. If the fetal survives, there is risk of IUGR, oligohydramnios and late intrauterine death.

Suicide

Attempted suicides are as common in pregnancy as in non pregnant women, though rarely successful. They are more common among teenagers, primigravida, unmarried women and with no social support. Involvement of psychiatrist is necessary. Suicide attempts are again increased in the puerperium.

ASSESSMENT OF FETAL WELL-BEING

Antepartum Fetal Surveillance (AFS)

Antepartum fetal surveillance is the assessment of in utero fetal well-being prior to the onset of labor. AFS is intended to identify those fetuses that may be at risk for in utero death or hypoxic injury so that they can be delivered before death or injury occurs. It is based on the principle that progressive fetal hypoxia can be detected by changes in the fetal heart rate, amniotic fluid volume, fetal behavior and fetal umbilical artery blood velocity.

AFS is designed to detect those fetuses at risk due to uteroplacental insufficiency. It is less effective in detecting other types of fetal risk like cord accident or infection but is still useful.

Indications of Antepartum Fetal Surveillance

Common indications are as follows:

a. Pregnancy with obstetric complication like pre-eclampsia, IUGR, Poly or Oligohydramnios, Postdate pregnancy, Rh isoimmunization, multiple pregnancy.
b. Pregnancy with medical complication—Insulin dependent diabetes, hypertension, epilepsy, renal disease, systemic lupus erythematous.
c. Other: Advanced maternal age (>35 years), previous still birth, IUD, recurrent abortion, structural or chromosomal anomaly.
d. Clinical situation like patient who perceives decreased fetal movement, to detect umbilical cord compression in patient with oligohydramnios and to help diagnose intraamniotic infection in patients with ruptured fetal membrane.

Tests Used for Antepartum Fetal Surveillance

a. *Fetal movement record:* It is quantified by mother of number of fetal movement perceived within a given time.
b. *Nonstress test:* External fetal heart rate monitoring which allows evaluation of fetal heart rate, baseline heart rate, variability and response to fetal movement.
c. *Contraction stress test:* External fetal cardiac and uterine contraction monitoring which allows evaluation of the fetal heart rate in response to uterine contraction.
d. *Biophysical profile:* It is nonstress test with added ultrasound evaluation of several fetal biophysical parameters.
e. *Amniotic fluid index:* It is ultrasound estimation of amniotic fluid volume.
f. *Doppler velocimetry:* Doppler ultrasound evaluation of blood flow velocity in various fetal vessels.

Fetal Movement

Maternal perception of fetal movement is a simple, inexpensive and non invasive method of monitoring the fetus and should be explained to every pregnant woman in late pregnancy. Fetal movement is recorded daily. A daily total below a set threshold (10-15 fetal movement) or any drastic change in fetal activity perceived by mother prompts further evaluation. The main disadvantage is its high false positive rate. At least 90% of fetuses with perceived decreased movement are found to be well on further testing.

Nonstress Test

Nonstress test is based on the principle that a well oxygenated fetus responds to spontaneous or induced movement with fetal heart acceleration. It indirectly indicates a normally functioning autonomic nervous system and excludes cellular hypoxia.

Method: For this electronic cardiotocography is used which records fetal heart rate and uterine activity on a graph by means of external monitor. It is done for 20-40 minutes. An event marker is given to the patient to mark the perceived fetal movement (Figs 56.2A and B).

Interpretation: Three components of the fetal heart rate are assessed—baseline, variability, and response to fetal

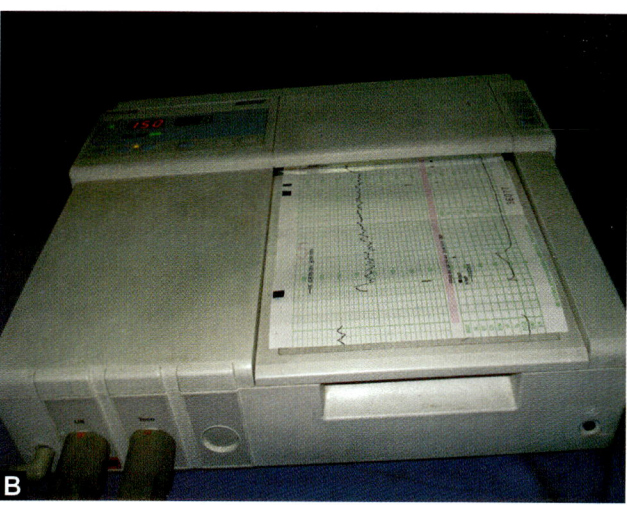

Figs 56.2A and B: Cardiotocography machine with printing and recording facility

movement. A reactive or normal NST is said when there is a normal baseline 120-160 bpm, heart rate variability of 6-10 bpm, 2-4 acceleration of the fetal heart rate with a peak of at least 15 bpm above baseline, lasting for at least 15 seconds and associated with fetal movement. It is not very informative in preterm fetus before 30-32 weeks because of central nervous system immaturity.

Computerized CTG: Computerized CTG has reduced testing time as well as the need for additional test of fetal surveillance and reduced the high inter and intra observer variability in conventional CTG.

Predictive value: Positive predictive value is less than 50% and negative predictive value is more than 90%. It means that a reactive test is more reliable in excluding fetal hypoxia than a non reactive test in predicting fetal compromise. But No abnormal test should be ignored and all abnormal test should be followedup with a second line test such as biophysical profile before any interventions.

Fetal Acoustic Stimulation Test (FAST)

Many NSTS are nonreactive by the criteria described, sometimes owing to fetal sleep cycle. In this test the vibroacoustic stimulus is used by artificial larynx or electronic tooth brush held briefly to the maternal abdomen. Accelerations in response to such acoustic stimuli have the same validity as an unprovoked reactive nonstress test.

Significance: It has been shown to shorten the amount of time necessary to obtain an NST and decrease number of falsely non reactive NSTS.

Contraction Stress Test (CST)

It is also called oxytocin challenge test. The basis of this test is to stimulate labor like condition and monitor the fetal heart rate (FHR) pattern in response to uterine contraction, because blood supply to the fetus is temporarily interrupted during uterine contraction. A healthy fetus with a good oxygen reserve is unaffected by this temporary hypoxia but a compromised fetus will manifest signs of fetal hypoxia in the form of fetal heart deceleration.

Method: Uterine contraction and fetal heart rate are monitored with the patient in a left lateral recumbent position. Uterine contraction may be spontaneous or induced with maternal nipple stimulation or intravenous oxytocin. Three uterine contraction of moderate intensity in 10 minutes must be achieved for an adequate CST.

Interpretation:

Positive CST: Late deceleration of fetal heart rate with more than half of the uterine contraction.

Negative CST: No late deceleration.

Equivocal CST: Deceleration with uterine hyperstimulation, isolated late deceleration, or technical artefacts like inability to achieve adequate contraction.

Predictive value: AT least 50% of patients with positive CST later deliver to have a healthy fetus. It has been largely replaced now by biophysical profile. Because it is more time consuming, inconvenient to the patient and contraindicated in:
a. Placenta previa
b. Previous uterine scar
c. Multiple gestation
d. Hydramnios
e. Incompetent cervix and history of preterm labor.

Biophysical Profile

The BPP score is a composite of four acute or *short term variable*—fetal tone, movements, breathing, and non stress test and one chronic or *long term variable*- amniotic fluid volume.

Principle of biophysical profile: All five parameters of the BPP are regulated by the fetal central nervous system. The fetal CNS is highly sensitive to the level of oxygenation and therefore these biophysical variables are directly influenced by the state of oxygenation of the fetus. The four short term variables respond to fetal hypoxemia in a predictable fashion —The BPP that appear earliest in the fetal life is the last to disappear with onset of fetal asphyxia. Fetal tone appears first followed by fetal movement then fetal breathing whereas fetal heart rate reactivity is controlled by the hypothalamus and medulla and appears late in the second trimester. They disappear in reverse order—reactivity of heart rate pattern, breathing followed by tone.

Method of BPP: The NST is performed first within 20-30 minutes with the patient in semi fowler's position. It is followed by sonographic evaluation of fetal biophysical activities including fetal tone, movement and breathing. Amniotic fluid volume is measured by holding the transducer perpendicular to the floor. The largest vertical pocket is selected and should at least be 1 cm in diameter. The composite of all four quadrant's deepest vertical pocket is termed as the amniotic fluid index (AFI). The normal range of AFI varies with gestational age. In general AFI <5 cm oligohydramnios 5-10 cm—decreased fluid 10-25 cm—normal. >25 cm—polyhydramnios. A total 30 minute is assigned for obtaining ultrasound variable.

Interpretation: A normal variable is assigned a score of 2 and abnormal variable a score of 0. Manning proposed a method using 5 fetal biophysical variable to assess the studies of fetal well-being antenatally.

And test should be repeated in 24 hours except in case of oligohydraminios with intact membranes – in that case delivery or close surveillance is indicated.

Score of 4, 2, or 0—indicate fetal compromise and delivery should be strongly considered.

Predictive value: Predictive value of all variable is not the same. Most important variables are NST and amniotic fluid volume. Intermediary Important are fetal breathing movement and least important are fetal tone and fetal body movement.

Table 56.2: Fetal biophysical profile—Manning score

Biophysical variable	Normal (Score - 2)	Abnormal (Score - 0)
Nonstress test	Reactive ≥ 2 acceleration of ≥ 15 b/min for > 15 sec in 20 minutes	Nonreactive < 2 acceleration of ≥ 15 b/min or ≥ 15 sec in 20 minutes
Fetal breathing movement	≥ 1 episode of ≥ 30 sec in 30 minutes	Absent or ≤ 30 sec in 30 minutes
Gross body movement	≥ 3 discrete body limb movement in 30 minutes	≤ 2 discrete body/limb movements in 30 minutes
Fetal tone	≥ 1 active extension/flexion of limb, trunk or hand	Slow or absent fetal extension flexion
Amniotic fluid volume	≥ 1 pocket of fluid ≥ 2 cm on two perpendicular line	No pocket > 1 cm in two perpendicular line
Score of	8-10 = normal – absent fetal acidemia 6 = Equivocal 5 or less = Abnormal	

BPP score correlate well with fetal acid base balance. A normal BPP score virtually rule out the possibility of fetal acidemia being present at the time of testing (Table 56.2).

Modified Biophysical Profile

Modified biophysical profile consists of NST and AFI. It is quicker than a complete BPP and appears to have the same sensitivity for detecting fetal compromise. So full BPP can be reserved for nonreassuring or equivocal NST's.

Significance of BPP and modified BPP

a. It is noninvasive, easily performed test of fetal well-being that is highly accurate in detecting fetal hypoxemia. There is inverse relationship between the last BPP score before delivery and adverse long term outcome that is cerebral palsy, mental retardation, cortical blindness, deafness and learning disabilities.
b. The use of BPP provides reassurance in a setting of a non reactive NST.
c. It serves as a mean to decrease fetal morbidity and mortality by timely intervention.
d. NST has a 50% false positive rate (meaning proportion of non reassuring test when fetus is well). BPP has false positive rate of 20%. NST has false negative rate of 1.4 per 1000 test (means proportion of reassuring test when the fetus is at imminent risk). The BPP has slightly lower false negative rate of 0.6 per 1000.

The common conditions where false negative NST or BPP are commonly observed are:
a. Insulin dependent diabetes
b. Postdate pregnancy
c. Pre-eclampsia with intrauterine growth retardation, *so twice weekly monitoring has been advocated in these situation.*

Doppler Velocimetry

a. *Doppler velocimetry of umbilical artery:* The umbilical artery Doppler wave from is used to measure the peak systolic (S) peak diastole (D) and mean (M) values. From these values S/D ratio and Pulsatility Index PI (PI = S-D/m) calculated. In a *normal pregnancy* the S/D ratio and the Pulsatility Index decrease as the gestational age advances. Higher values of S/D and PI means reduced diastolic velocities and increased placental vascular resistance found in IUGR, hypertensions. Absent or reverse diastolic flow predicts acidemic fetus and increased perinatal morbidity and mortality of 15-30% (Figs 56.3A to C).
b. *Middle cerebral artery Doppler:* The fetal circulation responds to a fall in oxygen saturation by vasoconstriction of the somatic, renal and hepatic vessels and increased blood supply to the vital organs like the brain, heart and adrenals. This preferential blood flow to brain during hypoxia can be detected by middle cerebral artery Doppler which shows increased end diastolic flow and fall in PI and RI. Middle cerebral artery Doppler velocimetry is not recommended in routine practice but it provides further information on fetus in high risk pregnancy.
c. *Doppler of fetal venous circulation:* Venous velocimetry can provide additional information in high risk pregnancies when abnormal umbilical or middle cerebral artery Doppler indices are detected. It helps in deciding the timing of delivery. The commonly studied veins are— umbilical vein, inferior vena cava and ductus venosus. **Principal**—In fetal hypoxia initially, there is redistribution of blood flow. But if hypoxia remains uncorrected, fetal decompensation occurs at the same time which results in increase in central venous pressure. This leads to abnormal Doppler wave form in fetal venous system. In healthy fetus the venous circulation is essentially non pulsatile. *Appearance of pulsatile flow in the venous system is associated with increased morbidity and mortality.* The further away from heart that the veins demonstrating the abnormality are the worse is the prognosis. The perinatal mortality is highest when pulsations are seen in the umbilical vein. The ductus venosus connects the umbilical vein with inferior vena cava causing highly oxygenated blood to the heart. In healthy fetus there is continuous forward flow throughout the cardiac cycle so called **Monophasic** flow. If there is reverse flow (**biphasic**), it indicates raised CVP and imminent cardiac failure and increased perinatal mortality.

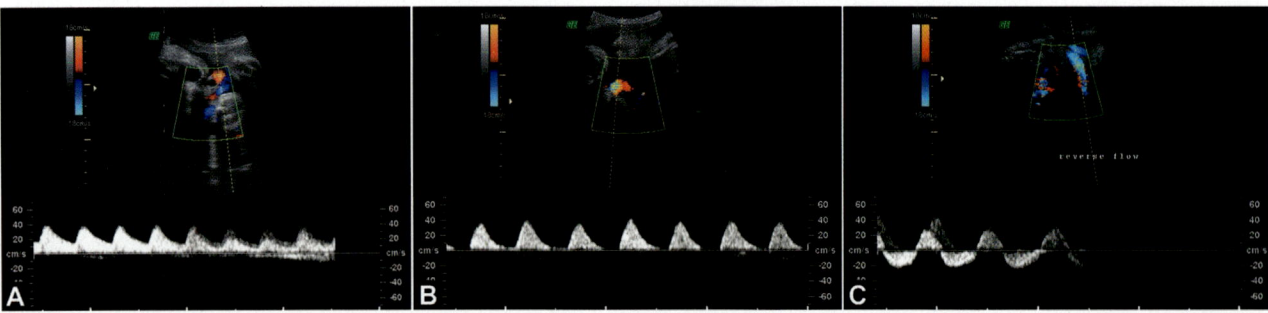

Figs 56.3A to C: Ultrasonography image showing: (A) Normal diastolic flow; (B) Absent diastolic flow; (C) Reverse diastolic flow

Formulation of Antepartum Fetal Surveillance

Antepartum fetal surveillance is often initiated at least 1-2 weeks before fetal risk is perceived to begin. Patients at relatively low risk might receive a daily fetal movement count and weekly NSTS. Patients at high risk should have daily fetal movement count. Twice weekly NSTS, and a weekly AFI. BPP and/or Doppler velocimetry can be added for patients at very high risk. Patients beyond 40 weeks gestation are typically followed with twice weekly NST and weekly AFI, starting at or before 41 weeks gestation.

INTRAPARTUM FETAL SURVEILLANCE

General Considerations

Intrapartum fetal monitoring (IFM) means to observe fetal behavior during labor. The aim of intrapartum fetal monitoring is to detect early fetal response to intrauterine hypoxia, so that timely intervention can prevent irreversible neurological damage and death. Labor is the most stressful period of human life, because oxygen supply to the fetus is interrupted at each contraction. There is head compression which affects the function of the vital centres of the brain. A healthy fetus has inbuilt mechanism to tide over these short periods of hypoxia without any lasting damage. But a fetus with borderline reserve due to chronic uteroplacental insufficiency may decompensate and show signs of overt asphyxia during labor. *The aim of intrapartum monitoring is to identify early signs of developing hypoxia, so that timely intervention can prevent irreversible brain damage and death.*

Method of IFM

a. Intermittent auscultation by Doppler or stethoscope.
b. Continuous electronic fetal heart rate monitoring.

Other Methods of Fetal Scalp Stimulation

i. Fetal scalp pH
ii. Fetal pulse oximetry (investigational)

Intermittent Auscultation

Guidelines for intermittent auscultation in labor are:
a. The nurse to patient ratio should be 1:1 and intermittent auscultation should be performed by trained and experienced personnel.
b. Fetal heart rate auscultation should be done after a contraction for 1 minute at interval of 15 minutes in 1st stage of labor and every 5 minutes in 2nd stage of labor in presence of risk factors.
c. In the absence of risk factor, no data determines the frequency of auscultation. Usual recommendation is to auscultate the fetal heart rate at least every 30 minutes during the active phase of the first stage of labor and at least every 15 minutes during the second stage of labor.

Electronic Fetal Monitoring (EFM)

It is performed using a cardiotocography machine with transducers attached for fetal heart as well as the uterine activity. Principles of CTG machine are as follows:

External Fetal Monitoring

It is base on the Doppler principle of ultrasound which state that frequency of sound waves shifts as the sensor move related to receiver. This method aims to pickup the mechanical activity of fetal heart. For this ultrasonic transducer aquasonic gel and abdominal belt is required.

Internal Fetal Monitoring

It is accomplished by obtaining a direct fetal echo by picking up the electrical activity of fetal heart directly from the fetal body through placement of electrode on it. Internal method can only be applied during labor with minimal of 2 cm dilatation of the cervix and ruptured membranes. In this a metal hook is required to penetrate and anchor the electrode on the skin of the presenting part of fetus and act as one of the electrical poles of ECG. A plastic body incorporates the second pole of ECG which is termed as reference electrodes. Electrodes wires usually red and white are to be connected to the connector cable through its "clamp block" (Fig. 56.4).

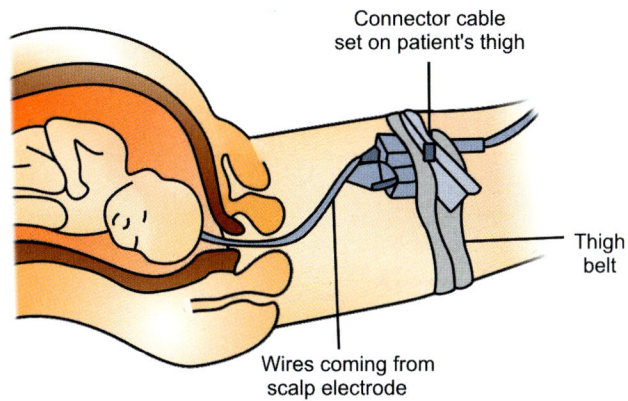

Fig. 56.4: Connection of scalp electrode

The frequency of electronic fetal heart rate monitoring: The fetal heart rate tracing should be evaluated and recorded in the chart at regular interval. In the presence of risk factors, it should be evaluated at least every 15 minutes during the active phase of the first stage of labor and at least every 5 minutes during the second stage of labor.

Risk Factors Which Warrant Intensive Intrapartum Fetal Surveillance

a. *Antepartum:* Pre-eclampsia, chronic hypertension, maternal diabetes, IUGR, multiple gestation.
b. *Intrapartum:* Placental abruptio, induction for non-reassuring fetal status, prematurity, meconium stained amniotic fluid, chorioamnionitis, documentation of non-reassuring fetal heart rate pattern when using the low risk auscultation period.
c. *Intervention in labor:* Use of analgesia or anesthetic, use of oxytocin.

Advantages of EFM

a. It allows reliable determination of the presence of fetal well-being.
b. It allows with a high degree of reliability, determination of the presence of early fetal problem.
c. It is objective and independent of human factor.
d. It gives amplitude of uterine contraction and hypotonic or hypertonic status.
e. CTG graph provides hard evidence of the event which has medicolegal importance.

Sensitivity and specificity of CTG: Continuous electronic fetal heart rate monitoring has quiet good sensitivity in detecting fetus at risk for asphyxia (hypoxia with metabolic acidosis). False negative are rare which means that a normal FHR tracing confirms reassuring fetal well-being in almost all cases. However specificity of continuous electronic fetal heart monitoring is poor. The false positive rate is high ≥ 50%. So the largest risk of continuous fetal heart rate monitoring is increase in cesarean section rate.

Parameters of Fetal Heart Monitoring and Its Interpretation

A. Baseline heart rate
B. Baseline FHR variability
C. Presence of FHR acceleration
D. Periodic or episodic FHR deceleration
E. Change or trends of FHR pattern over time.

A. *Baseline fetal heart rate:* It is approximate mean FHR rounded to increment of 5 beat/minute during at least 10 minutes segment excluding periodic or episodic changes, periods of marked fetal heart rate variability. In order to deduce baseline FHR the minimum baseline duration must be 2 minutes out of 10 minutes segment. The normal baseline FHR is 110-160 beats/minute. Bradycardia defines FHR < 110 beats/minute. Tachycardia defines baseline FHR > 160 beats/minute.

Causes of fetal tachycardia
 i. *Maternal:* Pyrexia, hypovolemia, hyperthyroidism, use of β agonist drug, Nifedipine.
 ii. *Fetal:* Prematurity, chorioamnionitis, fetal anemia, fetal arrythmia and hypoxia.

Causes of fetal bradycardia
 i. Maternal intake of drugs like beta blockers
 ii. Paracervical anesthetic
 iii. Postdate fetus
 iv. Fetal hypoxia: Fetal bradycardia may supervene on Chronic hypoxia or may be a manifestation of acute fetal distress in response to uterine hyperstimulation or acute maternal or cord accidents like placental abruption, cord prolapse, scar dehiscence.

B. *Baseline variability (beat to beat variation)* — Baseline fetal heart rate variability is fluctuation on the baseline FHR of two cycles per minutes or greater. They are visually quantified as the amplitude of the peak to trough in beats/minute. It is an important *index of cardiovascular function and regulated by sympathetic and parasympathetic control of the sinoatrial node* – significance of variability is assessed broadly as follows:
 i. Less than 5 BPM —Omnius
 ii. Between 5-10 BPM —Normal but needs observation
 iii. Between 10-20 BPM—Healthy fetus
 iv. More than 25 BPM—Needs critical observation

Causes of minimal or absent FHR variability
 i. Fetal hypoxia
 ii. Maternal administration of narcotic drug
 iii. Magnesium sulphate
 iv. Congenital anomalies of central nervous system
 v. Fetal sleep cycle
 vi. Extreme prematurity

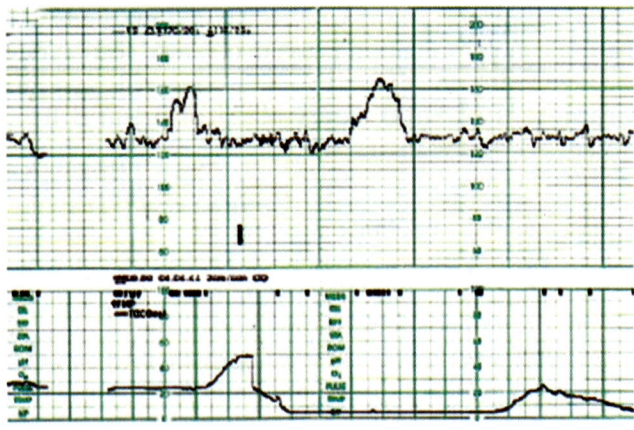

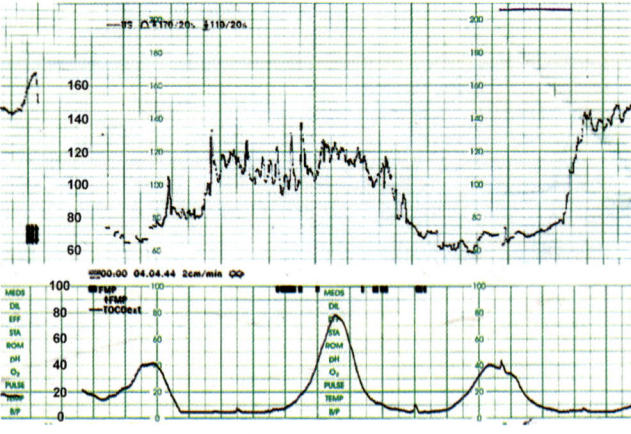

Fig. 56.5: Fetal acceleration

Fig. 56.6: Late deceleration

C. **Fetal heart rate acceleration:** An acceleration is defined as a visually apparent, abrupt increase (onset of acceleration to peak in less than 30 seconds) in FHR above the baseline. The peak is ≥ 15 beats seconds and < 2 minutes from the onset to return to baseline. Before 32 weeks of gestation acceleration are defined as having a peak ≥ 10 beats/ minute and duration > 10 seconds. An acceleration that last ≥ 10 minutes is a change in baseline (Fig. 56.5).

Significance of acceleration: Acceleration can occur spontaneously or be associated with fetal movements or uterine contraction. The presence of acceleration means an intact nervous system and normal pH that is healthy fetus. Therefore they are reassuring, but their absence is not a sign of fetal compromise as long as other reassuring parameters are present such as normal beat to beat variation.

D. **Fetal heart rate deceleration:** If there is sudden decrease in fetal heart rate from the baseline by more than 15 BPM, lasting for more than 15 seconds but less than two minutes is considered as deceleration. Classically deceleration is classified into three types:

  i. **Early deceleration:** It is a visually apparent, gradual decrease (onset of deceleration to nadir < 30 seconds) and return to baseline FHR associated with uterine contraction. In most cases the onset, nadir and recovery of the deceleration are coincident with the beginning, peak and ending of the contraction respectively.

  Causes of significance of early deceleration: Early deceleration are thought to be caused by fetal head compression leading to a vagal response. Early deceleration is not associated with fetal hypoxia or acidosis. Since they are presumed to be benign, no intervention is required when they are present.

  ii. **Late deceleration:** Late deceleration is similar to an early deceleration except the deceleration is delayed in timing and the nadir of deceleration occurs after the peak of the contraction. In most cases, the onset, nadir and recovery of the deceleration occur after the beginning, peak and ending of the contraction respectively (Fig. 56.6).

  Cause and significance of late deceleration: Late deceleration are thought to be caused by hypoxia and acidosis due to uteroplacental insufficiency. It is caused by following mechanism:
  i. Central reflex caused by hypoxia
  ii. Direct myocardial depression caused by acidosis. The most common causes are hypotension from epidural analgesic and uterine hyperactivity due to oxytocin stimulation. Maternal diseases as hypertension, diabetes and collagen vascular disease can cause chronic placental dysfunction. Placental abruption can cause acute and severe late deceleration. When late deceleration are recurrent (in 50% or more of uterine contraction) fetal hypoxia and/or acidosis is suspected. Intervention like expedite delivery or further testing (fetal scalp pH) is considered.

  iii. **Variable deceleration of FHR:** Variable deceleration of the fetal heart rate is defined as a visually apparent abrupt decrease (onset of deceleration to nadir lasting less than 30 seconds) in rate. This decrease in FHR below the baseline is ≥ 15 beat/minutes and last ≥ 15 seconds but < 2 minutes from of return to baseline. They are not always associated with uterine contraction, and if they recur, their onset, depth and duration vary with successive uterine contraction (Fig. 56.7).

  Cause and significance of variable FHR: They are the most common deceleration seen in labor especially during the second stage of labor. They are caused by umbilical cord compression usually due to uterine contraction or fetal movement.

  Significant variable deceleration: Have been defined as those decreasing to less than 70 bpm and lasting more than 60 seconds. Isolated variable decelerations are not omnius but fetal hypoxia and acidosis should

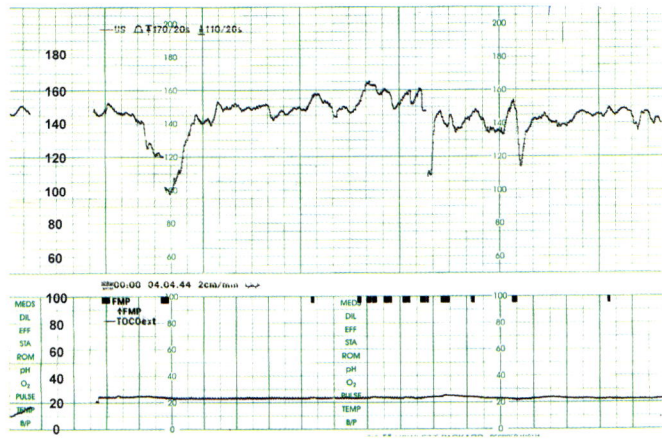

Fig. 56.7: Variable deceleration

be suspected when they are associated with non reassuring changes on fetal heart rate pattern.

iv. **Prolonged deceleration:** A prolonged FHR deceleration is visually apparent decrease in FHR below the baseline. The decrease is ≥ 15 beats/minutes and last ≥ 2 minutes but < 10 minutes from onset to return to baseline. A deceleration that last ≥ 10 minutes is change in the baseline.

Cause and significance of prolonged deceleration: Prolonged deceleration are usually caused by prolonged umbilical cord compression (caused by hyperstimulation, umbilical cord compression or fetal hypoxia (maternal hypotension). They can also be seen with rapid descent of the fetal head during the second stage. If isolated they may not require intervention, but if other non reassuring fetal heart rate pattern are seen as tachycardia, decreased variability, warrant intervention.

v. **Sinusoidal fetal heart rate pattern:** A sinusoidal fetal heart rate pattern is a smooth wave like pattern of regular frequency (usually 3-5 cycle/minute) and amplitude (usually 5-20 beat/minute). Short episodes (<5-10 minutes) of a sinusoidal pattern may be a variant of normal. A prolonged period of a sinusoidal fetal heart rate pattern has been associated with moderate to severe fetal anemia as in alloimmunization or fetomaternal hemorrhage) and severe fetal hypoxia, or twin to twin transfusion. Insignificant sinusoidal patterns have been reported following maternal administration of narcotic.

Reassuring and Nonreassuring Fetal Heart Rate Tracing

Reassuring

Normal baseline rate, moderate fetal heart rate variability, absence of late deceleration, presence of acceleration.

Nonreassuring

Fetal tachycardia or bradycardia, minimal or absent fetal heart rate variability, late deceleration, repetitively variable deceleration especially if associated with changes in baseline FHR and FHR variability, absence of acceleration (spontaneous or elicited).

Treatment of Nonreassuring Fetal Heart Rate Pattern

1. **General measures to improve uterine blood flow** and fetal oxygenation. So named intrauterine resuscitation:
   a. Lateral recumbent position
   b. Maternal oxygen administration
   c. Increase in intravenous hydration
   d. Discontinuation of oxytocin infusion.
2. **Correction of any identified etiology:**
   a. **Amnioinfusion** has been tried in oligohydraminios
   b. In thick meconium presence amnioinfusion is tried with aim to dilute meconium. In this 500-800 ml bolus of warmed normal saline is given in bolus by catheter inserted in uterine cavity followed by a continuous infusion of approximately 3 ml/hour. The results are variable and there is risk of infection, uterine hypertonus.
3. **Tocolytic agent:** Terbutaline can be used if non reassuring fetal heart rate tracing is caused by excessive uterine activity. Terbutaline 0.25 ml subcutaneous or 0.125-0.25 mg intravenously can be given followed by close observation or while preparing patient for cesarean section or transfer to patient.
4. Further test can be added to assess fetal well-being as fetal scalp pH, fetal scalp stimulation.
5. **Terminate delivery:** If the FHR pattern is omnius or fetus does not respond to intrauterine resuscitation or if fetal well-being is nonreassuring with further testing, the fetus should be delivered by cesarean section or assisted vaginal delivery.

Other Methods for Fetal Monitoring Adjunct to EFM

i. *Fetal scalp stimulation:* Acceleration of the heart rate in response to stimulation has been associated with a normal scalp blood pH. Conversely, failure to provoke acceleration is not uniformly predictive of fetal acidemia. It has high false positive rate.

ii. *Fetal scalp blood sampling (FBS):* It is performed with the patient in the lithotomy position. Under direct visualization the fetal scalp is punctured and capillary blood obtained for pH assessment.

Interpretation is as follows—
   a. pH ≥ 7.25—reassuring – No intervention is required.
   b. pH ≥ 7.20—Indeterminate fetal scalp blood pH should be repeated immediately to confirm the value.

c. pH < 7.20 —Nonreassuring delivery.
Intervention delivery is performed promptly if the low pH is confirmed otherwise labor is allowed to continue and scalp blood samples are repeated periodically.

Limitation because of cumbersome nature of the procedure fetal scalp sampling is commonly not used.

iii. **Fetal pulse oxymetry:** Using technology similar to that of adult pulse oxymetry, a sensor placed on the fetus cheek determines oxyhemoglobin saturation after rupture of membranes. Fetal pulse oxymetry was shown to assess fetal oxygenation safely and effectively, but when used as an adjunct to FHR monitoring when fetal heart rate tracing was non reassuring, fetal pulse oxymetry did not lead to a decrease in the overall cesarean section rate. ACOG has not endorsed its adaptation in clinical practice.

Presence of Meconium in the Amniotic Fluid

12-22% of human labors are complicated by meconium passage by fetus. It is a potential warning of fetal asphyxia.

Pathophysiology of meconium: Three theories have been suggested to explain fetal passage of meconium:
a. Fetus pass meconium in response to hypoxia
b. In uterus passage of meconium may represent normal gastrointestinal tract maturation under neural control.
c. Meconium passage could follow vagal stimulation from transient umbilical cord entrapment. So in some situation fetal release of meconium may also represent physiological process.

Meconium aspiration: The aspiration of some amniotic fluid before birth can be considered a physiological event. In meconium stained fluid, it can lead to respiratory distress and hypoxia. Meconium aspiration syndrome is associated with fetal acidemia at birth.

OBSTETRIC ULTRASOUND

Ultrasound is today an integral part of the obstetrician's armamentarium. It has profound effect on obstetric practice. A carefully performed ultrasound examination can reveal vital information about fetal anatomy as well as fetal environment, growth and well-being. It contributes significantly to identify the fetus at risk and alert the obstetrician to implement timely correction measures or intervention to improve the obstetric outcome.

Basics of Equipment of Obstetric Ultrasound

Ultrasound equipment uses sound waves delivered at high frequency, usually >20000 cycles per second (Hz). In most diagnostic application 2-10 million cycles per second frequency (2-10 Mhz) is used. The best resolution is obtained

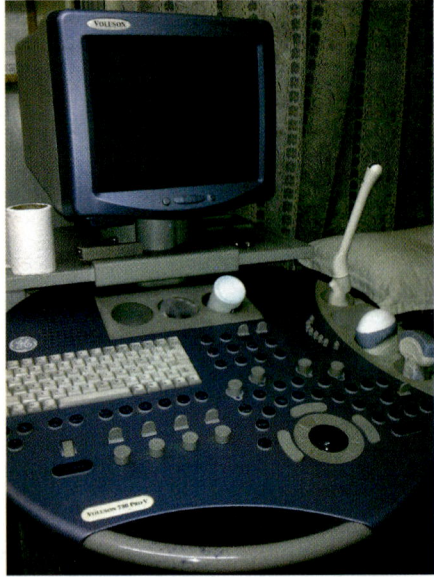

Fig. 56.8: Ultrasound machine

with highest frequency ultrasound, though depth of visualization is compromised. Abdominal ultrasound transducer have a linear array with a rectangular image, sector scanner have pie shaped images, or curvilinear scanner that combine both principles. Abdominal transducer operate at 3.5-5 Mhz, vaginal scanner operates at 5-10 Mhz (Fig. 56.8).

Types of Scans

a. **A mode:** It consists of graph indicating reflectors at the level of their depth. They are no longer used in obstetric.
b. **B mode:** The conventional ultrasound scan today is a real time gray scale B mode study. It is also known as 2D study.
c. **3D ultrasound:** Now a third dimension can be added to the image by special transducer and computer software arrangement.
d. **4D ultrasound:** Real time 3D ultrasound is known as 4D ultrasound.
e. **M mode:** It refers to a motion mode in B mode studies. It is currently employed in obstetrics to evaluate fetal cardiac motion to assess heart rate and rhythm as well for studying the excessive of the cardiac values and the myocardium.
f. **Doppler:** This term is used to indicate blood flow information. It is based on the Doppler Effect, which says that returning frequency of waves is altered by the movement of a target. The moving target is the red blood cells in the blood vessel in region of observation. The returning signals are mapped in two ways. A map of vessels can be obtained which can be superimposed on the gray scale image. It is known as **Color flow mapping**, which indicates direction and velocity of flow.

g. **Doppler spectrum:** It consists of a graph showing flow characteristics as a wave form. It has an equivalent simultaneous audio signal as well and waves form which can be quantified as velocities, ratio and indices.
h. **Power Doppler:** It is a newer form of flow imaging. It quantifies and displays flow information as amplitude of scatter of the ultrasound multidirectional slow flow. It is useful in studying placental angiogenesis and assessing vascular details of some fetal malformation.
i. **Fetal echocardiography:** It is detailed evaluation of fetal cardiac anatomy and flow pattern. This includes a 2D evaluation of the configuration and connection, color flow mapping of flow in the chambers and outflow tract and a Doppler spectral analysis of flow across the values and outflow tract. This can be suggested by 3D and 4D studies.

Safety of ultrasound examination in obstetrics: There has been no confirmed adverse biologic effect on patients, fetus or instruments operators.

Patient Consideration in Obstetric Ultrasound

a. Women must be reassured about the painlessness and safety of examination particularly regarding fetus.
b. Appropriate clinical information and consent forms should be completed as per institutional and legal requirements. In current Indian PNDT Act there must be signature of doctor as well patient implying that sex of fetus has not been communicated in any form to patient by doctor.
c. Transabdominal scan is done in supine position. In last trimester if patient feels faint or uncomfortable, she should be put in a lateral position for a few minute before resuming the scan.
d. In transvaginal scan operator must use gloves for transvaginal procedure. A condom should be used to cover the transducers.
e. Ultrasound gel should be used as necessary to permit smooth transducer movements. Ultrasound gel may be warmed in the winter months by placing the bottle in a container of warm water.

First Trimester Ultrasound Scan

Component of 1st trimester ultrasound scan are:
a. Location of the gestational sac.
b. Identification of embryo.
c. Measurement of crown rump length.
d. Presence or absence of cardiac activity.
e. Fetal number.
f. Condition of uterus, cervix and maternal adnexa.
g. Presence, size and shape of the yolk sac.

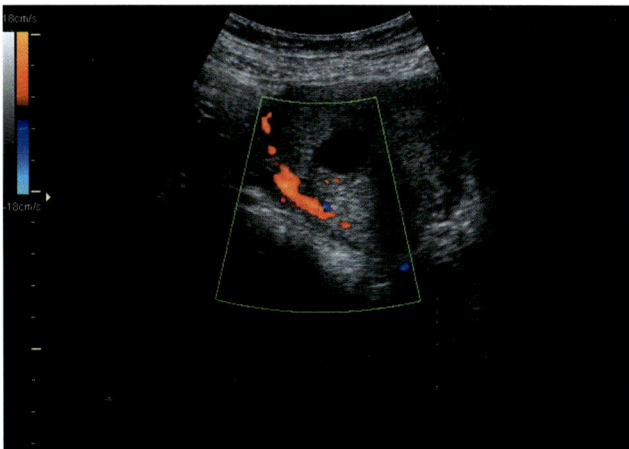

Fig. 56.9: Ultrasound image of blighted ovum (Empty gestational sac without embryo)

Helpful Landmark of Early Pregnancy

a. When the mean sac diameter measures > 25 mm by transabdominal scan, a living embryo should be **identified in a viable pregnancy**. It occurs generally by 7-8 weeks of gestation. By transvaginal ultrasound, fetal cardiac activity should be documented by 6.5 weeks, when the mean sac diameter is approximately 18 mm. At HCG level of 1000 mIU a normal gestational sac can be visualized transvaginally.
b. Ultrasound can help in diagnosis of **blighted ovum (Anembryonic pregnancy).** The absence of fetal pole in a gestational sac with a diameter of 3 cm or more is consistent with diagnosis of blighted ovum (Fig. 56.9).
c. Ultrasound helps in differentiating missed abortion, incomplete abortion, threatened abortion, vesicular mole and ectopic pregnancy which are **causes of 1st trimester bleeding.**
d. **Identification of multiple pregnancy** can be done in 52-63% of cases.
e. **Dating the pregnancy:** Measure of crown rump length (CRL) in the first trimester (between 7-12 weeks) is most accurate (± 5 days) for assessing the gestational age of the fetus. After 12 weeks accuracy of CRL decreases due to progressive curvature of the fetus.
f. **Nuchal translucency:** Nuchal translucency (NT) is a translucent area behind the fetal neck in first trimester ultrasound. **An enlarged NT more than 3 mm by transvaginal ultrasound is a strong marker for chromosomal anamolies.** Increased nuchal thickness in first trimester is a screening test for chromosomal anamolies in first trimester.
g. **Nasal bone:** Absence or delayed development of the nasal bone can be studied in a sagittal plane of the fetus and is *marker for trisomy 9, 18, 21 and Turner syndrome. It*

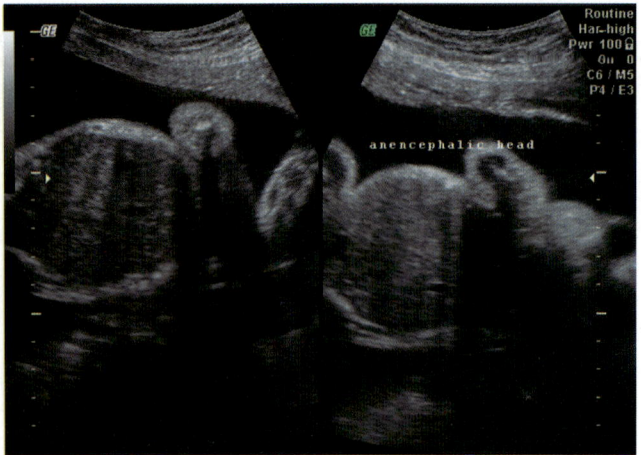

Fig. 56.10: Ultrasound image showing anencephaly

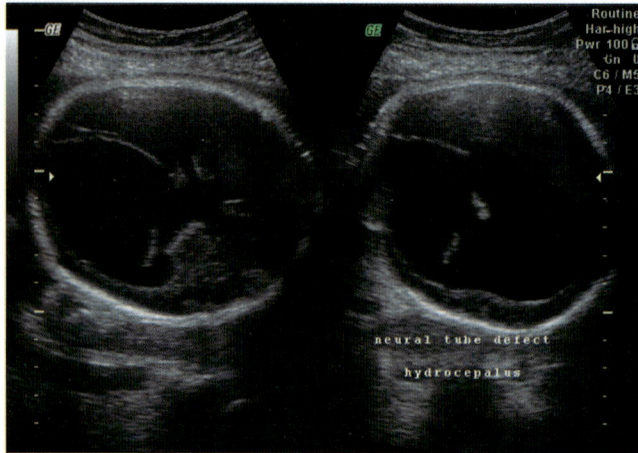

Fig. 56.11: Ultrasound image showing hydrocephalus

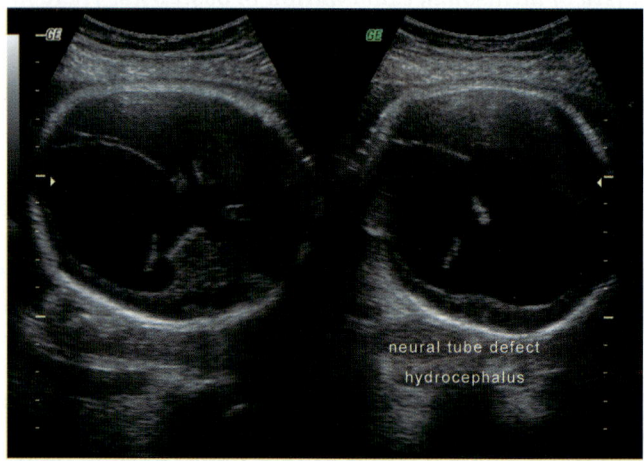

Fig. 56.12: Ultrasound image showing cystic hygroma

is independent of Nuchal Translucency and have 90% sensitivity and 3% false positive rate.

Second and Third Trimester Ultrasound Scan

Following things should be demonstrated and documented in a second or third trimester scan:
a. Fetal number
b. Fetal cardiac activity
c. Fetal presentation
d. Assessment of amniotic fluid volume
e. Fetal biometry and gestational age
f. Appearance of the placenta and its location especially with reference to the cervical os
g. Condition of maternal uterus and adnexa
h. Fetal anatomic examination should include but is not limited to evaluation of the cerebral ventricles, four chamber view of the heart, spine, stomach, bladder, cord insertion, kidney and limbs. BPD is measured in a transverse axial plane at the level of the falx cerebri, the thalamic nuclei and cavum septum pellucidi. Three axial views of the fetal brain are usually imaged.

Ultrasound Diagnosis of Common Fetal Anomalies

Anencephaly: It is characterized by absence of the brain and cranial vault above the base of the skull and orbits (Fig. 56.10).

Encephalocele: It is herniation of meninges and often brain through a defect in the cranium. *Cranial signs suggestive of neural tube defects—banana and lemon signs* are two sonographic signs of the Arnold Chiari malformation seen in spina bifida. The frontal bones of the skull are scalloped giving a **lemon like configuration**. The cerebellum is flattened and centrally curved, obliterating the posterior fossa and giving the cerebellum **banana like appearance**. Ventriculomegaly can also be seen. **Spina bifida** consists of hiatus in the vertebrae through which a meningeal sac may protrude forming a meningocoele. If sac contains neural element, the anomaly is called **meningomyelocele**. **Hydrocephalus** is the presence of excessive cerebrospinal fluid within the intracranial cavity. The ventricles become enlarged and dangling of the choroid plexus within the lateral ventricle is a characteristic finding (Fig. 56.11).

Cystic hygroma: It is a congenital malformation of the lymphatic system in which fluid filled sac extends from the posterior neck. Approximately 60-70% are associated with fetal aneuploidy (Fig. 56.12).

Heart: The basic anatomic survey includes evaluation of the four chamber view of heart, rate, and rhythm. The four chamber view is a transverse image through the thorax just above the level of the diaphragm. *Indications for targeted fetal electrocardiography include suspected anomaly or arrythmia, extracardiac anomaly, parent or sibling with heart defect, maternal pregestational diabetes, teratogen exposure and nonimmune hydrops.*

Thorax: The lungs are best visualized after 20-25 weeks of gestation and appears as homogeneous structure surrounding the heart, occupying approximately two third of the area of chest is four chamber view.

Diaphragmatic hernia: It complicates 1 in 2000 to 5000 birth. Classically the four chamber cardiac view shows the heart pressed to the middle or to the right of the thorax by the stomach or bowel which appears as cystic structure behind the left atrium. Pulmonary hypoplasia and Hydrops may results.

Gastrointestinal tract: Most atresia are characterized by obstruction with proximal bowel dilatation. **Esophageal atresia** is suspected when the stomach can not be visualized. It is encountered in about 1 in 3000 births. **Duodenal atresia** occurs 1 in 10000 live births. It may be detected prenatally by **demonstration of the double bubble sign,** which represents distension of proximal duodenum adjacent to the stomach. The diagnosis of duodenal atresia generally is difficult before 24 weeks. *About 30% of cases of duodenal atresia have Trisomy 21, and other associated anomalies.*

Gastroschisis: It occurs in approximately 1 per 5000 birth. It is a full thickness defect in the abdominal wall through which bowel can herniate into the amniotic cavity.

Omphalocele: It is extrusion of the abdominal content into the base of the umbilical cord, so in omphalocele the herniated mass is covered with parietal peritoneum, amnion and Wharton's jelly (Fig. 56.13).

Genitourinary tract: The fetal bladder can be visualized by the early trimester and kidneys are routinely visualized by 18 weeks. Renal agenesis complicates 1 in 4000 births. No kidneys are visualized sonographically and adrenal glands typically enlarge and occupy the renal fossae. Without kidneys there is no urine production and severe oligohydramnios leads to pulmonary hypoplasia, limb contracture and ultimately fetal death.

Potter syndrome: *Multicystic renal dysplasia* results from obstruction/atresia at the level of renal pelvis or proximal ureter prior to 10 weeks. Most cases are unilateral though contralateral renal anomalies occurs in 40%, the most common being uteropelvic junction obstruction. Sonographically there is abnormally dense renal parenchyma with multiple peripheral cysts of varying sizes, which do not communicate with each other or renal pelvis.

Ultrasound features of hydrops fetalis: It is a condition of excessive fluid accumulation within the fetus. It is characterized by varying degree of ascites, pleural effusion, skin edema, placental edema and polyhydramnios.

Fetal weight: Estimated fetal weight is determined from the average of these reading for each of the following—FL, AC and BPD. AC is most important. Estimated fetal weight has an error risk of 15-20%. The later in gestation the examination is performed, the greater the standard deviation.

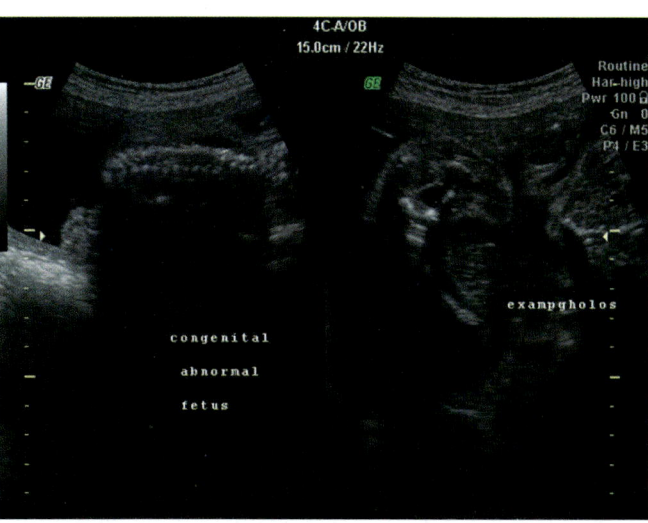

Fig. 56.13: Ultrasound image showing omphalocele

Amniotic fluid index: It is a quantitative technique to assess amniotic fluid volume. The maternal abdomen is divided into four quadrants, using the umbilicus and linea nigra as reference points. The transducer head is maintained perpendicular to the floor and the largest vertical pocket in each quadrant is measured. The sum of the four measurements (in cm) is the AFI in singleton pregnancy. In multiple pregnancy the single largest pocket is used.

Placenta and umbilical cord: Placenta is an echogenic discoid mass. Placenta thickness at term is about 30 mm. *Placental thickness more than 45 mm at any period of gestation is considered abnormal.* The relationship of placenta to internal cervical os is important to define low lying placenta.

Fetal biophysical profile: It is a sonographic assessment of multiple fetal biophysical activities or components, including fetal body movements, fetal breathing movement, fetal tone and amniotic fluid volume. The non stress test is also included as part of profile **(details in AFS Part).**

Doppler ultrasound: Doppler ultrasound and velocimetry is useful in predicting fetal anemia, especially which are associated with isoimmunization.

Use of USG in Detection of Chromosomal Anomalies or Down Syndrome

Ultrasound can detect many of the malformations associated with chromosomal abnormalities. Fetus with Trisomy 13 and 18 tend to have major malformation, most of which can be detected sonographically. In Down syndrome many fetus have either no major malformation or malformation that tends to be detected late in pregnancy such as duodenal atresia, so only 30% down syndrome fetus are detected by routine USG. Subtle biometric or morphologic abnormalities are noted in screening for fetal Down syndrome following:

a. Nuchal fold > 5 mm
b. Echogenic bowel
c. Short Humerus
d. Short femur
e. Echogenic intracardiac focus
f. Pyelectesis
g. Any two minor markers.

Integrated screening: It is a two step screening protocols between 10-13 weeks – Nuchal translucency with screening assay for PAPP – A are obtained. Between 15-16 weeks gestation. AFP, HCG, µ E3, Inhibin A is obtained. A single risk assessment is then calculated at 16 weeks gestation.

Causes of abnormal alpha fetoprotein in relation with ultrasound: Maternal serum alpha feto protein is elevated in multiple gestation, fetal death, cystic hygroma, and other conditions associated with fetal edema, anterior abdominal wall defects and other fetal skin defect. Low serum maternal alpha feto protein is associated with chromosomal abnormalities, e.g. Down's syndrome, Trisomy 18, dating errors, molar pregnancy, fetal death.

Ultrasound markers in twin pregnancy: In sonographic assessment, evaluation of chorionicity is important component. Evidences of dichorionicity are:
a. Separate sac in the first trimester
b. Separate placenta
c. Different genders
d. Thick intertwine septa
e. Presence of chorionic peak (didi sign, twin peak sign). It is a projecting zone of tissue extending from the chorionic surface of the placenta and tapering within the intertwine membrane.

57. Critical Care Obstetric

When fear ceases to scare you, it cannot stay.

SHOCK IN OBSTETRICS

General Consideration

Shock is defined as a state of circulatory inadequacy with poor tissue perfusion resulting in generalized cellular hypoxia. The basic underlying defect is a significant reduction in the supply of oxygenated blood to various tissues due to inadequate perfusion. The physiologic compensation to all shock state involves tachycardia and peripheral vasoconstriction to maximize cerebral and cardiac perfusion by way of sympathetic nervous system. Failure of these compensatory mechanisms will lead to predominance of anaerobic metabolism of lactic acidosis, which can be potentially devastating to the patient and fetus.

Classification of Shock

a. **Cardiogenic:** Pump failure as cardiac arrhythmias, myocardial infarction.
b. **Peripheral circulatory failure:**
   i. Hypovolemic shock
   ii. Normovolemic shock
   iii. Bacteremic
   iv. Anaphylactic
   v. Neurogenic
   vi. Adrenal insufficiency

Hypovolemic Shock

It can be of following types:

- Hemorrhagic shock associated with postpartum or postabortal hemorrhage, ectopic pregnancy, placenta previa.
- Fluid loss shock: Associated with excessive vomiting, diarrhea, diuresis or too rapid removal of amniotic fluid.
- Supine hypotension syndrome: Caused by compression of inferior vena cava by the pregnant uterus.
- Shock associated with disseminated intravascular coagulation in cases of intrauterine dead fetus syndrome and amniotic fluid embolism.

Pathophysiology

a. *Early phase (Compensatory phase):* In the early phase there is mild vasoconstriction and with compensatory sympathetic mechanism operating, the patient has relatively normal blood pressure, tachycardia and diaphoresis. Extremities are warm, patient is restless and anxious—**this phase is easily managed by volume replacement.**

b. *Intermediate phase (Reversible phase):* If the early phase is not managed, the patient passes into stage of hypotension. Patient gradually become pale, tachycardia persist and due to intense vasoconstriction the periphery become cold and there is excessive sweating. In this stage there is preferential blood flow to vital organs. So the patient is conscious and urine output is within limits. With **adequate management the shock state can be reversed.**

c. *Late stage (Irreversible):* If intermediate stage is also not managed, hypotension continues and there is stagnation of blood at the microvascular level. In this stage it can not be reversed by fluid replacement. Extremities become cold and clammy because of intense vasoconstriction caused by sympathetic stimulation. Color of skin is ashen gray. There is low volume pulse, oliguria, mental confusion because of circulatory failure and anaerobic metabolism. There is multiple organ failure. **Mortality in this stage is 3-100%.**

Complications

Electrolyte imbalance, acidosis, acute tubular necrosis and stress induced gastric ulceration, pulmonary edema and ARDS are common complications associated with hemorrhagic shock.

Management of Hemorrhagic Shock

Basic management of hemorrhagic shock is to stop the cause of bleeding.
i. **Replace** the blood volume and optimize cardiac performance.
ii. **Cause** of bleeding should be controlled. Uterine atony, genital tract laceration. Uterus rupture should be looked for and treated appropriately.

Infusion and Transfusion

Crystalloid: Typically 1-2 liter of ringer lactate solution should be administered as rapidly as possible. Ringer lactate solution more closely approximates plasma and metabolism of lactate to bicarbonate provides some buffering capacity for acidosis. So it is considered better than normal saline.

Colloids: Polygelatin solution (hemocele) are isosmotic with plasma. They do not interfere with coagulation system and promote osmotic diuresis. Large volumes can be administered.

Dextran: They are polymolecular polysaccharides. They interfere with crossmatching and to be avoided.

Blood: Blood should be transfused as early as it is available. A guide to transfusion requirements should be based on clinical responses. The blood should be warmed to 35°C and given rapidly. If large quantities of stored blood are given the clotting factors-platelets, calcium, factors V and VIII lowered. The chances of this can be minimized by giving *500 ml of fresh blood for every 2-3 liter of stored blood infused. 10 ml of 10% calcium gluconate is given for every unit of blood transfusion.* The metabolic acidosis present in shock may be worsened by the acidity (pH 6.6-6.8) of stored blood in large amount. *If more than 3 liter of stored blood is given, 50 ml of 4.2% sodium bicarbonate solution should be given.*

Maintenance of Cardiac Efficacy

When a large volume of fluid or blood is to be administered, the efficacy of cardiac competence should be ascertained, otherwise there is a risk of overloading the circulation and cardiac failure. Six liter of crystalloid may be needed for loss of 1 liter of plasma volume. Hemodynamic monitoring should be aimed to maintain systolic BP > 90 mm Hg, mean arterial pressure ≥ 60 mm of Hg, CVP 12-15 cm H_2O and pulmonary capillary wedge pressure 14-18 mm Hg.

Oxygen Administration

Administration of oxygen by face mask at rate of 6-8 liter per minute is given. Oxygen delivery is continued to maintain oxygen saturation ≥ 92%. In late phase sometimes endotracheal intubation may be necessary for ventilation.

Pharmacologic Agent

Vasopressors drug should be kept to minimum because there is already peripheral vasoconstriction. Vasodilators are occasionally used but close monitoring of CVP and adequate blood volume replacement is required. **Phenoxylbenzamine** (Dibenzyline) is alpha receptor blocker and drug of choice. It is given as 1 mg/ kg over 1 hour intravenously. *Oliguria refractory to volume loading may be improved by the addition of intravenous Dopamine in low dose (2-5 μg / kg/ minute) to improve renal perfusion.*

Monitoring

Hemodynamic Monitoring

a. *Fluid balance:* From intravenous infusion and urine output should be meticulously recorded. Urine output > 300 ml/hour is useful guide. Arterial blood pressure is a poor indication to assess tissue perfusion. In some cases measurement of CVP (central venous pressure) is needed to assess adequacy of patient's circulatory volume and contractility state of the myocardium. Pulse oximetry and blood gas analysis are useful to assess tissue perfusion. In selected cases measurement of left atrial pressure by pulmonary artery catheterization is needed.
b. *Hematocrit monitoring:* Blood test for complete blood count, serum electrolytes, serum creatinine, and arterial blood gas analysis and coagulation profile is done. Frequent serial hematocrit may provide an index of acute blood loss. A baseline hematological profile – PT, partial thromboplastin time, fibrinogen and platelet count is necessary to evaluate the possibility of coagulopathy.
c. *A baseline chest radiography and ECG is desirable.*

Prognosis

Maternal and fetal survival rates are directly related to the magnitude of volume depletion and duration of shock. If cause of hemorrhage is controlled and blood volume is restored rapidly, prognosis is generally good in the absence of complication. But in delayed shock or irreversible shock prognosis is bad with mortality rate of 3-100%.

SEPTIC SHOCK (ENDOTOXIC SHOCK)

Septic shock is a life-threatening disorders secondary to bacterial infection or bacterial products in the bloodstream. **ACOG defines septic shock as a sepsis with hypotension despite adequate fluid replacement with the presence of perfusion abnormalities including lactic acidosis and oliguria.**

Incidence: Incidence of septic shock is 0.7-10% in obstetric patients.

Etiopathogenesis

The most common cause of obstetric septic shock is infected abortion and postoperative endometritis (85%). Other causes are antepartum pyelonephritis, chorioamnionitis. Causative organisms are usually gram-negative bacteria. *E. coli* have been implicated in 25-50% cases. Other organisms are *Klebseilla, Enterobacter, Proteus, Pseudomonas, Staphylococcus, Clostridium* and *Bacteriodes*.

Endotoxin is a complex lipopolysaccharides present in the cell wall of gram-negative bacteria. The active component of endotoxin, lipid A is responsible for initiating activation of the coagulation, fibrinolysis, complement and prostaglandin and kinin system. Activation of coagulation and fibrinolysis system may lead to consumptive coagulopathy. Complement activation leads to release by leukocytes of mediators which cause damage to vascular endothelium, platelet aggregation and intensification of coagulation cascade and degranulation of mast cells, which release histamine and cause increased capillary permeability are hypotension.

In early stage: There is low SVR and high cardiac output with a relative decrease in intravascular volume.

Late and cold shock: In this phase there is myocardial depression. Pathogenesis of sepsis and septic shock are summarized in Flow charts 57.1 and 57.2.

Symptoms and Signs

a. **Preshock:** There is tachypnea, respiratory alkalosis, normal blood pressure and elevated cardiac output. Response to therapy is best at this stage.
b. **Early shock (warm shock):** It is more hyperdynamic state. Blood pressure drops (SBP < 60 mm Hg) and there is altered mental status, temperature instability and sinusoidal fluctuation in arterial blood pressure.

Flow chart 57.1: Pathogenesis of sepsis

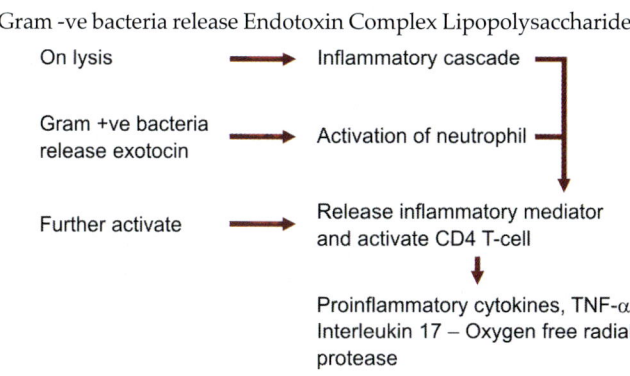

Flow chart 57.2: Pathogenesis of septic shock

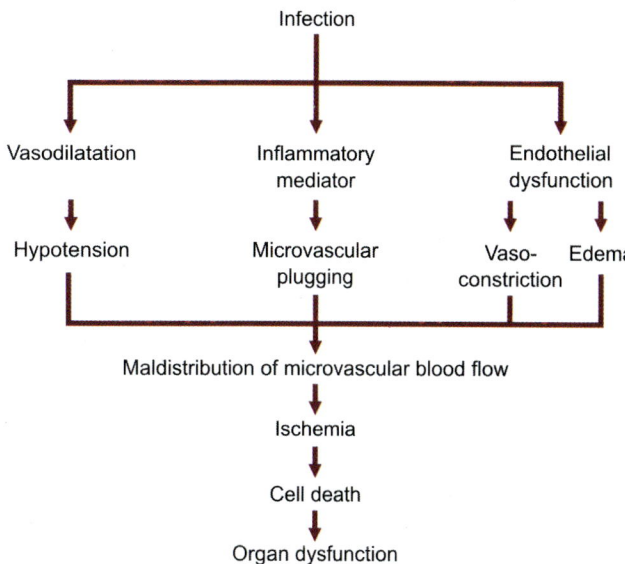

c. **Late shock:** There is intense vasoconstriction which reverts to shunt blood from the peripheral tissue to heart and brain. The compensatory vasoconstriction results in increased cardiac work, lactic acidosis, poor coronary perfusion and myocardial depression.

The common cause of death in septic shock is respiratory insufficiency secondary to adult respiratory distress syndrome.

Fetus is more resistant to effect of endotoxin than the mother. There can be fetal hypoxia, acidosis, placental abruption and fetal death.

Laboratory Investigation

a. **Complete blood count, serum electrolyte, and urinalysis.** They may be significant anemia, thrombocytopenia, and leukocytosis. Serum electrolytes are abnormal, urinalysis permits evaluation of renal involvement.
b. **Urine culture, aerobic and anaerobic blood culture should be taken.**
c. **Chest X-ray and arterial blood gas level** to assess ventilatory and oxygenation status.
d. **A baseline ECG** is done to rule out myocardial infarction or cardiac dysrhythmia.
e. **Ultrasound and X-ray abdomen** is done to rule out intrapelvic or intra-abdominal source of obstetric sepsis like uterus or bowel perforation, tubo-ovarian abscess.
f. **Coagulation factor test** for diagnosis of DIC.

Complications

Complications depend on the target organ involved:
a. ARDS (Adult respiratory distress syndrome)
b. Congestive heart failure

c. Dysrhythmia
d. Hepatic failure
e. Renal insufficiency
f. Intrauterine fetal death
g. Maternal mortality

Treatment

General Measurement

a. Broad spectrum antibiotic regimen is started as Ampicillin, Gentamycin and Clindamycin. Newer antibiotic as Vancomycin, extended spectrum penicillin as Ticarcillin, Cilastin, Vancomycin are also proving to be effective therapies.
b. Careful search for infected or necrotic foci and surgical intervention to remove that cause, like removal of infected products of conception. In cases of chorioamnionitis prompt delivery is necessary.
c. Supportive treatment is control of fever with antipyretic and cooling.

Cardiovascular Support

a. **Volume therapy** begins with 1-2 liter of Ringer lactate solution infused over approximately 15 minutes. The total amount of crystalloid administered should be guided by presence or absence of maternal hypoxia. PCWP of 14-16 mm Hg is maintained.
b. **Blood component therapy** is an important adjuvant if there has been associated significant hemorrhage and an associated coagulopathy.
c. **Inotropic agent:** If shock persists despite volume replacement, myocardial performance and vascular tone should be improved. Inotropic agents as dopamine, dobutamine or isoterenol are excellent choice.

   Dopamine is first line drug of choice. Dopamine is a chemical precursor of norepinephrine which has alpha adrenergic, beta adrenergic and dopaminergic receptor stimulating actions. The dopamine infusion is started at 2-5 µg/kg/minute and titrated against its effect on improving cardiac output and blood pressure. At low doses (0.5-5.0 µg/kg/minute) dopamine acts primarily on dopaminergic receptors leading to vasodilatation and improved perfusion of renal and mesenteric vascular beds. Higher dopamine dose (5.0 or 14.0 µg/kg/minute) is associated with predominant effects on the β receptors of the heart, which improves myocardial contractility, stroke volume and cardiac output. Much higher dose (15-20 µg/kg/minute) will have an alpha adrenergic effect, like norepinephrine and cause vasoconstriction which can be detrimental to organ perfusion.

   Dobutamine is an inotropic agent. It can be added to dopamine at rate of 2-20 µg/kg. It is direct myocardial α1 stimulant which increases cardiac output with only minimal tachycardia. *Isoproterenol* is third line agent, which is given at rate of 1-2 µg/kg/minute. It acts primary on beta adrenergic receptors to increase contractility and heart rate. But side effect can be ventricular ectopy, excessive tachycardia. *Digitalis* – it is commonly added to above requirement to improve the force and velocity of myocardial contraction. This is given in a loading dose of 0.5 mg I/V followed by 0.25 mg every 4 hours for a total dose of 1.0 mg. I/V digoxin should always be given with continuous ECG monitoring with special attention to serum potassium level which should be maintained at 0.25-0.37 mg/dl. Peripheral vasoconstrictor *Phenylephrine* in dose of 1-5 µg/kg/minute is given if there is reduced systemic vascular resistance index with systolic blood pressure of less than 80 mm Hg despite ionotropic therapy. *Norepinephrine* is only indicated for septic shock patients with decreased after loads, who do not respond to volume replacement, inotropic therapy and phenylephrine.

d. **Corticosteroid:** It can be given 3-4 gm intravenously daily for 24-48 hours but its efficacy is inconclusive.
e. **Newer agents:** Anti endotoxin therapy.

Prognosis

The overall maternal mortality rate in septic shock is approximately 50%. The prognosis is worsened by the presence of ARDS or pre-existing medical problem.

AMNIOTIC FLUID EMBOLISM

It is a rare, life-threatening complication of pregnancy with high mortality rate. This is a complex disorder characterized by the abrupt onset of hypotension, hypoxia and consumption coagulopathy.

Incidence and Facts

There is no definitive diagnostic test for this condition even at postmortem. Incidence is 1.5-2/10000 childbirth. The syndrome is uncommon in absolute sense but it is one of the important causes of maternal death. The interval between collapse and death is generally sudden with 85% maternal mortality rate and with 25% of women dying within first hour. The women who survive, most of them develop DIC and perinatal mortality rate is 40%.

Pathogenesis

Amniotic fluid probably enters the maternal venous circulation through a breech in the barrier between maternal vasculature and amniotic fluid either from placental site or at site of uterine trauma after rupture of membrane. The amniotic fluid contains particulate constituent of liquor amni such as epithelial squamous, fat, lanugo hairs, and meconium, which provoke immunological and humoral reaction in mother. This results in an inflammatory cascade which leads to multi organ failure and disseminated coagulopathy. It is now being suggested that it is not an embolic episode but an anaphylactic type reaction to amniotic fluid. **It is a combination of left ventricular failure and acute lung injury accompanied by activation of clotting factors**.

Symptoms and Signs

Risk factors are multiparity, tumulous labor, hypertonic uterine contractions.

Patient can present as: (a) Sudden hypotension and shock, (b) Sudden onset of acute fetal distress, (c) Pulmonary edema or adult respiratory distress syndrome, (d) Cardiopulmonary arrest, (e) Maternal cyanosis, (f) Coagulopathy, (g) Convulsion.

Differential Diagnosis

a. Pulmonary thromboembolism
b. Congestive heart failure
c. Severe postpartum hemorrhage
d. Pulmonary aspiration
e. Myocardial infarction
f. Anaphylaxis
g. Uterine rupture
h. Transfusion Reaction
i. Local anesthetic toxicity

Laboratory Findings

a. Arterial blood oxygen level show severe hypoxemia.
b. Coagulapathy is evident if present, by hypofibrinogenemia, prolonged clotting and bleeding time and elevated fibrin split product.
c. Chest X-ray is nonspecific though pulmonary edema can be seen.
d. ECG reveals sinus tachycardia and nonspecific ST-T changes.

Treatment

AFE remains one of the most devastating and unpreventable condition complicating pregnancy. It requires coordinated care of anesthetist, obstetrician, midwives and hematology team. Treatment is directed to:

a. Cardiopulmonary resuscitation.
b. Immediate oxygen and intubation.
c. Vasopressor like dopamine, Derbutamine or Phenylephrine.
d. Blood transfusion.
e. Treatment of coagulopathy. If mother survives, usually require intensive care management for development of complications.

PULMONARY THROMBOEMBOLISM

Incidence and Facts

It is a rare complication of pregnancy (0.09%) but it is a significant cause of maternal morbidity and mortality in western world. In untreated case mortality is 12.8% and in treated case 0.7%.

Etiopathogenesis

Women are at higher risk of venous thromboembolic disease in pregnancy and puerperium because of following reasons:

a. Maternal circulation becomes hypercoagulable from alteration in the coagulation and fibronolytic systems. Fibrinogen and factors II, VII, VIII, IX and X increase during pregnancy. At the same time there is decreased fibrinolytic activity.

b. There is venous stasis especially in lower extremities because the enlarging uterus reduces blood return to the inferior vena cava by direct mechanical factors. Hormonal factors also add to vasodilatation and stasis during pregnancy. Stasis secondary to prolonged bed rest for a medical or obstetric complication predispose a pregnant women to increased venous stasis and formation of vascular thrombin.

c. Women with congenital or acquired Thrombophilias are at increased risk for thrombosis. The most commonly recognized Thrombophilia are factor V Leiden mutation (5%).

Once the venous thrombosis is formed, it may dislodge from its peripheral vascular origin and enter the central maternal circulation. There can be propagation of original venous clot or recurrent pulmonary emboli.

Diagnosis

a. The diagnosis is easier in women with clinical suspicion of deep vein thrombosis (DVT). Signs suggestive of DVT are redness, swelling and tenderness over a vein in one of the legs.

b. PTE can occur with asymptomatic DVT so high risk factors should be screened early in pregnancy like screen for Thrombophilia.

c. *Classic symptoms of PTE* are—hemoptysis, chest pain and dyspnea/chest pain and apprehension. **Physical findings** are tachycardia, tachypnea (rate >16/min), pulmonary rates, wheezing and pleural friction rub.

Laboratory findings: There is no specific routine laboratory finding associated with PTE. ECG may reveal unexplained tachycardia associated with cor pulmonale. A chest X-ray may be normal or may show infiltrates, atelectesis or effusion but 30% of patients with PTE will have normal X-ray. **Non invasive Doppler studies should be considered as an initial diagnostic test for suspected DVT involving lower extremities.** Sensitivity is 95%. **Venography with pelvic shield can be done to confirm the extent of the original thrombotic event.**

Differential Diagnosis

a. Amniotic fluid embolism
b. Air emboli
c. Spontaneous pneumothorax
d. Septic shock
e. Pre-existing heart disease.

Treatment

Preventive Measure

In high risk patients measures should be taken to prevent venous stasis like:

a. Raising leg 15° to horizontal, keeping the leg straight rather then bent.
b. Heparin prophylaxis 5000 IU S/C 2 hours before surgery and every 12 hours until routine ambulation is achieved. Low Molecular Weight Heparin (LMWH) can also be used.

Treatment of Documented PTE

a. Correction of arterial hypoxemia and hypotension by fluid replacement and oxygen by face mask to achieve arterial oxygen tension of at least 70 mm Hg.
b. A loading dose of 5000-10000 IU of heparin should be given intravenously by continued infusion followed by a maintenance dose of approximate 1000 unit/hour. PTT should be maintained at 1.5-2.5 times control values. Heparin level may be measured on every 3rd and 4th day and should be about 0.2 µg/ml.
c. Leg elevation and local heat and I/V sedation for symptomatic relief and alleviate anxiety.
d. Postpartum patients receiving heparin may be switched over to warfarin once oral intake is tolerable. Heparin should be continued for the first 5-7 days of warfarin therapy. Alternatively, it may be desirable to continue moderate doses of subcutaneous heparin (10,000 units twice daily) especially in nursing mothers. Postpartum anticoagulation should be continued for at least 3 months if the patient has developed pulmonary embolism in the third trimester.

Complications of Treatment

The major potential complications of anticoagulant therapy is maternal or fetal hemorrhage. Heparin does not cross the placenta due to its large molecular weight, but it has been associated with maternal thrombocytopenia and osteoporosis. These effects can be avoided with low molecular weight heparin. Warfarin is known to cross the placental barrier and its use in the first trimester has been associated with embryopathy (nasal hypoplasia and stippled epiphysis).

Alternative Treatment

A small percentage of patients will experience recurrent pulmonary emboli despite full anticoagulation. **These patients may be candidate for venocaval ligation by a transabdominal approach under general or regional anesthetic.** If the pelvis is suspected as the source of embolus, the right ovarian vein also should be ligated. It has been estimated that approximately 95% of patients with pulmonary embolism massive enough to cause hypotension eventually die. In this context pulmonary artery embolectomy may be life saving.

Section Four

Appendices

Appendix 1: Investigations in Gynecology

I attribute my success to this—I never gave or took any excuses.

GENERAL CONSIDERATION

Detailed history and clinical examination often clinch the diagnosis or limits the differential diagnosis to a few possibilities. However, investigation may be necessary to confirm the diagnosis and to have a baseline for patient's general health status and future options for treatment.

Common Investigations in Gynecological Diagnosis

Certain common investigations and procedures used in gynecological diagnosis are described below:

1. **Blood investigation:** Hemoglobin assessment is important in all cases of excessive bleeding for any causes. Total and differential leukocytes count (TLC, DLC) and ESR are helpful in diagnosis of pelvic inflammation and infection. Platelet count and bleeding time, clotting time is important in puberty menorrhagia.
2. **Urine analysis:** Urine is routinely examined for presence of protein and sugar. A microscopic examination is done for detection for pus cell and counts. Urine culture is required if microscopy shows more than 5 cells per high power field.
3. **Other blood test** done in preoperative evaluation or directed by clinical picture are:
   a. Fasting and postprandial blood sugar.
   b. Kidney function test – blood urea, serum creatinine, and uric acid.
   c. Test for STD like VDRL for syphilis, Australia antigen, HIV I and II.
   d. Serum electrolytes Na, K, Ca and HCO_3.
   e. Blood group and Rh factor.
4. **Special blood test like tumor markers:** CA–125 in suspected neoplasm of ovary, Beta hCG in gestational trophoblast disease.
5. **Bacterial examination of genital tract:** For this vaginal discharge is taken and examined with one drop of normal saline, covered with cover slip and microscopic examination is done to look for *Trichomonas vaginalis* and *Candidial hyphae*. For collection of vaginal discharge, Sims or Cusco's speculum is introduced without lubrication and without prior per vaginal examination. The material collected in the posterior blade is taken. From cervical canal discharge can be taken either by platinum loop or swab stick. For sending culture, the sterile prepared cotton swab stick is put in a sterile container with the stopper and sent immediately to the laboratory.

Special Tests in Gynecological Practice

a. ***Papanicolaou test:*** This test was first described by Papanicolaou and Traut in 1943 and often referred to as Pap test or surface biopsy. It forms a part of the routine gynecological examination in women. Details of method of taking Pap smear is described in chapter of Intraepithelial Lesion of Cervix.

b. ***Colposcopy:*** The colposcope is a binocular microscope giving a 10-20 times magnification. It is useful in locating abnormal areas and obtaining accurate guided biopsy from the suspicious areas on the cervix. Details of this technique are described in chapter of Intraepithelial Lesion of Cervix (Fig. A1.1).

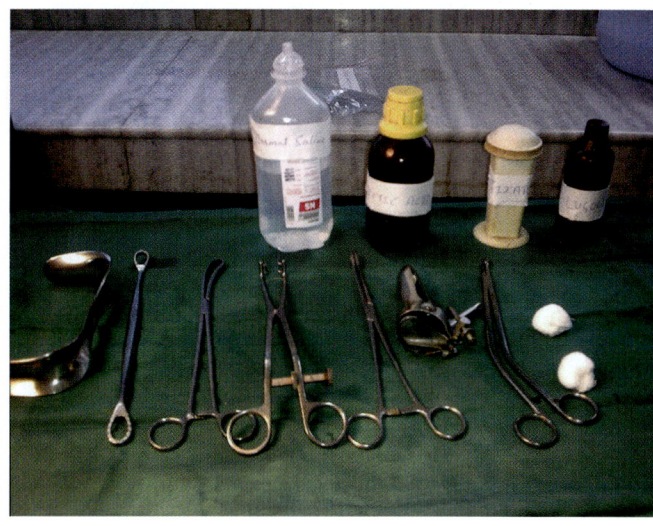

Fig. A1.1: Instruments for colposcopic directed biopsy

c. *Cytohormonal evaluation:* The ovarian hormones estrogen and progesterone influence the vaginal mucosa. So the epithelial cells exfoliated in the vagina reflect the influence of the prevailing dominant hormone in the system at that time.

Karyopyknotic index or KPI (Maturation index): It is the ratio of mature squamous cells over the intermediate and basal cells. It is more than 25% in estrogenic phase (Proliferative phase), low in progestogenic phase (secretory) and during pregnancy. Normally peak value of KPI reaches on the day of ovulation (2 days after serum E_2 peak).

d. *Uterine aspiration cytology:* Perimenopausal and postmenopausal women on hormone therapy or having complaint of abnormal uterine bleeding, endometrial aspiration cytology is done with uterine aspiration syringe. Details are in chapter of Endometrial Hyperplasia (Fig. A1.2).

e. *Endometrial biopsy:* It is an office or outpatient procedure. **It is done in suspected case of tubercular endometritis, secondary amenorrhea, abnormal uterine bleeding and to diagnose endometrial hyperplasia in patients of postmenopausal bleeding and in some cases of infertility.** In this procedure fine curette is introduced into the uterine cavity to obtain a small strip of endometrial lining for histopathological examination (Fig. A1.2).

f. *Cervical biopsy:* In suspected malignant lesion cervical biopsy is mandatory. It can be done as office procedure. Details are described in chapter of Cervical Cancer.

g. *Culdocentesis:* Culdocentesis is the transvaginal aspiration of peritoneal fluid from the cul-de-sac or pouch of Douglas. **It is done in diagnosis of – Pelvic abscess, Ectopic pregnancy in Hematocele. The only therapeutic indication is to drain the pus in pelvic abscess.**

In the procedure patient is placed in lithotomy position, and posterior lip of cervix is drawn forward and downward with volsellum forceps while the Sim's speculum retracts back the posterior vaginal wall. The procedure is done with full aseptic precaution. An 18-gauge spinal needle with aspiration syringe is inserted at point 1 cm below the cervicovaginal junction in the posterior fornix. After inserting needle to a depth of about 2 cm, aspiration is done. The procedure should be best done in Operation Theater under full aseptic precaution with all preparation to perform laparoscopy or laparotomy if needed (Fig. A1.3).

h. *Pregnancy test:* Sample to confirm the pregnancy by rapid immunological test is tabin in outpatient by performing first morning sample of urine to confirm pregnancy and in suspected pregnancy related complication like ectopic pregnancy, miscarriage.

i. *Hormonal assay:* In present clinical practice, levels of many hormones like FSH, LH, Prolactin, T_3, T_4, TSH, estradiol, progesterone, testosterone can be measured by using radioimmunoassay or ELISA test. *These assays are used in management of infertility, polycystic ovarian disease, amenorrhea, menopause, prolactinoma.*

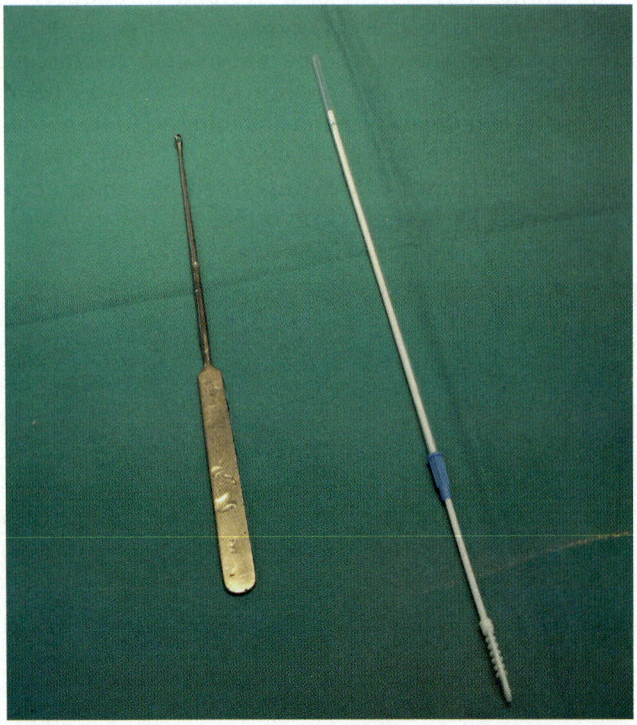

Imaging Techniques

Fig. A1:2: Endometrial biopsy curette and Vabra Aspirator

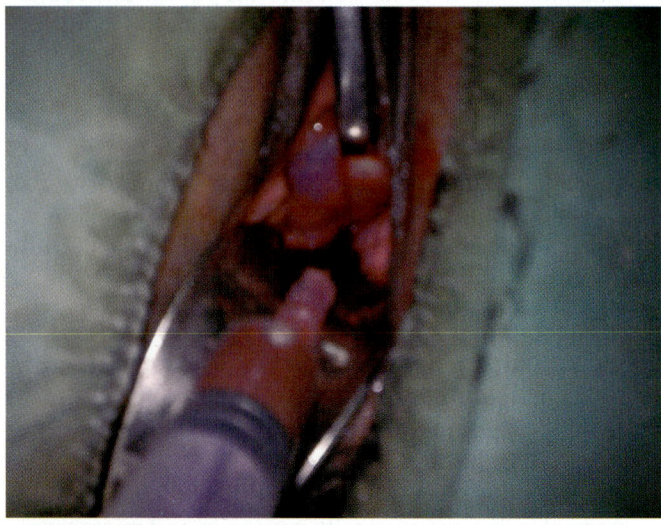

Fig. A1.3: Culdocentesis procedure

APPENDIX – 1 ♦ Investigations in Gynecology

X-ray

Plain radiograph have a minor role in gynecology practice. However, its use are as follows:

a. **To locate misplaced intrauterine contraceptive device (IUCD) or foreign body** when ultrasound fails to locate IUCD. In this situation plain X-ray of abdomen in erect position with uterine sound in situ helps in diagnosis of uterine or extrauterine location of IUCD or foreign body.

b. **Plain X-ray chest** is required in suspected cases of tuberculosis and to determine metastasis in gynecological malignancies and as part of routine work up before any major gynecological surgery.

Special X-ray

Hysterosalpingography

In this X-ray is taken after injection of radiopaque die through the cervix into uterus and fallopian tubes. Dye can be water soluble – Renograffin 60, cornay dye or low viscosity oil based dye – Ethidol. Usually 2-4 radiographic views are taken. The first one shows the filling of uterine cavity, other two shows filling of fallopian tube and last view is taken on completion of procedure usually taken after 10-15 minutes. The passage of dye in the uterus and fallopian tube can be observed by using X-ray image intensifier and video display unit.

Indications of Hysterosalpingography

i. In infertile women to test the patency of fallopian tubes.
ii. To evaluate result of tuboplasty postoperatively.
iii. To detect uterine abnormalities like fibroid, polyps in menorrhagia, uterine anomalies in cases of habitual abortion.
iv. To diagnose Asherman's syndrome.

Contraindications of Hysterosalpingography

i. Presence of genital tract infection. HSG should be performed after full treatment of genital tract infection.
ii. Suspected or previous genital tract tuberculosis.
iii. Suspected pregnancy or secretory phase of menstrual cycle.
iv. Patient is allergic to radiopaque dye.

Complications of HSG can be:
i. Pelvic pain and peritoneal irritation.
ii. Vasovagal attack.
iii. Extravasations of dye within venous and lymphatic channel which is common in tubercular endometritis.
iv. Flaring up of pelvic infection in 1-3% of cases.

Intravenous Urography

Urography outlines the urinary tract following the administration of an intravenous iodinated contrast medium. Indications of intravenous urography in gynecologic practice are as follows:

i. **In gynecological malignancy** to determine the normality of urinary tract. In cancer cervix there can be hydroureter, hydronephrosis. In cancer ovary the ureter may get displaced.
ii. **Confirmation of ectopic kidney.** In malformation of genital tract, it is wise to perform intravenous pyelography to exclude urinary tract abnormalities.

In young girls **urinary incontinence** can be due to ectopic ureter. Intravenous urogram is useful in diagnosis.

In **genital urinary fistula**, the relationship of the ureteric orifice to the site of fistula is important in planning any surgical repair.

Contraindications of Intravenous Urogram

i. It is mandatory to do sensitivity test prior to investigation. In women with iodine sensitivity it should be undertaken with caution.
ii. Women with impaired renal function.
iii. Suspicion of pregnancy.

Cystourethrography

It is useful in certain cases of urinary incontinence: It permits the evaluation of disorder of bladder neck and proximal urethral displacement and inappropriate detrusor contraction.

Gastrointestinal Studies

Barium meal and follow through, barium enema are some times needed in ovarian malignancy, pelvic inflammatory disease, endometriosis. Large bowel inflammation, Crohn's disease, chronic amoebiasis, etc. can confuse clinical picture and these studies can give clue to diagnosis.

Arteriography and Arterial Embolization

In selected cases arteriography can establish cause of unexplained heaving abnormal uterine bleeding. Embolization of the anterior division of iliac artery has been successfully used in treatment of bleeding from advanced cervical cancer, secondary hemorrhage after hysterectomy, cervical ectopic pregnancy and for embolization of uterine artery in menorrhagia and in fibroids.

ULTRASONOGRAPHY IN GYNECOLOGY

The use of ultrasound was first pioneered by Ian Donald (1974) in gynecology and obstetrics. Sonography is generally the first and only imaging modality used to demonstrate physiological and pathologic changes in pelvic anatomy. Ultrasound is cheap, easily available, noninvasive technique and there is no danger of radiation exposure. Besides imaging of soft tissue is possible (Fig. A1.4).

Methods of Ultrasound

1. *Transabdominal:* In this 3.5–5.0 Mhz sector or curvilinear probe is used to obtain a panoramic view of pelvis and abdominal organs. For gynecological scan full bladder is required which displaces the bowel loops and provides window for visualizing pelvic structures. Following full scan, it is advisable to examine the patient on an empty bladder particularly if there has been any difficulty in interpreting between the bladder and cystic mass in the pelvis. It also gives useful information about fixity of pelvic structure and volume of residual urine present in the bladder after voiding.
2. *Transvaginal ultrasound:* In this higher frequency 5.0-7.5 MHz of ultrasound waves and vaginal probe is used. Bladder should be empty. Proximity of vaginal probe to pelvic organ and higher frequency gives higher resolution images. In virgin and menopausal women transvaginal scan can not be used, but perineal or labial ultrasound can be done by use of vaginal probe.
3. *Sonography or sonosalpingography:* In this normal saline with or without antibiotic is inserted in uterine cavity via use of pediatric foley's catheter no 5 or 8, and balloon of catheter is filled with 2-2.5 ml of fluid. Uterine cavity is observed. In cases of infertility tubal patency is evaluated by observing water fall sign (fluid shower from fallopian tubes) and Sion test (presence of fluid in pouch of Douglas). The common indications of sonohysterography/sonosalpingography are:
   a. In infertility workup.
   b. Abnormal uterine bleeding, especially to diagnose endometrial polyp or submucous fibroid.
   c. Recurrent miscarriage.

Indications of Ultrasound

Diagnostic

i. Obstetrical indication (chapter – Obstetric Ultrasound)
ii. Use of infertility workup for follicles monitoring, ovulation and endometrial pattern.
iii. In dysfunctional uterine bleeding.
iv. In pelvic adnexal mass.
v. In suspected ectopic pregnancy and first trimester bleeding.
vi. To diagnose genital tract abnormalities, hematocolpos and hematometra.
vii. Location of misplaced IUCD.
viii. In evaluation of postmenopausal bleeding.
ix. In male infertility work up to diagnose testicular size, varicocele and if needed ultrasound guided fine needle aspiration cytology.
x. In some cases of gynecological malignancy, ultrasound guided fine needle aspiration cytology.

Therapeutic

a. **In IVF program** oocyte is retrieved under ultrasound guidance. Embryo transfer is also facilitated by use of ultrasound.
b. **Ultrasound guided drainage of pelvic abscess.** Sometimes residual cyst can be aspirated.
c. **Retrieval of embedded intrauterine contraceptive device** under ultrasound guidance.
d. **Injection of methotrexate in ectopic gestational sac** in unruptured ectopic pregnancy under ultrasound guidance.
e. **All fetal diagnosis and procedure** like cord blood sampling, intrauterine transfusions are done under ultrasound guidance.
f. **Selective termination of anomalous fetus or selective reduction of fetus** is done under ultrasound guidance.

Computed Tomography Scan

It provides high resolution two dimensional image. In this cross-sectional image of the body are taken at very close interval in form of multiple slices which are read on television monitor or X-ray film. Contrast CT scan can be done with use of 600-800 ml of dilute oral contrast media

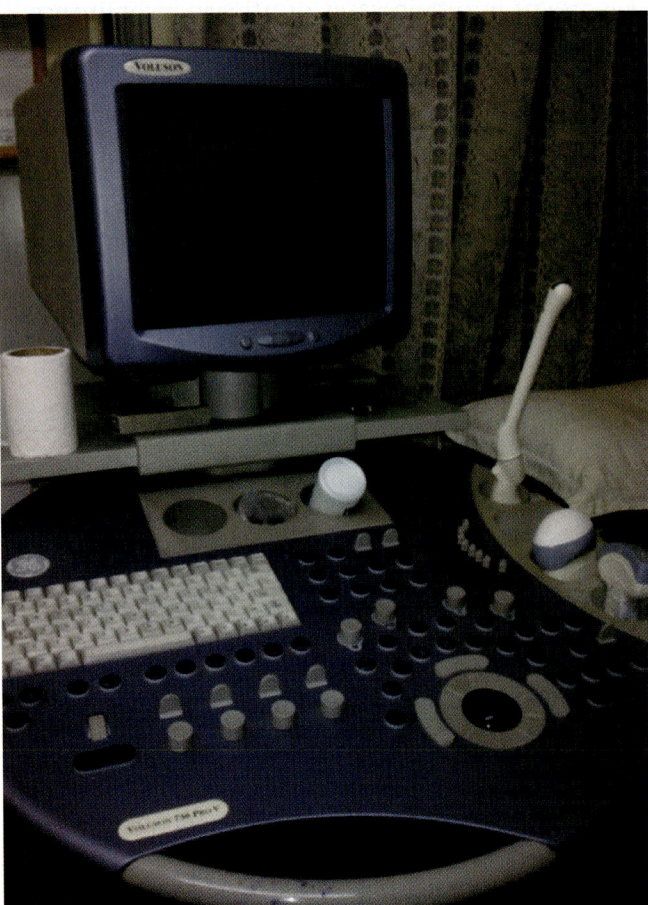

Fig. A1.4: Ultrasound machine

about 1 hour prior to procedure. The contrast media helps to differentiate bowel loops from other pelvic organs. In gynecological malignancies, intravenous injection of iodinated contrast medium is recommended to improve tumor delineation, characterization of vascularity and lymph node identification. Lymph nodes must be enlarged by 2 cm to be detected by CT.

Indications of CT Scan

a. *In gynecological malignancy*: In cancer cervix local recurrence, parametrical infiltration and enlarged lymph nodes are seen. In endometrial cancer myometrial invasion can be seen. In ovarian cancer intrahepatic metastasis and para-aortic lymph nodes are identified.
b. In detecting pituitary tumors and brain metastasis in Choriocarcinoma.

Advantages and Disadvantages

CT Scan supplements the information obtained on ultrasound examination and helps in management of gynecological malignancies and adnexal masses. But it is expansive and radiation exposure up to 2-10 CGY. So it is not used in obstetric situations.

Magnetic Resonance Imaging

The phenomenon of nuclear magnetic resonance was first described by Felix Block and Edward Purcell in 1946.

Principle

It provides multiplanar imaging capability with high soft tissue contrast resolution without interference from air or bone. **In this combination of non ionizing radiation and combination of magnetic field are used.** Biologic tissues nuclei with protons or neutrons have got magnetic properties. When a pulse of radio waves is imposed on the nuclei, a strong resonance will occur and energy is absorbed by nuclei. A signal is detected in receiver coil when energy is emitted by nuclei. The strength of emitted signal varies directly with proton densit y. Sagittal and coronal views can be obtained without moving the patients.

Indications

MRI is found superior to CT scan in gynecology. It can also be used selectively in obstetrics. The indications and use of MRI are:
  i. To assess pelvic anatomy and endometriosis.
 ii. To evaluate Müllerian anomalies.
iii. Localize the position and size of fibroid, adnexal mass and assessment of malignant changes.
 iv. To assess depth of myometrial invasion in case of endometrial cancer.
  v. Staging of cervical cancer.
 vi. Assess recurrent pelvic disease and metastasis.
vii. In obstetrics it can pick up fetal anomalies but it should not be employed in first trimester.

Contraindications

a. It cannot be used in patients with pacemaker or cochlear implant.
b. Metallic foreign body in eye, or paramagnetic aneurysm clip.
c. Epileptic women and women with atrial fibrillation because electroconvulsion can occur because of rapidly changing magnetic field.

Radionuclide Imaging

It is used for specific clinical situation. Bone scans using technetium-99 m methylene diphosphonate are used to detect *bone metastasis* in patients with malignancies. *Ventilation perfusion* scans are used for detecting pulmonary emboli. *Radio leveled white cells scans* can be used for locating abscesses.

Dual Photon Densitometry

It is used to determine risk of osteoporosis in postmenopausal women. The lumbar spines and hip are scanned with a dual photon densitometer which provides computerized graphs and measurement of bone density and relates them to age related normal values.

Positron Emission Tomography (PET)

It is a functional diagnostic imaging technique, based on the fact that malignant cells have a greater glycolysis as compared to normal tissue. Imaging is based on tissue uptake of 18 F fluoro 2 deoxyglucose (FDG) given I/V. FDG – PET scan is then done and the images are interpreted. FDG PET scan is more sensitive for detection of metastatic disease and recurrence of ovarian malignancy than MRI. It is also useful to assess responses following tumor therapy. PET CT combines the anatomical details with metabolic status of the lesion.

ENDOSCOPY IN GYNECOLOGY

Endoscopy has become an essential armamentarium in the diagnostic evaluation of gynecologic lesions as well for operative procedures. Endoscopes are telescopes designed to view the interior of body spaces or viscera. When used in appropriate selected situation by experts, endoscopic surgery offers the advantages of a more accurate diagnosis, less invasiveness, reduced pain, faster recovery and shortened hospital stay or daily care. With advances in instrumentation and techniques now endoscopist can accomplish several operative procedure through endoscopes.

Hysteroscopy

Hysteroscopy involves passing a small diameter telescope either flexible or rigid through the cervix to directly inspect the uterine cavity. Excellent images can be obtained through camera and television system. A flexible hysteroscope may be used in outpatient setting with carbon dioxide as a filling medium. Rigid instruments employ circulating fluid like normal saline or glycine (when electric current is used) and therefore can be used to visualize the uterine cavity even if women is bleeding (Figs A1.5A to C).

Indications

Diagnostic

1. **Any abnormal uterine bleeding** from the uterus can be investigated by hysteroscopy like:
   a. Postmenopausal bleeding.
   b. Irregular menstruation.
   c. Persistent menorrhagia.
2. **In suspected uterine malformation,** confirm uterine synechia, types and extent of adhesions.
3. Suspected Asherman's syndrome.
4. **In endometrial tuberculosis:** The presence of caseous areas, ulcers or tubercles on endometrial lining suggests tuberculosis. Selective biopsies for histology or polymerase chain reaction test for tuberculosis confirms the diagnosis.
5. **Misplaced IUCD:** Hysteroscope determines if IUCD is embedded in uterine endometrium and allows its safe retrieval under direct vision.
6. **Infertility evaluation:** Hysteroscopy helps in detecting:
   a. Endocervical abnormalities.
   b. Endometrial synechia.
   c. Any polyps.
   d. Evaluation of cornuotubal junction.

Therapeutic

In therapeutic procedure cervical dilatation up to 8-10 may be required to insert the operating channel. In this because of prolonged surgery general anesthetic is needed. Glycine is required for uterine cavity distention and electrolyte level are to be monitored.

1. **Uterine septum removal:** Uterine septum is cut with scissor or resectoscope. If done under laparoscopic vision, uterine perforation can be avoided.
2. **Asherman's syndrome:** Hysteroscopic adhesiolysis under laparoscopic view can be done. It can be followed by insertion of IUCD for 3 months and hormone therapy to prevent re adhesion and helps to regenerate endometrium.
3. **Removal of embedded IUCD.**
4. **Removal of submucous fibroid:** Type 0 pedunculated fibroid or type I fibroid with 50% intramural location can be morcellated or destroyed by coagulation.*
5. **Dysfunctional uterine bleeding:** Transcervical resection of endometrium (TCRE) in premenopausal women can be offered for DUB in appropriately selected cases.
6. **Tubal cannulation:** In cornual tubal block tubal cannulation and breaking up of flimsy adhesion of cornual end can be offered.
7. **New technique of tubal sterilization:** Uterine sclerosing agents, cautery or intratubal rings are under research trials.

Complications of Hysteroscopy

Immediate

i. Perforation of uterus.
ii. Cervical damage if cervical dilatation is necessary.
iii. If there is genital infection, hysteroscopy can cause ascent of infection.
iv. Anesthetic complication.

---

* Classification of uterine myomas (European Society of Laparoscopy)
  Gr – Degree of intramural development of myoma
  Go – Myoma limited to uterine cavity (Pedunculated)
  G1 – Myoma, endocavitory component (>50%)
  G2 = Myoma, endocavitory component (<50%)

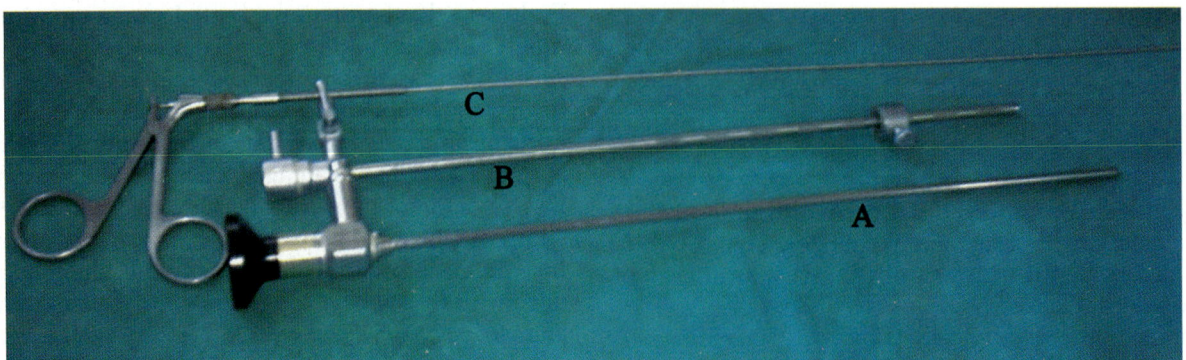

Figs A1.5A to C: Hysteroscopic instruments: (A) Hysteroscope; (B) Trocar; (C) Hysteroscopic biopsy forceps

v. Organ injury to bowel and bladder: rare.
vi. Thermal injury to bowel with cautery and laser.
vii. Allergic reaction is noted with glycine.
viii. Postoperative bleeding in 1-2% of cases.
ix. Fluid overload in 4% of cases. It can lead to pulmonary edema if deficit of fluid is more than 1000 ml and electrolyte disturbance can occur.
x. Distending media complication: CO_2 embolism can be avoided by using the proper instrument, not increasing the flow to more than 70 ml/ minute, the pressure less than 100 mm of Hg. Distending media can increase the procedure morbidity like hyponatremia, neurological symptoms, ammonia toxicity.

Laparoscopy

Laparoscopy was developed during 1970 and operative laparoscopy started gaining ground and popularity in the last two decades. Laparoscopy allows visualization of the peritoneal cavity. *Laparoscopic surgery has benefits of being minimally invasive, lowered incidence of adhesion formation and infection.*

The **limitations** of laparoscopy are:
a. Reduced exposure to the operating field.
b. Restricted manipulation of viscera.
c. More risk of iatrogenic complication like organ injury.
d. More operating time.
e. Less accurate tissue apposition during suturing.
f. Expensive instruments and experienced training is required.

Instruments

Basic Instruments

Following basic instruments are required for laparoscopic surgery:
a. **Laparoscope:** It is rigid telescope varying in diameter 4-10 mm and 30 cm long. It incorporates optical system as a medium of illumination.
b. **Verre's needle:** It is used for creating pneumoperitoneum by carbon dioxide. It is spring loaded which prevents visual injury. The blunt tip point springs out when it enters the peritoneal cavity.
c. **Trocar and cannula:** After pneumoperitoneum trocar and cannula is inserted through a small incision. The trocar is removed and telescope is introduced through the cannula or sleeve.
d. **Light source:** High intensity light (xenon or halogen source) beam (cold light) is transmitted to the telescope for excellent visualization. Fibroptic cables are used to transmit the cold light from source to the telescope.
e. **CO_2 insufflators:** It is used to create controlled pneumoperitoneum. CO_2 cylinder is attached to CO_2 insufflators, which provides CO_2 at controlled rate and pressure through different ports. Low flow rate (0.5-1 lit/ml) or high flow rate is used depending on the need.

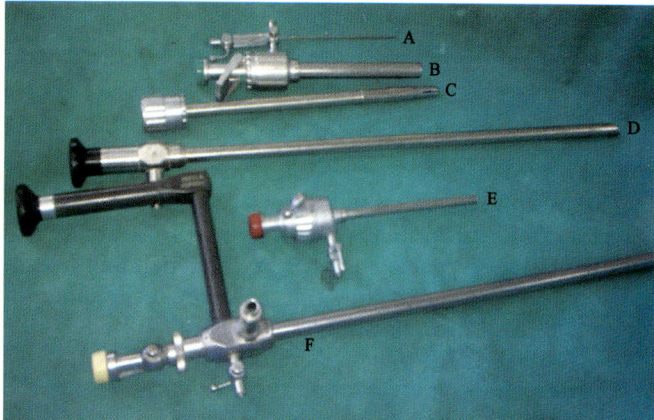

Figs A1.6A to F: Laparoscopic basic instrument; (A) Verre's needle for pneumoperitoneum; (B) Trocar; (C) Cannula; (D and F) Laparoscope straight and angled; (E) Small trocar for other entry

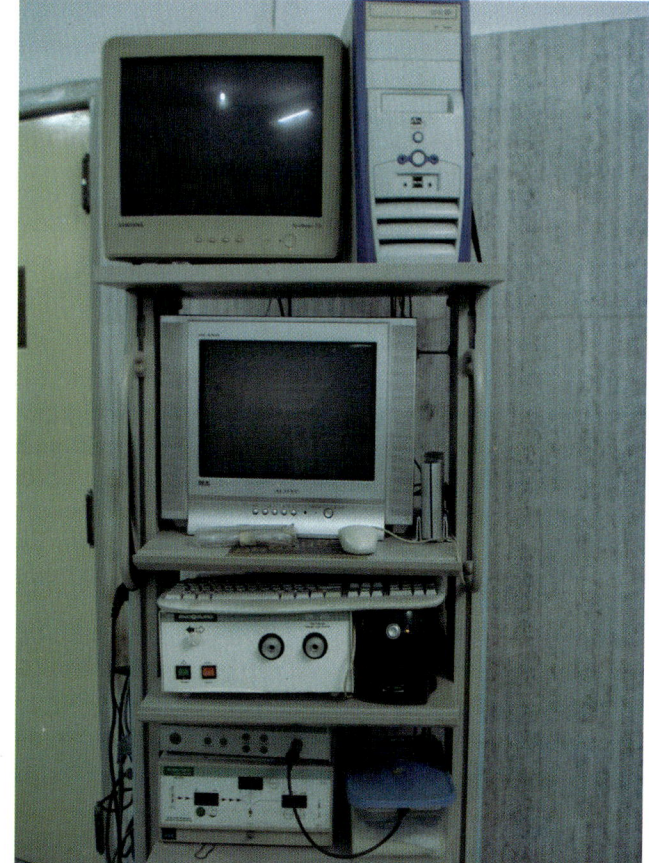

Fig. A1.7: Equipment for endoscopic surgery

f. **Cameras:** The telescope is connected with camera lens and pictures are obtained from the monitor (Figs A1.6 and A1.7).

Accessory Instruments

Different accessory instruments especially designed for laparoscopic surgery are used during diagnostic or operative endoscopy:

a. *Scissors.*
b. *Grasping forceps.*
c. *Probes.*
d. *Aspirator and irrigator.*
e. *Morcellator.*
f. *Uterine manipulator.*
g. *Electrosurgical unit for cutting and coagulation of tissues.* Monopolar or bipolar cautery is used. In monopolar cautery the current is pushed from the generator through active electrode to the contact tissue, so chance of undetected burn to tissue is more. In bipolar cautery, the current flows from the generator between two jaws of the forceps or scissors holding the target tissue. So chance of thermal damage to tissue is less.
h. *Suturing instrument:* Intracorporeal knot tying, extracorporeal knot tying or roedor loops are available for laparoscopic suturing.
i. *Mechanical clips*, staples are used for hemostasis by suturing blood vessels.
j. *Harmonic blade* is used which cuts tissue and at the same time secure hemostasis.
k. *Laser*: Laser used in gynecologic surgery for cutting are CO_2, 532 mm KTP and Nd: YAG laser. The depth of tissue penetration depends on type of laser used – In CO_2 laser which is most commonly used is 0.1 mm, KTP – 532 – 0.4-0.8 mm and ND: YAG is 0.6-4.2 mm.

Indications of Laparoscopic Surgery

Diagnostic Laparoscopy

a. **Infertility evaluation:** Laparoscopy is indicated if hysterosalpingography reveals abnormal or ambiguous findings. Laparoscopy is helpful in overall evaluation of female infertility factors as external characteristics of adnexa and uterus, presence of endometriosis, adhesion, bands, feature suggestive of tuberculosis or *Chlamydia* can be visualized directly. Beside biopsy can be taken from suspected lesions to confirm the diagnosis. At the same time fertility enhancing surgery like adhesiolysis, excision of endometriotic cyst can be done at the same time.
b. To confirm diagnosis of endometriosis.
c. In evaluation of chronic pelvic pain.
d. In suspected adnexal mass.
e. In suspected ectopic pregnancy.
f. **Ovarian malignancy:** Laparoscopic evaluation can help in staging the disease.
g. Detection of uterine abnormalities.
h. **To confirm genital tuberculosis:** Genital tuberculosis can cause infertility, chronic pelvic pain, and adnexal mass and menstrual abnormality. Laparoscopy can help in confirming the diagnosis. The features suggestive of genital tract tuberculosis are presence of tubercles on the serosa, multiple constrictions, thick rigid tubes, presence of flimsy as well violin string adhesions, presence of tubercles on the bowel serosa or peritoneal surface.

Operative Laparoscopy

Nowadays minimal access surgery that is laparoscopic surgery is replacing conventional surgery as the procedure of choice in selected gynecological surgeries. Some of the surgeries which are routinely done via laparoscope are as follows:

1. **Adhesiolysis.**
2. **Ovaries:**
   a. **In polycystic ovarian** disease laparoscopic drilling of ovary by cautery or laser improves the response to hormonal ovulation stimulation and avoids the hyperstimulation. But there is also risk of adhesion formation and thermal damage to the ovary.
   b. **Cystectomy.**
   c. **Endometriotic cyst** is incised; the content aspirated and cyst wall is either ablated or excised.
   d. **Second look laparoscopy** in ovarian malignancy.
   e. **Pelvic lymphadenectomy** in cases of early cancer cervix can be performed via laparoscope.
3. **Uterus:**
   a. **Myomectomy:** In women desirous to retain reproductive capacity, laparoscopic myomectomy can be performed in selected cases.
   b. **Laparoscopic assisted vaginal hysterectomy (LAVH)** can be done. The purpose of LAVH is to convert an abdominal hysterectomy to vaginal hysterectomy or difficult vaginal hysterectomy to easy surgery.
4. **Fallopian tube:**
   a. The most common operation performed is tubal sterilization for permanent contraception by Electrocoagulation of two cut end of fallopian tube or by use of Falope ring or Hulka's clip.
   b. An early unsuspected ectopic pregnancy can be treated by laparoscope, with conservation of fallopian tube.
   c. Hydrosalpinx of tube can be treated by lateral salpingostomy and fimbrioplasty.

Contraindications of Laparoscopy

a. **Cardiac and respiratory disease** which contraindicates Trendelenburg position and CO_2 pneumoperitoneum.
b. Diaphragmatic hernia and umbilical hernia.
c. **Acute pelvic infection** which can flare up during laparoscopy.
d. Intestinal obstruction.
e. Significant hemoperitoneum.
f. Large pelvic tumor.

g. Extreme obesity.
h. **Previous surgery** is relative contraindication.

Complications of Laparoscopy

Complications in minor procedures are less than 0.5-1% but incidence in major procedure is 5-15%.

Major complications in laparoscopy can be:
a. Cardiopulmonary arrest and gas embolism.
b. Hemorrhage due to injury of epigastric vessels during insertion of Verre's needle, injury to aorta, inferior vena cava, iliac vessels and mesenteric vessels.
c. Cautery burns to various viscera.
d. Injury to bowel, small intestines, blood vessels, bladder and ureter with instruments.

Late and other complications:
a. Postoperative peritoneal adhesions.
b. Hernia at site of portals, though it is rare.
c. Failed procedure due to adhesions, extensive pelvic lesions or uncontrolled hemorrhage. In these situations laparoscopy need to be abandoned and converted to laparotomy.

Salpingoscopy and Falloscopy

In salpingoscopy a fine salpingoscope, 1 mm in diameter is introduced through the fimbrial end of the fallopian tube via the laparoscope and ampullary portion of fallopian tube is distended with saline. This is recently added to detect pathology of lumen of fallopian tube and consideration of tuboplasty.

APPENDIX 2

Polycystic Ovarian Syndrome (PCOS)

Things don't change, you change your way of looking, that's all.

INTRODUCTION

Polycystic ovarian syndrome (PCOS) is a common endocrinopathy characterized by oligo-ovulation or anovulation, signs of androgen excess, and ultrasound evidence of polycystic ovaries.

Incidence

Polycystic ovarian syndrome is the most common endocrine disorder of reproductive aged women and affects approximately 4-12%.

Definition and Diagnostic Criteria

As to recent consensus the diagnostic criteria of polycystic ovarian syndrome is that affected individual must have two out of the following criteria:
a. Oligo-and or anovulation.
b. Hyperandrogenism: Clinical and/or biochemical.
c. Polycystic ovaries on sonographic examination.

The Rotterdam criteria defines PCOS by ovulatory dysfunction with clinical and or biochemical hyperandrogenism without regard to ovarian sonographic appearance.

Differential Diagnosis of PCOS

It is important to remember that other causes like *congenital adrenal hyperplasia, androgen secreting tumor* and *hyperprolactinemia* may also lead to oligo-ovulation and androgen excess which must be excluded before diagnosis of PCOS.

Box A2.1 summarizes differential diagnosis of polycystic ovarian syndrome.

Etiopathophysiology

1. *Genetic factor:* Though underlying cause of PCOS is unknown, a genetic basis which is both multifactorial and polygenic is suspected because there is increased prevalence of PCOS between affected individuals and their sisters. The recent research has suggested following:
   a. Dysregulation of CYP II a gene which encodes the cholesterol side chain cleavage enzyme.
   b. Upregulation of other enzyme in androgen biosynthesis pathways.
   c. Insulin receptor gene on chromosome 19p13.2 may be involved. Studies also imply autosomal dominant mode of inheritance.

2. *Gonadotropins:* In PCOS there is alteration in gonadotropin releasing hormone (GnRH) which causes preferential production of luteinizing hormone (LH) compared with FSH. So LH:FSH ratio is elevated and rises more than 2 in approximately 60% of PCOS patient. It causes arrest in follicular development and later stage of maturation which is required for successful ovulation.

3. *Insulin resistance:* Insulin resistance is defined as reduced glucose response to a given amount of insulin. Insulin may function as a secretogogue for ovarian androgens, which disrupt the normal delicate balance among ovarian steroid hormones with an increase in androgen secretion. Androgen is peripherally aromatized to the weak estrogen estrone. Estrone by feedback to pituitary leads to an increase in LH hormone, which binds to ovarian theca cells, which further elicits productions of androgens. When there is

Box A2.1: Differential diagnosis of polycystic ovary syndrome

1. Exogenous androgenic steroid ingestion
2. Thyroid disease
3. Hyperprolactinemia
4. Androgen secreting tumor or adrenal tumor
5. Late onset CAH (21 α hydroxylase deficiency)
6. Cushing's syndrome
7. Ovarian hyperthecosis*

* Ovarian hyperthecosis is a rare condition which is characterized by nest of luteinized theca cells distributed throughout the ovarian stroma. In this there are signs of severe hyperandrogenism.

increased circulating androgen, there is decrease SHBG (Sex hormone binding globulin) which increases further androgen concentration and perpetuate the vicious cycle. *Long-term health consequences of PCOS are explained on basis of insulin resistance as it can cause. Type 2 diabetes mellitus, hypertension, dyslipidemia, and cardiovascular disease.*

4. *Anovulation:* Hypersecretion of LH level, insulin resistance has been implicated for anovulation. The stunted development of numerous graafian follicle leads to the characteristic ultrasound appearance of ovaries containing multiple small follicle usually smaller than 8 mm. These cystic ovaries can maintain the ability to convert androgens to estrogen. Thus, there is a continuous state of mild hyperestrogenism. **In absence of progesterone due to anovulation, elevated estrogen level lead to constant stimulation of uterine lining, which causes increased risk of endometrial hyperplasia, endometrial cancers in PCOS patient.**

5. *Androgens:* Both insulin and LH stimulate ovarian theca cell androgen production. So women with PCOS have clinical evidence of hyperandrogenism. The most common finding is hirsutism, other are acne, male pattern baldness, voice deepening, etc.

Flow chart A2.1 summarizes the initiation and maintenance of PCOS.

Clinical Presentation

The classic description of patient with PCOS is *an obese, hirsute woman with oligomenorrhea or amenorrhea.* The women can present with menstrual disorder or infertility. Menstrual problems can be amenorrhea, oligomenorrhea with episodic menometrorrhagia with anemia. Characteristically *oligomenorrhea* (defined as less than 8 menstrual cycles in one year) or *amenorrhea* (defined as absence of menstruation for 3 or more consecutive months), starting at age of adolescence. Hyperandrogenism can be manifested by acne, hirsutism and androgenic alopecia. If there is virilization like cliteromegaly or increased muscle mass, investigation for androgen producing tumor or adrenal gland should be done immediately. *Acne* is caused by androgen induced increased sebaceous gland secretion, resulting in increased oil production. *Hirsutism* is caused by conversion of DHEA, androstenedione and testosterone in hair follicle by 5 α reductase is dihydrotestosterone which is a potent androgen and promotes increased hair growth.

Other Endocrine Dysfunction

Associated with PCOS are insulin resistance, impaired glucose tolerance, type 2 diabetic mellitus, dyslipidemia and obesity. *Metabolic syndrome* is reported in approximately 45% of women with PCOS. It is characterized by insulin resistance, obesity, thermogenic dyslipidemia and hypertension.

Infertility

Infertility is one of common presentations and accounts for 80-90% of cases of anovulatory infertility.

Pregnancy Complications

In women with PCOS there is increased rate (30-50%) of early pregnancy loss compared with 15% in general population. Cause of RPL can be insulin resistance and increased LH level. There is 2-3 fold higher risk of gestational diabetes, pregnancy induced hypertension, preterm birth and increased perinatal mortality.

Diagnostic Evaluations

1. *History:* Careful questioning of menstrual history, co-morbidities like diabetes, thyroid disorders, and use of medication, lifestyles and history of PCOS, infertility or diabetes, dyslipidemia should be taken carefully.

2. *Physical examination:* Body mass index should be calculated by measuring patient height and weight. Evidence of hirsutism or other signs of hyperandrogenism should be looked for. Abdomen is inspected for striae and vulva for cliteromegaly. Signs of Cushing's syndrome like elevation of blood pressure, assessment of presence of dorsocervical fat pad, peripheral muscle wasting and centripetal obesity should be sought. *Acanthosis nigricans* condition characterized by thickened velvety and hyperpigmented skin is sign of insulin resistance which may be seen in back of neck, axillae, beneath breast or on vulva.

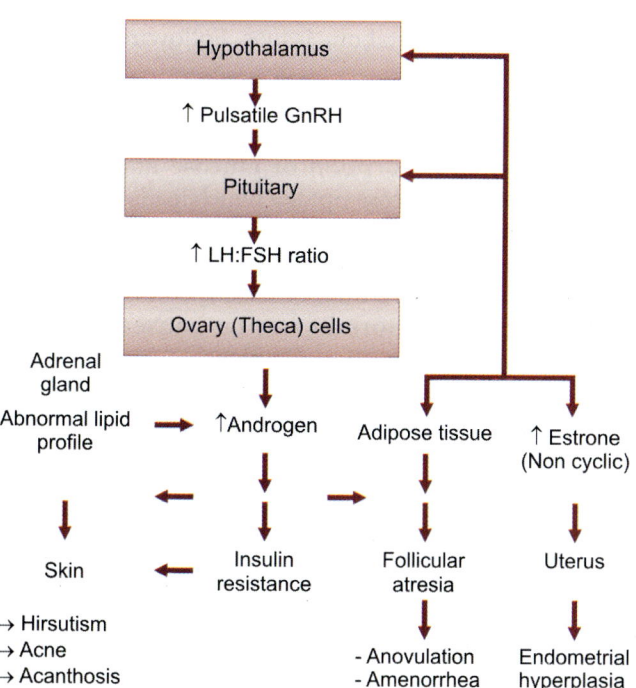

Flow chart A2.1: Summarizes the initiation and maintenance of PCOS

3. *Laboratory investigations:* Following laboratory test in evaluation of PCOS guided by clinical presentation should be done.
   a. Urine pregnancy test: If patient presents with amenorrhea.
   b. Total testosterone.
   c. Free testosterone.
   d. DHEAS.
   e. Prolactin.
   f. Thyrotropin (TSH).
   g. Basal 17 α hydroxyprogesterone
   h. ACTH stimulation test if elevated 17 hydroxyl progesterone level.
   i. 2 hours oral glucose tolerance test.
   j. Fasting lipid profile.
   k. Endometrial biopsy: It is recommended in women older than 35 years with abnormal bleeding and in younger women with anovulatory bleeding refractory to hormonal treatment and ultrasound showing persistent endometrial hyperplasia.
4. *Sonography: Sonographic criteria for PCO are ≥12 small cysts (2-9 mm) and increased ovarian volume >10 ml or both.* There can be increased stroma relative to number of follicles. Finding in only one ovary is sufficient to define PCOS. It is important to note that 23% of young women can exhibit ultrasound feature of PCO without other symptoms of PCOS (Fig. A2.1).

Treatment

The choice of treatment for each symptom of PCOS depends upon women's age, priorities, concern and severity of endocrine dysfunction. Following therapeutic intervention can be done depending on clinical situations:

1. *Observation:* In women with mild symptoms, like 8-10 menstrual cycles per year and mild hyperandrogenism may not require any treatment. But screening for dyslipidemia and diabetes should be done.

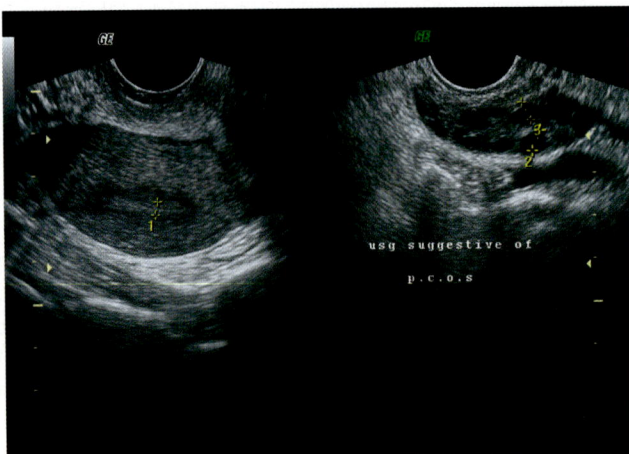

Fig. A2.1: Ultrasound image showing polycystic ovaries

2. *Lifestyle modification:* For obese women with PCOS lifestyle focused on diet and exercise are very important to treatment at each stage of life. Even a modest amount of weight loss (5% of body weight) can result in resumption of normal ovulatory cycles in same women. Well balanced hypocaloric diet with regular exercise offers most benefit.
3. *Combined oral contraceptive pills:* When fertility is not desired, the first line treatment of oligo-ovulation and oligomenorrhea is combined oral contraceptive pills. COCS suppress gonadotropin secretion, which result in decreased ovarian estrogen production. COCS also increase SHBG level. The progestin component antagonizes the endometrial proliferative effect of estrogens which reduces the risk of endometrial hyperplasia due to unopposed estrogen. The COCS containing newer progestin like drosperinone or third generation progestin like norgestinate or desogesterol are preferred to COCS but no pill has shown superiority over other in reducing hirsutism. In start of therapy, if a women's last menstrual period is delayed more than 4 weeks, a pregnancy test is done. If negative, progesterone is given to produce a withdrawl bleeding prior to COC initiation.
4. *Cyclic progestin:* In patient, where estrogen is not indicated or contraception is not desired, progesterone withdrawl is recommended every 1-3 months. Dosage is Medroxyprogesterone 5-10 mg orally daily for last 12 days, or micronized progesterone 200 mg orally each evening for 12 days. This regimen does not correct acne, hirsutism and not provide contraception.
5. *Insulin sensitizing agents:* Though the use of insulin sensitizers has not been approved by FDA, they have been found increasingly beneficial for both gynecological as well metabolic issues. Following drugs can be used:
   a. *Metformin:* It is Biguanide oral hypoglycemic agent which reduces hepatic glucose production and intestinal absorption of glucose and improves peripheral glucose uptake which leads to increased insulin sensitivity. **Dose** of Metformin is started at 500 mg orally per day with increased gradually to usually effective dose of 1500-2550 mg daily. **Side effect** of Metformin can be nausea, diarrhea, vomiting, indigestion, flatulence. A normal serum creatinine should be documented before initiating therapy to avoid lactic acidosis which is uncommon complication of Metformin.
   b. *Thiazolidinediones:* Are another class of drugs which include rosiglitazone and pioglitozone. These agents bind to insulin receptors on cells throughout the body and make them more responsive to insulin. But glitazones are category C drugs and should be discontinued in care of pregnancy.

6. **Induction of ovulation:** In women who desire conception following ovulation induction regimen can be treated:
   a. *Clomiphene citrate*: It is a weak antiestrogenic compound that stimulates FSH secretion. It is first line therapy for ovulation induction in PCOS coming for infertility. The drugs exert antiestrogenic effect on the hypothalamus leading to increased GnRH hormone release which cause increased LH and FSH output and pulsatility which lead to progressive development of ovarian follicles. Increased estradiol level give positive feedback to HP axis and result in LH surge which triggers ovulation. **Dose** of Clomiphene is started with 50 mg/day orally and can be increased up to 150-200 mg/day. Dosage increase is monitored by ultrasound and hormone monitoring of follicle development and ovulation. Ovulation occurs in 75% of patient with Clomiphene and 50-70% of women achieve pregnancy within six cycles.
   b. *Aromatase inhibitor:* They suppress the biosynthesis of estrogen by blocking the conversion of androgen to estrogen in ovarian granulosa cells. So they reduce the negative feedback effect at the hypothalamic pituitary level and increased FSH secretion.
      Dosages: Letrozole is given from 3 days to day 7 of menstrual cycle in dose of 2.5 mg. The efficacy of Letrozole and Aromatase inhibitor over clomiphene is still not proved.
   c. *Gonadotropin*: Women with PCOS who fail to ovulate with maximum dose of clomiphene poses a difficult challenge. In these cases low dose gonadotropin regimen is advocated. Conventional dose of exogenous gonadotropin are associated with lower rate of ovulation and pregnancy but increased risk of ovarian hyperstimulation. In PCOS exogenous gonadotropin either human menopausal gonadotropin or recombinant FSH preparation are administered daily intramuscular or subcutaneously after the onset of spontaneous or progesterone induced menstrual cycle. Serial transvaginal ultrasound and serum estradiol level monitoring is done, when dominant follicle of 18-20 mm emerges, ovulation is triggered by intramuscular dose of human chorionic gonadotropin.
      With above regimen ovulation is achieved in 70% of women with repeated pregnancy rate of 20%.
   d. *ART procedure*: If woman fails to conceive by 6 cycle of above regimen intrauterine insemination can be offered or to transit to *in vitro* fertilization. Successful *in vitro* pregnancy rate with IVF are similar to women with PCOS compared with women without PCOS.
   e. *Laparoscopic ovarian drilling:* Laparoscopic ovarian drilling can be a therapeutic option for women with PCOS who fail to achieve medical ovulation induction alone. Laparoscopic ovarian drilling can be done as day care surgery. It results in postoperative decreased serum androstenedione and testosterone concentration. But effect is usually transient. *Drilling can be done with low voltage electro surgery 50-80 watts depending upon ovaries size and number of cyst.* Three-four punctures are made 1 cm apart in each ovary. Suction irrigation can be done to minimize adhesion formation. Laser Nd/YAG device can be used if facility is available (Fig. A2.2).
      The benefit of laparoscopic ovarian drilling can be:
      a. Helps to release of androgen rich follicular fluid and decrease the androgen providing stroma.
      b. Crowding of cortex decreases which allows progress of normal follicles to the surface resulting in normal ovulation.
      c. There is reduction in inhibin and precipitous fall in LH, which results in increased secretion of FSH. Reported ovulation and pregnancy rate after laparoscopic ovary drilling is 80 and 50% respectively.
7. **Hirsutism:** Hirsutism associated with PCOS can be treated by following modalities.
   a. Combined oral contraceptive pills.
   b. *Spironolactone*: It is a diuretic with aldosterone antagonist action and cause inhibition of ovarian and adrenal androgen synthesis. It is given in dose of 50-200 mg daily. Maximum effect is observed after 6 months of treatment. Side effects are hypotension and hyperkalemia but they are rare. Though the treatment is effective but reserved for difficult or resistant case as drug can rarely cases hepatotoxicity.
   c. *Flutamide*: It is given as 250 mg daily with periodic monitoring of liver enzyme. Flutamide may be used in conjunction with oral contraceptive for maximum effect.

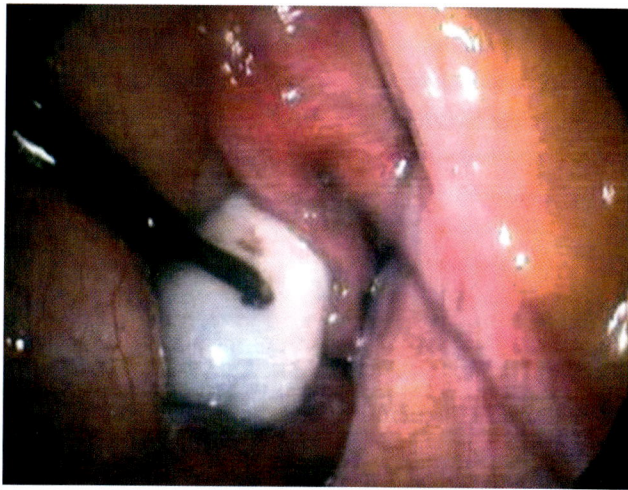

Fig. A2.2: Laparoscopic ovarian diathermy for polycystic ovaries

d. *Cyproterone acetate*: It is an androgen receptor antagonist with reported efficacy of 50-70%.
e. *Gonadotropin hormone releasing agonist*: These agents lower androgen level but it is not a preferred long-term treatment method due to associated bone loss, high cost and menopausal side effect for treatment of hirsutism.
f. *Eflornithine hydrochloride:* This is antimetabolic topical cream applied twice daily to areas of facial hirsutism. It acts by irreversibly inhibiting ornithine decarboxylase enzyme which is necessary for hair follicle division and function.
g. *Cosmetic* like hair removal, depilation, epilation can be adjuvant therapy.

8. **Acne:** Therapy for acne may include:
   a. Combined oral contraceptive pills.
   b. Antiandrogen like spironolactone or Flutamide.
   c. Five α reductase inhibitor as Finasteride.
   d. Other therapies–with consultation with dermatologist:
      i. Topical and systemic antibiotic: Erythromycin, Doxycycline and Clindamycin can be used.
      ii. Topical benzyl peroxide: It is an excellent antimicrobial and anti-inflammatory agent.
      iii. Topical retinoid: It is derived from Vitamin A, which regulates the follicular keratinocyte and normalize its desquamation. The cream agent is tretinoin (Retin A) and tazarotene.
      iv. Isoretinon: Oral isoretinon is an analog of vitamin A that is highly effective for treatment of severe acne. It is teratogenic. So its use should be combined with reliable contraception.

Long-term Risk in PCOS

Long-term risk to patient with PCOS are development of type 2 diabetes and increased risk of cardiovascular problem. So the women will PCOS should be regularly screened for above disorder by biochemical test. These women should always be encouraged to opt for life style modification. As there is increased risk of endometrial hyperplasia and endometrial cancer, oral contraceptive pills or intermittent progesterone induced withdrawl bleeding should be administered to reduce risk of endometrial hyperplasia. **Endometrial biopsy should be performed in all patients with long-standing anovulation and amenorrhea regardless of age.**

APPENDIX 3

Fetal Medicine

I am an artist at living
My work of art is life.

GENERAL CONSIDERATION

Although prenatal treatment is currently not feasible for most fetal abnormalities, some interventions developed in last decade have altered the course of selected fetal anomalies and certain fetal conditions. The 2000 NIH sponsored multidisciplinary workshop on fetal treatment was designed to develop a plan for evaluation of such *in utero* therapy.

The following interventions can improve the fetal outcome.

Fetal Transfusions

The intrauterine transfusions of red blood cells (RBCs) has radically improved the natural history of fetal anemia. Fetal anemia can be caused by alloimmunization, infection, genetic disease like thalassemia and fetomaternal hemorrhage. Fetal anemia is diagnosed by fetal blood sampling and Doppler evaluation of fetal middle cerebral artery peak systolic velocity.

Technique of Fetal Transfusion

Under sonographic guidance, O, D-ve Cytomegalovirus negative, with hematocrit of 80% and leukocyte poor, irradiated red blood cells are transfused into umbilical vein of fetus under sonographic guidance. The volume of transfused red blood cells is calculated by multiplying the estimated fetal weight by .02 for each 10% increase in hematocrit needed. Prior to intrauterine blood transfusion a paralytic agent like vecuronium may be gives to the fetus to minimize movements and potential trauma. In severely anemic fetus less blood is transfused initially and the next transfusion is planned 2 days later. Subsequent transfusions are given every 2-4 weeks, depending on the hematocrit.

Fetal Medicine Therapy

There are several clinical situations where maternal fetal therapy improves the fetal outcome. In such cases medication administered to mother is transported transplacentally and give benefit to the fetus. The conditions are:

a. **Thyrotoxicosis**: In maternal thyroid disease fetal thyroid status can be assessed by cord blood sampling in selected cases (details thyroid disorder in pregnancy). If there is fetal hyperthyroidism, prophylthiouracil given to mother suppress fetal thyroid and correct fetal hyperthyroidism.

b. **Congenital adrenal hyperplasia**: Severe autosomal recessive enzyme deficiencies cause congenital adrenal hyperplasia (CAH) which is characterized by impaired synthesis of cortisol from cholesterol by adrenal cortex. In 90% of CAH, the deficient enzyme is 21 hydroxylase deficiency. The incidence is 1:15000. In this there is excessive fetal adrenal androgen production which can cause virilization of female fetus. Newborn is at risk for salt wasting adrenal crises.

   Maternal treatment to prevent fetal virilization must be started early, ideally prior to 9 weeks before it is known whether the fetus will be affected or even the gender. Dexamethasone orally to mother is given at a dose of 20 µg/kg/day in 3 divided dose. Treatment is started and later prenatal diagnosis with chorion villous sampling (CVS) or amniocentesis is done. If test show the male karyotype, Dexamethasone is stopped. If fenale karyotype is detected, treatment is continued till term.

c. **Fetal arrhythmia:** Approximately 1% of pregnancies are complicated by fetal arrhythmia. Fetal arrhythmias are diagnosed by M-Mode sonography. Most are benign atrial extrasystole which usually resolves before delivery with maturity of conduction system. Sustained tachyarrhythmia can lead to cardiac failure and Hydrops if not treated. Maternal administration of anti-arrhythmic drug which cross the placenta can improve fetal heart rate and rhythm. Drugs are digoxin, sotalol, flecainide and procainamide. Before drug administration maternal electrocardiogram should be done. If fetus has become hydropic, the drugs may have to be administered via umbilical vein.

d. **Congenital infection:** A number of infectious organisms affect the fetus transplacentally. Prompt maternal treatment of infection may prevent or reduce fetal morbidity. For example, timely treatment of maternal syphilis.
e. **Metabolic disorder:** Some inherited metabolic disorders can been treated *in utero*, like fetal methylmalonic acidemia can be treated with maternal oral and intramuscular vitamin B_{12} therapy, which is continued after birth.

Fetal Stem Cell Transplantation

Fetal stem cell transplantation has been tried to treat a variety of hematological, metabolic and immunological disease. In fetal period the fetus in first and early second trimester does not have adaptive immune response to foreign antigens and so termed perimmune.

Till date human fetal stem cell transplantation has been successfully done in treatment of immunodeficiency syndrome. Like base lymphocyte syndrome, chronic granulation disease.

Fetal Gene Therapy

With advancement in genetic technologies efforts are being focused on therapeutic gene transfer. Early gene therapy has the potential of requiring only one treatment which will be definitive and would span for lifetime. Still there is no definite opinion about timing of procedure, ideal recipient or target cells and method of gene transfer. Till now it has only been attempted in animal models.

Fetal Surgery

In few fetal conditions, only in few places fetal surgery *in utero* has been tried. Because it has substantial fetal and maternal risk, these procedures are considered only when reasonable fetal outcome is expected. Type of fetal surgery can be:
  a. Open.
  b. Fetoscopic.
  c. Percutaneous.
  d. *Ex utero* intrapartum treatment (Exit).

a. **Open fetal surgery:** In this procedure, under GA and uterine tocolytic, hysterotomy incision is given and fetus is gently manipulated under close monitoring. After fetal surgery hysterotomy is closed and tocolysis is continued. Later in pregnancy delivery is completed by cesarean section.
b. **Fetoscopic surgery:** In this fibroptic endoscope of 1-2 mm are used for selected fetal conditions like twin to-twin transfusion, congenital diaphragmatic hernia.
c. **Percutaneous procedure:** In this under sonographic guidance shunt, radiofrequency ablation needle or angioplasty catheter is used in highly specialized center for CCAM, posterior urethral valve; twin reversed arterial perfusion (TRAP) sequence or Acardiac twin.
d. ***Ex utero* intrapartum treatment (EXIT):** The procedure is designed to allow the fetus or infant to remain prefused by the placental circulation after being partially delivered so that lifesaving treatment can be performed prior to complete delivery. The technique has been used to treat airway obstruction after fetal surgery or which is caused by neck masses and laryngeal or tracheal atresia or stenosis.

APPENDIX 4

Recurrent Pregnancy Loss and Bad Obstetrical History

Learning without thought is labor
But thought without learning is perilous.

GENERAL CONSIDERATION

Human reproduction is an inefficient process, only 15-30% of fertilized oocyte result in viable pregnancy. Approximately 13% of all recognized first pregnancies are lost. The risk of second consecutive miscarriage is only slightly increased to 17%. However, the risk of miscarriage after two consecutive pregnancy losses rises to 35-40% and continues to rise with each subsequent miscarriage. Approximately 1% of women have recurrent miscarriage.

Recurrent pregnancy loss (RPL) is a devastating medical problem with far reaching physical and emotional effect on the couple, their support system and caregivers. So that it is essential for physician to have clear information about recurrent pregnancy loss.

Definition

Recurrent pregnancy loss is classically defined as *three or more consecutive pregnancy losses at 20 weeks or less or with fetal weight less than 500 gm*. Although the definition includes three or more miscarriage, many agree that evaluation should at least be considered following two consecutive losses. It also depends on age of patient and concern of patient and relatives.

Recurrent miscarriage should be differentiated from:

Sporadic pregnancy loss: Sporadic loss implies that intervening pregnancy have resulted in healthy fetus.

Primary recurrent miscarriage: It denotes that there is no successful pregnancy.

Secondary recurrent miscarriages: It denotes when couple has one prior live birth.

Etiology of Recurrent Pregnancy Loss

A. Chromosomal
B. Anatomical/uterus
C. Immunologic
D. Thrombophilia
E. Endocrine
F. Infectious
G. Environmental
H. Unexplained

Chromosomal Cause

Although parental chromosomal abnormalities account for only 2-4% of recurrent pregnancy losses, karyotype evaluation of both parents remain critical part of evaluation. Among chromosomal abnormalities includes balanced reciprocal translocation which account for approximately 50% of identified abnormalities, Robertsonian translocation for 24%, X chromosomal mosaicism like 47XXY — Kleinfelter syndrome for 12%.

The etiology of chromosomal abnormalities is not completely understood. Abnormalities that arise during the first meiotic division account for majority of aneuploidy. Reproductive ageing in women is associated with increased prevalence of oocyte aneuploidy. Translocation can be of two major types — *Reciprocal* in which two segments from different chromosomes are exchanged, and *Robertsonian* in which there is fusion at the centromere of two acrocentric chromosomes. Balanced translocation may result in normal carriers but can lead to unbalanced rearrangement in offspring and threatened miscarriage. Pregnancy loss is more common with maternal translocation. Nutritional factors such as abnormal folate metabolism, elevated homocysteine level (>18 μ mol/lit) and low vitamin B_6 level (<49 μ mol/lit) are all linked to RPL.

Karyotyping of abortus: It is useful as:
a. It can explain the cause of abortion, e.g. it can show aneuploidy.
b. Provide evidence for chromosomal translocation in a parent.

c. If karyotype is normal it suggests a nongenetic cause. However, a normal karyotype does not entirely exclude genetic cause for miscarriage. Besides routine karyotyping of products of conception is costly and may not accurately reflect the fetal karyotype.

Anatomical Factors

Approximately 15% of women with RPL have congenital or acquired uterus anomaly (Devi, 2006). Anatomical defect can be: (a) Müllerian tract anomalies, (b) Cervical in competence, (c) Uterine fibroids, (d) Abnormalities due to DES exposure, (e) Asherman's syndrome.

Approximately 50% of women with uterine defects have no reproductive problem. Septate uterus accounts for majority of women with uterine malformation and RPL. Unicornuate and bicornuate uterus are less commonly associated. Submucous leiomyomas are responsible for much smaller percentage of recurrent pregnancy pregnancy loss. Generally losses from anatomic abnormalities occur in the second trimester. Possible mechanisms for recurrent loss are interference with implantation, lack of adequate blood supply and growth restriction.

Diagnosis

Diagnosis of uterine anomalies can be done by **hysterosalpingography, ultrasound, or hysteroscopy.** Magnetic resonance imaging may be required to accurately differentiate septate and bicornuate uterus.

Treatment

a. Hysteroscopic metroplasty is indicated in women with RPL and septate uterus.
b. ACOG does not recommend any surgical correction on women with Müllerian tract anomalies unless attempt at pregnancy has been made and has failed.
c. Hysteroscopic lysis is preferred in cases of uterine-synechia and Asherman's syndrome. Hysteroscopic adhesiolysis reduces miscarriage rate from 79 to 22%.
d. **Cervical circlage** may help to improve pregnancy in congenital abnormalities due to DES exposure and trauma of cervix due to previous D & C cone biopsy. Outcome in women are improved by cervical circlage with bicornuate or unicornuate uterus who have previous preterm delivery and exhibit progressive cervical shortening in early pregnancy.

Cervical circlage is recommended between 12 and 14 weeks gestations. Cervical circlage can be done by *McDonald* circlage to which number 2 monofilament suture is placed in body of uterus near the level of internal os. In *Shirodkar* circlage the bladder is pushed anteriorly after dissection in mucosa over cervix and Mersilene tape on Mayo' needle is passed anteriorly to posteriorly.

e. Uterine leiomyomas are often identified with RPL, but only submucous myoma and larger intramural fibroid which clearly encroach upon or displace uterine cavity should be considered for myomectomy.

Immunologic Factor

Approximately 15% of women with RPL has recognized immunological factor. Two primary pathophysiological models are recognized.
a. **Autoimmune theory:** Immunity against self.
b. **Alloimmune theory:** Immunity against other persons.

Autoimmune factors: Autoimmune disease like systemic lupus erythematosus and the antiphospholipid syndrome are identifiable and treatable immunologic disorders associated with recurrent pregnancy loss. Antiphospholipid antibodies are family of autoantibodies that bind to negatively charged phospholipids, phospholipid binding protein or combination of two. The antiphospholipid antibodies predispose to placental thrombosis and interfere with normal development of the uteroplacental circulation to cause both early as well as late pregnancy losses.

Diagnosis: At the present time assays for the lupus anticoagulant and anticardiolipin antibodies are the only validated immunologic test having clinical utility in evaluation of women with RPL.

Treatment: Low combined dose aspirin and heparin therapy has proven to be effective treatment for women with recurrent pregnancy loss associated with antiphospholipid syndrome. ACOG 2005 recommends low dose aspirin 75-80 mg orally per day along with unfractionated heparin 5000 unit subcutaneously twice daily. The therapy is begun with diagnosis of pregnancy and continued till delivery. This treatment improves overall pregnancy success, but there is increased risk of preterm labor, premature rupture of membrane, fetal growth restriction, pre-eclampsia, and placental abruptio.

Alloimmune Disorder

It is suggested that normal pregnancy requires the formation of blocking factors that prevent maternal rejection of foreign fetal antigen that are paternally derived. A woman will not produce these serum blocking factors if she has human leukocyte antigens (HLAs) similar to those of her partner. These alloimmune disorders may be cause of otherwise unexplained recurrent pregnancy loss. At present cytokine deregulation of immune mechanism operating at the maternal fetal interface is the most likely pathophysiologic mechanism involved.

Diagnosis: All current method for evaluation of suspected alloimmune pathology including HLA testing, natural killer cell assays and cytokine testing are considered investigational.

Treatment: Paternal leukocyte immunization and intravenous immunoglobin has been tried for alloimmune disorder but has not proven effective.

Inherited Thrombophilia

These are genetically determined abnormal clotting factors which can cause pathological thrombosis from an imbalance between clotting and anticoagulation pathways. The most widely studied factors are resistance to activated protein (α Pc) caused by factor V Leiden mutation and decreased or absent antithrombin III activity — the prothrombin gene mutation and mutation in the gene for methylene tetrahydrofolate reductase which causes elevated serum level of homocysteine — hyperhomocysteinemia.

Diagnosis: Evaluation for inherited thrombophilia is still unanswered questions. Selective screening for most common abnormality in women with otherwise unexplained RPL can be advised but routine screening of all women with RPL is not justified.

Treatment: Recent studies (Kandorp, 2009) conclude that women with recurrent miscarriage and inherited thrombophilia do not benefit from aspirin or heparin therapy.

Endocrine Factors

Several endocrinologic conditions have been implicated in RPL, including luteal phase defect (LPD), polycystic ovary syndrome (PCOS), hyperandrogenism, increased gonadotropin, hyperprolactinemia, thyroid abnormalities and diabetes mellitus. In some cases, it is possible to correct the endocrinopathy and improve pregnancy outcome.

Luteal Phase Defect

Ovarian progesterone is required for implantation and maintenance of early pregnancy. Some investigators believe that 20-25% of RPL results from progesterone deficiency during the luteal phase, which is termed luteal phase defect. But no properly controlled trials have proved that LPD cause RPL.

Diagnosis of LPD is made by *out of phase endometrial biopsy* specimen, when histologic dating lagged behind menstrual dating by at least 3 days and *serum progesterone level*. But no method gives substantial evidence of LPD, because a low progesterone level detected during early pregnancy can reflect a defective corpus luteum, an intrinsically abnormal conceptus or both. It is difficult to assess loss after 8 weeks gestation to LPD because the placenta begins to synthesize progesterone and ovarian progesterone is no longer required. **Consistently short luteal phase duration is most reliable diagnostic criticism.**

Management: Recent evidence indicates that luteal phase deficiency is a subtle form of ovulation dysfunction which can be corrected by protocol for ovulation induction and monitoring for prolactin and TSH level. Oral or vaginal progesterone and hCG injection are given by some clinician, Cochrane review suggest that this therapy may reduce risk of pregnancy loss, but more research are needed to confirm role of exogenous progesterone in RPL. If the corpus luteum is removed surgically, as for ovarian tumor, progesterone replacement is indicated in pregnancy less than 8-10 weeks.

Thyroid Disease

Severe iodine deficiency is associated with excessive early pregnancy losses. Untreated thyroid disorders are associated with infertility and recurrent miscarriage. But RPL is not associated with subclinical hypothyroidism or adequately treated thyroid disease. ACOG recommends that there is no indication for screening asymptomatic women. But initial screening by TSH in RPL should be done, as test is inexpensive and treatment is highly effective.

Hyperprolactinemia

Elevated prolactin levels have been associated with RPL. Treatment with bromocryptine can be useful.

Diabetes Mellitus

Poorly controlled diabetes mellitus has been consistently associated with early pregnancy loss. High hemoglobin A_{IC} values are associated with higher rates of miscarriage. Optimal metabolic control of diabetes substantially reduces pregnancy loss.

Polycystic Ovarian Syndrome Disease (PCOS and PCOD)

PCOS is a disorder characterized by acyclic production of estrogen via peripheral aromatization of circulating androstenedione, because of oligo or anovulation. These women are subfertile. If pregnancy occurs there may be increased risk of miscarriage. The possible mechanisms are elevated luteinizing hormone (LH) and direct effect of hyperinsulinemia on ovarian function.

Management: Metformin is the best initial treatment before and during pregnancy. Continuing metformin throughout pregnancy has been shown to be effective. It significantly reduce incidence of insulin dependent gestational diabetes and intrauterine growth restriction.

Infectious Cause

Very few infections are firmly proven to cause early pregnancy loss. Moreover, if any infections like TORCH are associated with miscarriage, they are even less likely to cause recurrent miscarriage because maternal antibodies usually develop with the primary infection.

Management: Routine serologic testing, tissue culture and endometrial biopsy to detect genital infection in women with RPL is not justified. Evaluation for infection should be done only in women with clinical cervicitis, chronic or recurrent bacterial vaginosis or other symptoms of pelvic infection. Likewise antibiotic treatment in women suspected of having a genital *Mycoplasma* (*Chlamydia*) infection is less costly and less complicated than serial cultures.

Environmental Factors

Smoking increases the risk of miscarriage and should be discouraged prior to conception and throughout the pregnancy. **Alcohol** consumption exceeding two drinks per day and caffeine consumption exceeding 300 mg/day may increase risk for pregnancy loss and are best avoided. **Imaging radiation** is abortificient in sufficient doses (>5 rads). The average chest X-ray administering 8 m rads and a barium enema delivers 800 m rads. Therapeutic radiation delivers 360-500 rads and almost always causes miscarriage.

Maternal hyperthermia resulting from fever or hot tub use is teratogenic and results in neural tube defect and spontaneous abortions. Hot tub and sauna bath use should be avoided during pregnancy. **High exposure to bromodichloromethane** in tap water has been associated with a two-fold increase in spontaneous abortion. *Lead and mercury, formaldehyde, ethylene oxide and nitrous oxide increase the risk of miscarriage.*

Unexplained Recurrent Pregnancy Loss

Even after a thorough and systematic evaluation, more than 50% of women with RPL have no identified predisposing factor. In these patients frequent communication, optimum caution and emotional support during first trimester and throughout pregnancy have their own distinct therapeutic value. Many clinicians offer empirical **exogenous progesterone** supplementation during early pregnancy in women with unexplained RPL.

Low dose aspirin treatment is also commonly prescribed drug. But both treatments have no clear evidence of their effectiveness. With determined efforts, 70-75% of women with unexplained recurrent pregnancy loss ultimately achieve successful pregnancy. Careful monitoring is warranted throughout pregnancy for fetal growth, anomalies of preterm labor.

Table A4.1 summarizes basic cause, evaluation and treatment in recurrent pregnancy loss.

BAD OBSTETRICAL HISTORY

Bad obstetrical history defines when obstetrical future is likely to be modified by the nature of previous disaster. Recurrent pregnancy loss has already been discussed. Other aspects of bad obstetrical history include the following points.

Table A4.1: Causes, evaluation and treatment in recurrent pregnancy loss

Category	Evaluation	Treatment
Genetic	• Karyotype both parents • Ovarian reserve test	• Counseling • Donor genetic where appropriate • PGD
Anatomic	• Sonohysterography • HSG • MRI • IVP and renal USG	• Hysteroscopic metroplasty • Hysteroscopic myomectomy • Hysteroscopic adhesiolysis, cervical circlage • Abdominal myomectomy
Immunologic	• Lupus anticoagulant • Anticardiolipin antibody	• Aspirin and heparin
Thrombophilia	• Factor V Leiden • Prothrombin gene mutation • Activated C protein • Homocysteine • Protein SC • Antithrombin III	• Aspirin and heparin
Endocrine	• TSH • Luteal phase duration • Blood glucose • HgBA1c • Prolactin	• Thyroxine • Clomiphene citrate • Metformin • Dopamine agonist
Infectious	• As indicated by symptoms	• Empirical antibiotic
Environmental	• History	• Behavior modification

Appendix –4 ♦ Recurrent Pregnancy Loss and Bad Obstetrical History

1. *History taking:* The fullest information should be taken about previous deliveries and abortion.
   a. If there is history of **stillbirth**, all records should be seen to see whether it was fresh stillbirth or intrauterine death. What was the gestational age at time of delivery and whether labor was spontaneous or induced. Autopsy details if available are important especially about excessive moulding of skull bones, intracranial hemorrhage.
   b. In case of **neonatal death**, maturity and weight of fetus, any fetal abnormality, duration of life and cause of fetal death should be ascertained. Previous ultrasound seen or infantogram should be reviewed.
   c. **Indication of cesarean section** should be reviewed. If there is history of puerperal sepsis, the integrity of scar is in doubt, the trial for vaginal delivery should be deferred in next pregnancy. Likewise if cesarean was after failed trial of labor or major degree cephalopelvic disproportion, trial of vaginal birth is not indicated.
2. *Evaluation and management options:*
   a. If there has been previous intrauterine death, screening for PIH and gestational diabetes should be done. Beside investigating and treating the probable cause of intrauterine death, close fetal monitoring using biophysical profile and Doppler flow studies should be done and timely interventions is done to effect delivery of fetus to prevent fetal morbidity and mortality.
   b. *Maternal syphilis* gives typical picture of mid-trimester abortion progressing in successive pregnancies to intrauterine death at advancing period of gestation until the women delivers a live baby with signs of congenital syphilis. Though, nowadays it is rare cause of BOH but VDRL test in pregnancy should not be omitted.
   c. *TORCH* testing is usually recommended in BOH but opinion is divided on the role of these infections in causing recurrent problems.
   d. *Antiphospholipid syndrome: It* is now recognized as an important factor is recurrent pregnancy loss. It may present as recurrent first trimester abortion to early onset severe pre-eclampsia resulting in preterm delivery or intrauterine death. The two main antibodies of this syndrome are anticardiolipin (ACL) and lupus anticoagulant (LAC).
   e. *History of fetal abnormality* is important as incidence of fetal abnormality increases after each incident. After one congenital abnormal baby the chances next time are about 6-8 times as great and after 2 consecutive incidences the chance of third are in range of 60-70%. In these cases prepregnancy counseling, history of maternal diabetes, substance abuse, thyroid disorders should be elicited and should be properly treated before conception. *In woman with any history of previous fetal abnormality, targeted ultrasonography with fetal echocardiography is indicated to search for any fetal abnormality*. If there has been history of chromosomal abnormality, chorion villous sampling or amniocentesis should be offered.
   f. If there is previous history of *pre-eclampsia, hypertensive disorder, nephritis, disease should* be appropriately treated. In cardiac patient full detailed history should always be obtained of previous pregnancies and labors. In Rh negative women the previous history of neonatal jaundice, need of exchange transfusion, Rh anti D vaccination should be meticulously sought and management lines decided accordingly, according to Rh antibody titer and middle cerebral artery Doppler studies.
   g. *Details of labor should* be taken regarding place of delivery, duration of labor, any operative intervention required like forceps, ventouse. History of third stage complication is important and adherent placenta can be recurrent. In case of history of manual removal of placenta or adherent placenta, specialized hospital delivery is recommended as there can be recurrence.
   h. If there is *history of previous injury to bladder,* cesarean section is indicated. In history of third degree perineal tear, careful assessment for appropriate mode of delivery is required.

Good history-taking in obstetrics with attention to important details is important to identify causes of bad obstetrical history. Identification of bad obstetrical history warrants appropriate line of management in pregnancy and labor.

APPENDIX 5

Drug Use in Pregnancy

The best decision makers are those who are willing to suffer the most over their decisions
But still retain their ability to be decisive.

INTRODUCTION

Medication during pregnancy and lactation should be prescribed judiciously, because their efficacy and responses may be altered due to physiological change of pregnancy and possibility of adverse effect on the growing fetus or the infant. Obstetrician should be familiar with potential unwanted effects of the commonly prescribed and non prescription drug of pregnancy and growing fetus.

Drug Categories in Pregnancy

The Food and Drug Administration (FDA) has classified drugs into different categories based on their potential adverse effect on the fetus and safety of their use in pregnancy in following categories:

Category A: Studies in pregnant women have not shown an increase risk for fetal abnormalities, if administered during any trimester of pregnancy.

Category B: Animal studies have revealed no evidence of harm to the fetus but are no adequate and well controlled studies in pregnant women or animal studies have shown an adverse effect but adequate and well controlled studies in pregnant women have failed to demonstrate risk to the fetus.

Category C: Animal studies have shown an adverse effect and there are no adequate and well controlled studies in pregnant women or no animal studies have been conducted and there are no adequate and well controlled studies in pregnant women.

Category D: Studies adequate well controlled or observational in pregnant women have demonstrated a risk to the fetus. However, the benefit of therapy may outweigh the risk.

Category X: Studies adequate well controlled or observational in animal or pregnant women have demonstrated positive evidence of fetal abnormalities. The use of product is contraindicated in women who are or may become pregnant.

Categories for Drug Use During Breastfeeding

Pediatric academies and World Health Organization monitors and updates the effects of maternal ingestion of drugs during lactation. WHO has classified following classification to categorize drugs in breastfeeding.

1. *Compatible with breastfeeding:* There is no known or theoretical consideration for the use of drug and considered safe for mother.
2. *Compatible with breastfeeding, monitor infants for side effects:* There can be theoretically side effects in the infants but have either not been observed to do so or have only occasionally mild side effects. If there are side effects, the medicine should be stopped or breastfeeding should be discontinued temporarily.
3. *Avoid if possible—monitor infant for side effects:* Side effect reported in the infant especially serious side effects. The drug should only prescribed for mother, only if it is essential for mother's treatment and no safer alternative is available. Breastfeeding can be continued with close observation of the baby. If side effects occur, either the medicine should be stopped or breastfeeding should be discontinued temporarily until treatment is completed.
4. *Avoid if possible—may inhibit lactation:* Drug classified in this category may reduce breast milk production and if possible they should be avoided.
5. *Avoid:* Serious side effects reported and drug should not be given to mother while she is breastfeeding.

Though the above classification is meant to clear the ambiguities about prescribing in pregnancy but apart from A and X drug, other classification (B,C,D) is not so clearly helpful and still leaves the responsibility on the treating doctor for prescribing or not prescribing a particular drug. Because of these problems, the FDA has proposed new rules for labeling drugs for use by pregnant women. The center for drug evaluation and research has replaced A-X category with a narrative fetal risk summary, clinical consideration and inadvertent exposure in registry. **This** evidence based rating system is currently under development. Meanwhile the most current and accurate information can be obtained through online reproductive toxicity services such as Reprotox and Teris.

Teratogenicity

Teratogens act by disturbing specific physiological process which leads to cell death, altered tissue growth or abnormal cellular differentiation. Teratogen can act by following ways:

a. *Disruption of folic acid metabolism:* Folic acid is essential for production of methionine which is required for methylation reaction and thus production of protein, lipids and myelin. Hydantoin, Carbamazepine, Valproic acid and Phenobarbitone impair folate absorption or act as antagonist.

b. *Fetal genetic composition:* Many multifactorial anamolies are caused by the interaction of environment and certain altered genes, that is mutation of gene for methylene Tetrahydrofolate Reductase (MTHFR). Thus mutation is associated with neural tube defects and other malformation.

c. *Homeobox genes:* Homeobox genes are highly conserved genes which share a region of hemology. Example of homeobox gene teratogenicity is retinoic acid and Valproic acid. During embryogenesis retinoids such as vitamin A activates genes essential for normal growth and tissue differentiation. Retinoic acid is potential teratogen that can activate gene prematurely; resulting in chaotic gene expressions at sensitive stage of develo-pment. Valproic acid preferentially alters the expression of homeobox Hox genes.

d. *Paternal exposure:* In some cases paternal exposure to drug or environmental influence may increase the risk of adverse fetal outcome.

Counseling for Teratogen Exposure

Questions regarding medication and illicit drug use should be part of routine preconceptional and prenatal care. It is also important to keep in mind that with few notable exceptions most commonly prescribed drugs and medication can be used with relative safety during pregnancy. For the few drugs believed to be teratogenic, counseling should emphasize only relative risk. Concept of risk verses benefit also should be introduced.

APPENDIX 6
Psychological Aspects in Obstetrics and Gynecology

We know nothing higher than goodness.

GENERAL CONSIDERATION

Human sexual behavior and reproduction have long been influenced by culture, taboos, religions and civic forces. That's why psychological aspect of obstetrics and gynecology deserve special consideration.

A woman is likely to experience a variety of changes in her body throughout her life — puberty, menstrual cycle, pregnancy and menopause are all life states which are defined by physical and psychological changes. If psychological aspect in obstetrics and gynecology is not looked after, it can have effect on women's ability to function in other areas of her life. So it is important that clinician should have a holistic approach integrating physical, psychological and cultural dimensions.

Adolescence

In adolescence, the growing girl has to adapt to changing body shape, menstruation and awareness of femininity and sexuality. In phase of adolescence, there is formation of identity, separation from the family, decision about relationship, and sexual behavior. In adolescence, there is tendency to risk taking behavior, some remain dependent and insecure and some become rebel against significant adult in their lives.

Menstrual Problems

Emotional problems can affect the menstrual cycle, like missing a period during examination, or can be more protracted like amenorrhea in anorexia nervosa. Menorrhagia and psychosomatic factors may interact like heavy menstrual bleeding and consequent anemia can lead to distress and lethargy. Chronically, anxious or depressed women may be less tolerant of menstrual bleeding and report menorrhagia or dysmenorrhea more frequently.

So psychological factors from the history should alert the gynecologist to the possibility of an emotional disturbance. A nonjudgmental approach between psychological distress and physical illness should be made if there are multiple social problems, recent life stress, history of abuse or symptoms suggestive of chronic anxiety or depression. It is important to refer the woman to a counselor or psychologist and not to report to early surgical treatment. Likewise in women with premenstrual syndrome psychological approach can help the women in understanding the cyclic patterns of premenstrual syndrome.

Menopause

Attitude of women to menopause varies and ranges from relief to acute anxiety. It depends also largely on social and cultural environment. For many women, menopause also coincides with variety of stressful life events like leaving of children, retirement, elderly parents or moving home. Short-term use of hormone replacement therapy can be used for alleviation of unpleasant symptoms. Psychological rapport between physician and women, life style modification in diet, exercise, cultivation of hobbies can help the women to adapt to reality of aging and motivate the elder women to lead meaningful life.

Subfertility

Subfertility is related to personal, emotional, social, and psychological stress with cycles of continued hope and disappointments. Life centers on having a baby. With advancement of technology in field of infertility, it is becoming more confusing and stressful for couples to accept subfertility. Gynecologist can help a lot in resolving or reducing psychological stress associated with infertility. Apathetic evaluation and transparent explanation of role and limitation of different treatment of infertility can help couples in making decision of trying advanced technology, adoption or acceptance of infertility.

Fertility Choice

The responsibility of use and choice of contraception ideally should be of couple but usually women have the sole responsibility towards it. Social, cultural and ethical taboos have conflict with physician's advice about use of different type of contraception like use of intrauterine contraceptive device and oral contraception is linked to many side effects by elder members of women and friends. Gynecologist can help a lot again making the women understand about need and advantage of contraceptive methods and finally in choosing one of the contraception method.

Chronic Pelvic Pain

Chronic pelvic pain is a common symptoms presenting in gynecology outpatient clinic. Chronic pelvic pain is often associated with psychologic issues like marital disharmony, family conflict, etc. Psychological work-up should be an integral part of evaluation of chronic pelvic pain.

Sexual Problem

Sexual intimacy is a fundamental to humanity. Sexual problem in women can be primary, secondary or situational. Precipitating factor in causing sexual problem can be parenthood, illness, life stress, performance pressure, traumatic sexual experience and psychiatric illness. Gynecologist should be able to offer first line education, advice and guidance.

Psychological Aspect of Pregnancy

Pregnancy affects nearly all aspect of women's life — her body, family, relationships, job, financial status and life plans. Good obstetric and gynecologic care requires consideration of each woman as an individual with a biopsychosocial approach by the clinician treating a person and not a disease. Objective compassion and nonbiased approach are essential principles that encourage appropriate care. The following factors are to be understood by doctor while caring the women in pregnancy:

a. **Motivation for pregnancy:** Pregnancy may be enjoyable and fulfilling experience for many but not for all. Motivations for pregnancy are varied and complex and only some of them are conscious. The desire of pregnancy is not always the same as the wish for a child. For example, desire for a pregnancy may be wanted to confirm ones sexual identity, or reproductive integrity, or response to loneliness, or response to family or cultural pressure. Besides regardless of multifactorial forces play in women's reproductive choices, many women face similar stress as stage of pregnancy advances.

b. **Pregnancy as a developmental transition:** Pregnancy is a major developmental step in the lives of women, which gives sense of creativity, self-realization and opportunity for new growth. But at the same time, it is stressful experience. A women response to pregnancy is related to her early childhood experience, coping mechanism, personality style, life situation and physical problems. The father to be is also presented with challenges and conflicts. Men may envy their partner's new condition, have conflicts with sexuality and pregnancy or may feel threatened by the baby's potential to replace them as the mother's focus of attention. With a full understanding of the psychological aspects of pregnancy, an insightful physician can identify these issues and help a patient in passing through this developmental stage.

c. **Normal psychological process during pregnancy and puerperium:** The psychological reaction to pregnancy vary with stages of pregnancy. **During the first trimester** there is anxiety and heightened emotion and a woman tends to corporate the fetus as an integral part of her body. Ultrasonography has led to earlier maternal and paternal bonding. In the **second trimester** separate entity of fetus is recognized. In **third trimester** and postpartum, the patient comes to see herself as a mother and begin to establish nurturing relationship with the infant. **Labor** is a stressful experience and there is fear about bodily injury, loss of control, even death. Hospital environment should strive to provide a more homelike and less institutional atmosphere for the birthing experience.

In **puerperium**, the bonding between mother and child develops, bonding refers to sensitive period after birth, during which interaction between mother and infant facilitate a powerful connection. Early visual and physical contact, breastfeeding and fondling increase bonding. Factors which can interfere the bonding are— psychological problem, inadequate preparation, physical illness in mother or baby and hospital practices that separate mothers and infant.

d. **Transition to motherhood:** Mothering has instinctive roots but is largely a learned behavior. Endocrinal, psychological and body changes contribute to make pregnancy and puerperium time of stress. It is helpful for a woman to review her labor and delivery experience with her physician.

Domestic Violence and Sexual Assault: General Consideration

For many victims of domestic violence and sexual assault, the first contact with the healthcare system is with obstetrician and gynecologist or primary care doctors. So it is critical that their physician be knowledgeable in the identification, evaluation and treatment of such patients. Domestic violence can be psychological, physical or sexual. All violent relationships are characterized by exertion of power and control by perpetrator against the victim. Although victims of domestic violence may be male or female, 90-95% of victims are women. As assaults are significantly underreported, it is difficult to compare the data but we have come to appreciate that domestic violence is an epidemic that has to be addressed by clinicians. Violence by an intimate partner accounts for approximately 21% of all the violence crimes experienced by women.

Cycle of Domestic Violence

Domestic violence frequently includes verbal abuse, threats, throwing objects, pushing, kicking, hitting, sexual assault and threatening with or using weapon. The violence typically occurs in *predictable, progressive cycle. The tension building phase* is characterized by argument and blaming. It leads to the *battering phase* that may involve verbal threats, sexual abuse, physical battering and use of weapons. The battering phase is followed by a honeymoon phase during which abuser may deny the violence, make excuses, apologize and promises never to do it again. Until the next cycle begins, domestic violence often occurs within a frame work of family violence that can include child abuse, elder abuse or abuse of adults who are disabled. It is estimated that child abuse occurs in 33-77% of families where adults are abused.

Causes of Domestic Violence

Domestic violence crosses racial, socioeconomic and cultural lines. A woman may stay in an abusive relationship because she is even more fearful, about what will happen to her and her children if she leaves. In fact if this fear is justified, abused women are at the highest risk for serious injury and death when leaving or after leaving an abuser. Women or abused child, adolescent, or elder may be economically dependent on her partner or may not be able to support herself or children if they leave. Women may feel a religious or cultural obligation to keep the family intact and finally women may blame herself for abuse.

Clinical Presentation

Clinical presentation can be recurrent chronic pelvic pain, sexual dysfunction, multiple bodily complaints like headache, palpitation, sleep and appetite disturbance. They may have symptoms of depression or can even be suicidal. These women can have post-traumatic stress disorder (PTSD), which occurs in individuals, who have experienced psychologically disturbing events. **Symptoms** are re-experiencing the traumatic event through intrusive memories, dreams, flashbacks. They also exhibit a psychic numbing that is they are detached from other people and have difficulty feeling emotions. Other clinical syndromes include personality disorder characterized by maladaptive character traits. In very extreme cases, patient may have maladaptive personality disorder.

Domestic Violence in Pregnancy

It merits special attention because it is threat to both mother and developing fetus. Incidence of domestic violence can be 1-20%, so it is more common problem than Pre-eclampsia, gestational diabetes for which women are screened in pregnancy. Domestic violence or abuse in pregnancy is associated with increased physical and psychological stress, inadequate prenatal care utilization, poor nutrition and weight gain. It can lead to problem in fetal growth and development. Physical trauma can cause abruptio placenta, preterm labor and preterm premature rupture of membrane, maternal and fetal injury and demise.

Diagnosis and Treatment

Although abused women seek medical care, but only 1 in 20 to 1 in 100 are identified by the doctor to whom they turn for help. Barrier to diagnosis are the practitioner's lack of knowledge or training, lack of recognition of the widespread prevalence of the problem, time constraints, fear of offending the patients and feeling of powerlessness in the area of treatment.

Research suggest that use of abuse assessment questionnaires and asking patients directly about prior or ongoing victimization increases the likelihood of disclosure. For example, has anyone close to you ever threatened to hurt you, or are you afraid at home. It is important to ask the patient questions in private apart from male partner and children, family or friends.

Intervention

Offering the abused women a nonjudgmental compassionate response can in itself be a powerful form of intervention. Assuring immediate safety and establishing safety plans, providing patient education and referral of available to community support service are effective and efficient strategy.

The physician must resist the impulse to urge the patient to leave her abuser partner at once. As leaving an abusive relationship is a process, not an event. As one expects that life style changes as smoking cessation take time, and require multiple messages and strategies, this is the case with addressing violence as well. Doctor should assure the patient that she does not deserve to be abused and help is available. Helping the patient to be safer is of paramount importance.

Legal Issues in Domestic Violence

Up to now laws do not mandate physician reporting of domestic violence. There is evidence that mandatory reporting, in addition to further eroding victim's confidence and autonomy, may even increase her risk for additional violence in the future.

Documentation of Domestic Violence

Patient's own words should be used as far as possible. Name of perpetrator and description of nature of the violence and any weapon should be documented. A standard consent form is adequate for taking photograph to document violence. Good documentation can provide crucial evidence for the patient at a later time particularly if there are child custody issues as there are seldom any evidence to corroborate abuse.

Referral in Domestic Violence

Clinician should assure the patient that she does not deserve to be abused and situation, is likely to get worse if continued. She can take help and support from social workers, organization, government as well non-government like women's right organization. Routine referral for couple counseling is not recommended. If the patient discloses feelings of angers, e.g. in counseling session, her partner's abuser behavior may escalate. After the violence and threat of violence has ceased, then in some cases joint counseling can be one option. While clinician are not expected to be domestic violence experts, they should have access to names and phone numbers of local hotline, shelters and other resources.

Sexual Assault

Sexual assault is any sexual act performed by one person on another without the person's consent. Sexual assault includes genital, oral, or anal penetration by a part of accused body or by any object. It may result from force, the threat of force either on victim or another person or victims inability to give appropriate consent.

Variant of Sexual Assault

a. Marital rape is defined as forced sexual act within a marital relationship without the consent of partner.
b. Acquaintance rape refers to those sexual assault committed by some one known to victim. More than 75% of adolescent rapes are committed by acquaintance.
c. Statutory rape refers to sexual intercourse with a female under age 14-18 years of age.
d. Child sexual abuse is defined as contact or interaction between a child and an adult.

Our society has many misperceptions about sexual assault. The victims are often blamed for having encouraged the assault by their behavior; dress, for being promiscuous, or for having ulterior motives for pressing charged. This explains victim's reluctance to report the violent crime to the authorities. Another misperception is that it is an impulsive or aggressive extension of normal sex drive on the part of rapist, while usually the motivation for most sexual assault is degradation, terrorization and humiliation of victim.

Clinical Presentation

The majority of rape victims coming to emergency room do not openly admit to, having fear, sexually assaulted. They, can concern for AIDS or STD.

Rape trauma syndrome often occurs, the **initial response acute phase** is characterized by paralysis or distortion of coping mechanism, uncontrolled emotion or total detachment. **Next phase occur many years** after incident and characterized by chronic anxiety, self blame, loss of control.

Documentation

The physician evaluating the victims has both medical and legal responsibilities and should be aware of state laws. **Informed consent** must be obtained prior to examination of sexual assault victims. A **careful history** and physical examination should be performed in the presence of chaperon or victims advocate. History should include last menstrual period, contraceptive use, preexisting pregnancy, infection one last consensual intercourse. Careful **examination** of entire body for bruises, laceration, should be noted. Injury should be documented with photograph and drawing in medical records.

A pelvic examination for injury to genitalia is noted. The speculum must be inserted with saline, nonabsorbent cotton swab should be used to sample fluid from vaginal pool. Air dried, nonfixed smear of some fluid is placed in glass slide. Motile sperm may be noted in vagina for up to 8 hours after intercourse and nonmotile sperm for 24 hours. Acid phosphatase enzyme is found in high concentration, seminal fluid. It can be detected even in absence of sperm. DNA evaluation may be performed from the vaginal swab. A wet mount or vaginal swab is obtained for organism like Trachomatis, test should be done for gonorrhea and *Chlamydia trachomatis*. Baseline serologic test for hepatitis B virus, HIV and syphilis should be offered.

Collection of sample for forensic purpose is an important part of physician legal responsibility. Pubic hair combing, finger nail scrapping, skin washing, clothing are investigated for presence of blood or semen. All colleted specimens are placed in larger sealed container and sending and receiving should be verified.

Treatment

Treatment of physical injury sustained at the time of assault should be started immediately. Prophylactic medical treatment like Ceftriaxone 125 mg I/M single dose + Metronidazole 2 gm orally single dose and Doxycycline 100 mg orally two times a day for 7 days is one of the regimens offered to victim of sexual assault.

It is recommended that hepatitis B immunoglobulin should be administered intramuscularly as early as possible but certainly within 14 days of exposure followed by standard 3 dose active immunization of hepatitis B vaccine at 0, 1 and 6 month. Prophylaxis against HIV is contraindicated. **Emergency contraceptive** can be offered as prophylaxis against pregnancy. **A urine pregnancy test** prior to administration of emergency contraception is done. Emergency contraceptive should be given within 72 hours of assault though it is effective up to 120 hours.

Psychological follow-up counseling should be offered by primary care provider or experienced counselor. A follow-up visit should be scheduled approximately 15 days after assault for repeat examination and collection of addition samples, and again after 12 weeks. At the visit serology test for antibodies against *T. pallidum*, hepatitis B (if vaccine not given) and HIV test (repeated after 6 month is done). During each visit, assessment of the patient's psychological symptoms should be performed and referral for further counseling is made as indicated.

APPENDIX 7
Ethicolegal Issues in Obstetrics and Gynecology

The person who believe in justice remains clam through all trials and difficulties.

GENERAL CONSIDERATION

The word 'Ethics' is derived from Greek word meaning manner and habit of a man. Ethical means principles that govern right conduct. Medical ethics means values and guidelines that should drive decision making in medical practice. Medical ethics upholds, fosters and guarantees the mode of conduct and behaviors of the members of medical profession to the patient, fellow doctors and state. **Ethics differs from law or legalization because ethics is governed and guided by moral sense, conscience and medical council, and not by any state or act of legalization.** Ethical code though is not law, yet is equally forceful because it has the approval of profession at large. In all actions conscience guides the doctor to do what is good and not to do what is bad.

The Hippocratic Oath written in 5th century BC was intended to be affirmed by each doctor on entry to medical profession. World medical association established in 1914, made a modern restatement of Hippocratic Oath known as Geneva declaration and international code of medical ethics.

Hippocratic Oath

It is oath, or declaration by every medical personnel to register of state medical council. It states as follows with affixing his signature:

a. I solemnly pledge myself to consecrate my life to the service of humanity.
b. I shall give to my teachers the respect and gratitude which is their due.
c. I will practice my profession with conscience and dignity.
d. The health of my patient will be my first consideration.
e. I will respect the secrets which are confided to me by the patients.
f. I will maintain by all means in my power, the honor and noble tradition of medical profession.
g. My colleagues will be my brothers and sisters.
h. I will not permit consideration of religion, nationality, race, party, politics or social standing to intervene between my duty and my patient.
i. I will maintain the utmost respect for human life from the time of conception until death.
j. Even under threat, I will not use my medical knowledge contrary to the laws of humanity.

The medical person affirms that "I make these promises solemnly, freely and upon my honor."

Code of Medical Ethics

Each country has its own code of ethics. As per Medical Council Amendment Act no. 24 of 1964, the council has prescribed standard of professional conduct and etiquette, a code of ethics for medical practitioners, specifying a warning notice that violation of this code of ethics shall constitute **professional misconduct**.

a. **Malpractice:** Substandard management of the patient due to incompetence, negligence, carelessness, monetary or other ulterior motive constitute breech of contractual duty and called malpractice.
b. **Incompetence:** Quality of service by doctors has to be sound by experience, expertise, diligence and sincerity. The physician can help in improving competence by participation in continuing medical education.
c. **Negligence:** Doctor-patient relationship is a form of implied contract established between patient and medical practitioner. It is built on mutual trust, confidence, goodwill and proper understanding between the doctor and the patient. Doctor's primary concern will be his/her patients to whom he/she will owe utmost loyalty. While treating, doctor is not to make experimentation on the patient or use any medication without strict therapeutic or prophylactic indication. Treating a patient without taking any fees does not absolve the doctor from his duties and obligations to the patients.

Legal Problems in Medical Practice

The allegation and accusation against doctors can be classified under three broad heading:

1. **Ethical:** Professional misconduct as described above.
2. **Civil wrong:** Medical negligence. It includes:
   a. Error of judgment
   b. Therapeutic misadventure that is experimental misadventure and calculated risk.

   In above situation, the task of proving negligence generally is on the patient or plaintiff petitioner under the civil procedure code, standard of proof is taken as the balance of probabilities. It means that the alleged event has more than 50% chance of probability and is more likely to happen.

   Damages are monetary compensation for the damage or loss of injury caused by treatment. The amount of damages depends on the degree of negligence and assessment of other factors and it is fixed by judicial discretion.

   No fault compensation: It basically means the patient gets compensation irrespective of doctor's negligence. Like sterilization operation has certain failure rates but if a woman gets pregnant after sterilization of herself or her husband in a government setup or registered place, patient may claim compensation from government health authority.

3. **Criminal offense:** It can be in two categories: (a) Criminal negligence, (b) Criminal malpractice.
   a. *Criminal negligence* is sort of gross negligence act which causes serious irreparable bodily harm or death of a patient and the treating doctors is liable to be punished under Indian Penal Code Section 304A. Lately Supreme Court has given clear instruction not to make doctor punishable only by prima facie, but only after proper investigation by experts.
   b. *Criminal malpractice* includes illegal abortion, false certificate regarding birth and death, manipulation of records of history.

Ethicolegal Issues for Obstetrician and Gynecologist

The obstetricians are especially vulnerable to the greatest number of legal cases for medical negligence because of the emotionally charged sensitivity involving the well-being of two lives—mother and baby. It is necessary that obstetrician and gynecologist should be aware of the constantly changing concept and technology in the field. The Table A7.1 summarizes the possible act of omission and commission in obstetrics and gynecology.

Medicolegal Problems in Specialized Field of Obstetrics and Gynecology

Obstetrics and Gynecology is terminal subject till now but in last decade there has been many technical advancement in field of endoscopic surgery, assisted reproductive technology and imaging.

Endoscopic Surgery

In case of endoscopic surgery still the rules and norms of training period, learning centers, quality control of operation theater, equipment and assistant are not clear. Beside types of surgery which can be performed by varying level of experts also differs. Endoscopic surgery has many advantage of short hospital stay, fast recovery, but has potential inherent grave complication like gas embolism, electrolyte imbalance, organ injury and anesthetic related

Table A7.1: Possible acts of omission and commission in field of obstetrics and gynecology

Obstetrics

I. Act of omission
   a. Failure to provide antenatal care.
   b. Failure to diagnose fetal anomaly.
   c. Failure to attend at time of delivery.
   d. Maternal perineal or rectal, bladder injury.
   e. Failure to remove placenta completely.
   f. Failure to repair birth canal injury.
   g. Failure to use aseptic technique.
   h. Forgotten packs in abdominal cavity or vagina.
   i. Failure to treat life threatening condition like eclampsia properly.
   j. Use of drug, vaccine or investigation which can be harmful to fetus.

II. Act of commission
   a. Unnecessary cesarean section operation.
   b. Instrumental injury to mother and child.
   c. Hemorrhage from the cord.
   d. Diagnosis of pregnancy as tumor and vice versa.
   e. Failure to assess CPD or malpresentation and difficult vaginal delivery resulting in maternal and neonatal complications.

III. Accidental complication
   a. Anesthetic complication.
   b. Fresh stillbirth.
   c. Failure to detect intrapartum fetal risk.
   d. Neonatal physical or mental handicap.

Gynecology

I. Act of omission
   a. Failure to obtain informed consent before performing abortion or sterilization or artificial insemination.
   b. Failure to use aseptic technique in surgery.
   c. Failure to inform about mishap.
   d. Failure to diagnose certain problem like premalignant condition, ectopic.
   e. Improper indication and improper type of surgery.

II. Act of commission
   a. Operation resulting in sterility done without prior consent.
   b. Perforation of uterus during minor operation like D & C.
   c. Fistula formation with ureter, bladder, rectum.
   d. Failed tubectomy.

complications. There has been number of litigation by the patient due to improper, incomplete or complicated endoscopic surgery. To avoid medical litigation following endoscopic surgery the following measures should be followed:

a. Training of surgeon and selection of patient should be proper.
b. Informed consent with possibility of open surgery should be taken.
c. Proper technique should be used.
d. Endoscopic surgeon should know their capacity and limitation and take up only those cases which can be managed by them efficiently.

Assisted Reproduction

Assisted reproductive technology (ART) is newer development in management of infertility. Beside *in vitro* fertilization, there are techniques like ICSI (Intracytoplasmic sperm injection) which involve direct manipulation of human genetic material. Third party donation includes insemination of donor sperm, oocyte donation and surrogacy. There are certain legal guidelines which have to be followed in these cases like proper screening for all transmissible disease like HIV, hepatitis B, syphilis, proper selection of donor and receiver, proper technique, and protection of right of donor and receiver.

In developed countries, ART centers are under strict regulatory bodies. In India though many ART centres and experts are there, there is still no licensing authority or regulatory bodies. Recently MCI, Government of India and doctors associations are framing guidelines for standard practice in ART. ART experts and clinics should closely follow these guidelines.

Measures to Minimize Medicolegal Problem

a. ***Communication:*** Communication is the art of sharing. Information communication between doctor and patient may be necessary for imparting knowledge, communicating probable diagnosis and treatment option and follows up. In busy schedule of obstetrics and gynecology lack of proper communication is the major cause of litigations. The good communicator doctors face less chance of litigation in their practice. It is important always to say truth. This builds reputation of doctor and become important when one has some mishap in obstetric surgery. One has to be apathetic and approach the main point directly. In critical situation doctor should always tell a responsible person and should be transparent in explaining sequence of events, limitation of procedures and prognosis.

b. ***Informed written consent:*** Informed written consent gives patient and its relative the power of participating in decision concerning their own management. The consent should be orally explained and written in patient's language. It should give honest, unbiased, up-to-date information about their illness, mode of surgical intervention and its inherent risk and complications. According to laws, the informed consent can be given by the patient or person mentally competent to make the decision, have adequate information and can reach a decision voluntarily. Clear conversation at a time convenient to the patient and the doctor goes a long way in reducing litigation. In a critically life threatening situation, when immediate intervention is necessary to save life, doctor can provide medical treatment and take decision. Doctor should talk with the patient and relative about procedures and treatment done as soon as the condition is settled.

c. ***Case note documentation:*** Good medical records are critical to the delivery of quality medical care. Accurate medical records are doctor's best defense against litigation. Clinical records should be correct, clear, comprehensive and chronological. Photocopies of outdoor prescription should be with doctor otherwise doctors have no record of their own and they are at mercy of patients to provide the paper. In case of emergency situations one should be given responsibility to document in time wise manner what treatment is given chronologically and patient's status.

d. ***Adherence to established management protocol:*** It is essential as law wants doctors the give due, desired care to the patient, not any heroic measures. The doctors should keep themselves updated in recent guidelines for treatment. Doctors should also be careful in maintaining standard quality of care, sterilization and equipments in labor room, operation theater, intensive care unit and wards.

e. ***Adequate training and supervision of junior staff, paramedicals*** which are involved in labor room, indoor patient care. Senior must be available for consultation or direct involvement, when asked for.

f. ***Proper investigation:*** Right investigation at right time can save lot of litigation. One should not hesitate to perform any noninvasive or invasive procedures provided the risk and benefits are well judged and are duly informed.

g. ***Adequate supervision:*** Adequate supervision by a well organized graded system is highly recommended in hospital setup. Early detection of complication by junior doctors and timely notification of consultant may prevent a lot of mishap.

h. ***Surgical intervention:*** Operation itself can be cause of litigation. Surgical procedures should always be performed in places where there are adequate facilities and personnel. Proper pre and postoperative management and record is important to reduce complication as well litigation.

i. ***Timely referral:*** Early detection of the complication and timely referral to higher center can be life saving and can avoid legal hazards.
j. ***Professional auditing:*** Auditing is defined as systemic and critical analysis of the quality of medical care. Mortality and morbidity audits are important mainly for the maintainence of standard of patient care. Regular meetings of all staff to discuss their work and results, analysis and constructive criticism of errors and decisions would be beneficial to everyone involved in patient care.
k. ***Medical indemnity insurance:*** The doctor must cover himself in every possible way for his protection. Indemnity insurance is one of them. The premium for medical indemnity insurance varies widely and is quite high for obstetrician and gynecologist, and for hospital setups. In developed countries, there are medical defense organizations. In India, we need such organization for protection of doctors against litigation and malpractice plan.
l. ***Medical defense procedure:*** The efficiency of ***defense attorney*** is important to defend against litigation. The doctors must provide its attorney all clinical details, records, scientific knowledge and treatment guidelines. The doctor must go through the patient records before a court appearance because giving a different answer contrary to record can be disastrous. Another important issue is ***expert witness***. In this one has to take opinion of an up-to-date practicing doctor who will give their expert opinion in the particular situation to the best of his ability.

CONCLUSION

Medical profession, especially obstetrician and gynecologist is always exposed to the threat of litigation, but defensive medical practice is not the solution for minimizing medicolegal problems. Defensive approach not only hampers their professional confidence but can also bring out other legal problems. The three main points to prevent litigation are adoption of all preventive precaution and professional updating by healthcare personnel. At one end generalized improvement of healthcare infrastructure including health education to the community plays significant role in preventing complications. If mishaps occur despite utmost health care, service and sincerity; they are unlikely to end in court as long as doctor patient relationship is good. A doctor who is well conversant with current trends in medical practice, meticulous, vigilant and at the same time courteous and sympathetic towards patient is less likely to have litigation or to be proved negligent by court of law.

Section Five

Annexures

Annexure 1

Medical Eligibility Criteria for Initiation and Continuation of Intrauterine Devices (IUD)

WHO Category 4: Not to be used (absolute contraindications)

- Immediate postseptic abortion
- Vaginal bleeding suspicious/unexplained
- Management of trophoblast disease
- Cervical cancer
- Endometrial cancer
- Uterine fibroids with distortion of uterine cavity

The following criterias are special for LNG IUD only
- Ovarian cancer
- Current breast cancer

- Distorted uterus (congenital and/or after operation)
- Current pelvic inflammatory disease (PID)
- Current STDs
- Pelvic tuberculosis

WHO Category 3: Risks outweigh advantages

- Postpartum (48 hours to <4 weeks)
- Benign trophoblast disease

The following criterias are special for LNG IUD only
- Postpartum breastfeeding or not
- Current or history of ischemic heart disease
- Current breast cancer

- Ovarian cancer
- Increased risk of STDs
- AIDS

- Viral hepatitis
- Cirrhosis
- Liver tumors

WHO Category 2: Advantages outweigh risks

- Age: menarche to <20 years
- Parity: nulliparous
- Postpartum breastfeeding or not
- Postabortion: Second trimester
- Complicated valvular heart disease
- Vaginal bleeding (heavy and prolonged)
- Severe dysmenorrhea
- Endometriosis

The following criteria are special for LNG IUD only
- Hypertension Systolic >160 or diastolic >100
- Stroke
- Valvular heart disease
- Multiple risk factors (e.g. old age, smoking, diabetes, hypertension)
- Major surgery with prolonged immobilization

- STDs excluding HIV
- Vaginitis
- HIV infection
- Thalassemia (1 for LNG)
- Sickle cell disease (1 for LNG)
- Iron deficiency anemia (1 for LNG)
- Antiretroviral (ARV) therapy

- Cervical intraepithelial neoplasia

- Diabetes
- Cholecystitis (past/present)
- Hyperlipidemia

WHO Category 1: No restriction of use

Criteria not mentioned in category 2-4.

In general, criteria for women who can use IUDs safely and effectively include

- Smoking any age, light/ heavy smoker
- Obesity
- Breastfeeding
- Ischemic heart disease
- Stroke
- Hypertension
- Having antibodies (including rifampicin and griseofulvin)
- Postabortion first trimester
- Migraine with or without aura
- Diabetes
- Thyroid disorders
- Liver/gallbladder disease

Source: WHO, Medical Eligibility Criteria for Contraceptive Use (3rd Ed) Geneva, WHO 2004.

ANNEXURE 2

Medical Eligibility Criteria for Initiation and Continuation of Combined OCs/Combined Injects/Transdermal Patches and Vaginal Rings

WHO Category 4: Not to be used (absolute contraindications)

- Age: >35 years taking ≥35 cigarettes/day
- Postpartum: breastfeeding women <6 weeks' postpartum
- Multiple disorders (old age, smoking, diabetes, hypertension)
- Rare factors (past thrombin mutations, protein D, protein C, antithrombin deficiencies)
- Cardiovascular disorders
  1. Hypertension (systolic ≥160 or diastolic ≥100)
  2. Deep vein thrombosis/pulmonary embolism (DVT/PE)
  3. Major surgery with prolonged immobilization

WHO Category 3: Risks outweigh advantages

- Age: ≥ 35 years having <35 cigarettes/day
- Postpartum:
  1. Breastfeeding women ≥ 6 weeks to < 6 months
  2. Non-breastfeeding women < 21 days
- Multiple disorders (old age, diabetes, smoking, hypertension)
- History of hypertension
  1. Where BP can be evaluated
  2. Adequately controlled BP
  3. Systolic 140-159 or diastolic 90-99
- Hyperlipidemia

WHO Category 2: Advantages outweigh risks

- Age: <35 years
- Obesity: More than 90 kg weight
- Cardiovascular disorders
  1. History of hypertension
  2. Family history of DVT/PE
  3. Superficial thrombophlebitis
  4. Hyperlipidemia
  5. Uncomplicated cardiovascular disease
  6. Major surgery with prolonged immobilization

WHO Category 1: No restriction of use

- Age: Menarche to <40 years
- Parity: Nulliparous/parous
- Postpartum: Non-breastfeeding ≥ 21 days
- Postabortion: 1st/2nd trimester—immediate postseptic abortion
- Past ectopic pregnancy
- Cardiovascular disorders
  1. History of hypertension
  2. Varicose veins
  3. Minor surgery

Source: WHO, Medical Eligibility Criteria for Contraceptive Use (3rd Ed.) Geneva, WHO 2004.

ANNEXURE 3
Medical Eligibility Criteria for Emergency Contraceptive Pills

Contraindication or delay
No such condition

WHO Category 2: Caution—extra precautions

· History of severe cardiovascular complications (ischemic heart disease, cerebrovascular attack or thromboembolism)	· Angina pectoris · Migraine · Severe liver disease

WHO Category 2: Accept—no reason to prevent use

· Breastfeeding · History of ectopic pregnancy	· Repeated ECP use

Source: WHO, Medical Eligibility Criteria for Contraceptive Use (3rd Ed.) Geneva, WHO 2004.

ANNEXURE 4

Normal Values in Pregnancy

Noninvasive Monitoring (Cardiovascular)

Measure	10-18 weeks	18-26 weeks	26-34 weeks	34-42 weeks
Cardiac output (L/min)	7.26 ± 1.56	7.60 ± 1.63	7.38 ± 1.63	6.37 ± 1.48
Stroke volume (mL)	85 ± 21	85 ± 21	85 ± 21	70 ± 14
SVR (dyne cm second^{-5})	966 ± 226	901 ± 224	932 ± 240	1118 ± 325
Heart rate (beats/min)	87 ± 14	90 ± 14	92 ± 14	92 ± 7
Mean arterial pressure (mm Hg)	87 ± 7	84 ± 7	84 ± 7	86 ± 7

Pulmonary Function Tests

	8-11 weeks	20-23 weeks	28-31 weeks	36-40 weeks
Respiratory Rate (br/min)	15 (14-20)	16 (15-18)	18 (15-20)	17 (16-18)
Tidal volume (mL)	640 (550-710)	650 (625-725)	650 (575-720)	700 (660-755)

Liver Function Tests

	12 weeks	32 weeks	Intrapartum
Total alkaline phosphatase (IU/L)	42 (17-88)	82 (46-165)	97 (48-249)
Gamma glutamyl transferase (IU/L)	7 (2-18)	6 (3-20)	9 (5-79)
Aspartate transaminase (AST, IU/L)	9 (4-18)	9 (5-21)	11 (5-103)
Alanine transaminase (ALT, IU/L)	9 (4-30)	8 (2-22)	12 (5-115)
Total bilirubin (IU/L)	4 (1-12)	4 (2-9)	4 (2-10)

Metabolic Markers and Lipids

	4-16 weeks	16-24 weeks	24-34 weeks	Term
Uric acid (mg/dl)	3.21 ± 0.10	3.48 ± 0.13	3.49 ± 0.11	4.72 ± 0.13
Creatinine (mg/dl)	0.58 ± 0.03	0.50 ± 0.04	0.50 ± 0.03	0.57 ± 0.03
Total cholesterol (mg/dl)	153.5 ± 3.8	194.0 ± 5.2	218.3 ± 6.4	220.4 ± 8.4
Triglycerides	70.1 ± 4.5	109.6 ± 5.8	139.6 ± 6.9	159.0 ± 8.1
Free fatty acids (mEq/L)	0.42 ± 0.03	0.34 ± 0.02	0.21 ± 0.02	0.67 ± 0.04

Umbilical Cord Blood at Delivery

	Artery	Vein
pH	7.06-7.36	7.14-7.45
PCO_2 (mm Hg)	27.8-68.3	24.0-56.3
PO_2 (mm Hg)	9.8-41.2	12.3-45.0
Base deficit (mmol/L)	0.5-15.3	0.7-12.6

Reference: Eskes TKAB, Jongsma HW, Houx PCW: Percentiles for gas values in human umbilical cord blood. Eur Jr Obst Gynecol Reprod Biol 14:341, 1983.

24 Hour Urinary Protein (mg/24 hrs)

First trimester	80.0 ± 60.6
Second trimester	116.7 ± 69.3
Third trimester	115.3 ± 69.2

ANNEXURE 5
Indications and Risks of Common Vaccines During Pregnancy

Infective agent	Nature of vaccine	Indications	Vaccination schedule
BCG	Live attenuated virus	Contraindicated	
Tetanus	Toxoid	Lack of primary series or no booster within 10 years	For previously unimmunized. Two doses IM at 1-2 months interval in second/ third trimester. Third dose 6-12 months after the second. Booster after 10 years.
Influenza	Inactivated (live attenuated influenza virus vaccine should not be given in pregnancy)	All women in second and third trimester during flu season. Women at high risk of pulmonary complications in any trimester	One dose IM
Typhoid	Parenteral VI polysaccharide vaccine (ViCPS). Oral. Live attenuated	Oral vaccine contraindicated. Parenteral can be given. Not indicated routinely except for close continuous exposure or travel to endemic area	ViCPS. Single injection IM
Yellow fever	Live attenuated virus	Contraindicated. Administered only if travel to endemic area is unavoidable	Single dose SC
Anthrax	Cell free filtrate from B. anthracis	Indicated if high risk of infection. No studies on safety of vaccination in pregnancy	Six dose primary vaccination SC, then annual booster
Rabies	Killed virus vaccine	As in nonpregnant	
Measles	Live attenuated virus	Contraindicated in pregnancy. Pregnancy should be avoided for 4 weeks after vaccination. Recommended postpartum in susceptible women, breastfeeding not contraindicated	Postpartum. Single dose SC, preferably as measles, mumps, rubella
Mumps	Live attenuated virus	Contraindicated in pregnancy. Pregnancy should be avoided for 4 weeks after vaccination. Recommended postpartum in susceptible women	Postpartum. Single dose SC, preferably as measles, mumps, rubella
Rubella	Live attenuated virus	Contraindicated in pregnancy. Pregnancy should be avoided for 4 weeks after vaccination. Recommended postpartum in susceptible women.	Postpartum, single dose SC, preferably as measles, mumps, rubella

Contd...

Contd...

Infective agent	Nature of vaccine	Indications	Vaccination schedule
Hepatitis A	Inactivated virus	Pre-exposure and post-exposure prophylaxis in women at high risk	Two doses at 6 months interval
Hepatitis B	Purified recombinant surface antigen	Pre-exposure and post-exposure prophylaxis in women at high risk	Three doses IM at 0, 1, 6 months
Herpes zoster	Live attenuated virus	Contraindicated	

INDEX

A

Abdominal
    incision infection 220
    sacrocolpopexy 164
Aberrations of pubertal development 91
Ablatio placenta 416
Ablation
    therapy 255
    treatment 289
Abnormal
    androgen synthesis 99
    bleeding 139
    course of labor 527
    pattern of labor 532
    puerperium 572
    uterine bleeding 125, 127
Abnormalities of renal position 75
Abortions 359
Abruptio placenta 416
Absence of estrogen 242
Absolute contraindication of pregnancy 337
Accessory
    genital glands 74
    instruments 615
Accidental hemorrhage 416
Acid-base equilibrium 342
Acquired
    hypothalamic dysfunction 105
    pituitary dysfunction 106
Acrochordon 116
Acute
    abdominal pain 466
    complications 265
    cystitis 208, 470
    fatty liver of pregnancy 465
    HIV infection 204
    morbidity 265
    pelvic inflammatory disease 212
    pyelonephritis 209, 470
    renal failure 471
Adenocarcinoma 259, 295
Adenomyosis 131
Adherent placenta 547
Adjuvant
    chemoradiation 263
    chemotherapy 283
    therapy 272, 274, 331
Administration of GnRH analog 34
    infection 220
    mass in pregnancy 482
Adolescence 90, 632
Adolescent gynecology 89
Adult polycystic kidney disease 472
Advantage of
    partograph 508

    colposcopy 252
    EFM 593
    ventouse over forceps application 559
Alloimmune disorder 626
Alteration in function of pituitary gland 106
Alternative
    medicine for menopause 245
    parenteral regimen 214
    regimen 198, 199
    treatment 606
Ambulatory uterine monitoring 379
Amenorrhea 106
Amnion 67
Amniotic fluid 67
    embolism 604
    index 431
Amniotomy 508
Anal
    canal 13
    sphincter 14
Analgesia for episiotomy 552
Anatomic destruction 106
Anatomy of
    external genitalia 3
    female genital tract 3
Androgen insensitivity syndrome 98
Anemia 444
Anemia in pregnancy 445
Anesthetic option for cesarean delivery 586
Anovulatory bleeding 140
Antenatal care in twin pregnancies 426
Antepartum
    fetal surveillance 588
    management 429, 440, 515
Anterior
    abdominal wall 21
    fontanelle 497
    vaginal wall defect 157
Anti D immunoglobulin 392
Antibiotics 379, 382
Antibody test 206
Anticholinergic medication 171
Anticonvulsant therapy 474
Antiviral treatment 200
Anus and rectum 21
Aortic stenosis 456
Apgar score 576
Apical vaginal repair 164
Aplastic anemia 448
Apocrine sweat gland cyst 116
Arrest disorders 533
Arteriography and arterial embolization 611
Artificial rupture of membrane 508
Ascites 185
Asphyxia 579

Assessment of fetal well-being 588
Assisted reproductive techniques 155
Asthma in pregnancy 477
Asymptomatic bacteriuria 469
Asymptomatic fibroid 128
Atrophic vaginitis 195, 244
Attachment of placenta 69
Atypical endometrial hyperplasia 268
Atypical vascular pattern 253
Autonomic nerves 21
Axial rotation 185
Axis of
    pelvic brim 25
    pelvis 27

B

Backache 347
Bacterial vaginosis 190, 485
Baden-Walker-Halfway system 157
Bandl's ring 538
Barrier methods 306
Bartholin's gland adenocarcinoma 292
Basal cell carcinoma 292
Basics of equipment of obstetric ultrasound 596
Benign
    and malignant tumors of reproductive tract 144
    breast condition 324
    degeneration 124
    disorders of uterine corpus 123
    neoplasm of cervix 119
    solid tumors of vulva 116
Bethseda system 246
Bilateral uterosacral ligament suspension 164
Bimanual
    examination of uterus and adnexa 86
    pelvic examination 184
    pelvic examination 217
Biology of trophoblast 50
Biophysical profile 590
Birth environment 504
Bisphosphonates 241
Bladder
    and urethra 71
    injury during gynecological surgery 176
Blighted ovum 361
Blood flow 69
    in individual organs 338
Blood
    pressure 338, 444
    transfusion and fluid replacement 545
    vessels 323
        of pelvis 17
    volume and composition 339

Botox injection 173
Bowel habits 346
Brain metastasis 302
Breast
    abscess 327, 573
    cancer 329, 486
    condition requiring evaluation 326
    examination 87, 327
    imaging mammography 328
    feeding 479
Breech
    delivery 519
    presentation 514
Bringing down leg 519
Burn victim in pregnancy 588
But thought without learning is perilous 625
By amount of placental involvement 547
By degree of adherence 547

C

Calcitonin 241
Calcium 342
Calculation of date of labor 495
Cancer of
    cervix 258
    vagina 293
Carbohydrate metabolism 341
Carcinoma
    cervix during pregnancy 484
    of cervical stump 264
    of cervix during pregnancy 264
    ovary 483
Cardiac
    catheterization 454
    disease in
        evaluation 337
    output 444
Cardinal movement of labor 502
Cardiovascular
    changes 403, 584
    disease 242
    support 604
    system 338
Care during puerperium 571
Care of teeth 347
Categories for drug use during breastfeeding 630
Cause and location of
    labor pain in
        pain in 1st stage of labor 583
Cause of
    iron deficiency anemia 445
    maternal hypothyroidism 461
    occipitoposterior position 527
    onset of labor 495
    pain during labor 583
    postpartum and puerperal fever 572
    post-term pregnancy 385
    seizure in pregnancy 473
Causes of
    abnormal uterine bleeding 137
    compromised neonatal infant 579
    contracted pelvis 534
    delayed puberty 91
    domestic violence 634
    failure of IVF 235
    hirsutism 237
    jaundice in pregnancy 463
    malpresentation 514
    polyhydramnios 432
    prolonged latent phase 532
    protracted disorders 532
    recurrent pregnancy loss 363
    thrombocytopenia 451
    trauma 587
Cautions in insulin therapy 441
Central
    nervous system 301
    thermoregulation change 240
Cephalopelvic disproportion 533
Cervical
    cancer incidentally diagnosed after simple hysterectomy 265
    cap 307
    circlage 379
    dystocia 537
    ectopy (erosion) 121
    factor 229
    length assessment 378
    mucorrhoea or vaginal epithelial discharge 195
    polyp 120, 485
    stenosis 122
    tears 119
Cervicitis 196
Cervix 7, 20, 161, 190, 216
Cesarean section 524, 563, 564, 567
    delivery in breech presentation 521
Chancroid 201
Chemical resuscitation 581
Chemoprophylaxis for pregnant women 480
Chemotherapy 274, 283, 302
    in SCST 284
    of germ cell neoplasm 284
Chest X-ray 454
    film 217
Childhood 397
Chimera 353
Chlamydial infection 198
Choice of drugs 474
Cholecystitis and cholelithiasis 468
Cholelithiasis in pregnancy 466
Choriocarcinoma 278, 298
Chorion 66
Chorionic villus sampling (cvs) 355
Chromosomal
    abnormalities 353
    cause 625
Chromosomes 351
Chronic
    cervicitis 196
    hypertension in pregnancy 409
    inversion of uterus 127
    morbidity 265
    pelvic pain 633
    renal disease 471
Cigarette smoking 249
Classification and
    nomenclature of abnormal sexual differentiation 97
    pathophysiology 123
Classification
    based on quantification of blood loss 541
    of asthma 477
    of forceps delivery 555
    of perineal laceration 553
    of placenta previa 412
    of postpartum hemorrhage 540
    of shock 601
Clear cell
    adenocarcinoma 295
    carcinoma (mesonephroid tumors) 278
Cleavage of embryo—the morula and blastocyst 49
Climacteric 239
Clinical
    features of ovarian tumors 183
    history and physical examination 535
    latency 204
    management of IUD 309
    manifestation and complication 471
    pelvimetry 535
    staging of cervical cancer 261
Clomiphene citrate challenge test (CCCT) 228
Clotting factors 339
CO_2 laser ablation 255
Coagulation
    defects 541
    disorder 417
Coarctation of aorta 457
Code of medical ethics 637
Coitus 347
    interruptus 305
Colposcope 252
Colposcopic grading 252
Colposcopy 251
Columnar epithelium 247
Combined oral contraceptive
    and parity 249
    pills 237
Combined spinal epidural block 586
Common
    clinical conditions of menopause and postmenopausal women 242
    complaint and maternal concerns during prenatal visits 346
    iliac glands 20
    investigations in gynecological diagnosis 609
    problems in pediatric gynecology 88
    site of ureteric injury 176
Complete abortion 359
Complication in pregnancy 450
Complication of
    cesarean section 566
    chemotherapy 283
    forceps application 558
    induction of labor 554
    ventouse 560
Complications and
    management of abruptio 419
    risk of HRT 244
Complications
    following mid trimester MTP 367
    in antepartum period 396
    in breech delivery 521
    in pregnancy 436

INDEX

Complications of
    abortion 362
    anemia 446
    art 234
    diabetes in pregnancy 442
    episiotomy 552
    hysteroscopy 614
    IUFD 387
    IUGR 396
    laparoscopy 617
    macrosomia 399
    menstruation 144
    multiple pregnancies 425
    ovarian tumor 185
    placenta previa 414
    polyhydramnios 432
    PPROM 383
    pre-eclampsia 407
    pregnancy 435
    pregnancy in elderly primigravida 435
    radical surgery 265
    radiotherapy 265
    therapy 265
    treatment 292, 606
    related to trauma 587
Composition of amniotic fluid 67
Compound presentation 525
Compression suture 545
Computed tomographic (CT)
    scanning 536
    scan 612
Conception, fertilization and implantation 47
Concluding remark 23
Conduct of labor and delivery 382
Confirmation of diagnosis 261
Congenital
    adrenal hyperplasia (adrenogenital syndrome) 97
    uterine anomalies 481
    ventricle septal defect or atrial septal defect 456
Conservative measures 162
Constriction ring 537
Contraception in India—past, present and future 304
Contracted pelvis 533
    and cephalopelvic disproportion 533
Contraction stress test (CST) 590
Contraindication to estrogen replacement therapy 244
Contraindications of
    COC's 313
    epidural anesthetic 586
    hysterosalpingography 611
    of induction of labor 554
    intravenous urogram 611
    laparoscopy 616
    tocolysis 381
Contraindications to
    trial of labor 537
    use of IUCD 310
Conventional temporal classification 540
Cord
    pH and blood gases 382
    prolapse 525
    structure 68

Core needle biopsy 329
Corpus
    body of uterus 6
    luteum 40
        granulosa lutein cyst 178
        of pregnancy 40
Correction of
    cervical factors 233
    identified cause 230
    uterine factors 233
Correlation of mammographic findings 328
Cough stress test 170
Counseling for teratogen exposure 631
Course of
    disease 259
    labor in contracted pelvis 536
Couvelaire uterus 417
Craniopharyngioma 106
Critical care obstetric 601
Cryotherapy 255
CT and MRI 184
Culdocentesis 213
Cycle of domestic violence 634
Cyproterone acetate 238
Cystectomy vs oophorectomy 186
Cystic vulvar tumors 115
Cystosarcoma phyllodes 326
Cystourethrography 611
Cytogenetics 351
Cytologic examination 138
Cytology 184
Cytomegalovirus—general consideration 489

D

Death of one fetus *in utero* 427
Decidual blood supply 52
Decidual
    changes 70
    reaction 52
    structure 52
Defense
    mechanism 190
    mechanisms of genital tract 189
Deficient flexion of head 527
Definition and
    classification of hypertensive disorders in pregnancy 401
    diagnostic criteria 618
Degree of uterine inversion 548
Delay in descent of breech 519
Delayed or interrupted puberty workup 91
Delivery room management 576
Dependent diabetes mellitus 438
Descent of ovary into pelvis 73
Design of forceps 555
Determination of gestational age 344
Development of
    amnion 67
    cord 68
    external genitalia 74
    hypogonadotropic hypogonadism 106
    ovary 73
    uterus 74
    vagina 74
    villous system 53

Dexamethasone 238
Diabetes mellitus 627
    and pregnancy 439
Diabetic pregnancy 438
Diagnosis and
    evaluation of patient with possible preterm labor 379
    management 96, 326, 492
        of placenta accreta 415
    treatment 634
    breech presentation 514
    carcinoma cervix 260
    chlamydia infection 198
    contracted pelvis 535
    fetal growth restriction 397
    GTN 301
    infection 248
    iron deficiency anemia 445
    ovarian cancer 279
    pregnancy 347
    prom 382
    twin pregnancy 424
    evaluation 169
Diagnosis, symptoms and signs 273, 415
Diagnostic
    conization in stage IA 264
    consideration 467
    criteria 440
    pregnancy 439
    evaluation 301
    laparoscopy 616
    studies 454
    test 325
Diagonal conjugate 25
Dialysis during pregnancy 472
Diameter of
    anatomical outlet 26
    narrow pelvic plane 27
Diameters and circumference of fetal head 497
Diameters of
    mid cavity 26
    pelvic brim 25
Dietary
    deficiency 249
    recommendation 440
Differential diagnosis of PCOS 618
Differentiation of trophoblast 51
Difficulty in
    delivery of after-coming-head 521
    spontaneous breech delivery 516
Dilatation and curettage 139
Dilemma of vaginal birth after cesarean 568
Direct extension 270, 282
Disadvantages of ventouse over
Disorder of
    uterus 78
    amniotic fluid 431
    anterior pituitary gland 106
    development of müllerian system 75
    gonadal development 99
    hypothalamus 105
Disseminated intravascular coagulation 419
Distribution of lesion 149
DNA assays 225

Documentation 635
    and litigation 563
    of domestic violence 634
    of POP-Q 159
Domestic violence
    and sexual assault
        in pregnancy 634
Doppler velocimetry 591
Drug
    categories in pregnancy 630
    interaction 312
Dual photon densitometry 613
Ductal lavage cytology 329
Duplication of upper ureter and renal pelvis 75
Duration of
    second stage of labor 501
    third stage 502
Dynorphin 34
Dysfunctional uterine bleeding 140
Dysgerminoma 278
Dysmenorrhea 132, 145
Dyspnea of pregnancy 477
Dystocia 532
    and cephalopelvic disproportion 532

E

Early
    detection and screening program 330
    pregnancy factor (EPF) 66
    reproductive period (15-25 years) 324
    trophoblast invasion 53
Echocardiography 454
Eclampsia 408
Ectopic
    gestation 185
    pregnancy 368
Edema 111
Effect of
    asthma on pregnancy 477
    chronic renal disease in
        fibroids on pregnancy 482
    hypothyroidism of pregnancy 461
    ICP on pregnancy 465
Effect of pregnancy in asthma 477
Effect of pregnancy on
    chronic renal disease 472
    fibroids 482
    Graves' disease 461
    malaria and vice versa 492
    prolapse 485
    tuberculosis 479
Effect of
    seizure disorders on
        tuberculosis on pregnancy 479
Effect on
    pregnancy 469
    pregnancy and complication 470
Effectiveness 308
Efficacy of contraception 304
Eisenmenger's syndrome 456
Elaborate criteria 212
Elderly primigravida 435
Elective cesarean section 537

Electrical injury 588
Electrocardiography 454
Electronic
    cardiotocography (CTG) 508
    fetal monitoring (EFM) 592
ELISA test 206
Embryology 71
Embryonic carcinoma 278
Emergency
    contraception 315
    measures 128, 274
Employment 347
Encysted peritonitis 185
Endocrine
    disorders 104
    factors 627
    system 62
Endodermal sinus tumor 106, 278
Endogenous opioids and effects on GnRH 34
Endometrial
    ablation 131
    biopsy 138
    cancer 268
    screening 267
    hyperplasia 268
    intraepithelial neoplasia (EIN) 268
    polyp 123, 133
    lesions 182
Endometrioid neoplasm 277
Endometrioma 179
Endorphins 34
Endoscopic surgery 638
Endoscopy in gynecology 613
Endotracheal intubation 581
Engagement 502
Enkephalin 34
Enterobiasis (pinworm, seatworm) 113
Environmental factors 360, 628
Epidemiological factors 377
Epidemiological risk factors for CIN 247
Epigenetics 351
Epilepsy and seizure disorder 473
Episiotomy 551
Epithelial
    neoplasm 277
    tumors 180
Epoophoron (organ of Russell Miller) 10
Erysipelas 113
Erythropoiesis 444
Erythropoietin 447
Essential of normal newborn assessment and care 576
Estrogen 43, 65, 241
    component 311
    progestin contraceptive 140
    replacement 108
    therapy and risk of thromboembolism 141
Ethical issues in neonatal resuscitation 582
Etiology of
    postpartum hemorrhage 541
    recurrent pregnancy loss 625
Etiopathogenesis
    and risk factors 289
Etiopathophysiology 618

Evaluation
    for specific causes of infertility 227
    in case of amenorrhea 106
Evaluation of
    abnormal bleeding
    abnormal uterine bleeding 138
    breast mass 327
    cytology results 250
    female factor 226
    male factors 223
persistent bleeding 544
    pregnancy with isoimmunization 390
    pregnant patient with vaginal bleeding 359
Eversion (ectropion) 119
Examination of
    female patient 226
    male patient 226
    patient in labor 504
Exercise stress testing 454
Exogenous hormone replacement therapy 143
Expectant management 152, 186
    in mild PIH 404
    of severe preeclampsia 406
External
    cephalic version (ECV) 515, 524
    fetal monitoring 592
    rotation 503

F

Face presentation 522
Facts of obstetrical significance 498
Failed forceps delivery 558
Fallopian tube 8, 215, 285
    and ovary 20
Fascia of pelvic diaphragm 15
Fat necrosis of breast 327
Features of
    asymmetrical IUGR 396
    symmetrical IUGR 396
Female
    ageing and ovulatory dysfunction 227
    condom (vaginal pouch) 306
    factor infertility 231
    genital tract
anomalies 75
    differentiation 73
    pelvis 495
    sterilization 316
    urological system 11
Ferrokinetic studies 446
Fertility awareness based methods 305
Fertility choice 632
Fertilization 49
Fetal
    acoustic stimulation test (FAST) 590
    adrenal gland 62
    and maternal
        blood circulation
        risk 525
    attachment of umbilical cord 69
    blood 59
        cells 61
        volume 60

Index

cells in maternal circulation 356
complications in placenta previa 415
consideration 466
dimension and disposition 495
effects in isoimmunization 389
erythropoiesis 60
fibronectin 378
gastrointestinal tract 62
gene therapy 624
glucose homeostasis
growth, placenta and umbilical cord 57
heart rate tracing 595
hemoglobin 59
hemopoiesis 59
indication 556
medicine therapy 623
membrane, amniotic fluid and umbilical cord 66
monitoring 460
  in labor 508
movement 589
nervous system 64
physiology and organ system 59
pituitary 62
position and denominator 498
presentation 496
pulmonary system 61
respiration 61
risk factor 378
skin 62
skull 496
stem cell transplantation 624
surgery 624
surveillance 441
transfusions 623
urinary system 61
Fetomaternal surface 55
Fibroadenoma 326
Fibrocystic disease of breast 325
Fibroid 185
  in pregnancy 482
Fibroma 117, 182
Finasteride 238
Fine needle aspiration cytology (FNAC) 329
First
  stage of labor 500
  trimester ultrasound scan 597
  trimester vaginal bleeding 359
Flexion 503
  and version 6
Flutamide 238
Follicular
  atresia 41
  development 36
  phase 35
Follow-up visits 572
Fontanelles 497
Foramina and canals in pelvis 24
Forceps application 559
  in direct occipitoposterior position 558
  in face presentation 558
  after coming head of breech 558
Forceps operations 555
Foreign bodies 195
Formulation of antepartum fetal surveillance 592

Fothergill's repair (Manchester operation) 165
Fourth stage of labor 502
Fox Fordyce disease 116
Friedman curve 500
Full
  bladder 184
  blown aids 204
Function of
  amniotic fluid 68
  fallopian tube 9
Functional
  cyst 178
  disorders of hypothalamic amenorrhea 105
Function—mechanism of action of GnRH on pituitary cells 33
Functions of placenta 64

G

Gastrointestinal
  changes 584
  studies 611
  system 340
General
  feature of bony pelvis 24
  management of antepartum hemorrhage 411
  management of mother 506
  measurement 604
  principle of management 139
  risk of incontinence surgery 173
Generalized tonic contraction (uterine tetany) 538
Genesis of twins 423
Genetic
  amniocentesis 355
  disease 336
  testing 226
Genital
  ambiguity at birth 96
  prolapse in pregnancy 485
  system 72
  tract changes in pregnancy 342
  tract tuberculosis 214
Genital
  trauma 89, 541
  ulcer disease 199
Genitourinary fistula 173
Genomic imprinting 351
Germ cell tumor 183
Germinomas 106
Gestational
  diabetes mellitus 439
  hypertension 409
Glucocorticoids 451
GnRH
  agonist 93, 238
  independent precocious puberty 93
  agonist and antagonist (structure and function) 33
Gonadal
  differentiation 72
  dysgenesis 99
Gonadoblastoma 278
Gonadotropic releasing hormones 32

Gonadotropin 35
Gonadotropins releasing hormone agonist 142
Gonorrhea in pregnancy 493
Grading of CIN of uterine cervix 246
Grand multipara 435
Grandmother theory 393
Granular cell myoblastoma (schwannoma) 117
Granuloma
  inguinale (donovanosis) 201
  pyogenicum 111
Granulosa stromal cell tumors 279
Graves' disease 460
Gross anatomy of term placenta 69
Group B streptococcal 492
Growth problem in normal adolescents 94
Guidelines of treatment issued by CDC 191
Guiding principles in evaluation of infertility 223
Gynecological history and clinical examination 83

H

Headache 476
Heart
  burn 346
  disease in pregnancy 453
Hellp
  syndrome 408
  syndrome 466
Helpful landmark of early pregnancy 597
Hemangioma 111
Hematogenous
  dissemination 271
  spread 282
Hematologic changes 403
Hematological disorders
Hematoma 111
Hemodynamic monitoring 602
Hemoglobinopathies 449
Hemorrhagic disorders 451
Hemorrhoids in pregnancy 468
Hepatic 301
Herpes simplex 199
  virus—general consideration 490
High-grade squamous intraepithelial lesions (HSIL) 246
High-risk GTN 302
Hilus cell tumor 183
Hippocratic oath 637
Hirsutism 180, 237
Histogenesis and classification 272
Histologic analysis 329
Histologic characteristics 371
Histologic classification of endometrial carcinoma 270
Histology of vagina 5
Histopathologic categories of ovarian cancer 277
HIV infection 258
  during pregnancy 206
Homeostasis in diabetic mother 439
Hormonal
  contraception 310
  evaluation of male 225
  function and regulation 40

Hormone
    receptor sites 331
    releasing IUD 308
    replacement therapy 243
    therapy 94
    variation and correlation of endometrial and ovarian cycle 43
HRT preparation and use 243
Human
    chorionic gonadotropin (HCG) 66
    immune deficiency virus 491
    immunodeficiency virus infection 203
    papilloma virus 247
    placental lactogen (HPL) 65
Hydatidiform mole 297, 299
Hydradenitis 113
Hypergonadotropic hypogonadism (premature ovarian failure) 104
Hyperpigmentation 341
Hyperprolactinemia 627
Hyperthecosis 179
Hyperthyroidism in pregnancy 459
Hypogonadotropic hypogonadism 105
Hypothalamic like releasing hormones 66
Hypothalamus—functional anatomy 31
Hypothyroidism in
    iodine deficient area 462
    pregnancy 461
Hypovolemic shock 601
Hysterectomy 130, 133, 136, 256, 545
Hysterosalpingography 217, 611
Hysterosalpingography (HSG) 228, 611
Hysteroscopy 139, 229, 614

I

Iatrogenic 378
Identification 176
Idiopathic 378
IInd meiotic division 353
Ileococcygeal vaginal suspension 164
Immature teratoma 278
Immediate 367, 614
    care 571
Immunologic factor 626
Immunology of HPV 248
Imperforate hymen 76
Implantations of blastocyst and early development of placenta and embryo 50
In
    cervical cancer 258
    mature placenta 54
    menopause 240
    menstrual cycle 41
    more advanced stage 483
    normal pregnancy 439
    pregnancy 200
    severe PIH 407
Incarceration of prolapse 161
Incidence and
    general consideration 289
    genetics of RH factor 388
    risk factors 561
    risk factors
        for pre-eclampsia 401
        of placenta accreta 414

    types of cardiac disease in pregnancy 453
Incidence of
    abortion 360
    PROM 382
    RPL 363
    twin pregnancy 423
Incomplete
    abortion 359
    androgen insensitivity 98
    or foot ling presentation 519
Incoordinate uterine action 537
Increased abdominal pressure 160
Indication and contraindication of ventouse 559
Indication of
    cesarean section 455
    cesarean section in trauma 588
    induction of labor 553
    prenatal diagnosis 350
    surgery 483
Indications of
    antepartum fetal surveillance 589
    cesarean section 388
    CT scan 613
    forceps delivery 556
    hysterosalpingography 611
    laparoscopic surgery 616
    ultrasound 612
Induced abortion 364
Induction of labor 386, 388, 553
    and augmentation 555
Inevitable abortion 359
Infection during pregnancy 488
Infectious cause 627
Infectivity of genital herpes 201
Infertility 126, 180, 223, 619
Infestation of vulva 112
Infiltrative disease 106
Inflammatory bowel disease 466
Inflammatory vaginitis 194
Infusion and transfusion 602
Inguinal rings and canal 22
Inhalational analgesia 585
Inherited
    abnormalities of pituitary gland 106
    thrombophilia 627
Inhibin 45
Initial visit (first prenatal visit) 343, 345
Injectable progestin contraceptives 314
Inspection of external genitalia 85
Instrument design 558
Insulin like growth factor 46
Insulin therapy 441
Intermediate type 396
Intermittent auscultation 592
Internal
    fetal monitoring 592
    genital organs 5
    podalic version 524
    pudendal artery 18
    rotation 503
Interpretation of test of ovarian reserve 228
Intersex 96
Interstitial
    and cervical pregnancy 375
    or intramural 124
    tuberculous salpingitis 215

Intervention 634
Intervillous space 70
Intrahepatic cholestasis of pregnancy 465
Intralesional injection 118
Intramuscular administration 314
Intrapartum 396
    care 475
    fetal surveillance 592
    management 386, 429, 442
        of pre-eclampsia 407
Intrapartum risk factor 561
Intrauterine
    device (IUD, IUCDs) 307
    fetal death (IUFD) 386
    growth restriction 395
Intravenous
    immunoglobulin 451
    urography 611
Invasive
    diagnostic test 356
    mole 297
Investigation for specific disorders 107
Investigations for etiology of anemia 446
Iron 339
    deficiency anemia 445
Ischemic necrosis of distal organs 419
Isochromosomes 354
Isoimmunization and other blood group incompatibility 388

J

Jaundice
    and hepatitis in pregnancy 463

L

Lab
    finding 120
    testing 243
Labia majora 116
Labial adhesion 88
Labor
    and conduct of delivery 509
    by partogram 508
    in face presentation 522
    management 451
Laboratory
    and radiological investigation 93
Lactational
    abscess 327
    amenorrhea 305
    mastitis 327
Laparoscopic approach 318
Laparoscopy 184, 186, 213, 217, 215
Laparoscopy vs laparotomy 375
Laparoscopy with chemopertubation 229
Laparotomy 184, 187
Laparotomy vs laparoscopy 154
Laparotomy vs minilaparotomy vs laparoscopy 186
Large for gestational age and fetal macrosomia 398
Late pregnancy and labor 447
Lea's shield 307
Learning without thought is labor 625

Legal
    issues in domestic violence 634
    problems in medical practice 638
Leiomyoma, fibroma and lipoma 117
Leprosy in pregnancy 493
Leukocyte 60
Leukorrhea 347
Levator ani (pelvic diaphragm) 14
Levonorgesterel IUD 142
Lichen planus 115
Lichen
    sclerosis 113
    simplex chronicus 115
Life table analysis 305
Lifestyle
    changes 170
    modification 144
    therapies 230
Ligament of uterus 16
Lipid 341
Lipoma 117
Liver
    disease unrelated to pregnancy 463
    problems unique to pregnancy 465
Local
    abnormalities 481
    analgesia 585
    gynecological abnormalities associated
Localization of placenta 413
Long-term
    complications 320
    prognosis 385
    risk 397
        in PCOS 622
Lower gastrointestinal tract 13
Low-grade squamous intraepithelial 246
Low-risk GTN 302
Lumbar
    epidural block 585
    group 20
Lung 300
Luteal
    phase 35
    phase 39
    phase defect 627
Luteoma of pregnancy 180
Lymphatic
    dissemination 282
    drainage of pelvis 19
    spread 270
Lymphatics 9, 324
Lymphogranuloma venereum (LGV) 202

M

Macromastia 327
Magnetic resonance
    guided focused ultrasound surgery 131
    imaging 329, 613
Maintenance of cardiac efficacy 602
Maintenance therapy 141
Major causes of anovulation 140
Malaria—general consideration 492
Male
    condom 306
    infertility 230
    sterilization—vasectomy 320

Malformation
    and maldevelopment of genital tract 75
    of breast 327
Malignant
    change 121
    neoplasm of
Malposition 514
Malpresentation 514
    and malposition 514
Mammographic abnormalities 328
Management
    during labor 515
        and delivery 478
Management in
    deep transverse arrest 530
    labor 433
    postpartum hemorrhage 541
    Rh negative pregnancy 389
    severe pre-eclampsia 405
Management of
    advanced ovarian cancer 283
    benign ovarian tumors 186
    cardiac disease in pregnancy 454
    delayed puberty 92
    dysmenorrhea 145
    epithelial ovarian cancer 282
    erosion 122
    first stage 529
        of labor 455, 506
    fourth stage of labor 510
    germ cell neoplasm 284
    GTN 301
    hemorrhagic shock 602
    histologic cin 254
    in multiple pregnancies 427, 428
    IUGR 397
    labor 504, 529
        delivery 455
    labor in
        CPD 536
        vertex breech 428
    last report 562
    malignant sex cord tumors 284
    menopause 243
    mild PIH 404
    oligohydramnios 433
    patients in remission 283
    persistent occipitoposterior position 529
    postpartum hemorrhage 541
    PPH after delivery of placenta 542
    PPROM 383
    precocious development 93
    pregnancy with RH isoimmunization 391
    second stage of labor 455, 529
    specific
        anomalies 76
        condition 467
    specific situations 427
    thalassemia in pregnancy 449
    third stage 529
    unsensitized Rh negative pregnancy 389
    vaginal birth after cesarean 568
    vulvodynia 117
Manual removal of placenta 542
Masculinization due to elevated androgen in
    maternal circulation 98

Masculinized female 97
Mastalgia 325
Mastitis 573
Maternal
    and fetal risk 528
        gain during pregnancy 341
    glucose homeostasis in normal pregnancy 438
    immunization during pregnancy 347
    indication 556
    medical condition 337
    mortality 567
    outcome 420
    serum alpha fetoprotein 415
    weight 345
Mature
    reproductive period (25-40 years) 324
    teratoma — dermoid 183, 278
Measurement 577
    of amniotic fluid by ultrasound 431
Measures to minimize medicolegal problem 639
Mechanical
    heart valves 457
    method 554
Mechanism for formation of trisomy 353
Mechanism of
    action 307
        of only progestin preparation 311
    action of oral contraception pills 311
    labor 502
        in occipitoposterior position 527
Medical
    measures 218
    methods—induction of labor 366
    termination of pregnancy 364
Medicolegal problems in specialized field of obstetrics and gynecology 638
Megaloblastic anemia 447
Meiosis 352
Meiotic arrest of oocyte and resumption 36
Menopausal ovary 40
Menopause 239, 632
Menorrhagia 132
Menstrual
    disturbance 240
    phase 42
    problems 632
Metabolic changes 341
Metabolism of estrogen 43
Metaplastic epithelium 247
Metastatic
    gestation trophoblastic tumors (disease) 300
    lesion 106
Metformin 180
Method of
    assessment of cervical length 378
    cervical
        ripening 554
        screening 249
    contraception 305
    establishing zygosity 423
    IFM 592
    induction 386, 388
        of labor 554

terminating pregnancy between 16-20 weeks of gestation 367
termination of pregnancies 364
between 13-15 weeks of gestation 366
ultrasound 612
Microchimerism 55
Microcystic disease 116
Microglandular hyperplasia of endocervical mucosa 119
Microscopic appearance 149
of lesion 216
Mid pelvis (pelvic cavity) 26
Migraine headache 476
Mild
intermittent asthma 478
persistent asthma 478
Milky discharge (galactorrhea) 326
Minilaparotomy 186
Minimum criteria 212
Missed
abortion 359
pill 316
Mitosis 352
and meiosis 352
Mitral
regurgitation 456
stenosis 456
Mixed
cervical carcinoma 259
germ cell tumors 279
gonadal dysgenesis (mosaicism) 100
Mode of
action of progestins 140
delivery in Rh negative women 392
Moderate persistent asthma 478
Modified
biophysical profile 591
radical hysterectomy 262
Molluscum contagiosum 203
Monitoring
of women on antithyroid drug 460
progress of labor 506
protocol in expectant treatment 406
Monosomy 353
Mons pubis 116
Morphologic and genetic abnormalities 360
Morphological changes 403
Mortality and cause of death 368
Mosaic 253, 353
Mother 489
Mucinous tumor 181, 277
Müllerian duct (paramesonephric duct) 72
Multiple marker screen 355
Multiple pregnancy 423
Muscles of anterior abdominal wall 22
Musculoskeletal system 342
Myolysis 131
Myoma and pregnancy 127
Myomectomy 129

N

Narrow pelvic plane 27
of least pelvic dimension syn 26
Natural history
and management 288
of disease 204

Natural methods 305
Nausea and vomiting in pregnancy (NVP) 346
Nebothian cyst 119
Neisseria gonorrhoeae 197
Neonatal
assessment 461
complications 396
effects 389
exchange transfusion 392
infection 490
resuscitation 579, 580
risk 528
Neoplasm metastatic to ovaries 279
Nerve and vessels 23
Nerve supply of vulva 4
Nerves supply 324
Nervous system disorders in pregnancy 473
Neuroendocrine tumors of cervix 259
New patient assessment 223
Newborn screening and prophylaxis 577
Newer tocolytics 381
Nipple discharge 326
Nonatypical endometrial hyperplasia 268
Nondysjunction 353
Nonepithelial ovarian cancers 278
Nonlactational abscess 327
Non-neoplastic findings 251
Non-nucleoside reverse transcriptase inhibitor 207
Nonpharmacological method of pain relief 584
Nonreassuring 595
Nonspecific treatment for abnormal menstrual bleeding 141
Nonsteroidal anti-inflammatory drugs (NSAIDS) 128, 141
Nonstress test 589
Nonvertex twin 428
Normal
fetal growth 395
labor 495
menstrual cycle 35
puerperium 571
Nucleoside reverse transcriptase inhibitor 207
Nutrition in pregnancy 345
Nutritional requirement 346

O

Obesity 436
Objective of intranatal care 504
Oblique
diameter 26
internus muscle 22
Obliterating vaginal operation (colpocleisis and Le Fort operation) 165
Obstetric
anesthesia and analgesia 583
conjugate 25
problem in congenital uterine anomaly 481
ultrasound 596
Obstetrical
axis 28
factors 377
outlet 26
Occipitoposterior position 526

Oligohydramnios 433
in late pregnancy 433
Oogenesis 47
Open excisional biopsy 329
Operative
laparoscopy 616
obstetrics 551
vaginal delivery 555
Opioids injection 585
Option for termination of pregnancy 440
Oral
contraceptives 142
Organization of placenta 53
Organ-wise lymphatic drainage of female reproductive system 20
Origin and circulation of amniotic fluid 67
Osteopenia and osteoporosis 240
Other
blood group isoimmunization 389
complications unique to twin 426
endocrine dysfunction 619
genital infections 492
infections of vulva 113
lesions of cervix 484
malignancies during pregnancy 486
methods for fetal monitoring
methods of fetal scalp stimulation 592
obstetrical related risk 160
obstetrical significant landmarks 27
treatment option 145
vulvar carcinomas 292
Outcome of
active management of labor 511
HPV infection 248
Outflow tract 104
Outlet of pelvis 26
Outpatient
care 214
therapy-criteria for
treatment regimen 214
Ovarian
abscess, infected pelvic hematoma 220
artery 18
cyst and adnexal torsion 468
follicular development 35
neoplasm 180
plexus 21
pregnancy 375
reserve 227
steroidogenesis 43
torsion 185
tumor and pregnancy 89, 186
Ovaries 9, 216
Ovulation 39
Ovulatory
dysfunctional uterine bleeding 140
factor 227, 231
Oxygen administration 602

P

Pain 125, 219
Palliative care 264
Pancreatitis 468
Paracervical block 585
Parameters of fetal heart monitoring and its interpretation 593

Index

Parasitic infection 195
Parathyroid hormones (PTHS) 241
Parenteral
    iron 447
    tocolytic agents 381
Parietal obliquity 498
Paroophoron 11
Partial breech extraction (assisted breech extraction) 516
Pathogenesis
    and natural history 258
    of CIN 247
    of tubal pregnancy 369
Pathogens
    causing mass lesions 203
    causing suppurative cervicitis 197
Pathological amenorrhea 103
Pathology of pelvic organs 215
Pathophysiology
    changes during pregnancy 466
Patient
    consideration in obstetric ultrasound 597
    education 108
    evaluation for menopause 242
    selection 309
    with physiologic delay 92
Patterns of abnormal uterine bleeding 137
Pearl index 305
Pediculosis pubis 112
Pelvic
    abscess 220
    cellulitis 219
    colon 21
    contraction 527
    examination 280
    floor 14
    inflammatory disease 185
    mass 127
    nerves 21
    organ prolapse 157
    organ prolapse (POP) 157
    peritoneum 216
        quantification (POP-Q) 158
    shapes 28
    skeleton 23
    ultrasound scan 138
    veins 19
    X-ray abdomen 184
Pendulous abdomen 481
Peptic ulcer 466
Peptide—inhibin and activin 45
Peravaginal repair 163
Perforation of uterus 265
Performing Pap test 249
Perimenopause or menopausal transition 239
Perinatal care and guidelines of delivery in HIV positive women 207
Perinatal
    morbidity 567
    mortality 567
    outcome 419
Perineal
    body (central tendon of perineum) 15
    laceration 553
Perineum 15
Peripartum cardiomyopathy 457

Peritoneal covering and relation 13
Peritoneum and ligaments of pelvis 16
Persistent gestational trophoblastic tumor (gtt) 300
Pessary and urethral inserts 171
Phantom β-hCG 302
Pharmacologic agent 602
Pharmacologic method 554
    of obstetric analgesia and anesthesia 585
Pharmacological treatment 145
Phases of labor (parturition) 499
Physical changes associated with menopause 239
Physiological changes during pregnancy: general consideration 337
Physiological changes in
    liver during pregnancy 463
    pregnancy and effect of cardiac disease on pregnancy 453
    pulmonary system in pregnancy 477
    renal hemodynamics in pregnancy 469
Physiological
    hemodynamic changes in pregnancy and erythropoiesis 444
    vaginal discharge of pregnancy 485
Physiology of
    amniotic fluid 431
    androgen 236
    iron metabolism in pregnancy 445
    menstruation 35
    micturition 168
        and continence 13
    spermatogenesis 223
    third stage of labor 540
Pigmented nevus 116
Pituitary
    hormone secretion 34
    anatomy and embryology 32
Pityalism 346
Placenta 339
    accreta
    previa 411
Placental
    ageing 70
    attachment of umbilical cord 69
    examination 424
    factors 378
    site trophoblastic tumor 302
    site trophoblastic tumors (PSTTS) 298
Plane of mid cavity 26
Polycystic ovarian syndrome (Stein-Leventhal syndrome) 179
Polycystic ovaries 108
Polyembryoma 279
Polygenic inheritance 351
Polyhydramnios 432
Polymerase chain reaction (PCR) 206
POP-Q examination 161
Position for cesarean section 565
Positive
    emission tomography scanning 329
    manifestation 349
Positron emission tomography (PET) 613
Possible adverse effects 312
Post-treatment surveillance 302
Post void residual volume 169

Postcoital test 225
Posterior
    fontanelle 497
    fontanelle 497
    pituitary gland (neurohypophysis) 34
    vaginal prolapse 163
    vaginal wall 157
Postmenopausal bleeding 143
Postnatal care 475
Postoperative
    complication 566
    infection 219
    management 79
Postpartum 390
    care 442
    hemorrhage 540
    neuropsychiatric complications 574
    psychosis 574
    thyroiditis 462
    thyroiditis 574
Post-renal type 471
Post-term pregnancy 385
Potential long-term complications of PID 213
Practice recommendation/maneuvers 562
Precaution in ventouse application to avoid complication 560
Precaution with pessary 162
Precipitate labor 533
Precocious puberty 92
Preconception counseling 335
Preconceptional
    counseling 335
    counseling 474
Preconceptual risk factors 561
Prediction 399
    of preeclampsia 403
    of preterm labor 378
Pre-eclampsia 401
Pregnancy
    after renal transplantation 472
    and vice versa 473
    associated plasma protein (PAPP) 66
    between 24 and 34 weeks 405
    complications 619
    outcome 472
    specific β-1 glycoprotein (PS β-1g) 66
    test 349
Preimplantation genetic diagnosis (PGD) 356
Preinduction cervical assessment 554
Preinvasive disease and cancer of vagina 293
Premalignant and malignant
    disorders of uterine corpus 267
    lesions of cervix 484
Premalignant lesions 484
Premature
    induction of labor 537
    separation of placenta 416
    thelarche 89
Premenstrual syndrome 144
Prenatal
    care 343
    counseling 450
    diagnosis 349
    records 343
    screening and diagnostic test 354
    testing 424

Preoperative
    evaluation 78
    preparation 564
    procedure 317
Preparation for forceps delivery 556
Prepregnancy counselling 440, 454
Prepubertal period 90
Prerequisites for forceps applications 556
Presence of meconium in amniotic fluid 596
Presenting part of fetus 496
Pressure effect 126
Presumptive manifestation 347
Preterm
    breech 521
    labor 377, 427
    neonate 384
    premature rupture of membrane (PPROM) 382
Prevention and
    prophylaxis 465
    treatment for osteoporosis 240
Prevention of
    ovarian cancer 276
    PID 213
    POP 162
    pre-eclampsia 404
    preterm labor 379
    SSI 220
Prevention strategies 492
Preventive measure 606
Primary
    and secondary apnea 579
    protection 336
    pulmonary hypertension 457
    radiation therapy 263
    therapy 272
    treatment 162, 199
Principle 613
Principle of
    genetic disorders and sex chromosome anomalies 350
    induction of labor 553
    management in occipitoposterior position 529
    neonatal exchange transfusion 392
    surgical management 467
Probable manifestation 348
Procedure of
    vacuum application 559
    vaginal hysterectomy 166
Progestational agents 180
Progesterone 45, 65, 379
    contraceptive 314
Progestin
    component 311
    estrogen therapy 244
    implants 315
    therapy 140
Proliferative phase 41
Prolonged latent phase 532
Prophylactic vaccines 248
Prophylaxis 446
    for postpartum hemorrhage 541
Protein 341

Protocol of neonatal resuscitation 579
Protracted disorders 532
Pseudomyxoma peritonei 186
Psychological aspect of pregnancy 633
Psychological factors influencing labor pains 584
Psychosocial
    factors 377
    problem 94
Puberty 89
    period 90
Pudendal
    arteries 18
    block 585
Puerperal
    care and contraception 451
    fever 572
    venous thrombosis 574
Puerperium 456, 570
Pulmonary
    disorders in pregnancy 477
    system adaptation in pregnancy 339
    thromboembolism 605
Pulsatile secretion 32
Punctation 253
Purulent discharge 326

Q

Quality of life measures 169

R

Race 160
Radiation 272, 274
Radical hysterectomy 262
    type III 262
    trachelectomy 263
Radionuclide imaging 613
Radiotherapy 284
Rapid test 206
Reassuring 595
Rectal examination 87
Rectum 13
Rectus
    abdominis 22
    sheath 23
Recurrent and metastatic breast cancer 332
Recurrent
    cystitis 209
    disease 263
    pregnancy loss (RPL) 363
        and bad obstetrical history 625
    vulvovaginal candidiasis 193
Red blood cells 339
Reductase deficiency 98
Referral in domestic violence 635
Reflux esophagitis 466
Regeneration 43
Regional anesthetic technique 585
Regular exercise 440
Reinfection 471
Release pressure on cord 526

Remote
    complication 553
    complications 368, 567
Renal
    agenesis 75
    disorders in
    function 340
    system 340
    type 471
Repair
    and sterilization 421
Repair of
    episiotomy 552
    laceration 543
    scar 421
Repeat cervical cytology 251
Reproductive
    hormones 32
    physiology 31
    tract 239
Requisites of ideal analgesia and anesthesia in labor 584
Resource poor settings 254
Respiratory
    changes 584
    tract infection 574
Restitution 503
Retained
    placenta 546
    placental tissue or blood clot 541
Retrograde transtubal transport 271
Retroversion uterus 481
Risk factors
    vain 293
    associated with preterm labor 377
    for development of macrosomia 398
    for nulliparous prolapse 160
    for uterus rupture 420
    which warrant intensive intrapartum fetal surveillance 593
Risk of
    epilepsy in child 475
    inversion 548
    prolonged pregnancy 385
    tubal sterilization 319
    scoring system 378
Risks of
    antiepileptic drugs 475
    general anesthesia 587
    anti-hypertensive 409
Role of
    chemoradiation 292
    epoxide hydrolase enzyme in development of congenital malformation 475
    gynecologic oncologist 187
    myomectomy in pregnancy 482
    preconceptional counseling 335
    surgical treatment 461
Route of transmission 204
Routine
    antepartum administration of anti D immunoglobulin 392
    care of newborn 578
Rubella (german measles) 488
Rupture 185
    of uterus 420

Index

S

Sacral group 20
Sacral neuromodulation 173
Sacrospinous ligament fixation 164
Safety of hormonal contraception 312
Salient features of pelvic blood vessels 19
Salivary estriol 379
Salpingoscopy and falloscopy 617
Sarcoma botryoides 296
Scabies 112
Scarring of cervix 484
Screening 293
    and diagnosis for gestational diabetes 439
    guidelines 249
    test 237
Second
    and third trimester ultrasound scan 597
    look surgery 284
    stage of labor 501
    trimester termination (13-20 weeks) 366
Secondary
    change in POP 161
    changes 124
    changes in polyp 133
    disease 264
    postpartum hemorrhage 546
    tumors 302
Secretory phase 41
See and treat options 256
Selective
    estrogen receptors modulator 241
    reduction in multiple pregnancies 429
    termination 429
Semen analysis 225
Separation of placenta 70
Septic
    abortion 359, 364
    pelvic thrombophlebitis 573
    shock (endotoxic shock) 602
Sequelae 196
    of bacterial vaginosis 191
Serous tumors 181, 277
Sertoli-Leydig tumors 279
Severe persistent asthma 478
Sex cord stromal tumor (mesenchymoma) 182
    of ovary 279
Sexual
    assault 635
    dysfunction 241
    problem 633
Sexually transmitted disease (STD) 190
Shock in obstetrics 601
Short stature management 94
Shoulder dystocia 561
Sickle cell disease 450
Side effects of
    GnRH 34
    regional anesthesia 586
    tocolytics 381
Sigmoid colon 13
Signs of pregnancy 348
Silent pelvic inflammatory disease 211
Simple test 169
Single gene defect 350
Site and causes 176
Sites of injury 176
Skin 341
Skin and hair changes 242
Smoking, caffeine and alcohol 347
Solitary thyroid nodule during pregnancy 462
Somatic nerves 21
Sonohysterogram 228
Spastic lower segment 537
Special
    cases in obstetrics 435
    clinical form of breast carcinoma 330
    consideration for contraception 316
    maneuvers for delivery of head 517
    postoperative care 176
    risk status 390
    situation 257, 264, 310
    tests in gynecological practice 609
    topics in obstetrics 583
    X-ray 611
Specific
    heart disease during pregnancy and management 456
    measures 128
    postoperative infections 219
Speculum examination 85
Sperm
    antibodies 225
    penetration assay 225
Spermatogenesis 47, 224
Spermicidal preparation 307
Spinal block 586
Spironolactone 238
Splenectomy 451
Spontaneous abortion 126
Spontaneously vaginal delivery 516
Squamous cell
    carcinoma 259
    hyperplasia 114
Squamous columnar junction 247
Stages of pubertal development in girls 90
Staging of
    endometrial cancer 271
    ovarian neoplasm 282
    vaginal cancer 294
    vulvar cancer 290
Steps of cesarean section 565
Sterilization 316
Steroid pharmacology 311
Stress
    incontinence 171
    urinary incontinence 168
Structure 11
    amnion 67
    mature ovum 47
Struma ovary 183
Subacute complications 265
Subareolar abscess 327
Subfertility 632
Submucous leiomyoma 124
Subsequent
    pregnancy outcome 302
    prenatal visit 345
    visit 345
Subserous or subperitoneal 124
Success of assisted reproductive technique 234
Suicide 588
Superficial and deep external
Supportive treatment 200
Surgical
    condition with left upper quadrant pain 468
    management of septate uterus 79
    measures in dysfunctional uterine bleeding 142
    site infection (SSI) classification 219
    treatment of
        anatomic stress incontinence 172
        detrusor overactivity 173
        intrinsic sphincter deficiency 172
    options 154
Surveillance of maternal diabetes 440
Syphilis 202, 491

T

Tall stature 94
Tanner staging 91
Technique of
    endotracheal intubation 581
    fetal transfusion 623
    insertion 310
Techniques used in prenatal diagnosis 354
Tension headache 476
Teratogenicity 631
Teratogens 96
Term placenta 69
Testicular biopsy 226
Testosterone (androgen) 45
Tests used for antepartum fetal surveillance 589
Thalassemia in intermediate and minor 449
Thalassemia major 449
Theca lutein cyst 179
Thecoma 182
Therapeutic 612, 614
Therapeutic 614
Third stage 528
    labor 455, 501
Threatened abortion 359, 361, 362
Thrombocytopenia 451
Thyroid
    disease 627
    dysfunction with pregnancy 459
    physiology during normal pregnancy 459
    physiology in fetus and neonate 62
    storm 461
Time and mode of delivery 441
Timing and persons for preconceptional counseling 335
Timing for infertility evaluation 222
Timing of
    episiotomy 551
    insertion 310
    puberty 89
Topical treatment 289
Torch infection—general consideration 488
Torsion of adnexa 483
Total
    breech extraction 519
    duration of labor 502
Toxic shock syndrome 195
Toxoplasmosis 488
Traditional repair 163

Transcoelomic 282
Transdermal hormonal contraception 311, 313
Transformation zone 247
Transfusion of
    blood and other components in obstetrical hemorrhage 548
    platelet and whole blood 451
Transitional cell (Brenner)
    carcinoma 278
    tumor 182
Translocation 353
Transmission 248
Transvaginal
    administration 314
    ultrasound (TVUS) 132
Transverse diameter 26
    of fetal skull 498
Transverse
    lie/oblique and shoulder presentation 523
    abdominis 22
Trauma in pregnancy 587
Treatment for recurrent HSV outbreaks 200
Treatment in
    hypogonadism 92
    pregnancy 198
Treatment of
    acute asthmatic attacks 478
    complicated VVC 193
    iron deficiency anemia 447
    nonreassuring fetal heart rate pattern 595
    peritoneal disease 233
    pituitary adenoma 106
    preterm labor 380
    prolonged labor 532
    recurrent vulvovaginal candidiasis 193
    Turner's syndrome 100
    uncomplicated VVC 193
Treatment
    plan for CIN 254
    plan for infertile couple 230
    problem 98
Trial of
    forceps 558
    labor 537
Trichomonas vaginitis 193, 485
Triplets and higher order multiples 429
Trisomy 353
True hermaphroditism 99
Tubal and pelvic factor evaluation 228
Tubal damage 368
Tubercular
    endosalpingitis 215
    exosalpingitis 215
Tuberculosis 478
Tubo-ovarian abscess 214
Tumor
    markers 184
    spread 258
Turner's syndrome 99
Twin locking 428
Twin to twin transfusion syndrome (TTTS) 427
Type
    I or symmetrical or intrinsic IUGR 395
    II noninsulin

II or asymmetrical IUGR 396
Types and causes of osteoporosis 240
Types of
    breech presentation 514
    chronic renal diseases 471
    dysmenorrhea 145
    epileptic seizures 473
    episiotomy 551
    forceps 555
    intrauterine growth restriction 395
    invasive vulvar cancer 289
    malpresentation 514
    presentation 416
    scans 596
    surgery 154
    surgery 218
    vaginal breech delivery 516

U

Ultrasonography 328
    in gynecology 611
Ultrasound 179, 184, 212, 228, 280, 355
    diagnosis of common fetal anomalies 598
    examination 424
Under suturing placental bed 545
Undifferentiated carcinoma 278
Unexplained
    infertility 233
    recurrent pregnancy loss 628
Unstable lie 524
Ureter 11
Ureteric injury 176
Urethra 12
    and bladder 21
Urethrovaginal fistula 176
Urge incontinence 169
    and overactive bladder 171
Urinary
    bladder 11, 340
    calculi 471
    system 71, 161
    tract 240
        anomalies 75
        infection 208, 469, 573
Urine analysis 169
Urodynamics 170
Urogenital triangle 15
Use of
    HRT 171
    USG in detection of chromosomal anomalies or down syndrome 599
Uterine
    appendages 8
    arteries 17
    atony 541
    cervix 119
    factors 360
    fibroid embolization 130
    inversion 548
    leiomyoma 468
    sarcoma 272
Uterus 6, 190, 216, 342

V

Vagina 5, 20, 161, 189
Vaginal 301
    adenosis 295
    aplasia (agenesis of lower vagina/segmental vaginal agenesis) 78
    arteries 18
    atrophy and vaginal and vulvar lesions 143
    birth after cesarean 568
    bleeding 89, 359
    diaphragm 306
    discharge in pregnancy 485
    examination 527
    hysterectomy 165
Vaginitis 190
Vaniqua (eflornithine hydrochloride) 238
Variant of sexual assault 635
Variants of endometrial cancer 267
Variation of female pelvis 533
Varicella
    vaccination 490
    zoster 490
Varicosities 347
Varieties of presentation and positions 498
Various
    tocolytic agents 380
    types of IUDS 307
Vasa previa 415
Vascular connexion of vulva 4
Veins 323
Ventouse (vacuum extractor) 558
Verrucuous carcinoma 259
    of vagina 295
Vertex-vertex twins 427
Vessels, lymphatic and nerves 323
Villi changes 70
Viral
    1-24 antigen CD4 count 206
    hepatitis 463
    infection 112
Vitamin
    'A' and pregnancy 337
    B_{12} deficiency 448
    K administration to mother and neonate 475
Vitamins 342
Vulva 3, 189
Vulva and
    perineum 20
    vagina 216
Vulvar
    biopsy 114
    cancer 289
    disorders 110
    intraepithelial neoplasia (VIN) 288
    manifestation of systemic disease 112
    non-neoplastic epithelial disorders 113
    Paget's disease 292
    pain syndrome (vulvodynia) 117

sarcoma 292
  varicosity 111
Vulvovaginitis 89
Vulvovaginal candidiasis 192, 485

W

Waste space of Morris 27
Water metabolism 341

Weight
  gain 242
  loss 180
Western blot or immunoblot 206
White blood cell 339
Window period 204
With
  menopause 240
  pregnancy 481

Wolffian duct 11
Workup of patients with precocious puberty 93
Wound infection 574

X

X-ray 611
  findings 217
  pelvimetry 536